GOLDSMITH'S

Assisted Ventilation
of the Neonate

7th Edition

An Evidence-Based Approach to Newborn Respiratory Care

MARTIN KESZLER, MD, FAAP

Professor of Pediatrics
Warren Alpert Medical School
Brown University
Director of Respiratory Services
Department of Pediatrics
Women and Infants Hospital
Providence, Rhode Island

K. SURESH GAUTHAM, MD, DM, MS, FAAP

Chair of Pediatrics and Pediatrician-in-Chief
Nemours Children's Health System
Professor of Pediatrics
University of Central Florida College of Medicine
Orlando, Florida

ELSEVIER

Elsevier
1600 John F. Kennedy Blvd.
Ste 1800
Philadelphia, PA 19103-2899

GOLDSMITH'S ASSISTED VENTILATION OF THE NEONATE,
SEVENTH EDITION

ISBN: 978-0-323-76177-2

Notices

Knowledge and best practice in this field are constantly changing. As new research and experience broaden our understanding, changes in research methods, professional practices, or medical treatment may become necessary.

Practitioners and researchers must always rely on their own experience and knowledge in evaluating and using any information, methods, compounds or experiments described herein. Because of rapid advances in the medical sciences, in particular, independent verification of diagnoses and drug dosages should be made. To the fullest extent of the law, no responsibility is assumed by Elsevier, authors, editors or contributors for any injury and/or damage to persons or property as a matter of products liability, negligence or otherwise, or from any use or operation of any methods, products, instructions, or ideas contained in the material herein.

Previous editions copyrighted 2017, 2011, 2003, 1996, 1988, and 1981.

Library of Congress Control Number: 2021937544

Content Strategist: Sarah Barth
Content Development Manager: Kathryn DeFrancesco
Content Development Specialist: Ann Anderson
Publishing Services Manager: Deepthi Unni
Project Manager: Janish Ashwin Paul
Design Direction: Renee Duenow

Printed in India

Last digit is the print number: 9 8 7 6 5 4 3 2 1

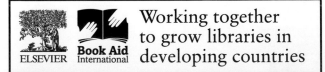

Kabir Abubakar, MD
Professor of Clinical Pediatrics
Director, Neonatal ECMO Program and Respiratory Services
Division of Neonatology, M3400
MedStar Georgetown University Hospital
Washington, DC

Namasivayam Ambalavanan, MBBS, MD
Professor
Department of Pediatrics
University of Alabama at Birmingham
Birmingham, AL

Robert Mason Arensman, BS, MD
Jayant Radhakrishnan Emeritus
Professor of Pediatric Surgery
Department of Surgery
University of Illinois at Chicago
Chicago, IL

Nicolas Bamat, MD, MSCE
Assistant Professor of Pediatrics
Perelman School of Medicine at the University of Pennsylvania
Division of Neonatology
Children's Hospital of Philadelphia
Philadelphia, PA

Eduardo H. Bancalari, MD
Professor
Department of Pediatrics
University of Miami
Miami, FL

Keith J. Barrington, MB, ChB
Professor
Department of Paediatrics
Université de Montréal
Montréal, Québec, Canada

Monika Bhola, MD
Medical Director
Professor of Pediatrics
Division of Neonatology
Rainbow Babies and Children's Hospital
University Hospitals of Cleveland
Cleveland, OH

David M. Biko, MD
Assistant Professor
The Children's Hospital of Philadelphia
Pediatric Radiologist
Pennsylvania Hospital
The University of Pennsylvania Health System
Philadelphia, PA

Laura D. Brown, MD
Associate Professor
Department of Pediatrics, Section of Neonatology
University of Colorado School of Medicine
Aurora, CO

Waldemar A. Carlo, MD
Edwin M. Dixon Professor of Pediatrics
University of Alabama at Birmingham
Codirector
Division of Neonatology
University of Alabama at Birmingham
Birmingham, AL

Robert L. Chatburn, MHHS, RRT-NPS, FAARC
Clinical Research Manager
Respiratory Care
Cleveland Clinic
Professor
Department of Medicine
Lerner College of Medicine of Case Western Reserve University
Cleveland, OH

Nelson Claure, MSc, PhD
Professor of Pediatrics and Biomedical Engineering
Director Neonatal Respiratory Physiology Laboratory
Department of Pediatrics, Division of Neonatology
University of Miami Miller School of Medicine
Miami, FL

Clarice Clemmens, MD
Associate Professor
Department of Otolaryngology
Medical University of South Carolina
Charleston, SC

Christopher E. Colby, MD
Professor of Pediatrics Neonatal Medicine – Division Chair
Mayo Clinic
Rochester, MN

Sherry E. Courtney, MD, MS
Professor of Pediatrics
University of Arkansas for Medical Sciences
Little Rock, AR

Peter G. Davis, MBBS, MD
Professor of Neonatology
The Royal Women's Hospital
University of Melbourne
Melbourne, Victoria, Australia

Eugene M. Dempsey, FRCPI
Professor
Department of Paediatrics and Child Health
University College Cork
Professor
Irish Centre for Fetal and Neonatal Translational Research (INFANT)
University College Cork
Cork, Ireland

Robert M. DiBlasi, RRT-NPS, FAARC
RT Research Manager
Respiratory Therapy
Seattle Children's Hospital and Research Institute
Seattle, WA

Matthew Drago, MD, MBE
Assistant Professor of Pediatrics
Division of Newborn Medicine
The Icahn School of Medicine at Mount Sinai
New York, NY

Eric C. Eichenwald, MD
Professor of Pediatrics
Perelman School of Medicine
University of Pennsylvania
Chief, Division of Neonatology
Children's Hospital of Philadelphia
Philadelphia, PA

Jonathan M. Fanaroff, MD, JD
Professor of Pediatrics
Case Western Reserve University School of Medicine
Director
Rainbow Center for Pediatric Ethics
Rainbow Babies & Children's Hospital
Cleveland, OH

Maria V. Fraga, MD
Attending Neonatologist
Children's Hospital of Philadelphia
Associate Professor of Pediatrics
Perelman School of Medicine
University of Pennsylvania
Philadelphia, PA

Debbie Fraser, MN, CNeoN(C)
Associate Professor
Faculty of Health Disciplines
Athabasca University
Athabasca, Alberta, Canada
Neonatal Nurse Practitioner
NICU
St Boniface Hospital
Winnipeg, Manitoba, Canada

K. Suresh Gautham, MBBS, MD, DM, MS, FAAP
Chair of Pediatrics and Pediatrician-in-Chief
Nemours Children's Health System
Professor of Pediatrics
University of Central Florida College of Medicine
Orlando, FL

Jay P. Goldsmith, MD
Clinical Professor of Pediatrics
Tulane University
New Orleans, LA

Peter H. Grubb, MD
Clinical Professor of Pediatrics
University of Utah
Salt Lake City, UT

Malinda N. Harris, MD
Assistant Professor of Pediatrics
Knoxville, TN
East Tennessee Children's Hospital

Helmut Hummler, MD, MBA
Professor of Pediatrics
Ulm University
Hagnau, Germany

Erik B. Hysinger, MD, MS
Assistant Professor
Department of Pediatrics
Cincinnati Children's Hospital Medical Center
Cincinnati, OH

Robert M. Insoft, MD, FAAP
Professor of Pediatrics
Brown University Alpert Medical School
Chief Medical Officer
Women and Infants Hospital
Providence, RI

Erik Allen Jensen, MD, MSCE
Assistant Professor
Department of Pediatrics
University of Pennsylvania
Attending Neonatologist
Children's Hospital of Philadelphia
Philadelphia, PA

Jegen Kandasamy, MBBS, MD
Assistant Professor
Department of Pediatrics
University of Alabama at Birmingham
Birmingham, AL

Lakshmi I. Katakam, MD, MPH
Associate Professor of Pediatrics
Division of Neonatology, Baylor College of Medicine
Medical Director of NICU, Texas Children's Hospital
Houston, Texas

Martin Keszler, MD
Professor
Department of Pediatrics
Alpert Medical School of Brown University
Director of Respiratory Services
Pediatrics
Women and Infants Hospital
Providence, RI

Haresh Kirpalani, BM, MSc
Professor of Neonatology
Department of Pediatrics
The Children's Hospital of Philadelphia
Philadelphia, PA
Emeritus Professor
Clinical Epidemiology
McMaster University
Hamilton, Ontario, Canada

Nathaniel Koo, BS, MD
Assistant Professor of Pediatric Surgery
University of Illinois at Chicago
Chicago, IL

Satyan Lakshminrusimha, MBBS, MD, FAAP
Professor and Dennis and Nancy Marks Chair
Department of Pediatrics
Pediatrician-in-Chief
University of California Davis Children's Hospital
Sacramento CA

Krithika Lingappan, MD, MS
Assistant Professor
Department of Pediatrics
Baylor College of Medicine
Houston, TX

Akhil Maheshwari, MD
Professor of Pediatrics
Johns Hopkins University
Baltimore, MD

Mark Crawford Mammel, MD
Professor of Pediatrics
University of Minnesota
Minneapolis, MN

Brett J. Manley, MBBS (Hons), FRACP, PhD
Neonatologist
Newborn Research
The Royal Women's Hospital
Associate Professor
Department of Obstetrics and Gynecology
The University of Melbourne
Honorary Fellow
Murdoch Children's Research Institute
Melbourne, Victoria, Australia

Camilia R. Martin, MD, MS
Associate Director, NICU
Department of Neonatology
Beth Israel Deaconess Medical Center
Associate Professor of Pediatrics
Harvard Medical School
Boston, MA

Richard John Martin, MBBS
Professor
Department of Pediatrics, Reproductive Biology, and
    Physiology & Biophysics
Case Western Reserve University School of Medicine
Drusinsky/Fanaroff Professor of Pediatrics
Rainbow Babies & Children's Hospital

Bobby Mathew, MBBS
Associate Professor of Pediatrics
Division of Neonatology, Department of Pediatrics
Oishei Children's Hospital
Buffalo, NY

Mark R. Mercurio, MD, MA
Professor of Pediatrics
Chief, Division of Neonatal-Perinatal Medicine
Director, Program for Biomedical Ethics
Yale University School of Medicine
New Haven, CT

Andrew Mudreac, BS
Resident Physician
Department of Surgery
New York Presbyterian—Weill Cornell Medicine
New York, NY

Leif D. Nelin, MD
Chief
Division of Neonatology
Nationwide Children's Hospital
Professor and Chief of Neonatology
The Ohio State University
Columbus, OH

Louise S. Owen, MBChB, MRCPCH, FRACP, MD
Neonatologist,
Newborn Research,
Royal Women's Hospital,
Melbourne
Associate Professor, Principal Research Fellow,
Department of Obstetrics and Gynaecology,
University of Melbourne
Research Fellow,
Murdoch Children's Research Institute,
Melbourne, Australia

Allison Hope Payne, MD, MS
Assistant Professor of Pediatrics/Neonatology
Rainbow Babies and Children's Hospitals/Case Western Reserve
    University
Cleveland, OH

Jeffrey M. Perlman, MB, ChB
Professor of Pediatrics
Weill Cornell
New York, NY
Division Chief
Newborn Medicine
New York Presbyterian Hospital
New York, NY

Joseph Piccione, DO, MS
Pulmonary Director
Center for Pediatric Airway Disorders
The Children's Hospital of Philadelphia
Associate Professor of Clinical Pediatrics
Division of Pediatric Pulmonary Medicine
University of Pennsylvania School of Medicine
Philadelphia, PA

J. Jane Pillow, BMedSci(Dist), MBBS, FRACP, PhD(Dist)
Professor, NHMRC Leadership Fellow
School of Human Science
University of Western Australia
Lead, Cardiorespiratory Health
Telethon Kids Institute
Associate Editor, Neonatology
School of Human Sciences
Perth, Western Australia, Australia

Richard Alan Polin, BA, MD
Director Division of Neonatology
Department of Pediatrics
Morgan Stanley Children's Hospital
William T Speck Professor of Pediatrics
Columbia University College of Physicians and Surgeons
Executive Vice Chair
Department of Pediatrics
Columbia University
New York, NY

Francesco Raimondi, MD, PhD
Professor of Pediatrics
Neonatal Intensive Care Unit and Regional Transport Program
Università Federico II di Napoli
Naples, Italy

Tonse N.K. Raju, MD, DCH, FAAP
Program Officer
Office of the Director
Environmental Influences on Child Health Outcomes (ECHO)
National Institutes of Health
Bethesda, MD,
Adjunct Professor of Pediatrics
Uniformed Services University, Bethesda, MD,

Lawrence Rhein, MD, MPH
Associate Professor
Department of Pediatrics
University of Massachusetts Medical School
Chief, Division of Neonatology
Chair, Department of Pediatrics
UMass Memorial Health
Worcester, MA

Guilherme Sant'Anna, MD, PhD, FRCPC
Professor of Pediatrics
Neonatal Division McGill University Health Center
Associate Member of the Division of Experimental Medicine
McGill University
Montreal, Quebec, Canada

Georg Schmölzer, MD, PhD
Associate Professor
Faculty of Medicine & Dentistry, Department of Pediatrics,
Division of Neonatal-Perinatal Care (NICU)
University of Alberta
Neonatologist
Northern Alberta Neonatal Program, AHS
Director
Centre for the Studies of Asphyxia & Resuscitation
Royal Alexandra Hospital
Edmonton, Alberta, Canada

Andreas Schulze, MD
Professor Emeritus of Pediatrics
University of Munich Perinatal Center
Department of Pediatrics
Division of Neonatology
Munich, Germany

Grant Shafer, MD, MA
Neonatologist
Division of Neonatology
Children's Hospital of Orange County
Orange, CA
Assistant Professor of Pediatrics
Division of Neonatology
University of California Irvine School of Medicine
Irvine, CA

Wissam Shalish, MD, FRCPC
Assistant Professor
Department of Pediatrics
Division of Neonatology
McGill University Health Center
Montreal, Quebec, Canada

Edward G. Shepherd, MD
Chief
Section of Neonatology
Nationwide Children's Hospital
Associate Professor of Pediatrics
Department of Pediatrics
The Ohio State University College of Medicine
Columbus, OH

Billie Lou Short, MD
Chief of Neonatology
Children's National Hospital
Professor
Department of Pediatrics
The George Washington University School of Medicine
Washington, DC

Thomas L. Sims Jr., MD
Assistant Professor
Department of Surgery
University of Illinois at Chicago
Chicago, IL

Nalini Singhal, MBBS, MD, FRCP
Professor of Pediatrics
Alberta Children's Hospital Cumming School of Medicine
University of Calgary
Calgary, Alberta, Canada

Roger F. Soll, MD
H. Wallace Professor of Neonatology
Department of Pediatrics
University of Vermont
Burlington, VT

Amuchou Singh Soraisham, MBBS, MD, DM, MS, FRCPC, FAAP
Professor of Pediatrics
Department of Pediatrics, Cumming School of Medicine
University of Calgary, Alberta, Canada
Medical Director,
NICU Foothills Medical Centre, Calgary, Alberta, Canada

Nishant Srinivasan, MD
Assistant Professor of Clinical Pediatrics
Associate Program Director
Neonatal-Perinatal Fellowship
Director for Neonatal Simulation
Division of Neonatal-Perinatal Medicine
Department of Pediatrics
Children's Hospital at the University of Illinois (CHUI)
Chicago, IL

Raymond C. Stetson, MD
Assistant Professor of Pediatrics
Neonatal Medicine
Mayo Clinic
Rochester, MN

Sarah N. Taylor, MD, MSCR
Associate Professor
Department of Pediatrics
Yale School of Medicine
New Haven, CT

Colm P. Travers, MD
Assistant Professor
Department of Pediatrics
University of Alabama at Birmingham
Birmingham, AL

Payam Vali, MD
Assistant Professor
Department of Pediatrics
University of California Davis
Sacramento, CA

Anton H. van Kaam, MD, PhD
Professor of Neonatology
Emma Children's Hospital
Amsterdam UMC
Amsterdam, the Netherlands

Maximo Vento, MD, PhD
Professor
Division of Neonatology
University & Polytechnic Hospital La Fe
Professor
Neonatal Research Group
Health Research Institute La Fe
Valencia, Spain

Michele Walsh, MD, MSEpi
Professor
Department of Pediatrics
UH Rainbow Babies & Children's Hospital
Professor
Department of Pediatrics
Case Western Reserve University
Cleveland, OH

Gary Weiner, MD
Associate Clinical Professor
Neonatal-Perinatal Medicine
University of Michigan
Ann Arbor, MI

Gulgun Yalcinkaya, MD
Assistant Professor of Pediatrics
Division of Neonatology
Medical Director of Transitional Care Nursery
UH Rainbow Babies and Children's Hospital
Case Western University School of Medicine
Cleveland, OH

Vivien Yap, MD
Associate Professor of Clinical Pediatrics
Pediatrics
New York Presbyterian–Weill Cornell Medicine
New York, NY

Bradley A. Yoder, MD
Professor
Department of Pediatrics
University of Utah School of Medicine
Salt Lake City, UT

Huayan Zhang, MD
Attending Neonatologist
Director, The Newborn and Infant Chronic Lung Disease Program
Division of Neonatology, Department of Pediatrics
Children's Hospital of Philadelphia
Philadelphia, PA
Associate Professor of Clinical Pediatrics
University of Pennsylvania Perelman School of Medicine
Philadelphia, PA
Chief, Division of Neonatology and Center for Newborn Care
Guangzhou Women and Children's Medical Center
Guangzhou, Guangdong, China

FOREWORD

Assisted Ventilation of the Neonate is one of the few textbooks in our subspecialty that I consider iconic. The first edition of this book was published 40 years ago, and at least two generations of trainees and practicing neonatologists have considered it the "bible" of respiratory management of critically ill infants.

As I think back to the beginning of my training in the 1970s, I am amazed how much progress has been made in respiratory support of the newborn infant. The first large case series of "near-terminal" preterm neonates with "hyaline membrane disease" by Papadopoulos and Swyer in 1964 provided a framework for ventilation to reverse acid–base disturbances but was associated with almost 100% mortality. It is noteworthy that Patrick Bouvier Kennedy (President John F. Kennedy's son) born at 34 weeks' gestation was treated with hyperbaric oxygen rather than positive-pressure ventilation and is a prime example of the skepticism surrounding ventilation of the newborn infant in the mid-1960s. The problem was twofold. First, there was a general lack of understanding of neonatal respiratory physiology and disease pathophysiology, including the importance of positive end expiratory pressure and surfactant in maintaining alveolar stability. Second, most neonatal intensive care units were using ventilators designed for adults in modes that were never meant for newborns. Beginning in the 1970s, a new generation of ventilators designed for neonates became commercially available. However, those ventilators were still not refined. They did not allow infants to breathe when the ventilator was not cycling (intermittent mandatory ventilation was not available) or were associated with difficult regulation of delivered tidal volumes, resulting in pneumothoraces and chronic lung injury. Since the initial publication of *Assisted Ventilation of the Neonate*, the mortality rate for infants with respiratory distress syndrome has plummeted. The improvement in mortality is multifactorial but is likely secondary to a variety of clinical advancements (including widespread administration of surfactant), greater use of noninvasive ventilation strategies, a better understanding of transitional and postnatal physiological disturbances, smarter clinicians, and increasingly sophisticated ventilators. However, increasingly complex ventilators allowing multiple modes of ventilation has increased the opportunity for operator errors because of the number of ventilator decisions clinicians must make. As with every edition of this textbook, the editors and authors provide a clear way forward to take much of the guesswork out of mechanical ventilation.

The seventh edition of this textbook has the subtitle of "an evidence-based approach." The editors have successfully integrated the "art" of ventilation with current best evidence. As a foundation to those sections, there are in-depth discussions of respiratory physiology and control of breathing, pulmonary function testing, newer radiographic techniques to assess lung pathology, use of oxygen, and delivery room stabilization. Each of the newest strategies for ventilating neonates is presented in great detail along with how to manage infants with diverse respiratory diseases. Finally, the editors have wisely chosen to include chapters on home ventilation, transport, intraoperative management of the neonate, ethical and medical-legal issues, pharmacotherapies, nursing care, and respiratory care in resource-limited setting.

The seventh edition of *Goldsmith's Assisted Ventilation of the Neonate*, edited by Martin Keszler and K. Suresh Gautham, is an outstanding compendium of well-written chapters, which not only guides care providers in how to care for neonates with respiratory diseases but also provides the basis for their recommendations. The editors of this book and authors of the chapters are to be congratulated for producing another superb edition.

Richard A. Polin, MD
William T. Speck Professor of Pediatrics
Columbia University, College of Physicians and Surgeons

In 1978, before there were exogenous surfactants, inhaled nitric oxide, high-frequency ventilators, and other modern therapies, a young overly confident neonatologist (JPG) thought that there needed to be a primer on newborn assisted ventilation for physicians, nurses, and respiratory therapists entrusted with treating respiratory failure in fragile neonates. In the preceding decade, ventilation of neonates was undertaken only in major medical centers, and in 1963, the late preterm son of the President of the United States, John F. Kennedy, died of lack of adequate respiratory support. As the first edition of this text was being written, assisted ventilation had become widely available in hundreds of hospitals in the United States and around the world. Even in the early days of this new subspecialty called neonatology, respiratory support was an essential part of neonatal intensive care. However, there was little guidance in standard neonatal textbooks regarding the proper techniques in neonatal ventilatory support. The initial publication was conceived to fill a void and provide a reference to the caretakers in this new and exciting field but was not intended as a "license in assisted ventilation" for the novice. The neonatologist, only 2 years out of his fellowship, recruited his young partner (EHK) and they prevailed upon their former teachers and mentors to write most of the chapters of the text, while they served mostly as organizers in this initial project. The result exceeded their most optimistic expectations in creating a "how to" guide for successful ventilation of the distressed newborn. The first edition, published in 1981, was modeled after the iconic text of Marshall Klaus and Avroy Fanaroff, *Care of the High-Risk Neonate*, which was the standard clinical reference for practicing neonatal caregivers at the time. Dr. Klaus wrote the foreword, and the first edition of *Assisted Ventilation of the Neonate* was born.

The preface to the first edition started with a quotation from Dr. Sydney S. Gellis, then considered the Dean of Pediatrics in the United States:

"As far as I am concerned, the whole area of ventilation of infants with respiratory distress syndrome is one of chaos. Claims and counterclaims about the best and least harmful method of ventilating the premature infant make me lightheaded. I can't wait for the solution or solutions to premature birth, and I look forward to the day when this gadgetry will come to an end and the neonatologists will be retired."

Year Book of Pediatrics (1977)

After over four decades and seven editions of the text, we are still looking for the solutions to premature birth despite decades of research on how to prevent it, and neonatal respiratory support is still a mainstay of neonatal intensive care. Initially, there were concerns regarding the experience and competence of those managing these new ventilation devices with an unacceptable rate of complications such as bronchopulmonary dysplasia (BPD), pulmonary air leaks (especially with high frequency ventilation), unplanned extubations, plugged endotracheal tubes, nasal trauma with continuous positive airway pressure (CPAP) devices, and others. In the past 40 plus years, pharmacological, nutritional, technological, and philosophical advances in the care of newborns, especially the extremely premature, have continued to refine the way we manage neonatal respiratory failure. Microprocessor-based machinery, information technology, an emphasis on safety, quality improvement, and evidence-based medicine have affected our practice as they have all of medical care. However, the wide variance in outcomes of this most vulnerable population is striking among even the most sophisticated university-based neonatal intensive care units (NICUs). The Vermont Oxford Network, through their Nightingale data collecting system, reports that in the most advanced NICUs (Type C, $n = 158$), BPD secondary to assisted ventilation varied in 2020 from a median of 20.7% in the first quartile to 38% in the third quartile in neonates born under 1500 g or 32 weeks' gestation. Literature reports of BPD vary even more widely, documenting a reported incidence of 5% to 6% in one institution to as high as 50% to 60% in others.

Mere survival is no longer the only goal; the emphasis of neonatal critical care has changed to improving functional outcomes of even the smallest premature infant. While the threshold of viability has been lowered only modestly in the past decade, there have been decreases in morbidities, even at the smallest weights and lowest gestational ages. However, the large institutional variation in morbidities such as BPD, even in the era of widespread administration of antenatal corticosteroid administration to mothers, can no longer be attributed to differences in the populations treated. The uniform application of evidence-based therapies and quality improvement programs has shown significant improvements in outcomes, but unfortunately, not in all centers. We have recognized that much of neonatal lung injury (i.e., ventilator induced lung injury) is due to our ventilatory techniques and occurs predominantly in the most premature infants. Our perception of the ventilator has shifted from that of a lifesaving machine to a tool that can also cause harm—a double-edged sword. However, the causes of this morbidity are multifactorial, and its prevention remains controversial and elusive. This is not a new concept. As early as 1745, Fothergill cautioned regarding the deleterious effects of mechanical ventilation: "Mouth to mouth resuscitation may be better than using a mechanical bellows to inflate the lung because . . . the lungs of one man may bear, without injury, as great a force as those of another can exert, which by the bellows cannot always be determined" (*J Philos Trans R Soc, Lond.* 1745). Specifically, attempts to decrease the incidence of BPD have concentrated on ventilatory approaches such as earlier and more extensive use of CPAP, noninvasive ventilation, volume-targeted modes, various devices to synchronize ventilator and spontaneous breathing, and adjuncts such as caffeine and vitamin A. Yet, some of these therapies remain unproven in large clinical trials, and the national incidence of BPD in large databases for very low birth weight infants exceeds 30%. Thus, until there are social, pharmacological, and technical solutions to prematurity, neonatal caregivers will continue to be challenged to provide respiratory support for the smallest premature infants without causing lifelong pulmonary or central nervous system injury.

In this, the seventh edition, the transition to two new editors, Dr. Keszler and Dr. Gautham, has been completed. Martin Keszler, MD, Professor of Pediatrics and Medical Director of Respiratory Care at Brown University, is internationally renowned for his work in neonatal ventilation. Kanekal Suresh Gautham, MD, DM, MS, is the Chairman of Pediatrics and Pediatrician-in-Chief at Nemours Children's Hospital and a Professor of Pediatrics at the University of Central Florida College of Medicine, Orlando, FL. He is a Deputy Editor of The Joint Commission Journal on Quality and Safety, is a Senior Editor for the Neonatal Review Group of the Cochrane Collaboration, and is regarded as one of the foremost authorities on quality improvement in neonatal care.

Since the sixth edition, new ventilatory devices have been introduced, and support has continued to shift from an invasive to a noninvasive approach, which has resulted in significant improvements in some outcomes, but also new challenges for providers. Recent improvements to ventilatory devices have also not come without cost. The new generation of ventilators has added a new level of complexity as well as expense to neonatal care. While some clinicians may be attracted to the advanced features of new devices, the new technology may pose risks to patients as devices may not be fully understood or misapplied by multiple caretakers at the bedside. More commonly, many of the new ventilator features are infrequently used in clinical practice. Unfortunately, many providers do not use or understand how to apply important adjuncts to care, such as pulmonary graphics. Hopefully, these deficiencies can be addressed by texts such as this.

The seventh edition of *Assisted Ventilation of the Neonate* has been extensively updated and rewritten, with many new contributors and several new chapters. The text is divided into six sections. The first section covers general principles and concepts and includes chapters on physiologic principles, ethical and medical-legal aspects of respiratory care, and quality and safety. The second section reviews assessment, diagnosis, and monitoring methods of the newborn in respiratory distress, including chapters on physical assessment, imaging, blood gas monitoring, and pulmonary function and graphics. Essential aspects of respiratory support are covered in the third section with discussions on delivery room management, oxygen therapy, and all types of ventilatory modes and strategies. A new chapter on respiratory gas conditioning has been added to this section. Adjunctive interventions such as pulmonary and nursing care, nutritional support, and pharmacologic therapies are the subjects of the fourth section. The fifth section reviews special situations and outcomes, including chapters on BPD care, surgical and medical considerations of the airway, intraoperative management, and new chapters on persistent pulmonary hypertension and congenital diaphragmatic hernia. Finally, the sixth section reviews complications, transition from hospital to home, pulmonary and neurologic outcomes, care in resource limited settings, and a new final chapter on gaps in knowledge and future directions.

During the four-plus decade and seven-edition life of this text, neonatology has grown and evolved in the nearly 1000 NICUs in the United States. The two young neonatologists, now past-due for retirement, have turned over the leadership of this and future editions of the text to the new editors. We have seen new and unproven therapies come and go, and despite our frustration at not being able to prevent death or morbidity in all our patients, we continue to advocate for evidence-based care and robust clinical trials before the application of new devices and therapies. We hope this text will stimulate its readers to continue to search for better therapies as they use the wisdom of these pages in their clinical practice. We are honored to have Dr. Richard Polin, the American Academy of Pediatrics 2021 Apgar Award winner and editor/author of his own classic text on *Fetal and Neonatal Physiology*, favor us with the foreword to this edition. And as we wait for the solution(s) to prematurity, we should heed the wisdom of the old *Lancet* editorial: "The tedious argument about the virtues of respirators not invented over those readily available can be ended, now that it is abundantly clear that the success of such apparatus depends on the skill with which it is used" (*Lancet*. 1965;2:1227).

Jay P. Goldsmith, MD, FAAP
November 2021

CONTENTS

Introduction and Historical Aspects

Jay P. Goldsmith and Tonse N. K. Raju

KEY POINTS

- The birth and early death of a premature son to President John F. Kennedy and Jacqueline Kennedy in 1963 focused the world's attention on prematurity and the treatment of hyaline membrane disease (HMD), leading to the research and development of pulmonary surfactants, ventilatory devices and improved ventilatory techniques that heralded the modern era of neonatology.
- Although the first reference to providing assisted ventilation to a child is found in the Old Testament, the first 15 centuries AD of recorded attempts to ventilate the neonate or child were crude and generally unsuccessful.
- The early understanding of general cardiorespiratory physiology in the fifteenth through nineteenth centuries led to some anecdotal success of basic ventilatory devices that improved neonatal resuscitation efforts and offered some long term respiratory support to children.
- The first half of the twentieth century witnessed the introduction of many devices that proved mostly unsuccessful in the respiratory treatment of neonates with respiratory failure. In the second half of this century, improved understanding of the physiology of respiratory distress syndrome, the application of end expiratory pressure, and enhancing pulmonary maturation with antenatal steroids and pulmonary surfactant therapy were major advances in the treatment of premature lung disease.
- The major reduction in morbidity and mortality from respiratory failure of newborns seen from 1970 to 2010 has been followed by only modest improvement in the last decade. Further gains in reducing chronic pulmonary morbidities associated with assisted ventilation will depend on translational research and quality improvement initiatives from the bench to the bedside.

The birth of a premature son to President John F. Kennedy and Jacqueline Kennedy on August 7, 1963, focused the world's attention on prematurity and the treatment of hyaline membrane disease (HMD), then the current appellation for respiratory distress syndrome (RDS). Patrick Bouvier Kennedy was born by cesarean section at 34 weeks' gestation at Otis Air Force Base Hospital in Massachusetts. He weighed 2.1 kg and was transported to Boston's Massachusetts General Hospital, where he died at 39 hours of age (Fig. 1.1).[1] The Kennedy baby was treated with the most advanced therapy of the era, hyperbaric oxygen,[2] but he died of progressive hypoxemia. There was no neonatal-specific ventilator in the United States to treat the young Kennedy at the time. In response to his death, *The New York Times* reported: "About all that can be done for a victim of hyaline membrane disease is to monitor the infant's blood chemistry and try to keep it near normal levels."[1] The Kennedy tragedy, followed only 3 months later by the president's assassination, stimulated a heightening of interest and research in neonatal respiratory diseases and the treatment of prematurity. This interest resulted in increased federal funding in these areas as well as the proliferation of special areas (neonatal intensive care units [NICUs]) for the care of sick and premature infants at birth in hospitals around the country.

With the possible exception of pediatric oncology, no branch of medicine has seen such dramatic progress in the last half century as has the field of neonatal-perinatal medicine. Less than five decades ago, many centers would not routinely resuscitate infants under 28 weeks of gestation and, in some cases, even those under 1500 g birth weight. A dramatic shift in the physician response and public expectations of care to the very (<1500 g) and extremely low birth weight (<1000 g) newborn occurred largely because of significant advances in perinatal and neonatal care during this period. The improvements in the neonatal areas of respiratory, nutritional, and cardiac care as well as other technological advances gave support to the perception that most preterm infants can be treated effectively and saved from the disorders of prematurity, but also that an overwhelming majority survive without significant long-term disabilities. Specifically, the major technologic advances in ventilatory support, especially over the past two decades, have helped push the concept of the borderline of viability well into the mid second trimester of pregnancy.[3] Improved perinatal care also helped contribute to improved neonatal outcomes, especially the improved assessment of fetal wellbeing, enhancing fetal lung maturation and optimizing the time and method of delivery. The results of these advances have made death from respiratory failure relatively infrequent in the neonatal period

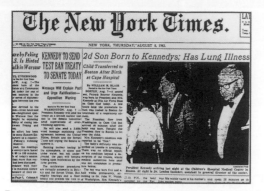

Fig. 1.1 Front page of *The New York Times*. August 8, 1963. (Copyright 1963 by The New York Times Co. Reprinted by permission.)

unless there are significant underlying conditions such as severe sepsis, necrotizing enterocolitis, major intraventricular hemorrhage, or pulmonary hypoplasia. Thus, there is little doubt that had Patrick Bouvier Kennedy been born today, he would have survived without significant long-term sequelae.

Nonetheless, the long-term consequences of respiratory support continue to be a major issue in neonatal intensive care. Chronic lung disease (CLD), also known as bronchopulmonary dysplasia (BPD), oxygen toxicity, and ventilator-induced lung injury (VILI), continue to afflict a significant number of babies, particularly those with birth weights less than 1500 g.

The focus today is not only to provide respiratory support, which will improve survival, but also to minimize the pulmonary and neurologic complications of these treatments. Quality improvement programs to reduce the unacceptably high rate of CLD and other morbidities of prematurity are an important part of translating the improvements in our technology to the bedside. However, many key issues in neonatal respiratory support still need to be answered and many knowledge gaps persist. These include the optimal ventilator strategy for those babies requiring respiratory support; the role of noninvasive ventilation; the best use of pharmacologic adjuncts such as surfactants, inhaled nitric oxide, methylxanthines, and others; the management of the ductus arteriosus; and many other controversial questions. The potential benefits and risks of many therapies represent dilemmas which are discussed in subsequent chapters and will hopefully assist clinicians in their bedside management of newborns requiring respiratory support.

The purpose of this chapter is to provide a brief history of neonatal assisted ventilation with special emphasis on the evolution of the methods devised to support the neonate with respiratory insufficiency to provide the reader with a perspective of how this field has evolved over the past several thousand years.

HISTORY OF NEONATAL VENTILATION: EARLIEST REPORTS

The exact purpose of breathing for survival remained elusive to ancient physicians although cessation of breathing, or respiratory failure, was well recognized as a cause of death for all age groups, including newborn infants. Hwang Ti (2698–2599 BC),

the Chinese philosopher and emperor, noted that respiratory failure occurred more frequently in children born prematurely.[4] Moreover, the medical literature of the past several thousand years contains many references to early attempts to resuscitate infants at birth.

The Old Testament contains the first reference to providing assisted ventilation to a child (II Kings 4:32–35, King James version). "And when Elisha was come into the house, behold the child was dead, and laid upon his bed…. He went up, and lay upon the child and put his mouth upon his mouth, and his eyes upon his eyes, and his hands upon his hands: and he stretched himself upon the child; and the flesh of the child waxed warm…and the child opened his eyes."[5] This description of the first reference to mouth-to-mouth resuscitation suggests that we have been fascinated with resuscitation for millennia.

The Ebers Papyrus from sixteenth century BC Egypt reported increased mortality in premature infants and the observation that a newborn crying at birth will probably survive but the one with an expiratory grunt will die.[6]

Descriptions of artificial breathing for newly born infants and inserting a reed in the trachea of a newborn lamb can be found in the Jewish Talmud (200 BC to 400 AD).[7] Hippocrates (c. 400 BC) first recorded his experience with intubation of the human trachea to support pulmonary ventilation.[8] Soranus of Ephesus (98–138 AD) described signs to evaluate the vigor of the newborn (possibly a medieval precursor to today's Apgar score) and criticized the immersion of the newborn in cold water as a technique for resuscitation.[4]

Galen, who lived between 129 and 199 AD, used a bellows to inflate the lungs of dead animals via the trachea and reported that air movement caused chest "arises." The significance of Galen's findings was not appreciated for many centuries thereafter.[9]

Around 1000 AD, the philosopher and physician Avicenna (980–1037 AD) described the intubation of the trachea with "a cannula of gold or silver." Maimonides (1135–1204 AD), the famous rabbi and physician, wrote about how to detect respiratory arrest in the newborn infant and proposed a method of manual resuscitation. In 1472 AD, Paulus Bagellardus published the first book on childhood diseases and described mouth-to-mouth resuscitation of newborns.[4]

During the Middle Ages, the care of the neonate rested largely with midwives and barber surgeons, delaying the next significant advances in respiratory care until 1513 when Eucharius Rosslin's book first outlined standards for treating the newborn infant.[6] Contemporaneous with this publication was the report by Paracelsus (1493–1541), who described using a bellows inserted into the nostrils of drowning victims to attempt lung inflation and using an oral tube in treating an infant requiring resuscitation.[6]

SIXTEENTH AND SEVENTEENTH CENTURIES

In the sixteenth and seventeenth centuries, advances in resuscitation and artificial ventilation proceeded sporadically with various publications of anecdotal short-term successes, especially in animals. Andreas Vesalius (1514–1564 AD), the famous Belgian anatomist, performed a tracheostomy, intubation, and ventilation on a pregnant sow. Perhaps the first documented trial of "long-term" ventilation was performed by the English scientist Robert Hooke (1635–1703 AD), who kept a dog alive for over an hour using a fireside bellows attached to the trachea.

The scientific renaissance in the sixteenth and seventeenth centuries rekindled interest in the physiology of respiration and in techniques for tracheostomy and intubation. By 1667, simple forms of continuous and regular ventilation had been developed.[9] A better understanding of the basic physiology of pulmonary ventilation emerged with the use of these new devices. However, even at this early stage, some physicians recognized the potential for lung injury by mechanical devices with inspired pressures or volumes too great for the human lung to withstand. In 1745, John Fothergill (1712–1780 AD), an English physician, noted in a lecture to the Royal Society: "Mouth to mouth resuscitation may be better than using a mechanical bellows to inflate the lung because…the lungs of one man may bear, without injury, as great a force as those of another can exert, which by the bellows cannot always be determined."[10]

Various descriptions of neonatal resuscitation during this period can be found in the medical literature. These anecdotal descriptions by midwives included a variety of interventions to revive a depressed neonate, such as giving a small spoonful of wine into the infant's mouth in an attempt to stimulate respirations (first described by Bourgeois in 1609) as well as some more detailed descriptions of mouth-to-mouth resuscitation.[11]

EIGHTEENTH AND NINETEENTH CENTURY

In Europe, medical teaching was dominated by the Church until the French Revolution. The physician Cangiamila was appointed inquisitor by Benedict XIV and wrote a comprehensive textbook describing improved efforts to resuscitate newborns before baptism was allowed.[6] Three different types of crude ventilators were described by Hunter (1755), Chaussier (1780), and Gorcy (1790) in the second half of the eighteenth century.[6] In the early 1800s, there were sporadic attempts to resuscitate and offer mechanical ventilation to the newborn. In 1800, Fine from Geneva described nasotracheal intubation as an adjunct to mechanical ventilation.[12] At about the same time, a better understanding of the principles for mechanical ventilation in adults was evolving. This included the concept of offering rhythmic support of breathing using mechanical devices and, on occasion, passing tubes into the trachea to provide ventilatory support.

In 1806, Vide Chaussier, professor of obstetrics in the French Academy of Science, described his experiments with the intubation and mouth-to-mouth resuscitation of asphyxiated and stillborn infants.[13] The work of his successors led to the development in 1879 of the Aerophore Pulmonaire (Fig. 1.2), the first device specifically designed for the resuscitation and short-term ventilation of newborn infants.[8] This device was a simple rubber bulb connected to a tube. The tube was inserted into the upper portion of the infant's airway, and the bulb was alternately compressed and released to produce inspiration and passive expiration. Subsequent investigators refined these early attempts by designing devices that were used to ventilate laboratory animals.

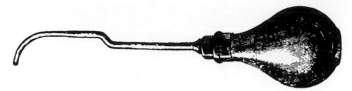

Fig. 1.2 Aerophore pulmonaire of Gairal. (From DePaul. *Dictionnaire Encyclopédique*. XIII, 13th series.)

Charles-Michel Billard (1800–1832) wrote one of the finest early medical texts dealing with clinical-pathologic correlations of pulmonary disease in newborn infants. His book, *Traite des maladies des enfans nouveau-nes et a la mamelle*, was published in 1828.[14]

Billard's concern for the fetus and intrauterine injury is evident, as he writes: "During intrauterine life man often suffers many affectations, the fatal consequences of which are brought with him into the world…children may be born healthy, sick, convalescent, or entirely recovered from former diseases."[14] His understanding of the difficulty newborns may have in establishing normal respiration at delivery is well illustrated in the following passage: "…the air sometimes passes freely into the lungs at the period of birth, but the sanguineous congestion which occurs immediately expels it or hinders it from penetrating in sufficient quantity to effect a complete establishment of life. There exists, as is well known, between the circulation and respiration, an intimate and reciprocal relation, which is evident during life, but more particularly so at the time of birth…. The symptoms of pulmonary engorgement in an infant are, in general, very obscure, and consequently difficult of observation; yet we may point out the following: the respiration is labored; the thoracic parietals are not perfectly develop(ed); the face is purple; the general color indicates a sanguineous plethora in all the organs; the cries are obscure, painful and short; percussion yields a dull sound."[14] It is remarkable that these astute observations were made nearly 200 years ago.

Arguably, James Blundell (1790–1878), the British obstetrician, was perhaps the first to successfully resuscitate apparently stillborn newborn infants by intubation of the trachea using a silver pipe. In his brilliant 1834 paper, he describes how, using the left forefinger as a guide, one can introduce the pipe into the trachea and inflate the infant's lungs by blowing into it.[15]

The advances made in the understanding of pulmonary physiology of the newborn and the devices designed to support a newborn's respiration undoubtedly were stimulated by the interest shown in general newborn care that emerged in the latter part of the nineteenth century and continued into the first part of the twentieth century.[16] The reader is directed to multiple references that document the advances made in newborn care in France by Dr. Étienne Tarnier and his colleague Pierre Budin. Budin may well be regarded as the "father of neonatology" because of his contributions to newborn care, including introducing gavage feeding, publishing survival data, and establishing follow-up programs for high-risk newborn patients[16] (Fig. 1.3).

In Edinburg, Scotland, Dr. John William Ballantyne, an obstetrician working in the latter part of the nineteenth and early

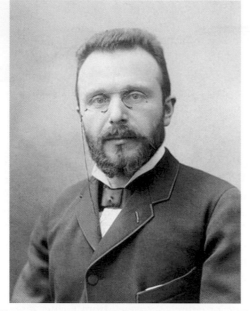

Fig. 1.3 Pierre Budin (1846–1907), Professor of Obstetrics, Hospital de la Charite, Paris, France, the "Father of Neonatology."

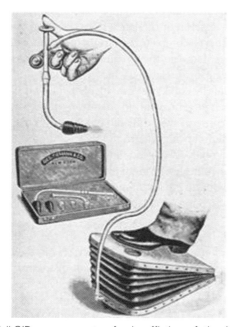

Fig. 1.4 Fell-O'Dwyer apparatus for insufflation of the lungs. (From Mushin WW, Rendell-Baker L (eds): The Principles of Thoracic Anesthesia. Springfield, IL, Charles C Thomas, 1953, with permission. Copyright Wiley-Blackwell.)

twentieth centuries, emphasized the importance of prenatal care and recognized that syphilis, malaria, typhoid, tuberculosis, and maternal ingestion of toxins such as alcohol and opiates were detrimental to the development of the fetus.[16]

O'Dwyer[17] in 1887 reported the first use of long-term positive-pressure ventilation in a series of 50 children with croup. The best known of the early American devices for positive-pressure insufflation on the lungs was described by Fell in 1889. This device became known as the Fell-O'Dwyer apparatus (Fig. 1.4).

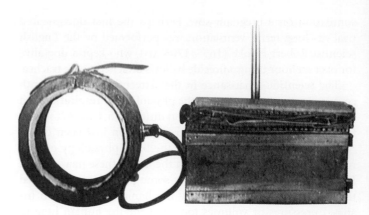

Fig. 1.5 Alexander Graham Bell's negative-pressure ventilator, c. 1889. (From Stern L, Ramos AD, Outerbridge EW, Beaudry PH: Negative pressure artificial respiration: use in treatment of respiratory failure of the newborn. Can Med Assoc J 102(6):595–601, 1970.)

Shortly thereafter, Egon Braun and Alexander Graham Bell independently developed intermittent body-enclosing devices for the negative-pressure/positive-pressure resuscitation of newborns (Fig. 1.5).[18] One might consider these seminal reports as the stimulus for the proliferation of work that followed and the growing interest in mechanically ventilating newborn infants with respiratory failure.

TWENTIETH CENTURY

A variety of events occurred in the early twentieth century in the United States, including most notably the improvement of public health measures, the emergence of obstetrics as a full-fledged surgical specialty, and the assumption of care for all children by pediatricians.[16] In Europe, there were multiple attempts to create a mechanical respirator that would treat respiratory failure in children. A short-term mobile respirator ("the Pulmonator") using alternating positive and negative pressure was introduced by Draeger and Blume in 1907, but the neonatal version received mixed reviews.[6] In 1914, the use of continuous positive airway pressure (CPAP) for neonatal resuscitation was described by Von Reuss.[4] Henderson advocated positive-pressure ventilation via a mask with a T-piece in 1928.[19] In the same year, Flagg recommended the use of an endotracheal tube with positive-pressure ventilation for neonatal resuscitation.[20] The equipment he described was remarkably similar to that in use today.

Modern neonatology was born with the recognition that premature infants required particular attention with regard to temperature control, administration of fluids and nutrition, and protection from infection. In the 1930s and 1940s, premature infants were given new stature, and it was acknowledged that of all of the causes of infant mortality, prematurity was the most common contributor.[16]

Similar advances were being made in basic science and physiology. Sir Joseph Barcroft (1872–1947) of Cambridge inaugurated the modern era in the study of fetal physiology. After an illustrious career studying high-altitude cardiorespiratory physiology, Barcroft began a new line of research when he turned age

60 years—the study of mammalian fetal physiology. He adopted a method reported by A. St. Huggett of exteriorizing fetal sheep delivered into a saline bath and maintaining an intact placental circulation. With this and other models, Barcroft and colleagues studied the mechanisms of fetal-placental gas exchange; placental blood volume; fetal cardiovascular reflexes; cardiac output and distribution; the nutrient functions of oxygen, glucose, fat, proteins, and amino acids; and many facets of fetal growth and growth restriction.[21] He also trained future scientists from around the world, including Clement Smith of Boston and Donald Baron of Gainesville, Florida. These efforts helped establish a firm foundation for the study of cardiorespiratory physiology of the newborn—a welcome addition to the early and fledging efforts by his junior contemporaries trying to develop methods of support for breathing in newborn infants.

The years following World War II were marked by soaring birth rates, the proliferation of labor and delivery services in hospitals, the introduction of antibiotics, positive-pressure resuscitators, miniaturization of laboratory determinations, X-ray capability, and microtechnology that made intravenous therapy available for neonatal patients. These advances and a host of other discoveries heralded the modern era of neonatal medicine and set the groundwork for developing better methods of ventilating neonates with respiratory failure.

Improvements in intermittent negative-pressure and positive-pressure ventilation devices in the early twentieth century led to the development of a variety of techniques and machines for supporting ventilation in infants. In 1929, Drinker and Shaw[22] reported the development of a technique for producing constant thoracic traction to produce an increase in end-expiratory lung volume. In the early 1950s, Bloxsom[23] reported the use of a positive-pressure air lock for resuscitation of infants with respiratory distress in the delivery room. This device was similar to an iron lung; it alternately created positive and negative pressure of 1 to 3 pounds per square inch at 1-minute intervals in a tightly sealed cylindrical steel chamber that was infused with warmed humidified 60% oxygen.[24] Clear plastic versions of the air lock quickly became commercially available in the United States in the early 1950s (Fig. 1.6). However, a study by Apgar and Kreiselman in 1953[25] on apneic dogs and another study by Townsend involving 150 premature infants[26] demonstrated that the device could not adequately support the apneic newborn, which is not surprising, because the infant's face was enclosed in the device and thus there was no pressure gradient between the outside air and the infant's lungs. The linkage of high oxygen administration to retinopathy of prematurity and a randomized controlled trial of the air lock versus care in an Isolette® incubator at Johns Hopkins University[27] revealed no advantage to either study group and heralded the rapid decline in the use of the Bloxsom device.

In the late 1950s, body-tilting devices were designed that shifted the abdominal contents to create more effective movement of the diaphragm. Phrenic nerve stimulation[28] and the use of intragastric oxygen[29] also were reported in the literature but had little clinical success and did not gain wide acceptance.

In the first half of the twentieth century, multiple devices were designed by Flagg, Kreiselman, and others including the Engström device using volume control, but none was particularly effective

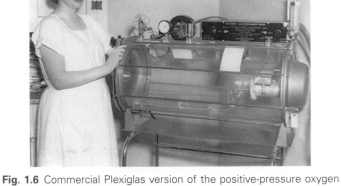

Fig. 1.6 Commercial Plexiglas version of the positive-pressure oxygen air lock. Arrival of the unit at the Dansville Memorial Hospital, Dansville, NY, June 1952. (Photo courtesy of James Gross and the *Dansville Breeze*. June 26, 1952.)

for the ventilation of preterm neonates. By 1960, Abramson listed 21 ventilators designed for neonates in his text on newborn resuscitation.[6]

In the 1950s and early 1960s, many centers also used bag and tightly fitting face mask ventilation to support infants for relatively long periods of time. Unfortunately, there was a high complication rate of intracranial hemorrhage which curtailed the use of these devices.

To the best of our knowledge, Professor Ian Donald and his group from Glasgow, UK, were among the first scientists who successfully provided assisted ventilation for prolonged periods of time for newborn infants with respiratory distress. In 1953, Donald reported the results of "augmented respiration" given to 28 infants from Cape Town, South Africa. Three of the 28 infants lived at least for three or more hours.[30] In 1958, they followed this reporting with pulmonary function test results (using transesophageal electromanometry and spirometry) in 38 infants, 16 of whom had respiratory distress. They also reported that of the 151 newborn infants treated with "augmented respiration," 50 survived, including 11/62 infants with a birth weight ranging between 2 lb and 2 lb 15 oz[31] (907 g and 1332 g).

Two other historical milestones approximately overlapped the efforts of Donald and colleagues in providing assisted ventilation to preterm newborn infants in respiratory distress. In the fall of 1961, Dr. Mildred Stahlman at Vanderbilt University devised a negative pressure ventilator and treated her first patient with severe HMD.[32] In a talk given in 1980, she said, "After placing an umbilical venous catheter in the left atrium, the baby was sealed in the tank where she remained for five very tiring, but enormously instructive days…" The infant survived, and currently, at age 59, she is a registered nurse working at the same institution where she was cared for as a newborn.[33] In 1965, Delivoria-Papadopoulos and colleagues from Canada reported that of the 18 patients offered assisted ventilation using positive-pressure ventilation, one infant who weighed 1.8 kg at 34 weeks' gestation survived, was discharged on the 47th day and appeared to be doing well at age 6 months.[34] These efforts, besides being of historical significance, should be viewed as great success stories because they attempted to treat infants who were extremely ill, and in some cases, "terminal" or "near-terminal."[35]

Partially in response to the Kennedy baby's death in 1963, several intensive care nurseries around the country (most notably at Yale, Children's Hospital of Philadelphia, Vanderbilt, and the University of California at San Francisco) began programs focused on respiratory care of the premature neonate and the treatment of HMD. The initial success with ventilatory treatment of HMD reported by Delivoria-Papadopoulos[34] and Stahlman[32] resulted in the use of modified adult ventilatory devices in these and other medical centers across the United States. However, these successes also led to the emergence of a new disease, BPD, first described in a seminal paper by Northway et al.[36] in 1967. Initially, Northway attributed BPD to the use of high concentrations of inspired oxygen, but subsequent research by others demonstrated that the cause of BPD was much more complex. Besides high concentrations of inspired oxygen, intubation, barotrauma, volutrauma, infection, and other factors were involved, superimposed on the immature lungs and airways of premature infants. Chapters 21 and 36 discuss the current theories for the multiple causes of BPD or VILI.

Advances in ventilatory support for the neonate also influenced improvement in neonatal resuscitation. Varying techniques in the United States were published from the 1950s to the 1980s, but the first systematic approach was created by Bloom and Cropley in 1987 and adopted by the American Academy of Pediatrics and American Heart Association as a standardized teaching program.[37] A synopsis of the major events in the development of neonatal resuscitation is shown as a timeline in Box 1.1.

In the decades following Donald's pioneering efforts, the field of mechanical ventilation made dramatic advances; however, the gains were accompanied by several temporary setbacks. Because of the epidemic of poliomyelitis in the 1950s, experience was gained with the use of the tank-type negative-pressure ventilators of the Drinker design.[32] The success of these machines with children encouraged physicians to try modifications of these ventilators for use in the treatment of newborn infants and some anecdotal success was reported. However, initial efforts to apply intermittent positive-pressure ventilation (IPPV) to premature infants with RDS were disappointing overall. Mortality was not demonstrably decreased, and the incidence of complications, particularly that of pulmonary air leaks, increased.[38] During this period, clinicians were hampered by the available types of ventilators and by a lack of physiologically based approaches for their use.

In accordance with the findings of Cournand et al.[39] in adult studies conducted in the late 1940s, standard ventilatory technique often required that the inspiratory positive-pressure times be very short. Cournand et al. had demonstrated that the prolongation of the inspiratory phase of the ventilator cycle in patients with normal lung compliance could result in impairment of thoracic venous return, a decrease in cardiac output, and the unacceptable depression of blood pressure. To minimize cardiovascular effects, they advocated that the inspiratory phase of a mechanical cycle be limited to one-third of the entire

---

BOX 1.1   Neonatal Resuscitation Timeline

1300 BC: Hebrew midwives use mouth-to-mouth breathing to resuscitate newborns.

460–380 BC: Hippocrates describes intubation of trachea of humans to support respiration.

200 BC–500 AD: Hebrew text (Talmud) states, "we may hold the young so that it should not fall on the ground, blow into its nostrils and put the teat into its mouth that it should suck."

98–138 AD: Greek physician Soranus describes evaluating neonates with a system similar to present-day Apgar scoring, evaluating muscle tone, reflex or irritability, and respiratory effort. He believed that asphyxiated or premature infants and those with multiple congenital anomalies were "not worth saving."

1135–1204: Maimonides describes how to detect respiratory arrest in newborns and describes a method of manual resuscitation.

1667: Robert Hooke presents to the Royal Society of London his experience using fireside bellows attached to the trachea of dogs to provide continuous ventilation.

1774: Joseph Priestley produces oxygen but fails to recognize that it is related to respiration. Royal Humane Society advocates mouth-to-mouth resuscitation for stillborn infants.

1783–1788: Lavoisier terms oxygen "vital air" and shows that respiration is an oxidative process that produces water and carbon dioxide.

1806: Vide Chaussier describes intubation and mouth-to-mouth resuscitation of asphyxiated newborns.

1834: James Blundell describes neonatal intubation.

1874: Open chest cardiac massage reported in an adult.

1879: Report on the Aerophore Pulmonaire, a rubber bulb connected to a tube that is inserted into a neonate's airway and then compressed and released to provide inspiration and passive expiration.

1889: Alexander Graham Bell designs and builds body-type respirator for newborns.

Late 1880s: Bonair administers oxygen to premature "blue baby."

1949: Dr. Julius Hess and Evelyn C. Lundeen, RN, publish *The Premature Infant and Nursing Care*, which ushers in the modern era of neonatal medicine.

1953: Virginia Apgar reports on the system of neonatal assessment that bears her name.

1961: Dr. Jim Sutherland tests negative-pressure infant ventilator.

1971: Dr. George Gregory and colleagues publish results with continuous positive airway pressure (CPAP) in treating newborns with respiratory distress syndrome.

1987: American Academy of Pediatrics publishes the Neonatal Resuscitation Program (NRP) based on an education program developed by Bloom and Cropley to teach a uniform method of neonatal resuscitation throughout the United States.

1999: The International Liaison Committee on Resuscitation (ILCOR) publishes the first neonatal advisory statement on resuscitation drawn from an evidence-based consensus of the available science. The ILCOR publishes an updated Consensus on Science and Treatment Recommendations (CoSTaR) for neonatal resuscitation every 5 years thereafter. The NRP published every 5 years based on the ILCOR CoSTaR recommendations.

2020: Over 4 million health care providers trained in the NRP program by over 21,000 active instructors over the history of the NRP program.

---

cycle.[39] Some ventilators manufactured in this period were even designed with the inspiratory-to-expiratory ratio fixed at 1:2.

However, the recommendations by Cournand et al. were not applicable to patients with significant RDS, who had a complex combination of abnormal pulmonary mechanics. The dramatically reduced lung compliance and the highly compliant chest wall, combined with a tendency for terminal airways and alveoli to collapse, were factors that led to poor responses to IPPV techniques without positive end-expiratory pressure (PEEP) that worked well in adults and older children. Clinicians were initially disappointed with the outcome of neonates treated with assisted ventilation using these adult oriented techniques.

BREAKTHROUGHS IN VENTILATION

The important observation of Avery and Mead in 1959 was that babies who died of HMD lacked a surface-active agent (surfactant), which increased surface tension in lung liquid samples and resulted in diffuse atelectasis.[40] This finding paved the way toward the modern treatment of respiratory failure in premature neonates by suggesting the constant maintenance of functional residual capacity through some form of end expiratory pressure and the eventual creation of surfactant replacement therapies.

A major breakthrough in neonatal ventilation occurred in 1971 when Gregory et al.[41] reported on clinical trials with CPAP for the treatment of RDS. Recognizing that the major physiologic problem in RDS was the collapse of alveoli during expiration, they applied continuous positive pressure to the airway via an endotracheal tube or sealed head chamber ("the Gregory box") during both expiration and inspiration; dramatic improvements in oxygenation and ventilation were achieved. Although infants receiving CPAP breathed spontaneously during the initial studies, later combinations of IPPV and CPAP in infants weighing less than 1500 g were not as successful.[38] Nonetheless, the concept of CPAP was a major advance. It was later modified by Bancalari et al.[42] for use in a constant distending negative-pressure chest cuirass and by Kattwinkel et al.,[43] who developed nasal prongs for the application of CPAP without the use of an endotracheal tube.

The observation that administration of antenatal corticosteroids to mothers prior to premature delivery accelerated maturation of the fetal lung was made in 1972 by Liggins and Howie.[44] Their randomized controlled trial demonstrated that the risks of HMD and death were significantly reduced in those premature infants whose mothers received antenatal steroid treatment. However, this therapy did not gain wide acceptance for over 2 decades.

Meanwhile, Reynolds and Taghizadeh,[45,46] working independently in Great Britain, also recognized the unique pathophysiology of neonatal pulmonary disease. Having experienced difficulties with IPPV similar to those noted by clinicians in the United States, Reynolds and Taghizadeh suggested prolongation of the inspiratory phase of the ventilator cycle by delaying the opening of the exhalation valve. The "reversal" of the standard (i.e., short) inspiratory-to-expiratory ratio (advocated by Cournand), or "inflation hold," allowed sufficient time for the recruitment of atelectatic alveoli in RDS with lower inflating pressures and gas flows, which, in turn, decreased turbulence and limited the pulmonary effects on venous return to the heart. The excellent results of Reynolds and Taghizadeh shown in the United Kingdom could not be duplicated uniformly in the United States, perhaps because their American colleagues used different ventilators.

Until the early 1970s, ventilators used in NICUs were modifications of adult devices; these devices delivered intermittent gas flows, thus generating IPPV. The ventilator initiated every mechanical breath, and clinicians tried to eliminate the infants' attempts to breathe between IPPV breaths ("fighting the ventilator"), which led to rebreathing of dead space air. In 1971, a new prototype neonatal ventilator was developed by Kirby and colleagues.[47] This ventilator used continuous gas flow and a timing device to close the exhalation valve modeled after Ayre's T-piece used in anesthesia (Fig. 1.7).[47,48] Using the T-piece concept, the ventilator provided continuous gas flow and allowed the patient to breathe spontaneously between mechanical breaths. Occlusion of the distal end of the T-piece diverted gas flow under pressure to the infant. In addition, partial occlusion of the distal end generated PEEP. This combination of mechanical and spontaneous breathing and continuous gas flow was called intermittent mandatory ventilation (IMV).

IMV became the standard method of neonatal ventilation and has been incorporated into all infant ventilators since then. One of its advantages was the facilitation of weaning by progressive reduction in the IMV rate, which allowed the patient to gradually increase spontaneous breathing against distending pressure. Clinicians no longer needed to paralyze or hyperventilate patients to prevent them from "fighting the ventilator." Moreover, because patients continued to breathe spontaneously and lower cycling rates were used, mean intrapleural pressure was reduced and venous return was less compromised than with IPPV.[48]

Meanwhile, progress was also being made in the medical treatment and replacement of the cause of RDS, the absence or lack of adequate surfactant in the neonatal lung. Building on the observations of Avery and Meade in 1959, Fujiwara et al.

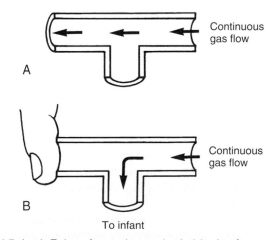

Fig. 1.7 Ayre's T-piece forms the mechanical basis of most neonatal ventilators currently in use. **(A)** Continuous gas flow from which an infant can breathe spontaneously. **(B)** Occlusion of one end of the T-piece diverts gas flow under pressure into an infant's lungs. The mechanical ventilator incorporates a pneumatically or electronically controlled time-cycling mechanism to occlude the expiratory limb of the patient circuit. Between sequential mechanical breaths, the infant can still breathe spontaneously. The combination of mechanical and spontaneous breaths is called intermittent mandatory ventilation. (From Kirby RR: Mechanical ventilation of the newborn. Perinatol Neonatol 5:47, 1981.)

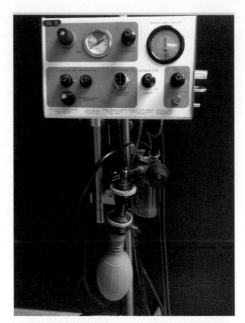

Fig. 1.8 Babybird Neonatal Ventilator (circa 1970).

reported in 1980 on the beneficial effect of exogenous surfactant in a small series of premature infants with HMD.[49] Thereafter, several large randomized studies of the efficacy of surfactant were conducted, and by the end of the decade, the use of surfactant was well established. However, controversies continued for decades concerning surfactant treatment regiments, such as prophylactic versus rescue therapy, types of surfactants, and dosing schedules.[50]

From 1971 to the mid-1990s, a myriad of new ventilators specifically designed for neonates were manufactured and sold. The first generation of ventilators included the Babybird 1® (Fig. 1.8), the Bourns BP200®, and a volume ventilator, the Bourns LS 104/150®. All operated on the IMV principle and were capable of incorporating CPAP into the respiratory cycle (known as PEEP when used with IMV).[51] The first edition of this text published in 1981 described these ventilators in detail.

The Babybird 1® and the Bourns BP200® used a solenoid-activated switch to occlude the exhalation limb of the gas circuit to deliver a breath. Pneumatic adjustments in the inspiratory-to-expiratory ratio and rate were controlled by inspiratory and expiratory times, which had to be timed with a stopwatch. A spring-loaded pressure manometer monitored peak inspiratory pressure and PEEP. These early mechanics created time delays within the ventilator, resulting in problems in obtaining short inspiratory times (<0.5 seconds).

In the next generation of ventilators, electronic controls, microprocessors, and micro-circuitry allowed the addition of light-emitting diode monitors and provided clinicians with faster response times, greater sensitivity, and a wider range of ventilator parameter selection. These advances were incorporated into ventilators such as the Sechrist 100® and Bear Cub® to decrease inspiratory times to as short as 0.1 second and to increase ventilatory rates to 150 inflations per minute. Monitors incorporating microprocessors measured pinspiratory and expiratory times and calculated inspiratory-to-expiratory ratios

and mean airway pressure. Ventilator strategies abounded, and controversy regarding the best (i.e., least harmful) method for assisting neonatal ventilation arose. High-frequency positive-pressure ventilation using conventional ventilators was also proposed as a beneficial treatment of RDS.[52]

Meanwhile, extracorporeal membrane oxygenation and true high-frequency ventilation (HFV) were being developed at a number of major medical centers.[53,54] These techniques initially were offered as a rescue therapy for infants who did not respond to conventional mechanical ventilation. The favorable physiologic characteristics of HFV led some investigators to promote its use as an initial treatment of respiratory failure, especially when caused by RDS in very low birth weight (VLBW) infants, in the hopes of decreasing lung injury.[55]

A third generation of neonatal ventilators began to appear in the early 1990s. Advances in microcircuitry and microprocessors, developed as a result of the space program, allowed new dimensions in the development of neonatal assisted ventilation. The use of synchronized IMV, assist/control mode ventilation, and pressure support ventilation—previously only used in the ventilation of older children and adults—became possible in neonates because of the very fast ventilator response times. Although problems with sensing a patient's inspiratory effort sometimes limited the usefulness of these new modalities, the advances gave hope that ventilator complications could be limited and that the need for sedation or paralysis during ventilation could be decreased. Direct measurement of some pulmonary functions at the bedside became a reality and allowed the clinician to make ventilatory adjustments based on physiologic data rather than on an educated "hunch."

Since the turn of the century, an even newer generation of ventilators has been developed. These are microprocessor based, with a wide array of technological features, including several forms of patient triggering, volume targeting, and pressure support modes and the ability to monitor many pulmonary functions at the bedside with ventilator graphics. As clinicians become more convinced that VILI was secondary to volutrauma more than barotrauma, the emphasis to control tidal volumes especially in the "micropremie" resulted in major changes in the technique of ventilation. The chapters in Section III elaborate more fully on these advances and ventilatory strategies.

Concurrent with these advances came an increased complexity related to controlling the ventilator and, thus, more opportunity for operator error. Some ventilators are extremely versatile and can function for patients of extremely low birth weight (<1000 g) to 70-kg adults. Although these ventilators are appealing to administrators who purchase expensive machines for different categories of adult and pediatric patients in the hospital, they add increased complexity and patient safety issues in caring for neonates. Chapter 6 discusses some of these issues.

Respiratory support in the present-day NICU continues to change as new science and new technologies point the way to better outcomes with less morbidity, even for the smallest premature infants. However, as the technology of neonatal ventilators advanced, a concurrent movement away from intubation and standard ventilation was gaining popularity in the United States. In 1987, a comparison of eight major centers in the

National Institute of Child Health and Human Development Neonatal Research Network by Avery et al. reviewed oxygen dependency and death in VLBW babies at 28 days of age.[56] Although all centers had comparable mortality, one center (Columbia Presbyterian Medical Center) had the lowest rate by far of CLD among the institutions. Columbia had adopted a unique approach to respiratory support of VLBW infants, emphasizing nasal CPAP as the first choice for respiratory support, whereas the other centers were using intubation, surfactants, and mechanical ventilation. Other centers were slow to adopt the Columbia approach, which used bubble nasal CPAP, but gradually institutions began using noninvasive techniques for at least the larger VLBW infants. A Cochrane review of multiple trials in 2012 concluded that the combined outcomes of death and BPD were lower in infants who had initial stabilization with nasal CPAP, and later rescue surfactant therapy if needed, compared with elective intubation and prophylactic surfactant administration (relative risk, 1.12; 95% confidence interval, 1.02 to 1.24).[57] In recent years, "noninvasive" respiratory support with the use of nasal CPAP, synchronized noninvasive intermittent positive pressure ventilation, and neurally adjusted ventilatory assist (NAVA) have become more widely used techniques to support premature infants with respiratory distress in the hope of avoiding the trauma associated with intubation and VILI. Using a noninvasive approach as one potentially better practice is attractive, but quality improvement programs to lower the rate of BPD have had mixed success. Noninvasive ventilation has been supported by a number of retrospective and cohort studies, and reports suggest that the earlier use of noninvasive therapies such as CPAP started in the delivery room has a role in treating neonates with respiratory disease and preventing the need for intubation to treat respiratory failure.

RECENT ADVANCES AND OUTCOMES

The advances in neonatal ventilation over the past five decades has resulted in the mortality from HMD, later called RDS, to decrease dramatically from 1971 through 2019. The rate in the United States dropped from 268 per 100,000 live births in 1971 to 98 per 100,000 live births by 1985 and continued to drop further through the final decades of the twentieth century and into the twenty-first century.[58] By 2007, the rate had decreased to 17 per 100,000 live births.[59]

In an epidemiological study of over 1.5 million preterm live births under 34 weeks' gestation born between 2003 and 2014 reported by Donda et al., RDS was diagnosed in around 36% (554,409 cases). The all-cause mortality in this group decreased from 7.6% to 6.1%. The mortality among those under 28 weeks of gestation dropped from 21.7% to 16.8%, and among 29 to 34 weeks' gestation, from 1.6% to 1.4% between 2003 and 2014, respectively.[60]

The late preterm infant (34 to 36 and 6/7 weeks' gestation) has shown even more compelling improvements as compared with the state-of-the-art medical care available to Patrick Bouvier Kennedy in 1963. In the antenatal steroid trial for women in labor during late preterm gestation (defined in this study as 34 weeks 0 days to 36 weeks 5 days), the incidence of RDS was around 6% (168/2827 in the total cohort). There were only two deaths before hospital discharge, both from non-RDS causes.[61] Similarly, Sekar et al. reported in 2019 that the RDS-related mortality was 2% among the 13,240 preterm infants, 25 to 36 weeks of gestation, born between 2010 and 2013.[62] Based on the available data, we can safely conclude that the mortality from RDS occurs extremely rarely in the modern NICU, mostly confined to extremely preterm infants.

Thus, over a period of five decades, the mortality attributed to RDS has approached less than 2% owing in part to the improvements in ventilator technology, the development of medical adjuncts such as antenatal steroids and exogenous surfactants, and the skill of the physicians, nurses, and respiratory therapists using these devices while caring for these fragile infants.[58-64]

Although the advances made in providing assisted ventilation to our most vulnerable patients have improved survival (85%–90% in premature infants <28 weeks' gestation and/or 1000 g), morbidities remain troublesome. In recent years, the emphasis has shifted from just survival to survival without significant neurologic deficit, BPD, or retinopathy of prematurity. Nonetheless, benchmarking groups such as the Vermont-Oxford Network have shown a wide variance in these untoward outcomes that cannot be explained by variances in the patient population alone. BPD in infants born at less than 1500 g birth weight (i.e., VLBW infants) varies from 6% to over 50% in various NICUs. Thus, it appears that overall advances in the morbidity and mortality rates of the VLBW infant group as a whole will be made from more uniform application of technology already available rather than the creation of new devices or medications. Moreover, despite continued technological advances in respiratory support in the last decade, the reduction in morbidity and mortality rates in high-resource countries has only seen modest improvement. Many of the large organizations of hospitals (Vermont-Oxford Network, Neonatal Research Network) as well as physician organizations (Perinatal Section of the American Academy of Pediatrics, Mednax) have played a major role in disseminating improved aspects of care to the nearly 1000 NICUs in this country. Perhaps entirely new approaches are necessary to produce major leaps forward in the treatment of neonatal respiratory failure. However, in resource-limited areas throughout the world, the use of basic respiratory support technologies (i.e., CPAP, resuscitation techniques) has begun to have a major impact on the outcomes of newborns (see Chapter 40).

Despite the wide array of technology now available to the clinician treating neonatal respiratory failure, there are still significant limitations and uncertainty about our care. We continue to research and discuss issues such as conventional ventilation versus HFV, noninvasive ventilation versus the early administration of surfactant, the best ventilator mode, the optimum settings, and the most appropriate approach to weaning and extubation. There are very few randomized controlled trials that demonstrate significant differences in morbidity or mortality related to new ventilator technologies or strategies. This is owing to the difficulty in enrolling neonates into clinical trials, the large number of patients needed to detect statistical differences in outcomes, the reluctance of device manufacturers to support expensive studies, and the rapidly changing software, which make it difficult for research to keep up with the technological advances. Perhaps the main reason is the fact that outcomes of studies comparing complex interventions, such as ventilator modalities, depend greatly on the skill with which the device or intervention is employed and the appropriateness of the strategies for the population under study. It is the editors' expectations that this book will provide some more food for thought in these areas and the necessary information for the physician, nurse, or respiratory therapist involved in the care of neonates to provide the best possible care based on the information available in 2020 and beyond.

A complete reference list is available at https://expertconsult. inkling.com/.

KEY REFERENCES

X3. Rysavy MA, Horbar JD, Bell EF et al; Eunice Kennedy Shriver National Institute of Child Health and Human Development Neonatal Research Network and Vermont Oxford Network. Assessment of an updated neonatal research network extremely preterm birth outcome model in the Vermont Oxford Network. JAMA Pediatr 2020 Mar 2:e196294. doi: 10.1001/jamapediatrics. 2019.6294. [Epub ahead of print.]

X9. Raju TNK: History of neonatal resuscitation: tales of heroism and desperation. Clin Perinatol 26:629–640, 1999.

X30. Donald I, Lord J: Augmented respiration: studies in atelectasis neonatorum. Lancet 1:9, 1953.

X36. Northway WH Jr., Rosan RC, Porter DY: Pulmonary disease following respiratory therapy of hyaline-membrane disease. Bronchopulmonary dysplasia. N Engl J Med 276:357, 1967.

X41. Gregory GA, Kitterman JA, Phibbs RH, et al: Treatment of the idiopathic respiratory-distress syndrome with continuous positive airway pressure. N Engl J Med 284:1333, 1971.

X44. Liggins GC, Howie RN: A controlled trial of antepartum glucocorticoid treatment for prevention of the respiratory distress syndrome in premature infants. Pediatrics 50:515–525, 1972.

X47. Kirby R, Robison E, Schulz J: Continuous flow ventilation as an alternative to assisted or controlled ventilation in infants. Anesth Analg 51:871, 1972.

X55. Frantz ID 3rd, Werthammer J, Stark AR: High-frequency ventilation in premature infants with lung disease: adequate gas exchange at low tracheal pressure. Pediatrics 71:483, 1983.

X56. Avery ME, Tooley WH, Keller JB, et al: Is chronic lung disease in low birth weight infants preventable? Pediatrics 79(1): 26–30, 1987.

X63. Reese CN, Reese J. Reflections on the early years of neonatology. Paul R. Swyer: the beginnings of Canadian neonatology at The Hospital for Sick Children in Toronto and insights into his early career. J Perinatol 2018; 38:297–305.

2

Physiologic Principles

Martin Keszler and Kabir Abubakar

A good understanding of the unique physiology and pathophysiology of the newborn respiratory system is necessary to provide individualized care that optimizes pulmonary and neurodevelopmental outcomes. It is the responsibility of those who care for critically ill infants to have a sound understanding of respiratory physiology, especially the functional limitations and the special vulnerabilities of the immature lung. The first tenet of the Hippocratic Oath states, "Primum non nocere" ("First do no harm"). That admonition cannot be followed without adequate knowledge of physiology. In daily practice, we are faced with the difficult task of supporting adequate gas exchange in an immature respiratory system, using powerful tools that by their very nature can impair ongoing developmental processes, often resulting in alterations in end-organ form and function.

In our efforts to provide ventilatory support, the infant's lungs and airways are subjected to forces that may lead to acute and chronic tissue injury. This results in alterations in the way the lungs develop and the way they respond to subsequent noxious stimuli. Alterations in lung development result in alterations in lung function as the infant's body attempts to heal and continue to develop. Superimposed on this is the fact that the ongoing development of the respiratory system is altered by the healing process itself.

This complexity makes caring for infants with respiratory failure both interesting and challenging. To effectively provide support for these patients, the clinician must have an understanding not only of respiratory physiology but also of respiratory system development, growth, and healing. Although the lung has a variety of functions, some of which include the immunologic and endocrine systems, the focus of this chapter is its primary function, that of gas exchange.

BASIC BIOCHEMISTRY OF RESPIRATION: OXYGEN AND ENERGY

The energy production required for a newborn infant to sustain metabolic functions depends upon the availability of oxygen and its subsequent metabolism. During the breakdown of carbohydrates, oxygen is consumed and carbon dioxide and water are produced. The energy derived from this process is generated as electrons, which are transferred from electron donors to electron acceptors. Oxygen has a high electron affinity and therefore is a good electron acceptor. The energy produced during this process is stored as high-energy phosphate bonds, primarily in the form of adenosine triphosphate (ATP). Enzyme systems within the mitochondria couple the transfer of energy to oxidation in a process known as *oxidative phosphorylation*.[1]

For oxidative phosphorylation to occur, an adequate amount of oxygen must be available to the mitochondria. The transfer of oxygen from the air outside the infant to the mitochondria, within the infant's cells, involves a series of steps: (1) convection of fresh air into the lung, (2) diffusion of oxygen into the blood, (3) convective flow of oxygenated blood to the tissues, (4) diffusion of oxygen into the cells, and finally, (5) diffusion into the mitochondria. The driving force for the diffusion processes is an oxygen partial pressure gradient, which, together with the convective processes of ventilation and perfusion, results in a cascade of oxygen tensions from the air outside the body to intracellular mitochondria (Fig. 2.1). The lungs of the newborn infant transfer oxygen to the blood by diffusion, driven by the oxygen partial pressure gradient. For gas exchange to occur efficiently, the infant's lungs must remain expanded, the lungs must be both ventilated and perfused, and the ambient partial pressure of oxygen in the alveolar space must be greater than the partial pressure of the oxygen in the blood. The efficiency of the newborn infant's respiratory system is determined by both structural and functional constraints; therefore, the clinician must be mindful of both aspects when caring for the infant.

The infant's cells require energy to function. This energy is obtained from high-energy phosphate bonds (e.g., ATP) formed

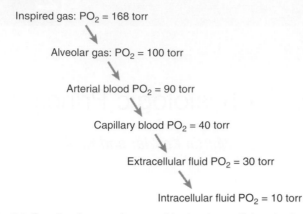

Inspired gas: PO_2 = 168 torr

Alveolar gas: PO_2 = 100 torr

Arterial blood PO_2 = 90 torr

Capillary blood PO_2 = 40 torr

Extracellular fluid PO_2 = 30 torr

Intracellular fluid PO_2 = 10 torr

Fig. 2.1 Transfer of oxygen from outside air to intracellular mitochondria via an oxygen pressure gradient: oxygen tension at various levels of the O_2 transport chain.

during oxidative phosphorylation. Only a small amount of ATP is stored within the cells. Muscle cells contain an additional store of ATP, but to meet metabolic needs beyond those that can be provided for by the stored ATP, new ATP must be made continuously by phosphorylation of adenosine diphosphate (ADP). This can be done anaerobically through glycolysis, but this is an inefficient process and leads to the formation of lactic acid. Long-term energy demands must be met aerobically, through ongoing oxidative phosphorylation within the mitochondria, which is a much more efficient process that results in the formation of carbon dioxide and water.

There is a hierarchy of how energy is used by the infant. During periods of high energy demand, tissues initially draw upon the limited stores of ATP, then use glycolysis to make more ATP from ADP, and then use oxidative phosphorylation to supply the infant's ongoing energy requirements. Oxidative phosphorylation and oxygen consumption are so closely linked to the newborn infant's energy requirements that total oxygen consumption is a reasonably good measure of the total energy needs of the infant. When the infant's metabolic workload is in excess of that which can be sustained by oxidative phosphorylation (aerobic metabolism), the tissues will revert to anaerobic glycolysis to produce ATP. This anaerobic metabolism results in the formation of lactic acid, which accumulates in the blood and causes a decrease in pH (acidosis/acidemia). Lactic acid is therefore an important marker of inadequate tissue oxygen delivery.

ONTOGENY RECAPITULATES PHYLOGENY: A BRIEF OVERVIEW OF DEVELOPMENTAL ANATOMY

Lung Development

The tracheobronchial airway system begins as a ventral outpouching of the primitive foregut, which leads to the formation of the embryonic lung bud. The lung bud subsequently divides and branches, penetrating the mesenchyma and progressing toward the periphery. Lung development is divided into five

sequential phases.[2] The demarcation of these phases is somewhat arbitrary with some overlap between them. A variety of physical, hormonal, and other factors influence the pace of lung development and maturation. Adequate distending pressure of fetal lung fluid and normal fetal breathing movements are some of the more prominent factors known to affect lung growth and development.

Phases of Lung Development

- Embryonic phase (weeks 3 to 6)
- Pseudoglandular phase (weeks 6 to 16)
- Canalicular phase (weeks 16 to 26)
- Terminal sac phase (weeks 26 to 36)
- Alveolar phase (week 36 to 3 years)

Embryonic Phase (Weeks 3 to 6): Development of Proximal Airways

The lung bud arises from the foregut 21 to 26 days after fertilization.

Aberrant development during the embryonic phase may result in the following:

- Tracheal agenesis
- Tracheal stenosis
- Tracheoesophageal fistula
- Pulmonary sequestration (if an accessory lung bud develops during this period)

Pseudoglandular Phase (Weeks 6 to 16): Development of Lower Conducting Airways

During this phase, the first 20 generations of conducting airways develop. The first eight generations (the bronchi) ultimately acquire cartilaginous walls. Generations 9 to 20 comprise the nonrespiratory bronchioles. Lymph vessels and bronchial capillaries accompany the airways as they grow and develop.

Aberrant development during the pseudoglandular phase may result in the following:

- Bronchogenic cysts
- Congenital lobar emphysema
- Congenital diaphragmatic hernia (CDH)

Canalicular Phase (Weeks 16 to 26): Formation of Gas-Exchanging Units or Acini

The formation of respiratory bronchioles (generations 21 to 23) occurs during the canalicular phase. The relative proportion of parenchymal connective tissue diminishes. The development of pulmonary capillaries occurs. Gas exchange depends upon the adequacy of acinus–capillary coupling.

Terminal Sac Phase (Weeks 26 to 36): Refinement of Acini

The rudimentary primary saccules subdivide by formation of secondary crests into smaller saccules and alveoli during the terminal sac phase, thus greatly increasing the surface area available for gas exchange. The interstitium continues to thin out, decreasing the distance for diffusion. Capillary invasion leads to an increase in the alveolar–blood barrier surface area. The development and maturation of the surfactant system occur during this phase.

Birth and initiation of spontaneous or mechanical ventilation during the terminal sac phase may result in the following:

- Pulmonary insufficiency of prematurity (because of reduced surface area, increased diffusion distance, and unfavorable lung mechanics)
- Respiratory distress syndrome (RDS) (owing to surfactant deficiency and/or inactivation)
- Pulmonary interstitial emphysema (PIE) (owing to tissue stretching by uneven aeration, excessive inflating pressure, and increased interstitium that traps air in the perivascular sheath)
- Impairment of secondary crest formation and capillary development, leading to alveolar simplification, decreased surface area for gas exchange, and variable increase in interstitial cellularity and/or fibroproliferation (bronchopulmonary dysplasia [BPD]).

Alveolar Phase (Week 36 to 3 Years): Alveolar Proliferation and Development

Saccules become alveoli as a result of thinning of the acinar walls, dissipation of the interstitium, and invagination of the alveoli by pulmonary capillaries with secondary crest formation during the alveolar phase. The alveoli attain a polyhedral shape.

MECHANICS

The respiratory system is composed of millions of air sacs that are connected to the outside air via airways. The lung behaves like a balloon that is held in an expanded state by the intact thorax and will deflate if the integrity of the system becomes compromised. The interior of the lung is partitioned so as to provide a large surface area to facilitate efficient gas diffusion. The lung is expanded by forces generated by the diaphragm and the intercostal muscles. When the diaphragmatic and intercostal muscle contraction stops, it recoils secondary to elastic and surface tension forces. This facilitates the inflow and outflow of respiratory gases required to allow the air volume contained within the lung to be ventilated. During inspiration, the diaphragm contracts. The diaphragm is a dome-shaped muscle at rest. As it contracts, the diaphragm flattens, and the volume of the chest cavity is enlarged. This causes the intrapleural pressure to decrease and results in gas flow into the lung.[3] During unlabored breathing, the intercostal and accessory muscles serve primarily to stabilize the rib cage as the diaphragm contracts, countering the forces resulting from the decrease in intrapleural pressure during inspiration. This limits the extent to which the infant's chest wall is deformed inward during inspiration.

Although the premature infant's chest is very compliant, the rib cage offers some structural support, serves as an attachment point for the respiratory muscles, and limits lung deflation at end expiration. The elastic elements of the respiratory system—the connective tissue—are stretched during inspiration and recoil during expiration. The air–liquid interface in the terminal air spaces and respiratory bronchioles generates surface tension that opposes lung expansion and promotes lung deflation. The conducting airways, which connect the gas exchange units to the outside air, provide greater resistance during exhalation than during inspiration, because during inspiration, the tethering elements of the surrounding lung tissue increase the airway diameter, relative to expiration. The respiratory system is designed to be adaptable to a wide range of workloads; however, in the newborn infant, several structural and functional limitations make the newborn susceptible to respiratory failure.

Differences between the shape of a newborn infant's chest and that of an adult put the infant at a mechanical disadvantage. Unlike the adult's thorax, which is ellipsoid in shape, the infant's thorax is more cylindrical and the ribs are more horizontal, rather than oblique. Because of these anatomic differences, the intercostal muscles in infants have a shorter course and provide less mechanical advantage for elevating the ribs and increasing intrathoracic volume during inspiration than do those of adults. Also, because the insertion of the infant's diaphragm is more horizontal than in the adult, the lower ribs tend to move inward rather than upward during inspiration. The compliant chest wall of the infant exacerbates this inward deflection with inspiration. This is particularly evident during rapid eye movement (REM) sleep, when phasic changes in intercostal muscle tone are inhibited. Therefore, instead of stabilizing the rib cage during inspiration, the intercostal muscles are relaxed. This results in inefficient respiratory effort, which may be manifested clinically by intercostal and substernal retractions associated with abdominal breathing, especially when lung compliance is decreased. The endurance capacity of the diaphragm is determined primarily by muscle mass and the oxidative capacity of muscle fibers. Infants have low muscle mass and a low percentage of type 1 (slow twitch) muscle fibers compared to those of adults.[4] To sustain the work of breathing, the diaphragm must be provided with a continuous supply of oxygen. The infant with respiratory distress is thus prone to respiratory muscle fatigue leading to respiratory failure.

During expiration, the main driving force is elastic recoil, which depends on the surface tension produced by the air–liquid interface, the elastic elements of the lung tissue, and the bony development of the rib cage. Expiration is largely passive. The abdominal muscles can aid in exhalation by active contraction if required, but they make little contribution during unlabored breathing. Because the chest wall of premature infants is compliant, it offers little resistance against expansion upon inspiration and little opposition against collapse upon expiration.

This collapse at end expiration can lead to atelectasis. In premature infants, the largest contributor to elastic recoil is surface tension. Pulmonary surfactant serves to reduce surface tension and stabilize the terminal airways. In circumstances in which surfactant is deficient, the terminal air spaces have a tendency to collapse, leading to diffuse atelectasis. Distending airway pressure in the form of positive end-expiratory pressure (PEEP) or continuous positive airway pressure (CPAP) may be applied to the infant's airway to counter the tendency toward collapse and the development of atelectasis. The application of airway-distending pressure also serves to stabilize the chest wall.

Lung compliance (a measure the volume of gas the lungs accommodate per unit of pressure applied) and airway resistance are related to lung size. The smaller the lung, the lower the compliance and the greater the resistance. If, however, lung compliance is corrected to lung volume (specific compliance), the values are nearly identical for term infants and adults.[5] In term infants, immediately after delivery, specific compliance is low but normalizes as fetal lung fluid is absorbed and a normal functional residual capacity (FRC) is established. In premature infants, specific compliance remains low, due in part to diffuse microatelectasis and failure to achieve a normal FRC, because the lung recoil forces are incompletely opposed by the excessively compliant chest wall.

Resistance is the result of friction. Viscous resistance is the resistance generated by tissue elements moving past one another. Airway resistance is the resistance that occurs between moving molecules in the gas stream and between these moving molecules and the wall of the respiratory system. The fact that the newborn's bronchial tree is short and the inspiratory flow velocities are low are teleologic advantages for the newborn because both of these factors decrease airway resistance.

Overcoming the elastic and resistive forces during ventilation requires energy expenditure and accounts for the work of breathing. The normal work of breathing is essentially the same for newborns and adults when corrected for metabolic rates.[5] When the work of breathing increases in response to various disease states, the newborn is at a decided disadvantage. The newborn infant lacks the strength and endurance to cope with a significant increase in ventilatory workload; thus, a large increase in ventilatory workload can easily lead to respiratory failure.

Elastic and resistive forces of the chest, lungs, abdomen, airways, and ventilator circuit oppose the forces exerted by the respiratory muscles and/or ventilator. The terms *elastic recoil*, *flow resistance*, *viscous resistance*, and *work of breathing* are used to describe these forces. Such forces may also be described as *dissipative* and *nondissipative* forces. The latter refers to the fact that the work needed to overcome elastic recoil is stored like the energy in a coiled spring and will be returned to the system upon exhalation. Resistive and frictional forces, on the other hand, are lost and converted to heat (dissipated). The terms *elasticity*, *compliance*, and *conductance* characterize the properties of the thorax, lungs, and airways. The static pressure–volume curve illustrates the relationships between these forces at various levels of lung expansion. Dynamic pressure–volume loops illustrate the pressure–volume relationship during inspiration and expiration (Figs. 2.2 to 2.4).

Elastic recoil refers to the tendency of stretched objects to return to their original shape. When the inspiratory muscles relax during exhalation, the elastic elements of the chest wall, diaphragm, and lungs, which were stretched during inspiration, recoil to their original shapes. These elastic elements behave like springs (Fig. 2.5). The surface tension forces at the air–liquid interfaces in the distal bronchioles and terminal airways decrease the surface area of the air–liquid interfaces (Fig. 2.6).

At some point, the forces that tend to collapse are counterbalanced by those that resist further collapse. The point at which these opposing forces balance is called the *resting state of the respiratory system* and corresponds to FRC (Fig. 2.7; see also Fig. 2.2). Because the chest wall of the newborn infant is compliant, it offers little opposition to collapse at end expiration. Thus, the newborn, especially the premature newborn, has a

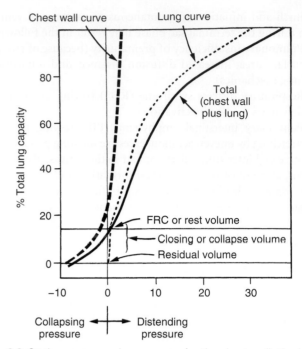

Fig. 2.2 Static pressure–volume curves for the chest wall, the lung, and the sum of the two for a normal newborn infant. Functional residual capacity (*FRC*) or rest volume (less than 20% of total lung capacity) is the point at which collapsing and distending pressures balance out to zero pressure. The lung would empty to residual volume if enough collapsing pressure (forced expiration) was generated to overcome the chest wall elastic recoil in the opposite direction. The premature infant has an even steeper chest wall compliance curve than that shown here, whereas his or her lung compliance curve tends to be flatter and shifted to the right, depending on the degree of surfactant deficiency.

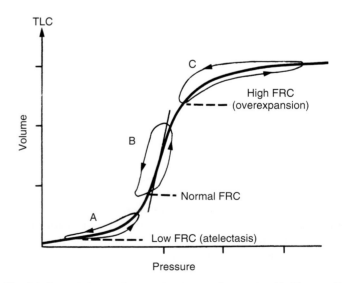

Fig. 2.3 Extended compliance or lung expansion curve with "flattened" areas (*A* and *C*) at both ends. Area *A* represents the situation in disease states leading to atelectasis or lung collapse. Area *C* represents the situation in an overexpanded lung, as occurs in diseases involving significant air trapping (e.g., meconium aspiration) or in the excessive application of distending pressure during assisted ventilation. *FRC*, Functional residual capacity; *TLC*, total lung capacity.

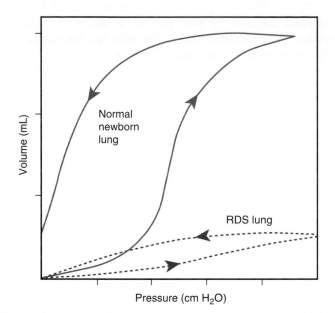

Fig. 2.4 Comparison of the pressure–volume curve of a normal infant (*solid line*) with that of a newborn with respiratory distress syndrome (*dotted line*). Note that very little hysteresis (i.e., the difference between the inspiratory and the expiratory limbs) is observed in the respiratory distress syndrome curve because of the lack of surfactant for stabilization of the alveoli after inflation. The wide hysteresis of the normal infant's lung curve reflects changes (reduction) in surface tension once the alveoli are opened and stabilized. *RDS*, Respiratory distress syndrome.

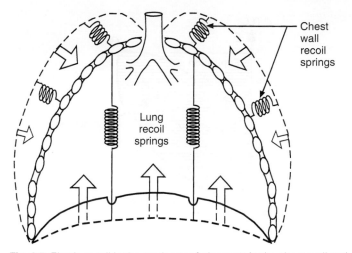

Fig. 2.5 Elastic recoil is the tendency of elements in the chest wall and lungs that are stretched during inspiration to snap back or recoil (*arrows*) to their original state at the end of expiration. At this point (functional residual capacity or rest volume), the "springs" are relaxed and the structure of the rib cage allows no further collapse. Opposing forces of the chest wall and elastic recoil balance out, and intrathoracic and airway pressures become equal (this further defines functional residual capacity or rest volume; see also Fig. 2.2).

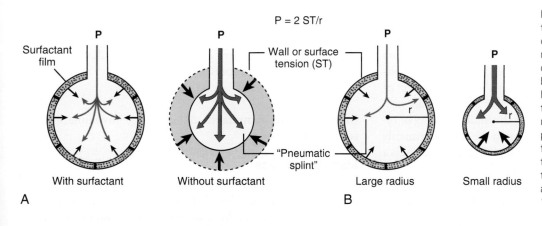

Fig. 2.6 Diagrammatic illustration of the Laplace relationship and the effects of **(A)** surfactant film and **(B)** alveolar radius on wall or surface tension. The degree (reflected in the size of the brown arrows) of airway or intra-alveolar pressure (*P*) needed to counteract the tendency of alveoli to collapse (represented by the black arrows) is directly proportional to double the wall or surface tension (*ST*) and inversely proportional to the size of the radius (*r*). Distending airway pressure applied during assisted ventilation can be likened to a "pneumatic splint."

relatively low FRC and thoracic gas volume, even when the newborn does not suffer from primary surfactant deficiency. Clinically, this manifests as a mild degree of diffuse microatelectasis and is referred to as *pulmonary insufficiency of prematurity*. This low FRC and the relative underdevelopment of the conducting airway's structural support explain the tendency for early airway closure and collapse, with resultant gas trapping in premature infants.

The respiratory system's resting volume is very close to the closing volume of the lung (the volume at which dependent lung regions cease to ventilate because the airways leading to them have collapsed). In newborns, closing volume may occur even above FRC (see Fig. 2.2).[6] Gas trapping related to

airway closure has been demonstrated experimentally by showing situations in which the thoracic gas volume is greater than the FRC. For this to occur, the total gas volume measured in the chest at end expiration is greater than the amount of gas that is in communication with the upper airway (FRC).

The main contributor to lung elastic recoil in the newborn is surface tension. The pressure required to counteract the tendency of the bronchioles and terminal air spaces to collapse is described by the Laplace relationship:

$$P = \frac{2ST}{r}$$

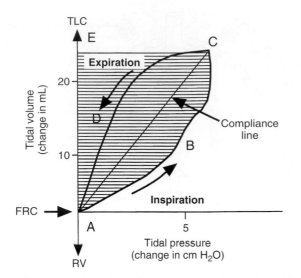

Fig. 2.7 Pressure–volume loop showing the compliance line (*AC*, joining points of no flow); work done in overcoming elastic resistance (*ACEA*), which incorporates the frictional resistance encountered during expiration (*ACDA*); work done in overcoming frictional resistance during inspiration (*ABCA*); and total work done during the respiratory cycle (*ABCEA*, or the entire *shaded area*). *FRC*, Functional residual capacity; *RV*, residual volume; *TLC*, total lung capacity.

Simply stated, this relationship illustrates that the pressure (*P*) needed to stabilize the system is directly proportional to twice the surface tension (*2 ST*) and inversely proportional to the radius of curvature (*r*). In infants, the relationship should be modified, because, unlike in a soap bubble, there is an air–liquid interface on only one side of the terminal lung unit, so $P = ST/r$ probably describes the situation more accurately in the lung.

In reality, alveoli are not spherical but polyhedral and share their walls with adjacent alveolar structures, making strict application of Laplace's law suspect. Nonetheless, the basic concept of the law does apply to both terminal air sacs and small airways, and it provides a crucial framework for the understanding of respiratory physiology. The surface tension in the lung is primarily governed by the presence or absence of surfactant. Surfactant is a surface-active material released by type II pneumocytes. It is composed mainly of dipalmitoyl phosphatidylcholine but contains other essential components, such as surfactant-associated proteins A, B, C, and D, as well.

Surfactant has a variety of unique properties that enable it to decrease surface tension at end expiration and thereby prevent further lung deflation below resting volume and allow an increase in surface tension upon lung expansion that facilitates elastic recoil at end inspiration. In addition, surfactant reduces surface tension when lung volume is decreased.[7] A reduction in the quantity and quality of surfactant results in an increase in surface tension and necessitates the application of more distending pressure to counter the tendency of the bronchioles and terminal air spaces to collapse (see Fig. 2.6A).

As can be seen from Laplace's law, the larger the radius of curvature of the terminal bronchioles or air spaces, the less pressure is needed to hold them open or to expand them further (see Fig. 2.6B). The smaller the radius of curvature (e.g., in

premature infants), the more pressure is required to hold the airways open. Surfactant helps this situation throughout the respiratory cycle. As the radii of the air–liquid interfaces become smaller during exhalation, the effectiveness of surfactant in reducing surface tension increases; as the radii become larger, its effectiveness decreases.

RDS imposes a significant amount of energy expenditure on the newborn infant, who must generate high negative intrapleural pressures to expand and stabilize the distal airways and alveoli (see Fig. 2.4). In untreated RDS, each breath requires significant energy expenditure because lung volumes achieved with the high opening pressures during inspiration are rapidly lost as the surfactant-deficient lung collapses to its original resting volume during expiration. The burden imposed by this large work of breathing may quickly outstrip the infant's ability to maintain this level of output and lead to respiratory failure.

The infant with RDS may need a relatively high inflation pressure to open atelectatic alveoli, and provision of adequate end-expiratory pressure will help keep the lung open. However, once the lung is expanded, the radii of the bronchioles and terminal air spaces are larger, and therefore, less pressure is required to hold them open or to expand them further. Attention should be paid to tidal volume and overall lung volume after initial alveolar recruitment to avoid overdistention and volutrauma, which are major factors in the development of BPD.[8] Failure to reduce inflation and end-expiratory pressures appropriately and thus avoid lung overdistention once normal lung volume has been achieved may lead to air-leak complications such as PIE and pneumothorax (see Chapter 22).

Compliance

Compliance is a measure of the change in volume resulting from a given change in pressure:

$$C_L = \Delta V / \Delta P$$

where C_L is lung compliance, ΔV is change in volume, and ΔP is change in pressure.

Static Compliance

When measured under static conditions, compliance reflects only the elastic properties of the lung. Static compliance is the reciprocal of elastance, the tendency to recoil toward its original dimensions upon removal of the distending pressure required to stretch the system. Static compliance is measured by determining the transpulmonary pressure change after inflating the lungs with a known volume of gas. Transpulmonary pressure is the pressure difference between alveolar pressure and pleural pressure. It is approximated by measuring pressure at the airway opening and in the esophagus. To generate a pressure–volume curve, pressure measurements are made during static conditions after each incremental volume of gas is introduced into the lungs (see lung curve in Fig. 2.2). If one measures the difference between pleural pressures (esophageal) and atmospheric pressures (transthoracic) at different levels of lung expansion, the plotted curve will be a chest wall compliance curve (see chest wall curve in Fig. 2.2). This kind of plot shows the elastic properties of the chest wall. In the newborn, the chest wall is very compliant; thus, large volume changes are achieved with small pressure changes. Taking the lung and chest wall compliance curves together gives the total respiratory system compliance (see the total curve in Fig. 2.2).

Dynamic Compliance

If one measures compliance during continuous breathing, the result is called *dynamic compliance*. Dynamic compliance reflects not only the elastic properties of the lungs but, to some extent, also the resistive component. It measures the change in pressure from the end of exhalation to the end of inspiration for a given volume and is based on the assumption that at zero flow, the pressure difference reflects compliance. The steeper the slope of the curve connecting the points of zero flow, the greater the compliance. Dynamic compliance is the compliance that is generally measured in the clinical setting, but its interpretation can be problematic.[9]

At the fairly rapid respiratory rates common in infants, the instant of zero flow may not coincide with the point of lowest pressure. This is because dynamic compliance is rate dependent. For this reason, dynamic compliance may underestimate static compliance, especially in infants who are breathing rapidly and those with obstructive airway disease. Two additional factors further complicate the interpretation of compliance measurements. In premature infants, REM sleep is associated with paradoxical chest wall motion, so pressure changes recorded from the esophagus may correlate poorly with intrathoracic or pleural pressure changes. Chest wall distortion generally results in underestimation of esophageal pressure changes.[10] Also, because lung compliance is related to lung volume, measured compliance is greatly affected by the initial lung volume above which the compliance measurement is made. Ideally, comparisons should be normalized to the degree of lung expansion, for example, to FRC. Lung compliance divided by FRC is called *specific lung compliance.*

Dynamic pressure–volume relationships can be examined by simultaneous recording of pressure and volume changes. The pressure–volume loop allows one to quantify the work done to overcome airway resistance and to determine lung compliance (see Figs. 2.4 and 2.7). Fig. 2.3 shows a static lung compliance curve upon which three pressure–volume loops are superimposed. Each of the loops shows a complete respiratory cycle, but each is taken at a different lung volume. The overall compliance curve is sigmoidal. At the lower end of the curve (at low lung volume), the compliance is low; that is, there is a small change in volume for a large change in pressure (see Fig. 2.3A). This correlates with underinflation. Pressure is required to open up terminal airways and atelectatic terminal air spaces before gas can move into the lung. The lung volume is starting below critical opening pressure. At the center of the curve, the compliance is high; there is a large change in volume for a small change in pressure. This is where normal tidal breathing should occur (see Fig. 2.3B). This is the position of maximum efficiency in a mechanical sense, the best ventilation/perfusion matching and lowest pulmonary vascular resistance. At the upper end of the curve (at high lung volume), the compliance is low; again, there

is a small change in volume for a large change in pressure (see Fig. 2.3C). This correlates with a lung that already is overinflated. Applying additional pressure yields little in terms of additional volume but may contribute significantly to airway injury and compromises venous return because of increased transmission of pressure to the pleural space. This is the result of the chest wall compliance rapidly falling with excessive lung inflation. Thus, it is important to understand that compliance is reduced at both high and low lung volumes. Low lung volumes are seen in surfactant deficiency states (e.g., RDS), whereas high lung volumes are seen in obstructive lung diseases, such as BPD. Reductions in both specific compliance and thoracic gas volume have been measured in infants with RDS.[11,12]

The rapid respiratory rates of premature infants with surfactant deficiency can compensate for chest wall instability to a certain extent because the short expiratory time results in gas trapping that tends to normalize their FRC. They also use expiratory grunting as a method of expiratory braking to help maintain FRC. In infants with RDS treated in the presurfactant era, serial measurements of FRC and compliance have been shown to be sensitive indicators of illness severity.[13]

Dynamic lung compliance has been shown to decrease as the clinical course worsens and to improve as the recovery phase begins. When mechanical ventilation is used in infants with noncompliant lungs resulting from surfactant deficiency, elevated distending pressures may be required initially to establish a reasonable FRC. Fig. 2.4 shows the pressure–volume loop of a normal infant and that of an infant with RDS. A higher pressure is required to establish an appropriate lung volume in the infant with RDS than in the normal infant. However, this lung volume will be lost if the airway pressure is allowed to return to zero without the application of PEEP. Mechanical ventilation without PEEP leads to surfactant inactivation resulting in worsening lung compliance, and the repeated cycling of the terminal airways from below critical opening pressure leads to cellular injury and inflammation (atelectotrauma). This results in alveolar collapse, atelectasis, interstitial edema, and elaboration of inflammatory mediators.

Once atelectasis occurs, lung compliance deteriorates, surfactant turnover is increased, and ventilation/perfusion mismatch with increased intrapulmonary right-to-left shunting develops. A higher distending pressure and higher concentrations of inspired oxygen (FiO_2) will be required to maintain lung volume and adequate gas exchange, resulting in further injury. Early establishment of an appropriate FRC, administration of surfactant, use of CPAP or PEEP to avoid the repeated collapse and reopening of small airways (atelectotrauma), avoidance of overinflation caused by using supraphysiologic tidal volumes (volutrauma), and avoidance of use of more oxygen than is required (oxidative injury) all are important in achieving the best possible outcome and long-term health of patients.[14]

The level of PEEP at which static lung compliance is maximized has been termed the best, or optimum, PEEP. This is the level of PEEP at which O_2 transport (cardiac output and O_2 content) is greatest. If the level of PEEP is raised above the optimal level, dynamic compliance decreases rather than increases.[15] Additionally, venous return and cardiac output are compromised by excessive PEEP. The explanation for this reduction in dynamic lung compliance is that some alveoli become overexpanded because of the increase in pressure, which puts them on the "flat" part of the compliance curve (see Fig. 2.3C). Therefore, despite the additional pressure delivered, little additional volume is obtained. The contribution of this "population" of overexpanded alveoli may be sufficient to reduce the total lung compliance. It has been shown that dynamic lung compliance was reduced in patients with CDH even though some of the infants had normal thoracic gas volumes.[11] The reduction in dynamic lung compliance in patients with CDH is attributed to overdistention of the hypoplastic lung into the "empty" hemithorax after surgical repair of the defect. Because CDH infants have a reduced number of alveoli, they develop areas of pulmonary emphysema that persist at least into early childhood.[16]

Based on available evidence, it seems prudent to avoid rapid expansion of the lungs in the treatment of CDH. Clinicians must be alert to any sudden improvement in lung compliance in infants receiving assisted ventilation (i.e., immediately after administration of surfactant or recruitment of lung volume). If inflation pressure is not reduced as compliance improves, cardiovascular compromise may develop because proportionately more pressure is transmitted to the mediastinal structures as lung compliance improves. The distending pressure that was appropriate before the compliance change may become excessive and lead to alveolar overexpansion and ultimately air leak.[17] The use of volume-targeted ventilation would be ideal in these circumstances, because in this mode, the ventilator will decrease the inflation pressure as lung compliance improves to maintain a set tidal volume.[18]

Because the chest wall is compliant in the premature infant, use of paralytic agents to reduce chest wall impedance is rarely necessary. Little pressure is required to expand the chest wall of a premature infant (see chest wall curve in Fig. 2.2). In studies investigating the use of paralytic agents in premature infants at risk for pneumothoraces, no change in lung compliance or resistance was demonstrated after 24 or 48 hours of paralysis, and many of the infants studied required more rather than less ventilator support after paralysis.[19,20]

In the past, paralysis was often used in larger infants who were "fighting the ventilator" or who were actively expiring against it despite the use of sedation and/or analgesia.[19] It should be noted that poor gas exchange (inadequate support) is usually the cause rather than the result of the infant's "fighting" the ventilator, and heavy sedation or paralysis masks this important clinical sign. The use of synchronized mechanical ventilation modes such as assist/control will obviate the need to paralyze or heavily sedate infants because they will then be breathing in synchrony with the ventilator.[21-23]

During positive-pressure ventilation, the relative compliance of the chest wall and the lungs determines the amount of pressure transmitted to the pleural space. Increased intrapleural pressure leads to impedance of venous return and decreased cardiac output, a well-documented but largely ignored complication of positive-pressure ventilation. The relationship is described by the following equation:

$$P_{PL} = \overline{P}_{aw} \times (C_L / C_L + C_{CW})$$

where P_{PL} is pleural pressure, $\overline{P}_{aw}$ is mean airway pressure, C_L is compliance of the lungs, and C_{CW} is compliance of the chest wall.

Thus, it can be seen that in situations of good lung compliance but poor chest wall compliance, transmission of pressure to the pleural space and hemodynamic impairment are increased. This situation commonly arises in cases of increased intra-abdominal pressure with upward pressure on the diaphragm, as may be seen in infants with necrotizing enterocolitis or after surgical reduction of viscera that had developed outside the abdominal cavity—for example, large omphalocele, gastroschisis, or CDH.

Resistance

Resistance is the result of friction. Viscous resistance is the resistance generated by tissue elements moving past one another. Airway resistance is the resistance that occurs between moving molecules in the gas stream and between these moving molecules and the wall of the respiratory system (e.g., trachea, bronchi, bronchioles). The clinician must be aware of both types of resistance, as well as the resistance to flow as gas passes through the ventilator circuit and the endotracheal tube (ETT). In infants, viscous resistance may account for as much as 40% of total pulmonary resistance.[24] The relatively high viscous resistance in the newborn is caused by relatively high tissue density (i.e., a low ratio of lung volume to lung weight) and the higher amount of pulmonary interstitial fluid. This increase in pulmonary interstitial fluid is especially prevalent after cesarean section delivery[25] and is associated with conditions such as transient tachypnea of the newborn or delayed absorption of fetal lung fluid.

A reduction in tissue and airway resistance has been shown after administration of furosemide.[26] Airway resistance (R) is defined as the pressure gradient (P1 − P2) required to move gas through the airways at a constant flow rate ($\dot{V}$ or volume per unit of time). The standard formula is as follows:

$$R = (P1 - P2)/\dot{V}$$

Airway resistance is determined by flow velocity, length of the conducting airways, viscosity and density of the gases, and especially the inside diameter of the airways. This is true for both laminar and turbulent flow conditions.

Although in absolute terms airway resistance is elevated in the newborn infant, when corrected to lung volume (specific conductance, which is the reciprocal of resistance per unit lung volume), the relative resistance is lower than in adults. It is important to remember that because of the small diameter of the airways in the lungs of the newborn infant, even a modest narrowing will result in a marked increase in resistance.

Resistance to flow depends on whether the flow is laminar or turbulent. Turbulent flow results in inefficient use of energy, because the turbulence leads to flow in random directions, unlike with laminar flow, in which molecules move in an orderly fashion parallel to the wall of the tube. Therefore, the pressure gradient necessary to drive a given flow is always greater for turbulent flow but cannot be easily calculated. The Reynolds number is used as an index to determine whether flow is laminar or turbulent.[27] It is a unitless number that is defined as follows:

$$Re = 2r \cdot v \cdot d / \eta$$

where r is the radius, v is the velocity, d is the density, and η is the viscosity. If the Reynolds number is greater than 2000, then turbulent flow is very likely. According to this equation, turbulent flow is likely if the tube has a large radius, a high velocity, a high density, or a low viscosity.

When flow is laminar, resistance to flow of gas through a tube is described by Poiseuille's law:

$$R \propto L \times \eta / r^4$$

where R is the resistance, L is the length of the tube, η is the viscosity of the gas, and r is the radius. In the following paragraphs we will consider each factor in more detail.

Flow Rate

Average values for airway resistance in normal, spontaneously breathing newborn infants are between 20 and 30 cm H_2O/L/s,[28] and these values can increase dramatically in disease states. Nasal airway resistance makes up approximately two-thirds of total upper airway resistance; the glottis and larynx contribute less than 10%; and the trachea and first four or five generations of bronchi account for the remainder.[29] Average peak inspiratory and expiratory flow rates in spontaneously breathing term infants are approximately 2.9 and 2.2 L/min, respectively.[28] Maximal peak inspiratory and expiratory flow rates average about 9.7 and 6.4 L/min, respectively.[30] The range of flow rates generated by spontaneously breathing newborns (including term and premature infants) is approximately 0.6 to 9.9 L/min. Turbulent flow is produced in standard infant ETTs whenever flow rates exceed approximately 3 L/min through 2.5-mm internal diameter (ID) tubes or 7.5 L/min through 3.0-mm ID tubes.[31] Flow rates that exceed these critical levels produce disproportionately large increases in airway resistance. For example, increasing the rate of flow through a 2.5-mm ID ETT from 5 to 10 L/min raises airway resistance from 32 to 84 cm H_2O/L/s, more than twice its original value.[31]

The resistance produced by infant ETTs is equal to or higher than that in the upper airway of a normal newborn infant breathing spontaneously. The increased resistance caused by the ETT poses little problem as long as the infant receives appropriate pressure support from the ventilator, because the machine can generate the additional pressure needed to overcome the resistance of the ETT. However, when the infant is being weaned from the ventilator or if the infant is disconnected from the ventilator with the ETT still in place, the infant may not be capable of generating sufficient effort to overcome the increase in upper airway resistance created by the ETT.[32] LeSouef et al.[33] measured a significant reduction in respiratory system expiratory resistance after extubation in premature newborn infants recovering from a variety of respiratory illnesses, including RDS, pneumonia, and transient tachypnea of the newborn.

Airway or Tube Length

Resistance is linearly proportional to tube length. The shorter the tube, the lower the resistance; therefore, it is good practice to cut ETTs to the shortest practical length. Shortening a 2.5-mm ID ETT from 14.8 cm (full length) to half its length is feasible, because the depth of insertion in a small premature infant is usually about 6 cm. This would reduce the resistance of the tube to half. Cutting the tube to 4.8 cm reduces the flow resistance in vitro to essentially that of a full-length tube of the next size (3.0-mm ID ETT). These relationships are consistent for the range of flows generated by spontaneously breathing newborns.[34]

Airway or Tube Diameter

The radius of the tube is the most significant determinant of resistance. As previously described, Poiseuille's law states that resistance is inversely proportional to the fourth power of the radius. Therefore, a reduction in the radius by half results in a 16-fold increase in resistance and thus the pressure drop required to maintain a given flow. It is important to fully appreciate that resistance to flow increases exponentially as ETT diameter decreases. This is one of the reasons extremely low birth weight infants are difficult to wean from mechanical ventilation. In a multiple tube system, like the human lung, resistance depends on the total cross-sectional area of all of the tubes. Although the individual bronchi decrease in diameter as they extend toward the periphery, the total cross-sectional area of the airway increases exponentially.[35]

Because resistance increases to the fourth power as the airway is narrowed, even mild airway constriction can cause significant increases in resistance to flow. This effect is exaggerated in newborn infants compared to adults because of the narrowness of the infant's airways. Resistance during inspiration is less than resistance during expiration because the airways dilate upon inspiration (Fig. 2.8). This is true even though gas flow during inspiration usually is greater than that during expiration, because as we saw earlier, the relationship between resistance and flow is linear, whereas that to radius is geometric. There is an inverse, nonlinear relationship between airway resistance and lung volume, because airway size increases as FRC increases.

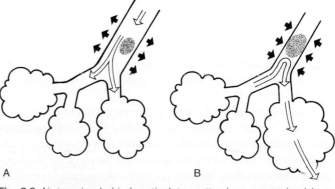

Fig. 2.8 Air trapping behind particulate matter (e.g., meconium) in an airway, which leads to alveolar overexpansion and rupture. This illustrates the so-called ball–valve mechanism, in which **(A)** tidal gas passes the particulate matter on inspiration, when the airways naturally dilate but **(B)** does not exit on expiration, when the airways naturally constrict. (From Harris TR, Herrick BR: Pneumothorax in the Newborn. Tucson, AZ, Biomedical Communications, Arizona Health Sciences Center, 1978.)

Lung volume recruitment therefore reduces resistance to airflow. Any process that causes a reduction in lung volume, such as atelectasis or restriction of expansion, results in increased airway resistance. At extremely low volumes, resistance approaches infinity because the airways begin to close as residual volume is approached (see Fig. 2.2).

Consistent with the earlier physiologic principles, the preponderance of evidence indicates that the application of PEEP and CPAP decreases airway resistance.[36-38] ETT resistance is of considerable clinical importance. It has been shown that successful extubation is accomplished more often in infants coming directly off intermittent mandatory ventilation than after a 6-hour preextubation trial of endotracheal CPAP.[32] Nasal CPAP circuit design, specifically its resistance, and the means by which nasal CPAP is attached to the patient are the most important determinants of CPAP success or failure.[39]

Viscosity and Density

Gas viscosity is negligible relative to the viscosity of fluids. However, gas density can be of clinical significance. The relationship between airway resistance and the density of the gas in turbulent flow is directly proportional and linear. Decreasing the density of the gas by two-thirds, such as occurs when heliox, a mixture of 80% helium and 20% O_2, is administered, reduces airway resistance to one-third compared to that when room air is breathed. Heliox can be useful for reducing upper airway resistance (and work of breathing) in patients with obstructive disorders such as laryngeal edema, tracheal stenosis, and BPD,[40] but its effectiveness is reduced if higher oxygen requirement reduces the proportion of helium in the mixture. Gas density is influenced by barometric pressure, so airway resistance is slightly decreased at high altitudes, although this has little clinical significance.

Work of Breathing

Breathing requires the expenditure of energy. For gas to be moved into the lungs, force must be exerted to overcome the elastic and resistive forces of the respiratory system. This is referred to as work of breathing and is mathematically expressed by the following equation:

Work of breathing = Pressure (force) × Volume (displacement)

where pressure is the force exerted and the volume is the displacement. Work of breathing is the integrated product of the two, or simply the area under the pressure–volume curve (see Fig. 2.7).

The workload depends on the elastic properties of the lung and chest wall, airway resistance, tidal volume (V_T), and respiratory rate. Approximately two-thirds of the work of spontaneous breathing is the effort to overcome the static elastic forces of the lungs and thorax (tissue elasticity and compliance). Approximately one-third of the total work is applied to overcoming the frictional resistance produced by the movement of gas and tissue components (airflow and viscous).[41]

In healthy infants, exhalation is passive. A portion of the energy generated by the inspiratory muscles is stored (as potential energy) in the lungs' elastic components; this energy is returned during exhalation, hence it is also referred to as *nondissipative work*, in contrast to the frictional forces that are lost or dissipated as heat. If the energy required to overcome resistance to flow during expiration exceeds the amount of elastic energy stored during the previous inspiration, work must be done not only during inspiration but also during expiration; thus, exhalation is no longer entirely passive.

In infants, energy expenditure correlates with oxygen consumption. Resting oxygen consumption is elevated in infants with RDS and BPD.[42] Mechanical ventilation reduces oxygen consumption by decreasing the infant's work of breathing.[13,43] Work of breathing is illustrated in a dynamic pressure–volume loop (see Fig. 2.7). Pressure changes during breathing can be measured with an esophageal catheter or balloon, and volume changes can be measured simultaneously with a pneumotachograph. During inspiration (ascending limb of the loop) and expiration (descending limb of the loop), both elastic and frictional resistance must be overcome by work. If only elastic resistance needed to be overcome, the breathing pattern would follow the compliance line; however, because airway resistance and tissue viscous resistance must also be overcome, a loop is formed (hysteresis). The areas ABCA and ACDA in Fig. 2.7 represent the inspiratory work and the expiratory work, respectively, performed to overcome frictional resistance. The area ABCEA represents the total work of breathing during a single breath.

The diaphragm is responsible for the majority of the workload of respiration. The most important determinant of the diaphragm's ability to generate force is its initial position and the length of its muscle fibers at the beginning of a contraction. The longer and more curved the muscle fibers of the diaphragm, the greater the force the diaphragm can generate. In situations in which the lung is hyperinflated (overdistended), the diaphragm is flattened and thus at a mechanical disadvantage.

The application of PEEP or CPAP (continuous distending pressure [CDP]) may reduce the work of breathing for an infant whose breathing is on the initial flat part of the compliance curve secondary to atelectasis (see Fig. 2.3A). In this situation, CDP should reduce the work of breathing by increasing FRC and bringing breathing to a higher level on the pressure–volume curve where the compliance is higher (see Fig. 2.3B). Reductions in respiratory work with the application of CDP have been shown in newborns recovering from RDS[44] and in babies after surgery for congenital heart disease.[37]

If the lung already is overinflated, increasing CDP will not result in a decrease in the work of breathing (see Fig. 2.3C). The one exception here is when lung overinflation is the result of airway collapse, as can be seen in infants with BPD. In this unique situation, higher CDP will maintain airway patency and relieve air trapping, reducing lung volume to a more normal level. Alveolar overdistention caused by any reason is often accompanied by an increase in $PaCO_2$ (indicating decreased alveolar ventilation) and a decrease in PaO_2, despite an increase in FRC.[36,45]

Time Constant

The time constant of a patient's respiratory system is a measure of how quickly his or her lungs can inflate or deflate—that is, how long it takes for alveolar and proximal airway pressures to equilibrate. Passive exhalation depends on the elastic recoil of the lungs and chest wall. Because the major force opposing exhalation is airway resistance, the expiratory time constant (K_t) of the respiratory system is directly related to both lung compliance (C_L), which is the inverse of elastic recoil, and airway resistance (R_{aw}):

$$K_t = C_L \times R_{aw}$$

The time constants of the respiratory system are analogous to those of electrical circuits. One time constant of the respiratory system is defined as the time it takes the alveoli (capacitor) to discharge 63% of its V_T (electrical charge) through the airways (resistor) to the mouth or ventilator (electrical) circuit. By the end of three time constants, 95% of the V_T is discharged. When this model is applied to a normal newborn with a compliance of 0.005 L/cm H_2O and a resistance of 30 cm H_2O/L/s, one time constant = 0.15 seconds and three time constants = 0.45 seconds.[46] In other words, 95% of the last V_T should be emptied from the lung within 0.45 seconds of when exhalation begins in a spontaneously breathing infant. In a newborn infant receiving assisted ventilation, the exhalation valve of the ventilator would have to be open for at least that length of time to avoid air trapping. Inspiratory time constants are roughly half as long as expiratory, largely because airway diameter increases during inspiration. This relationship between inspiratory and expiratory time constants accounts for the normal 1:2 inspiratory/expiratory (I:E) ratio with spontaneous breathing.

The concept of time constants is key to understanding the interactions between the elastic and the resistive forces and how the mechanical properties of the respiratory system work together to modulate the volume and distribution of ventilation. A working understanding of time constants is essential for choosing the safest and most effective ventilator settings for an individual patient at a particular point in the course of a specific disease process that necessitates the use of assisted ventilation. It must be recognized that compliance and resistance change over time, and therefore, the optimal settings need to be reevaluated frequently.

Patients are at risk of incomplete emptying of a previously inspired breath when their lung condition involves an increase in airway resistance with no or only a modest reduction in lung compliance. They also are at risk when the pattern of assisted ventilation does not allow sufficient time for exhalation—that is, the lungs have an abnormally long time constant—or there is a mismatch between the time constant of the respiratory system (time constant of the patient + that of the ETT + that of the ventilator circuit) and the expiratory time setting on the ventilator. In these situations, the end result is gas trapping. This gas trapping is accompanied by an increase in lung volume and a buildup of pressure in the alveoli and distal airways referred to as *dynamic PEEP, inadvertent PEEP,* or *auto-PEEP.*[47]

Important clinical and radiographic signs of gas trapping and inadvertent PEEP include (1) radiographic evidence of overexpansion (e.g., increased anteroposterior diameter of the thorax, flattened diaphragm below the ninth posterior ribs, intercostal pleural bulging), (2) decreased chest wall movement during assisted ventilation, (3) hypercarbia that does not respond to an increase in ventilator rate (or even worsens), and (4) signs of cardiovascular compromise, such as mottled skin color, a decrease in arterial blood pressure, an increase in central venous pressure, or the development of a metabolic acidosis. Such late signs of air trapping should never occur today because all modern ventilators give us the ability to monitor flow waveforms, which allow us to graphically see whether expiration has been completed before the next inflation begins.

Time constants are also a function of patient size because total compliance is proportional to size. The much shorter time constants of an infant are reflected in the more rapid normal respiratory rate, compared with adults. To keep the concept simple, remember that whales and elephants have very large lungs and very long time constants; hence, they breathe very slowly. Mice and hummingbirds have tiny lungs with extremely short time constants and have a very rapid respiratory rate to match. Everything else being equal, large infants have longer time constants than "micropreemies." Any decrease in compliance makes the time constant shorter, and therefore tachypnea is the usual clinical sign of any condition leading to decreased compliance.

Extremely low birth weight infants with RDS have decreased compliance but initially relatively normal airway resistance. This means that the time constants are extremely short. Equilibration of the airway and alveolar pressures occurs very quickly (i.e., early in the inspiratory cycle). Reynolds[48] estimated that the time constant in RDS may be as short as 0.05 seconds. This means that 95% of the pressure applied to the airway is delivered to the alveoli within 0.15 seconds, a value consistent with clinical observation. Short time constants make rapid-rate conventional ventilation feasible in these infants and makes them ideal candidates for high-frequency ventilation (HFV).

Term infants with meconium aspiration or older growing preterm infants with BPD have elevated airway resistance and correspondingly longer time constants; therefore, they are most at risk of inadvertent PEEP. They should be ventilated with slower respiratory rates and longer inspiratory and, especially, expiratory times. Evidence of air trapping should be actively sought by examining ventilator waveforms before clinical signs of CO_2 retention and hemodynamic impairment develop. It should be noted that the proximal airway PEEP level does not indicate the level of alveolar PEEP, nor does it demonstrate the occurrence of alveolar gas trapping. Even under conditions of zero proximal airway PEEP, alveolar PEEP levels and the degree of gas trapping may be dangerously high if the baby has compliant lungs, increased airway resistance, or both (i.e., a prolonged time constant).[49]

Although it is useful clinically to think of the infant's respiratory system as having a single compliance and a single resistance, we know this is not really the case. The resistance and compliance values we obtain from pulmonary function measurements are essentially weighted averages for the respiratory system. There are populations of respiratory subunits with a range of discrete compliance and resistance values, whereas what we measure at the airway are averaged values for those populations of subunits.

GAS TRANSPORT

Mechanisms of Gas Transport

Ventilation or gas transport involves the movement of gas by convection or bulk flow through the conducting airways and then by molecular diffusion into the alveoli and pulmonary capillaries. This makes possible gas exchange (O_2 uptake and CO_2 elimination) that matches the minute-by-minute metabolic needs of the patient. The driving force for gas flow is the difference in pressure at the origin and destination of the gases; for diffusion, it is the difference in the concentrations between gases in contiguous spaces. Gas flows down a pressure gradient and diffuses down a concentration gradient. The predominant mechanism of gas transport by convection is bulk flow, whereas the predominant mechanism of gas transport by diffusion is Brownian motion.

Ventilation of the alveoli is an intermittent process that occurs only during inspiration, whereas gas exchange between alveoli and pulmonary capillaries occurs throughout the respiratory cycle. This is possible because a portion of gas remains in the lungs at the end of exhalation (FRC); the remaining gas provides a source for ongoing gas exchange and maintains approximately equal O_2 and CO_2 tensions in both the alveoli and the blood returning from the lungs.

During spontaneous breathing, inspiration is achieved through active contraction of the respiratory muscles. A negative pressure is produced in the interpleural space, a portion of which is transmitted via the parietal and visceral pleura through the pulmonary interstitial space to the lower airways and alveoli. A pressure gradient between the outside atmospheric pressure and the airway and alveolar pressures results in gas flowing down the pressure gradient into the lungs (Fig. 2.9). Interpleural pressure is more negative than alveolar pressure, which is more negative than mouth and atmospheric pressures.

When an infant receives negative-pressure ventilation, pressure is decreased around the infant's chest and abdomen to supplement the negative-pressure gradient used to move gas into the lungs, mimicking the normal physiologic function. During positive-pressure ventilation, the upper airway of the infant (Fig. 2.10) is connected to a device that generates a positive-pressure gradient down which gas can flow during inspiration. The pressure in the ventilator circuit and in the upper airway is greater than the alveolar pressure, which is greater than the interpleural pressure, which is greater than the atmospheric pressure. The negative intrathoracic pressure during spontaneous or negative pressure respiration facilitates venous return to the heart. Positive-pressure ventilation alters this physiology and inevitably leads to some degree of impedance of venous return, adversely affecting cardiac output.

The amount of gas inspired in a single spontaneous breath or delivered through an ETT during a single cycle of the ventilator is called the *tidal volume*. V_T in milliliters (mL) multiplied by the number of inflations per minute, or respirator frequency (*f*), is called *minute ventilation* (V_E):

$$V_E = V_T \times f$$

The portion of the incoming V_T that fails to arrive at the level of the respiratory bronchioles and alveoli but instead remains in

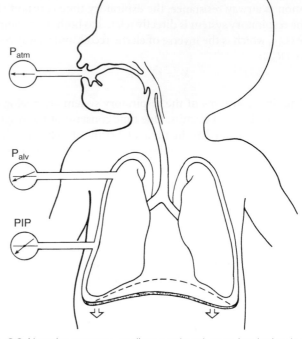

Fig. 2.9 Negative-pressure gradient produced upon inspiration by the descent of the diaphragm in a spontaneously breathing infant. Pressures are measured in the interpleural space (*PIP*), in the alveoli (P_{alv}), and at the opening of the mouth, or atmosphere (P_{atm}). PIP < P_{alv} < P_{atm}.

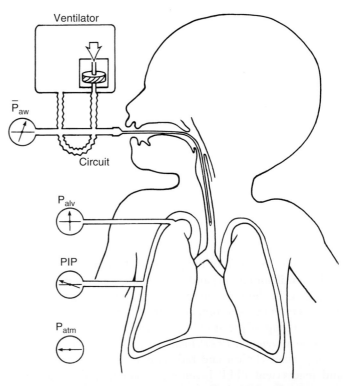

Fig. 2.10 Positive-pressure gradient produced by a ventilator. Pressures are measured in the airway (Paw) and as shown in Fig. 2.9. Paw > P_{alv} > PIP > P_{atm}. Abbreviations as in Fig. 2.9.

the conducting airways occupies the space known as the *anatomic dead space*. Another portion of V_T may be delivered to unperfused or underperfused alveoli. Because gas exchange does not take place in these units, the volume that they constitute is called *alveolar dead space*. Together, anatomic dead space and alveolar dead space make up *total* or *physiologic dead space* (V_{DS}). The ratio of dead space to V_T (V_{DS}/V_T) defines *wasted ventilation*, which reflects the proportion of tidal gas delivered that is not involved in gas exchange. In general, rapid shallow breathing is inefficient because of a high V_{DS} to V_T ratio.

A number of mechanisms of gas transport other than bulk convection and molecular diffusion have been described, particularly as they relate to HFV. They include axial convection, radial diffusive mixing, coaxial flow, viscous shear, asymmetrical velocity profiles, and the pendelluft effect.[50]

The concept of anatomic dead space is a useful one and does apply under conditions of relatively low flow velocities. It assumes that the fresh gas and exhaled gas move as solid blocks without any mixing. However, in small infants, with their rapid respiratory rates and small airways, the concept begins to break down. In 1915, Henderson et al.[51] noted that during rapid shallow breathing or panting in dogs, adequate gas exchange was maintained even though the volume of gas contained in each "breath" was less than that of the anatomic dead space. They hypothesized that low-volume inspiratory pulses of gas moved down the center of the airway as axial spikes and that these spikes dissipated at the end of each "breath" (Fig. 2.11). The faster the inspiratory pulse, the farther it penetrated down the conducting airway and the larger the boundary of mixing between the molecules of the incoming gas (with high O_2 and low CO_2) and the outgoing gas (with high CO_2 and low O_2).

During this kind of breathing, both convection and molecular diffusion are enhanced or facilitated. The provision of a greater

interface or boundary area between inspiratory and expiratory gases with their different O_2 and CO_2 partial pressures is known as *radial diffusive mixing*. During HFV, with each inspiration, gas molecules near the center of the airway flow farther than those adjacent to the walls of the airway, because the gas traveling down the center of the airway encounters less resistance. Fig. 2.12A illustrates the velocity profiles using vectors that demonstrate the airway flow patterns of gas molecules in a representation of the airway during inspiration. At the end of the inspiratory phase, the contour of the leading edge of the inspired gas is cone shaped (Fig. 2.12B), having a larger diffusion interface with the preexisting gas than would be present if the leading edge were disk

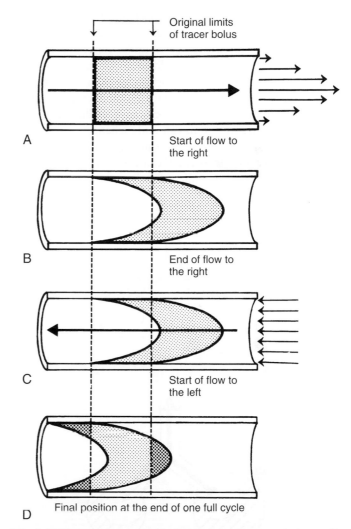

A — Original limits of tracer bolus / Start of flow to the right

B — End of flow to the right

C — Start of flow to the left

D — Final position at the end of one full cycle

Fig. 2.12 Viscous shear and inspiratory-to-expiratory velocity profiles associated with respiratory cycling. **(A)** During inspiration or movement toward the right, the gas molecules of a cylindrical tracer bolus that are situated near the center of the tube travel farther and faster than the gas molecules near the wall, as represented by the velocity profile arrows at the right. **(B)** At the end of the inspiratory half of the respiratory cycle, a paraboloid front has formed. **(C)** During exhalation or movement toward the left, the velocity profiles are essentially uniform across the lumen. **(D)** The end result after a complete respiratory cycle (with zero net directional flow) is displacement of axial gas to the right and wall gas to the left. (Modified with permission from Haselton FR, Scherer PW: Bronchial bifurcations and respiratory mass transport. Science 208:69, 1980. © 1990 by the American Association for the Advancement of Science.)

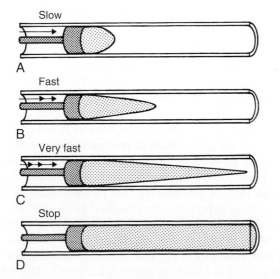

Slow — A

Fast — B

Very fast — C

Stop — D

Fig. 2.11 Spike theory of panting or high-frequency ventilation. **(A–C)** The quicker or more "energy dense" the puff (or inspiratory pulse), the sharper the spike and the farther it extends into the airway. **(D)** If the pulse is suddenly stopped at end inspiration, mixing occurs instantaneously. (Modified from Henderson Y, Chillingworth FP, Whitney JL: The respiratory dead space. Am J Physiol 38:1, 1915.)

shaped. During exhalation, the flow velocity is lower (assuming the usual 1:2 I:E ratio) and the velocity profiles are more uniform across the entire lumen rather than being cone shaped (Fig. 2.12C).[52] The pulse of gas originally occupying the lumen of the airway is displaced to the right (i.e., toward the patient's alveoli), and an equal volume of gas is displaced to the left (Fig. 2.12D). This occurs even though the net displacement of the piston at the end of a cycle of high-frequency oscillatory ventilation (HFOV) is zero. Although these mechanisms have mostly been recognized to be operative with HFV, evidence suggests that they are present to some degree even at conventional respiratory rates in small preterm infants with narrow ETTs.[53,54]

The back-and-forth currents of gas through lung units with unequal time constants are called *pendelluft*.[50,55] This gas flow is produced because of local differences in airway resistance and lung compliance that are accentuated under conditions of high-velocity flow. This leads to regional differences in rates of inflation and deflation. "Fast units" with short time constants inflate and deflate more rapidly, emptying out into the conducting airways to be "inhaled" by "slow units" still in the process of filling (Fig. 2.13). Pendelluft thus improves gas mixing and exchange.

Carbon dioxide diffuses more easily than oxygen across the alveolar/capillary wall, an essential characteristic given the relatively low concentration gradient between the alveoli and the

capillary blood. The effectiveness of CO_2 removal is primarily determined by the effectiveness of alveolar ventilation, that is, the process by which CO_2 that has diffused into the alveoli is removed, so that the maximal diffusion gradient is maintained. The movement of any gas across a semipermeable membrane is governed by Fick's equation for diffusion:

$$dQ / dt = k \times A \times dC/dl$$

where dQ/dt is the rate of diffusion in mL/min, k is the diffusion coefficient of the gas, A is the area available for diffusion, dC is the concentration difference of molecules across the membrane, and dl is the length of the diffusion pathway. It is evident from the earlier that both atelectasis, which will reduce the area available for gas exchange, and interstitial pulmonary edema, which will increase the diffusion pathway, will reduce the effectiveness of CO_2 removal. Very immature infants whose lungs have not yet undergone thinning of the interstitium also have less efficient diffusion across the alveolar capillary membrane. Alveolar minute ventilation is, of course, the most critical element, because it maintains the concentration gradient that drives diffusion.

OXYGENATION

Oxygen transport to the tissues depends on the oxygen-carrying capacity of the blood and the rate of blood flow. The amount of oxygen in arterial blood is called *oxygen content* (CaO_2).

$$CaO_2 = (1.34 \times Hb \times SaO_2) + (0.003 \times PaO_2)$$

where Hb is the hemoglobin concentration and SaO_2 is the arterial oxygen saturation. Oxygen is contained in the blood in two forms: (1) a small quantity dissolved in the plasma and (2) a much larger quantity bound to hemoglobin. The total O_2 content of the blood is the sum of these two quantities. The contribution of hemoglobin to oxygen content is described in the first term of the equation, which states that each gram of hemoglobin will bind 1.34 mL of O_2 when fully saturated with oxygen. The second term of the equation describes the contribution of oxygen dissolved in the plasma.

The dissolved portion of O_2 in blood is linearly related to PO_2, such that an increase in PO_2 is accompanied by an increase in O_2 content. Oxygen content increases 0.003 mL per 100 mL of blood with every 1–mm Hg increase in PO_2. For an infant breathing 21% O_2, the dissolved portion of the blood's O_2 content is only 1.5% of the total, assuming normal hemoglobin (Hb). However, for a healthy infant breathing 100% O_2, with a very high PaO_2 of 500 mm Hg (not recommended because of the dangers of hyperoxia), the dissolved portion of the blood's O_2 content can be as much as 7.5% of the total. Oxygen binds reversibly to hemoglobin. Each hemoglobin molecule can bind up to four molecules of O_2. The hemoglobin-bound portion of the O_2 content is nonlinear with respect to PO_2. This relationship is illustrated by the oxyhemoglobin dissociation curve, which is sigmoid in shape (Fig. 2.14).

The amount of O_2 that binds to hemoglobin increases quickly at low PO_2 values but begins to level off at PO_2 values greater than 40 mm Hg. After PO_2 exceeds 90 to 100 mm Hg,

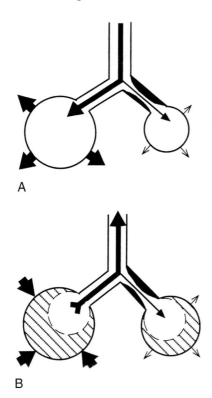

A

B

Fig. 2.13 Effects of different time constants on the uneven distribution of ventilation and the production of pendelluft. **(A)** On inspiration, the fast unit receives the majority of ventilation, whereas the slow unit fills slowly (owing to local increase in airway resistance). **(B)** At the beginning of expiration, the slow unit may still be filling and actually "inspires" from the exhaling fast unit. These effects are accentuated at higher frequencies, with gas "pedaling" back and forth between neighboring units with inhomogeneity of time constants. (Modified from Otis AB, McKerrow CB, Bartlett RA, et al: Mechanical factors in distribution of pulmonary ventilation. J Appl Physiol 8:427, 1956.)

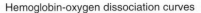

Hemoglobin-oxygen dissociation curves

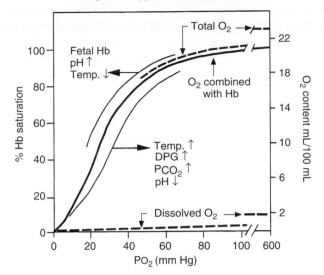

Fig. 2.14 Nonlinear or S-shaped oxyhemoglobin curve and the linear or straight-line dissolved O_2 relationships between O_2 saturation (SaO_2) and O_2 tension (PO_2). Total blood O_2 content is shown with division into a portion combined with hemoglobin and a portion physically dissolved at various levels of PO_2. Also shown are the major factors that change the O_2 affinity of hemoglobin and thus shift the oxyhemoglobin dissociation curve to either the left or the right (see also Appendix 12). *DPG*, 2,3 Diphosphoglycerate; *Hb*, hemoglobin. (Modified from West JB. Respiratory Physiology: The Essentials. 2nd ed. Baltimore, Williams & Wilkins, 1979, pp. 71, 73.)

the curve flattens. Once the hemoglobin is saturated, further increases in PO_2 do not increase the content of bound oxygen. The total amount of O_2 carried by hemoglobin depends on the hemoglobin concentration of the blood and the blood's oxygen saturation. Several factors affect hemoglobin's affinity for oxygen. These factors include the (1) percentages of fetal and adult hemoglobin present in the patient's blood, (2) effect of 2,3-diphosphoglycerate, (3) pH, and (4) temperature. A greater percentage of fetal hemoglobin (as seen in premature infants), a decrease in 2,3-diphosphoglycerate content (as occurs in premature infants with RDS), alkalization of the pH (as in metabolic alkalosis), a reduction in PCO_2 (secondary to hyperventilation), and a decrease in body temperature (as occurs during open heart surgery or therapeutic hypothermia for neuroprotection) all increase the O_2 affinity of hemoglobin (shift the oxyhemoglobin dissociation curve to the left without changing its shape). This means that the same level of hemoglobin saturation can be achieved at lower PO_2 values. In contrast, increased production of 2,3-diphosphoglycerate (as occurs in healthy newborns shortly after birth or with adaptation to high altitudes), a reduction in the percentage of fetal hemoglobin (e.g., after transfusion of adult donor blood to a newborn infant), a more acidic pH, CO_2 retention, and febrile illness each result in a reduction in O_2 affinity (shift of the oxyhemoglobin dissociation curve to the right) (see Fig. 2.14).

These shifts in the oxyhemoglobin dissociation curve promote O_2 uptake in the lungs, O_2 release at the tissue level, or both. For example, when pulmonary arterial blood (which is rich in CO_2 and poor in O_2) passes through the lung's capillaries,

it releases its CO_2; this raises the local pH, which increases O_2 affinity. This allows more of the incoming O_2 to be bound to hemoglobin, thus maximizing the concentration gradient down which O_2 diffuses from the alveoli into the pulmonary capillary plasma. Also, when systemic arterial blood (which is rich in O_2 and low in CO_2) enters the tissue capillaries, it picks up CO_2 (which is in high concentration in the tissues). As a result, pH and O_2 affinity are lowered; this allows hemoglobin to release its O_2 without significantly decreasing PO_2 and thus helps to maintain the concentration gradient down which O_2 diffuses into the tissues.[56] This remarkable evolutionary adaptation is known as the Bohr effect. The Haldane effect refers to a related phenomenon whereby increased oxygen tension in the pulmonary capillary blood enhances the release of CO_2 from Hb and enhances its diffusion into the alveoli.[57-59]

SaO_2 as monitored clinically with pulse oximetry (SpO_2) shows the percentage of hemoglobin in arterial blood that is saturated with O_2 and therefore more closely reflects blood oxygen content than does PaO_2, especially in the newborn infant with predominantly fetal hemoglobin. The greater affinity of fetal hemoglobin for oxygen, together with the relative polycythemia normally seen in newborns, allows the fetus to maintain adequate tissue oxygen delivery in the relatively hypoxemic environment in utero. The PaO_2 and SaO_2 in the healthy fetus are only about 25 mm Hg and 60%, respectively. This is, of course, why normal newborn infants emerge from the womb quite cyanotic. It has been demonstrated that SpO_2 in the healthy newborn infant increases gradually after birth and does not normally reach 90% until 5 to 10 minutes of life.[60]

Rapid increases in PaO_2, such as occur when delivery room resuscitation is carried out with 100% oxygen, appear to result in a variety of adverse consequences, including delayed onset of spontaneous breathing and increased mortality.[61] The normal range of SaO_2 in newborn infants is different from that in adults; instead of the SaO_2 levels of 95% or greater in adults, SaO_2 levels of 85% to 92% appear to be adequate for newborns, and higher values may predispose the antioxidant-deficient preterm infant to the dangers of hyperoxia. It has been shown that the O_2 demands of most extremely premature infants can be met by maintaining PaO_2 levels just above 50 mm Hg or SaO_2 levels just above 88%.[62] There is currently insufficient evidence to recommend a definite range of optimal SpO_2 values, but there is mounting evidence that some complications of prematurity in which damage from reactive oxygen species is implicated can be reduced by the use of lower SpO_2 targets in the range of 85% to 92%.[63,64] However, while there was a reduction in retinopathy with lower oxygen saturation targets between 85% and 89% compared to 91% to 95%, mortality was increased in a series of large oxygen-targeting randomized trials[65] (see Chapter 16).

Tissue oxygen delivery depends not only on blood oxygen content but also on cardiac output and tissue perfusion. Positive-pressure ventilation impedes venous return to various degrees and therefore can adversely affect cardiac output and pulmonary blood flow. These important cardiorespiratory interactions are often not fully appreciated but nevertheless deserve close attention during mechanical ventilation.

The partial pressure of O_2 in arterial blood (PaO_2) is the tension or partial pressure of O_2 physically dissolved in the arterial blood plasma and is expressed in millimeters of mercury (mm Hg), or torr. This oxygen is in equilibrium with the oxygen that is bound to hemoglobin, which as we saw earlier constitutes the bulk of the total. PaO_2 is measured directly as part of the blood gas analysis. PaO_2 is a useful indicator of the degree of O_2 uptake through the lungs. The fraction of inspired O_2 (FiO_2) is the proportion of O_2 in the inspired gas. FiO_2 is measured directly with an O_2 analyzer and is expressed as a percentage (e.g., 60% O_2) or, preferably, in decimal form (e.g., 0.60 O_2). The FiO_2 in room air is approximately 0.21. The partial pressure of O_2 in alveolar gas (PAO_2) is the tension of O_2 present in the alveoli.

Alveolar gas typically contains oxygen, nitrogen, CO_2, and water vapor. PAO_2 represents the amount of O_2 available for diffusion into the pulmonary capillary blood. The partial pressure of CO_2 in the alveoli, or $PACO_2$, is nearly identical to partial pressure of CO_2 in the arterial blood, or $PaCO_2$. The partial pressure of water vapor at 100% relative humidity at body temperature and normal atmospheric pressure is 47 mm Hg. One additional correction factor must be used. This is called the *respiratory quotient* (RQ), which is the ratio of CO_2 excretion to O_2 uptake. The respiratory quotient ranges from approximately 0.8 to slightly greater than 1.0, depending on diet. To calculate the partial pressure of O_2 in alveolar gas or PAO_2, we use the alveolar gas equation:

$$PAO_2 = [(\text{barometric pressure} - \text{partial pressure of water vapor}) \times FiO_2] - (PaCO_2/RQ)$$

At sea level, with normal $PaCO_2$ of 40 mm Hg and respiratory quotient of 0.8, the alveolar gas equation for breathing room air is as follows:

$$PAO_2 = [(760 - 47) \times 0.21] - 40/0.8$$

Therefore,

$$PAO_2 \text{ is approximately } 150 - 50 = 100$$

A high-carbohydrate diet raises the respiratory quotient, thus increasing CO_2 production. It is important to remember that $PACO_2$ is decreased by hyperventilation and that the decrease in $PACO_2$ is matched by an equal increase in PAO_2. Barometric pressure varies with weather conditions and altitude. To demonstrate the effect of altitude on the absolute amount of oxygen available at the alveolar level, let us consider an infant with $PACO_2$ of 40 mm Hg and respiratory quotient of 0.8 who is breathing room air in Denver, Colorado, which is located 5280 ft above sea level and has an average barometric pressure of approximately 600 mm Hg. Subtracting 42 mm Hg (the partial pressure of water vapor is also reduced proportionally at altitude, although this fact is often ignored) from 600 mm Hg yields 558 mm Hg, which, when multiplied by 0.21, gives a value of around 117 mm Hg. After subtracting the dividend of 40 mm Hg/0.8, or 50 mm Hg, from 117 mm Hg, a PAO_2 value in Denver of only 67 mm Hg is obtained (instead of the approximately 100 mm Hg that would be expected at sea level). Therefore, the infant has

about one-third less available oxygen in the alveoli when breathing room air in Denver compared to when breathing room air at sea level. The alveolar gas equation is useful in calculating a variety of indexes of oxygenation, as well as, for example, the FiO_2 need of an infant with compromised gas exchange who must travel to a home at higher altitude or in a commercial aircraft cabin pressurized to 7000 or 8000 ft above sea level.

Some important values derived from blood gas measurements are useful as clinical indicators of disease severity and are commonly used as criteria for initiation of invasive or costly therapies. They include the following:

1. Arterial–alveolar O_2 tension ratio (PaO_2:PAO_2, or the a:A ratio). The a:A ratio should be close to 1 in a healthy infant. A ratio of less than 0.3 indicates severe compromise of oxygen transfer.
2. Alveolar–arterial O_2 gradient or difference ($AaDO_2 = PAO_2 - PaO_2$). In healthy infants, $AaDO_2$ is less than 20 in room air. Calculating $AaDO_2$ allows the clinician to estimate disease severity and estimate appropriate FiO_2 change when PaO_2 is high.
3. Oxygenation index $(P_{aw} \times FiO_2 \times 100)/PaO_2$

The oxygenation index factors in the pressure cost of achieving a certain level of oxygenation in the form of $\overline{P}_{aw}$. An oxygenation index greater than 15 signifies severe respiratory compromise. An oxygenation index of 40 or more on multiple occasions has historically indicated a mortality risk approaching 80% and continues to be used as an indication for extracorporeal membrane oxygenation (ECMO) in most ECMO centers.[66] When PaO_2 is unavailable, the oxygen saturation index can be used instead,[67] provided the oxygen saturation is between approximately 60% and 95%, that is, on the relatively linear portion of the oxyhemoglobin dissociation curve.

Effects of Altering Ventilator Settings on Oxygenation

Oxygen uptake through the lungs can be increased by (1) increasing PAO_2 via increasing the FiO_2 (increasing the concentration gradient), (2) optimizing lung volume (optimizing ventilation-to-perfusion [V/Q] matching and increasing the surface area for gas exchange), and (3) maximizing pulmonary blood flow (avoiding lung over-expansion that increases pulmonary vascular resistance and preventing blood from flowing right to left through extrapulmonary shunts). There are functionally two ventilator changes available to the clinician:

1. Alter $\underline{Fi}O_2$
2. Alter $\overline{P}_{aw}$

Fig. 2.15 is a graphic representation of the factors that affect proximal airway pressure for conventional mechanical ventilation. It has been demonstrated that, regardless of how the increase in $\overline{P}_{aw}$ is achieved, it has a roughly equivalent effect on oxygenation.[68] Although increasing each of these variables will increase $\overline{P}_{aw}$, the relative safety and effectiveness of these maneuvers have not been systematically evaluated. Prolongation of the inspiratory time to the point of inverse I:E ratio is potentially the most dangerous measure and is no longer used today. Higher frequency and higher peak inflation pressure (PIP) both may result in inadvertent hyperventilation, which is also undesirable. The rate of upstroke (also known as rise time) has a relatively

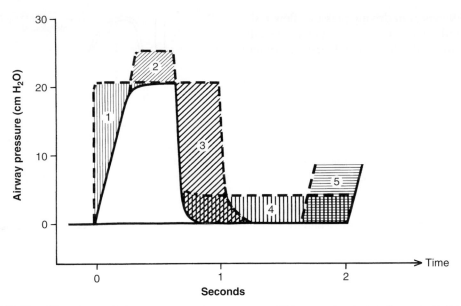

Fig. 2.15 Five different ways to increase mean airway pressure: (1) increase inspiratory flow rate or rise time, producing a square-wave inspiratory pattern; (2) increase peak inspiratory pressure; (3) reverse the inspiratory-to-expiratory ratio or prolong the inspiratory time (I-time) without changing the rate; (4) increase positive end-expiratory pressure; and (5) increase ventilatory rate by reducing expiratory time without changing the I-time. (Modified from Reynolds EOR: Pressure waveform and ventilator settings for mechanical ventilation in severe hyaline membrane disease. Int Anesthesiol Clin 12:259, 1974.)

minor impact. In practice, increasing PEEP appears to be the safest and most effective way to achieve optimal P_{aw}, in part because normally, the greatest proportion of the respiratory cycle is the expiratory phase. However, sufficient PIP is transiently needed to open atelectatic alveoli.

Although general principles and guidelines for ventilator management can be developed, it is important to recognize that individual infants may at times respond differently under apparently similar circumstances. Therefore, individualized care based on these principles is the best approach. To optimize care, the clinician should formulate a hypothesis based on a physiologic rationale, make a ventilator change, and observe the response. This provides the clinician with feedback that either confirms or refutes the hypothesis. The response of biological systems is never entirely predictable and occurs against a background of continuing change in the infant's condition. Additionally, there are complex interactions among the various organ systems. Otherwise, appropriate ventilator changes may have adverse hemodynamic effects. Opening of a ductus arteriosus may alter hemodynamics and lung compliance, the infant's own respiratory effort may change because of neurologic alterations, and so on. In addition, it is important to keep in mind that, because ventilators are powerful tools, they can cause significant damage even under the best of circumstances, but especially if they are not used judiciously. We must learn from experience (our own and that of others) and apply that knowledge when making ventilator setting changes during assisted ventilation of the newborn.

VENTILATION

For gas exchange to occur efficiently, ventilation and perfusion must be well matched. Gas is distributed through the lung via the airways. The volume of gas moved into and out of the lung with each normal breath is the *tidal volume* (V_T). The largest volume that can be inhaled after a full exhalation is the *vital capacity*. The volume of gas that remains in the lung after a normal expiration is the FRC. The volume that remains in the lung after a maximal expiration is the *residual volume*. Residual volume and vital capacity together are the *total lung capacity* (see also Chapter 12). The product of V_T and breathing frequency is the minute volume. As previously discussed, only a portion of the minute volume actually reaches the alveoli; this is known as *alveolar minute ventilation*.

As respiratory rate and/or V_T is increased, minute ventilation increases. When V_T is increased, alveolar minute ventilation increases even more than total minute ventilation because the anatomic dead space remains constant at about 2 mL/kg. Thus, an increase in V_T from 3 mL/kg to 4 mL/kg, a 25% increase, will increase alveolar tidal volume by 50% (from 1 mL/kg to 2 mL/kg). In contrast, with increases in respiratory rate, alveolar minute ventilation and total minute ventilation increase proportionally. Despite the fact that increasing the V_T has a greater impact on alveolar minute ventilation, increasing the V_T may not always be the optimal choice, because excessive V_T has been shown to be the most important determinant of lung injury, and increasing the V_T appears to be more injurious to the lung than a faster rate.[69,70] The dimensions of the airway system influence ventilation. With progressive dichotomous branching moving toward the lungs' periphery, the overall cross-sectional area of the airways increases, so airflow velocity decreases, as does resistance.

With each breath, inspired gas is distributed by bulk flow to the distal airways, depending on the length of the conducting airways and the rate of flow through them. Gas flow rates are determined by local differences in driving pressure, flow resistance, tissue elasticity, and compliance. For spontaneous breathing, the driving pressure is the interpleural pressure swings generated during inspiration; during assisted ventilation, the transpulmonary pressure swings are produced by the forces exerted by the ventilator combined with the patient's own respiratory effort, if present (see Figs. 2.9 and 2.10). Therefore, with synchronized (assisted) ventilation, the negative inspiratory effort of the infant and the positive pressure generated by the ventilator are additive and together form the *transpulmonary pressure* that determines the V_T. It should be noted that in routine ventilator-based pulmonary mechanics measurement, only the ventilator contribution to the transpulmonary pressure is measured, ignoring the infant's contribution. Therefore, in actively breathing infants, ventilator-based lung mechanics measurements are not accurate.

In the healthy lung, gravity-dependent differences in interpleural or transpulmonary pressure are responsible for most of the regional differences in ventilation. In the sick lung, local differences in compliance and airway resistance (time constants) are the major contributors to uneven distribution of ventilation. Bryan et al.[71] showed that the dependent lung regions in normal subjects have a greater regional volume expansion ratio (change in volume per unit of preinspiratory volume) than do the nondependent regions of lung. When a patient is upright, the basal regions of the lung are ventilated to a greater extent than are the apical regions. When a patient is supine, the basal and apical regions are ventilated to similar extents, but the posterior (dependent) regions are ventilated to a greater extent than the anterior regions (nondependent).

It is important to remember, however, that at the end of a normal exhalation (at FRC), the volume in the uppermost regions of the lung is greater than that of the dependent regions. This may appear contradictory, but these differences can be explained on the basis of regional interpleural pressure differences (Fig. 2.16). Interpleural pressure at end expiration is more negative in the uppermost portions than in the dependent portions of the lung. Converting the interpleural pressures to transpulmonary pressures, one can plot a pressure–volume curve (lower right of Fig. 2.16). When the lungs are inflated starting from FRC, the dependent lung units will receive proportionately more of the inspired gas, and the nondependent units will receive proportionately less as the height above the dependent units increases. The basilar units are stretched proportionately more than the higher units because they are operating on a steeper slope of the volume–pressure curve. Compliance increases progressively from the highest portion of the lung to the most dependent portion or from high starting lung volumes to lower volumes. At the beginning of a gradual inflation from FRC, the more dependent lung regions operate on a steeper part of the compliance curve than the less dependent regions, so ventilation is greater in the dependent regions. However, because of the small size of newborn infants, the gravity-dependent regional differences are not nearly as large as they are in adults.

Lung units that contain collapsed airways require large pressure changes before the airways open to permit gas transfer.

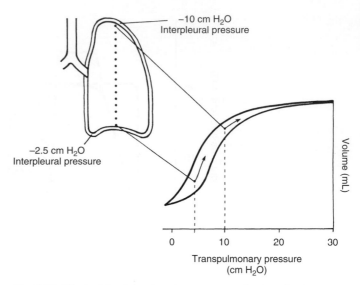

Fig. 2.16 Effect of the interpleural pressure gradient up the lung upon the distribution of ventilation. The greatest negative pressure is at the top owing to the gravitational tug (weight) of the lung through its visceral pleura on the parietal pleura. Because the upper and lower areas are on different parts of the pressure–volume curve, different amounts of volume (ventilation) are achieved by the two areas given the same pressure change. The steeper compliance line for the lower area means a greater increase in volume per unit pressure change. (Modified from West JB: Respiratory Physiology: The Essentials. 2nd ed. Baltimore, Williams & Wilkins, 1979, p. 96.)

These units are not ventilated as well as units in which the airways are patent from the start. Units with high resistance are ventilated poorly regardless of their position because these units have low compliance for any given transpulmonary pressure. In newborn infants, airway closure may be present in the resting V_T range, unlike in older individuals in whom pleural surface pressure at FRC is substantially subatmospheric throughout the lung, thus preventing airway closure while the lung is at operational volume.[72] Starting inspiration from a lung volume that is below FRC or rest volume actually reverses the pattern of the distribution of ventilation.[73] If inspiration is started from a low level of lung volume, interpleural pressures are less negative overall (because elastic recoil is minimal at these low lung volumes) and even may be positive in the more dependent regions of the lung.

When regional interpleural pressure exceeds (is more positive than) airway pressure, then airway closure occurs and no gas enters that segment for the first portion of inspiration or until regional interpleural pressure decreases to below airway pressure further along into inspiration. Thus ventilation is reduced in dependent regions and is redirected to the upper lung regions, making them the better ventilated areas; this is a reversal of the usual pattern.

During assisted ventilation, inflation at end inspiration is uniform, as evidenced by the observation of alveoli of equal size throughout the lung.[74] At end expiration or FRC level, however, alveoli in the uppermost regions of the lung are found to have a volume fourfold that of alveoli at the base. Moderate levels of PEEP increase FRC more in dependent regions than in upper regions of the lung because the former are less well expanded initially and are at a lower and more favorable point on their compliance curve. If significant basilar atelectasis preexists, the addition of PEEP or CPAP should help the most in the more dependent areas, opening them for improved regional ventilation. All forms of CDP favor uniformity of ventilation because they expand airways and thus lower resistance and because they prevent airway closure and gas trapping during forced exhalation.

Gravitational effects on the distribution of ventilation have been exploited in adult patients with or without ventilatory assistance who have unilateral lung disease[75] or who have undergone thoracotomy.[76] Improved gas exchange in these patients can be accomplished if they are positioned with their "good" side down. This technique increases ventilation to the dependent lung regions, which also receive relatively greater blood flow, resulting in better V/Q matching in the good lung. Body position affects ventilation and gas exchange in infants in the opposite way.

When infants with unilateral lung disease are placed in the lateral decubitus position, the uppermost "good" lung receives a greater portion of ventilation than the dependent lung. This may be the case for infants with restrictive lung disease such as unilateral PIE. In cases of unilateral PIE, one sees ideal circumstances for the occurrence of airway closure in the "bad" lung when it is placed in the dependent position. In patients with unilateral tension PIE, interpleural pressure on the bad side already is elevated secondary to the presence of high (positive) interstitial pressure because of gas trapping outside of the terminal air spaces. Positioning patients with the PIE side down adds the additional weight of the mediastinal structures, which causes the interpleural pressure to exceed local airway pressure and results in airway collapse. This airway closure in the dependent (bad) lung often facilitates resolution of unilateral PIE, while the infant's gas exchange needs are met by the nondependent lung.[77,78]

The pattern of diaphragmatic motion plays a role in the distribution of ventilation in the newborn infant. When the diaphragm is paralyzed and the patient is supine, mechanical ventilation tends to produce greater motion of the superior than of the inferior portion of the diaphragm because the superior portion is less constrained by the abdominal contents and mediastinal structures. Therefore, ventilation of the upper (anterior) segments of the lung is preferential.[79] Because perfusion still is likely to be better in the dependent regions secondary to gravitational effects, paralysis may result in V/Q mismatch with hypoxemia. The improvement in oxygenation achieved after adults with acute respiratory failure[80] or premature infants with respiratory insufficiency[81] are switched from the supine to the prone position is attributable to the enhancement of V/Q matching (or an increase in ventilation to a level that better matches the existing degree of perfusion). In premature infants, the prone position affords better distribution of ventilation throughout the lung, especially to the dependent regions that are better perfused.[81]

During assisted ventilation, to minimize risk to the infant, the most minimal amount of pressure required to achieve adequate tidal volume and alveolar ventilation should be used. Enough distending pressure should be applied to optimize lung volume and the homogeneity of lung expansion and prevent airway collapse. Enough driving pressure should be applied so as to achieve an appropriate V_T.

PERFUSION

Before delivery, only 8% to 10% of cardiac output flows to the lungs. In the fetus, pulmonary vascular resistance is high and systemic vascular resistance is low.[82] Most of the blood coming from the fetal inferior vena cava flows from right to left through the foramen ovale and much of the right ventricular output shunts through the ductus arteriosus, thus bypassing the lungs. Under normal circumstances after delivery, a relatively rapid transition to the adult pattern of circulation occurs, after which virtually all right-heart output goes through the lungs, then through the left side of the heart, and out the aorta.

Key to this transition is a decrease in pulmonary vascular resistance and an increase in pulmonary blood flow preceding closure of the fetal shunts. Experiments carried out on fetal lambs and investigations into the actions of certain mediators, including nitric oxide (NO) (Table 2.1), have demonstrated a number of factors that contribute to the decrease in pulmonary vascular resistance that occurs at birth. These include (1) expansion of the lung with a gas,[83] (2) increase in PAO_2,[84] (3) increase in PaO_2,[85] (4) increase in pH,[86] and (5) elaboration of vasoactive substances such as bradykinin,[87] the prostaglandins (PGE_1, PGA_1, PGI_2 [prostacyclin],[88,89] and PGD_2[90]), and NO.[91,92] Blood flow through the pulmonary circuit is directly proportional to the pressure gradient across the pulmonary vessels and the total cross-sectional area of the vessels that make up the pulmonary vascular bed. Blood flow is inversely proportional to the blood's viscosity. Increased blood viscosity interferes with gas exchange by reducing pulmonary perfusion.

As the lung expands after birth, pulmonary vascular resistance decreases and pulmonary blood flow increases.[83] With inflation of the lungs, some "straightening out" of pulmonary vessels occurs. The larger vessels are pulled open by traction of the lung parenchyma that surrounds them. The perialveolar capillary lumens enlarge because of the action of surface tension produced by the newly established air–fluid interfaces. There are two types of pulmonary blood vessels: alveolar vessels, which are

TABLE 2.1 Factors Affecting Pulmonary Blood Flow

Increasing Flow	Decreasing Flow
Optimization of lung volume	Lung atelectasis
Increase in PAO_2	Decrease in PAO_2
Increase in PaO_2	Hypoxemia (reduction in PaO_2)
Alkalosis (respiratory or metabolic)	Acidosis (respiratory or metabolic)
Release of mediator substances (e.g., bradykinin, prostaglandins)	Mast cell degranulation with release of histamine
Left-to-right shunting (intracardiac or ductal)	Right-to-left shunting (intracardiac or ductal)
Endogenous production of NO	Systemic hypotension (when right-to-left shunting is already present)
Inhalation of exogenous NO	Lung overexpansion

NO, Nitric oxide; *PaO_2*, partial pressure of oxygen in arterial blood; *PAO_2*, partial pressure of oxygen in the alveoli.

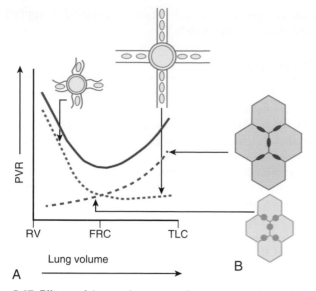

Fig. 2.17 Effects of lung volume on pulmonary vascular resistance (*PVR, solid curved line*). **(A)** "Extra-alveolar" vessels pose high resistance (*dotted curved line*) at low and high lung volumes, at the former because they become narrow and at the latter because they become stretched. **(B)** "Alveolar" vessels pose the least resistance (*dashed curved line*) when they are open widest at the functional residual capacity (*FRC*) lung volume level, but they become compressed under conditions of lung overinflation. *RV,* Residual volume; *TLC,* total lung capacity. (Modified from West JB: Respiratory Physiology: The Essentials. 2nd ed. Baltimore, Williams & Wilkins, 1979, p. 39.)

composed of capillaries and the slightly larger vessels in the alveolar walls (these vessels are exposed to alveolar pressure), and extra-alveolar vessels, which include the arteries and veins that run through the lung parenchyma but are surrounded by interstitial tissue rather than alveoli (Fig. 2.17).[93]

The diameter of alveolar vessels is determined by the balance between the alveolar pressure and the hydrostatic pressure within the vessel. The vessel walls contain little elastic tissue and virtually no muscle fibers. Alveolar vessels collapse if alveolar pressure exceeds pulmonary venous pressure. Extra-alveolar vessels have structural support in their walls and are not significantly influenced by alveolar pressure. The vessel diameter of extra-alveolar vessels is affected by lung volume, because expanding the lung tends to pull these vessels open. If an airless lung is inflated to total lung capacity, pulmonary vascular resistance shows a U-shaped response, with high resistance at the low and high ends of inflation and low resistance in the middle (see Fig. 2.17). Resistance is high at low lung volumes because the extra-alveolar vessels are narrowed (they are not being pulled open). Resistance is high at high inflation volumes because the alveolar vessels are narrowed by compression, sometimes to the point of collapse. The lowest pulmonary vascular resistance, as well as the best lung compliance, is found when the lung is neither underinflated nor overinflated.

The rapid rise in oxygen tension in the alveoli (PAO$_2$) and in the arterial blood (PaO$_2$) perfusing the pulmonary vessels plays a major role in the circulatory adaptation that occurs during transition to extrauterine life. It is the influence of PaO$_2$ on adjacent arteries that exerts the greatest effect on decreasing

pulmonary vascular resistance with the initiation of breathing air.[85] With the initiation of breathing air, the lung is exposed to a PO$_2$ of approximately 100 mm Hg. PaO$_2$ in the central circulation of the newborn infant rises from the fetal range between 25 and 30 mm Hg to greater than 60 mm Hg within the first hours after birth.

Many mediators have been implicated in the pulmonary vasodilation seen in the newborn infant. Bradykinin is a vasoactive peptide that produces pulmonary vasodilation in fetal lambs.[87] Bradykinin concentration increases transiently in blood that has passed through the lungs of fetal lambs ventilated with oxygen, but it does not increase if the lungs are ventilated with nitrogen. Bradykinin stimulates the local production of prostacyclin, which is also a potent pulmonary vasodilator.[88] PGA$_1$, PGE$_1$, and prostacyclin decrease pulmonary vascular resistance by dilating both pulmonary veins and arteries.[88,89,94] Prostacyclin production is stimulated by lung expansion with air and by mechanical ventilation.

The decrease in pulmonary vascular resistance associated with mechanical ventilation can be attenuated by prior administration of a prostaglandin synthesis inhibitor (indomethacin).[89] PGD$_2$, another prostaglandin, is a semiselective pulmonary vasodilator. It promotes pulmonary vasodilation without causing the systemic vasodilatory effect produced by other prostaglandins.[90] The pulmonary vasodilatory effect of PGD$_2$ is present only during the first few days after birth; thereafter, it becomes a pulmonary vasoconstrictor. This observation suggests that PGD$_2$ plays a role in the transition from fetal to adult-type circulation after birth. PGD$_2$, like histamine, is released through mast cell degranulation. The number of mast cells in the lungs increases just before birth and then declines after delivery.[95] Mast cells play an important role in the pulmonary vasoconstrictive response to hypoxia.[96] Mast cells are abundant in the lung and are ideally located for modulation of vascular tone. Mast cell degranulation has been demonstrated to occur after acute alveolar hypoxia.[97] Pretreatment with cromolyn sodium (a mast cell degranulation blocking agent) prevents the pulmonary vasoconstriction normally induced by alveolar hypoxia.[98]

Nitric oxide plays an important role in regulating pulmonary vascular resistance. Its action reduces pulmonary vasoconstriction, thereby increasing pulmonary blood flow.[99-101] Endogenous NO is generated in vascular endothelial cells by enzymatic cleavage of the terminal nitrogen from L-arginine; production is accelerated at birth owing to the increase in PO$_2$. NO diffuses into the vascular smooth muscle cells and stimulates the production of cyclic guanosine monophosphate, which causes smooth muscle relaxation.

The primary factor keeping pulmonary vascular resistance high in the fetus is relative hypoxemia. Because of the preferential perfusion of the pulmonary circuit with the most desaturated blood (venous blood returning from the fetus's upper body), the PaO$_2$ of blood perfusing the lungs of a fetal lamb is around 18 to 21 mm Hg. Profound fetal hypoxemia causes further pulmonary vasoconstriction. A decrease in pulmonary arterial PO$_2$ to about 14 mm Hg diminishes pulmonary blood flow in the fetus to approximately 50%, its base level.[102] Hypoxemic stress produces progressively greater increases in pulmonary vascular resistance as the gestational age of a fetus advances.[103] Chronic hypoxemia in the fetus produces an increase in the medial smooth muscle of the pulmonary arterioles, which may lead to pulmonary hypertension and increased pulmonary vasoreactivity.[104] This may contribute to the development of persistent pulmonary hypertension of the newborn (PPHN) in some newborn infants and may explain why infants born through meconium-stained fluid are at high risk for PPHN (see Chapter 34). Passage of meconium is thought to be a sign of fetal intolerance of labor, which is more likely to occur in infants whose placental function is compromised and who may have had prolonged fetal hypoxemia.

For these same reasons, infants living at high altitudes have an increase in pulmonary vascular resistance that persists into childhood. They have relative pulmonary hypertension and are at increased risk for developing cor pulmonale.[105] Infants with cyanotic congenital heart disease and chronic hypoxemia are also at risk for developing pulmonary hypertension and cor pulmonale, as are oxygen-dependent infants with BPD. The vasoconstriction response to alveolar and arterial hypoxemia is potentiated by acidosis.[86]

Inhaled NO causes a decrease in pulmonary vascular resistance and an increase in pulmonary blood flow, without affecting systemic arterial pressure.[106-108] It is a selective pulmonary vasodilator, because it is inactivated by being bound to hemoglobin upon entering the systemic circulation.[109] When used at low concentrations, inhaled NO also improves ventilation–perfusion matching by selectively vasodilating the well-ventilated areas of the lung (see Chapter 34).[110]

The pulmonary arteries, like the airways, form a treelike structure. The pulmonary circulation is perfused by the entire cardiac output. Blood flow is determined by the pressure difference between pulmonary arteries and veins and by the vascular resistance. The pulmonary circulation is a low-pressure, low-resistance system. The distribution of blood flow to the gas exchange units depends on the distribution of resistances, which are affected by contraction of the smooth muscle walls of the arteries. In hypoxia, resistance increases, owing to hypoxic pulmonary vasoconstriction.[111]

There are regional differences in ventilation and perfusion. The dependent portions of the lung are better ventilated and better perfused than the upper portions. Hypoxic vasoconstriction shunts blood away from poorly ventilated acini, which helps preserve V/Q matching. Ideally, ventilation and perfusion are evenly matched, with a V/Q ratio of 1. When a lung or lung unit is relatively underventilated but normally perfused or is normally ventilated but overperfused, it is said to have a low V/Q (less than 1). When a lung unit is overventilated and normally perfused or is normally ventilated and underperfused, the resultant V/Q is high (>1).

The more dependent the lung region, the greater its perfusion.[112] The vessels in dependent regions of the lung are more distended and thus present less resistance to flow because their transmural pressure (the difference between the hydrostatic pressure inside and the pressure outside the vessel wall, i.e., pleural pressure) is greater. Interpleural pressure decreases the more dependent the lung region is. Because the hydrostatic pressure increase (inside the vessel) is greater than the interpleural pressure decrease (outside the vessel), the transmural pressure increase is greater the more dependent the lung region.

Regional hypoventilation produces local pulmonary vasoconstriction that diverts blood flow away from underventilated areas. This is a protective mechanism that decreases the perfusion of nonventilated or poorly ventilated areas of the lung. Term newborn and premature lambs are capable of redirecting blood flow away from hypoxic regions produced by atelectasis or bronchial obstruction.[111,113] The flow directed away from atelectatic and hypoxic lung segments is directly proportional to the amount of lung volume loss.[114] Lung scans in infants have identified perfusion deficits in areas of atelectasis.[115] Alveolar overdistention secondary to air trapping may reduce area blood flow by collapsing surrounding capillaries.

When CPAP or positive-pressure ventilation is used to recruit atelectatic lung units, improvement in both local ventilation and perfusion may result in those regions. However, those areas of the lung, which already are well expanded, may be further inflated, which can increase rather than decrease pulmonary vascular resistance in those areas. The overall effect on pulmonary blood flow produced by positive-pressure ventilation depends on the initial lung volume status of the various functional lung regions and the net result of the therapy on global pulmonary blood flow.

CONTROL OF VENTILATION

The respiratory control center in the newborn infant is immature compared to that of adults and therefore more easily influenced by changes in acid−base status, temperature, sleep state, hypoxia, medications, and other variables. Because of this relative immaturity, the central and peripheral chemoreceptors that respond to changes in arterial O_2 and CO_2 tensions act both quantitatively and qualitatively differently compared to those in adults. Additionally, a set of chest wall stretch proprioceptors is able to reflexively inhibit or drive respiration.[116] REM sleep also has a significant effect on the control of respiration in the newborn infant. During REM sleep, the normal phasic tone changes in the intercostal muscles, which are important for stabilizing the rib cage during inspiration, are inhibited. Because the intercostal muscles fail to tighten with inspiration, the infant's chest wall deforms during inspiration. Contraction of the diaphragm worsens the paradoxical movement, increases its O_2 consumption measured during REM sleep, and may lead to fatigue-induced apnea.[117]

Application of CPAP or PEEP causes the infant's respiratory rate to slow and his or her respiratory efforts to become more regular with a reduction in periodic breathing and apneic episodes.[118,119] The distending pressure stabilizes the infant's compliant chest wall by providing a "pneumatic splint" that counters the tendency of the chest wall to collapse during inspiration. The application of CDP shortens and intensifies inspiratory effort while prolonging expiration. Methylxanthines such as caffeine and aminophylline (or theophylline) increase alveolar ventilation through central stimulation.[120] Methylxanthines cause an increase in diaphragmatic contractility and resistance to fatigue with a shift of the CO_2 response curve to the left so that an increase in V_T occurs in response to an increase in CO_2.[121,122] A more detailed discussion on the control of ventilation can be found in Chapter 3.

CONCLUSION

Based on an understanding of the physiologic principles of assisted ventilation, we know that ventilation strategies must be individualized for each patient. It is also clear that the use of the appropriate strategy to provide mechanical ventilatory support and the skill with which this is done are more important than the specific type of device used to deliver that support. Each time we encounter an infant in respiratory distress, we must determine the specific pathophysiology of the infant's condition and then decide what level of support is required, addressing the infant's specific condition. The least invasive level of support that is adequate to accomplish the task should be selected, and the infant's response to therapy must be closely monitored.[123] We must be cognizant of how our strategies and techniques of providing assisted ventilation to infants influence their long-term outcomes. Despite many years of diligent research, there are still more questions than answers. However, we do know that mechanical ventilation causes lung injury that leads to inflammatory response;[124] excessive oxygen exposure is harmful;[125,126] lung overdistention (volutrauma) causes lung injury;[127] lung injury and inflammation exacerbate the deleterious effects of oxygen toxicity and volutrauma;[128] and finally, atelectotrauma is a source of lung injury.[129]

Establishment of an appropriate FRC (optimization of lung volume), administration of surfactant, avoidance of mechanical ventilation (if possible), use of adequate PEEP to avoid the repeated collapse and reopening of small airways, avoidance of lung overinflation caused by using excessive distending airway pressure or supraphysiologic V_Ts, and avoidance of the use of more oxygen than is necessary all are important in achieving the best possible outcomes and long-term health of our patients.[123,130] While caring for your patients, always remember the words of the Hippocratic Oath, "First do no harm."

ACKNOWLEDGMENTS

We wish to acknowledge gratefully the important contribution of Brian Wood, MD, who was the author of this chapter in the early editions of this book.

A complete reference list is available at https://expertconsult.inkling.com/.

SELECTED READINGS

22. Greenough A, Milner AD, Dimitriou G: Synchronized mechanical ventilation for respiratory support in newborn infants. Cochrane Database Syst Rev 1:CD000456, 2001.

25. Milner AD, Saunders RA, Hopkin IE: Effects of delivery by caesarean section on lung mechanics and lung volume in the human neonate. Arch Dis Child 53:545–548, 1978.

33. LeSouef PN, England SJ, Bryan AC: Total resistance of the respiratory system in preterm infants with and without an endotracheal tube. J Pediatr 104:108, 1984.

38. Saunders RA, Milner AD, Hopkin IE: The effects of continuous positive airway pressure on lung mechanics and lung volumes in the neonate. Biol Neonate 29:178–186, 1976.

46. Bancalari E: Inadvertent positive end-expiratory pressure during mechanical ventilation. J Pediatr 108:567, 1986.

64. SUPPORT Study Group of the Eunice Kennedy Shriver NICHD Neonatal Research Network, Carlo WA, Finer NN, Walsh MC, et al: Target ranges of oxygen saturation in extremely preterm infants. N Engl J Med 362(21):1959–1969, 2010.

81. Balaguer A, Escribano J, Roqué M: Infant position in neonates receiving mechanical ventilation. Cochrane Database Syst Rev 18(4):CD003668, 2006.

83. Einhorning G, Adams FH, Norman A: Effect of lung expansion on the fetal lamb circulation. Acta Paediatr Scand 55:441, 1966.

128. Jobe AH, Ikegami M: Mechanism initiating lung injury in the preterm. Early Hum Dev 53:81–94, 1999.

129. Muscedere JG, Mullen JB, Gan K: Tidal ventilation at low airway pressures can augment lung injury. Am J Respir Crit Care Med 149:1327–1334, 1994.

3

Control of Ventilation

Richard J. Martin and Eric C. Eichenwald

INTRODUCTION

The transition from fetal to neonatal life requires a rapid conversion from intermittent fetal respiratory activity not associated with gas exchange to continuous breathing upon which gas exchange is dependent once the baby is born. This encompasses the development of neural circuitry that regulates respiratory control and serves as a unique link between the maturing lung and the brain. The frequent apneic events exhibited by preterm infants may be akin to the episodic pauses in respiratory movements that characterize fetal breathing. However, after birth, frequent apnea—often associated with bradycardia and oxygen desaturation events—may be one of the most troublesome problems in neonatal intensive care. The problem of vulnerable neonatal respiratory control is typically enhanced by the mechanical disadvantages of a compliant chest wall and unfavorable lung mechanics. This is compounded by the clinical observation that neonatal respiratory control is vulnerable to a diversity of pathophysiologic conditions (Fig. 3.1). Understanding the maturation of neonatal respiratory control is essential to providing a rational approach to ventilatory support for neonates.

PATHOGENESIS OF APNEA OF PREMATURITY

Our understanding of the pathogenesis of apnea of prematurity is hampered by our limited understanding of the integration of chemo- and mechanosensitive inputs to the autonomic control circuitry of the developing human brainstem. Neonatal animal models, such as rodents, are immature at birth compared with the human trajectory but do not typically exhibit apnea. Nonetheless, we are clearly dependent on animal models to characterize the maturation of neuroanatomic architecture and neurochemical transmitter changes in the brain-stem. Undoubtedly there are significant changes in adenosine, γ-aminobutyric acid (GABA), and serotonin content and corresponding receptor subtypes in respiratory-related brain-stem regions.[1]

Central Carbon Dioxide Chemosensitivity

Carbon dioxide (CO_2) is sensed primarily at or near the ventral medullary surface, but also by the carotid bodies, and is the major chemical driver of respiration at all ages. It has been recognized for several decades that preterm infants exhibit a diminished ventilatory response to CO_2 compared with more mature infants.[2] The response to CO_2 in preterm neonates results in an increase in tidal volume with little, if any, increase in frequency.[3] Furthermore, apneic preterm infants have a diminished CO_2 response compared with nonapneic preterm controls.[4] In preterm and term infants, the baseline partial pressure of carbon dioxide ($PaCO_2$) has been shown to be only up to 1.5 mm Hg above the apneic threshold; this narrow margin might predispose these children to apnea in the face of only minor oscillations in $PaCO_2$.[5] Breathing patterns tend to be more irregular in rapid eye movement (REM) than in quiet sleep, and it is possible that the closeness of the eupneic and apneic CO_2 thresholds may contribute to greater breath-to-breath respiratory irregularity in REM sleep. Unfortunately, REM sleep, quiet sleep, transitional sleep, and even wakefulness are often difficult to distinguish in preterm infants. This complicates the ability to draw conclusions about sleep state and respiratory control in the preterm population.

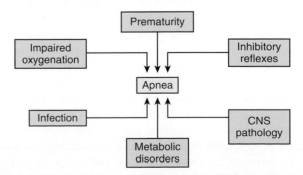

Fig. 3.1 Specific contributory causes of apnea. *CNS,* Central nervous system.

Peripheral (Hypoxic) Chemosensitivity

The peripheral chemoreceptors are located primarily in the carotid body and are responsible for stimulating breathing in response to hypoxemia. Both enhanced and reduced peripheral chemoreceptor functions have been proposed as contributors to apnea of prematurity.[6] In utero, carotid chemoreceptor oxygen sensitivity is adapted to the normally low partial pressure of oxygen (PaO_2) of the mammalian fetal environment ($\sim$23–27 mm Hg). After birth, in response to the increase in PaO_2 with the establishment of breathing, the peripheral chemoreceptors are silenced, followed by a gradual increase in hypoxic chemosensitivity. Once peripheral chemosensitivity is established, hyperoxic resuscitation rapidly elicits apnea, as clearly shown in rat pups.[7] It follows that inappropriate hyperoxic ventilatory support of an apneic infant may hinder recovery of the respiratory drive. Interestingly, infants with bronchopulmonary dysplasia seem to exhibit blunted peripheral chemoreceptor responses compared with controls,[8] which may increase their vulnerability to apnea.

Excessive peripheral chemoreceptor sensitivity in response to repeated hypoxemia may also destabilize breathing patterns in the face of significantly fluctuating levels of oxygenation. This is consistent with an earlier finding in preterm infants that a greater hypoxemia-induced increase in ventilation correlates with a higher number of apneic episodes.[9] Data from rat pups indicate that conditioning with intermittent hypoxic exposures results in facilitation of carotid body sensory discharge in response to subsequent hypoxic exposure. This effect appears to persist into adult life, raising questions about a longer lasting effect of early apnea in human respiratory control.[10]

In the neonatal period, it is well known that the ventilatory response to hypoxemia, an initial increase in minute ventilation, is followed by a posthypoxemia decline in frequency of breathing. This so-called hypoxic ventilatory depression is seen in less dramatic form in later life and may be an appropriate response to sustained hypoxemia when coupled with a decrease in metabolic rate. Descending inhibition from the midbrain and other structures appears to cause this hypoxic depression rather than a decline in peripheral chemoreceptor firing, although a contribution from the latter cannot be excluded. The role of hypoxic depression in contributing to apnea of prematurity is unclear; however, low baseline oxygenation is associated with more episodic desaturation in preterm infants.[11]

Role of Mechanoreceptor (Laryngeal) Afferents

Activation of the laryngeal mucosa elicits a potent airway-protective reflex, which, in preterm and term neonates and immature animals of various species, results in a host of autonomic perturbations including apnea, bradycardia, hypotension, closure of upper airways, and swallowing movements. Although this strong inhibitory reflex, termed the laryngeal chemoreflex, is thought to be an important contributor to apnea and bradycardia associated with excessive suctioning or aspiration, its relationship to apnea of prematurity is less clear. The pronounced inhibitory effect on ventilation in early life may be the result of enhanced central inhibitory pathways, and GABA has been proposed to mediate this effect.[12] Despite the

physiologic rationale for a relationship between stimulation of laryngeal afferents and apnea of prematurity, a temporal relationship between apnea of prematurity and gastroesophageal reflux is rare in preterm infants, as discussed later. Of interest are the data from piglets, confirmed in infants, showing that respiratory inhibition may precede a loss of lower esophageal sphincter tone and theoretically predispose to reflux.[13,14]

GENESIS OF CENTRAL, MIXED, AND OBSTRUCTIVE APNEA

Apnea is classified into three categories traditionally, each based upon the absence or presence of upper airway obstruction: (1) central, (2) obstructive, and (3) mixed. Central apnea is characterized by total cessation of inspiratory efforts with no evidence of obstruction. In obstructive apnea, the infant tries to breathe against an obstructed upper airway, resulting in chest wall motion without airflow throughout the entire apneic episode. Mixed apnea consists of obstructed respiratory efforts, usually following central pauses. The site of obstruction in the upper airways is primarily in the pharynx, although it also may occur at the larynx and possibly at both sites. Interestingly, upper airway closure may also occur during central apnea.

Unlike adult sleep apnea, which is primarily obstructive, apnea of prematurity has a predominantly central etiology with loss of respiratory drive initiated in the brainstem. During mixed apnea, it has been assumed that there is an initial loss of central respiratory drive and the resumption of inspiration is accompanied by a delay in activation of the upper airway muscles superimposed upon a closed upper airway.[15] This may be the result of a lower CO_2 threshold for activation of chest wall versus upper airway muscles. Mixed apnea typically accounts for more than 50% of long apneic episodes, followed in decreasing frequency by central and obstructive apnea.[16] Purely obstructive spontaneous apnea in the absence of a positional problem (such as neck flexion) is probably uncommon. As standard impedance monitoring of respiratory efforts via chest wall motion cannot recognize obstructed respiratory efforts, mixed (or obstructive) apnea is frequently identified by the accompanying bradycardia or desaturation, although these are not the initiating events.

RELATIONSHIP BETWEEN APNEA, BRADYCARDIA, AND DESATURATION

Cessation of respiration or hypoventilation is almost invariably the event that initiates various patterns of apnea, bradycardia, and desaturation in preterm infants. There is no clear consensus as to when a respiratory pause, which is universal in preterm infants, can be defined as an apneic episode. It has been proposed that apnea may be defined by its duration (e.g., >15 seconds) or by accompanying bradycardia and/or desaturations. However, even the 5- to 10-second pauses that occur in periodic breathing may be associated with bradycardia or desaturation. Periodic breathing—ventilatory cycles of 10- to 15-second duration with pauses of 5- to 10-second duration—is considered a "normal" breathing pattern in infants who should not require therapeutic intervention, as discussed earlier. Periodic breathing is speculated to be the result of dominant peripheral chemoreceptor activity responding to fluctuations in arterial oxygen tension. The rapidity of the fall in oxygen saturation after a respiratory pause is directly proportional to baseline oxygenation, and this, in turn, is related to lung volume and severity of lung disease.

Bradycardia is a prominent feature in preterm infants with apnea. The mechanism underlying bradycardia associated with apnea in preterm infants is not entirely clear. A significant correlation between decrease in oxygen saturation and heart rate has been noted, and the bradycardia during apnea might be related to hypoxic stimulation of the carotid body chemoreceptors, especially in the absence of lung inflation. On the other hand, bradycardia may occur simultaneously with apnea during stimulation of laryngeal receptors, suggesting a vagally mediated central mechanism for the production of both. Data in preterm infants indicate that isolated bradycardic events (<70/min) in the absence of accompanying hypoxemia are unlikely to significantly affect tissue oxygenation measured by near-infrared spectroscopy.[17]

CARDIORESPIRATORY EVENTS IN INTUBATED INFANTS

If apnea is the precipitant of episodic bradycardia and desaturation in spontaneously breathing events, what is the etiology of such events in intubated and ventilated infants? The likely answer is that mechanical ventilation does not always result in effective ventilation in intubated infants. Loss of lung volume and excessive abdominal expiratory muscle activity have been shown to accompany desaturation events in such infants, which might be ameliorated by an increase in positive expiratory pressure.[18] Loss of spontaneous ventilatory effort may also occur under these conditions. The presence of episodic desaturation and bradycardia in ventilated infants reinforces the need to synchronize spontaneous and ventilator inflations in infants. Extubation to continuous positive airway pressure (CPAP), if feasible, may effectively decrease the frequency of such events.

THERAPEUTIC APPROACHES

Impaired respiratory control is clearly a major contributor to the need for neonatal assisted ventilation. Our ability to enhance neonatal respiratory control will therefore probably diminish potential morbidity induced by ventilation. Aggressive therapy for apnea may be beneficial in avoiding intubation, enhancing extubation, and decreasing any adverse effects of apnea or gas exchange. To achieve these goals we have both nonpharmacologic and pharmacologic and ventilatory strategies. Many of the latter are addressed elsewhere in this book.

Optimization of Mechanosensory Inputs

The respiratory rhythm-generating circuitry within the central nervous system depends on intrinsic rhythmic activity and

sensory afferent inputs to generate breathing movement. Bloch-Salisbury et al. have demonstrated that their novel technique of stochastic mechanosensory stimulation, using a mattress with embedded actuators, is able to stabilize respiratory patterns in preterm infants as manifest by a decrease in apnea and an almost threefold decrease in percentage of time with oxygen saturations less than 85%.[19] Interestingly, the level of stimulation employed was below the minimum threshold for behavioral arousal to wakefulness, thus inducing no apparent state change in the infants, and the effect could probably not be attributed to the minimal increase in sound level associated with stimulation. A similar small study of vibratory stimulation of an extremity of premature infants showed a reduction of measured apneic events during periods of vibration.[20] Such an approach is clearly still a research tool but worthy of future study. It points to the important consideration that environmental stimulation of the infant must be optimized. Similarly, skin-to-skin care is a highly desirable practice in the neonatal intensive care unit (NICU) to encourage parental attachment and potentially influence respiratory control.[21] Data have shown that this practice is not only safe but also associated with decreased electrical diaphragm activity, potentially benefiting energy expended on respiratory efforts.[22]

Optimization of Blood Gas Status

Intermittent hypoxic episodes are almost always the result of respiratory pauses, apnea, or ineffective ventilation, aggravated by poor respiratory function (Fig. 3.2). Targeting lower baseline oxygen saturation has been associated with persistence of intermittent hypoxic episodes.[11] It is unclear whether this lower baseline oxygen saturation increases the incidence of apnea

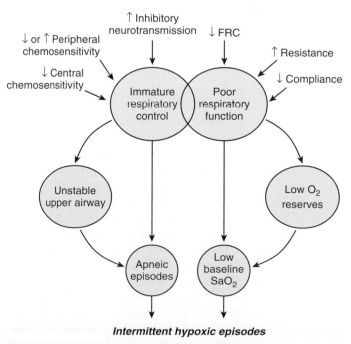

Fig. 3.2 Mechanisms whereby immature respiratory control superimposed upon poor respiratory function contributes to episodic desaturation. *FRC,* Functional residual capacity.

with resultant hypoxemia (via hypoxic depression of breathing) or whether the incidence of apnea is comparable between oxygen targets, but the lower oxygen saturation baseline predisposes to more frequent or profound intermittent hypoxemia. Regardless of mechanism, a low baseline oxygen saturation (e.g., <90%) should be avoided in the face of immature respiratory control superimposed upon poor respiratory function. It is also unclear whether the beneficial effect of packed red cell transfusion is secondary to improved respiratory control or decreased vulnerability to hypoxemia in the face of apnea.[23,24] These studies demonstrate that improvement in intermittent hypoxic episodes after red cell transfusion is manifest only after the first weeks of postnatal life and that nursing reports significantly underestimate the frequency of such cardiorespiratory events.[23,24] Obviously, any benefit of packed cell transfusion on apnea, bradycardia, and desaturation must be balanced against the potential hazards of transfusion.

Automated control of inspired oxygen is under study. This automated technique has been compared with routine adjustments of inspired oxygen as performed by clinical personnel in infants of 24 to 27 weeks' gestation.[25,26] During the automated period, time with oxygen saturation within the intended range of 87% to 93% increased significantly, and times in the hyperoxic range were significantly reduced. This was not associated with a clear benefit for hypoxic episodes; nonetheless, future refinement of this technology may prove useful to minimize intermittent hypoxemia. Finally, a novel approach is supplementation of inspired air with a very low concentration of supplemental CO_2 to increase respiratory drive.[27] Although of interest from a physiologic perspective, and likely to be successful in decreasing apnea, it is doubtful that this would gain widespread clinical acceptance as most preterm infants have residual lung disease and are prone to baseline hypercarbia, which may make clinicians reluctant to administer supplemental inspired CO_2.

Role of Gastroesophageal Reflux

Although pharyngeal and laryngeal stimulation may trigger apnea, caution should be exercised before apnea is attributed to gastroesophageal reflux. Despite the frequent coexistence of apnea and gastroesophageal reflux in preterm infants, investigations into the timing of reflux in relation to apneic events indicate that they are rarely temporally related.[28] Monitoring studies demonstrate that when a relationship between reflux and apnea is observed, apnea may precede rather than follow reflux.[14] This finding suggests that loss of respiratory neural output during apnea may be accompanied by a decrease in lower esophageal tone and resultant gastroesophageal reflux. Such a phenomenon is supported by data from a newborn piglet model, in which apnea was accompanied by a fall in lower esophageal sphincter pressure. Although physiologic experiments in animals reveal that reflux of gastric contents to the larynx induces reflex apnea, no clear evidence is available showing that treatment of reflux will affect frequency of apnea in most preterm infants.[29] Therefore the pharmacologic management of reflux with agents that decrease gastric acidity or enhance gastrointestinal motility generally should be reserved

for infants at specific risk (e.g., those with neurodevelopmental disability or following surgical repair of gastrointestinal anomalies). Use of these agents in preterm infants should be discouraged, even for those who exhibit signs of emesis or regurgitation of feedings, regardless of whether apnea is present because acid suppression therapy is associated with increased risk of neonatal sepsis, necrotizing enterocolitis, and death. If initiated in occasional preterm infants, such treatment should be promptly discontinued in the absence of clear clinical benefit.[30]

Xanthine Therapy

Xanthine therapy has had a remarkable impact on neonatal care over the past 40 years. Questions remain about its mode of action in enhancing neonatal respiratory control, but its efficacy and safety are widely accepted. Of interest is its remarkable ability to decrease apnea of prematurity, which is probably not the case for apnea in later life when the generalized stimulating effect of caffeine would not be well tolerated. It appears that the neonate exhibits a selective caffeine (or theophylline)-induced stimulation of respiratory neural output without a generalized stimulant effect.

Both caffeine and theophylline can be used to treat apnea of prematurity, although caffeine is preferred because of its broader therapeutic profile and longer half-life, allowing once-a-day dosing. Xanthines have multiple physiologic and pharmacologic mechanisms of action. The ability of xanthine therapy to enhance respiratory neural output in early life is manifested by an increase in minute ventilation, improved CO_2 sensitivity, and decreased hypoxic depression of breathing. The precise pharmacologic basis for this increase in respiratory neural output is still under investigation; however, competitive antagonism of adenosine receptors is a well-documented effect of xanthines.[31] Although adenosine acts as an inhibitory neuroregulator in the central nervous system via activation of adenosine A_1 receptors, activation of adenosine A_{2A} receptors appears to excite GABA-ergic interneurons, and released GABA may contribute to the respiratory inhibition induced by adenosine.[32] The xanthines also inhibit phosphodiesterase, which normally breaks down cyclic adenosine monophosphate (cAMP), although the relationship of cAMP accumulation with relief of apnea in infants is questionable.

These complex neurotransmitter interactions elicited by caffeine led to concerns regarding its safety. This concern was addressed in a large, randomized placebo controlled multicenter trial of caffeine citrate with a primary outcome of the incidence of neurodevelopmental impairment at 18 to 22 months. Of note, apnea density was not assessed in this study. The results clearly demonstrated that caffeine treatment in the doses used (used to treat apnea or enhance extubation) is safe and improved the neurodevelopmental outcome at 18 to 22 months, especially in those receiving respiratory support. Additionally, the study found that treatment with caffeine resulted in a decrease in the rate of bronchopulmonary dysplasia (BPD), perhaps owing to a shorter duration of mechanical ventilation in infants receiving caffeine.[33,34] There is also evidence for a reduction in developmental coordination disorder in the

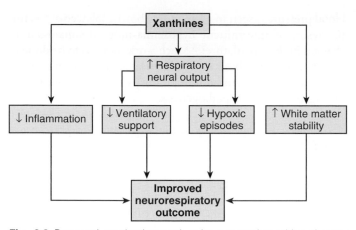

Fig. 3.3 Proposed mechanisms whereby neonatal xanthine therapy benefits later outcomes.

caffeine-treated cohort at 5 years of age, which persisted to school age.[35,36] Subsequent analysis of these data and further observational studies suggest that the neurologic benefits of caffeine may be highest in infants in whom caffeine is initiated in the first 3 days after birth.[37] It is possible that this benefit is secondary to a decrease in apnea and resultant intermittent hypoxic episodes, or a direct pharmacologic neuroprotective effect of caffeine; however, this remains speculative (Fig. 3.3).

Data in neonatal rodents demonstrate an anti-inflammatory effect of caffeine in proinflammatory states elicited by postnatal hyperoxia or antenatal endotoxin exposure.[38,39] In these studies, improved lung pathology and respiratory system mechanics were observed after caffeine treatment. In contrast, other data raise concerns about potential adverse effects of neonatal caffeine exposure in various animal models. Data on the effects of caffeine on the developing brain are also conflicting and include no effect in an ovine model, a protective effect in hypoxemia-induced perinatal white matter injury, and an adverse effect on brain imaging.

Caffeine is traditionally administered at a 10- to 12.5-mg/kg caffeine base (20–25 mg/kg caffeine citrate) loading dose followed by 2.5- to 5-mg/kg caffeine base (5–10 mg/kg caffeine citrate) maintenance dose every 24 hours. Changes in dosing that deviate from proven beneficial protocols should proceed with caution and be the subject of prospective clinical trials. Several small trials of higher loading and maintenance doses of caffeine have suggested a further reduction of apnea at higher doses; however, the safety of these higher doses has not been assessed.[40] Indeed, one study that used a loading dose of 80 mg/kg of caffeine citrate showed an association with an increased risk of cerebellar hemorrhage and seizure burden.[41,42] Based on the studies available to date, the timing of xanthine administration has changed, and caffeine use is now widespread in a prophylactic mode.[23] As noted earlier, initial studies suggest that very early initiation (within the first 3 days after birth) of caffeine therapy results in improved outcome; however, these findings are based on retrospective review with potential confounders.[37,43] Finally, the extended use of caffeine to 40 weeks' postmenstrual age was associated with a decrease in

intermittent hypoxemia among a cohort of preterm infants.[44,45] Higher doses of caffeine may be required if infants are treated beyond 36 weeks postmenstrual age (PMA) because of higher clearance of the drug at more advanced age.[45] Clearly more work is needed to further optimize caffeine therapy.

Continuous Positive Airway Pressure

CPAP has also proven to be a relatively safe and effective therapy for over 40 years and, together with caffeine, has revolutionized apnea management in infants. It has a dual function to stabilize lung volume and improve airway patency by limiting upper airway closure. Because longer episodes of apnea frequently involve an obstructive component, CPAP appears to be effective by "splinting" the upper airway with positive pressure and decreasing the risk of pharyngeal or laryngeal obstruction.[46] At the lower functional residual capacity that accompanies many preterm infants with residual lung disease, pulmonary oxygen stores are probably reduced, and there is a very short time from cessation of breathing to onset of desaturation and bradycardia. Therefore, CPAP is likely to reduce this vulnerability to episodic desaturation. Nasal CPAP is well tolerated in most preterm infants; however, as discussed elsewhere in this book, low- or high-flow nasal cannula therapies are being increasingly used as an equivalent treatment modality that may allow CPAP delivery while enhancing the mobility of the infant. Some studies suggest that synchronous nasal intermittent positive pressure ventilation (NIPPV) may be more effective than CPAP alone in some infants and could be considered as an adjunctive therapy in very preterm infants with significant apnea while on CPAP, particularly in the immediate postextubation period.[47] It is less clear whether asynchronous NIPPV, which is more commonly available, is equally as effective.

LONG-TERM CONSEQUENCES OF NEONATAL APNEA

Fortunately, apnea of prematurity generally resolves by about 36 to 40 weeks' postmenstrual age, although in more immature infants, apnea can persist beyond this time. This is of particular relevance in those who develop BPD. Available data indicate that cardiorespiratory events in most infants return to the baseline normal level at about 43 to 44 weeks' postmenstrual age.[48] In other words, beyond 43 to 44 weeks' postmenstrual age, the incidence of cardiorespiratory events in preterm infants does not significantly exceed that in term babies. For a subset of infants, the persistence of cardiorespiratory events may delay hospital discharge. For a few of these infants, home cardiorespiratory monitoring with or without persistent caffeine therapy until 43 to 44 weeks' PMA is offered in the United States as an alternative to a prolonged hospital stay. The absence of an obvious relationship between persistent apnea of prematurity and sudden infant death syndrome (SIDS) has significantly decreased the practice of home monitoring, with no increase in the SIDS rate.

Infants born prematurely experience multiple problems during their time in the NICU, and many of these conditions,

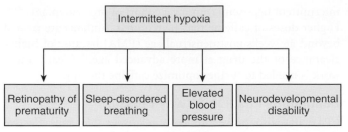

Fig. 3.4 Proposed morbidities attributable to intermittent hypoxia in the neonatal period, childhood, or adolescence.

such as apnea and resultant intermittent hypoxemia, may contribute to poor neurodevelopmental outcomes. The problem of correlating apnea with outcome is compounded by the fact that nursing reports of apnea severity may be unreliable, and impedance monitoring techniques often fail to identify mixed and obstructive events. Despite these reservations, available data suggest a link between the number of days apnea and assisted ventilation were recorded during hospitalization and the impaired neurodevelopmental outcome.[49] A relationship has also been shown between a delay in resolution of apnea and bradycardia beyond 36 weeks' corrected age and a higher incidence of unfavorable neurodevelopmental outcome, although these associations are fraught with potential confounding clinical issues.[50]

Studies might better focus on the incidence and severity of desaturation events, as techniques for long-term collection of pulse oximetry data are now advanced and can provide higher resolution of desaturations in monitored patients. Furthermore, it is likely that recurrent hypoxemia is the detrimental feature of the potential longer-term abnormalities exhibited by preterm infants. The incidence of intermittent hypoxic episodes in preterm infants is relatively low during the first week of life and then increases rapidly and is sustained over several weeks and may be persistent in many infants even after hospital discharge.[51] This time course may correspond to a postnatal rise in peripheral chemosensitivity and resultant respiratory instability as discussed earlier. Fig. 3.4 summarizes the proposed morbidities that might be attributable to intermittent hypoxic episodes in early life.[52] These proposed clinical consequences of neonatal intermittent hypoxemia need to be correlated with physiology studies that document any modulatory effects upon neuronal plasticity related to peripheral and/or central respiratory control mechanisms. We are currently learning a lot from ongoing studies in cohorts of former preterm infants. For example, the incidence of sleep-disordered breathing is exceedingly high in children born prematurely regardless of whether they were randomized to caffeine vs placebo therapy.[53] Elevated blood pressure is seen in prematurely born adolescents.[54] Is this the result of intermittent hypoxemia-induced inflammatory changes in the vasculature?[55] Much work remains to be done to elicit the biological basis for the sequelae we observe in preterm infants and the roles of both respiratory control and ventilatory management in their pathogenesis.

A complete reference list is available at https://expertconsult. inkling.com/.

KEY REFERENCES

6. MacFarlane PM, Ribeiro AP, Martin RJ: Carotid chemoreceptor development and neonatal apnea. Respir Physiol Neurobiol 185:170–176, 2013.
9. Nock ML, Di Fiore JM, Arko MK, et al: Relationship of the ventilatory response to hypoxia with neonatal apnea in preterm infants. J Pediatr 144:291–295, 2004.
11. Di Fiore JM, Walsh M, Wrage L, et al, on behalf of the SUPPORT Study Group of the Eunice Kennedy Shriver National Institute of Child Health and Human Development Neonatal Research Network: Low oxygen saturation target range is associated with increased incidence of intermittent hypoxemia. J Pediatr 161: 1047–1052, 2012.
14. Omari TI: Apnea-associated reduction in lower esophageal sphincter tone in premature infants. J Pediatr 154:374–378, 2009.
18. Bolivar JM, Gerhardt T, Gonzalez A, et al: Mechanisms for episodes of hypoxemia in preterm infants undergoing mechanical ventilation. J Pediatr 127:767–773, 1995.
24. Zagol K, Lake DE, Vergales B, Moorman ME, et al: Anemia, apnea of prematurity, and blood transfusions. J Pediatr 161:417–421, 2012.
27. Alvaro RE, Khalil M, Qurashi M, et al: CO_2 inhalation as a treatment for apnea of prematurity: a randomized double-blind controlled trial. J Pediatr 160:252–257, 2012.
28. Di Fiore J, Arko M, Herynk B, et al: Characterization of cardiorespiratory events following gastroesophageal reflux in preterm infants. J Perinatol 30:683–687, 2010.
34. Schmidt B, Roberts RS, Davis P, et al, Caffeine for Apnea of Prematurity Trial Group: Long-term effects of caffeine therapy for apnea of prematurity. N Engl J Med 357:1893–1902, 2007.
36. Schmidt B, Roberts R, Anderson P, et al. Academic performance, motor function, and behavior 11 years after neonatal caffeine citrate therapy for apnea of prematurity: an 11-year follow-up of the CAP randomized clinical trial. JAMA Pediatr 171(6): 564–572, 2017.
37. Lodha A, Lentz R, Synnes A, et al. Early caffeine administration and neurodevelopmental outcomes in preterm infants. Pediatrics 143(1):e20181348, 2019.
43. Lodha A, Seshia M, McMillan DD, et al, for the Canadian Neonatal Network: Association of early caffeine administration and neonatal outcomes in very preterm neonates. *JAMA Pediatr* 169:33–38, 2015.

4

Ethical Issues in Assisted Ventilation of the Neonate

Matthew Drago and Mark R. Mercurio

KEY POINTS

- Decisions regarding the provision, withholding, and withdrawal of assisted ventilation for a newborn should be based on an assessment of the goals of that therapy being reasonably achievable without intolerable side effects and, thus, in the newborn's best interest.
- Clinicians must recognize the subjective nature of quality of life assessments in determining what is in a newborn's best interest.
- Parents should be engaged in shared decision making with clinicians regarding the use of assisted ventilation. The right of parental authority must be balanced with the child's right both to certain treatments and to mercy.
- Withdrawing and withholding of life sustaining medical therapy are distinct acts but are ethically equivalent.

INTRODUCTION

Providing safe and effective assisted ventilation to critically ill newborns requires a great deal of knowledge, technical skill, and decision-making abilities. Much of this textbook is dedicated to the foundations of respiratory physiology, pathophysiology, and technical knowledge needed for clinical decision making. Given the gravity and complexity of these decisions, it is also important to have an understanding of the ethical reasoning necessary for responsible implementation of assisted ventilation for the neonate.

Although advances in obstetrical and neonatal care over the past decades have improved overall infant survival, the majority of pediatric deaths in the United States still occur in the neonatal intensive care unit (NICU) setting.[1] Of deaths that occur in the NICU, an increasing percentage are attributed to withdrawal or withholding of life-sustaining medical treatment (LSMT). Singh et al. published a retrospective review of deaths in a tertiary level NICU between 1988 and 1998, which showed that the number of infants who had a do not resuscitate (DNR) order placed before any episode of cardiopulmonary resuscitation rose from 36% in 1988 to 85% in 1998.[2] The same study also showed that, among patients who died in the NICU, withdrawal of LSMT rose from 10% in 1988 to 49% in 1998. A decade later, a 2008 study from another unit showed that withdrawal of LSMT preceded 61.6% of all NICU deaths, and another 20.8% of deaths were attributed to withholding of such treatment.[1]

Withdrawal of life-sustaining treatment in hospitalized patients can involve various interventions, such as discontinuation

of assisted ventilation, cessation of medically administered nutrition and hydration, turning off a ventricular assist device, stopping dialysis, and others. In the NICU population, withdrawal of LSMT is most often associated with removal of an endotracheal tube and cessation of mechanical ventilation. Thus initiation or discontinuation of assisted ventilation often involves not just a clinical decision but an ethical one as well. This ethical decision can be particularly challenging because discussions about the provision, withholding, or withdrawal of life support often occur when the prognosis, anticipated course, or range of choices for a given patient may be unclear.[3]

The goal of this chapter is to improve the reader's ability to navigate ethical challenges in caring for ventilated newborns through consideration of four key ethical questions:

1. What is the ethical basis for decisions regarding provision, withholding, and withdrawal of assisted ventilation for a newborn?
2. Who has, or should have, the authority to make these decisions?
3. What is the relevance of anticipated quality of life to decisions regarding assisted ventilation?
4. When might it be ethically permissible, or even advisable, to withhold or withdraw assisted ventilation?

Exploration of these questions will include discussion of the concepts of the patient's best interest, beneficence, nonmaleficence, futility, moral distress, relevant rights, and physicians' ethical obligations, all of which play into decisions regarding the provision of mechanical ventilation for the newborn.

AN ETHICAL BASIS FOR DECISION MAKING

Effective ventilatory support of newborns came into common use in the United States in the 1960s and early 1970s. Ethical consideration and debate of appropriate limitations on the utilization of this technology in newborns followed soon thereafter and have accompanied its use ever since. Neonatologists, philosophers, and bioethicists have long grappled with the fundamental questions of when it is appropriate to apply this technology and when it might be best to remove it.

Duff and Campbell initially described withdrawal of life support in the neonatal population in 1973.[4] Their article was published at a time when advances in neonatology had reduced infant mortality by 58% from 1940 to 1970. They were the first to openly discuss the anguishing ethical dilemma of whether to continue life support for infants that had survived the first days of life, but now faced severe chronic medical problems and a worrisome prognosis for future quality of life. Over the following decades, parents, clinicians, and public officials struggled with this concern both at the bedside and with public policy.[5,6] Some have argued that there are newborn patients with too grave a prognosis, or who are too costly to treat, to justify ongoing provision of intensive care measures such as assisted ventilation. However, translating this into practice or policy remains problematic, in part because of the wide spectrum of outcomes within certain diagnoses. [7,8] Categorically defining which newborns should or should not be treated with assisted ventilation because of poor prognosis for survival, or profound disability, is beyond the scope of this chapter. The focus, rather, is on elements of ethical decision making that the clinician should employ when deciding whether to use assisted ventilation in the care of a specific patient.

Assisted ventilation, like any treatment, should be provided if the goal of that therapy is reasonably achievable, and without intolerable side effects that would negate that goal. Put another way, a treatment should be initiated or continued if the benefits to the patient clearly outweigh the anticipated burdens. This, essentially, describes the widely accepted ethical principle of beneficence—the obligation of the clinician to act for the good of the patient.[9] If the benefit to the patient of a proposed treatment outweighs the burden, it is considered "in the patient's best interest" to be provided with that treatment. For the vast majority of newborns treated with assisted ventilation, the benefit of increased likelihood of survival clearly outweighs the burdens of the treatment itself and the potential long-term morbidities. For them, assisted ventilation is in their best interest, and there is rarely debate regarding its provision. There may be some, however, for whom the likelihood of survival is so low, or the anticipated burden of ongoing treatment and/or survival is so high, that assisted ventilation is not in the patient's best interest. The first, and most crucial, ethical assessment regarding provision of assisted ventilation, as with any treatment in the NICU, is this assessment of anticipated benefits and burdens to the newborn, both short-term and long-term.

The decision that best supports the child's interests is not always obvious, as the relative importance of various benefits and burdens will be a subjective assessment. And, there are at least two additional aspects of the standard worthy of consideration.[10] The best interest standard, strictly interpreted, perhaps sets an unrealistic expectation that parents must always choose what is best for their child. It may be best, for example, for parents of a given child to send him or her to an expensive private school, but this is not an expectation to which society holds parents. If providing it meant the parents and/or other members of the family would be required to sacrifice to an unfair or unrealistic extent, it might not be an appropriate expectation. Moreover, even if such things were in the best interest of a child and were not burdensome to the family, society still does not require it.

Rather than requiring parents to always decide based on the child's best interest, it has been suggested that parents are, and should be, free to choose and decide for their child, provided that care remains above some threshold of harm.[11] A parent is not, for example, required to choose a private school but is required to provide their child with an adequate education. Similarly, in medical decision making, it has been suggested that a parental decision should be honored even if that decision is not, in the eyes of the clinician, clearly the best choice for the child—until some threshold of harm is reached. Locating that threshold of harm is not obvious, and good clinicians, parents, and ethicists might disagree, but a standard set forth by the American Academy of Pediatrics seems a reasonable place to start; children, including newborns, "deserve effective medical treatment that is likely to prevent substantial harm or suffering or death."[12]

Another concern regarding the patient's best interest standard involves its scope. This standard, strictly interpreted, suggests decision making based upon the interests of the patient alone. Thus, it excludes consideration of others affected by the decision, such as family members. In practice, the interests of the parents, siblings, and others are likely being balanced by parents and clinicians alike as they grapple with difficult decisions in the NICU setting. It seems best, then, for clinicians and parents to openly discuss this aspect of deliberations. Although it seems right that some consideration should be given to the interests of others, parents and physicians should still prioritize the patient's best interest. To do this, they must evaluate the risks and benefits of assisted ventilation, including the infant's chance of survival, the anticipated difficulty of the treatment course, and the burdens the child may experience in the long term. Those burdens are often addressed under the general heading of quality of life, to be discussed later in this chapter.

WITHDRAWING AND WITHHOLDING ASSISTED VENTILATION

Consideration of the ethical basis for decision making regarding assisted ventilation requires an understanding of two separate specific actions: withholding assisted ventilation, most commonly by not employing it from the time of delivery or at the onset of respiratory failure, and withdrawing assisted ventilation, after a patient has been provided with this support for a period of time. These two acts are widely viewed by bioethicists as being ethically equivalent.[13] That assessment seems correct, in that the decisions to withhold or to withdraw both involve an assessment at a point in time that, based on the information available, provision of assisted ventilation is not in the patient's best interest. Both involve substituting a life-sustaining therapy with other treatment, perhaps comfort measures only, or other forms of palliative therapy.[14] Put simply, if it is acceptable not to start it based on consideration of anticipated benefits and burdens, then it is equally acceptable not to continue it for that same reason. Despite this common and reasonable view of moral equivalence, however, there are noticeable and clinically relevant differences between withholding and withdrawing life support.

Withholding assisted ventilation from a newborn usually means forgoing a trial of intensive care, including intubation and mechanical ventilation, and allowing natural death from apnea or respiratory failure. This, too, is sometimes considered for a patient having a very poor prognosis. And, as with withdrawal of ventilatory support, the decision should be based on an assessment of potential benefits and burdens to the child. A decision to withhold (e.g., not intubate during resuscitation in the delivery room) is a decision to forgo intensive intervention that could potentially keep the infant alive through a critical window of time. That time could allow for a trial of therapy, to see if the newborn can be adequately oxygenated and ventilated with available technology. For extremely premature newborns with questionable viability at the time of birth, for example, it is known that if they can survive the early days and weeks, the likelihood of survival to discharge increases significantly.[15]

A trial of therapy could also afford the opportunity to see if certain morbidities manifest, such as severe neuropathology, that might be determined by physical examination over time and/or with imaging, and that could inform the assessment of the benefits and burdens of ongoing treatment. A trial of therapy thus does not preclude withdrawal of ventilation at a later time as prognosis changes. Withdrawal in the NICU may occur in the face of imminent and unavoidable death, perhaps to provide more peaceful final minutes or hours for the infant and family. There is no significant ethical debate on the permissibility of this act, and it is not here questioned. Withdrawal might also, however, involve extubating an infant who is not actively dying, to allow death from respiratory failure or apnea. This might be considered because of a very poor prognosis regarding long-term survival. Withdrawal might also be considered in the setting of anticipated profound neurological impairment, if requested by informed parents. The ethical acceptability of this may be largely informed by the degree of anticipated impairment, but it is here suggested that for some cases of profound impairment, parents would be within their rights to decline initiation or continuation of mechanical ventilation based on their perceived best interests of their child.

Thus, some argue that withdrawal of life support is preferable to withholding because more clinical information upon which to base a decision has become available.[16] On the other hand, withholding might result in a lower overall burden (e.g., pain) to the child than a difficult and unsuccessful trial of therapy. But there is yet another factor that will exert significant influence in the clinical setting, related to psychological effect.

Withholding assisted ventilation represents an act of omission. Withdrawing, on the other hand, involves an act of commission, or actively taking away a therapy that had at one time been believed to be of potential benefit. Arguments for ethical equivalence aside, it could, for many, be psychologically more difficult to decide to withdraw ventilatory support from an infant in the NICU, than to decide not to intubate an infant who has not yet been born. The evolution of the relationships between the patient and parents, or patient and staff, over the first days of life can be complex and is beyond the scope of this chapter. It must be considered, however, that having seen and touched a newborn over time can have a profound effect on the emotional impact of a decision to forgo ongoing respiratory support. The ethical equivalence of withholding and withdrawing is not here refuted; if it is permissible in some settings to withhold assisted ventilation based on benefits and burdens to the newborn (as is widely accepted), then it is permissible on the same basis to withdraw it. That said, however, the potential for a very different emotional impact must nevertheless be recognized.

NONESCALATION AND "HEROIC MEASURES"

In addition to providing, withholding, and withdrawing assisted ventilation, there is yet another option, less often written about, but occasionally invoked in practice: nonescalation. When a patient's prognosis appears to be very poor despite ventilatory assistance, and clinicians have recommended withdrawal of respiratory support, but the parents wish to continue, some have settled on a compromise of sorts, to continue but not increase the level of support. This might reduce invasive interventions such as blood gas testing, and avoid worsened prolonging of the dying process, yet give parents time to process and accept the inevitability of a bad outcome without forcing a decision on them with which they are not yet comfortable. DNR orders commonly include chest compressions, intubation, and medications to maintain circulation, but nonescalation here refers to interventions not commonly included in DNR discussions, such as progression to alternative ventilatory strategies. If information is shared honestly, and the patient's pain is adequately addressed, this may be an acceptable option. One needs to be cognizant of the risk, however, that the patient could survive with worsened morbidity because, for example, of prolonged hypoxia. Thus the acceptability of this approach is linked to the degree of prognostic certainty.

When considering or proposing nonescalation, unhelpful or misleading terminology should not be part of the discussion. Physicians in this situation might suggest that ventilatory assistance be continued, but no "heroic" or "extraordinary" treatments be provided. However, "heroic" is poorly defined and subjective, and a treatment that one physician would consider heroic or extraordinary might not be described as such by another. To change from a conventional ventilator to high-frequency oscillatory ventilation could be viewed by one as an escalation, and another as simply switching modes of ventilation. And, interestingly, one rarely hears a physician describe a treatment they favor and recommend as being "heroic" or "extraordinary." Perhaps these words are code, or shorthand, for a further step that should not be taken. In the interest of honesty and clarity, if a plan to continue the current form and extent of respiratory support seems permissible to the physician based on benefits, burdens, and the anticipated outcome, it would be preferable to avoid such code words and instead simply suggest that no further increases or changes in ventilatory support be made, along with providing the rationale for that plan.

MORAL DISTRESS

Moral distress is another psychological factor associated with decisions regarding withholding or withdrawing assisted ventilation. The term "moral distress" describes the anguish felt when one believes one should act in a certain way but is unable to do so because of constraints beyond their control.[17] The definition has also been broadened to include distress felt when there is uncertainty about the rightness or wrongness of an action. It was initially described in nurses, perhaps owing to having less decisional authority in the intensive care setting than physicians and more direct interaction with patients and families at the bedside. It is, however, a relevant concern for all health care providers in the NICU setting, particularly within a framework of shared decision making between parents and professionals. This can be seen, for example, when ventilatory support is continued at parental request for a newborn whom the clinicians feel strongly is suffering and cannot survive long-term. Staff may feel complicit in ongoing treatment perceived as being cruel. It can also be seen, although perhaps less often, when staff feel strongly that respiratory support should be provided but a decision has been made to withhold or withdraw, allowing a newborn to die who, at least in the eyes of some, could have and should have been given a chance at survival. Health care providers can be negatively impacted from prolonged or repeated exposure to moral distress, leading to stress and burnout. Coping mechanisms such as an openness to, and flexibility with, moral subjectivity, and moral resilience through engaging in dialogue and self-care, can help staff members deal with the moral distress that often accompanies the provision of ongoing ventilatory support in the care of a critically ill newborn with a poor prognosis.[18] Although it might not eliminate moral distress, it can be helpful for physicians, practitioners, and nurses to engage in a frank and open dialogue about their concerns, and the reasoning behind the treatment plan, however troubling.

Decisions regarding the provision, withholding, or withdrawal of assisted ventilation are often made more difficult by the psychological and stressful nature of their context, and it is important to openly acknowledge these factors both among clinicians and in discussion with families. The ethical basis for the decisions, however, should remain primarily centered on an assessment of the benefits and burdens to the child of the treatment under consideration and, based on that assessment, judgment on what is in the patient's best interest. Undoubtedly, there will be some degree of subjectivity in such assessments, leading at times to disagreement between physicians and parents. This too, should be openly acknowledged and discussed. Adult patients have the right to forego medical therapies or stop medical therapies that they feel fall short of their therapeutic goals and thus are not in their own best interest. Neonates, obviously unable to decide or speak for themselves, rely on others to provide the assessment of their interests and direct decisions related to intensive care measures such as assisted ventilation. Who should have that authority?

Who Makes the Call? Shared Decision Making in the Neonatal Intensive Care Unit

Patient autonomy, or "self-rule," is widely considered a cornerstone of medical ethics. Whenever a patient is incapacitated and unable to exercise their right to autonomy, the medical community seeks to respect the patient's right to autonomy via either an advanced directive wherein the patient has already explicitly expressed their wishes, or a surrogate decision maker. This surrogate is expected to decide based upon substituted judgment. That is, they are not expected to choose what they themselves would want, or even what they feel is best, but rather what they believe that the patient would want if they could speak on their own behalf. [9,19] Neonates, of course, have no previously voiced preferences on which a substituted judgment could be made. Instead, surrogate decision making on behalf of infants should rely on an assessment of the patient's best interest, as described earlier, as an assessment of the benefits and burdens of the proposed treatment.

It is widely accepted in our society, going back to antiquity, that parents have a right to decide what is done to and for their children.[19] Justification for this right includes acknowledgement that, aside from the child himself or herself, the family will be the ones most likely to bear the burdens resulting from the decision, although this will not always be the case. Additionally, parents are generally felt to be in the best position to determine what is in their child's interest.[20] This right to decide is sometimes referred to as a right to "parental autonomy," but this is a misnomer, as one cannot have "self-rule" over another person, even one's own child. "Parental authority" is a better term, referring to the parental right to authority over what is done to and for their children.

Parents are granted wide latitude by society in their authority to raise their children in a manner consistent with their own values, and to shape their child into an autonomous adult. Parental authority, however, is recognized as being strong, but not absolute.[21] It may be overridden by society in extreme cases based on a consideration of the rights of the child. In the medical setting, the right to refuse an intervention, even LSMT, is essentially absolute for adults of sound mind, based on understanding of the right to autonomy. A parental refusal on behalf of their child, however, may be overridden when their decision is seen to clearly conflict with the rights or interests of that child. This is consistent with widely accepted pediatric ethical standards.[22] The American Academy of Pediatrics nearly three decades ago declared that all children have a right to treatment likely to prevent significant harm, suffering, or death.[11] Moreover, the newborn may also be seen to have a "right to mercy," described as the right not to be subjected to painful and invasive interventions that offer virtually no chance of benefit to the child.[23] This may become relevant when parents request or demand such an intervention, and in such cases, the child's right to mercy may also override the parents' right to decide. Such an assessment is consistent with the fundamental medical ethical principle of nonmaleficence, the obligation not to cause harm to the patient unless there is a larger benefit for the patient associated with it.

Ultimately, the parents' right to decide based upon their values and goals for their child and the child's right both to certain treatments and to mercy are interwoven with the physician's obligations to provide the relevant information in a clear and unbiased fashion to assist parents in their decision making and to demonstrate respect for each of these rights. This is, at times, a difficult balance to strike, requiring time and patience, consistent with a model of shared decision making in pediatrics, wherein parents and providers work together to determine the plan of care.[24]

Quality of Life Considerations

An assessment of benefits and burdens should take into account all significant burdens to the patient, which includes the possibility of long-term disability. NICU patients are often left with some degree of developmental delay or permanent disability and, sometimes, although thankfully rarely, profound disability. "Quality of life" considerations are thus sometimes invoked in determining the best course of action regarding provision of ventilatory support.

Quality of life can be defined as a subjective interpretation of one's own satisfaction with life.[25] Some describe a minimal requirement of an acceptable quality of life as the ability to interact with others, especially loved ones, and to express and perceive emotion.[26] Biological functions such as vision, hearing, motor function, or intellectual ability do not represent objective measures of quality of life. Parental perceptions of a child's quality of life, although important, also do not represent an objective measure. With regard to an individual's perception of their own quality of life, a disability paradox exists in which those individuals with mild disabilities may be more aware of them.[27] Being aware of one's own limitations may make one more prone to sense a lower quality of life. Profound cognitive impairment, on the other hand, could reduce or eliminate a person's perception of their own limitations, thus removing distress about the disability. Thus, with regard to cognitive function, some more severely affected individuals might have a higher perception of their quality of life than those with lesser impairment.

However one chooses to define quality of life, it is essential to recognize that it will be a subjective assessment. Individuals with disabilities might perceive their own lives and burdens very differently than others see them, including family members and physicians. It is known, for example, that parents of adolescents who were born at very low birth weight rate the quality of life for their children much higher than do their pediatricians. And, the patients themselves rate their quality of life still higher, higher than do their parents.[28] When determining whether ventilatory assistance should be provided, continued, or withdrawn, it is reasonable to consider all potential burdens to the patient, including the possibility of long-term disability. However, one should keep in mind that the assessment of another's quality of life is a dangerously subjective undertaking. Moreover, although it might be the case for the most extreme examples in the NICU, there should be a very high threshold for the assessment that the anticipated quality of an individual's life is so poor as to outweigh the benefit of survival.

Finally, there may be a unique psychological factor at play specifically in the NICU population with regard to anticipated disability and its influence on decisions regarding provision of ventilatory support. Former NICU patients, who were kept alive with critical care measures and later have significant disability, may be viewed differently from other patients. When an older child or adult experiences an illness or accident requiring ventilatory support, and is then left with a significant impairment

(e.g., from near drowning, or stroke), one might reasonably perceive that the medical team has saved this person, who is now left with a disability. When a decision is made to provide a neonate with life-sustaining therapy, and later the child has a significant disability (e.g., from periventricular leukomalacia or hypoxic ischemic encephalopathy), there may be a greater sense of moral responsibility—a perception among clinicians or others that, rather than having saved someone who is left with an impairment, they have in some sense "created" a disabled person. Clinicians might then not only perceive a poor quality of life for these children but might also feel a moral culpability, more so than physicians caring for critically ill older children and adults. That perception may well be shared by others, such as parents or colleagues, although the perception itself seems off the mark. NICU physicians do not "create" a disabled person any more than an emergency physician who intubates a patient after near drowning. Nevertheless, neonatologists should be aware of the potential for that unconscious or unspoken fear of moral culpability, and its possible influence on decisions. Although perhaps understandable, it does not represent an ethical justification for treating neonates differently than older patients, with regard to predicted disability and the possible provision of life-sustaining treatment.[29]

COMING TO A CONSENSUS: WHEN IS WITHHOLDING OR WITHDRAWAL OF ASSISTED VENTILATION ETHICALLY PERMISSIBLE?

Taking into account the principles, rights, and other factors outlined previously, neonatologists must then sometimes confront the important question: is it ethically permissible to withdraw mechanical ventilation in this patient?[30] The initiation or continuation of assisted ventilation, as with any treatment under consideration, can be viewed as ethically impermissible, permissible, or obligatory, depending largely upon the anticipated benefits and burdens to the patient.[31] Any feasible critical treatment that will bring a benefit to the patient that clearly outweighs risks or burdens should be considered ethically obligatory and should be provided. This is the case for most patients with respiratory failure in the NICU, about whom there is rarely ethical controversy regarding provision of assisted ventilation. If, on the other hand, the burdens to the patient clearly outweigh the benefits, it should be viewed as ethically impermissible, and neither provided nor offered. This, too, is sometimes seen in the NICU, such as with patients born with virtually no chance of survival or those with imminent unavoidable death. Conversely, one could view the acts of withholding and withdrawing assisted ventilation through this same lens, wherein it is impermissible, permissible, or obligatory to perform either of these, depending on the anticipated benefits and burdens to the patient of that act. It is essential to recognize that such an assessment requires an understanding of the most recent outcomes data. The likelihood of survival for neonates with some disorders, notably but not limited to those at the lowest gestational ages, has improved in recent years, and it is incumbent upon the clinician to be up to date when considering the potential benefit of assisted ventilation.[32]

Determination of whether assisted ventilation in a given situation should be viewed as impermissible, permissible, or obligatory will depend primarily upon the prognosis with and without that therapy—consideration of all anticipated benefits and burdens. The most challenging ethical dilemmas typically occur in the care of newborns for whom the prognosis is uncertain, and/or the relative weight that should be assigned to anticipated benefits and burdens is unclear, or a matter of disagreement. The significance of the burden imposed by long-term disability, for example, is a highly subjective assessment, as discussed earlier. When the provision of a critical treatment such as ventilatory assistance is not clearly consistent with, or clearly opposed to, the child's interests, and it does not reach a threshold of harm either to withhold or provide it, then that treatment may be considered ethically permissible. That is, it could be acceptable either to provide it or to withhold it.

Within this zone of ethical permissibility, the role of the physician is to inform parents about the options, provide guidance on what they feel is the best choice, and then respect parental preference. For the most uncertain cases, a physician may have no clear preference or recommendation, and that information should also be shared with parents. If ventilatory support is impermissible, for example, for an extremely premature infant at 20 weeks' gestation, or obligatory, such as for a term infant with meconium aspiration syndrome, parents should not be presented with a disingenuous offer of a choice, but rather be given a clear explanation of the situation and reasoning behind the decision. If the treatment is perceived as ethically permissible, then flexibility on the part of the physician is appropriate. A parental decision might not be what the physician would recommend, but if it does not reach a threshold of harm such that it should be overridden, then it should be supported. The hard ethical work, then, comes down to determining whether ventilatory support for a given child at a given point in time should be viewed as impermissible, permissible, or obligatory. Professional guidelines describe processes that may be helpful in this judgment and for engaging in these dialogues with parents.

The Royal College of Pediatrics and Child Health has proposed five circumstances in which withholding or withdrawing life-sustaining therapy would be considered allowable: brain death, permanent vegetative state, a "no chance" situation, a "no purpose" situation, and an "unbearable" situation.[33] The no chance situation is a case in which an infant has such severe disease that life-sustaining treatment only delays death without relieving suffering. The no purpose situation is seen with a patient who may be able to survive with treatment, but the degree of physical or mental impairment would be so great that it would be unreasonable to continue therapy. The unbearable situation is that in which a child for whom, irrespective of medical opinion about whether the treatment would be successful, it is felt that it would be unbearable to endure in the face of progressive and irreversible disease. For at least some of these conditions, withdrawing or withholding would presumably be allowable even over parental objection—brain death being the most clear example.

The American Academy of Pediatrics and American Heart Association resuscitation guidelines acknowledge that when available evidence to predict the chance of mortality and morbidity is insufficient, respecting parental wishes is encouraged. Providing parents with clear, consistent, understandable medical evidence in an unbiased fashion, and eliciting parental values and concerns, becomes the clinician's chief objective.[23,34,35] No single approach can suffice for all, because these nuanced situations involve diverse patient and family details and values that must be accounted for during counseling.[36] Individualized approaches are encouraged, and open communication to clarify misunderstandings and seek an agreed-upon course of action is preferred.[37]

The conflicts that arise when families and providers do not agree on whether assisted ventilation should be provided are commonly disagreements about values, or misunderstandings of the situation. Regardless of their origin, when conflicts arise, clinicians are encouraged to enlist the aid of others such as ethics committees, social workers, other support staff, and clergy to help facilitate a shared understanding. Despite these efforts, families may still request their infant be intubated and ventilated when physicians perceive this intervention be of no benefit to the infant, or futile. "Futile," in common language, refers to an act that serves no useful purpose, or is ineffective.[38] The term is sometimes used by clinicians as a means of justifying a refusal to comply with a parental request for a certain treatment, such as mechanical ventilation. Unfortunately, the term is sometimes invoked to close off conversation, or to avoid a more helpful and thorough explanation.[39] Moreover, even the understanding of what is a "useful purpose" is subjective and may differ between parents and clinicians. For example, keeping a terminally ill newborn alive with a ventilator for a few more days may be perceived as useful or valuable to one person but not another. Thus, a shared understanding of goals is essential to shared decision making. Although it may be appropriate to withhold a treatment that cannot be effective, it is preferable to avoid using the concept of futility as a means of obviating dialogue, and instead provide the data and/or physiological explanation as to why it cannot work and thus will not be done. If neither relevant outcomes data nor a reasonable physiological explanation can be identified that justify a refusal to provide a requested treatment, the physician should reconsider that refusal.

Some suggest that it is appropriate to provide a treatment at parental request even if the physician feels it cannot be effective, if it will provide a benefit to the family without further harming the infant. This argument has been made specifically in the setting of cardiopulmonary resuscitation where death seems inevitable (i.e., offering parents the option of attempted resuscitation)[40] but could also be extended specifically to assisted ventilation. Families may well derive some measure of comfort in feeling that every effort was made to save their child. However, it has also been suggested that to offer a specific therapeutic option, when there is no possibility that it would alter the child's outcome, would be providing parents with a false choice.[41] If a treatment, including intubation and assisted ventilation, truly holds no hope of success, it could be unkind or misleading to offer it. Some parents might understandably, but incorrectly, believe that the willingness to provide any specific treatment signals some hope for success on the part of the clinical team. It would be preferable for a physician to clearly and compassionately explain why the treatment in question cannot help and, on that basis, will not be provided. Physicians should provide parents with options that may benefit the patient, and should respect parental decisions, but be clear when intensive medical support can no longer achieve the goals that the parents hold for their child.[42] Such a statement and unilateral decision would not be appropriate, however, without a high degree of certainty that the treatment cannot be successful. It is critical at that point to emphasize that although curative therapy is no longer an option, palliative care will remain robust, and neither the patient nor the family will be abandoned.[43] Finally, although it may in certain extreme situations be appropriate to withdraw assisted ventilation without parental agreement, it must be recognized that this is controversial. Such a decision should not be made by a single physician acting alone and is best considered through a conscientious practice algorithm and/or ethics committee consultation, in addition to legal counsel.[44,45]

Among the best strategies for parent-physician conflict in critical cases is to anticipate it, and work to prevent it. Discussions early in a newborn's course, not limited to immediate resuscitative options, are helpful in preparing families for difficult and complex decisions. These should include the anticipated course and future timepoints where care might be reassessed and ventilatory support possibly withdrawn. By keeping families informed throughout the course, providers create an alliance and trust that will be vital to helping them navigate difficult and uncomfortable decisions. Palliative care teams can be introduced early, not to coerce toward a plan of withdrawal of ventilatory support or comfort measures only, but rather as a resource to help families think about and support their child's comfort, regardless of their wishes for intensive therapy.

CHRONIC VENTILATION AND TRACHEOSTOMY

Some neonates will become dependent on assisted ventilation and require long-term ventilation, often via tracheostomy. Those with bronchopulmonary dysplasia now represent the largest group of infants that receive tracheostomies compared with other airway anomalies such as laryngotracheal stenosis, and most children who undergo tracheostomy require it in the first year of life.[46] Infants who require tracheostomy often have experienced multiple morbidities during their NICU stay associated with worse long-term survival and neurodevelopmental outcomes that tracheostomy does not mitigate.[47]

It is therefore important that counseling and decision making regarding tracheostomy and long-term assisted ventilation openly address comorbidities and potential long-term disabilities, in addition to anticipated respiratory outcome and overall survival. As with all therapeutic decisions in the NICU, the discussion should be centered on short-term and long-term benefits and burdens to the child that can reasonably be anticipated from the procedure. Lastly, the financial cost of long-term dependence

on ventilation is often a concern to parents and others. These are valid concerns regarding health care justice that the authors feel are usually best addressed on a societal rather than individual basis. Interventions with little chance of benefit and exorbitant costs may rightly be withheld in certain circumstances, but interventions felt to provide significant net benefit to the child should be made available when feasible.

CONCLUSION

Assisted ventilation in the newborn portends the possibility of ethical conflict around decision making for critically ill newborns. In deciding whether this potentially life-saving treatment should be provided, withheld, or withdrawn, clinicians should focus primarily on the relative benefits and burdens to the newborn patient. This assessment will require as accurate a prognosis as possible and an honest acknowledgment when the prognosis is unclear. Provision of assisted ventilation may reasonably be perceived as either ethically impermissible, permissible, or obligatory, depending on the specifics of the patient and the anticipated outcomes associated with that intervention. All permissible options should be made known and, when feasible, available to parents. Within the preferred model of shared decision making, informed parental preference should generally be determinative, unless or until a clear threshold of harm to the child would be reached. Then, it is the physician's duty to oppose critical decisions that are clearly and significantly inconsistent with the newborn's best interest, and thus ethically impermissible. When considering the impact of possible or anticipated disabilities on decisions in the NICU, clinicians are cautioned to recognize that quality of life assessments are subjective, and parental values must be taken into account. Moreover, the best judge of an individual's quality of life is ultimately that individual herself, and these judgments may differ significantly from those of health care professionals.

Understanding these ethical concepts will aid clinicians in ethical decision making with families regarding assisted ventilation. Applying them properly will require knowledge of current relevant outcomes data (national and local). This information should be shared with families as part of the ongoing discussions of goals of care, therapeutic options, and potential time points when the goals and plan may need to be reassessed. The clinician should also be familiar with relevant professional guidelines and potential legal restrictions. When clear, frank, and frequent communication cannot achieve consensus on the best way forward, multidisciplinary involvement including representatives from palliative care, social services, chaplaincy, ethics, and legal consultation provides rich resources that may be used.

KEY REFERENCES

2. Singh J, Lantos J, Meadow W: End-of-life after birth: death and dying in a neonatal intensive care unit. Pediatrics 114(6): 1620–1626, 2004. doi:10.1542/peds.2004-0447
4. Duff R, Campbell AGM: Moral and ethical dilemmas in the special-care nursery. New Engl J Med 289(17):890–894, 2010.

9. Beauchamp T, Childress J: Principles of Biomedical Ethics. 5th ed. New York, NY, Oxford University Press, 2001.

10. Mercurio MR: Parental authority, patient's best interest and refusal of resuscitation at borderline gestational age. J Perinatol 26(4):452–457, 2006.

11. Diekema DS: Revisiting the best interest standard: uses and misuses. J Clin Ethics 22(2), 128–133, 2011.

21. Paris JJ, Schreiber MD: Parental discretion in refusal of treatment for newborns: a real but limited right. Clin Perinatol 23:573–581, 1996.

25. Brunkhorst J, Weiner J, Lantos J: Seminars in fetal & neonatal medicine infants of borderline viability: the ethics of delivery room care. Semin Fetal Neonatal Med 19(5):290-295, 2014. doi:10.1016/j.siny.2014.08.001

30. Mercurio MR, Cummings CL: Critical decision-making in neonatology and pediatrics: the I-P-O framework. J Perinatol 41(1):173–178, 2021.

33. Royal College of Paediatrics and Child Health: Withholding or Withdrawing Life Sustaining Treatment in Children: A Framework for Practice. 2nd ed. London, RCPCH, 2004.

35. Haward MF, Murphy RO, Lorenz JM: Message framing and perinatal decisions. Pediatrics 122(1):109–118, 2008. doi:10.1542/peds.2007-0620

5

Evidence-Based Respiratory Care

Krithika Lingappan and K. Suresh Gautham

KEY POINTS

- Clinical decisions for infants with respiratory disease should be based on the best evidence available (using primary sources or systematic reviews), while still using clinical judgment, patient values, and knowledge of the local circumstances.
- Evidence-based medicine (EBM) can be used to make decisions about the care of an individual patient, or for creating a guideline or protocol for the unit or practice, for the care of a defined category of patients (such as preterm infants with respiratory distress syndrome, or infants with air-leak syndromes).
- The steps of practicing EBM are framing a PICOT question; searching for evidence; critically appraising the evidence; deriving quantitative estimates of the effects of a diagnostic test or therapeutic intervention; weighing the risks, benefits, and costs; and implementation. In addition, several cognitive tools—critical thinking, clinical reasoning, decision making, and functioning under uncertainty—are also required to practice EBM.
- The quality (certainty) of evidence is best evaluated by the GRADE (grading of recommendations, assessment, development, and evaluation) system, which incorporates risk of bias, imprecision, indirectness, inconsistency of results, and publication bias.

BACKGROUND

Clinicians caring for infants with respiratory disease should make diagnoses, choose treatments, and counsel parents based on the best evidence available (preferably from high-quality research studies) while still using clinical judgment, patient values, and knowledge of the local circumstances. This approach, known as evidence-based medicine (EBM), discourages the sole use of less reliable "sources of truth" such as reasoning based on anatomy or pathophysiology, extrapolation from animal data, expert opinion that is not based on evidence, or adoption of a practice because peers and colleagues use it. Although the principles and steps of evidence-based practice are well described, it is common for diagnostic tests and treatments to be overused, underused, or misused. Therefore, clinicians providing respiratory care should become proficient in using the tools and skills of evidence-based practice. The technical skills for EBM, listed in the order they are used, are framing a question; searching for evidence; assessing its quality; weighing the risks, benefits, and costs; and implementation. In addition to these technical skills, several cognitive tools are also required to practice EBM, such as critical thinking, clinical reasoning, and decision making, particularly decision making in the face of uncertainty. EBM can be used to make decisions about the care of an individual patient, or for creating a guideline or protocol for the unit or practice, for the care of a defined category of patients (such as preterm infants with respiratory distress syndrome, or infants with air-leak syndromes).

THE TECHNICAL STEPS OF EVIDENCE-BASED MEDICINE

Formulating the Question

The first step in practicing EBM is to clearly delineate the clinical question. The components of a well-formulated question are patients, population, or problem (P); the intervention (I); the control or comparison (C); the outcomes of interest (O); and the type of study or time frame (T). These can be remembered with the acronym PICOT.[1] An example of a PICOT question is "In preterm infants of less than 28 weeks' gestation with respiratory distress syndrome (P), does the prophylactic use of vitamin A (I) compared to placebo (C) reduce the risk of bronchopulmonary dysplasia (BPD) (O) at 36 weeks postmenstrual age (T)? The best type of study (T) to answer this question is a randomized controlled trial."

Searching for the Evidence

Once a clear question is formulated, the clinician should then perform a search for all the relevant evidence. Collaborating with a medical librarian can ensure that the search is efficient and comprehensive, identifying all key published articles, abstracts, and reviews. The search can be performed using several electronic databases. The best known of these is MEDLINE (a bibliographic database of life sciences with a concentration on biomedicine), which can be accessed either using the free interface, PubMed (www.pubmed.gov), or through a proprietary interface such as Ovid. A particularly useful feature in PubMed is the "Clinical Queries" tab, which allows a user-friendly, quick, and focused search on a given topic that can help the clinician make informed decisions. There are three search filters available in Clinical Queries: clinical study categories (etiology, diagnosis, therapy, prognosis, and clinical prediction guides), systematic reviews, and medical genetics. Although MEDLINE contains millions of articles, it may still not contain all the relevant articles, and if an exhaustive search is essential, other databases such as CINAHL (an index of journal articles in nursing, allied health, biomedicine, and health care) and EMBASE (a biomedical and pharmacologic database of published literature) should also be searched. To identify unpublished abstracts (an important but often overlooked source of evidence), the proceedings and published abstracts (usually available online) of pediatric or neonatology conferences such as the Pediatric Academic Societies Meeting or the American Academy of Pediatrics National Conference and Exhibition should also be searched. Google Scholar is another Web-based search tool that searches the World Wide Web. In addition to published articles, it also identifies conference proceedings, books, and institutional repositories. It may serve as an adjunct but cannot replace a systematic search of a more comprehensive database such as MEDLINE.[2] Finally, the reference lists of full-text articles obtained from the electronic search should also be hand-searched to identify additional relevant articles.

Evidence identified through the search may fall into one of two categories: primary sources (i.e., original articles and abstracts) and reviews or summaries ("predigested sources") of existing evidence on a given topic or question. Among such reviews, conventional narrative reviews (similar to textbook chapters) can provide useful background information about the topic but are subject to the biases and viewpoints of the authors. Therefore, systematic reviews are preferred because their explicit methodology and transparency allow readers to replicate the methods and draw their own conclusions and inferences. The Cochrane Database of Systematic Reviews is a particularly useful source of high-quality systematic reviews in neonatology, and the full text of these reviews is available freely on the website of the National Institute of Child Health and Human Development (www.nichd.nih.gov/Cochrane). Only human studies/trials are included in Cochrane reviews—they do not cover studies in animal or mechanical models. For other primary articles and reviews, the full text of each article can be obtained from the journal's website, without a fee in some cases, and in other cases by an individual subscription or an institutional library subscription.

The search is typically performed by entering keywords (e.g., using the Medical Subject Headings [MeSH] database in PubMed) and using Boolean operators ("OR," "AND," and "NOT") to restrict the results to the most relevant articles. Custom search filters can be used to narrow the search by criteria such as study type, publication period, or type of journal.

In addition to performing searches for the evidence around specific clinical questions, clinicians should also develop good habits of keeping up to date with emerging evidence. With several thousand medical articles published each year, it is impossible for any clinician to read or even skim each published article or its abstract. Clinicians can keep up to date by subscribing to periodic updates from databases such as PubMed, RSS feeds, listservs managed by universities or scientific organizations, and table of content (TOC) alerts from journals.

Once the search is completed and the relevant articles have been obtained, the next task is to evaluate the evidence to determine whether and how it can be used in decision making.

Evaluating Evidence About Therapy
Evaluating the Quality (Certainty) of Evidence

Determining the quality (certainty) of evidence requires each article or abstract to be critically appraised, and to do this, the clinician should be aware of the strengths and weaknesses of different study designs. Table 5.1 summarizes the most common types of study designs and the advantages and disadvantages of each. Observational studies are useful for hypothesis generation, and randomized trials are best for hypothesis testing. Most of

TABLE 5.1	**Study Designs**		
Type of Study	**Description**	**Advantages**	**Disadvantages**
Intervention Studies (Trials)			
Randomized controlled trial	Subjects are allocated to either the intervention (experimental) group or a comparison (control) group by a pure chance process. The two groups are followed prospectively for a specified period of time and then compared in terms of outcome measures specified at the outset. Can be a parallel group trial or crossover trial. Useful to study the efficacy of an intervention in preventing or altering the course of a disease and to identify causes or risk factors or subjects at high risk.	Controls for major biases. Likely to yield valid results. Useful to detect small differences between groups.	Results may sometimes not be generalizable. Complex and expensive to conduct.
Cluster randomized trial	Instead of individual subjects, an entire group or a neonatal unit or a community is randomly assigned to intervention and control groups.	Avoids inadvertent exposure of control subjects to intervention ("contamination").	Usually unblinded. Potential for recruitment bias. Can generate difficult ethical challenges. Requires statistical analysis that adjusts for non-independence of observations within a cluster. Can suffer from selection bias.
Nonrandomized trial	Allocation of subjects to experimental intervention and control group occurs by nonrandom methods. Useful to study the efficacy of an intervention in preventing or altering the course of a disease and to identify causes or risk factors or subjects at high risk. However, can be subject to bias.		

TABLE 5.1 Study Designs—cont'd

Type of Study	Description	Advantages	Disadvantages
Observational Studies			
Cohort study	The course of a group of individuals is followed forward over time to monitor the natural history of a disease, to determine prognosis, or to identify the causes of disease. Can be prospective or retrospective. The researcher does not influence the exposure of the subjects to treatment or other interventions; exposure is not intentional. Good design to determine the natural history of the disease and to identify causes or risk factors or subjects at high risk.	Can establish causation, determines incidence. Can match for known confounders.	Needs considerable time and resources (although less expensive than randomized trials), controls may be difficult to find, difficult to study rare disorders, subject to bias.
Case-control study	Subjects with the disease or outcome of interest (cases) are compared to a group of subjects without the disease (controls). The frequency of causal or risk factors (exposures) in cases relative to controls is determined and expressed as the odds ratio. Always retrospective. Careful selection of controls is required to avoid bias. Useful to identify causes or risk factors or subjects at high risk.	Less expensive, can be performed quickly, requires fewer patients, useful for rare diseases, and when interval between exposure and outcome is long, can study multiple exposures.	Improper selection of controls can introduce bias, inefficient for rare exposures, temporal relationship may be difficulty to establish, cannot derive incidence, subject to recall bias.
Cross-sectional study	Individuals with a defined disease, risk factor, or other condition of interest are identified at a point in time (a "snapshot"). Exposure and outcome are determined simultaneously. Good design to estimate prevalence of the condition, which is calculated as the number of individuals with the condition divided by the total number in the sample. Useful to identify causes or risk factors or subjects at high risk.	Inexpensive and easy to perform.	Cannot establish causation. Exposure and outcome may depend on recall. Sample sizes or groups could be unequal.
Ecologic study	An observational study is conducted at a population level rather than an individual level. Differences in outcome between populations or over time are related to population characteristics that could be risk (or preventive) factors.	Inexpensive. Can potentially use data from existing databases.	Unable to assess how many exposed subjects actually develop the outcome. Tends to overestimate the degree of correlation.
Case series	Description of features of a coherent/consecutive set of cases.	Provides useful description of rare conditions. May be followed by clinical trials.	In the absence of controls, cannot assess risk factors and exposures or draw inferences about the efficacy of treatments.
Case report	Reports a rare or interesting finding in a single patient.	Useful to raise awareness of a potential complication of treatment or an unusual presentation or course of a disease.	Does not provide generalizable knowledge.

our current knowledge about risk factors and exposures that result in disease or poor outcomes comes from observational studies. Most of our current knowledge about therapies comes from trials.

Earlier systems of grading the quality of evidence relied almost exclusively on overall study design and ranked the evidence in a pyramid based on study design, with systematic reviews occupying the apex of the pyramid (and comprising the best evidence) and reasoning from physiology or expert opinion occupying the base of the pyramid (the least reliable form of evidence).

Currently, the quality (certainty) of evidence is best evaluated using the criteria of the GRADE (grading of recommendations, assessment, development, and evaluation) system (Table 5.2). In this system, study design remains a critical, but not the sole, factor in judging the certainty of evidence. Additional criteria are incorporated into a judgment of the certainty of the evidence. Also, the certainty of evidence is assigned for each outcome, not

for each study. Importantly, the GRADE system is applied to the collective body of evidence for a specific outcome, not to individual studies.

Applying the GRADE method to the evidence from therapeutic interventions involves five distinct steps:[3]

Step 1: Assign an a priori ranking of "high certainty" to randomized controlled trials (RCTs) and "low certainty" to observational studies.

Step 2: Downgrade or upgrade initial ranking.

Reasons to downgrade the certainty of evidence for RCTs include:

- Risk of bias—caused by lack of clearly randomized allocation sequence, lack of blinding, lack of allocation concealment, failure to adhere to intention-to-treat analysis, large losses to follow-up, early cessation of the trial, or selective outcome reporting.
- Imprecision—wide confidence intervals (CIs).

TABLE 5.2	**GRADE System**
Quality of Evidence	**Definition**
High	Further research is very unlikely to change our confidence in the estimate of effect. • Several high-quality studies with consistent results • In special cases: one large, high-quality multicenter trial
Moderate	Further research is likely to have an important impact on our confidence in the estimate of effect and may change the estimate. • One high-quality study • Several studies with some limitations
Low	Further research is very likely to have an important impact on our confidence in the estimate of effect and is likely to change the estimate. • One or more studies with severe limitations
Very low	Any estimate of effect is very uncertain. • Expert opinion • No direct research evidence • One or more studies with very severe limitations

GRADE, Grading of Recommendations, Assessment, Development, and Evaluations.

- Indirectness—extrapolation of results from a different population, outcome, or intervention or indirect comparison of two interventions (i.e., not a head-to-head comparison).
- Inconsistency of results—when the results vary significantly across trials without explanation.
- Publication bias—when studies with negative results are not published (this can bias the results of the review).

The certainty of evidence for an observational study can be upgraded if there was a large magnitude of effect, a dose–response relationship is noted, and all plausible biases would only reduce the treatment effect noted in the study (suggesting that the actual effect is likely to be larger than the study results suggest).

Step 3: Assign a final grade for the certainty of evidence as high, moderate, low, or very low.

Step 4: Consider other factors, such as side effects of therapy, patient preference, and cost-effectiveness, that affect the strength of recommendation.

Step 5: Make the recommendation for the actual implementation of the therapy in the form of a strong or weak recommendation to either use or not use the therapy.

Determining the Quantitative Effects of a Therapy

The p value: Clinical studies that use hypothesis testing rely on tests of statistical significance and often derive a p value to answer the question "Are the observed results purely owing to chance?" The p value indicates the probability of obtaining a result as extreme as or more extreme than the result noted in the study if the null hypothesis were true. If the p value is smaller than the threshold set by the investigators (conventionally chosen to be 0.05 or 5%) the null hypothesis is rejected in favor of the alternate hypothesis, and the result is said to be "statistically significant." A large p value indicates that the null hypothesis cannot be rejected.

Statistical versus clinical significance: Even if the results in a study are *statistically* significant, they may not necessarily be *clinically* significant. For example, in trials with a large sample size, statistical testing may show significance, but the results may not be clinically significant—the overall impact may be minuscule, the benefits may not outweigh the risks, and the costs of intervention may not be justifiable. Conversely, a lack of statistical significance (a high p value) could be the result of an inadequate sample size that led to a true effect not being detected in the study.

CIs: The CI represents the degree of uncertainty in estimating the population parameter owing to sampling error. Because the results of almost all studies are derived from sample data (and not from the entire population), the sample parameter may vary from the true population parameter and may vary in its degree of precision. The CI quantifies this imprecision. It indicates the range of values that is likely to include the "true" result of a study. It is most commonly reported as 95% CI. The values for the 95% CI imply that if a study were repeated 100 times, the measured statistical parameter would fall within the interval 95 of 100 times. Narrow CIs indicate greater precision in the results. If the CI is wide, it implies that the "true value" lies somewhere within a large range of values. Therefore, if a study found no differences in outcomes between groups being compared, examination of the CIs can help clinicians assess whether there was indeed no true difference between the two groups or whether the lack of difference noted was the result of a small sample size. The value that shows "no effect" for ratios (odds ratio, relative risk [RR]) is 1 and for differences (risk difference, etc.) is 0. If the value of the measured outcome that signifies "no effect" (1 for ratio and 0 for absolute difference) lies outside the CI, then it represents statistical significance.

Composite endpoints: Composite endpoints (in which multiple types of undesirable outcomes are combined into a single measurement) are commonly used in neonatology, either to jointly measure multiple negative outcomes or because one negative outcome such as death does not allow the other adverse outcome to occur (also known as a competing outcome, as when a baby dies before 36 weeks' postmenstrual age and cannot be assessed for the presence or absence of BPD). The results of trials reporting composite outcomes can sometimes be confusing to interpret and apply in clinical decision making, particularly when one of the included negative outcomes is increased and the other is decreased. In such a case, the clinician must weigh the severity of each of the outcomes and estimate the net benefit or harm before making clinical decisions. In addition, the multiple components of a composite outcome may not have the same significance for patient (adult survivors), family, and the clinician; for example, death or severe BPD.

Example: In an RCT, Bassler et al.[4] evaluated the effects of early inhaled budesonide compared to placebo in neonates at 23 0/7 to 27 6/7 weeks of gestation with a primary outcome of death or BPD.

For the primary outcome (death or BPD), the control event rate (CER) (placebo group) was 46.3%, and the experimental (budesonide group) event rate was 40%. The RR for inhaled budesonide was 40/46.3 = 0.86, with a 95% CI of 0.75–1 and a *p* value = 0.05. This is an example of a composite primary outcome with two components. However, when the investigators looked at the incidences of death and BPD individually, the effects were in opposite directions. For BPD, the CER (placebo group) was 38%, and the experimental event rate (EER) (budesonide group) was 27.8%. The RR for BPD was therefore 27.8/38 = 0.73, with a 95% CI of 0.6–0.91 and a *p* value of 0.004. This was a statistically significant reduction in BPD. For death, the CER (placebo group) was 13.6%, and the experimental (budesonide group) event rate was 16.9%. The RR for inhaled budesonide was therefore 16.9/13.6 = 1.24, with a 95% CI of 0.91–1.69 and a *p* value of 0.17. In other words, there was an increased incidence of death in the budesonide group, but this was not statistically significant. These results suggest that the risks of budesonide therapy (a possible increase in mortality up to 1.69 times higher, based on the upper limit of the CI) may outweigh the benefit (a reduction in BPD).

Once the clinician is satisfied with the internal validity of a study, the next step is to analyze the quantitative results of the study and assess the effect size.

Measures of treatment effect (effect size): The following measures of association are commonly reported in therapeutic trials that use dichotomous measures of outcome (examples are yes/no outcomes such as mortality, retinopathy of prematurity, or intraventricular hemorrhage [IVH]) (for definitions, see Table 5.3):

CER: The incidence of the outcome in the control group (e.g., the placebo group in an RCT).

EER: The incidence of the outcome in the experimental group.

RR: EER/CER.

RR reduction: 1 − RR.

Absolute risk reduction (ARR): CER − EER, the absolute difference in the incidence of the outcome in the control and experimental groups.

Number needed to treat (NNT): 1/ARR, the number of patients who need to be treated to achieve one therapeutic success. The lower the NNT, the stronger the therapeutic effect and the fewer nonresponders who need to be exposed to the therapeutic intervention and to its risks and costs. When the outcome is an undesirable one, the term used is number needed to harm (NNH).

RR and RR reduction measure the strength of the association. To determine the actual number of patients affected, the absolute risk difference (ARD) and NNT are more useful.

Example: The SUPPORT (Surfactant, Positive Airway Pressure, and Pulse Oximetry) study group compared outcomes in extremely preterm infants[5] (infants born between 24 0/7 and 27 6/7 weeks of gestation) maintained in a lower target range of oxygen saturation (85%–89%) versus a higher (91%–95%) range. In this study, for the primary outcome (severe retinopathy or death before discharge), the event rate was 28.3%

TABLE 5.3 Definitions

CER: This is the control event rate, the rate or incidence of event or disease in the control group.

EER: This is the experimental event rate, the rate or incidence of event or disease in the experimental group.

Relative risk (RR) = EER/CER. If RR <1, then the therapy decreased the risk of outcome; if RR = 1, then the treatment had no effect; if RR >1, then the treatment increased the risk of outcome.

Absolute risk reduction (ARR) or risk difference = CER − EER. An ARR of 0 signifies no treatment effect.

Relative risk reduction = 1 − RR.

Number needed to treat (NNT) = 1/ARR.

Odds ratio (OR): If *a* is the number of exposed cases, *b* is the number of exposed noncases, *c* is the number of unexposed cases, and *d* is the number of unexposed noncases, then:

OR = (*a*/*c*)/(*b*/*d*) = *ad*/*bc*.

Disease Test	Present	Absent
Positive	*a*	*c*
Negative	*b*	*d*

Sensitivity (true positives): *a*/*a* + *b*

Specificity (true negatives): *d*/*c* + *d*

Positive predictive value: *a*/*a* + *c*

Negative predictive value: *d*/*b* + *d*

Positive likelihood ratio (LR+) = sensitivity/(1 − specificity)

Negative likelihood ratio = (1 − sensitivity)/specificity

Posttest odds = pretest odds × LR

---

in the lower saturation group and 32.1% in the higher saturation group. The RR with lower saturation was 28.3/32.1 = 0.9 with a 95% CI of 0.76–1.06 (which crossed 1, the value of no effect) and the *p* value was 0.21; hence, the null hypothesis could not be rejected. For death alone, the event rate was 19.9% in the lower saturation group and 16.2% in the higher saturation group. The RR with lower saturation was 19.9/16.2 = 1.23, with a 95% CI of 1.01–1.60 (not crossing 1) and the *p* value was 0.04. This was a statistically significant result, raising the concern that there was increased mortality in the babies in the lower saturation group. The RR reduction (actually an increase in this case) was 1 − 1.23 − 0.23. This meant there was a 23% increased risk of death in the lower saturation group. The ARR, also known as ARD (a more appropriate term because the risk actually increased) was 19.9 − 16.2 = 3.7, or 0.037. The NNH in this case was (1/ARD) = (1/0.037) = 27. This would mean that of 27 babies maintained in the lower saturation range as opposed to the high range, there would be one additional death. For severe retinopathy, the event rate was 8.6% in the lower saturation group and 17.9% in the higher saturation group. The RR was 8.6/17.9 = 0.48 with a 95% CI of 0.37–0.73 (not crossing 1) and a *p* value of less than 0.001. This was a statistically significant result, showing that the risk of severe retinopathy was lower among babies in the lower saturation group. The RR reduction was 1 − RR = 1 − 0.48 = 0.52. This meant that there was 52% lesser risk of developing severe retinopathy in the lower saturation group. The ARR, also known as ARD, was 8.6 − 17.9 = 9.3, or 0.093 (absolute value). The NNH in this case, therefore, was

$(1/ARD) = (1/0.093) = 11$. This would mean that of 11 babies maintained in the lower saturation range as opposed to the high range, one additional case of severe retinopathy would be prevented.

Odds ratio: The odds ratio is a measure of association between an exposure and an outcome. In a cohort study, the odds ratio is the ratio of the odds of an event in exposed subjects to the odds of the same event in unexposed subjects. In a case-control study, the odds ratio is the ratio of the odds that a case (a subject experiencing an event) was exposed to a factor to the odds that a control (a subject not experiencing an event) was exposed to the same factor.

Null value: The "no effect" value (null value) for ratios (odds ratio, RR) is 1 and for risk difference is 0. In practice, the 95% CI is often used as a proxy for the presence of statistical significance if it does not overlap the null value. Specifically, when the control and experimental groups are compared, if the CI of the estimate of the difference between the two groups excludes 1 for RR and 0 for ARD, then the result is considered statistically significant.

All these measures are useful in describing dichotomous measures of outcome. In studies measuring continuous data (like duration of ventilation, length of hospital stay, FiO_2, etc.), the groups are compared using mean differences.

Noninferiority Trials

In recent years, the use of noninferiority trials has become common in the field of neonatal respiratory care. Randomized double-blind placebo-controlled trials are the gold standard for testing a new intervention to treat a certain disease. These trials are designed to show the efficacy and risks of a new intervention. In certain situations, when there is an effective intervention available for a condition, and another, new intervention is developed, it would be unethical to test the new intervention against a placebo because this would deprive patients receiving the placebo of an effective treatment. In such cases, the new intervention could be compared to the standard intervention, which then acts as an active comparator. Such studies can be designed to show that the new intervention is superior, equivalent, or noninferior to the active comparator. When the new intervention to be tested has some advantages over the active comparator, such as ease of administration, lower cost, better tolerability by patients, or shorter treatment regimens, clinicians and patients might be willing to accept the newer treatment even if it is slightly less effective than the active comparator in improving patient outcomes, that is, if it is "acceptably worse." If the clinical benefits of the new treatment are significantly lower than with the new comparator, then it is deemed to be "unacceptably worse"; that is, the advantages of easier administration and use, of costs, and of tolerability are not outweighed by the loss of clinical benefits. Thus, noninferiority trials seek to test whether or not the effect of the new intervention is unacceptably worse than that of the active comparator. A predefined noninferiority margin separates what is "acceptably worse" from what is "unacceptably worse." The noninferiority margin is the largest clinically acceptable difference between the new intervention and the active comparator. One common method to determine the noninferiority margin is to compare the estimated 95% CI of the difference between the new intervention and the active comparator to a predefined margin. If the limit of the CI does not cross the margin, it then demonstrates that even if the difference was in favor of the active comparator, it did not exceed the unacceptably worse criteria of noninferiority (i.e., the noninferiority margin). Therefore, noninferiority of the new intervention to the active comparator can be concluded. Defining the noninferiority margin is crucial, yet one of the most challenging aspects in the design of noninferiority trials. Ideally, the noninferiority margin should be defined based on statistical considerations and clinical judgment.

Systematic Reviews of Therapeutic Interventions and Meta-analyses

A systematic review is a review of a clearly formulated question that uses systematic, explicit, and transparent methods to identify, select, and critically appraise relevant research and to collect, pool, and analyze data from the studies that are included in the review. A well-performed, up-to-date systematic review is a quick, reliable source of evidence for a clinician. However, not all systematic reviews are of high quality, and systematic reviews also require critical appraisal.

Ideally, the systematic review should address a clearly formulated question (in the PICOT format), use multiple bibliographic databases, specify the search terms used (text and MeSH), include published as well as unpublished studies in all languages (not just English), specify a priori, the criteria to include and exclude studies, and use objective criteria to assess the quality of studies. Including all available studies avoids publication bias (negative studies tend not to get published and require special effort to be identified). The quantitative results of different studies may then be combined using a meta-analysis to derive the pooled effect size after assigning weights to each study based on its sample size. The results are displayed in the form of a forest plot. Before applying the findings of a systematic review in practice, the clinician should critically appraise it. The results of a systematic review should be trusted only if the review asked a focused research question, performed a comprehensive search to include all relevant studies, assessed the quality of the studies included, included only valid studies, combined studies only if there were reasonably similar, and included all important outcomes. A meta-analysis within a systematic review, for example, should not pool the results of studies with different devices, ventilator modes, populations or studies that span different epochs during which there were major changes in clinical practice (e.g., antenatal steroids, surfactant administration). The Neonatal Review Group of the Cochrane Collaboration creates and maintains a collection of high-quality systematic reviews. The full text versions of these reviews are available at Cochrane at VON—Vermont Oxford Network (https://public.vtoxford.org/).

Example: A good example of a systematic review related to ventilation is the analysis of volume-targeted ventilation versus pressure-limited ventilation in preterm infants. Peng et al. approached this question with a systematic review and meta-analysis.[6] The authors included 18 trials and concluded that the use of volume-targeted ventilation reduces the incidence of BPD with an RR for volume-targeted ventilation of 0.61 with a 95% CI of

0.46–0.82. They also concluded that volume-targeted ventilation decreased the length of mechanical ventilation (by 2 days), IVH, grade 3/4 IVH, pneumothorax, and periventricular leukomalacia compared with preterm infants who received pressure-limited ventilation.

Weighing Risks, Benefits, and Costs

After evaluating the certainty of evidence and determining the quantitative results, the clinician has to evaluate the risks, benefits, and costs of various therapeutic strategies. To weigh benefits against risks for a therapy, a simple method is the NNT/NNH ratio, or the use of a balance sheet.[7] The balance sheet format underlies the summary of findings tables that are included in most Cochrane reviews now, and these tables allow an easy quantitative comparison of important benefits and risks. More elaborate and detailed estimation of benefits and risks can also be derived using decision analysis. Formal descriptions of decision analysis, cost-effectiveness, and cost-benefit analyses are provided in other publications and are outside the scope of this chapter. Finally, when weighing benefits against risks, the values that parents of infants place on various health outcomes should be incorporated, because different families may value the same health outcome differently and this can affect the relative weight of benefits and risks.

Evaluating Evidence About Diagnostic Tests
Evaluating the Certainty of Evidence for Diagnostic Tests

To assess the evidence for a diagnostic test, the first question to address is whether the results of the study are valid (Can you believe the results of the study?). The answer to this question depends on the risk of bias in the study used to evaluate the diagnostic test, which is a function of the design of the study, and on how well the study was actually conducted. The study should be evaluated for the possibilities of bias from the way patients were selected, index tests were performed and interpreted, reference standards were applied and interpreted, and patients were recruited to the study groups. Ideally, a study used to assess a diagnostic test should include a wide spectrum of patients selected in an unbiased manner (this avoids "spectrum bias"), not exclude patients inappropriately, enroll consecutive patients or randomly selected ones, include all patients in the final analysis, and avoid a case-control design. The diagnostic test (index test) results should have clear prespecified criteria for abnormality and should be interpreted without knowledge of the results of the reference standard (gold standard). The reference standard used should correctly classify the target condition, be applied to all included patients irrespective of the results of the index test, be applied at an appropriate interval after the index test, and ideally be interpreted without knowledge of the results of the index test. The items listed previously can be formally assessed using a tool known as QUADAS 2 (Quality Assessment of Diagnostic Accuracy Studies).[8] This tool is applied in four phases: summarize the review question, tailor the tool and produce review-specific guidance, construct a flow diagram for the primary study, and judge bias and applicability. Specific GRADE criteria for diagnostic tests can also be applied to assign the certainty of evidence.

Determining Diagnostic Test Accuracy

Traditionally, the results of diagnostic tests are depicted in a 2×2 table that is used to calculate sensitivity, specificity, positive predictive value, and negative predictive value.

Sensitivity is the proportion of persons with a disease who have a positive diagnostic test. It is a measure of the true positives. A test with a high sensitivity is useful in ruling out a disease if the test result is negative.

Specificity is the proportion of persons without a disease in whom the diagnostic test is negative. It measures the true negatives. The false-positive rate of the test is $1 -$ specificity. A test with a high specificity is useful in ruling in a disease if the test result is positive.

By themselves, sensitivity and specificity cannot be used to estimate the probability of a disease in an individual patient.

Positive predictive value is the proportion of persons with a positive test who have the disease.

Negative predictive value is the proportion of persons with a negative test who do not have the disease.

Both the positive and the negative predictive values are dependent on the disease prevalence. Therefore, if published predictive values for a diagnostic test are available from one sample of patients, a clinician should not apply these values to patients in whom the prevalence of disease might be different from that of the sample of patients in the published study.

The calculations discussed earlier describe the accuracy of a diagnostic test. However, when faced with a patient, the task of the clinician is not to determine how well the test performs but to determine the probability that the patient does or does not have the disease, given a positive or negative diagnostic test. This can be determined using the likelihood ratio (LR), which is independent of the disease prevalence and can be used to calculate the probability of disease for individual patients.

LR: The LR is the ratio of the likelihood (probability) of a given result in patients with the disease to the probability in patients without the disease. It indicates how many times more (or less) likely patients with the disease are to have that particular result than patients without the disease. A positive LR (LR+) indicates how many times more likely persons with the disease are to have a positive diagnostic test than persons without the disease. A negative LR (LR−) indicates how many times more likely persons with the disease are to have a negative diagnostic test than persons without the disease.

Bayesian Reasoning in Diagnostic Testing

Using the estimated probability of the presence of a disease or condition before a diagnostic test is ordered (pretest probability) and the LR of a diagnostic test once a positive or negative result is obtained, we can calculate the posttest probability of the condition in question. To calculate the posttest probability, the pretest probability is converted to pretest odds, which is then multiplied by the LR to derive the posttest odds. This is then converted to posttest probability. Alternately, a nomogram (the Fagan nomogram)[9] can be used to derive posttest probability (Fig. 5.1).

If the LR is 1, then the posttest probability is exactly the same as the pretest probability. An LR much lower than 1 makes the

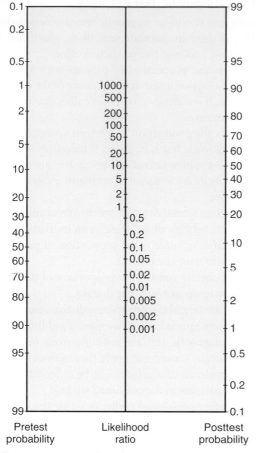

Fig. 5.1 Fagan nomogram. A straight line drawn through the pretest probability (*first column*) and the likelihood ratio (*second column*) provides the posttest probability (*third column*) of the disease or condition.

sensitivity and 61% specificity in babies of less than 34 weeks' gestation. The positive LR in this group of patients was 2.6, and the posttest probability was 72%.

Special Considerations in Applying Evidence to Respiratory Interventions

1. Respiratory interventions are often device based (ventilator, continuous positive airway pressure [CPAP], high-flow nasal cannula) and are thus difficult to blind. Inability to blind interventions may allow other biases (e.g., performance bias) to creep in and adversely affect the internal validity of the study.
2. The technology in the devices used for providing respiratory care constantly evolves with the development of better models/modes of ventilation, and so on. The comparison between these various devices/modes may be difficult.
3. Trials with respiratory intervention usually have short-term physiological outcomes (e.g., oxygen saturation) or short-term predischarge outcomes such as BPD as the primary outcome. Long-term outcomes such as lung function at school age and adolescence, and neurodevelopmental outcomes, may be better outcome measures, but they are difficult to gather because of logistic challenges and lack of resources for prolonged follow-up. Also, the commonly used outcome measure of BPD has multiple definitions and makes the comparison of trials challenging.
4. The effectiveness of a respiratory intervention depends on many other factors apart from the device itself, such as the clinical expertise and skills of physicians, nursing staff, and respiratory therapists using the device; consistency of care; presence of a champion; and closeness of monitoring. These subcomponents are often difficult to tease out in trials and may affect the external validity of the study.

COGNITIVE SKILLS FOR EVIDENCE-BASED PRACTICE

Critical Thinking

At its core, EBM is an application of critical thinking in medicine, which is defined as the ability to apply higher-order cognitive skills (conceptualization, analysis, evaluation) and the disposition to be deliberate about thinking (being open minded or intellectually honest), leading to action that is logical and appropriate.[11] Critical thinking allows a clinician to frame a problem appropriately; focus thinking around relevant issues; proceed systematically through analysis, evaluation, and decision making; and be self-aware of his or her own cognitive processes. Papp et al. postulate that milestones in critical thinking range from being an unreflective thinker (stage 1) to being an accomplished critical thinker (stage 5). As a developing critical thinker, the clinician should openly acknowledge his or her assumptions and accept uncertainty as the reason for further questions and research.[11] Instead of accepting established practices, the clinician should be able to ask appropriate questions and modify his or her practice based on new/emerging evidence. Good critical thinkers are open minded, are fair minded, search for the evidence, try to be well informed, are attentive to others' views and their reasons, hold beliefs in

posttest probability much lower (the disease is unlikely to be present in the patient). A very low LR of 0.1 or less virtually rules out the disease. An LR much higher than 1 makes the posttest probability much higher (the disease is much more likely to be present in the patient). A very high LR of 10 or greater virtually confirms ("rules in") the disease. The posttest probability of disease is the most useful estimate and helps the clinician decide whether to order additional diagnostic tests, to reassure the parents of an infant that the disease is unlikely to be present, or to initiate treatment for the disease. The posttest probability of a disease after one test becomes the pretest probability for the next diagnostic test if one is performed.

Example: Brat et al.[10] determined the diagnostic accuracy of a neonatal-adapted lung ultrasonography score (LUS) to predict the need for surfactant administration. The authors included all inborn neonates admitted to the neonatal intensive care unit with respiratory distress in the study and avoided a case-control design. The reference standard in this study for surfactant administration was according to the 2013 European guidelines. The criteria for abnormality were prespecified for the LUS. Neonatologists who were blinded to the clinical condition analyzed the results from the LUS. The authors reported that an LUS score cutoff of 4 predicted surfactant administration with 100%

proportion to the evidence, and are willing to consider alternatives and revise beliefs.[12]

Clinical Reasoning and Decision Making

Knowledge of the available evidence, its certainty, and the quantitative estimates of benefits, harms, and costs as described earlier should all be incorporated into a formal and explicit process of clinical reasoning that leads to a clinical decision or clinical guideline or protocol. In the GRADE method, either a strong or a weak recommendation to use or not use a diagnostic test or treatment can be generated. In reality, many decisions faced by clinicians have to be made under conditions of uncertainty. Uncertainty in decision making arises when:

- The evidence available is sparse,
- The available evidence lacks internal validity (poor study design or conduct),
- Study results are not important (small effect size or when a positive effect cannot be ruled out), or
- The study lacks external validity or applicability (different population or methodology from that in the clinician's practice).

In clinical situations, there is often pressure to act in the face of insufficient evidence. "Doing something" in such situations may not always be appropriate, and watchful waiting may be better than intervening. Acknowledging uncertainty of evidence in these situations is important, and involving colleagues (for brainstorming) and parents may be helpful for decision making. The clinician should also be clear about the distinction between a situation where sufficient evidence exists that proves an intervention is ineffective (i.e., there are multiple high-quality studies showing lack of efficacy) and one where insufficient or low-quality evidence exists for an intervention (i.e., the intervention is inadequately studied, and the possibility still exists that the intervention may be efficacious)—"absence of evidence of effect is not evidence of absence of effect."

TRANSLATING EVIDENCE INTO PRACTICE

Once the process of finding, appraising, and analyzing the evidence is completed, the clinician is now faced with the daunting task of converting this knowledge into practice. Knowledge translation is a dynamic and iterative process that includes synthesis, dissemination, exchange, and ethically sound application of knowledge to improve health, provide more effective health services and products, and strengthen the health care system.[13] The process of translating knowledge into action is not linear; considering the local context (policy and work culture) is an integral part of making this happen. Engaging stakeholders (leadership, bedside nurses, respiratory therapists) is important and it may entail education and training of all the team members involved in patient care before the research knowledge can be translated to clinical practice. The use of quality improvement methods allows systematic yet adaptive implementation of evidence-based practices.

SUMMARY

EBM encompasses both technical and cognitive skills that help the clinician to convert knowledge into practice and provide the best care to the neonate requiring respiratory care.

A complete reference list is available at https://expertconsult.inkling.com/.

SUGGESTED READINGS

1. Haynes RB: Clinical Epidemiology. Lippincott Williams & Wilkins, 2006.
3. Goldet G, Howick J: Understanding GRADE: an introduction. J Evid Based Med 6(1):50-54, 2013.
7. Eddy DM: Comparing benefits and harms: the balance sheet. JAMA 263(18), 1990.
8. Whiting PF, Rutjes AWS, Westwood ME, et al: QUADAS-2: a revised tool for the quality assessment of diagnostic accuracy studies. Ann Intern Med 155(8):529-536, 2011.
9. Fagan TJ: Letter: nomogram for Bayes theorem. N Engl J Med 293(5):257, 1975.
11. Papp KK, Huang GC, Lauzon Clabo LM, et al: Milestones of critical thinking: a developmental model for medicine and nursing, Acad Med 89(5):715-720, 2014.
12. Jenicek M, Hitchcock DL: Logic and Critical Thinking in Medicine. Chicago, American Medical Association, 2005.
13. Canadian Institutes for Health Research (CIHR): About knowledge translation. Available at: http://www.cihr-irsc.gc.ca/e/29418.html. Accessed December 26, 2015.

6

Quality and Safety in Respiratory Care

K. Suresh Gautham and Grant Joseph Dat Chiu Shafer

> ## KEY POINTS
>
> - Neonatal intensive care units should routinely assess and monitor the quality, safety, and value of the respiratory care they provide.
> - Based on the priorities identified through routine monitoring of quality, units should implement quality improvement projects to improve the processes and outcomes of respiratory care.
> - Participation in multicenter collaborative projects can boost a unit's level of engagement in quality improvement, increase the likelihood of success, and promote sustainability of results.

QUALITY AND SAFETY: BACKGROUND

The quality of health care is defined as "the degree to which health services for individuals and populations increase the likelihood of desired health outcomes and are consistent with current professional knowledge."[1,2] Many publications and expert reports[1,3-5] have emphasized that, in addition to widespread deficiencies of quality in health care, preventable harm to hospitalized patients from medical errors is frequent. A medical error is defined as the failure of a planned action to be completed as intended or the use of a wrong plan to achieve an aim.[5] An adverse event is defined as an injury resulting from a medical intervention.[5] Patient safety is defined as "prevention of harm to patients," and its practice "applies safety science methods toward the goal of achieving a trustworthy system of health care delivery."[6]

Another important concept that has been emphasized in the past decade is "value." Value in health care is the measured improvement in a patient's health outcomes per unit of cost of providing health care. This definition emphasizes the primary of improving health outcomes, rather than merely reducing costs of health care. Changes in health care delivery patterns and reimbursement methods, known as "value-based health care," are intended to achieve the "quadruple aim" of a health care system (a concept initially promulgated by the Institute for Healthcare Improvement as the triple aim and subsequently modified by other experts)—improving the patient experience of care, improving the health of populations, reducing the per capita cost of health care, and improving the work-life balance and satisfaction of health professionals.[7]

Institutions providing care for neonates with respiratory illness should continuously monitor and improve the quality, safety, and value of care provided to ensure that their patients receive the best care possible and that they attain the best clinical outcomes possible. To ensure this, each neonatal intensive care unit (NICU) should have a framework and approach for assessing, monitoring, and improving the quality of care in general and for neonates with respiratory illness in particular. Two frameworks are particularly useful—Donabedian's triad and the six domains of quality described by the Institute of Medicine.

Donabedian's Triad

An important framework for quality of care was proposed in the 1960s by Donabedian, who proposed that the domains of quality are structure, process, and outcomes.[8-10] *Structure* denotes the facilities, equipment, services, and labor available for care; the environment in which care is provided; the qualifications, skills, and experience of the health care professionals in that institution; and other characteristics of the hospital or system providing care. Therefore, for a neonatal unit, it encompasses aspects of quality such as space per patient, the layout of the unit, the nurse/patient ratio, the availability of radiology facilities around the clock, the types of respiratory equipment used, and the neonatology training and skills of the personnel. *Process* is defined as a "set of activities that go on between practitioners and patients." It refers to the content of care, that is, how the patient was moved into, through, and out of the health care system and the services that were provided during the care episode. Process is what physicians and other health care professionals do to and for patients. For a neonatal unit, process can include aspects of quality such as the percentage of personnel washing their hands before patient contact, the duration of time between birth and the first dose of surfactant, the average number of attempts to successful intubation, the percentage of infants in whom the examination for retinopathy of prematurity (ROP) is performed on time, the efficiency with which a neonate is transported from a referring hospital, the frequency of medical errors, and so on. Finally, *outcomes* are the end results of care. They are the consequences to the health and welfare of individuals and society or, alternatively, the measured health status of the individual or community. Outcomes of care have also been defined as "the results of care...[which] can encompass biologic changes in disease, comfort, ability for self-care, physical function and mobility, emotional and intellectual performance, patient satisfaction and self-perception of health, health knowledge and compliance with medical care, and viability of family, job and social role functioning."[11] For NICU patients and their parents, examples of outcome measures are mortality rate, the frequency of chronic lung disease, the number of nosocomial bloodstream infections per 1000 patient days, the percentage of NICU survivors who are developmentally normal, and parental satisfaction with the care of their baby. Box 6.1 demonstrates common quality measures in the field of neonatal respiratory care.

The Institute of Medicine's Domains of Quality

Six domains of quality were described by the Institute of Medicine in its 2001 report *Crossing the Quality Chasm*[1]—safety, timeliness, effectiveness, efficiency, equity, and patient-centeredness (these can be remembered by the acronym STEEEP). A neonatal unit should seek to optimize respiratory care in all these domains. *Safety* in particular is a high-priority domain that deserves specific emphasis and is defined as freedom from accidental injury (avoiding harm to patients from the care that is intended to help them). *Timeliness* is the reduction of delays and unnecessary waits for patients, their families, and health professionals. *Effectiveness* is the provision of health care interventions supported by high-quality evidence to all eligible patients and avoidance of those that are unlikely to be beneficial. *Efficiency* is avoiding waste, including waste of equipment, supplies, ideas, and energy. *Equity* is the provision of care that does not vary based on a patient's personal characteristics such as gender, ethnicity, geographic location, and socioeconomic status. *Patient-centered care* is the provision of care that is respectful of, and responsive to, an individual neonate's family preferences, needs, and values and ensuring that the family's values guide all clinical decisions.

ASSESSING AND MONITORING THE QUALITY OF CARE

The quality of respiratory care can be assessed and monitored using a set of quality indicators that measure different domains of quality. Individual units should choose the exact indicators to monitor based on local priorities, previously identified deficiencies of care, local patterns of practice, and ease of access to data and resources required to collect, analyze, and display data. Quality indicators should be collected both for (1) comparison and (2) improvement.

QUALITY INDICATORS FOR COMPARATIVE PERFORMANCE MEASURES

Such indicators are typically used to compare a unit's clinical performance (and not process measures) against comparators. Comparators can be the quality indicators of other similar units, national benchmarks, or targets. Ideally, these data should be risk-adjusted to make the comparisons valid. Risk adjustment applies statistical methods to differentiate intrinsic heterogeneity among patients (e.g., comorbid conditions) and institutions (e.g., available hospital personnel and resources). With risk adjustment, an outcome can be better ascribed to the quality of clinical care provided by health professionals and institutions. Several models of risk adjustment have been developed for the NICU setting and used to evaluate interinstitutional variation.

When quality indicators are monitored, although there is often a significant lag between the events being measured and the analysis, display, and comparison of the data, the discrepancy between an individual unit's performance and the comparators can be used to motivate change and launch improvement projects around specific topics. Quality indicators for such judgment may also be used by regulators and payers to rank neonatal units (sometimes publicly) according to the quality of care they provide (their performance), withhold payments, and provide incentive payments. They may also be used by families of patients, when choice is feasible (e.g., in an antenatally diagnosed fetal anomaly), to choose the neonatal unit where their infant will receive care. Many neonatal networks, such as the Vermont Oxford Network (VON), the Pediatrix neonatal database, and the Canadian Neonatal Network, collect predefined data items from member neonatal units and provide reports to these units that include quality indicators. For example, the VON provides member units quarterly and annually with a report that includes their rates of ventilation, use of postnatal steroids, use of surfactant, use of inhaled nitric oxide, pulmonary air leak, bronchopulmonary dysplasia (BPD), and mortality.

Published data from several neonatal networks reveal the existence of wide variations in neonatal process measures and neonatal outcomes (including respiratory outcomes) that persist after risk adjustment.[12-16] This suggests that the observed

---

BOX 6.1 Errors and Adverse Events Related to Mechanical Ventilation

Endotracheal intubation
Use of wrong size of endotracheal tube
Right mainstem bronchus intubation
Unplanned extubation
Obstruction of endotracheal tube because of inadequate suction
Airway injury leading to subglottic stenosis
Tracheal perforation from endotracheal tube suction catheter
Kinking of endotracheal tube
Initiation of mechanical ventilation
Improper setup of ventilator and accessories
Failure to add water to humidifier
Misconnection of ventilator tubing
Omission of safety limits on ventilator settings
Omission of alarm settings
Use of mechanical ventilation
Delay in changing ventilator settings in response to blood gas results
Inadvertent delivery of high or low ventilator pressures (e.g., auto-positive end-expiratory pressure)
Failure to wean inhaled oxygen when oxygen saturation is high
Ventilator-associated pneumonia and ventilator-associated events
Inadequate drainage of condensate in ventilator tubing leading to inadvertent pulmonary lavage
Ventilator failure because of poor maintenance by biomedical engineering
Overriding ventilator alarms
Ignoring ventilator alarms

differences in outcomes are the result of the quality of care provided to the patients and that the units with the poorer clinical outcomes have room to improve their quality of care.

A particularly important subset of quality indicators is that of patient safety events. Each neonatal unit should monitor medical errors and adverse events (patient safety events) related to respiratory care. These events are most commonly identified through reporting by health professionals involved in or witnessing the event, a method that is convenient and requires few resources.[16] Other concerted efforts to identify patient safety events include the use of trigger tools, chart review, random safety audits, mortality and morbidity meetings, autopsies, and review of patient family complaints or medical–legal cases.[17] These methods do not yield a true rate of these events, however, and therefore cannot be used to evaluate a unit's performance against comparators. The ideal method to identify these events is prospective surveillance.[18] This system yields accurate rates and can be used for comparison but is not widely used because it is laborious and requires many resources. Efforts to advance patient safety research related to neonatal respiratory care remain ongoing and neonatal units should prioritize endeavors to expand our understanding of the frequency and etiology of as well as harm caused by these adverse events. Particular emphasis should be given to studies employing prospective surveillance methods across multiple sites.

A variety of medical errors and adverse events related to neonatal respiratory care have been described in the literature (see Box 6.1).[19,20] In one study of 10 Dutch NICUs, 9% of patient safety incidents were related to mechanical ventilation. Of all recorded incidents, those related to mechanical ventilation and to blood products had the highest risk scores (an indicator of the likelihood of recurrence and likelihood of severe consequences).[21]

QUALITY INDICATORS FOR IMPROVEMENT

These indicators are used to monitor the progress of a specific quality improvement (QI) project. These usually are a combination of outcome measures and process measures. They are collected in real time and used by QI teams (see later) to monitor the progress of the project, identify unintended consequences, and draw inferences about the effects of their attempts to make change. Ideally, these data are disaggregated as much as possible (not lumped together) and displayed over time (with time on the x axis and the indicator on the y axis) in the form of either run charts or statistical process control charts as displayed in Fig. 6.1.[22]

IMPROVING THE QUALITY OF CARE

Since the mid-1990s, QI has emerged as a strong movement in the health care systems of developed countries. It reflects the effort to incorporate principles, tools, and techniques from other industries for improving product quality to meet their customers' needs and expectations into health care delivery. The basic premise of QI in health care is that improvements in patient care can be achieved by making a focused, conscious

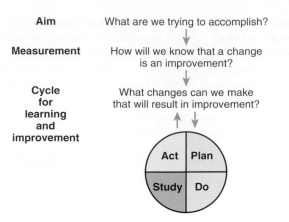

Fig. 6.1 The model for improvement.

effort, using a defined set of scientific methods and by constant reflection on the results of our attempts to improve care. It is based heavily on systems thinking and therefore emphasizes the organization and systems of care. Many approaches to QI have been described (IMPROVE, Model for Improvement, Lean or Lean-Six-Sigma [Define, Measure, Analyze, Improve, Control (DMAIC)], Toyota Production System, Rapid Cycle Improvement, Four Key Habits [VON], Advanced Training Program of Intermountain Healthcare, Microsystems approach) and all are broadly similar in their approaches. Of these, one simple and effective approach that can be used to improve the quality of care is the Model for Improvement (see Fig. 6.1) that was formalized by Langley et al.[23] and endorsed by the Institute for Healthcare Improvement.

THE IMPROVEMENT TEAM

To successfully carry out QI projects, it is important to have a core team of people in each unit. This is usually a multidisciplinary team composed of physicians, nurses, respiratory therapists, pharmacists, and others who are directly or indirectly involved in aspects of the topic that is targeted for improvement. The more disciplines represented, the better the QI efforts will be. The members of this team have to become skilled in several techniques, such as how to have productive meetings, how to work together as a team, how to bring about change in a unit, how to deal with barriers to improvement, and how to collect, analyze, and display data. The involvement of the entire NICU team in QI efforts should increase "buy-in" and heighten awareness of a problem, thereby possibly creating a Hawthorne effect, which is beneficial.

COLLABORATION

Improvement in patient care is impossible without cooperation—working together to produce mutual benefit or attain a common purpose. Collaboration and cooperation have to occur within each unit. Collaboration is a powerful force in motivating people toward improvement and in sustaining the momentum for change in each unit. The improvement team has to get buy-in from other members in their unit and get them to participate in the improvement effort. Collaboration and cooperation among units are also helpful. Different units can work together, share ideas, and help one another to improve care. Clemmer et al.[24] suggest five methods to foster cooperation: (1) develop a shared purpose; (2) create an open, safe environment; (3) include all those who share the common purpose and encourage diverse viewpoints; (4) learn how to negotiate agreement; and (5) insist on fairness and equity in applying rules.

AIM: WHAT ARE WE TRYING TO ACCOMPLISH?

The first step in any improvement project is to set a clear aim. This can be done in three stages. First, a list of problems faced by the unit or opportunities for change is created. The existence of quality indicators as described earlier will assist with the compilation of such a list. Second, the problems or opportunities for change that are listed are then prioritized using criteria such as the resources available, the probability of achieving change, emotional appeal, the importance to stakeholders (including patients and their families), and practicality. Third, one item is finally selected from this list as the aim for improvement. For those unfamiliar with QI, it is best to choose for the initial project a small and well-focused topic on which data are easy to obtain that will be more likely to generate interest among clinicians and nurses. Very low birth weight (VLBW) neonates have been the obvious target for QI in many QI initiatives. VLBW neonates contribute significantly to the mortality and morbidity burden in the neonatal units, consume the largest proportion of resources, are easily identified, and develop potentially preventable outcomes like nosocomial infections, intraventricular hemorrhage, BPD, and ROP. When an aim is selected, it should be specified as a SMART aim—that is, it should be specific, measurable, achievable, realistic, and time bound.

MEASUREMENT: HOW WILL WE KNOW THAT A CHANGE IS AN IMPROVEMENT?

Measurement is key to QI. Measuring the quality of care serves three purposes: (1) It indicates the current status of the unit or practice. This is called assessing "current reality." Without objective measurement, clinicians will be left guessing or relying on subjective impressions. Objective measurement of structures, processes, and outcomes provides strong motivation for a unit to embark on an improvement project. (2) Measurement of quality will inform QI teams whether they are actually making an improvement, without having to rely on subjective impressions or opinions, with the attendant risk of being misguided. (3) Measuring quality helps teams learn from attempts to make improvements and also learn from their successes as well as failures. Fig. 6.2 represents a statistical control chart—a common way of displaying measured metrics over time.

WHAT CHANGES CAN WE MAKE THAT WILL RESULT IN AN IMPROVEMENT?

The answers to this question come from many sources. Some of these include:

1. A detailed analysis and mapping of the process by which care is provided (process mapping). For medical errors and adverse events, a detailed systems analysis[25] is recommended. Such an analysis (the most extensive form of which is a root cause analysis [RCA][26]) attempts to identify workplace-related, human-related, and organizational factors[27] that contributed to the occurrence and propagation of the event. Box 6.2 details the steps involved in the RCA process. It is critical for the leader of the RCA process to be well versed in RCA methodology and also be focused on identifying system-related challenges rather than assignment of individual blame.

2. A review of published literature and using the principles of evidence-based medicine.

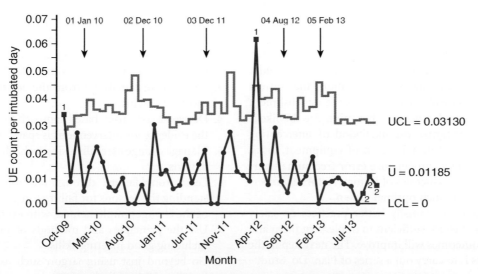

Fig. 6.2 Example of a statistical process control chart. *LCL,* Lower control level; *Ū,* average; *UCL,* upper control level; *UE,* unplanned extubation.

BOX 6.2 Steps in a Root Cause Analysis

Step 1: Identify a sentinel event.
Step 2: Assemble a multidisciplinary team including executive and operational leadership, quality improvement coaches, and providers who come into contact with the system.
Step 3: Verify facts surrounding the event and collect associated data.
Step 4: Chart causal factors using process maps, brainstorming, Pareto charts, fishbone diagrams, etc.
Step 5: Identify root causes by asking "why" five times for each issue, to get to the bottom of the cause.
Step 6: Develop strategies and make recommendations for process change.
Step 7: Present results to all stakeholders.
Step 8: Perform "tests of change."

---

3. Benchmarking—that is, learning from superior performers in the area chosen for improvement.
4. Advice from experts or others who have attempted improvement in similar topics.
5. Brainstorming, critical thinking, and hunches about the current system of care.
6. Use of "change concepts," a set of principles of redesign of process or work flow (such as "change the sequence of steps" or "eliminate unnecessary steps").[23]
7. Particularly for patient safety projects, use of knowledge of human psychology, the science of human factors engineering.

Through the use of one or a combination of these approaches, one or more interventions are identified that, if implemented, have the potential to result in improvements in patient care and outcomes. These interventions are variously known as "change concepts" or "potentially better practices"[28] or "key clinical activities,"[29] or for patient safety events, "safety practices." They are sometimes grouped into a set of synergistic or complementary interventions that are known as "bundles."

The well-known Swiss cheese model[30] depicts how an error reaches a patient despite a series of existing safety mechanisms because the "holes in the Swiss cheese line up" (multiple safety mechanisms fail concurrently or serially and allow propagation of the error). A key principle of improving patient safety and reducing medical errors is to focus not on individual health care providers as the cause of errors (the "person approach") but more broadly on the system of care (in which the provider is embedded) as the desired locus of prevention (the "system approach"). Ensuring patient safety involves the establishment of operational systems and processes that minimize the likelihood of errors and maximize the likelihood of intercepting them when they occur.[5] Optimal design of equipment, tasks, and the work environment can enhance error-free human performance, and the use of principles of human factors engineering can successfully guide such optimal design.

After the changes or potentially better practices or safety practices are selected, it is not sufficient to implement them and assume that patient outcomes will improve. The next step in the improvement process is to carry out a series of Plan–Do–Study–Act (PDSA) cycles.

PLAN–DO–STUDY–ACT CYCLES

No matter what the sources of our ideas for improvement are, there is no guarantee that these changes will improve the quality of care. The results of the implementation of these changes have to be studied, using the measures that have previously been set up when answering the question "How will we know that a change is an improvement?" In other words, the change has to be tested. This process also allows process-related obstacles to be identified and resolved. This process of testing a change is called a PDSA cycle. This is a critical step in the process of QI because it allows troubleshooting before widespread implementation. The PDSA cycles include planning an intervention (e.g., steps to enhance adherence to handwashing), carrying out the intervention, studying its effect (e.g., handwashing compliance rate, hospital-acquired infection rate), and finally implementing the intervention in day-to-day practice. Common questions the QI team should ask itself are as follows: Why did we succeed? Why did we fail? What further changes do we now need to make to succeed? By doing a series of PDSA cycles and thus learning from each effort at improvement, the team can achieve lasting improvements in the way they provide patient care. The apparent simplicity of the PDSA cycle is deceptive. The cycle is a sophisticated, demanding way to achieve learning and change in complex systems.[31]

Table 6.1 demonstrates the steps of the QI process using an example of a project designed to modify oxygen saturation guidelines in VLBW infants in a single tertiary NICU.

ENSURING THE SUCCESS OF QUALITY IMPROVEMENT PROJECTS

QI projects often are not completed as intended, are unsuccessful in achieving the desired results, or are unable to achieve sustained results. The following 10 tips can contribute to successful completion and sustained results:

1. Gain a deep understanding of the problem first using systems thinking[32] ("formulate the mess") before trying to implement solutions, and resist quick "off-the-shelf" solutions.
2. Avoid using solely a research mentality, especially with measurement. Successful QI requires a combination of rigorous scientific thinking and pragmatism. Particularly with measurement, seek usefulness, not perfection.[33]
3. Focus on sustainability from the beginning and not just on short-term wins.
4. Develop a consensus-based approach to decision making when the evidence for interventions is sparse, incomplete, or flawed.
5. Manage change carefully using published expert recommendations.[34,35]
6. Learn from "failure" through multiple PDSA cycles. Understanding the reasons for failure can guide future refinements of the changes implemented, with eventual success.
7. Use the principles and methods of project management,[36] including good meeting skills.
8. Go beyond just using jargon such as "silo," "low-hanging fruit," and "checklist."

TABLE 6.1   Steps in the Improvement Process With Example of a Project to Improve Compliance With New Oxygen Saturation Guidelines to Reduce Retinopathy of Prematurity[a]

Steps in the Improvement Process	Example
Evaluate indicators for improvement	Review of VON quality indicators for VLBW infants
Identify the "problem"	1. Poor compliance with oxygen saturation guidelines (based on sampling by volunteers)
	2. New evidence regarding oxygen saturation goals from the SUPPORT trial
Develop a multidisciplinary improvement team	Team comprising a physician, nursing respiratory therapy leadership, and end providers—physician, nursing RTs, QI coaches, trainees (medical residents, neonatal fellows, nursing students)
Develop a SMART aim	Increase compliance with O_2 saturation guidelines to >95% in 6 months in the NICU
Create process maps, brainstorming, and key driver diagrams	OWL task force met every week for a month to review the evidence surrounding oxygen saturation goals, create process maps, identify potential obstacles (e.g., tight staffing), brainstorm for potential solutions (e.g., use of an OWL nurse "buddy system") to help a nurse with a labile patient
Identify process, outcome, and balance measures	Process: Implement new oxygen saturation guidelines
	Outcome: Compliance with saturation guidelines
	Balance: BPD and ROP rates, staff satisfaction, alarm fatigue
Start continuous data collection immediately	Compliance audited by RTs during every shift for all patients on respiratory support
Plan and conduct PDSA cycles	Multiple cycles conducted on one to three patients, e.g., slight variations in alarm limits, the nurse OWL nurse buddy system
Receive and incorporate feedback regarding PDSA cycle	Verbal/written feedback (feedback forms provided at the bedside with space for open comments, option to stay anonymous) obtained from staff. Recommendations through feedback incorporated: change in saturation cycling time, change in amount of oxygen delivered by manual breaths through a ventilator
Implement changes	Once providers were satisfied with the new process, training was provided to staff through group sessions, one-on-one feedback, and newsletters
Monitor sustainability of process and outcomes	Initial compliance monitored through data collected by RTs on every shift and reviewed by task force weekly
	Ongoing random audits four or five times per week in random shifts
Share data continuously with providers	Data shared with providers through posters and staff meetings
Identify breaks in new process/system	Two-week time period when compliance was noted to drop below 90%
Perform RCA and modify system according to findings	RCA performed: outliers noted to be in cases with specific oxygen saturation compliance (complex heart disease)—staff noted confusion regarding guidelines because bedside sign was for regular alarm limits. Space was introduced on signs for special cases, which was to be approved by physician providers on a case-by-case basis

[a]Oxygen with Love (OWL).
BPD, Bronchopulmonary dysplasia; *NICU*, neonatal intensive care unit; *PDSA*, plan–do–study–act; *QI*, quality improvement; *RCA*, root cause analysis; *ROP*, retinopathy of prematurity; *RT*, respiratory therapist; *SMART*, specific, measurable, achievable, realistic, and time-bound; *SUPPORT*, Surfactant, Positive Airway Pressure, and Pulse Oximetry; *VLBW*, very low birth weight; *VON*, Vermont Oxford Network.

9. Use a QI coach if possible. Coaching can enhance the success of QI teams.[37]
10. Do not feel compelled to adhere rigidly to any one approach to QI.

LEADERSHIP AND UNIT CULTURE

Finally, the involvement, support, and encouragement of the leaders of the organization or the clinical unit, as well as a favorable organizational culture, are crucial elements for the success of quality and safety improvement efforts. Without such support, many improvement efforts will be doomed to failure. Leaders of neonatal units must focus on the quality of care as an important part of the mission of their units and must actively work to create an organizational culture in the unit that will encourage efforts to improve the quality of care. For patient safety in particular, this involves fostering a culture in which

staff members feel safe (i.e., not intimidated) in pointing out safety hazards, challenging authority, and stopping a work process or procedure if they feel it is unsafe ("stopping the line"[38]). Studies in the NICU have found a wide variation in the comfort level of NICU personnel at all levels in providing feedback or raising concerns if there are perceived deficiencies in care.[39,40] There are a multitude of factors that prevent this feedback from occurring, but one important component is psychological safety—belief that an environment is a safe place for risk-taking. When members of an organization feel that they can share potentially negative information, such as an adverse event, this fosters an environment that is more likely to lead to greater engagement in patient safety and QI work. One useful method to promote safety culture is "executive walk rounds,"[41] in which senior organizational leaders periodically walk through the neonatal unit and talk to frontline staff about their perceptions of patient safety problems, hazards, and requirements.

WHY IS QUALITY IMPROVEMENT IMPORTANT IN NEONATAL RESPIRATORY CARE?

Published literature on a wide variety of respiratory process measures and respiratory morbidity that persists after risk adjustment[12-16] suggests that the observed differences in outcomes are the results of the quality of care provided to the patients. That is to say, a significant proportion of neonates managed in NICUs suffer from preventable respiratory morbidity and the units with the poorer clinical outcomes have room to improve their quality of care. A particular concern is the high incidence in VLBW infants of chronic lung disease (BPD), a condition that has a major impact on long-term pulmonary function and is associated with high health care and societal costs and neurodevelopmental morbidity. Despite significant advances in neonatal pulmonary care since 1985, the rates of BPD in infants weighing under 1500 g have remained relatively unchanged since 2005 and also vary significantly across centers in the United States (despite adjustment for confounding factors). Neonatal health outcomes are influenced by a variety of endogenous and exogenous factors like birth weight, gestation, obstetric management during delivery, resuscitation practices, initial respiratory support, nutritional management, and measures to prevent nosocomial infections. Application of systematic QI efforts has the potential to reduce BPD and other forms of respiratory morbidity through reliable and consistent application of existing high-level evidence, without depending on new medications, technology, or innovations to be developed. Such efforts are described later.

EXAMPLES OF QUALITY AND SAFETY IMPROVEMENT IN NEONATAL RESPIRATORY CARE

Quality Improvement Projects in Individual Units

Birenbaum et al. reported a significant reduction in the rate of BPD as a result of a QI project in their unit.[42] The rate of BPD in VLBW neonates was reduced by more than half by avoidance of intubation, adoption of new pulse oximeter limits, and early use of nasal continuous positive airway pressure therapy (CPAP).

Nowadzky et al.[43] used QI methods to reduce BPD by implementing nasal bubble CPAP to reduce mechanical ventilation. Although the group was successful in implementing the use of bubble CPAP, the rate of BPD was unchanged and a concomitant increase in ROP rate was noted.

Merkel et al.[44] reduced unplanned extubations from 2.38 to 0.41 per 100 patient-intubated days by having at least two staff members participate in procedures such as retaping and securing endotracheal tubes; weighing and transferring the patient out of the bed; and placement of alert cards at the bedside indicating the risk level for an unplanned extubation, the security of the endotracheal tube, the depth of placement at the gums, and the proper care of the endotracheal tube. In addition to these measures, a commercial product was used to secure the endotracheal tube, education of staff by staff experts was initiated ("champions"),

the use of a real-time analysis form to identify causes of unplanned extubations was started, the use of a centrally located display of the days since last unplanned extubation was begun, and the nurses placed mittens or socks on the hands of intubated patients greater than 34 weeks' postmenstrual age. They suggest that the benchmark for unplanned extubation should be a rate of less than 1 per 100 patient-intubated days.

Collaborative Quality Improvement Projects

One successful approach that has been used in neonatology by the VON is that of collaborative QI in which a group of neonatal units collaborate for the purpose of improving the quality of neonatal care.[13,45] With this approach, a team of personnel from each hospital (from multiple disciplines involved in neonatal care, such as neonatologists, nurses, respiratory therapists, and others) meets periodically, with ongoing collaboration in between meetings carried on by the use of e-mail and telephone calls among these team members. The network acts as a coordinator, facilitator, and motivator of this collaborative effort and provides expert faculty members who work with individual sets of teams to facilitate their improvement efforts.

The VON has implemented a number of such collaborative projects, called the Neonatal Intensive Care Quality (NICQ) projects. The major components of NICQ projects included multidisciplinary collaboration within and among hospitals, feedback of information from the network database regarding clinical practice and patient outcome, training and QI methods, site visits to project NICUs, benchmarking visits to superior performers within the network, identification and implementation of potentially better practices, and evaluation of the results. In the first NICQ project, teams from the 10 hospitals worked together in cross-institutional improvement groups.[12] Six NICUs focused on reducing nosocomial infections, and four units focused on reducing BPD. The potentially best practices that were proposed were based on an evidence review and careful analysis of other practices at best-performing centers. During the project period from 1994 to 1996, the rate of infection with coagulase-negative *Staphylococcus* decreased from 22.0% to 16.6% at the six project NICUs in the infection group; the rate of supplemental oxygen at 36 weeks' adjusted gestational age decreased from 43.5% to 31.5% at the four NICUs in the BPD group. Another NICQ project evaluated how the adoption of "best practices" in 16 centers of the VON during 2001–2003 might reduce the incidence of BPD among VLBW neonates.[46] BPD rates dropped significantly in 2003 compared with the baseline year. In addition, severe ROP, severe intraventricular hemorrhage, and supplemental oxygen at discharge dropped significantly. The VON reported another QI project with an objective of promoting evidence-based surfactant treatment of preterm neonates.[47] Participating centers were randomized to a control or an intervention arm. Hospitals in the intervention arm received QI advice, including audit and feedback, evidence reviews, an interactive training workshop, and ongoing faculty support via conference calls and e-mail. Although there was no significant difference in the incidence of pneumothorax or mortality, neonates born in intervention hospitals were more likely to receive surfactant in the delivery room or within 2 hours of birth.

Payne et al.[48] reported the results over 9 years from eight NICUs that participated in a VON collaborative to reduce lung injury (the ReLI group). This group successfully decreased delivery room intubation, conventional ventilation, and the use of postnatal steroids for BPD. They increased the use of nasal CPAP, and survival to discharge increased. Nosocomial infections decreased. However, BPD-free survival remained unchanged, and the BPD rate increased.

In a cluster randomized trial done by the Canadian Neonatal Network,[49] six NICUs were identified to adopt practices to reduce nosocomial infections (infection group), and six units, to reduce BPD (pulmonary group). Practice change interventions were implemented using rapid-change cycles for 2 years. The incidence of BPD decreased in the pulmonary group, and the incidence of nosocomial infections decreased significantly in both the infection and the pulmonary groups.

In a cluster randomized QI trial, 14 centers of the National Institute of Child Health and Human Development Neonatal Research Network were randomized to intervention or control clusters.[50] Intervention centers implemented practices of the three best-performing centers of the network to reduce the rate of BPD. Although the intervention centers successfully implemented practices of the best performing centers, the rate of BPD was not reduced in intervention or control centers. Explanations given for the failure to reduce the rate of BPD were choosing interventions that were not evidence based and targeting a multifactorial disease with a single-prong strategy of reducing oxygen exposure.

More recently, statewide collaboratives have been developed in multiple US states where some or all NICUs in the state work collaboratively on the same clinical topics using QI methods, share data, and learn from one another to make improvements in clinical outcomes and processes. Such statewide collaboratives[51-54] have reported significant decreases in central line–associated bloodstream infections and are targeting other clinical outcomes as well.

In a systematic review, Healy et al.[55] summarized the results of 34 published reports of single-center and collaborative QI projects targeting a reduction in BPD. The primary intervention in many of these projects was a reduction in mechanical ventilation. Nearly 70% of these reported a reduction of BPD rates, and in several of the projects where BPD rates did not change, there was improvement in important respiratory care processes. These findings suggest that structured QI efforts can effectively reduce BPD.

CONCLUSION

Every NICU should monitor the quality of respiratory care provided and continuously work to improve the process measures and outcomes of infants in their unit. It is important to recognize that QI methods do not replace formal randomized controlled trials (RCTs) as a research method. Rather they complement RCTs by providing a framework for implementation of evidence-based practices to improve outcomes. The complex multifactorial nature of respiratory outcomes such as BPD often raises challenges in implementation of potentially better practices that have been successful elsewhere. It is thus imperative that changes be based on a review of the evidence when possible. Participation in a multicenter collaborative project may enhance the quality, scope, and effectiveness of such improvements. By employing evidence-based practices adapted to local context within structured QI projects, neonatal units can improve outcomes related to neonatal respiratory care.

A complete reference list is available at https://expertconsult.inkling.com/.

KEY REFERENCES

1. Institute of Medicine (US): Committee on Quality of Health Care in America. Crossing the Quality Chasm: A New Health System for the 21st Century. Washington, DC, National Academies Press, 2001.
5. Kohn LT, Corrigan JM, Donaldson MS (eds): To Err Is Human. Building a Safer Health System. Washington, DC, National Academies Press, 2000, pp. 28-29.
7. Teisberg E, Wallace S, O'Hara S: Defining and implementing value-based health care: a strategic framework. Acad Med 95(5):682-685, 2020.
9. Donabedian A: The quality of care. How can it be assessed? JAMA 260:1743-1748, 1988.
18. Thomas EJ, Petersen LA: Measuring errors and adverse events in health care. J Gen Intern Med 18(1):61-67, January 2003.
22. Gupta M, Kaplan HC: Using statistical process control to drive improvement in neonatal care: a practical introduction to control charts. Clin Perinatol 44(3):627-644, 2017.
25. Vincent C: Understanding and responding to adverse events. N Engl J Med 348(11):1051-1056, 2003.
31. Berwick DM: Developing and testing changes in delivery of care. Ann Intern Med 128:651-656, 1998.
45. Horbar JD: The Vermont Oxford Network: evidence-based quality improvement for neonatology. Pediatrics 103:350-359, 1999.
55. Healy H, Croonen LEE, Onland W, et al: A systematic review of reports of quality improvement for bronchopulmonary dysplasia. Semin Fetal Neonatal Med. 26(1):Article 101201, 2021.

7

Medical and Legal Aspects of Respiratory Care

Jonathan M. Fanaroff

KEY POINTS

- The medical malpractice system is a mechanism for injured patients to receive compensation for injuries resulting from medical errors.
- A number of strategies including maintaining competency, a focus on communication, and appropriate documentation can decrease the risk of liability.
- Alternative mechanisms to traditional malpractice lawsuits such as "Communication and Resolution" programs are promising but not yet widely adapted.

Caring for critically ill newborns takes years of training in which the clinician learns both the art and the science of the field. Relatively little time is spent learning about the legal system related to this discipline. The myriad regulations, unfamiliar language, and multimillion-dollar malpractice verdicts are hard to understand and comprehend. Consequently, most clinicians view the legal system with great mistrust and trepidation. Yet, it is essential that physicians, nurses, and other health care providers understand their rights, duties, and liabilities while practicing health care. Additionally, modern neonatal medicine is a team endeavor and is built on a number of relationships. Physicians must understand the legal relationship they have with their patients and families and must also understand the legal relationships they have with employers, the hospital and nurses, referring physicians, respiratory therapists, neonatal nurse practitioners, and physician assistants.

This chapter provides an overview of the legal system in the United States, including the way it is structured as well as basic vocabulary and concepts. The goal is to provide the clinician with a better comprehension of the legal principles that affect neonatal respiratory care on a daily basis. Although this chapter will center on the US legal system, legal issues and medical malpractice affect clinicians globally. In fact, some European countries are experiencing triple-digit increases in the number of cases presumed "malpractice or bad health care."[1] Accordingly, physicians who practice in any country must understand the particular laws and regulations where they practice.

DISCLAIMER

The purpose of this chapter is to provide an overview of legal issues to educate clinicians. This chapter does not create an attorney-client relationship and should not be taken as substantive legal advice. Medicine is regulated at both the state and the federal levels, and laws vary significantly from state to state. The outcome of a legal case is based upon a particular set of facts, witnesses, attorneys, judges, and juries. A clinician should never assume that his or her situation is exactly the same as that of any case mentioned in this chapter. For specific questions, the reader should consult a qualified attorney.

GENERAL LEGAL PRINCIPLES

If law is the system of rules upon which we live, then the US Constitution is the highest law of the land. Dating back to 1789, the Constitution sets up the framework of the federal and state governments. The federal government is divided into three separate but equal branches. Congress, composed of the Senate and House of Representatives, forms the legislative branch and is charged with making laws. The executive branch, led by the president and by far the largest branch, with approximately 4 million employed, carries out the laws. The judicial branch, which includes the US Supreme Court, reviews the ways in which laws are applied and mediates between the other two branches. State governments have the same organization as the federal government except the executive branch is led by the governor instead of the president.

Both the state and the federal government court systems have hierarchies that are shown in Fig. 7.1. Although both federal and state laws affect the practice of medicine, medicine is primarily regulated by the states. Thus, for example, a physician or respiratory therapist licensed in one state cannot practice in another state without obtaining an additional license to practice in that state. Similarly, the majority of legal cases involving medicine are adjudicated in the state court system. For this reason it is important for a clinician to understand the relevant laws affecting practice in the states in which he or she has a medical license.

SUPERVISION OF OTHERS

Modern neonatology is a team effort. The attending physician is generally considered to be the leader of the team and as such has traditionally been held responsible for the acts of other team members. This can even include situations in which the physician has had no contact, direct or indirect, with the patient

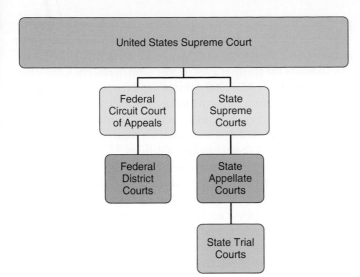

Fig. 7.1 State and federal government court system hierarchies.

filing the lawsuit. There have been a number of legal theories to justify this position. One analogy has held physicians, especially surgeons, to be analogous to the "captain of the ship" and thus responsible for all of the crew under his or her command.[2] As care models have evolved and health care systems expanded, courts have increasingly rejected the captain of the ship doctrine, recognizing that the "theory" that the attending "directly controls *all* activities of whatever nature…is not realistic in present day medical care."[3]

Although the attending neonatologist is no longer held responsible for all activities that occur in the neonatal intensive care unit (NICU), he or she still has authority over the actions of others in the unit. Consequently he or she may still be held liable under the legal theory of respondeat superior, which is Latin for "let the master answer."[4] When there is negligence by a nurse practitioner or resident who is within the legitimate scope of authority of the attending neonatologist, such as during an intubation, the attending may be held liable.

Attending physicians are also expected to provide appropriate supervision of residents and other health professionals and can be held liable for "negligent supervision." In one high-profile lawsuit, an attending anesthesiologist failed to respond to a resident physician's request to assist in an emergent cesarean section. The plaintiff alleged that the delay in timely supervision was the cause of permanent brain damage to the fetus, and the case settled for $35 million.[5]

MALPRACTICE

The cost of medical malpractice in the United States has been estimated at $50 billion per year.[6] These lawsuits have an impact on a large number of physicians. A study released by the American Medical Association noted that 68 liability claims were filed for every 100 physicians and that 28% of physicians 55 years and older have been sued.[7] Pediatricians, however, seem to have been sued less frequently in recent years. In a nationally representative random survey conducted for decades

by the American Academy of Pediatrics, the proportion of pediatricians who reported ever having been sued decreased from a peak of 33% in 1990 to 21% in 2015, the most recent survey.[8] Male pediatricians and hospital-based subspecialists such as neonatologists were more likely to have been sued. Relatively few cases went to trial, and in those cases, the defense prevailed the majority of the time. In the United States, however, each side pays its own costs, and the average defense costs can run tens of thousands of dollars for a claim and over $100,000 should the case go to trial.

Most medical malpractice cases are filed with the plaintiff claiming that the physician was negligent. Negligence lawsuits are part of the broader category of law known as torts, which is French for "wrong." Other broad legal categories include contracts, real property, and criminal law. Tort law is generally divided into intentional and unintentional torts. Most malpractice cases are considered unintentional torts, which is preferable as intentional torts such as defamation often carry broader penalties.

To prevail in a malpractice lawsuit, the plaintiff must prove that the clinician has failed to act as a reasonably prudent physician in the same or similar circumstances.[9] In practice, this requires the plaintiff to prove four elements: that the physician had a duty to the patient that was breached and that in turn caused measurable damages.[10]

Duty

The first element that must be shown in a malpractice case is that the physician had a duty or physician-patient relationship with the patient. If there is no duty to the plaintiff, then the physician has no obligation toward the patient and there is no negligence. For example, if a physician practices only at hospital A, he or she cannot be held liable for refusing to attend a delivery at hospital B. The existence of a duty, however, is usually not in dispute in most neonatal malpractice cases. Furthermore, it is possible for a physician who has cared for a pregnant woman to have a duty toward the newborn even if the baby is cared for by a separate physician. This was shown in the case of *Nold v Binyon*, in which a newborn became a chronic carrier of hepatitis B and the obstetrician had failed to inform the woman of her hepatitis B status.[11] The obstetrician claimed that there was no duty toward the newborn but the Kansas Supreme Court disagreed, stating that "A physician who has a doctor-patient relationship with a pregnant woman who intends to carry her fetus to term and deliver a healthy baby also has a doctor-patient relationship with the fetus." As discussed earlier, another situation in which a duty may attach even when the physician never saw the patient is in the context of supervising other clinicians such as residents and nurse practitioners.

Breach

Once a duty has been established, the plaintiff must next show that the clinician breached his or her duty by violating the "standard of care." There are misconceptions about "standard of care" that are important to clarify. First, physicians are not expected to be perfect but rather are expected to act as a "reasonably prudent" physician exercising "reasonable care and diligence." Second, "standard of care" is a legal concept that must be applied to a specific fact pattern of a case in litigation. The plaintiff's attorneys claim that the defendant has departed from an acceptable standard of care. The defense counters that the clinician has met the standard of care. Third, traditionally, physicians were compared with other physicians in their local community. With changes in communication (i.e., national meetings, national journals) and a move toward national board certification, physicians in specialties such as neonatology have increasingly been compared with other specialists nationally. Thus, a neonatologist in California can testify as an expert witness about the standard of care in Ohio.

The Expert Witness

In most areas of negligence, a jury can understand "reasonably prudent" behavior using common sense. A driver speeding 85 miles an hour in a snowstorm is obviously not using "due care." In most medical malpractice cases, however, lay juries do not know what a reasonably prudent practitioner would have done. So expert witnesses are used to explain it to a jury. Each state decides what "qualifies" an individual to serve as an expert witness. Expert witnesses testify under oath, and the American Academy of Pediatrics expects pediatricians who serve as experts to provide testimony containing "complete, accurate, and unbiased information."[12] Nevertheless, concerns remain that "hired gun" experts "fuel inappropriate litigation through testimony that is not well grounded in prevailing clinical standards or science."[13] Many states are taking proactive steps in an attempt to improve the quality of expert testimony. Florida, for example, now requires physician experts from out of state to obtain an expert witness certificate issued by the state.[14] By obtaining the certificate, the expert physician is then subject to discipline by the Florida Medical Board.

Causation

In addition to showing that the clinician breached his or her duty to the patient, the plaintiff must show that the breach in question was actually the cause of the injury for which the patient is suing for damages. It can be difficult to determine whether it was the breach of care rather than the underlying medical condition that led to the injury, especially in neonatal cases. Normal healthy newborns, for example, do not require resuscitation. So when an infant is born depressed and requires significant resuscitation it may be difficult to prove that it was the delay in intubation, for example, rather than the underlying pathology requiring intubation that led to a poor outcome. As with the element of breach, expert witnesses testify before the lay jury about causation issues.

Damages

The ultimate purpose of tort law is to "make whole" a party who has been injured through negligence. Accordingly, the final element a plaintiff must prove is that the injury led to measurable damages. There are two broad categories of damages: economic and noneconomic. Economic damages include items such as medical expenses, lost wages, home accommodations, and education expenses. Noneconomic damages include claims that are subjective and often more difficult to quantify, such as

pain and suffering, emotional distress, or loss of the parent-child relationship. Large jury awards are often associated with noneconomic damages, and thus, many state legislatures have placed limits on them as part of tort reform efforts. California, for example, has a $250,000 damage cap on noneconomic damages. The California Supreme Court ruled that such a cap was constitutional.[15] However, other states, including Georgia and Illinois, have decided that state caps on noneconomic damages are in violation of their state constitutions.[16,17]

If behavior is particularly egregious, courts may sometimes award punitive damages to the injured party. These are relatively rare in medical malpractice cases but can occur, for example, in cases in which the physician has behaved in a particularly reckless manner. An example would be if a physician practiced while under the influence of drugs or alcohol or intentionally altered or destroyed pertinent medical records in an effort to avoid liability.

Burden of Proof

The burden of proof refers to the "degree of belief" that the judge or jury must have to decide that a particular fact is true and find for one side over the other. In criminal cases, because of the injustice of jailing an innocent person, there is a very high burden of proof known as "beyond a reasonable doubt." Medical malpractice cases, on the other hand, have a much lower burden of proof. In general, the plaintiff must show for each element that it is "more likely than not," otherwise known as the preponderance of the evidence or the "51% test."

MALPRACTICE ISSUES SPECIFIC TO NEONATOLOGY AND NEONATAL RESPIRATORY CARE

Caring for sick newborns can be extremely rewarding, but unfortunately, there are a number of factors that increase the risk of a malpractice lawsuit. Babies in the NICU have among the longest stays in the hospital. During that time, they receive multiple medications that are individually dosed, and in fact, the same baby will have multiple dosages of the same medication over time owing to changes in weight. The requirement for round-the-clock care increases the number of caregivers involved and increases the risk of communication/hand-off errors. Additionally, many personal injury attorneys specialize in birth injury cases for a number of reasons. Economic damages for a brain-damaged infant can easily reach several million dollars, and juries tend to be very sympathetic toward the infant and his or her family.

Box 7.1 lists the common malpractice suits in neonatology. A number of areas specifically relate to neonatal respiratory care.

Resuscitation

Resuscitation of the depressed newborn is a relatively rare event that requires a combination of knowledge, teamwork, and technical skill. The Neonatal Resuscitation Program (NRP) provider course has been revised to incorporate teamwork and communication skills and an increasing emphasis on simulation.[18] Particular areas of medicolegal risk include timely attendance at delivery, giving medications without delay when indicated, and timely recognition of when the endotracheal tube is placed incorrectly. Additionally, as recognized by the NRP, prompt evaluation and referral for therapeutic hypothermia may help avoid a delay in establishing cooling within the 6-hour therapeutic window.

Prematurity/Periventricular Leukomalacia

Prematurity has not traditionally been a focus of medical malpractice litigation, and when lawsuits were filed, they usually were directed at obstetricians. As outcomes have improved, however, expectations have increased and prematurity has become a burgeoning area of malpractice lawsuits. Obstetricians remain at risk, as one recent case illustrates. A pregnant woman presented to the hospital in preterm labor. When the baby was born a few hours later in distress, the obstetrician and hospital were sued for failing to perform a cesarean section in a timely manner. The jury subsequently awarded the plaintiffs $229.6 million dollars, the largest medical malpractice verdict in United States history.[19]

The vast majority of extremely premature infants have a period of time during which their blood sugar, blood pressure, blood count, or blood gas is out of the "normal" range. When an adverse outcome occurs, the abnormal value can be cited as the proximate cause of the injury. Hypocarbia, for example, has been shown to be an independent predictor of periventricular leukomalacia.[20] As periventricular leukomalacia has in turn been associated with poor long-term neurodevelopmental outcomes (particularly cerebral palsy), it is advisable to respond to low CO_2 levels in a mechanically ventilated infant and document that response.

RESPIRATORY FAILURE/MECHANICAL VENTILATION

Although there is an increasing emphasis in neonatology on noninvasive ventilation, there are still situations in which surfactant is an appropriate therapy. Consequently, delay in giving surfactant leading to worsened respiratory failure with subsequent acidosis and potentially poor long-term neurodevelopmental outcomes can be an area of malpractice risk. Similar allegations can occur when there is delayed recognition and response to a pneumothorax, particularly tension pneumothorax, while an infant is mechanically ventilated. Clinicians should be vigilant and responsive to a number of complications associated with mechanical ventilation, including a plugged or displaced endotracheal tube, kinked ventilator tubing, and mechanical problems with the ventilator itself.

Patient Safety/Culture of Safety

Critically ill neonates require 24-hour care in a rapidly changing, complex, and technologically oriented environment. As in the delivery room, communication and teamwork are required to provide high-quality safe care. There has been an increasing focus on patient safety since a 1999 Institute of Medicine report estimated that preventable errors cause up to 98,000 patient deaths annually.[21] Efforts to improve patient safety have focused on adaptation of techniques from high-reliability industries including aviation and nuclear power. High-reliability organizations share a number of characteristics, including:

- Preoccupation with failure
- Reluctance to simplify interpretations
- Sensitivity to operations
- Commitment to resilience
- Deference to expertise[22]

Efforts to create a safer health care environment require more than updated policies and standards. Ultimately there must be a culture of safety as opposed to a culture of finger pointing and blame. Traditionally when, for example, a medication error occurred, the "solution" would be to fire the clinician who gave the medicine rather than look at potential system causes of the error. An institutional culture in which health care providers feel supported in efforts both to point out vulnerabilities in safe care delivery and to respond appropriately when an error occurs is much more likely to meet the World Health Organization vision of patient safety: A world where every patient receives safe health care, without risks and harm, every time, everywhere.[23]

DECREASING THE RISK OF A MALPRACTICE LAWSUIT

Being sued is an incredibly stressful experience. Unfortunately, the litigation can stretch out for years and cost thousands of dollars in defense costs alone. Additionally, it is common for physician defendants to suffer from a number of physical and emotional effects known as medical malpractice stress syndrome.[24] Just as adverse outcomes are not always preventable, physicians are always at risk of being named in a malpractice

---

BOX 7.2   Strategies to Avoid Tort Litigation

Stay current in the field
- Conference attendance
- Literature
- Textbooks

Communicate
- With other members of the team
- With the parents

Document
- Factually
- Professionally

Be aware of state laws that affect your practice.

---

lawsuit. It is important to involve risk management proactively when an unexpected adverse outcome occurs. A number of strategies (Box 7.2), however, may be helpful to avoid tort litigation.

Competency

Neonatology is a rapidly changing specialty, and it is important for clinicians to remain up-to-date in the field. There are a number of ways to achieve this goal, including attending local, regional, and national conferences and reading journals and textbooks. An example of the changing recommendations for the practice of neonatology is seen in the postnatal use of steroids in ventilator-dependent babies. Dexamethasone was widely used on ventilated preemies in the 1990s to enhance rapid weaning and extubation from ventilator support. In 2002, the American Academy of Pediatrics Committee on Fetus and Newborn recommended against the routine use of the drug owing to concerns over long-term neurologic effects. This position was reaffirmed in 2010 and again in 2014 with the advice that high-dose dexamethasone or other steroid use should be an "individualized decision…made in conjunction with the infant's parents."[25]

Communication

Communication is an important skill in providing safe and effective medical care. As The Joint Commission notes, "When communication is effective, it can help improve the care an organization provides. When it is poor it can lead to inconvenience, frustration, error, and sometimes tragedy."[26] Additionally, poor communication with patients and families is cited in more than 40% of malpractice cases.[27]

Documentation

There is an old saying that "if it was not documented, it was not done." This is not, of course, strictly correct. It may be several years, however, between the time care is provided and when a lawsuit is filed. The amount of time available to file a lawsuit, known as the statute of limitations, is determined by state law, and in many states, it can be as long as 20 or more years for minors. Accordingly, documenting the care provided in a factual and professional manner is important. It is important not to speculate or attribute causation when this is uncertain.

Communication with other team members as well as the family should also be documented, but the chart should not be used as a battleground between caretakers.

THE FUTURE OF MALPRACTICE LITIGATION

Few would disagree that the current malpractice system is expensive and inefficient. Malpractice premiums for obstetricians in New York City are more than $214,000 per year,[28] yet one study found that for every dollar spent on malpractice compensation, 54 cents went to administrative expenses such as lawyers, expert witnesses, and the courts.[29] Additionally, many victims of malpractice receive no compensation. For this reason, as well as increased efforts by health care in general to become both safer and more transparent, there are a number of "nontraditional" reform approaches that show some promise.[30] The University of Michigan Health System, for example, instituted a "Communication and Resolution" program in which they perform active surveillance for medical errors, fully disclose found errors to patients, and offer compensation when they are at fault.[31] Since implementing the program, they experienced fewer lawsuits, which were resolved more quickly and with dramatically lower legal costs. The states of Florida and Virginia have initiated Neurologic Injury Compensation Acts (or NICA laws), which allow newborns who are injured at birth to receive compensation through a "no fault"-type system.[32]

CONCLUSION

The field of neonatology has made tremendous progress over the past decades. With this progress have come greater expectations. Additionally, there is an increasing emphasis on transparency and creating a culture of safety with the goal of learning from both mistakes and near misses. The current adversarial malpractice system has been described as "prolonged, expensive, and inconsistent."[30] Nontraditional approaches to malpractice liability reform show promise but are mainly still in the testing phase. Clinicians will benefit from a greater understanding of the medical malpractice system, common areas of malpractice risk, and strategies to minimize the risk of being named in a malpractice lawsuit.

A complete reference list is available at https://expertconsult. inkling.com/.

KEY REFERENCES

8. Bondi SA, Tang SS, Altman RL, et al: Trends in pediatric malpractice claims 1987–2015. Results from the Periodic Survey of Fellows. Pediatrics 145(4):e20190711, 2020.
10. Turbow R, Fanaroff J: Legal issues in newborn intensive care. In: Sanbar SS (ed): Legal Medicine. 7th ed. Philadelphia, Mosby Elsevier, 2007.
12. Paul SR, Narang SK, Committee on Medical Liability and Risk Management: Expert witness participation in civil and criminal proceedings. Pediatrics 39:e20163862, 2017.

21. Kohn LT, Corrigan JM, Donaldson MS: To Err is Human: Building a Safer Health System. Washington, DC, Institute of Medicine, National Academies Press, 2000.

24. Sanbar SS, Firestone MH: Medical malpractice stress syndrome. In: Sanbar SS (ed): The Medical Malpractice Survival Handbook. Philadelphia, Mosby Elsevier, 2007.

29. Studdert DM, Mello MM, Gawande AA, et al: Claims, errors, and compensation payments in medical malpractice litigation. N Engl J Med 354(19):2024–2033, 2006.

30. Mello MM, Studdert DM, Kachalia A: The medical liability climate and prospects for reform. JAMA 312(20):2146–2155, 2014.

31. Kachalia A, Kaufman SR, Boothman R, et al: Liability claims and costs before and after implementation of a medical error disclosure program. Ann Intern Med 153(4):213–221, 2010.

32. Goldsmith JP: Programs offer alternative to malpractice suits when newborns suffer neurologic injury. AAP News Pediatr Law 33(2):10, February 2012.

8

Physical Examination

Edward G. Shepherd and Leif D. Nelin

KEY POINTS

- Despite the rapid proliferation of various laboratory and imaging modalities, the physical examination is the cornerstone of medical care.
- The physical examination is central to the care of the neonate and provides immediate information on the patient's status and how they are responding to therapy without the delays inherent in any diagnostic test.
- Effective physical examination can be performed on babies receiving any type of respiratory support.
- The physical examination can substitute effectively for invasive technology and noxious stimuli like lab draws; therefore, well-performed physical examinations may protect babies from long-term harms.

HISTORICAL ASPECTS

The physical examination, along with the history, is the oldest tool available to the physician to diagnose and assess response to treatment. Hippocrates and his contemporaries wrote about the importance of the physical examination, including inspection, palpation, and direct auscultation nearly 2500 years ago.[1] Leopold Auenbrugger first described the technique of percussion in 1761 and has been credited with the beginning of the modern physical examination. René Laennec invented the stethoscope and in 1819 published *On Mediate Auscultation*, which was essentially a manual on the stethoscope and included many terms still used today. The development of all components of the physical examination continued during the nineteenth century such that by the beginning of the twentieth century, the physical examination we perform today was fully established.[2]

The last half of the twentieth century saw a rapid development of diagnostic technology, which continues today. However, none of the currently available technologies has entirely supplanted the physical exam. Indeed, a study by Paley et al.[3] found that more than 80% of newly admitted internal medicine patients could be correctly diagnosed on admission based on the history and physical examination, and that basic clinical skills remain a powerful tool, sufficient for achieving an accurate diagnosis in most cases. In a study in a general medicine inpatient service, it was found that 26% of patients had physical findings by the attending physician that led to important changes in clinical management.[4] Thus, the physical examination remains the foundation upon which diagnosis and therapy are based.

IMPORTANCE OF THE PHYSICAL EXAMINATION

The physical examination is central to the care of the neonate, especially those requiring assisted ventilation. It provides immediate information on each patient's status and how he or she is responding to therapy without the delays inherent in any diagnostic test. Further, neonatal intensive care unit (NICU) patients are unique in that they are conscious and not routinely sedated while on positive pressure ventilation (PPV).[5] Thus the physical examination remains accurate in assessing both current status and immediate responses to changes in support. Finally, there is emerging evidence that the more noxious procedures (such as skin breaks that occur with lab draws) a baby undergoes during hospitalization, the worse their neurodevelopmental outcome.[6,7] Therefore, if the use of physical findings can replace at least some noxious procedures, then the physical examination may represent a potential means of improving long-term outcomes.

The physical examination then represents a low-cost and efficient guide to the care of the patient and can be particularly helpful in deciding what subsequent laboratory and imaging studies should be obtained, and which therapies to consider. In patients with evolving disease, physical examination should be frequently repeated as responses to therapy may be rapid. Indeed, the most reliable, most cost effective, and least invasive way to determine the success or failure of a change in therapy for any patient is to observe his or her response to that therapy by performing exams before and following institution of the therapy.

TECHNIQUE OF THE PHYSICAL EXAMINATION

Overview

The examiner should obtain the permission of the bedside nurse before the hands-on assessment, and the entire examination of the baby (including exposure to ambient light) should be done as gently and noninvasively as possible. Ideally, the examination should be clustered with other cares so that the baby is disturbed as little as possible. Physical examination of newborn infants is uniquely challenging as "normal" findings are dependent on a number of variables influenced by gestational age, age at examination, size, mode of respiratory support, and other factors.[8-10] In addition to these, a number of other examination findings change predictably with time and age. Skin color is blue or pale at birth but rapidly turns pink if transition occurs properly. Normal respiratory rates depend on gestational age, size, and mode of respiratory support, whereas normative goals for blood pressures depend on gestational age at birth and corrected gestational age at time of obtainment.[11-13] Blood pressure is low at the time of birth and gradually increases with each day and month until pediatric norms are achieved, whereas respiratory rate typically starts fast and slows until pediatric norms are achieved. In particular, physical examination findings in a newly born infant should be interpreted in light of the unique anatomic and physiologic changes that occur during transition from the intrauterine to the extrauterine environment. The following sections will therefore focus on the unique physiologic factors that influence the newborn respiratory physical examination and the specific examination techniques and findings most helpful in neonates at different ages and with specific conditions.

Performing the Neonatal Respiratory Physical Examination

The newborn respiratory examination begins with observation, followed by auscultation and palpation. Optimal physical examination of the respiratory system in the newborn requires both observation and hands-on assessment. Observation is focused on obtaining an overall impression of the infant's comfort, color, perfusion, movement patterns, respiratory effort, respiratory rate, and level of interaction with the environment. Hands-on assessment includes auscultation and palpation. Ideally, observation occurs before any hands-on assessment to obtain steady-state information, as hands-on assessments are likely to disturb the infant.

The respiratory physical examination can be divided into the following questions that the examiner should answer sequentially:

- How does the baby look?
- What am I hearing?
- What am I feeling?

The examination begins with an overall assessment of the baby's status and a rapid assessment of vital signs, keeping in mind that normal vital signs depend on gestational age at delivery and time in minutes and/or days of life.[13] The respiratory rate should be normal for age and gestation, and respiratory effort should be unlabored. For a period of time after birth up to 12 to 24 hours of age, mild retractions and tachypnea may be present as respiratory compliance improves (particularly in premature infants). The infant should be pink and resting comfortably, although acrocyanosis may persist well after delivery. The infant should be well perfused with brisk capillary refill and should have normal tone with a vigorous response to external stimuli. Respirations should be quiet, without stridor or stertor, and the infant must be able to breathe comfortably with a closed mouth. The thorax and abdomen should be normally shaped. The presence of a "barrel chest" suggests lung hyperinflation, and a bell-shaped chest may indicate poorly inflated lungs, whereas a scaphoid abdomen may suggest displacement of abdominal contents into the thorax. The rib cage and abdomen should move in synchrony during the respiratory cycle, but in the presence of lung disease, thoracoabdominal asynchrony may be marked. Specifically, movement of the rib cage lags behind movement of the abdomen on inhalation, so-called paradoxical movement, suggesting increased respiratory resistance or decreased compliance.[14]

A brief inspection of the infant should determine that the facies are normal in appearance, ears are properly placed and rotated, abdomen and chest are normal in appearance, and the extremities are supple with a full range of motion. Abnormalities in any of these observations should guide the subsequent examination and evaluation. For example, cyanosis out of proportion to respiratory distress should prompt a thorough cardiac evaluation, whereas contractures or other signs of Potter syndrome should prompt a careful respiratory, neurologic, and renal evaluation. This is followed by a detailed examination of the airway that includes examination of the palate and lip for possible clefts, the chin and tongue for possible airway obstruction, the neck for possible tracheal deviation or goiter, the nares for atresia or stenosis, the ear canals, and the eyes.

The initial observation should be followed by auscultation. This and all subsequent portions of the examination should be informed by any findings on initial observation; however, the examiner must ensure that a complete and thorough examination is performed on every newborn regardless of initial findings. Auscultation should begin with careful evaluation of heart and lung sounds, although the presence or absence of a murmur does not definitively include or exclude congenital heart disease, especially in the immediate postpartum period. Breath sounds both anteriorly and posteriorly should be clear and equal without wheezing or rhonchi; crackles are occasionally heard in the immediate postpartum period but should resolve quickly as lung water is resorbed. Audible bowel sounds in the chest suggest a congenital diaphragmatic hernia. The abdomen should be auscultated for the presence of bowel sounds, and the liver and head should be auscultated for the presence of bruits. In addition to auscultation with a stethoscope, the clinician should also listen for the presence of stridor (suggestive of upper airway obstruction) or audible wheezing (suggestive of bronchial constriction).

Once auscultation is completed, the examiner should palpate for determination of the presence or absence of crepitus; fractured clavicles, femurs, or humeri; hepatosplenomegaly; any intra-abdominal masses; hernias; or abdominal tenderness.

The chest should be palpated to determine heart position, as well as the presence of thrills or heaves. The abdomen should be soft and nondistended, and the liver edge should be even with the costal margin.

INTERPRETATION OF THE FINDINGS OF PHYSICAL EXAMINATION

General Physical Examination Findings

In the neonate with respiratory distress, hypoxemia, and/or respiratory failure, the physical examination may change with disease progression. The neonate often comes to the attention of the clinician with evidence of tachypnea, nasal flaring, retractions, and/or grunting. These signs on physical examination relate to pulmonary problems but are not pathognomonic for any particular neonatal respiratory disease. Thus, the spectrum of neonatal respiratory disease must be considered, and frequent reassessment of the patient is needed because the evolution of these symptoms can help to differentiate particular causes (Fig. 8.1). For example, if the symptoms improve within hours, then it is likely that the patient had transient tachypnea of the newborn (TTN). On the other hand, if the symptoms continue to worsen and the patient is a preterm infant, then surfactant deficiency (respiratory distress syndrome [RDS]) is the more likely diagnosis. It should be kept in mind that none of the currently available laboratory testing or imaging definitively differentiates the underlying causes of neonatal respiratory diseases due to parenchymal lung disease. For example, a low lung volume diffusely hazy chest x-ray in a preterm infant is likely to be RDS; however, other common causes of respiratory distress like neonatal pneumonia, TTN, and congestive heart failure cannot be ruled out. Thus, physical examination on admission and frequent reassessment are likely to be the best way to diagnose neonatal respiratory diseases. Furthermore, when a patient is improving and respiratory support is weaned, the first indication that a patient is not tolerating that wean is likely to come from the physical examination, particularly new findings of head bobbing, tachypnea, and nasal flaring.

There is a huge variety of potential abnormal findings on newborn examination, each of which may reflect a number of potential pathologies or normal variants. Asymmetric breath sounds, for example, may reflect pneumothorax, pneumonia, congenital diaphragmatic hernia, atelectasis, or malpositioned endotracheal tube or may be an artifact of the listener. Hepatosplenomegaly may reflect venous congestion, intrinsic liver disease, infection, platelet aggregation, or lung hyperinflation. Abdominal distention may reflect obstruction, atresia, malrotation, or swallowed air. The presence of abnormal findings, or the lack of normal findings, on physical examination should prompt and direct the ensuing laboratory and/or imaging diagnostic workup.

Although many of these examination findings will be static (e.g., once it is determined that the infant does not have a cleft palate, this portion of the examination may not need to be repeated daily), other aspects of an infant's examination will change with time, disease progression, and age. Retractions, for

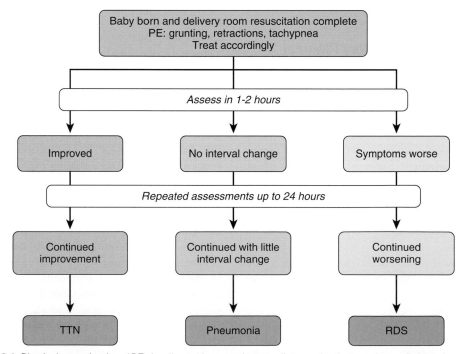

Fig. 8.1 Physical examination (*PE*) in diagnosing respiratory distress in the newborn. Babies born with transient tachypnea of the newborn (*TTN*) are sick at birth, but their signs and symptoms begin to resolve nearly immediately. Babies born with pneumonia will be sick at birth and show little improvement until the pneumonia begins to clear; with bacterial pneumonia, this can take 3–5 days. Babies born with respiratory distress syndrome (*RDS*), otherwise known as surfactant deficiency, continue to have worsening of symptoms until treated with exogenous surfactant or after about 48 to 72 hours of age. The key for physical examination of these infants is frequently repeated assessments.

instance, may be significant in the initial stages of both TTN and RDS, but they will improve steadily in the former and probably worsen in the latter if exogenous surfactant has not been given. Similarly, initial tachypnea by definition resolves in TTN but may not in RDS or pneumonia. Conversely, once compliance is improved after the administration of exogenous surfactant in RDS, both retractions and tachypnea tend to improve rapidly.

Special Technique of Examination: Transillumination

Pneumothorax is a potentially life-threatening complication in neonates and may be difficult to diagnose emergently; the chest x-ray remains the gold standard of diagnosis if time permits. Unfortunately, infants suffering this complication may require therapy well before a chest x-ray can be obtained. In such situations, transillumination may be helpful. The examiner places a cool, bright light source against the chest wall on the potentially involved side, and if a pneumothorax is present, the light will typically radiate across the chest and illuminate the entire hemithorax. Although this test can be helpful in emergent situations, it is prone to false-positive or -negative results and thus must be carefully considered in the context of all other available diagnostic information.

PHYSICAL EXAMINATION FINDINGS IN SPECIFIC CLINICAL SITUATIONS

Examination at Birth

The physiology of the newborn is uniquely adapted to the transition from intrauterine to extrauterine life. This transition leads to many of the physical examination findings noted at birth and is also the basis for a number of normal physical findings in neonates that would be atypical for older children and adults. Specifically, newborn infants are exiting a fluid-filled environment in which blood with relatively low oxygen tension (partial pressure of oxygen [PaO_2]) is supplied by the placenta to one in which blood with relatively high PaO_2 is supplied by the newly air-filled lungs; thus the neonate's skin color is often cyanotic even in the absence of deranged respiration. In addition, there are numerous hormonal surges associated with labor and delivery, such as antidiuretic hormone, that have an impact on the hypothalamic-pituitary axis, which can lead to the signs of hypoperfusion such as delayed capillary refill even in the absence of shock. Moreover, the newborn infant has a relatively compliant chest wall, especially if he or she is born prematurely. This increased chest wall elasticity may lead to decreased functional residual capacity, resulting in tachypnea and increased work of breathing even in the absence of pulmonary disease. Finally, newborn infants, especially those born prematurely, are at high risk for deranged control of breathing leading to apnea and bradycardia. Immediate observation at birth is well described in the Neonatal Resuscitation Program (NRP) and consists of a quick assessment of tone and respiratory effort followed by color. Subsequent assessments follow based on the results of this initial survey. Current NRP recommendations require placement of a pulse oximeter in the delivery room to follow oxygenation (SpO_2). Of note, during the immediate postpartum period,

SpO_2 will typically take more than 5 minutes to reach 80% and 10 min to reach 90%.[6] Once the infant is stabilized, a thorough respiratory examination should follow.

Examination of an Infant Receiving Face Mask or Laryngeal Mask Ventilation

Noninvasive ventilation may be provided to neonates via face mask or laryngeal mask airway (LMA) application. In most cases, such ventilation is adequate for neonatal resuscitation, and relatively few babies will need to proceed to intubation. Ventilation via either face mask or LMA, however, can be technically difficult, especially during stressful situations, and the examiner must be well attuned to the signs of proper noninvasive ventilation. Specifically, if ventilation is applied effectively, the baby should have a rapidly improving heart rate, tone should improve (unless the baby is hypotonic owing to extrinsic factors such as medication administration), color should improve, and, most important, the baby should have good chest rise with each bagged ventilation. If poor chest rise is noted, the patient's position should be readjusted to ensure the proper "sniffing" position, the seal between mask and face should be ensured, and the pressure applied via the bag should be evaluated to ensure adequacy. In those relatively few newborns and infants with highly significant lung disease, high pressures may be required to achieve adequate chest excursion.

Examination of the Ventilated Infant

The neonatal respiratory examination is further complicated because it is heavily influenced by the medical therapies and support many of these infants require as part of their care. Extremely low-birth-weight infants with very compliant chest walls, for instance, will all require positive pressure (nasal constant positive airway pressure [nCPAP], positive pressure ventilation [PPV], or high-frequency ventilation) in the first few weeks of life. Each mode of positive pressure support will interact with the infant's respiratory system in different ways and will create unique respiratory findings. Once the infant is stabilized on properly applied positive pressure, the physical examination should improve markedly, and failure to improve should conversely be taken as a warning that the infant may not be receiving adequate support. Typical signs of improvement include decreased respiratory rate; significant reduction in retractions; reduction in nasal flaring, grunting, and/or head bobbing; improved color; improvements in tone; and less agitation.

Conventional Ventilation

This section focuses on the essentials of the physical examination in ventilated neonates and how to interpret changes in the physical examination. Some key concepts to consider include (1) infants receiving synchronized intermittent mandatory ventilation (SIMV) will have both spontaneous and ventilator-assisted respirations, each of which will manifest distinctively; (2) infants with a large leak around the endotracheal tube will often have an audible air leak around the tube with each ventilator-delivered inflation; and (3) a patient on PPV whose delivered minute ventilation is too small (i.e., the patient is undersupported) will exhibit worsening physical examination findings as the patient "fights" the ventilator to try to improve minute ventilation.

The NICU is a unique environment for caring for patients with respiratory distress. Many NICU patients remain on PPV for long periods of time. A report from the Eunice Kennedy Shriver National Institute of Child Health and Human Development Neonatal Research Network (NRN) found that, in a cohort of appropriate-for-gestational-age infants born at less than 27 weeks' gestation admitted to NRN centers, the average duration of PPV was 26 ± 26 days.[15] In a population cohort of infants born at less than 27 weeks in Sweden, the median PPV days were 11, with a range of 1 to 134 days.[16] Therefore, it is no longer recommended to routinely sedate NICU patients on PPV, as this has been found to result in negative outcomes related to duration of PPV and neurodevelopment.[5] The majority of NICU patients on the ventilator for pulmonary disease will then be awake and alert, which allows the use of the physical examination to assess adequacy of support. If the ventilator support is adequate, the patient is likely to breathe comfortably and have normal awake and sleep states (Fig. 8.2). On the other hand, if the respiratory support is inadequate (i.e., the patient's needs are undersupported), the patient will exhibit signs of air hunger, including tachypnea, retractions, nasal flaring, and/or head bobbing, as well as being irritable, tachycardic, and difficult to console. Undersupported neonates often are given sedatives to try to control their irritability and movements, and yet what the undersupported patient really needs is an increase in respiratory support. It must also be kept in mind that our patients will do what they can via spontaneous respiratory effort to compensate when they are undersupported, such that, at least initially, the blood gases may not reflect the fact that the patient is undersupported. That is to say, if a patient has too low a minute ventilation (tidal volume times frequency), then the patient will compensate by tachypnea and an increased work of breathing such that the irritable, tachypneic, retracting patient may actually have a normal carbon dioxide tension (partial pressure of carbon dioxide [$PaCO_2$]) on the blood gas, until such time that the patient can no longer maintain those

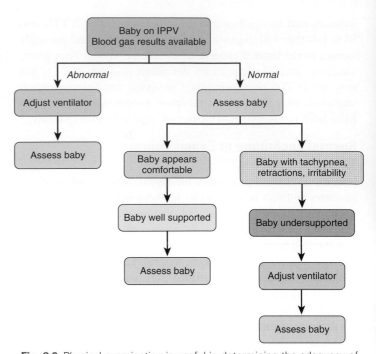

Fig. 8.3 Physical examination is useful in determining the adequacy of ventilator support for babies on positive pressure ventilation (PPV). Steady-state blood gases (i.e., those obtained from an indwelling vascular catheter) are often followed in these babies, particularly those with acute lung diseases in the first few days of life. When a blood gas is done on a baby on PPV and it is abnormal, then the ventilator has to be adjusted accordingly. If the blood gas is normal it is imperative to look at the baby. If the baby is well supported, then the baby will look comfortable on the ventilator—that is, breathing easily with minimal retractions, no tachypnea, and little evidence of "fighting" the ventilator. On the other hand, if the baby is undersupported and tachypneic with increased work of breathing, then he or she is likely to be compensating for the lack of adequate support such that the blood gas is normal but clearly the ventilator needs to be adjusted to improve the level of support. Once adjustments have been made, it is important to continue to frequently assess the baby on PPV as this will be the first evidence of changes in the patient's respiratory status. *IPPV,* Intermittent positive pressure ventilation.

spontaneous breaths (Fig. 8.3). Thus, it is likely that, at least for some patients, the physical examination may be a better indicator of acute patient status than the blood gases.

High-Frequency Ventilation: Oscillation

A patient placed on high-frequency oscillatory ventilation (HFOV) may not breathe regularly, and auscultation of the chest may not reveal breath sounds in a patient who is adequately supported. Properly applied HFOV will create a "wiggle" in the infant's chest that will be accompanied by vibratory sounds on auscultation. The presence of an adequate wiggle is a good sign, indicating that the ventilator is able to enhance gas exchange. A poor chest wiggle is a sign of low lung compliance (and is often associated with a wiggle of the abdomen that is more prominent than that of the chest). It will usually be impossible to hear typical breath sounds on a patient undergoing HFOV, so additional examination findings necessarily must be substituted to ensure proper placement of the endotracheal tube, symmetry of breath sounds, and so forth. Asymmetric oscillator sounds can

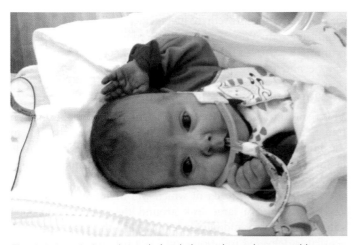

Fig. 8.2 A typical awake and alert baby on intermittent positive pressure ventilation. The patient is interactive with the environment, which allows for developmentally appropriate care to be successfully done.

indicate asymmetric lung expansion, which may be due to a main stem bronchus intubation (in which the right is most likely, given the anatomy) or a unilateral pneumothorax.

High-Frequency Ventilation: Jet Ventilation

A patient placed on the jet ventilator will have findings and interpretations similar to those on HFOV in terms of chest vibration. One difference with high-frequency jet ventilation (HFJV) is that it is used with a conventional ventilator to apply positive end-expiratory pressure and often to supply intermittent inflations (sighs). Thus during HFJV, when conventional sighs are used, auscultation can determine air entry and chest rise during the sigh inflations.

Examination of an Infant on Constant Positive Airway Pressure

Infants requiring nCPAP will typically have either "bubbling" breath sounds, if they are on properly applied bubble nCPAP, or a constant positive airway pressure "roar" if on properly applied infant-flow nCPAP. A preterm infant who has severe retractions, nasal flaring, and grunting and who is placed on nCPAP may quickly exhibit improvement or even resolution of symptoms.

CONCLUSION

The physical examination has been used in its current form for over a century. Despite the rapid proliferation of various laboratory and imaging modalities, the physical examination remains the cornerstone of medical care. Ventilated patients in the NICU are not routinely sedated, and modern ventilators allow for sensing of spontaneous breaths; therefore, the physical examination can be used as a rapid determinant of the adequacy of the support provided by the ventilator. Patients on PPV who are adequately supported should have normal sleep/wake cycles, should breathe comfortably while being supported, and should not be irritable. One should consider adjusting the ventilator of any patient in the NICU on PPV who is irritable, is tachypneic, or manifests increased work of breathing, rather than assuming that the patient requires sedation and/or paralysis. Although steady-state blood gases remain a mainstay of assessing adequacy of ventilator support, the physical examination remains the gold standard for assessing the neonate requiring mechanical ventilation.

KEY REFERENCES

1. Walker HK: The origins of the history and physical examination. In: Walker HK, Hall WD, Hurst JW (eds): Clinical Methods: The History, Physical, and Laboratory Examinations. 3rd ed. Boston, Butterworth, 1990.
4. Reilly BM: Physical examination in the care of medical inpatients: an observational study. Lancet 362:1100–1105, 2003.
5. American Academy of Pediatrics Committee on Fetus and Newborn, American Academy of Pediatrics Section on Surgery, Canadian Paediatric Society Fetus and Newborn Committee, Batton DG, Barrington KJ, Wallman C: Prevention and management of pain in the neonate: an update. Pediatrics 118(5): 2231–2241, November 2006.
6. Tortora D, Severino M, Di Biase C, et al: Early pain exposure influences functional brain connectivity in very preterm neonates. Front Neurosci 3:899, 2019.
8. Dawson JA, Kamlin COF, Vento M, et al: Defining the reference range for oxygen saturation for infants after birth. Pediatrics 125:e1340–e1347, 2010.
10. Dawson JA, Kamlin COF, Wong C, et al: Changes in heart rate in the first minutes after birth. Arch Dis Child Fetal Neonatal Ed 95:F177–F181, 2010.
12. Kent AL, Kecskes Z, Shadbolt B, et al: Normative blood pressure data in the early neonatal period. Pediatr Nephrol 22:1335–1341, 2007.
13. Martin RJ, Fanaroff AA, Walsh MC: Neonatal-Perinatal Medicine. 10th ed. Philadelphia, WB Saunders, 2015.
15. De Jesus LC, Pappas A, Shankaran S, et al: Outcomes of small for gestational age infants born at <27 weeks' gestation. J Pediatr 163(1):55–60, July 2013.
16. EXPRESS Group: Incidence of and risk factors for neonatal morbidity after active perinatal care: extremely preterm infants study in Sweden (EXPRESS). Acta Paediatr 99(7):978–992, July 2010.

9

Imaging: Radiography, Lung Ultrasound, and Other Imaging Modalities

Erik A. Jensen, María V. Fraga, David M. Biko, Francesco Raimondi, and Haresh Kirpalani

KEY POINTS

- Respiratory illnesses are among the most frequent and consequential conditions encountered in the newborn. Although the chest radiograph is an essential diagnostic tool for the evaluation of ill neonates and infants, other modalities such as ultrasound, computed tomography, and magnetic resonance imaging offer important advantages in certain clinical scenarios.
- Owing to the wide range of available imaging modalities, close communication between radiologists and clinicians is essential to select the most appropriate imaging technique to address the diagnostic question, minimize patient radiation exposure, and interpret imaging findings.
- Point of care ultrasound is an evidence-based diagnostic tool that can aid in the placement and surveillance of vascular catheters and facilitate rapid diagnosis of pneumothorax, pleural effusion, and congenital lung lesions.
- Computed tomography and magnetic resonance imaging provide detailed three-dimensional images of the lung that may improve diagnosis and inform care in conditions such as congenital lung lesions and bronchopulmonary dysplasia.

INTRODUCTION

Respiratory illnesses are among the most frequent and potentially life-threatening conditions encountered in the newborn. This makes the radiological examination of the infant chest a common and essential tool to guide the diagnosis and treatment of neonatal lung disease. Using and interpreting imaging studies well require teamwork and open lines of communication between clinicians (including obstetricians, surgeons, and pediatric subspecialists as appropriate) and radiologists. This is particularly true now as digital radiology and point-of-care ultrasound (US) make direct interaction between clinicians and radiologists less common. Although the plain radiograph remains the mainstay of neonatal chest imaging, other modalities such as US, computed tomography (CT), and magnetic resonance imaging (MRI) are increasingly used in the evaluation of ill neonates and infants. Technological advances in fetal imaging also permit improved prenatal diagnosis and, in some cases, fetal treatment of congenital chest lesions.

To provide high-quality care to acute and chronically ill infants, clinicians must understand the capabilities and limitations of available imaging tools and learn to identify the radiographic findings of common neonatal respiratory conditions. Although written materials aid in this educational process, pattern recognition can only be gained through regular review of films. This chapter highlights the important aspects of neonatal chest imaging and provides specific clinical examples directed toward trainees and practicing clinicians. More in-depth discussions of neonatal chest imaging can be found in other reviews.[1,2] Notably, the application of the imaging modalities discussed in this chapter will depend on the local availability of the necessary expertise and radiographic equipment. For each of the described indications for diagnostic imaging and respiratory conditions, we review multiple imaging techniques to help clinicians use this information within their own clinical practice as well as to understand the breadth of current and emerging imaging modalities.

RADIATION EXPOSURE

Several common imaging modalities, including plain radiography, CT, fluoroscopy, and nuclear medicine, use ionizing radiation to produce images. As radiation dose exposure is cumulative and even low total exposure in infancy is associated with a slight increase in the risk of later malignancy, clinicians must weigh the diagnostic advantage of an imaging modality with its expected radiation dose.[3,4] The typical dose from a single chest x-ray (CXR) is approximately 0.008 to 0.03 millisieverts (mSv) depending on the technique and equipment.[5,6] When combined with an abdominal radiograph, the dose is 1.5 to 2 times higher.[5,6] By comparison, the total natural radiation exposure from sources such as the sun and radioactive materials in the air and soil amount to about 3 mSv per year at sea level (roughly equivalent to one CXR per day) and 5 to 6 mSv at an elevation of 5000 feet.[7] The dose from a continuous digital fluoroscopic voiding cystourethrogram is approximately 0.45 to 0.59 mSv.[8] The use of pulsed fluoroscopy optimized for children reduces the dose to 0.05 to 0.07 mSv.[8] The effective dose received from an upper gastrointestinal series is 1.2 to 6.5 mSv.[9] For a chest CT taken without consideration of a patient's weight or dose lowering techniques, the radiation dose is approximately 4 to 7 mSv.[7,10] With low-dose, high-resolution CT, the dose is reduced to about 1 mSv with negligible loss in image quality.[10]

To minimize radiation exposure, clinicians and radiologists should adhere to the practice of "As Low As Reasonably

Achievable," which requires weight-based protocols, limiting the number of studies performed, and the use of nonradiation modalities such as US and MRI when appropriate.[11] The use of collimation (restriction of the x-ray beam to the desired anatomical area) and shielding of adjacent structures, particularly the gonads, are essential to reduce unnecessary radiation exposure. Health care workers also need to be aware of potential risks to themselves and take appropriate precautions to minimize exposure.

IMAGING MODALITIES

Chest Radiograph

The plain chest radiograph or CXR is the most widely used imaging modality in the neonatal intensive care unit (NICU). The CXR uses the natural contrast between air (dark or black on a standard radiograph) and fluid or tissue (white or gray). Appropriate positioning of the infant is essential to produce a high-quality radiograph. A "rotated" CXR may lead to a false diagnosis of cardiomegaly, mediastinal shift, atelectasis, or abnormal central line location (Fig. 9.1). When possible, the infant's arms should be extended away from the chest to prevent the scapulae from obscuring the upper lung fields.

In most cases, a single anterior-posterior (AP) view with the infant in a supine position is adequate to assess the chest wall, heart, airway and lungs, and any invasive lines or tubes. Lateral radiographs of the chest are not routinely necessary but can aid in specific circumstances such as assessment of the retrocardiac lung fields, diagnosis of air leak syndromes, and evaluation of pleural drain location. A systematic approach is recommended when evaluating a CXR to avoid missing potentially important findings. The "alphabet" approach reminds clinicians to assess the airway (trachea and its branches), bones (clavicles, ribs,

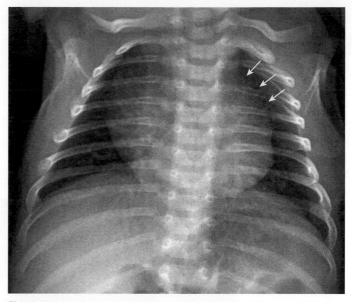

Fig. 9.2 Normal anterior-posterior radiograph of a 26-day-old full-term female. The lungs are clear. There is a left-sided aortic arch and the heart is normal in size. The prominent superior mediastinal contour with wavy borders (*arrows*) is compatible with a normal thymus.

scapulae, vertebrae, and humeri), cardiac structures (heart site, size, shape, border, and great vessels), diaphragm, effusions (small effusions blunt the costophrenic angle), fields and fissures (adequacy and symmetry of lung field expansion and thick or fluid filled fissures), gastric fundus (stomach bubble and other visible intra-abdominal structures), and the hilum and mediastinum.

In a normal, correctly positioned AP CXR, the neonatal chest is trapezoid in shape with horizontal ribs (Fig. 9.2). The diaphragm is domed bilaterally and lies at the level of the sixth to eighth rib. Both lungs should be symmetrically aerated with uniform radiolucency soon after birth. Air bronchograms in the lung bases, particularly in the lower left lobe behind the cardiac border, are normal. Pulmonary vascular markings are visualized centrally and become less prominent toward the periphery. The transverse cardiothoracic ratio should not exceed 60% to 65%.[12] Elimination of the normal border between the radiopaque thoracic structures (e.g., heart, great vessels) and the radiolucent lung, commonly referred to as the "loss of the silhouette" sign, suggests lobar atelectasis or pneumonia, a localized fluid collection, or intrathoracic mass. The thymus is often prominent after birth and may occupy the majority of the upper chest. It can involute during the first days of life, particularly in stressed infants. If a thymic shadow is not visualized on CXR, US may help evaluate for thymic aplasia.[13]

Ultrasound

US is an oscillating sound wave with a frequency outside the human hearing range. The most common form of US used in diagnostic imaging is the pulse echo technique with a brightness-mode (B-mode) display. B-mode involves transmission of a US pulse into the body. The advantages of US include its relative ease of use, noninvasive "real-time" point-of-care imaging capabilities, and lack of ionizing radiation. Although first introduced in

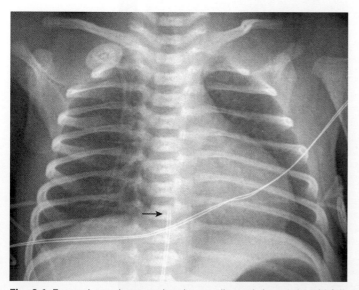

Fig. 9.1 Rotated anterior-posterior chest radiograph in a 4-day-old full-term infant. The right-sided ribs are foreshortened and the left are elongated. The mediastinum appears shifted to the left. An appropriately positioned umbilical venous catheter projects over the left of the spine, just above the diaphragm (*arrow*).

neonatology for imaging of the brain,[14] it is now applied to organ systems throughout the body. The application of US to chest imaging continues to expand as US technology and expertise improve. In the NICU, chest US is an evidence-based tool used for multiple indications including monitoring of lung fluid clearance after birth, diagnosis and management of pleural effusion, assessment of diaphragmatic movement (Fig. 9.3), evaluation of congenital lung lesions (CLLs), diagnosis of air-leak syndromes, and confirmation of endotracheal tube (ETT) and vascular catheter tip location.[15-18]

Lung US is preferably performed with a linear high-frequency probe.[19,20] However, unlike US of solid organs, the US beam does not penetrate in depth beneath the pleura owing to the high acoustic impedance of the air-filled lung. In the healthy neonate, the pleura appears as a regular, hyperechoic, linear structure moving in synchrony with respiration (the so-called "lung sliding sign"). Parenchyma in the normally aerated lung is represented by horizontal reverberations of the pleural line, known as A-lines (Fig. 9.4). With an increase in the fluid-to-air ratio such as in lung inflammation or edema,

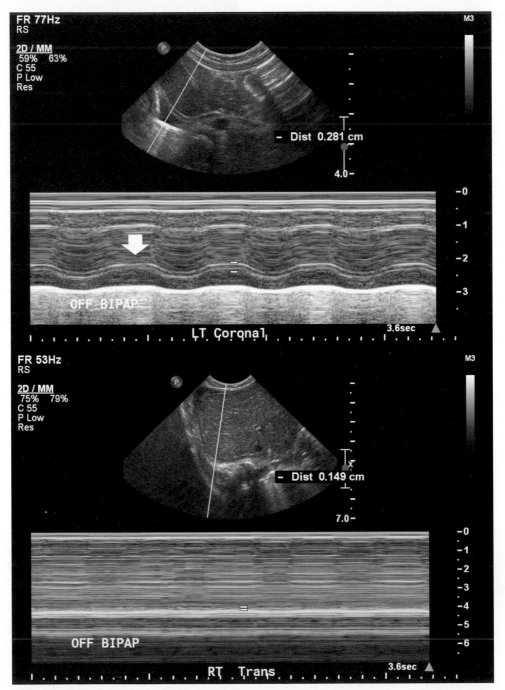

Fig. 9.3 M-mode ultrasound of the chest in a 1-month-old female who is status post repair of coarctation of the aorta. The top image demonstrates normal sinusoidal motion (*arrow*) of the left leaflet of the diaphragm. In the bottom image, there is no motion of the right leaflet of the diaphragm, compatible with paralysis.

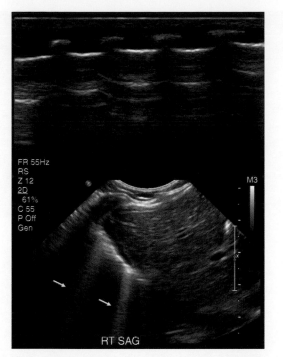

Fig. 9.4 Ultrasound images of the lung. In the top image of a normal lung, the pleura appears as a thin and regular hyperechoic line interrupted by the rib shadows. Horizontal reverberations below the pleural, known as A-lines (*red arrows*), are clearly visible. In the bottom image, long hyperechoic vertical lines, known as B-lines (*yellow arrows*), project from the pleural line adjacent to the diaphragm.

A-lines are replaced by vertical hyperechoic artifacts known as B-lines (Fig. 9.4). When a consolidation develops within the lung as seen in pneumonia or atelectasis, the loss in air content leads to a hypoechoic image with similar echodensity as the liver.

Computed Tomography

CT combines a series of x-rays performed helically around an axis of rotation to generate high-quality cross-sectional images of the body. Chest CT is useful for the identification and diagnosis of space-occupying lesions such as congenital pulmonary airway malformations (CPAMs), bronchopulmonary sequestration (BPS), and congenital or acquired lobar emphysema. CT and CT angiography (CTA) are also used in some centers in the evaluation and management of severe bronchopulmonary dysplasia (BPD) and pulmonary hypertension.[21-24] Emerging techniques such as dynamic airway imaging and dual-energy CT show promise as tools to evaluate the large airways and vascular perfusion of the lung parenchyma in these diseases.[25,26] Importantly, although these novel techniques may improve disease characterization and phenotyping in severe BPD and other cardiopulmonary diseases related to prematurity, the extent to which advanced CT imaging will augment clinical care and improve outcomes in these conditions is uncertain. Finally, although low-dose CT substantially reduces the effective radiation dose compared with previous techniques, clinicians should carefully assess the risks and benefits of this imaging modality before ordering any study.

Fluoroscopy

Fluoroscopy produces real-time, dynamic images using rapid, sequential x-rays. Fluoroscopy is most commonly used in neonates and infants to image the gastrointestinal and genitourinary tracts. In infants with respiratory distress of unclear etiology, fluoroscopy may aid in the identification of a tracheo-esophageal fistula or occult aspiration. Fluoroscopy can also assess diaphragmatic excursion and diagnose large airway diseases such as tracheobronchomalacia. As described earlier, fluoroscopy can result in substantial radiation exposure if dose-limiting procedures such as pulsed fluoroscopy, reduced pulse widths and pulse rates, appropriate beam filtration, increased source-to-skin distance, and proper collimation are not used appropriately.[27]

Magnetic Resonance Imaging

MRI uses the energy emitted by magnetically aligned protons to image anatomical structures within the body.[28] MRI does not require exposure to ionizing radiation; however, its use is limited in many centers by a lack of availability, expense, and the frequent need to administer anesthesia to infants to acquire high-quality images of the lung. Although the primary role of MRI in the neonate is to image the brain and heart, advances in pulmonary MRI such as ultrashort echo time and hyperpolarized gas techniques are expanding the utility of this imaging modality to infants and young children with respiratory disease.[29-31]

INVASIVE SUPPORT DEVICES

There is no evidence to support daily imaging to evaluate the position of invasive support devices. However, if malposition is suspected, imaging should be performed to prevent or ameliorate iatrogenic complications. Although x-ray is the most common imaging modality used to assess the position of invasive support equipment, point-of-care ultrasound (POCUS) is gaining popularity as a reliable bedside tool for this purpose. The choice of imaging technique will vary by center according to the availability of trained sonographers (clinicians, radiologists, or technicians) and the type and location of the support device under evaluation.

Endotracheal Tube

In ventilated infants, the ETT should be placed in the mid trachea between the second and fourth thoracic vertebral body and at least 1 cm above the carina. Deep positioning, typically into in the right mainstem bronchus, can result in unilateral baro- and volutrauma, pneumothorax, and collapse of the contralateral lung (Fig. 9.5). When performing a radiograph to determine ETT location, care should be taken to position the infant without rotation and with the neck in a neutral position. Extension of the neck will misleadingly suggest high placement of the ETT and the opposite during flexion.

The use of POCUS to visualize the ETT is hindered by the poor conductance of sound waves through air.[32] Nonetheless, the literature describes several US methods to identify esophageal intubation at the bedside. The quickest US technique for verifying ETT placement uses a transversely oriented transducer placed over the trachea above the sternal notch to visualize the

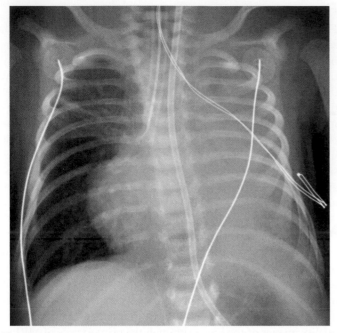

Fig. 9.5 Deep positioning of an endotracheal tube in a 19-day-old male with truncus arteriosus. The endotracheal tube (ETT) terminates in the right mainstem bronchus and there is resultant "white out" from atelectasis of the left lung. The streaky atelectasis seen in the right upper lobe suggests that this lobe is also under ventilated secondary to the malpositioned ETT.

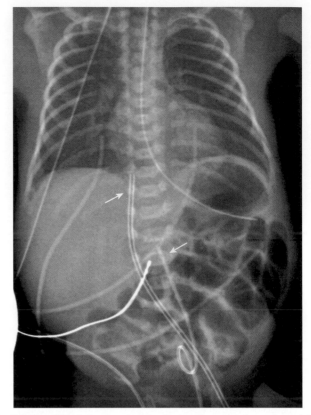

Fig. 9.6 Combined chest and abdominal radiograph of a preterm infant with acceptably positioned umbilical catheters. The tip of the umbilical venous line (*white arrow*) is in the inferior vena cava just above the diaphragm and the tip of a "low" lying umbilical arterial line (*yellow arrow*) is just above the L3 vertebral body.

airway and the esophagus. During intubation, observation of an empty esophagus and widening of the subglottis indicates successful tracheal intubation while the appearance of the ETT in the esophagus, referred to as "double trachea sign," indicates esophageal intubation.[33] Adult and pediatric literature shows a sensitivity and specificity of 98.5% to 100% and 75% to 100%, respectively, for this method.[33-36] Additional techniques for US-based verification of ETT position include distance from the ETT tip to the carina, aortic arch, right pulmonary artery, or thyroid, with or without bilateral sliding lung sign.[37-41]

Vascular Catheters

The umbilical artery and vein are commonly used to gain vascular access during the first days of life in preterm and ill neonates. On radiograph, an umbilical venous catheter (UVC) should lie at the junction of the inferior vena cava (IVC) and the right atrium (Fig. 9.6). Lateral CXR and thoracic vertebral level on AP CXR do not accurately identify UVC tip location.[42] Importantly, POCUS is now deemed superior to x-ray for identifying UVC tip position, especially in situations where abnormal anatomy, such as in congenital diaphragmatic hernia (CDH), hinder radiographic assessment.[42-45] UVC tip location is easily evaluated with US using a linear, curvilinear, or phased-array probe in a longitudinal IVC view (Fig. 9.7).

An umbilical artery catheter (UAC) can be placed in a "high" position, with the tip above the abdominal visceral arteries between the T7 and T9 vertebral bodies, or in a "low" position, with the tip between the L3 and L5 vertebral bodies (Fig. 9.6). Data from a small number of randomized infants

suggest that "high" placement of UACs is associated with a lower incidence of vascular complications (e.g., ischemic injury, aortic thrombosis).[43] When a "low" UAC is placed, a phased-array or curvilinear US transducer in a coronal abdominal view should be used to ensure the tip is positioned between the iliac bifurcation and the level of the renal arteries (Fig. 9.8A). The addition of color Doppler can highlight this area (Fig. 9.8B). For a "high" UAC, a longitudinal IVC view is obtained and the transducer fanned to the patient's left to visualize the descending aorta (Fig. 9.8C).

Peripherally inserted central catheters (PICCs) are optimally placed in an upper or lower extremity with the terminal end in a major vein near the heart (Fig. 9.9).[46,47] As a reference, the cavo-atrial junction is located approximately two vertebral bodies below the carina on AP CXR.[48] One of the most common applications for POCUS is to identify peripheral veins during PICC placement and assist with line positioning, mitigating the need for multiple readjustments and confirmatory radiographs (Fig. 9.10).[49-52] Because PICCs are prone to migration, periodic surveillance is recommended to prevent iatrogenic complications such as pleural effusion or cardiac tamponade (Fig. 9.9).[53,54] In particular, sudden worsening of respiratory status when an upper extremity PICC is present, and new onset limb swelling warrant prompt evaluation of the catheter's location and function. Arm positioning during

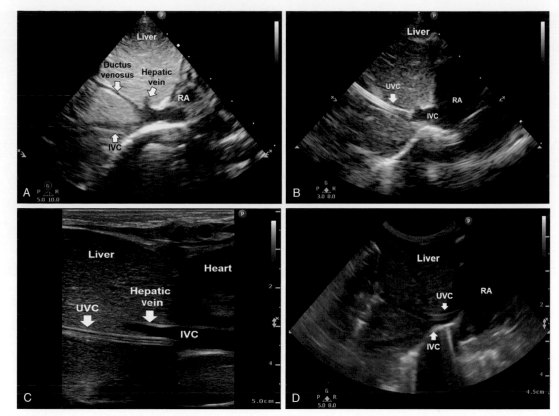

Fig. 9.7 A series of ultrasound images showing the position of an umbilical venous catheter (*UVC*) in the ductus venosus alongside adjacent landmarks. **(A)** A long axis view of the inferior vena cava (*IVC*) obtained by a phased array transducer demonstrates normal anatomy. **(B)** A long axis view shows the UVC in the ductus venosus terminating at the IVC junction. **(C)** A long axis view obtained with a linear transducer shows the UVC entering the IVC. **(D)** Visualization of the UVC entering the right atrium using a curvilinear transducer. *RA*, Right atrium.

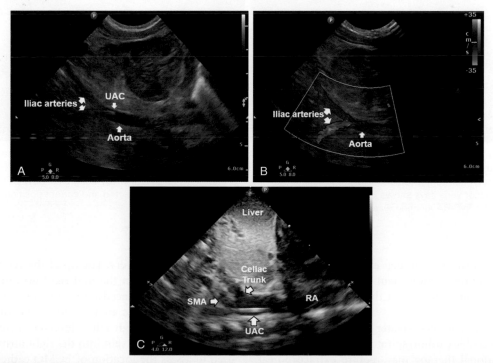

Fig. 9.8 A series of ultrasound images of an umbilical arterial catheter (*UAC*). **(A)** Curvilinear transducer in a left coronal abdominal view demonstrating the UAC tip in a low-lying position above the iliac bifurcation. **(B)** Visualization of the iliac bifurcation using color Doppler. **(C)** Long axis view of the descending aorta demonstrating high lying UAC. *SMA*, Superior mesenteric artery; *RA*, right atrium.

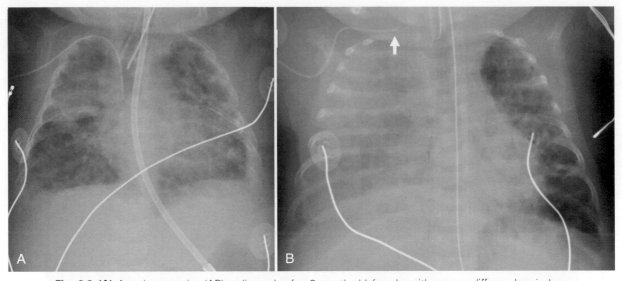

Fig. 9.9 (A) Anterior-posterior (AP) radiograph of a 3-month-old female with severe diffuse chronic lung disease. Patchy coarse opacities from atelectasis are present throughout the lung and are especially promi-nent and confluent in the right middle lobe. The right-sided peripherally inserted central venous catheter (PICC) is appropriately placed with the tip just proximal to superior caval-atrial junction. **(B)** AP radiograph of a 5-month-old male with severe bronchopulmonary dysplasia (BPD) who developed a large pleural effusion from extravasation of parenteral nutrition after inadvertent migration of a PICC (*arrow*). The scattered coarse opacities characteristic of severe BPD are seen throughout the right lung. The tip of the endotracheal tube is just below the thoracic inlet.

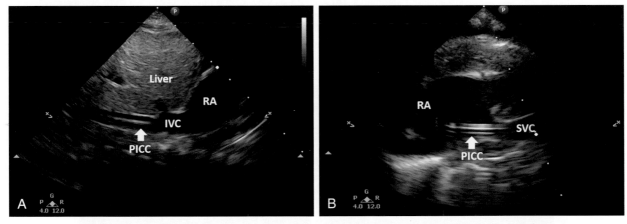

Fig. 9.10 Ultrasound (US) is used to confirm correct positioning of peripherally inserted central venous catheter (*PICC*) during placement. **(A)** Longitudinal view of the inferior vena cava (*IVC*) shows the PICC (*arrow*) correctly positioned near the junction of the IVC and right atrium (*RA*). **(B)** Long axis view of the superior vena cava shows the PICC (*arrow*) entering the RA. This line was retracted and correct positioning at the SVC-RA junction was subsequently confirmed by US.

placement and surveillance of upper extremity PICCs also requires specific attention as movement (flexion/extension at the elbow and abduction/adduction at the shoulder) can alter tip location.[55]

Infants with gestational ages greater than 34 weeks with early, severe, and reversible cardiorespiratory failure who do not respond to conventional therapy may require extracorporeal membrane oxygenation (ECMO). Venoarterial (VA) ECMO and venovenous (VV) ECMO are both used in neonates. In VA ECMO, catheters are inserted into the internal jugular vein and

common carotid artery. The tip of the venous cannula is most commonly placed in the mid right atrium and the tip of the arterial cannula is placed at the junction of the common carotid artery and the aortic arch.[56,57] In VV ECMO, blood is drained and reinfused through a dual-lumen catheter inserted although the internal jugular vein into the right atrium.[56,57] CXR can be used to assess the location of ECMO catheters (eFig. 9.1), but POCUS is a more reliable technique, especially when pulmo-nary edema develops and there is complete loss of anatomic landmarks (Fig. 9.11).[58]

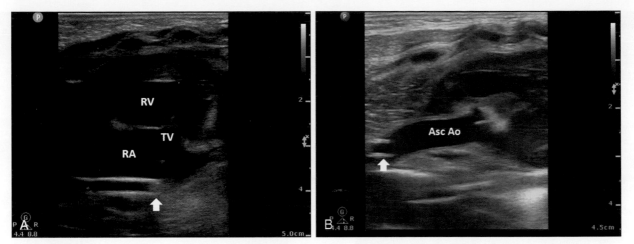

Fig. 9.11 Ultrasound is used to confirm correct positioning of venous and arterial cannulae used for extracorporeal membrane oxygenation in a full-term infant with hypoxemic respiratory failure. **(A)** The tip of the venous cannula (arrow) in shown in right atrium (*RA*). **(B)** The tip of the arterial cannula enters the aortic arch. *Asc Ao*, Ascending aorta; *RV*, right ventricle; *TV*, tricuspid valve.

COMMON ETIOLOGIES OF RESPIRATORY DISTRESS IN INFANTS

Respiratory Distress Syndrome

Primary respiratory distress syndrome (RDS) results from surfactant deficiency in the premature neonate and is the most common respiratory disorder among infants born less than 32 weeks' gestation.[59] Lower gestational age and birth weight, lack of exposure to antenatal corticosteroids, perinatal asphyxia, and maternal diabetes are important risk factors for RDS.[60,61] Clinical signs of RDS often present at or soon after birth and include tachypnea, grunting, chest wall retractions, nasal flaring, and hypoxemia.[61] Importantly, these signs may be indistinguishable from other causes of early respiratory failure such as congenital pneumonia (especially secondary to group B streptococcus), sepsis, and persistent pulmonary hypertension of the newborn (PPHN) in more mature infants. Secondary surfactant deficiency may also occur later in the neonatal period concomitant with episodes of hypoxemia, pulmonary edema, or infection (e.g., respiratory syncytial virus, bacterial pneumonia).

The CXR appearance in RDS depends on the severity of the disease. The classic findings are low lung volumes with a fine granular or "ground glass" appearance with air bronchograms (Fig. 9.12). In mild RDS, a diffuse, linear granular pattern is most common. Air bronchograms become more prominent as disease worsens and in severe cases the lungs are opaque, and the cardiac border is often difficult to identify (eFig. 9.2). These CXR findings are modified by the administration of positive airway pressure and exogenous surfactant. Exogenous surfactant typically distributes throughout the lung in a nonuniform way and can result in a heterogeneous radiographic appearance with asymmetrical multifocal opacities. This pattern may mimic the appearance of pneumonia and can be difficult to differentiate if earlier imaging is not available. When severe RDS is observed in more mature infants and fails to respond to conventional management, clinicians

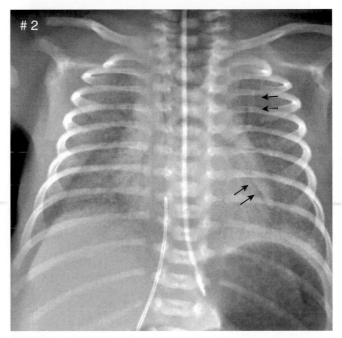

Fig. 9.12 Anterior-posterior radiographs of a newborn 26-week gestation female infant with respiratory distress syndrome. There are diffuse ground glass opacities throughout the lung fields with prominent air bronchograms (*arrows*). A nasogastric tube and a large stomach bubble are seen. The umbilical venous catheter is in good position.

should consider congenital etiologies such as surfactant deficiencies and alveolar capillary dysplasia.

RDS produces a "white lung image" on US with no spared areas. The pleural line is thick and coarse and small subpleural consolidations are often present (Fig. 9.13).[62] A lung US score has been validated to gauge the severity of RDS.[63] The score correlates well with the clinical and oxygenation status including subsequent likelihood of exogenous surfactant therapy.[64] International evidence-based recommendations suggest

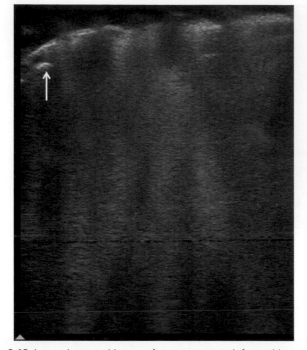

Fig. 9.13 Lung ultrasound image of a very preterm infant with respiratory distress syndrome. A "white lung image" with no spared areas is superiorly limited by a thick and coarse pleural image. A small subpleural consolidation is present (*white arrow*).

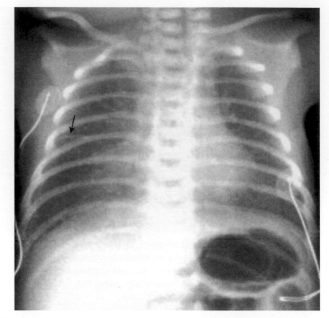

Fig. 9.14 Anterior-posterior radiograph of a 1-day-old full-term male born via cesarean section with moderate respiratory distress secondary to transient tachypnea of the newborn (TTN). Fine granular opacities, similar to respiratory distress syndrome, are seen throughout. The prominent perihalar streaking and small pleural effusion observed in the interlobar fissure on the right (*arrow*) are common findings in TTN.

comparable diagnostic accuracy for lung US and plain chest radiograph for the diagnosis of RDS; however, US may be superior for predicting failure of noninvasive respiratory support within the first 24 hours.[65,66] Notably, unlike CXR, lung US findings do not change soon after surfactant administration,[67] and the expected time until restoration of normal lung US findings is uncertain.

Transient Tachypnea of the Newborn

Transient tachypnea of the newborn (TTN) is characterized by mild to moderate respiratory distress that gradually improves during the first 48 to 72 hours after birth. TTN results from the delayed clearance of fetal lung fluid and is more commonly observed in infants with a history of maternal diabetes and those born via cesarean section.[68-70] The CXR shows normal to mildly overexpanded lungs with a diffuse hazy appearance and increased interstitial streaky shadowing extending to the periphery. Small pleural effusions, typically seen as prominence of the interlobar fissures, are common (Fig. 9.14). Early CXRs in TTN can appear similar to those of more serious conditions such as infection, surfactant deficiency, or cardiac failure. On US, TTN presents with variable densities of B-lines with a regular pleural image and no subpleural consolidations (Fig. 9.15).[71] Hyperechoic artifacts in the lower lung fields, the so-called "double lung point" sign, is an inconsistent finding that can also be observed in some RDS cases.[72] Consequently, at present, there is a lack of consensus regarding specific sonographic criteria that should be used to differentiate between infants with RDS and those with TTN.[72]

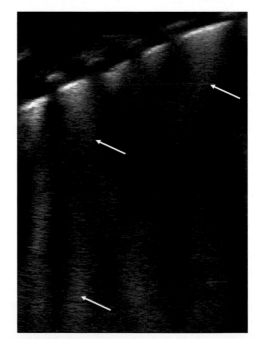

Fig. 9.15 Lung ultrasound of an infant with transient tachypnea of the newborn. Hyperechoic vertical artifacts (*arrows*), known as B lines, depart from a thin and regular pleural line. The number and the echodensity of B lines may be variable.

Meconium Aspiration Syndrome

Meconium is a viscous, hyperosmolar substance composed of water, mucous, gastrointestinal secretions, bile acids, pancreatic enzymes, lanugo, vernix caseosa, and blood.[73,74] Meconium stained fluid is present in approximately 10% to 15% of live births, but only 1% to 2% suffer significant respiratory compromise resulting from aspiration of meconium.[75,76] Fetal stress (e.g., hypoxemia, acidosis, infection) is a common antecedent of in utero passage of meconium and most infants with meconium aspiration syndrome (MAS) are born at or near full term.[77] Severe respiratory distress and hypoxemia are characteristic of MAS, and ventilation perfusion mismatch and acidosis can worsen PPHN.

The CXR findings in MAS range from lung hyperexpansion with or without heterogeneous patchy infiltrates to complete opacification of the thorax (Fig. 9.16). Pleural effusion can also develop and air trapping caused by a "ball-valve" phenomenon may lead to pneumothorax. Exogenous surfactant therapy is often beneficial, but similar to RDS, it can transiently increase the heterogeneous appearance of the lung parenchyma.[78]

The findings of MAS on POCUS are nonspecific with variable combinations of B-lines and consolidated areas that change over time potentially caused by evolving lung inflammation and meconium-induced lung injury.[79]

Pneumonia

Pneumonia is an important cause of neonatal morbidity and mortality. The estimated incidence ranges from 1.5 to 5 cases per 1000 live births.[80] Neonatal pneumonia is generally classified as early or late in onset. Early-onset pneumonia presents within the first week of life with respiratory distress and systemic signs of sepsis including poor perfusion, lethargy, and jaundice. Most early-onset pneumonias are acquired congenitally from transplacental inoculation or perinatally from the maternal vaginal tract. The presentation of early-onset pneumonia is similar to RDS, but a history of prolonged rupture of membranes, chorioamnionitis, or elevated inflammatory markers may help distinguish between the two. Pleural effusion is also more common in pneumonia than RDS (eFig. 9.3). The most common pathogens associated with early pneumonias are group B *Streptococci* and Gram-negative rods. Congenital viral infections and occasionally atypical bacterial (e.g., *Chlamydia trachomatis*) and fungal infections can also present as early pneumonia.

Late-onset pneumonia presents after the first week of life and is often a nosocomial complication of mechanical ventilation. Common pathogens include coagulase-negative *Staphylococci*, *Staphylococcus aureus*, Gram-negative rods (e.g., *Pseudomonas*), and *Candida*.[81] Viral infections such as rhinovirus, respiratory syncytial virus, and influenza can also cause late-onset pneumonia. The chest radiograph in late-onset pneumonia is diffusely hazy, similar to RDS, but in contrast to early-onset pneumonia, the lungs often exhibit normal or hyper-expansion with heterogeneously distributed densities (eFig. 9.4). Localized lobar pneumonias are uncommon in neonates but can develop in older infants and, when severe, result in lung necrosis and empyema. A chest CT can help confirm the diagnosis in these cases (eFig. 9.5).

Pneumonia appears on US as a hypoechoic area adjacent to an irregular and often fragmented pleural line (Fig. 9.17). With loss of aeration, the lung echodensity appears similar to the liver. The presence of dynamic bronchograms that appear as hyperlucent spots moving within the hypoechoic bronchial image may distinguish atelectasis from pneumonia.[66] Although a rare complication in infants, US may also help identify lung abscesses and determine whether higher-level imaging such as chest CT is indicated.

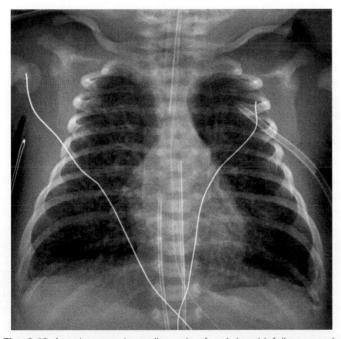

Fig. 9.16 Anterior-posterior radiograph of a 1-day-old full-term male with meconium aspiration syndrome (MAS). The lungs are hyperinflated (flattened diaphragms and 10–11 rib lung expansion) with patchy, rope-like opacities projecting from the hilum to the periphery. A "high" lying umbilical arterial catheter is seen at T6 and a malpositioned umbilical venous catheter is seen close to the right atrium. The percutaneous chest tube present on the left was placed to drain a large pneumothorax, a common complication in severe MAS.

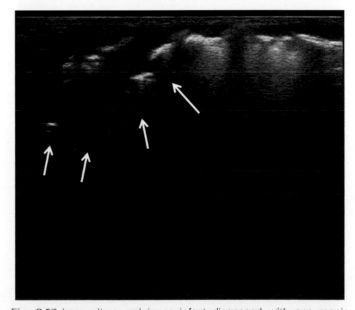

Fig. 9.17 Lung ultrasound in an infant diagnosed with pneumonia shows a thick, coarse, and vastly fragmented pleura beneath which are hypoechoic areas (*arrows*) with irregular lower margins.

Air Leak Syndromes

The application of positive airway pressure to poorly compliant or "stiff" lungs can result in leakage of air from the alveoli into the extra-alveolar space. The most common conditions that arise from alveolar air leak are pneumothorax, pulmonary interstitial emphysema (PIE), pneumomediastinum, and pneumopericardium. Rarely, pneumoperitoneum and subcutaneous emphysema can also develop.

Pneumothorax

Pneumothorax is the most common air leak syndrome in infants and occurs in approximately 2% to 10% of those with birth weights between 500 and 1500 g.[82-84] The clinical presentation of pneumothorax varies from an incidental finding on CXR to severe respiratory distress and cardiovascular collapse. A large pneumothorax is easily detected on AP CXR. The characteristic findings are air in the pleural space with compression of the affected lung, flattening of the diaphragm, and shift of the mediastinum to the contralateral side (Fig. 9.18, eFig. 9.6). In contrast, small pneumothoraces can be difficult to appreciate. In the supine infant, free air collects anterior to the lung and a collapsed edge may not be visible. Increased lucency on the affected side or a tiny lucent rim along the diaphragm may be the only findings. A lateral decubitus x-ray with the affected side up is often helpful in this situation. Large pneumothoraces generally require percutaneous decompression, whereas smaller ones that do not cause cardiorespiratory compromise may resorb spontaneously.[85]

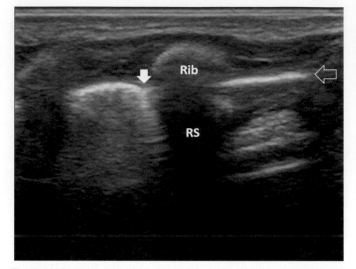

Fig. 9.19 Sagittal ultrasound view of the left chest in an infant with pneumothorax. The area where the visceral pleura begins to separate from the parietal pleura at the margin of the pneumothorax is the "lung point" (*closed arrow*). The pleural line (*open arrow*) is indicated adjacent to the rib shadow (*RS*).

Lung US offers a rapid and potentially more sensitive tool relative to x-ray and transillumination for diagnosing pneumothorax.[86-88] POCUS may be particularly valuable for detecting pneumothorax in settings where there are foreseeable delays in obtaining chest radiography. In one study, POCUS, relative to clinical assessment, reduced the time to diagnosis and drainage of pneumothorax by an average of approximately 15 minutes.[17] US signs of pneumothorax include absence of "pleural sliding," seen as movement of the visceral pleura on the parietal pleura with respiration, the "stratosphere" or "barcode" sign in M-mode, absence of lung pulse, absence of B-lines in the area of the pneumothorax, and the "lung point" sign (Fig. 9.19).[89] Lung point occurs at the border of the pneumothorax, where there is intermittent contact of the lung with the chest wall.[90]

Pneumomediastinum

Pneumomediastinum results from leakage of air into the mediastinal space. In most cases, affected infants are asymptomatic, but large collections of air may lead to respiratory or cardiac compromise. Similar to pneumothorax, pneumomediastinum most commonly occurs during positive pressure ventilation. On radiograph, a pneumomediastinum is most commonly seen as air surrounding the thymus above the cardiac shadow (Fig. 9.20). When large, it appears as a halo around the heart on AP view and as a retrosternal or superior mediastinal lucency on the lateral view.[91,92] The characteristic "spinnaker sail" sign is best appreciated on a left anterior oblique view, in which air is seen surrounding the thymus above the cardiac shadow (Fig. 9.21).[92]

Pneumopericardium

Pneumopericardium results from entrapment of air in the pericardial space and typically occurs only in infants with severe RDS who also have a pneumothorax or other air leak. Although it can be insidious in onset, the most common presentation is

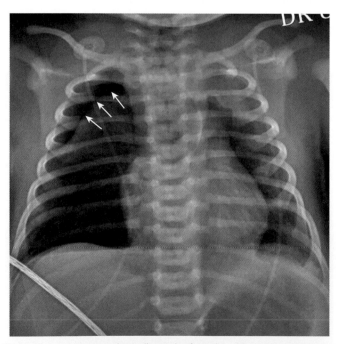

Fig. 9.18 Anterior-posterior radiograph of a 1-day-old, 41-week gestation female infant who developed a right-sided pneumothorax after receiving positive pressure bag-mask ventilation in the delivery room. The lateral edge of the right lung is displaced from the chest wall (*arrows*) and air within the pleural cavity outlines the right diaphragm.

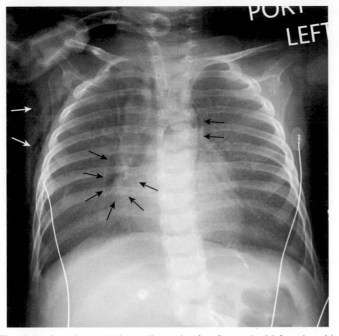

Fig. 9.20 Anterior-posterior radiograph of a 6-month-old female with pneumomediastinum. Streaky lucencies are seen along the upper mediastinum, outlining the thymus and descending thoracic aorta (*black arrows*). There is extension of air into the neck and subcutaneous emphysema is present along the right lateral chest wall (*white arrows*). The diffuse ground glass opacification of the lungs is from surfactant protein C deficiency.

abrupt hemodynamic compromise caused by cardiac tamponade. Pneumopericardium and pneumomediastinum share similar findings on AP CXR. A characteristic feature in pneumopericardium is air surrounding the cardiac border that does not extend beyond the reflection of the aorta or the pulmonary artery.[93] The presence of air under the heart is also diagnostic.[94] US detection of pneumopericardium is especially rapid and can be life-saving.[95]

Pulmonary Interstitial Emphysema

PIE is a consequence of alveolar rupture into the peribronchial space with subsequent spreading of air through the lymphatic vessels within the lung interstitium. PIE most commonly develops during the first week of life in preterm infants with moderate to severe RDS who are treated with high-pressure mechanical ventilation. The clinical presentation typically includes worsening hypoxemia and hypercarbia, which may trigger clinicians to increase ventilator settings and potentially exacerbate the disease. There is no definitive treatment for PIE; however, minimization of further baro- or volutrauma may help prevent additional air leak. Subsequent development of BPD is common in preterm infants with PIE.[96]

On CXR, PIE appears as small cystic or linear translucencies extending from the hilum to the periphery (Fig. 9.22, eFig. 9.7). Generally, both lungs are diffusely affected but unilateral and unilobar disease is also possible. Lung volumes usually appear increased in PIE and as a result may be mistaken for improvement in RDS as the lungs commonly appear darker and better

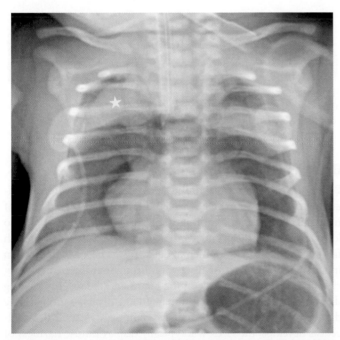

Fig. 9.21 Anterior-posterior radiograph of a 1-day-old, 34-week gestation male infant with pneumomediastinum. The lungs are diffusely hazy bilaterally with ground glass opacities consistent with respiratory distress syndrome. The thymus (*star*) is outlined by air and elevated away from the cardiac borders creating a "spinnaker sail sign." An anterior right-sided pneumothorax is also likely present.

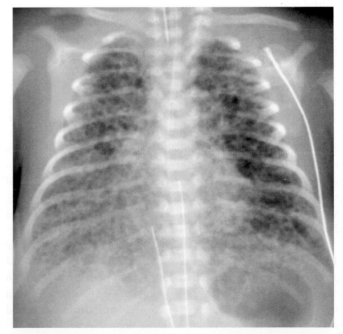

Fig. 9.22 Anterior-posterior radiograph of a 7-day-old, 26-week gestation male infant with bilateral pulmonary interstitial emphysema. The lungs are hyperinflated (flattened diaphragm and prominent posterior lung fields) with streaky lucencies throughout. The tip of the endotracheal tube is at the thoracic inlet and should be advanced. An umbilical venous catheter and "high" lying umbilical arterial catheter are appropriately positioned.

aerated in both cases.[97] Subpleural cysts can also develop and rupture causing a pneumothorax.

Pulmonary Hemorrhage

Pulmonary hemorrhage is an acute, often severe form of pulmonary edema that ranges in clinical presentation from a small amount of fresh, frothy blood from the airway to catastrophic bleeding and cardiopulmonary collapse. Prematurity is the most common risk factor. Other predisposing factors include asphyxia, patent ductus arteriosus, coagulopathy, infection, and severe respiratory distress. The findings on CXR range from patchy infiltrates to complete opacification of one or more lung fields (eFig. 9.8). Using a "splint" of high mean airway pressure may decrease bleeding in pulmonary hemorrhage while attempts are made to correct the underlying etiology. Mortality is 30% to 40%.

Lung US can aid in the identification of pulmonary hemorrhage. Findings include the "shred" sign, consolidation with air bronchograms, pleural line abnormalities, and disappearing A-lines.[98] The shred sign, which appears from a poorly demarcated border between the aerated and consolidated lung, may be the most sensitive and specific of these findings.[98]

Pleural Effusion

Pleural effusion is the accumulation of fluid between the visceral and parietal pleura. Pleural effusions are defined based on the timing of onset (congenital or acquired) and the content of the fluid (hydrothorax, chylothorax, or hemothorax). When sufficiently large, pleural effusions cause respiratory distress and hypoxemia caused by impaired lung expansion. Congenital pleural effusions can also cause pulmonary hypoplasia.

Congenital hydrothorax is often associated with hydrops fetalis. Congenital chylothorax results from malformation of the thoracic lymphatic vessels and may be syndromic (e.g., Turner, Down, or Noonan syndrome). Newborns with large congenital effusions present with severe respiratory distress at birth and emergent drainage is often necessary. Acquired hydrothorax is categorized as infectious or noninfectious in etiology. Common infectious organisms include Group B *Streptococcus*, *staphylococcus aureus*, and *Bacteroides fragilis*.[99] Noninfectious etiologies include RDS, TTN, MAS, congenital heart disease, and renal failure. Hydrothorax may also result from extravasation of parenteral nutrition from a central venous catheter (Fig. 9.9). Acquired chylo- and hemothorax are potential complications of thoracic surgery or misplacement of pleural drains.

On CXR, small pleural effusions blunt the costophrenic angle (Fig. 9.23). As the volume of pleural fluid increases, there is progressive opacification of the hemithorax (Fig. 9.9). Pleural effusion is easily identified on lung US as a hypoechoic collection between the parietal and visceral pleura (Fig. 9.24). Semiquantification and serial monitoring of effusion volume are well-established uses of POCUS.[100,101] Furthermore, when thoracentesis is indicated, POCUS can provide procedural guidance and help reduce the rate of complications.[102] Magnetic resonance lymphangiography may also aid in the diagnosis of congenital or acquired lymphatic abnormalities and permit simultaneous treatment with ethiodized oil embolization (eFigs. 9.9 and 9.10).[103]

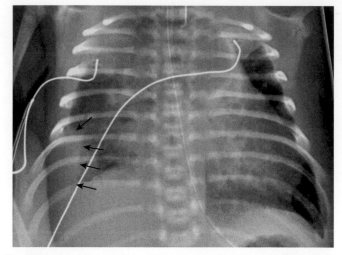

Fig. 9.23 Anterior-posterior radiograph of a 5-week-old full-term male with trisomy 21 with a moderate right-sided pleural effusion (*black arrows*). The appearance of cardiomegaly and diffuse vascular congestion is consistent with the complete atrioventricular canal defect.

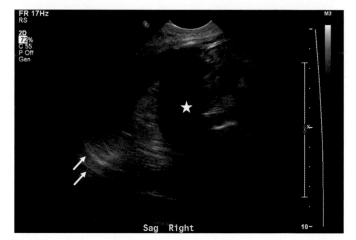

Fig. 9.24 Sagittal ultrasound image of the right lung. A-lines (*white arrows*) are the horizontal lines inferior to the atelectatic lung that is compressed by a surrounding, hypoechoic pleural effusion (*star*).

Bronchopulmonary Dysplasia

BPD is the most common chronic respiratory complication associated with preterm birth.[104] Affected infants suffer higher rates of neonatal and childhood mortality and survivors are predisposed to long-term respiratory and cardiovascular impairments, growth failure, and neurodevelopmental delay.[105,106] The CXR findings in infants with or at risk for BPD vary throughout the neonatal period and depend on the age of the infant and the severity of lung disease. Many infants born less than 1000 g display minimal lung disease right after birth and can have an initially clear CXR. If atelectasis develops, the CXR will typically display diffuse haziness of the lung fields. Once positive airway pressure is applied, the CXR shows a more heterogeneous pattern of lung collapse (Fig. 9.25A). If lung disease persists, coarse interstitial densities and small cyst-like areas can develop. This may progress over the subsequent weeks and months into generalized hyperinflation with larger

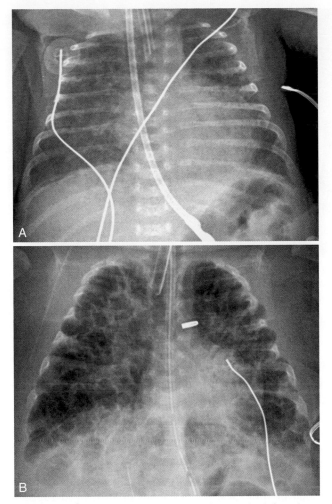

Fig. 9.25 Anterior-posterior radiographs of a male infant born at 23 weeks' gestation and 590 g who developed severe bronchopulmonary dysplasia. **(A)** At 6 weeks of age, there are coarse, diffuse interstitial markings consistent with subsegmental atelectasis and early chronic lung disease. **(B)** At 3 months of age, the lungs are hyperinflated with diffuse cystic disease in a "honeycomb" pattern. The heart appears small in comparison to the earlier radiograph (A) likely because of high intrathoracic pressure. A surgical clip from a patent ductus arteriosus closure is also seen in the later radiograph.

findings: hyperexpansion, emphysema, and fibrous/interstitial abnormalities.[23] When compared with CXR alone, the Ochiai CT score showed better correlation with the duration of oxygen therapy and clinical scoring of disease severity.[23] Studies of other scoring methods have also demonstrated an association between CT findings in BPD and the presence and severity of abnormalities detected on pulmonary function testing.[111-113] Despite these promising findings, the valid application of CT scoring systems may be reduced by the limited interrater reliability of some score components.[111]

In addition to assessment of lung disease severity, CT can be used to diagnose occult complications of BPD such as acquired lobar emphysema and focal atelectatic or infectious consolidations. Comparison of inspiratory and expiratory CT images and dynamic airway imaging may aid the diagnosis of airway disease such as tracheobrochomalacia.[114,115] However, the true diagnostic accuracy of these less invasive techniques relative to bronchoscopy in infants with BPD is uncertain. CTA may compliment echocardiography and cardiac catheterization detection of pulmonary hypertension (Fig. 9.26).[21,22] Dual-energy

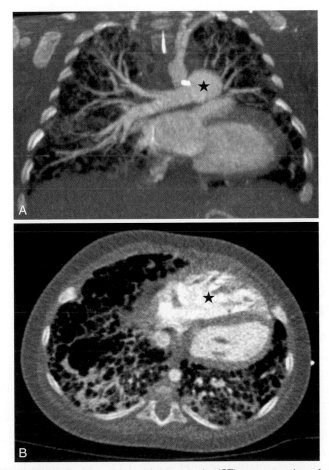

Fig. 9.26 (A) Coronal computed tomography (CT) reconstruction of an infant with severe BPD and pulmonary hypertension. Engorgement of the pulmonary arterial branches is seen centrally (*star*) with thinning and tapering ("pruning") of the vessels peripherally. **(B)** Axial image of a CT angiogram in an infant with pulmonary hypertension. The right ventricle is enlarged (*arrow*) and the intraventricular septum is bowed abnormally away from the right ventricle into the left ventricle. Although this is not a lung window, findings of chronic lung disease are noted throughout the parenchyma with cystic change and areas of architectural distortion.

cystic areas and increased linear densities (Fig. 9.25B).[107] Acquired lobar emphysema can develop as a sequelae of severe BPD and may require surgical resection if the emphysematous lobe prevents adequate aeration of the remaining lung (eFig. 9.11).[108] Right ventricular enlargement from cor pulmonale may also become apparent. The radiographic abnormalities seen in surviving infants with BPD often improve over time as new alveoli develop, but this process may take years in the most severely affected infants and residual scarring is seen even into adulthood.[109]

Chest CT provides greater detail than CXR to characterize lung structure and detect pulmonary lesions in BPD, and several CT scoring methods used to evaluate chest CT scans in infants with BPD have been proposed.[110,111] Almost all include assessment of lung hypoattenuation, linear or subpleural opacities, bronchial wall thickening or collapse, or the presence of consolidation or atelectasis.[111] One commonly used scoring system, developed by Ochiai et al., grades the presence and severity of the following three

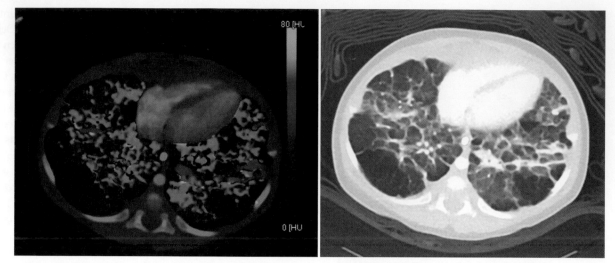

Fig. 9.27 Dual-energy computed tomography (CT) of a 12-week-old infant born at 29 weeks of gestation with BPD. **(A)** Axial CT angiogram image demonstrates heterogeneous aeration of the lung with thickened parenchymal bands. **(B)** Color map of the lung in the same region shows heterogeneous perfusion because of the dysplastic lung.

CT can also characterize the presence and severity of heterogeneous perfusion abnormalities within the lungs (Fig. 9.27).[25]

Lastly, new techniques for MRI are expanding the application of this modality to imaging the lungs. In recent years, there has been particular focus on studying the airway and lung architecture in infants and young children with BPD using this radiation-free technique.[29-31] For instance, one single-center study demonstrated greater than 80% accuracy of lung and airway three-dimensional MRI performed near term corrected gestation for predicting eventual tracheostomy.[116] Moreover, the use of MRI in conjunction with inhalation of a hyperpolarized noble gas (e.g., ^{3}He or ^{129}Xe) can provide functional and microstructural data down to the level of the alveolus.[117,118] These techniques have been especially useful for understanding the effects of BPD on later childhood lung growth.[119]

CONGENITAL AND SURGICAL CAUSES OF RESPIRATORY DISTRESS

Congenital Lung Lesions

The terms CLLs or congenital lung malformations refer to a broad range of developmental pulmonary abnormalities. The nomenclature of these lesions has evolved in recent years with the recognition that many share similar developmental origins and have overlapping radiographic and histological features.[120] The most common CLLs diagnosed in infancy are bronchial atresia (BA), CPAM, and BPS.[121] Other less common CLLs include congenital lobar emphysema (CLE) (or infantile lobar hyperinflation), bronchogenic cysts, pulmonary arteriovenous malformations, pulmonary agenesis/aplasia/hypoplasia, and tracheal bronchus.[121]

Pulmonary Agenesis, Aplasia, and Hypoplasia

Pulmonary agenesis is a rare congenital anomaly that results from failure of the primitive lung bud to develop and results in unilateral or bilateral absence of lung tissue. The lung parenchyma is also absent in pulmonary aplasia, but in contrast to pulmonary agenesis, there is a short, blind ending bronchus. Pulmonary hypoplasia is a condition of underdeveloped lungs and most often occurs secondary to another underlying abnormality. These secondary causes are categorized as malformations of the chest wall, space occupying lesions within the chest cavity (e.g., CDH, CPAM, pleural effusion), oligohydramnios because of renal or urological abnormalities or prolonged rupture of membranes (particularly with rupture before 20 weeks' gestation), and neuromuscular disorders that prevent normal fetal breathing. Primary pulmonary hypoplasia is rare. It occurs in congenital acinar dysplasia and can be a feature of Down syndrome.[122] PPHN is a common complication of both primary and secondary pulmonary hypoplasia and usually portends a poor prognosis.

The radiographic findings in pulmonary hypoplasia depend on the underlying etiology and severity of the disease. The typical features are small or absent lungs, crowded ribs, and an elevated diaphragm (eFig. 9.12). If unaffected, the contralateral lung may be overexpanded and the mediastinum shifted toward the affected side. A space-occupying lesion is often visible on CXR, but lung US or CT may be necessary to identify the specific etiology. CTA may also show a reduction in the size, number, and branching patterns of the pulmonary vessels and dual-energy CT perfusion can quantify the volume of pulmonary blood flow to help delineate the severity of lung hypoplasia within affected segments.[25,123]

Bronchial Atresia or Stenosis

Congenital BA results from focal interruption of a lobar, segmental, or subsegmental bronchus and may represent the underlying developmental abnormality in several CLLs including CPAM, BPS, and CLE.[124,125] BA typically affects a single segment, although multisegmental disease is possible. The left followed by the right upper lobes are the most common sites.[126] Postnatally, mucous collects in the distal portion of the affected bronchus and forms a mucocele (impacted mucous). There is no ball-valve effect, however, because of a lack of communication with the central airways.[127] The affected segment is aerated through collateral channels and is often only mildly overdistended.[127] Acquired bronchial stenosis can also develop from baro- and volutrauma to the cartilaginous airway and is associated with BPD.[128] BA appears on CXR as a tubular or nodular mass sometimes with an air-fluid level and an adjacent overinflated or cystic appearing lung. Small lesions may be difficult to detect on plain radiograph and chest CT is often necessary to distinguish between BA and other cystic lesions.[129]

Congenital Pulmonary Airway Malformation

CPAMs, previously known as congenital cystic adenomatoid malformations, are the most common form of CLL. The estimated incidence ranges from 1 in 10,000 to 1 in 30,000 live births.[130] Several classification schemes exist based on the embryologic origin, the appearance on prenatal imaging, and the size and epithelial lining of the resected cysts.[131-133] "Hybrid" lesions with histological features of both CPAM and BPS are also possible.[134] The most common CPAMs have multiple air-filled cysts that are greater than 2 cm in diameter. A CXR taken soon after birth may show a dense mass that is indistinguishable from other CLLs. Later radiographs show air-filled cysts and collapse of the surrounding parenchyma (Fig. 9.28). Microcystic and solid forms also exist and generally carry a poorer prognosis (eFig. 9.13). Overall, CXR has a low sensitivity for detecting CPAMs, and other imaging modalities such as CTA or MRI with angiography are recommended to define the anatomy and blood supply of the lesion (eFig. 9.14).[135]

Bronchopulmonary Sequestration

BPS is an isolated portion of lung tissue that does not communicate with the bronchial tree. Most sequestrations receive blood supply from a systemic artery, often the aorta, although this is not uniformly true. Venous drainage may be through pulmonary or systemic veins or both. Up to 50% of BPSs contain histologic areas of cystic adenomatous malformation.[136]

BPS is divided into two categories: intralobar and extralobar. Intralobar sequestrations are found within the normal lung tissue, predominately in basal segments of the lower lungs. Extralobar sequestrations are contained within a pleural covering distinct from the surrounding lung tissue. Most are located in the thoracic cavity but can also be found below the diaphragm. BPS appears on CXR as a dense mass, usually in the medial basal segment of the left lower lobe. Similar to CPAMs, identification of the blood supply can be done by US, CTA, or MRI with angiography (Fig. 9.29, eFig. 9.15). Additional congenital anomalies including diaphragmatic hernia and heart abnormalities can occur in infants with BPS, and chest imaging in these infants should be reviewed to assess for other lesions.

Congenital Lobar Emphysema

CLE results from air-filled distention of one or more lobes of the lung. CLE most commonly affects the left upper lobe (50%), followed by right middle lobe (30%) and right upper lobe (20%).[137] Lower lobe involvement is rare. The etiology of CLE is idiopathic in approximately half of cases.[138] The remaining cases are divided into intrinsic and extrinsic causes.[138] Intrinsic mechanisms include dysplasia of the bronchial cartilage, bronchial torsion or atresia, or extensive proliferation of the mucosa. Extrinsic etiologies usually result from bronchial compression or hypoplasia of the adjacent lung tissue. A chest radiograph obtained soon after birth may show opacification of the affected lobe as air more rapidly fills the surrounding, healthy lung. Once filled, however, the affected lung is overexpanded and hyperlucent and the adjacent lung appears dense

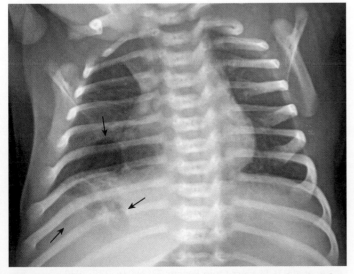

Fig. 9.28 Initial anterior-posterior radiograph of a full-term female infant with prenatally diagnosed right lower lobe macrocystic congenital pulmonary airway malformation (*arrows*). Consistent with retained fetal lung fluid, the remaining lung is diffusely hazy with air bronchograms and there is a small pleural effusion in the interlobar fissure on the right.

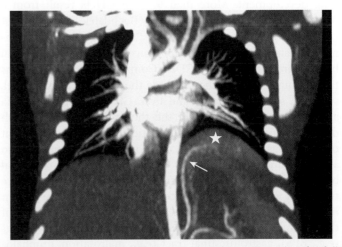

Fig. 9.29 Postnatal computed tomography with angiography of a full-term infant with a bronchopulmonary sequestration. Coronal reconstructed image demonstrates the feeding vessel (*arrow*) arising from the abdominal aorta to supply the lesion at the left lung base (*star*).

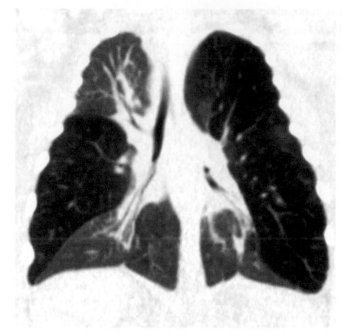

Fig. 9.30 Coronal reconstructed image of a chest computed tomography of a 6-month-old female (for the plain radiograph of the same infant see eFig. 9.16), with congenital lobar emphysema of the left upper and right middles lobes. There is marked hyperexpansion of the affected lobes with compression of the right upper lobe and bilateral lower lobes.

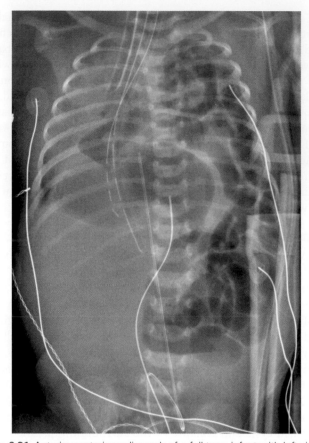

Fig. 9.31 Anterior-posterior radiograph of a full-term infant with left-sided congenital diaphragmatic hernia. Aerated loops of bowel are seen extending from the abdomen into the left hemithorax. The mediastinum is shifted to the right demonstrated by the cardiothymic silhouette, endotracheal tube, and gastric sump coursing through the esophagus all overlying the right hemithorax. This results in the visible compressive atelectasis of the right lung. A "high" lying umbilical arterial catheter terminates at T7 and umbilical venous catheter at T9.

and compressed (Fig. 9.30, eFig. 9.16). Mediastinal shift can also occur and large lesions may be confused with pneumothorax. CT may be necessary to identify which lobe is involved as unaffected structures are often too distorted to discern clearly on plain radiograph.

Congenital Diaphragmatic Hernia

CDH affects approximately 1 in 2500 infants and results from a failure of the pleural-peritoneal fold to close early in gestation. The diaphragmatic defect permits the abdominal contents to herniate into the thorax and creates a mass effect that impedes lung development. More than 95% of CDHs result from a posterolateral diaphragmatic defect (Bochdalek hernias). Most (80%–85%) occurs on the left side.[139] Morgagni hernias (anterior parasternal defect), septum transverse defects, and hiatal hernias are rare types of CDH. Common abdominal organs that herniate into the chest include the small and large bowel, stomach, spleen, pancreas, and liver. Greater lung hypoplasia and presence of the liver in the thorax are associated with decreased survival rates.[140] In addition to underdevelopment of the lungs, the peripheral pulmonary vasculature is also abnormal and hypermuscular.[139] As a result, pulmonary arterial hypertension complicates most CDH cases and may require treatment with ECMO. Other congenital anomalies are present in 20% of infants with CDH. These include abnormalities of the central nervous system (e.g., neural tube defects), lungs (e.g., BPS), gastrointestinal tract (e.g., malrotation, omphalocele), and cardiovascular and genitourinary systems. The typical postnatal CXR shows air-filled loops of bowel within the hemithorax, compression of the lung on the affected size, and contralateral displacement of the mediastinum (Fig. 9.31). The x-ray findings in diaphragmatic eventration, a disorder in which all or part of the diaphragm is replaced by fibroelastic tissue, can mimic those of a CDH if the weakened diaphragm is displaced into the thoracic cavity. US can help distinguish between these two entities and also determine what organs are herniated into the chest if not established prenatally. CT can also confirm the diagnosis of CDH if other imaging modalities are inconclusive.

KEY REFERENCES

17. Raimondi F, Rodriguez Fanjul J, Aversa S, et al: Lung ultrasound for diagnosing pneumothorax in the critically ill neonate. J Pediatr 175:74–78 e71, 2016.
18. Miller LE, Stoller JZ, Fraga MV: Point-of-care ultrasound in the neonatal ICU. Curr Opin Pediatr 32(2):216–227, 2020.
23. Ochiai M, Hikino S, Yabuuchi H, et al: A new scoring system for computed tomography of the chest for assessing the clinical status of bronchopulmonary dysplasia. J Pediatr 152(1):90–95, 95.e91–93, 2008.

29. Higano NS, Spielberg DR, Fleck RJ, et al: Neonatal pulmonary magnetic resonance imaging of bronchopulmonary dysplasia predicts short-term clinical outcomes. Am J Respir Crit Care Med 198(10):1302–1311, 2018.

45. Meinen RD, Bauer AS, Devous K, et al: Point-of-care ultrasound use in umbilical line placement: a review. J Perinatol 40(4):560–566, 2019.

49. Katheria A, Fleming S, Kim J: A randomized controlled trial of ultrasound-guided peripherally inserted central catheters compared with standard radiograph in neonates. J Perinatol 33(10):791–794, 2013.

51. Jain A, McNamara PJ, Ng E, El-Khuffash A: The use of targeted neonatal echocardiography to confirm placement of peripherally inserted central catheters in neonates. Am J Perinatol 29(2):101–106, 2012.

58. Thomas TH, Price R, Ramaciotti C, et al: Echocardiography, not chest radiography, for evaluation of cannula placement during pediatric extracorporeal membrane oxygenation. Pediatr Crit Care Med 10(1):56–59, 2009.

63. Brat R, Yousef N, Klifa R, et al: Lung ultrasonography score to evaluate oxygenation and surfactant need in neonates treated with continuous positive airway pressure. JAMA Pediatr 169(8):e151797, 2015.

65. Raimondi F, Migliaro F, Sodano A, et al: Use of neonatal chest ultrasound to predict noninvasive ventilation failure. Pediatrics 134(4):e1089–e1094, 2014.

88. Deng BY, Li N, Wu WS, et al: Use of neonatal lung ultrasound for the early detection of pneumothorax. Am J Perinatol 37(9):907–913, 2020.

92. Correia-Pinto J, Henriques-Coelho T: Images in clinical medicine. Neonatal pneumomediastinum and the spinnaker-sail sign. N Engl J Med 363(22):2145, 2010.

100. Conlon TW, Nishisaki A, Singh Y, et al: Moving beyond the stethoscope: diagnostic point-of-care ultrasound in pediatric practice. Pediatrics 144(4):e20191402, 2019.

111. van Mastrigt E, Logie K, Ciet P, et al: Lung CT imaging in patients with bronchopulmonary dysplasia: a systematic review. Pediatr Pulmonol 51(9):975–986, 2016.

116. Higano N, Adaikalam S, Hysinger E, et al: Clinically-relevant tracheostomy prediction model in neonatal bronchopulmonary dysplasia via respiratory MRI. Eur Respir J 56(suppl 64):4789, 2020.

119. Narayanan M, Beardsmore CS, Owers-Bradley J, et al: Catch-up alveolarization in ex-preterm children: evidence from (3)He magnetic resonance. Am J Respir Crit Care Med 187(10):1104–1109, 2013.

138. Durell J, Lakhoo K: Congenital cystic lesions of the lung. Early Hum Dev 90(12):935–939, 2014.

10

Blood Gases: Technical Aspects and Interpretation

Colm Travers and Namasivayam Ambalavanan

KEY POINTS

- Intermittent arterial blood gas measurement is the gold standard by which the adequacy of oxygenation and ventilation is assessed in sick neonates.
- Bedside continuous noninvasive monitoring devices, such as pulse oximeters, near-infrared spectroscopy, and transcutaneous carbon dioxide monitors, are commonly used to provide real-time approximations of blood gas values.
- Knowledge of methods of blood gas collection, technical aspects of blood gas analyzers, and how blood gas values are derived is fundamental to providing optimal patient care.
- Neonates have unique physiology and disorders that impact the clinical interpretation of data from blood gas testing and noninvasive monitors.

INTRODUCTION

Blood gas measurements estimate the magnitude of respiratory illness severity, diagnose respiratory failure, and also inform adjustments of respiratory support. In this chapter, we first discuss the physiology of gas transport in the blood, followed by a description of techniques of measurement of blood gases commonly used in the neonatal intensive care unit (NICU). Next, we will describe the technical aspects of blood gas estimation by commercially available devices. Finally, we will discuss the interpretation of blood gases, as well as some perils and pitfalls of blood gas measurement in clinical practice.

BLOOD GAS PHYSIOLOGY

Gas exchange occurs primarily in lung saccules in extremely preterm infants and in alveoli in more mature preterm and term infants, although a little gas exchange occurs through immature skin soon after birth.[1-3] Postnatally, deoxygenated systemic venous blood returns to the right atrium and then the right ventricle. This blood is pumped through the pulmonary arterial vasculature to the capillaries contiguous to saccules/alveoli. As the blood flows past ventilated alveoli, oxygen is added to the blood, and carbon dioxide is removed. In general, the oxygen concentration of arterial blood exiting the left ventricle reflects the matching of ventilation and perfusion. A decrease in oxygen content would occur if perfusion (blood) is not matched with ventilation (aerated alveoli).

Ventilation-perfusion mismatch results when blood passes from the right side of the heart to the left side of the heart without traversing the pulmonary circulation (extrapulmonary shunt) or when blood traverses parts of the lung that are atelectatic and/or underventilated (intrapulmonary shunt).

Carbon dioxide (CO_2) elimination is primarily dependent upon the magnitude of alveolar ventilation. As alveolar ventilation increases, the partial pressure of CO_2 in alveolar gas (P_ACO_2) decreases. The concentration gradient between partial pressure of CO_2 in arterial blood ($PaCO_2$) and P_ACO_2 increases so that more CO_2 diffuses from blood into the alveoli and is removed from the blood flowing through the lungs. Hence, the partial pressure of CO_2 in blood ($PaCO_2$) decreases. Conversely, a decrease in alveolar ventilation will increase the $PaCO_2$ in systemic arterial blood because of a decreased concentration gradient.

Aerobic metabolism of glucose for the production of adenosine triphosphate (ATP) is responsible for the consumption of oxygen and the production of CO_2. Aerobic metabolism produces approximately 38 ATP molecules for each molecule of glucose metabolized, although some of the ATP is consumed in the process, yielding a net of 30 ATP.[4] During conditions of insufficient oxygen delivery to cells, anaerobic metabolism occurs with conversion of glucose to pyruvate. This process is less efficient than aerobic metabolism and yields two molecules of ATP for each molecule of glucose consumed. Pyruvate is metabolized to lactic acid, which increases the base deficit of arterial blood. Base deficit is defined as the difference between the actual buffer capacity and the ideal buffer capacity.

An important concept is that although arterial PaO_2 and $PaCO_2$ provide important information about ventilation-perfusion matching and adequacy of alveolar ventilation, they do not provide direct information about the adequacy of oxygen delivery to the systemic vascular bed and peripheral tissues. To estimate if adequate oxygen has been delivered to tissues, blood returning from the systemic circulation to the heart (mixed venous blood) can be evaluated. Blood sampling from the right atrium using an umbilical venous catheter with its tip in the low right atrium, closely approximates mixed venous blood. Monitoring of mixed venous oxygenation is extremely helpful in assessing the adequacy of tissue oxygen delivery and consumption, particularly in neonatal extracorporeal membrane oxygenation (ECMO).

Oxygen Transport

Oxygen delivery to tissues depends upon the oxygen content of the blood as well as the cardiac output. In most neonates, cardiac output ranges from 120 to 150 mL/kg/min. Objective bedside assessment of cardiac output is neither easy nor accurate. Functional echocardiography and Doppler methods are typically used. Alternative methods such as pulse contour analysis, bioimpedance, or indicator dilution techniques (generally in larger and older infants) also exist.[5] The oxygen content of arterial blood (C_aO_2) consists of oxygen bound to hemoglobin and free dissolved oxygen. Hence, $C_aO_2 = (HbO_2) + (\text{dissolved } O_2)$, where C_aO_2 is the oxygen content, HbO_2 is the oxygen bound to hemoglobin, and dissolved O_2 is the oxygen in solution.

Normally, only a small amount of oxygen is dissolved in the plasma, unless the Pao_2 is extremely high (e.g., exposure to high FiO_2 or hyperbaric oxygen therapy). At 38° C, 0.3 mL of oxygen is dissolved in 100 mL of plasma (0.003 mL/dL/mm Hg of PaO_2, at an assumed PaO_2 of 100 mm Hg). This relationship is linear over the entire range of PaO_2 (see Fig. 10.1, curve B). Because the amount of oxygen that is dissolved in the blood is minimal, the oxygen content of blood typically approximates the amount of oxygen bound to hemoglobin alone (i.e., $C_aO_2 \sim HbO_2$).

Therefore, the amount of oxygen bound to hemoglobin depends on the hemoglobin concentration, the oxygen-carrying capacity of hemoglobin, and the percentage oxygen saturation of the hemoglobin, expressed mathematically as $C_aO_2 \sim (HbO_2) = (\text{grams of Hb}) \times (O_2 \text{ capacity}) \times (\% \text{ saturation})$. O_2 capacity represents the maximum amount of oxygen that can be carried by a gram of hemoglobin that is fully saturated. This value is 1.34 mL of O_2 per gram of 100% saturated hemoglobin.[6]

Assuming a hemoglobin level of 15 g/100 mL blood, and 100% saturation of arterial blood, and ignoring the small amount of dissolved oxygen in blood, the oxygen content of normal arterial blood is approximately $C_aO_2 = 15 \times 1.34 \times 1.0 = 20$ mL O_2 per 100 mL arterial blood or 0.2 mL O_2 per mL of blood. Using the same assumptions, and with the additional assumption that the normal cardiac output in a newborn is

approximately 120 mL/kg/min, the amount of O_2 that can be delivered to the systemic circulation can be calculated as follows:

$$O_2 \text{ delivered} = (\text{Cardiac Output}) \times (C_aO_2)$$
$$= (120 \text{ mL blood/kg/min}) \times (0.2 \text{ mL } O_2/\text{mL blood})$$
$$= 24 \text{ mL } O_2/\text{kg/min.}$$

Oxygen consumption for a neonate is approximately 6 mL/kg/min under normal circumstances.[7,8] Therefore, the body extracts 6 mL/kg/min of oxygen from the approximately 24 mL/kg/min that can be delivered via the systemic circulation. The amount of oxygen delivered is therefore usually higher than the amount required by tissues. When oxygen delivery falls below the threshold at which the delivered amount of oxygen is less than the amount required, tissue hypoxia and anaerobic metabolism ensue. Normally, about 25% of the oxygen is removed from the blood by the time it returns to the heart. In general, a mixed venous saturation of 70% to 75% represents adequate tissue oxygen delivery. Therefore, mixed venous saturations of 70% to 75% are targeted in patients in whom mixed venous saturations can be directly monitored (e.g., patients on ECMO).

Understanding the Oxyhemoglobin Dissociation Curve

Although the PaO_2 contributes very little to the overall oxygen content of blood, its physiologic importance cannot be overstated as only oxygen dissolved in plasma enters cells. Oxygen bound to hemoglobin is not available to tissues until released from heme and dissolved in plasma. The sigmoidal oxyhemoglobin dissociation curve (ODC) describes the percent of hemoglobin saturated with oxygen at a given PaO_2. Hemoglobin is almost fully saturated at a PaO_2 of 80 to 100 mm Hg (Fig. 10.1, curve A).

However, the concentration of red blood cell diphosphoglycerate (DPG), the ratio of adult hemoglobin (A) to fetal hemoglobin (HbF), temperature, $PaCO_2$, and hydrogen ion concentration (acidosis) shift the position of the dissociation curve. With increasing postnatal age, the concentration of DPG and the proportion of hemoglobin A increase, shifting the curve to the right (Fig. 10.2). DPG has a greater effect on oxygen binding for adult hemoglobin, as compared with HbF.[8a] Increases in temperature, $PaCO_2$, and hydrogen ion concentration (acidosis) also shift the curve to the right. As the curve shifts to the right, hemoglobin binds less oxygen at a given Pao_2 and therefore releases oxygen more easily to the tissues (Fig. 10.3). The fetus has a lower red blood cell DPG concentration and more HbF so that the dissociation curve is shifted to the left. This helps maintain a higher oxygen saturation at a lower Pao_2. Conditions such as alkalosis or hypothermia will also shift the dissociation curve to the left, resulting in a higher hemoglobin oxygen saturation for a given PaO_2.

Hemoglobin binds oxygen in the lungs and transports oxygen to the tissues. Oxygen is then released from the hemoglobin and enters a dissolved phase in the plasma, which is represented by the partial pressure of oxygen (PaO_2). As noted, hemoglobin increases the oxygen delivery tremendously as the amount of dissolved oxygen in blood is minimal. The relationship between

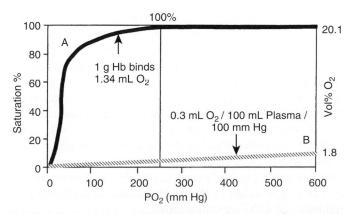

Fig. 10.1 Comparison between the dissociation curve of hemoglobin (*curve A*) and the amount of oxygen dissolved in plasma (*curve B*). Note that the hemoglobin is almost 100% saturated at PO_2 80 mm Hg. When fully saturated, 15 g Hb will bind 20.1 mL O_2. (From Duc G: Assessment of hypoxia in the newborn. Pediatrics 48:469, 1971.)

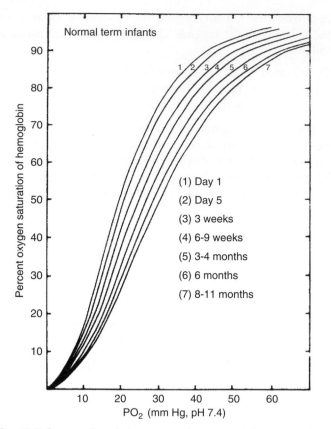

Fig. 10.2 Oxygen dissociation curves from term infants at various postnatal ages. (From Delivoria-Papadopoulos M, Roncevic NP, Oski FA: Postnatal changes in oxygen transport of term, premature and sick infants. Ped Res 5:235, 1971.)

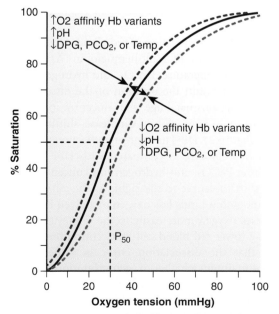

Fig. 10.3 Oxygen dissociation curve of hemoglobin. The percent saturation of hemoglobin with oxygen at different oxygen tensions is depicted by the sigmoidal curves. The P50, indicated by the dashed lines, is about 27 mm Hg in normal erythrocytes. Modifications of hemoglobin function that increase oxygen affinity shift the curve to the left, whereas those that decrease oxygen affinity shift the curve to the right. *DPG*, Diphosphoglycerate. (From Kelley's Textbook of Internal Medicine. 4th ed. Philadelphia, Lippincott Williams & Wilkins, 2000.)

oxygen saturation and PaO_2 is described by the sigmoidal ODC. The steep portion of the curve demonstrates that oxygen saturations change quickly during the loading and unloading of hemoglobin with oxygen. This reflects the relaxation of the hemoglobin structure that occurs with oxygen binding. As oxygen binds to heme, the hemoglobin molecule relaxes, thereby exposing further heme molecules, facilitating subsequent binding of oxygen. This process of relaxation is called allosteric modification and is governed by the Haldane effect. The reverse process occurs with oxygen unloading. As the oxygen binding sites on the hemoglobin molecule approach full saturation with oxygen, the ODC flattens. Therefore, at higher oxygen saturations, it is difficult to predict the PaO_2. An oxygen saturation of 100% can correspond to a PaO_2 ranging from 80 to over 300 mm Hg.

The position of the ODC is described by the P50, defined as the PaO_2 at an oxygen saturation of 50%. P50 is dependent on several factors. Increases in body temperature, hydrogen ion concentration (decreased pH), $PaCO_2$, 2,3-DPG, or adult hemoglobin concentration independently shift the ODC to the right. Conversely, decreases in any of these factors will shift the curve to the left. Therefore, the PaO_2 for any given oxygen saturation will vary within an individual as these factors change. For example, in the presence of a fever, the rightward shift of the curve results in a higher Pao_2 for the P50 value. Both adult hemoglobin concentrations and 2,3-DPG concentrations increase during infancy, causing a shift in the ODC position to the right.[9]

Considerations Regarding Fetal Hemoglobin

Neonates born at less than 30 weeks' gestation have nearly 100% HbF. The ratio of fetal to adult hemoglobin gradually diminishes so that by 40 weeks' gestation, HbF accounts for approximately 70% of all hemoglobin species, with adult hemoglobin accounting for the remaining 30%.[10] This shift to producing adult hemoglobin and away from producing HbF is related to postmenstrual age rather than chronological age.[11] Preterm birth does not directly affect the transition from fetal to adult hemoglobin production. A baby born at 24 weeks with nearly 100% HbF would be expected to have approximately 70% HbF at 16 weeks of age (40 weeks' corrected gestational age), similar to a baby born at 40 weeks' gestation, although the ratio will change more quickly following transfusion with adult blood.

The first observation that HbF has different oxygen binding properties than adult hemoglobin was reported in 1930.[12] HbF is composed of two α chains and two γ chains ($\alpha_2\gamma_2$), in contrast to adult hemoglobin, which contains two α and two β chains ($\alpha_2\beta_2$). HbF has a higher oxygen affinity (holds onto oxygen "more tightly") than adult hemoglobin, which promotes diffusion of oxygen from the maternal side to the fetal side of the placental circulation. This left shift of the ODC results in a P50 in term infants of approximately 21 mm Hg compared with a P50 of 27 mm Hg in adults (see Fig 10.2).[13,14] In preterm infants, the P50 may be as low as 18 mm Hg because of the higher HbF and lower 2,3-DPG concentrations.[15]

Therapies can alter the position of the ODC curve. Packed red blood cells administered to neonates are donated by adults and essentially contain 100% adult hemoglobin. Therefore, transfusion shifts the ODC to the right. Preterm babies have higher concentrations of HbF and are also more likely to be transfused. Blood transfusions among preterm infants cause a larger shift in the ODC compared with term infants.[16] There are other important factors to consider regarding the effect of blood transfusions on the ODC, such as the 2,3-DPG concentration, temperature, and type of preservative used.

Based on the position of the ODC, the oxygen saturation for a given PaO_2 may be quite different.[17] In practice, clinicians target specific oxygen saturation ranges to avoid the dangers of both hyperoxemia and hypoxemia. Oxygen saturation targets are not typically changed when the position of the ODC shifts posttransfusion, resulting in a higher PaO_2 for a given oxygen saturation. This is appropriate, because it is the oxyhemoglobin saturation rather than the PaO_2 that directly affects oxygen content of blood and tissue delivery.

Modern blood gas analyzers have two presets for HbF: 0% and 80%. Although not exact, using the 80% HbF preset is preferable for neonatal blood gas testing.[15] Errors in reporting uncorrected blood gas values may not always be obvious to the clinician. A blood gas result with an oxygen saturation of 100% corrected for HbF corresponds to an uncorrected oxygen saturation of 105%.[18] However, because blood gas machines do not report oxygen saturations greater than 100%, this would not be apparent to the clinician.

Hypoxemia and Hypoxia

Although hypoxemia and hypoxia often occur together, they are not synonymous. Hypoxemia is generally defined as low arterial blood oxygen content, whereas hypoxia refers to inadequate oxygen delivery to tissue. Hypoxemia occurs in any situation in which blood enters the systemic circulation without perfusing adequately ventilated alveoli (reduction in ventilation-perfusion matching). Blood can bypass adequately ventilated alveoli by extrapulmonary and/or intrapulmonary shunts. With persistent pulmonary hypertension of the newborn (PPHN) or cyanotic congenital heart disease, blood enters the aorta without passing through the pulmonary circulation (extrapulmonary shunt). In PPHN, a right-to-left shunt across the ductus arteriosus can often be detected by comparing the PaO_2 or oxygen saturation of preductal and postductal blood (Fig. 10.4). If the saturation of the preductal blood is significantly higher than the saturation of the postductal blood ($\geq 5\%$–10% difference), this indicates a clinically significant right-to-left shunt. However, equal pre- and postductal saturations do not exclude pulmonary hypertension. Right-left shunting may occur through the foramen ovale without any pre- and postductal difference. Hypoxemia associated with lung diseases characterized by atelectasis (e.g., respiratory distress syndrome, pneumonia) is primarily because of intrapulmonary shunting. Whenever alveoli are inadequately ventilated, the blood flowing to those alveoli may not be fully saturated. With worsening atelectasis, intrapulmonary shunting and subsequent hypoxemia increase.

Tissue hypoxia results when the amount of oxygen delivered to the tissues decreases below the critical threshold of oxygen consumption. Hypoxia can occur despite an apparently adequate PaO_2. It is helpful to conceptualize hypoxia in terms of imbalances in supply, delivery, and demand for oxygen. Decreased "supply" is

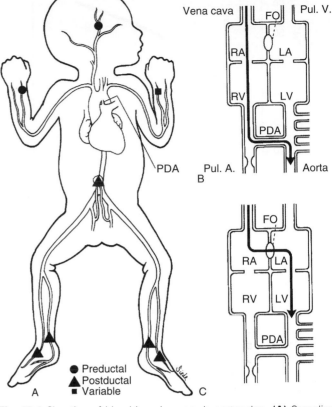

Fig. 10.4 Shunting of blood in pulmonary hypertension. **(A)** Sampling sites. **(B)** Right-to-left shunt across the ductus arteriosus. **(C)** Right-to-left shunt across the foramen ovale. *FO,* Foramen ovale; *LA,* left atrium; *LV,* left ventricle; *PDA,* patent ductus arteriosus; *RA,* right atrium; *RV,* right ventricle.

observed at high altitude because of a lower partial pressure of oxygen in the atmosphere, with inadequate respiratory effort, and with ventilation-perfusion mismatch. "Delivery" of oxygen is impaired in the settings of inadequate tissue perfusion (e.g., reduced cardiac output), anemia, and abnormal hemoglobin species (e.g., methemoglobin), where the unloading of oxygen to the tissues is negatively affected. The "demand" for oxygen will increase as tissue oxygen requirements rise in response to illness such as fever or sepsis.

Carbon Dioxide Transport

CO_2 transport is less complicated than oxygen transport. CO_2 is a by-product of aerobic metabolism of glucose. Carbon dioxide is transported in the blood to the lungs, where it is exhaled. Some 85% of the CO_2 in blood is transported as carbonic acid (bicarbonate buffer system), 10% is carried by hemoglobin as carbamate, and 5% is transported as dissolved gas.[19,20] Equilibrium is maintained between dissolved CO_2 and bicarbonate. Thereby, the relationship between the partial pressure of CO_2 in the blood ($PaCO_2$) and the total CO_2 content of blood is essentially linear over the physiologic range (Fig. 10.5). Carbon dioxide diffuses rapidly from blood into alveolar gas. Therefore, the partial pressure of CO_2 in blood ($PaCO_2$) leaving the lungs is essentially the same as the partial pressure of CO_2 in alveolar

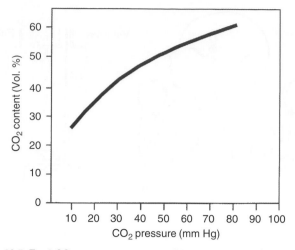

Fig. 10.5 Total CO_2 content versus partial pressure of CO_2 in blood. (From Comroe JH: The Lung. Chicago, Year Book Medical Publishers, 1962, pp. 44–49.)

gas (P_ACO_2). Increasing the minute alveolar ventilation decreases the P_ACO_2 and the $PaCO_2$. This is the reason $PaCO_2$ is dependent on the magnitude of alveolar ventilation.

Metabolic Acidosis

Metabolic acidosis can occur because of increased losses of base or increased production of acid. Anaerobic metabolism of glucose leads to the accumulation of lactic acid, resulting in metabolic acidosis. Lactic acid is buffered by bicarbonate (a base), causing the serum bicarbonate to fall, resulting in a base deficit. Lactic acidosis is most commonly caused by inadequate tissue oxygen delivery as a result of some combination of hypoxemia, severe anemia, and inadequate cardiac output. Other causes of metabolic acidosis in the newborn include sepsis, inborn errors of metabolism, and renal bicarbonate wasting. Iatrogenic causes, such as a large protein load in enteral or parenteral nutrition, especially when extra cysteine is added, also cause metabolic acidosis in very preterm infants.

In most healthy newborns, the base deficit is usually between $+3$ and -1. Although it may be logical to provide base to infants who have metabolic acidosis because of renal bicarbonate losses, there is evidence suggesting that bicarbonate administration may be deleterious to the patient with hypoxia and metabolic acidosis, and it should not be used routinely.[21–23] In patients with metabolic acidosis, therapy should target restoring tissue oxygen delivery by correcting the underlying problem. Sodium bicarbonate is no longer recommended during cardiopulmonary resuscitation.[21]

When metabolic acidosis is treated with exogenous base, the most commonly used drug is sodium bicarbonate. The number of milliequivalents of bicarbonate needed to half correct a base deficit can be approximated from the following equation:

$$\text{Bicarbonate (mEq) to be administered} = (\text{base deficit}) \times \text{body weight in kg} \times 0.3.$$

Owing to its hypertonicity, sodium bicarbonate (1 mEq/mL) should be diluted 1:1 with sterile water and administered slowly, preferably over 30 to 60 minutes.[24] Acetate may be added to parenteral nutrition in place of chloride to treat metabolic acidosis.[25] Bicarbonate and acetate should be administered with care among infants with a combined respiratory and metabolic acidosis because CO_2 is a by-product of bicarbonate and acetate metabolism. Therefore, $PaCO_2$ will increase unless there is also an increase in minute ventilation. Thus, the use of exogenous base should be limited to the few cases of renal tubular bicarbonate wasting or certain rare causes of congenital lactic acidosis.

Metabolic Alkalosis

The most common cause of relative metabolic alkalosis in neonates is a chronic compensation for respiratory acidosis. If a compensated respiratory acidosis is corrected by rapidly lowering the $PaCO_2$, an absolute metabolic alkalosis will result. Other causes of metabolic alkalosis in the newborn include hypochloremia from chronic diuretic therapy, or gastric secretion losses (drainage or frequent vomiting), and the administration of excess acetate in parenteral nutrition. Mild metabolic alkalosis can also occur following an exchange transfusion when the citrate in the anticoagulant is metabolized. It is rarely necessary to correct metabolic alkalosis with acidic compounds such as ammonium chloride or arginine hydrochloride or with bicarbonate-wasting diuretics such as acetazolamide. In most cases, treating metabolic alkalosis with these agents results in an uncompensated respiratory acidosis.

TECHNIQUES FOR OBTAINING BLOOD SAMPLES

Although it is possible to manage a sick newborn without arterial access, the presence of an arterial catheter often simplifies care significantly. Arterial access allows accurate measurement of arterial blood gases and direct measurement of arterial blood pressure and provides a route for obtaining other blood samples. Although valuable, umbilical catheters are not without risk; therefore, standardization of their usage is preferred.[26]

Umbilical Artery Catheters

Umbilical artery catheters (UACs) are the preferred route for arterial access in most NICUs. UACs can usually be quickly and easily placed soon after birth, with small risk of complications. The umbilical arteries are readily accessible during the first days of life. Although successful cannulation is considerably less likely after a few days, it may still be possible up to 2 weeks of age. Blood gas measurements performed on blood drawn from an umbilical catheter reflect postductal blood.

An umbilical catheter should be flexible, nonkinking, radiopaque, transparent, and nonthrombogenic and should have an end hole but no side hole.[27] There are two common catheter sizes, 3.5 and 5.0 F. Few data are available about the relative merits of the two catheter sizes. Some clinicians feel that the larger catheter should be used to minimize thrombus formation, making it less prone to "clotting off." Others feel that the smaller catheter is better because it minimizes changes in aortic blood flow.[28] The decision about which catheter size to use is usually based on personal preference and patient size. Our usual approach is to use a

3.5-F single-lumen catheter in infants weighing less than 1500 or 2000 g and a 5.0-F single-lumen catheter in infants who weigh more than 1500 or 2000 g. We only use single lumen catheters when cannulating the umbilical artery.

The procedure for cannulation of the umbilical vessels can be seen in a video by Anderson et al. in the *New England Journal of Medicine*.[29] Additional videos describing the method are also available through Pedialink, the American Academy of Pediatrics Online Learning Center (https://vimeo.com/57453941).

Before insertion, the catheter is attached to a three-way stopcock and syringe containing a heparinized saline solution and then flushed to remove bubbles. When the catheter has been inserted and is functioning adequately, the stopcock should be attached to a continuous infusion of heparinized fluid and to a pressure transducer. Care should be taken when tightening stopcock connections to minimize the possibility of accidental disconnection.

The catheter is inserted while the infant is maintained in a neutral thermal environment with vital signs monitored. The infant's legs should be loosely restrained, and it may be helpful to also loosely restrain the arms. UACs are inserted under sterile conditions after the umbilical cord is cleaned with povidone-iodine or chlorhexidine. Antiseptics should be removed immediately after insertion to reduce skin injury. In addition, iatrogenic hypothyroidism may occur if iodine is allowed to remain on the skin.[30] A sterile umbilical tie is placed around the lower portion of the cord and tied with a single knot. The tie is placed so it can be either tightened, if bleeding occurs when the cord is cut, or loosened, if it prevents passage of the catheter. Next, the cord is cut approximately 0.5 to 1.0 cm above the skin. Longer umbilical stumps make catheter insertion more difficult. Cut the cord using a scalpel in a single cut, rather than with a sawing motion. This results in a flat umbilical surface from which the umbilical arteries usually protrude. The two thick-walled arteries and the single, larger, patulous thin-walled vein (usually at a superior 12 o'clock position) can easily be identified.

One of the more important steps in the insertion of UACs is dilation of the arterial lumen. The goal of dilation is to open the lumen enough to allow smooth catheter passage without tearing the intima and creating a "false lumen." Once a false lumen is made, the UAC will rarely reenter the true lumen, leading to insertion failure. The dilation of the vessel starts with placing one arm tip of a small forceps into the lumen. Forceps with teeth should be avoided. Gentle rotation will help the vessel dilate until both arms of the forceps can be placed into the lumen (Fig. 10.6). Once both arms are placed, they can be slowly rotated and spread while withdrawing to gradually dilate the vessel to the caliber of the catheter. As the lumen dilates, the forceps are advanced with the goal of dilating at least 5 to 8 mm. Once the vessel has been adequately dilated, the catheter can be inserted. It is easier to pass the catheter if the vessel is stabilized with one or two small, curved forceps. Usually, the catheter passes with little resistance. If the catheter meets significant resistance, it usually means that the catheter has dissected through the intima and has created a false lumen. When this occurs, the catheter should be removed. Forcing the catheter may result in damage to the vessel and/or perforation of the peritoneum or bladder.

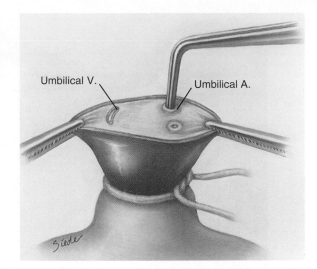

Fig. 10.6 Umbilical stump with two umbilical arteries and one vein. A small forceps is used to gently dilate one artery.

Rarely, a catheter will travel inferiorly into the external iliac artery, which becomes the femoral artery that perfuses the lower limb, rather than superiorly into the aorta. If this occurs, a second catheter can sometimes be inserted into the same umbilical artery without removing the first catheter. With the first catheter lodged in the external iliac artery, the second is often directed into the descending aorta.

Once the catheter enters the aorta, it should be advanced to either "high position" or "low position." These positions avoid placing the catheter tip adjacent to the origin of the renal, mesenteric, or celiac vessels. If a low position is chosen, the catheter tip should be between the levels of the third and fourth lumbar vertebrae (L3–L4) on a radiograph, safely below the renal and mesenteric arteries. If a high position is chosen, the catheter tip should be between the sixth and the tenth thoracic vertebrae (T6–T10, optimally T8), above the origin of the celiac vessels. Although both positions are commonly used, a meta-analysis of randomized trials comparing low versus high catheter placement found a greater rate of peripheral vascular complications among infants with catheters in the low position. However, most of these complications were minor.[31]

Several published graphs are available for estimating the distance that a catheter must be inserted to correctly place it in the lower position.[32,33] The simplest method is based on the infant's weight.[34] When a low position is targeted, for a 1-kg infant, the catheter should be inserted approximately 7 cm; for a 2-kg infant, it should be inserted approximately 8 cm; and for a 3-kg infant, it should be inserted approximately 9 cm. For a catheter to be placed in the high position, the formula "3 times the weight plus 9" gives a rough estimate of the required catheter insertion length in centimeters. A study suggests that the formula "4 times the weight plus 7" for very preterm infants gives a better estimate of the required catheter insertion length.[35] Surface measurements (umbilicus-nipple length minus 1 cm plus twice the distance from umbilicus to symphysis pubis) or graphs based on shoulder-umbilicus length may be used to estimate the correct insertion length, but randomized clinical trials suggest that using birth

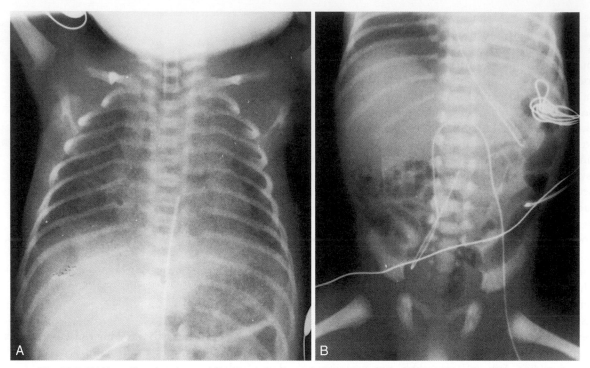

Fig. 10.7 **(A)** X-ray film showing umbilical artery catheter in "high" position. **(B)** X-ray film showing umbilical artery catheter in "low" position.

weight to estimate insertion depth is superior.[36] Regardless of the method used for calculating the depth of insertion, the length of the umbilical stump must be added to the estimated depth of insertion. Following insertion, the catheter position should be confirmed radiographically (Fig. 10.7) because these methods are not always accurate.[37] Ultrasound can also be used to check for catheter tip position.[38] Once correct positioning is confirmed, the catheter should be secured using sutures and tape. Generally, a 3-0 silk suture is tied to the umbilical cord, forming an "anchor," and then tied to the catheter. Special care must be taken not to puncture the catheter with the suture needle. The catheter can then be further secured with a tape bridge.

Subumbilical Cutdown

If attempts to cannulate both umbilical arteries and peripheral arteries are unsuccessful, and the patient cannot be adequately managed without an arterial catheter, the umbilical arteries can sometimes be cannulated via subumbilical cutdown.[39] This is a surgical procedure and should not be attempted by anyone other than a physician who has previous experience with the technique, as several complications can result, including entering the peritoneal cavity and subumbilical hernia.

Complications of Umbilical Artery Catheterization

Although umbilical artery catheterization is safe and well tolerated in most patients, it is important to remember that it is not without risks. Complications related to umbilical arterial catheters include vascular compromise, complications related to malposition, infection, bleeding, and catheter-related accidents (accidental disconnection, rupture, etc.). Rarely, catheter placement

is associated with severe thrombotic complications, including frank gangrene and necrosis of the buttocks or leg. Studies indicate that UACs in the first 5 days are not associated with a high risk of thrombosis. However, animal evidence suggests that even short-term use is associated with histological evidence of aortic thrombi and neointimal proliferation of the vascular wall that may not be clinically evident.[40,41]

Infants with UACs in place will occasionally develop dusky or purple discoloration of their toes, presumably from microemboli or vasospasm. Warming of the contralateral leg may cause reflex vasodilation and increased perfusion in the compromised extremity. Although this is a common practice, a study in normal infants without vasospasm showed that local warming has no effect on peripheral blood flow to the contralateral heel.[42] The compromised leg should not be warmed because of the possibility that this might increase the metabolic rate and increase hypoxic tissue injury of the warmed tissues. Although the majority of patients with dusky toes have adequate perfusion and suffer no ill effects, there is a risk of potentially significant vascular compromise with necrosis and tissue loss. If toes remain dusky, or worsens with poor capillary filling, or spread to involve more of the foot or leg, the catheter should be removed. In rare instances, an infant with a UAC will develop blanching of the foot or part of the leg representing severely compromised arterial blood flow, necessitating immediate catheter removal.

If perfusion to the limb does not immediately improve with removal of the catheter, this may indicate a severe thrombotic complication. Evaluation usually includes some combination of ultrasound or Doppler assessment, or possibly angiography.

Both systemic vasodilators and topical vasodilators have been described as having some efficacy in this situation, but definitive evidence for efficacy is lacking.[43,44] When a significant clot is identified, thrombolysis with tissue plasminogen activator, infused either directly into the affected vessel or systemically, has been attempted.[45,46] The potential advantages of thrombolytic therapy must be weighed against the risks of such therapy, particularly in the infant with a preexisting intracranial hemorrhage that could potentially extend. Unfortunately, there is little literature available regarding the optimal approach to infants with severe vascular obstruction.

The incidence of infection associated with UACs appears to be lower than the incidence of infections associated with central venous catheters. However, as with all central catheters, meticulous care must be taken to maintain sterility during catheter insertion and during subsequent access of hubs. We recommend minimizing line "breaks" to reduce the risk of central line infection. A Cochrane review suggests that there is inadequate evidence to recommend either for or against routine antibiotic use in infants with umbilical catheters in place, and it is recommended to not use prolonged empiric antimicrobial therapy with negative cultures in infants.[47] However, antibiotic locks may reduce catheter-related blood stream infections in neonates.[48]

A concern of UACs is the effect of blood sampling on cerebral blood flow. Ultrasonographic and near-infrared spectroscopy (NIRS) studies have shown that routine blood sampling from an umbilical catheter alters cerebral hemodynamics and oxygenation.[49] Although reducing the volume of blood withdrawn may reduce these changes, it is unclear whether a slower withdrawal is also beneficial.[50,51] Although it is unknown whether such changes in cerebral hemodynamics increase the risk of complications such as intraventricular hemorrhage, it is reasonable to minimize the volume of blood withdrawn and avoid rapidly withdrawing from or infusing into any umbilical catheter.

Concomitant enteral nutrition with UACs in place is considered safe, with most clinicians continuing to feed with umbilical catheters.[52] Superior mesenteric arterial flow is not affected by the presence of an umbilical catheter during trophic feeding.[53]

There is little published literature on which to base decisions about how long a UAC can remain safely in place. In most institutions, they are usually removed within several days, when the infant no longer requires significant respiratory support or frequent blood sampling. As with all therapies, the potential risks of UACs must be balanced against the potential advantages for each infant.

Other Indwelling Catheter Sites

In some infants, umbilical artery catheterization is unsuccessful. In these cases, percutaneous cannulation of a peripheral artery is the preferred alternative. Percutaneous arterial cannulation is also the best option for infants who no longer have a UAC but still require arterial access. Other techniques, such as umbilical artery or peripheral artery cutdown, are more difficult to perform and involve more risk. Although percutaneous cannulation of a peripheral artery is technically challenging, especially in infants weighing less than 1 kg, cannulation of the radial, dorsalis pedis, or posterior tibial artery is often possible.

Temporal artery cannulation should be avoided because cerebral emboli and stroke have been reported.[54,55]

If the radial artery is to be cannulated, an Allen test may be performed to ensure ulnar artery patency. However, the reliability of this test has been questioned.[56] Conversely, if the ulnar artery is to be cannulated, radial artery patency should be assessed. Begin the Allen test by gently squeezing the hand to empty it of blood. Apply pressure to both the radial and the ulnar arteries and then remove pressure from the hand and the artery that will not be cannulated. If the entire hand flushes and fills with blood, it is safe to proceed.[19] Doppler evaluation may also be used to document collateral circulation.

The artery can be localized by either palpation or transillumination. If the radial or ulnar artery is to be cannulated, the hand should be restrained in mild hyperextension. Systemic analgesia may be provided before cannulation. Local anesthesia with lidocaine is sometimes used, and the resulting wheal may require gentle massage and waiting a few minutes. The insertion site should be cleaned before proceeding with a povidone-iodine or chlorhexidine solution. The radial artery is usually most easily cannulated at the point of maximal pulsation over the distal portion of the radius, proximal to the superficial palmar branch of the artery. In this position, the artery lies between two tendons, superficial and lateral to the median nerve (Fig. 10.8).

The catheter can be used either dry or flushed with a heparinized saline solution to facilitate flashback of blood. The catheter and needle are advanced at an angle of approximately 30 degrees until the vessel is entered and a pulsatile blood return is encountered. The needle is held stationary and the catheter is threaded into the artery. The needle is then withdrawn.

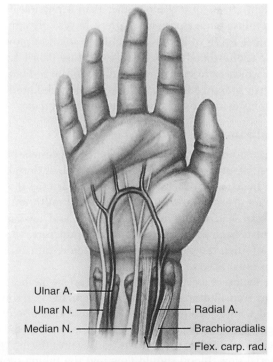

Fig. 10.8 Anatomy of the hand demonstrating radial and ulnar arteries and surrounding structures. *A.,* Artery; *Flex. carp. rad.,* flexor carpi radialis; *N.,* nerve.

An alternative technique is to puncture the artery through both the anterior and the posterior walls and then withdraw the needle. The catheter is then withdrawn until its tip reenters the vessel lumen and a brisk blood return is obtained, at which point it is threaded into the vessel. However, in our experience, this method is less successful in neonates.

Once in place, the catheter should be taped securely and connected to an infusion of heparinized saline with a T-connector and a three-way stopcock. The tape securing the catheter must allow for unobstructed view of all digits because hypoperfusion, potentially leading to ischemic necrosis, is a complication of peripheral arterial catheters. The limb chosen for insertion of the peripheral artery catheter will determine whether blood gas testing reflects pre- or postductal values.

Infusion of Fluids Through Arterial Catheters

The patency of both central and peripheral arterial catheters should be maintained with a heparinized solution. In most centers, the heparin concentrations range from 0.25 to 1.0 unit/mL. Heparinization of the infusate decreases the incidence of catheter occlusion but does not affect the frequency of aortic thrombosis, intracranial hemorrhage, death, or clinical ischemic phenomena.[57] Although there is little evidence on fluid infusion rates for arterial catheters, most clinicians use a minimal rate of 0.5 mL/h in very preterm infants or 1 mL/h in larger preterm or term infants.

Saline, glucose, and hyperalimentation solutions can all be infused into a UAC, and it has been shown that infusing an amino acid–containing solution of normal osmolarity causes less hemolysis than a quarter normal saline solution, while improving nutrition.[58] In contrast to umbilical arteries through which one can infuse a wide range of solutions, there is concern about the irritant effects of anything other than a physiologic saline solution infused into a peripheral artery. In very preterm infants for whom 1 mL/h of a physiologic saline solution provides an excessive sodium load, clinicians often infuse 0.45% saline. In cases in which extra base is required, we infuse sodium acetate rather than sodium chloride. Medications or blood products are not administered through a peripheral arterial catheter.

Arterial Puncture

Blood gas samples can be obtained from intermittent puncture of the radial, ulnar, temporal, posterior tibial, or dorsalis pedis arteries. In general, the femoral and brachial arteries should not be used for arterial puncture because significant thrombus formation can lead to loss of the extremity, and median nerve damage has been reported with brachial puncture.[59] As noted earlier, an Allen test may be performed before puncture of the radial or ulnar artery.

After the exact location of the desired artery has been determined by transillumination or by palpation, the skin should be prepared with a povidone-iodine or chlorhexidine solution. A small-gauge needle (e.g., 23–25 gauge) is inserted in the bevel-up position at an angle through the skin, against the direction of the arterial flow. Blood should flow into the tubing spontaneously or with gentle suction. After the needle is removed, continuous pressure should be applied for 5 minutes. If hematoma

formation is prevented, the same artery can be reaccessed several times.

The main drawback to arterial puncture is procedural pain. One study showed that venipuncture, generally regarded as less traumatic than arterial puncture, caused a 6-mm Hg decrease in $PaCO_2$ and a 17-mm Hg decrease in PaO_2.[60] Although subcutaneous administration of lidocaine (without epinephrine) over the artery before arterial puncture will provide partial analgesia, most infants still become agitated during the puncture. For this reason, arterial puncture to obtain blood gases is used infrequently.

Arterialized Capillary Blood

Arterialized capillary blood provides a crude estimate of arterial blood values. In theory, blood flowing through a dilated peripheral capillary bed has limited time for O_2 and CO_2 exchange to occur so that capillary blood gas values approximate arterial blood gas values. However, blood obtained simultaneously from the UAC and warmed heels of infants demonstrated that arterialized capillary blood was a poor predictor of arterial blood values including pH, $PaCO_2$, and PaO_2.[62] Arterialized capillary samples are probably most useful in chronically ventilated infants as they are moderately useful for tracking large changes in pH and $PaCO_2$.

To arterialize the capillary blood, the extremity should be warmed for several minutes. Warming should be performed with exothermic chemical packs specifically designed for arterializing capillary blood rather than with warm compresses. The site should be carefully cleaned, and a small lancet should be used to puncture the skin on the medial or lateral aspect of the plantar surface. The posterior curvature should not be used (Fig. 10.9).

There are multiple technical challenges to obtaining optimal capillary blood samples. Inadequate warming results in inadequate arterialization of the blood. Excessive squeezing will

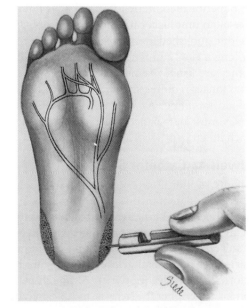

Fig. 10.9 Technique for obtaining an arterialized capillary heel sample. Stippled sections denote the correct areas for sampling.

cause contamination of the "arterialized" blood with venous blood and/or interstitial fluid. Exposure of blood to air during collection will falsely increase the PO_2 and falsely decrease the PCO_2 values. Low peripheral perfusion states lead to stasis and falsely elevated PCO_2 values. For this reason, a capillary specimen in a 2-hour-old infant with obvious acrocyanosis seldom yields useful information and risks unnecessary intubation for apparent respiratory acidosis because of stasis. Longer-term problems associated with frequent capillary samples include calcaneal osteochondritis and calcified heel nodules.[61] These calcified nodules may persist for several months to years but do not seem to cause permanent problems for the infant.

Continuous Invasive Monitoring

A number of devices have been developed for the direct intravascular or "inline" measurement of hemoglobin saturation, PaO_2, and $PaCO_2$.[63,64] However, despite their apparent advantages, these devices still have not made it into common use in most North American NICUs, both because of their cost and complexity and because of the ease of use of noninvasive technology. One study demonstrated a reduction in the need for blood transfusions in premature infants using an inline blood gas analyzer.[65]

Noninvasive Estimation of Blood Gases

The development of simple, safe, and noninvasive techniques for obtaining continuous estimates of blood gases is one of the most important advances in neonatal care. Pulse oximeters are ubiquitous in NICUs and oxygen saturations are now considered a vital sign. Although less widely used than pulse oximeters, both transcutaneous and end-tidal CO_2 monitors have an important role in the management of neonates. NIRS is another technology that is gradually moving from research to routine clinical use in selected infants.

Pulse Oximetry

Oxygen saturation monitoring via pulse oximetry (SpO_2) is standard practice in NICUs. Pulse oximeters work on the principle that saturated hemoglobin (oxyhemoglobin) is a different color from desaturated hemoglobin (deoxyhemoglobin) and thus absorbs light of a different frequency.[66–68] Oxyhemoglobin demonstrates higher absorbance of infrared light at a wavelength of 940 nm compared with deoxyhemoglobin, which demonstrates a higher absorbance of red light at a wavelength of 660 nm. A probe consisting of a light source and a photosensor is placed so that the light source and photosensor are on opposite sides of each other with tissue in between. As light passes through the tissues, the saturated hemoglobin and desaturated hemoglobin absorb different frequencies of light. By measuring the difference between the ratio of the different frequencies of light absorbed during systole and diastole, the amount of light absorbed because of arterial flow can be calculated. Then, by comparing light absorption at the two appropriate frequencies, the percentage of saturated hemoglobin is calculated. Refinements of this system include complex algorithms for calculating more exact saturation and for separating arterial pulsations from motion artifact. The so-called functional oxygen saturation measured by

pulse oximeters is represented by the equation $100 \times$ OxyHb/ (OxyHb + DeoxyHb), where OxyHb is oxyhemoglobin and DeoxyHb is deoxyhemoglobin.

In general, pulse oximeters provide excellent data about oxygenation in the physiologic range, but there are important limitations that should be considered. The calculation of saturation is dependent on sensing light so that ambient light striking the sensor can lead to a false reading. Poor perfusion and motion may interfere with the signal. By focusing only on oxyhemoglobin and deoxyhemoglobin, traditional pulse oximetry may provide misleading values in the setting of elevated levels of other hemoglobin species.

In the setting of elevated carboxyhemoglobin levels, pulse oximetry will overestimate oxygen saturation by 1% for every 1% increase in carboxyhemoglobin.[70] This occurs because carboxyhemoglobin absorbs light similar to oxyhemoglobin (Fig. 10.10). In contrast, methemoglobin absorbs equal amounts of red and infrared light (see Fig. 10.10). As the amount of methemoglobin increases, the ratio of light absorbance at both wavelengths approaches 1, which corresponds to an oxygen saturation of 85%.[71,72] With advancing technology, the number of wavelengths of light employed by some pulse oximeter manufacturers has increased, allowing the pulse oximeter to measure total hemoglobin and other hemoglobin species such as methemoglobin and carboxyhemoglobin.[69] However, this technology is not used routinely in newborn infants.

Co-oximetry is used in modern blood gas analyzers and differs from pulse oximetry in that it uses spectrophotometry to determine the relative concentrations of hemoglobin derivatives. Modern co-oximeters use over 100 different wavelengths of light.[73] In this manner, they directly measure several hemoglobin species including oxyhemoglobin, deoxyhemoglobin, carboxyhemoglobin, methemoglobin, and sulfhemoglobin. Therefore, they are less prone to error in reporting oxygen saturations compared with pulse oximetry. The "fractional" oxygen saturation measured by blood gas analyzers is represented by

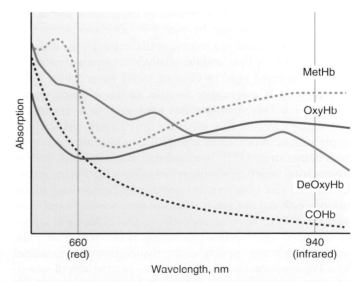

Fig. 10.10 Light absorption. *COHb*, Carboxyhemoglobin; *DeOxyHb*, deoxyhemoglobin; *MetHb*, methemoglobin; *OxyHb*, oxyhemoglobin.

the equation $100 \times OxyHb/(OxyHb + DeoxyHb + COHb + MetHb)$, where OxyHb is oxyhemoglobin, DeoxyHb is deoxyhemoglobin, COHb is carboxyhemoglobin, and MetHb is methemoglobin. In the setting of elevated concentrations of abnormal hemoglobin species, blood gas testing rather than pulse oximetry should guide therapy.

Different manufacturers use different algorithms that may give slightly different results. Manufacturers are constantly updating the software in their devices, making many published articles on the limitations of specific devices out of date. It should be noted that the presence of HbF, anemia, or hyperbilirubinemia has negligible effects on the accuracy of pulse oximetry.[74–76] Pulse oximeters are dependent on adequate pulsatile blood flow. In situations such as shock, or if severe edema obscures pulsatile flow, pulse oximeters may not function reliably. Similarly, in patients on total support from venoarterial ECMO, who have minimal arterial pulsations, many pulse oximeters do not function well if the pulse pressure is less than 10 mm Hg.

Pulse oximeters do not differentiate between degrees of hyperoxemia at the flat upper part of the ODC (see Fig. 10.1). For example, a PaO_2 of 80 and a PaO_2 of 180 mm Hg both represent essentially 100% oxygen saturations (SpO_2). Some clinicians suggest that this is a significant limitation of pulse oximetry compared with transcutaneous oxygen monitoring. Current recommendations target an SpO_2 of 91% to 95% in preterm infants to avoid hyperoxemia and thereby decrease the risk of retinopathy of prematurity.[77] Pulse oximeters are also less accurate at low SpO_2 (e.g., <70% saturation). Outside of the delivery room, this does not usually pose a clinically significant problem because the exact degree of low saturations may not alter clinical decision making.

One major advantage of pulse oximetry is that oxygen saturation is a better indicator of oxygen content than is PaO_2, as saturation is used to calculate oxygen carried by hemoglobin (the major contributor to oxygen content in blood), whereas PaO_2 represents dissolved oxygen, which is a minor component of oxygen transport.

Near-Infrared Spectroscopy

The light-absorbing characteristics of oxygenated and deoxygenated hemoglobin can be used for techniques other than pulse oximetry. NIRS is a technique that relies on the differential absorption of light and the relatively transparent nature of tissue to infrared light to estimate tissue oxygenation. NIRS may be used as a surrogate measure of tissue mixed venous oxygenation. This technique has been gaining acceptance in neonatology but its true value remains largely unknown, as improvement in outcomes with NIRS monitoring has not yet been demonstrated.[99–102] In a randomized clinical trial, cerebral oxygenation targeting was improved using NIRS but the reduction in the risk of severe intraventricular hemorrhage or the risk of death did not reach statistical significance,[101] and there were no differences in neurodevelopmental outcome at 2 years of corrected age.[102] NIRS monitoring is different from pulse oximetry in many aspects as the tissue saturation measured by NIRS represents a weighted average of arterial and venous saturations wherein the weighting factor cannot be precisely determined and varies from tissue to tissue and over time.

CHOICE OF MONITORING METHODS

Transcutaneous Monitoring

Transcutaneous oxygen and CO_2 electrodes allow continuous indirect estimation of PaO_2 and $PaCO_2$. Although pulse oximetry has largely replaced transcutaneous oxygen monitoring for estimating oxygenation, many centers routinely use transcutaneous CO_2 monitoring. Current transcutaneous CO_2 monitoring devices can be run at lower temperatures than previous generations of monitors to lower the risk of thermal injury to immature skin.[78,79] There are several good reviews of the theory and practice of transcutaneous monitoring.[68,79-81]

Transcutaneous PO_2 ($TcPO_2$) essentially measures the PO_2 of skin. Although the PO_2 of skin is usually lower than the PaO_2, heating of the skin directly under the $TcPO_2$ electrode causes local cutaneous vasodilation resulting in the skin PO_2 approaching PaO_2. Although heating the skin causes several effects other than vasodilation, these effects on the ODC, tissue oxygen consumption, and electrode oxygen consumption cancel out for most patients. Studies have shown that $TcPO_2$ approximates PaO_2 even in patients with poor perfusion; however, in older infants with chronic lung disease, $TcPO_2$ underestimates PaO_2.[82]

The relationship between $PaCO_2$ and transcutaneous PCO_2 ($TcPCO_2$) is more complex than between PaO_2 and $TcPO_2$. $TcPCO_2$ should always be greater than $PaCO_2$ because (1) heating causes increased local production of CO_2, (2) there is a significant arterial-cellular CO_2 gradient, and (3) the skin has a cooling effect on the electrode. These effects are fairly uniform at a given temperature and combine to create a linear relationship between $TcPCO_2$ and $PaCO_2$.[83] False readings may occur with $TcPCO_2$ monitors. Although extremely low $TcPCO_2$ readings may be caused by contact with air, false high $TcPCO_2$ readings typically necessitate blood gas correlation to ensure that the $PaCO_2$ is not truly elevated.

Despite its limitations, transcutaneous CO_2 measurement is helpful for trending $PaCO_2$ values, particularly in the absence of reliable clinical indicators of adequacy of ventilation. It may be particularly helpful in the management of infants in whom it is difficult to assess tidal volume. Many clinicians consider $TcPCO_2$ monitoring useful when initiating high-frequency ventilation because both jet and oscillatory ventilation can change $PaCO_2$ rapidly when transitioning from conventional ventilation.

Capnography

Capnography, also known as end-tidal CO_2 monitoring, is the measurement of exhaled CO_2. Because alveolar PCO_2 approximates $PaCO_2$, a sample of pure alveolar gas will provide an estimate of $PaCO_2$. Capnography measures the concentration of CO_2 in exhaled gas and displays this concentration as a function of time. If there is a good end-tidal plateau in exhaled PCO_2, this usually represents the alveolar PCO_2. End-tidal CO_2 monitoring can be done using mainstream, sidestream, or microstream techniques.[84–86] This technique has found widespread use in adult and pediatric intensive care units where patients receive relatively large tidal volumes and low respiratory rates so the alveolar plateau is readily measured. However, it has not been widely accepted into NICUs, primarily because it provides only a rough estimate of $PaCO_2$ among infants with significant lung disease.

In sick neonates, it is difficult to obtain a sample of alveolar gas that is not mixed with gas from the airways. Newborns typically use higher respiratory rates and lower tidal volumes that are too small to obtain an adequate end-tidal alveolar plateau sample. In addition, alveolar disease independently interferes with the relationship of end-tidal CO_2 compared with $PaCO_2$.[87] Capnography may be an accurate method of estimating $PaCO_2$ in healthy infants, or in ventilated postsurgical infants with normal lungs, but provides only a rough estimate of $PaCO_2$, which is usually underestimated in infants with significant lung disease.[85,88–91] One study of capnography during transport of infants found that the end-tidal PCO_2 significantly underestimated $PaCO_2$ but that the degree of underestimation was independent of either the $PaCO_2$ or the severity of lung disease.[92] Quantitative analysis of capnographic curves may indicate the magnitude of spontaneous compared with ventilator-assisted breaths.[93]

Capnography does have a number of advantages, including that it is relatively inexpensive, portable, noninvasive, and easy to use. One of the most useful applications of exhaled CO_2 monitoring is in rapidly confirming proper endotracheal tube placement.[94,95] Small, disposable colorimetric devices are attached to the hub of endotracheal tubes immediately after intubation to ensure that exhaled CO_2 is detected, indicating successful intubation. Moreover, the Neonatal Resuscitation Program recommends that a colorimetric CO_2 detector be used to verify the placement of endotracheal tubes. Infants with very low cardiac output may not exhale sufficient CO_2 to be detected reliably by CO_2 detectors. Although qualitative (colorimetric) detection is useful to confirm endotracheal tube placement, there is no strong evidence supporting quantitative monitoring of end-tidal CO_2 in the delivery room or during resuscitation.[96–98] Many bedside monitors have built-in end-tidal CO_2 monitoring as an option, making continuous monitoring of exhaled CO_2 a realistic option for ventilated infants, with the caveat that some end-tidal CO_2 monitors increase dead space substantially in very preterm infants.

There has been a gradual decline in the reliance on arterial blood gas samples. Efforts to reduce the number of blood tests, including blood gases, have been promoted to reduce the volume of iatrogenic blood loss. "Permissive hypercarbia" has led to a wider range of accepted $PaCO_2$ values and, therefore, less frequent blood gas measurements. The increased use of patient-triggered volume-targeted ventilation modes may have further reduced the frequency of blood gas sampling. Despite these trends, a reliable arterial blood gas sampling in unstable infants remains important. We routinely place a UAC in infants who require intubation or nasal continuous positive airway pressure with significant oxygen requirements and in most infants who weigh less than 1 kg. We usually remove UACs after a few days when frequent blood gas or continuous blood pressure measurements are no longer needed. In older infants who are critically ill peripheral arterial catheters can be placed.

We monitor all infants with continuous pulse oximetry until discharge, although some units switch to apnea monitors alone before discharge. Infants requiring significant respiratory support are followed with transcutaneous CO_2 monitoring in addition to pulse oximetry. Capnography is not widely used in our NICU but has been used in larger infants with minimal lung disease. We use NIRS monitoring routinely in very preterm infants requiring respiratory support during the first week after birth.

Continuous monitoring of ventilated infants is supplemented with intermittent measurements of blood gases. In our NICU, stable ventilated infants without arterial access usually have capillary blood gases performed every 24 to 48 hours, whereas less stable infants have them performed as frequently as two to four times per day. In critically ill infants without arterial access, we rarely use samples drawn from an umbilical venous catheter as the venous PCO_2 may be significantly higher than the arterial PCO_2. It may be occasionally preferable to use this crude measure than to perform repeated arterialized capillary blood gas samples or intermittent arterial punctures.[103,104]

BLOOD GAS ANALYZERS

Blood gas analyzers continue to evolve, offering more than basic blood gas measurement of pH, $PaCO_2$, and PaO_2. Modern blood gas analyzers are capable of measuring various forms of hemoglobin, serum electrolytes, and metabolites. Point-of-care blood gas analyzers facilitate analyzing of the blood sample near the bedside and in the delivery room, which can accelerate clinical decision making.[105,106] Arterial, venous, and capillary blood gas analyzed in the NICU may reduce pre– and post–sample collection errors and decrease time to results.[105,106] Analyzers come in a variety of sizes from handheld to portable desktop systems.

Measuring Principle of a Blood Gas Analyzer

Traditional blood gas electrodes for pH, $PaCO_2$, and PaO_2 measure changes in electrical current or voltage. Electrodes are constructed of a permeable membrane and are bathed in a solution that allows H^+, CO_2, or O_2 to pass through the membrane, react with the solution, and cause a current or voltage change that equates to the measurement of pH, $PaCO_2$, or PaO_2. Currently, analyzers use technologies such as potentiometry, amperometry, fluorescence, and ion-selective electrodes to measure blood gases, electrolytes, and metabolites.[106] The analyzer derives other variables such as base excess (BE)/deficit, bicarbonate, oxygen saturation of hemoglobin from the pH, $PaCO_2$, and PaO_2 measured values through algorithms and nomograms. Derived values are calculated and therefore may not be accurate compared with measured values.

The oxygen saturation of hemoglobin calculation fails to account for dyshemoglobins. A co-oximeter is preferable in this instance as it can directly measure different hemoglobin species. For this reason, some modern blood gas analyzers also incorporate a co-oximeter. Sample volumes required for capillary and arterial blood gas measurements are analyzer dependent and may range from 65 to 150 μL. Smaller sample volumes may provide fewer analytes or no co-oximeter values. The validity of blood gas results is dependent on analyzer function, sample collection, and sample handling techniques (pre- and postanalytical factors). Blood samples introduced into the analyzer must be collected in an appropriate syringe or capillary tube containing the correct anticoagulant.

TABLE 10.1	Analytical Methods for Measuring Oxygen Saturation				
Device	**Specimen**	**Measurement**	**Reported Data**	**Advantages**	**Disadvantages**
Arterial blood gas (ABG) analyzer	Blood	Partial pressure of oxygen dissolved in whole blood at an electrode	PaO_2, SO_2 (oxygen saturation) Some models available with CO-oximetry capabilities	Also measures pH and $PaCO_2$	Invasive, SaO_2 may be inaccurate if abnormal hemoglobin species present
CO-oximeter	Blood	Absorption of Hb derivatives using multiple wavelengths of light	SaO_2, FO_2Hb^a, $FHHb^a$, $FMetHb^a$, $FCOHb^a$, $FSHb^a$, total hemoglobin concentration	Measures the concentration of Hb species	Invasive, performed in laboratory
Pulse oximeter	Transcutaneous	Absorption at two wavelengths (660 nm and 940 nm) in blood	SpO_2	Noninvasive, continuous bedside monitoring	Inaccurate when interfering substances are present: MetHb, certain dyes

[a]The "F" preceding each acronym refers to "fractional," referring to the fractional concentration of each hemoglobin species.
Reproduced with modifications from Haymond S: Oxygen Saturation, A Guide to Laboratory Assessment. Clinical Laboratory News, February 10–12, 2006.

Blood Gas Analyzer Quality Assurance

To ensure consistent reliable results, the blood gas analyzer should be part of a quality assurance program that monitors, documents, and regulates the accuracy of the analyzer. Internal quality control measures may consist of calibration, quality control and maintenance schedules, comparing samples to lab equipment, and external proficiency testing.[107] The newest generation of point-of-care analyzers contains disposable sealed packs that include sensors, electrodes, quality control solutions, cleaning solutions, and waste containment. Advantages of these systems are less maintenance, better error detection, and consistent quality control.[108,109] Traditional analyzers are still in use today and require more maintenance, manual care of electrodes, quality control solutions, and waste management.[106,109] A comparison of different analytical methods for measuring oxygen saturation is presented in Table 10.1.

CLINICAL INTERPRETATION OF BLOOD GASES

Understanding the physiology of gas exchange makes the interpretation of blood gases a relatively straightforward process. Hypoxemia is most commonly the result of ventilation-perfusion mismatch or shunting. In many instances, hypoxemia can be treated by reversing atelectasis and/or decreasing pulmonary vascular resistance or, in infants with cyanotic congenital heart disease, improving pulmonary blood flow. Our goal in all infants should be to ensure optimal oxygen delivery to the tissues by targeting appropriate oxygen saturations, hemoglobin levels, and adequate cardiac output. Hypercarbia is treated by increasing minute ventilation by increasing the respiratory rate and/or tidal volume. However, it is uncertain what "normal" and "acceptable" ranges of $PaCO_2$ are, particularly in the premature infant.

In this section, we review the physiology that is relevant to interpreting the core elements of a blood gas analysis—the pH, $PaCO_2$, PaO_2, bicarbonate, and BE/base deficit. The blood gas analyzer directly measures the pH, $PaCO_2$, and PaO_2. Typically, these results are collected on either arterial blood or an arterialized capillary sample.

COMPONENTS OF BLOOD GAS TESTING THAT ARE MEASURED DIRECTLY

pH

The pH provides an overall assessment of acid-base. The pH reported on a blood gas result reflects the concentration of extracellular hydrogen ions: $pH = -\log[H^+]$. More accurately, the pH is equal to the negative log of the hydronium ion (H_3O^+), although we make reference to hydrogen ions by convention. Higher concentrations of hydrogen ions result in a low pH, and vice versa. Because pH is equal to the negative log of the hydrogen ion concentration, large changes in the concentration of hydrogen result in small changes in the pH.

The concentration of hydrogen ions in the blood is surprisingly low compared with other common ions. For example, the concentration of serum sodium is over 3 million times greater than the concentration of hydrogen ions.[110] Maintaining the pH within a normal range is important for normal cellular function throughout the body as pH affects the function of proteins and cell membranes. For this reason, the body maintains very tight control of hydrogen ion concentrations. Chemoreceptors in our arteries and the medulla adjust ventilation based on the pH (and also the PaO_2 and $PaCO_2$).[111–113]

Across the entire range of pH compatible with life (6.9–7.6), the observed difference in hydrogen ion concentration is less than 0.13 mmol/L.[110] This tight control is achieved through a series of buffering systems and compensatory mechanisms within the body. The most important buffering system is the carbonic acid–bicarbonate buffer, in which H^+ and HCO_3^- combine to form H_2CO_3, which is in equilibrium with water and CO_2. The normal ratio of bicarbonate to dissolved CO_2 is 20:1. Hemoglobin, proteins including albumin and globulin, and phosphate also have important acid-buffering functions. Disturbance of acid-base balance results is either an acidosis (low pH) or an alkalosis (high pH). The normal pH range is 7.35 to 7.45. Even in states of significant "acidosis" (e.g., pH 7.10), the blood is relatively alkaline, as acid-base neutrality is defined as a pH of 7.0.

In addition to buffering, or neutralizing acids, volatile acids can be removed from the body via the lungs, whereas the kidneys can excrete fixed acids and regulate the concentration of bicarbonate. Hasselbalch introduced the use of the term "compensation" to describe the means to correct acid-base disturbances in 1915.[114] Compensatory mechanisms restore the pH toward normal levels but usually do not result in full correction or overcorrection of the pH. This occurs as the stimulus driving the compensation is lost as the pH approaches normal levels. For example, a baby with metabolic acidosis and a pH of 7.30 may increase minute ventilation to remove CO_2 from the body, with a resulting increase in pH to 7.35 but not higher. However, more recent evidence citing correction of pH to more than 7.40 in adult patients with chronic respiratory acidosis raises questions about our understanding of this topic.[115–117]

Some clinicians believe that the term "compensation" is misleading and recommend referring to this process as a "secondary response."[118] The respiratory secondary response to acid-base derangements begins nearly immediately and affects the pH within minutes, whereas the renal response begins within 6 to 12 hours and takes 3 to 5 days.[111,112,119] The first step in assessing the acid-base status of the body is evaluating the pH to determine if it is normal. If the pH is abnormal, the next step is to determine whether the derangement is respiratory or metabolic.

Carbon Dioxide

The $PaCO_2$ is usually the next variable examined after evaluation of the pH. Carbon dioxide is a normal by-product of aerobic metabolism. $PaCO_2$ represents the partial pressure of CO_2 that is dissolved in the blood. Carbon dioxide is over 20 times more soluble than oxygen in blood. $PaCO_2$ is the best indicator of the respiratory contribution to acid-base control. The normal range of $PaCO_2$ is 35 to 45 mm Hg.[111,112,120]

Most of the CO_2 in blood is transported to the lungs in the form of bicarbonate, before converting it back to CO_2, which is exhaled and eliminated.[121] Hence, any maneuvers that increase alveolar ventilation will reduce the $PaCO_2$. Alveolar ventilation is represented by the following equation: respiratory rate × (tidal volume − dead space volume). Increasing the ventilator rate, increasing the tidal volume, and/or decreasing the dead space volume will lead to a decrease in $PaCO_2$. Dead space can account for up to 20% of tidal volume in an intubated extremely low–birth weight neonate. Maintenance of $PaCO_2$ within physiologic ranges is dependent both on alveolar ventilation and on the rate of CO_2 production.

Partial Pressure of Oxygen

The PaO_2 represents the oxygen dissolved within the plasma of the blood and offers an assessment of the patient's oxygenation status. By examining the equation for the oxygen content of the blood (oxygen content = 1.34 × hemoglobin concentration × oxygen saturation/100 + 0.003 × PaO_2), it is clear that the dissolved oxygen contributes very little to the total amount of oxygen in the body. However, it is critically important, as it is this dissolved form of oxygen that enters cells.

The PaO_2 can be accurately measured only from arterial blood. The site of arterial blood testing is important to consider in the newborn with a patent ductus arteriosus, especially in the setting of pulmonary hypertension with right to left shunting

in which preductal blood will have a higher PaO_2 than postductal blood. Arterial right upper extremity blood is preductal, whereas blood drawn from the lower limbs or from a UAC is postductal. Although the origin of the left subclavian artery is more likely to be preductal than postductal in location, an echocardiogram would be required to confirm this.[122] Therefore, it is not recommended to use blood drawn from the left radial or ulnar artery if possible.

Hypoxia is a qualitative term that refers to inadequate tissue oxygenation. It should not be confused with hypoxemia, which refers to a below "normal" PaO_2 in the blood. The definitions of normoxemia, hypoxemia, and hyperoxemia will depend on what is considered "normal" for PaO_2. Changing therapy in response to hypoxemia requires careful evaluation of the patient, as there are a wide variety of causes for hypoxemia. Evaluation of hypoxia includes assessment of clinical signs of illness including the adequacy of perfusion and chest rise, and the presence and type of acidosis including lactate, and investigation and treatment of the underlying disease. It is vital to direct therapy toward correcting the underlying cause before simply adjusting the oxygen concentration.

COMPONENTS OF BLOOD GAS TESTING THAT ARE NOT MEASURED DIRECTLY

The following values commonly reported on blood gas results are derived from other measured values or calculated using nomograms or algorithms.

Bicarbonate

Bicarbonate is a base, meaning that it is an acceptor of hydrogen ($HCO_3^- + H^+ \leftrightarrow H_2O + CO_2$). It is therefore "consumed" when neutralizing acids, resulting in a lower bicarbonate serum concentration in the setting of a metabolic acidosis. The normal concentration of bicarbonate in blood is 22 to 24 mEq/L. The kidneys play an important role in acid-base homeostasis through reabsorption of HCO_3^-, urinary excretion of ammonium, and titratable acid formation. The renal threshold of bicarbonate is typically 15 mEq/L. Extremely preterm infants often develop metabolic acidosis because of renal bicarbonate losses down to this threshold in the first weeks after birth. A chronic increase in $PaCO_2$, as seen in infants with bronchopulmonary dysplasia, will eventually lead to an increased HCO_3^- as the body attempts to maintain a 20:1 ratio of bicarbonate to dissolved CO_2. Increased HCO_3^- levels may be exacerbated by chronic diuretic use, as kidneys of infants with low chloride anions retain bicarbonate anions. Giving a patient sodium bicarbonate can transiently elevate the $PaCO_2$ levels until the lungs can correct them. Sodium bicarbonate was once commonly administered for the treatment of lactic acidosis.[123] However, this practice has been called into serious question and is no longer recommended.[21] The correction of the underlying cause should instead be the focus.

The HCO_3^- concentration reported on a blood gas result is not directly measured but rather calculated from the pH and $PaCO_2$. It reflects the inferred metabolic status of the acid-base balance. Various methods have been reported over the years to calculate the HCO_3^- level in a blood gas sample given a certain level of pH and $PaCO_2$. Standard bicarbonate is calculated with blood equilibrated to a $PaCO_2$ of 40 mm Hg at 37 °C. Calculated HCO_3^- values may not reflect a pure metabolic index during hypo- and hypercapnea and the clinicians should learn which method their own institution uses to calculate HCO_3^- values. We encourage the reader to explore publications that describe in greater detail the relationship between $PaCO_2$ and HCO_3^-.[110]

Base Excess

BE refers to the difference between the observed and the normal buffer base concentration or, expressed differently, the amount of acid or base required to return the pH to 7.4 in the setting of a normal $PaCO_2$.[124] The BE is commonly derived from nomograms. Because different models of blood gas analyzers use different methods of calculating the BE, the results may differ among manufacturers.[125]

Although the name implies an excess of base, a deficit can occur when the observed base concentration is below normal. Some clinicians prefer to use the term "base deficit" to refer to levels of base that have a negative value and to reserve the term "BE" for the opposite scenario. BE/base deficit is another indicator of the metabolic acid-base status. Some centers may measure standard BE or BE of extracellular fluid. The standard BE is calculated differently from BE and was developed as a $PaCO_2$-independent index.[110]

Normal BE values in newborns range from −3 to +1.[126] A negative BE, or a base deficit, is observed in the setting of a metabolic acidosis, whereas a positive BE occurs in metabolic alkalosis. The BE is interpreted along with the bicarbonate concentration.

Oxygen Saturation

A broader discussion of oxygen saturation is provided earlier in this chapter. The arterial oxygen saturation (SaO_2) reported by a standard blood gas machine is a calculated value. Because the calculation does not consider nonstandard hemoglobin species (e.g., carboxyhemoglobin, methemoglobin), it may provide an inaccurate estimate.

Blood gas machines that use co-oximetry measure multiple hemoglobin species directly and therefore provide a more accurate SaO_2. Co-oximetry directly measures the following types of hemoglobin:

1. Oxyhemoglobin: hemoglobin that is bound to oxygen
2. Deoxyhemoglobin: hemoglobin that is not bound to oxygen
3. Carboxyhemoglobin: hemoglobin that is bound to carbon monoxide
4. Methemoglobin: an oxidized form of hemoglobin
5. Sulfhemoglobin: an abnormal form of hemoglobin that cannot bind oxygen

Lactate

Lactate is not a traditional blood gas value. However lactate is routinely measured by many blood gas analyzers, so a brief basic discussion of its value is warranted. Analyzers equipped to measure lactate will directly measure the blood with a biosensor utilizing amperometric principles.[106] Lactate is the result of the metabolism of glucose during tissue hypoxia whereby lactate,

ATP, and water are produced.[127] Tissue hypoxia and/or poor tissue perfusion can lead to hyperlactatemia, which can also result from other mechanisms.[128] Blood lactate levels are a reflection of the difference between production and elimination, with the liver responsible for the majority of lactate clearance.[128] Normal blood lactate levels for the term infant depend on local established values and have been reported at less than 2.0 mmol/L.[129]

Arterial, venous, and capillary values for lactate levels have been used clinically, with most reporting good correlation between the sample types.[127,130] Samples should be run within 15 minutes to prevent lactate levels from increasing before testing.[127] Lactate values have a useful role in the assessment of the newborn. Lactate measured in umbilical cord blood was shown to agree with pH and BE and has similar predictive value for short-term morbidities compared with pH and BE.[131] A retrospective study of term infants with intrapartum asphyxia comparing the predictive value of pH, base deficit, and lactate for the incidence of moderate to severe hypoxic encephalopathy (HIE) showed that the highest lactate levels in the first hours of life are important predictors of moderate to severe HIE.[127] Measurement of serum lactate is very helpful in differentiating increased acid production (e.g., because of inadequate tissue oxygen delivery) from loss of bicarbonate, such as occurs in renal tubular acidosis.

ERRORS IN BLOOD GAS MEASUREMENTS

Even small air bubbles in a blood gas sample can cause significant errors. The air bubbles contain room air, which has four main components: nitrogen (78%), oxygen (21%), argon (1%), and CO_2 (0.04%). Room air has a P_ACO_2 that is nearly zero and a PAo_2 of approximately 150 mm Hg. Therefore, air bubbles lower the $PaCO_2$ and can either raise or lower the PaO_2, depending on whether the PaO_2 is below or above 150 mm Hg.[132] The amount of air that comes in contact with arterial blood drawn through a butterfly (scalp vein) infusion set is enough to alter the PaO_2 measurement.[133] Thus, it is important to expel air bubbles from the blood sample before placing it in the blood gas analyzer.

Dilution of a blood sample with intravenous fluids will typically lower the $PaCO_2$ and increase the base deficit without affecting the pH. This is probably because of the diffusion of CO_2 from blood into the intravenous fluid, which contains no CO_2.[132,134,135] Because of the buffering capacity of the blood, the pH changes little, despite the decrease in $PaCO_2$, giving the appearance of a combined metabolic acidosis and respiratory alkalosis. Dilution of a blood gas sample with a lipid emulsion does not appear to have any effect on the blood gas measurements.[136] Dry heparin also does not affect blood gas results.[134]

Blood gas results may be inaccurate if the specimen is not processed promptly, as the cells continue to consume oxygen and produce CO_2 after sampling. Therefore, samples are often placed on ice to slow down the metabolism of the cells in the sample. However, a bench study found that samples were stable for PaO_2 and SaO_2 for up to 30 minutes either at room temperature or when kept in iced water, and that changes after

60 minutes were small and unlikely to be clinically significant.[137] $PaCO_2$ showed a statistically significant increase after 20 minutes at room temperature, but the changes were not clinically significant.[137]

Most blood gas analyzers measure PaO_2 and then calculate the saturation with the assumption that the blood sample is from an adult. However, if the sample contains a significant amount of HbF, the calculated saturation will be inappropriately low (because of the leftward shift of the ODC with HbF). If it is important to exactly measure the patient's saturation, this should be done using co-oximetry.

ASSESSING THE ACCURACY OF A BLOOD GAS RESULT

Determining if a blood gas result is valid requires critical thinking on the part of the clinician. There are several potential errors that can adversely affect the accuracy of blood gas results. Broadly, the timing of these errors can be divided into preanalytical and analytical phases.

Preanalytical errors refer to errors that occur during the period of time before testing the sample in the blood gas analyzer. They include errors in sample collection and handling. The discussion below focuses on preanalytical errors as these are the errors that the clinician is most likely to encounter.

A note on temperature: Modern blood gas analyzers correct samples to 37° C. Although this is standard in modern NICUs, there are situations in which the clinician may wish to test a nontemperature-corrected sample. For example, infants with hypoxic-ischemic encephalopathy are treated with therapeutic hypothermia for a period of 72 hours. The target core body temperature is usually in the range of 33.5° C to 34.5° C. Should we correct this sample to 37° C? Doing so may not reflect the true acid-base status of the patient as it will change the reported PaO_2 (~15 mm Hg higher) and $PaCO_2$ (~6 mm Hg lower).[138,139] There is confusion regarding the best approach to temperature correction in these situations. Many clinicians in adult intensive care units do not correct blood gases to 37° C for this reason. The evidence in the pediatric population is less clear, leading some centers to advocate providing both temperature-corrected and nontemperature-corrected blood gas results for patients with body temperatures significantly outside the normal range.[139,140]

Clinicians are encouraged to critically evaluate blood gas results to determine their level of confidence in their accuracy. There are several accepted approaches. Below is a brief discussion of a few of these approaches:

1. Review the relationship between pH and acute changes in $PaCO_2$. Assuming a normal and constant metabolic rate, an acute increase in $PaCO_2$ of 1 mm Hg causes a corresponding decrease in pH of 0.006, whereas an acute decrease in $PaCO_2$ of 1 mm Hg leads to a 0.01 increase in pH. Understanding this relationship allows the clinician to compare the expected and measured pH. For example, following an acute increase in $PaCO_2$ of 15 mm Hg, the pH should decrease by 0.09 (15 × 0.006 = 0.09), leading to an expected pH of 7.31 (7.40 − 0.09 = 7.31). If the measured pH differs from the expected pH by ±0.03 units, a nonrespiratory or metabolic disorder must be present.
   a. In hypocarbia, expected pH
      = 7.40 + (40 mm Hg − $PaCO_2$) 0.01
   b. In hypercarbia, expected pH
      = 7.40 − ($PaCO_2$ − 40 mm Hg) 0.006
   This independent accuracy check aids the clinician in assessing the patient's metabolic condition without the need to refer to the HCO_3^- or BE values.[19]
2. Use formulas, nomograms, or a blood gas map to calculate or plot the acid-base variables.[19]
3. Compare the calculated plasma bicarbonate to total CO_2.
   a. Total CO_2 is a measure of CO_2 in all states, is measured with venous blood during lab electrolyte testing, and is an indicator of plasma bicarbonate.
   b. The total CO_2 value will be slightly higher than plasma bicarbonate because of the venous blood; however, it can be another check for blood gas accuracy.

Regardless of the methods used, it is critical to consider the patient's clinical status when interpreting the blood gas result.

FINAL THOUGHTS

Although arterial blood gas values are frequently invaluable in managing patients with respiratory distress, they should not be interpreted in the absence of clinical data. A blood gas result that is significantly different from previous results may indicate a major change in the patient's status or may represent an error in blood gas measurement. Neither a blood gas laboratory nor sophisticated noninvasive monitors can replace careful clinical observation.

There are several useful online and mobile-friendly tools for interpreting blood gases.

See Appendix 19 for a few apps related to blood gas evaluations in the newborn developed by a neonatologist from India, Dr. Satish Deopujari.

ACKNOWLEDGMENT

The authors acknowledge the contributions of Drs. David Durand, Nick Mickas, Yacov Rabi, and Mr. Derek Kowal, previous authors of this chapter.

A complete reference list is available at https://expertconsult. inkling.com/.

KEY REFERENCES

15. Whyte RK, Jangaard KA, Dooley KC: From oxygen content to pulse oximetry: completing the picture in the newborn. Acta Anaesthesiol Scand Suppl 107:95–100, 1995.
17. Wimberley PD, Helledie NR, Friss-Hansen B: Some problems involved in using hemoglobin oxygen saturation in arterial blood to detect hypoxemia and hyperoxemia in newborn infants. Scand J Clin Lab Invest 48:45–48, 1988.
21. Aschner JL, Poland RL. Sodium bicarbonate: basically useless therapy. Pediatrics 122:831–835, 2008.

29. Anderson J, Leonard D, Braner DA: Videos in clinical medicine. Umbilical vascular catheterization. N Engl J Med 359:e18, 2008.

66. Tin W, Lal M: Principles of pulse oximetry and its clinical application in neonatal medicine. Semin Fetal Neonatal Med 20(3):192–197, 2015.

79. Eberhard P: The design, use, and results of transcutaneous carbon dioxide analysis: current and future directions. Anesth Analg 105:S48–S52, 2007.

85. Singh BS, Gilbert U, Singh S, et al: Sidestream microstream end tidal carbon dioxide measurements and blood gas correlations in neonatal intensive care unit. Pediatr Pulmonol 48:250–256, 2013.

100. Wolf M, Greisen G: Advances in near-infrared spectroscopy to study the brain of the preterm and term neonate. Clin Perinatol 36:807–834, 2009.

124. Kellum JA: Determinants of blood pH in health and disease. Crit Care 4:6–14, 2000.

131. Armstrong L, Stenson BJ: Use of umbilical cord blood gas analysis in the assessment of the newborn. Arch Dis Child Fetal Neonatal Ed 92:F430–F434, 2007.

11

Noninvasive Monitoring of Gas Exchange

Bobby Mathew and Satyan Lakshminrusimha

KEY POINTS

- Gas exchange monitoring is of utmost importance in the management of preterm and sick term newborn infants.
- Arterial blood gas analysis is the gold standard for monitoring gas exchange but is limited in its utility because of the attendant risks of iatrogenic anemia and vascular injury.
- Noninvasive monitoring of gas exchange provides a reliable alternative, with continuous monitoring of gas exchange at the lung and the arterial capillary and tissue levels.
- It is critical that physicians have a sound understanding of available technology, its utility, and their own limitations, especially in tiny preterm neonates, to best use the many modalities that are available at their disposal.

Gas exchange is a dynamic process that is dependent on complex interactions among respiratory, cardiovascular, and central nervous systems. In a healthy individual breathing room air, the arterial blood levels of oxygen and carbon dioxide are maintained within a narrow range. In neonates receiving assisted ventilation, supplemental oxygen, or suffering from impaired respiratory control, gas exchange may be compromised and close monitoring of blood gases becomes imperative to maintain homeostasis. Analysis of an arterial blood gas (ABG) sample is the gold standard for assessment of gas exchange. However, the inherent risks associated with arterial access such as vasospasm, thrombosis, ischemia, and iatrogenic blood loss necessitate alternate noninvasive methods to assess gas exchange. Blood gas analysis provides only a snapshot of a dynamic process and results are frequently delayed unless performed using a point-of-care device. This chapter briefly describes the techniques, indications, strengths and limitations of the common noninvasive modalities used to monitor gas exchange (Fig. 11.1) in the neonatal intensive care unit (NICU). These monitors provide a large amount of data that, with careful interpretation, can guide therapeutic strategy and achieve the best possible outcome.[1]

NONINVASIVE MONITORING OF OXYGENATION

Pulse Oximetry

Oxygen has been widely used in the NICU since the mid-twentieth century. The misadventures with oxygen therapy and retinopathy of prematurity (ROP) are well documented in the neonatal literature. There is controversy surrounding the target saturations during intensive care of preterm infants despite multiple large randomized controlled trials.[2-6] In the premature infant blood flow, the amount and type of hemoglobin and the percentage of arterial oxygen saturation of hemoglobin (SaO_2) are the major determinants of tissue oxygen delivery (Fig. 11.2). Cyanosis is an unreliable assessment of oxygenation as it is detectable only by visual observation when deoxyhemoglobin (DeoxyHb) is above 5 g/dL.[7] Thus, continuous monitoring of saturation by pulse oximetry (SpO_2) is crucial to providing optimal care.

Pulse oximetry measures the percentage of hemoglobin saturated with oxygen. It provides a transcutaneous, noninvasive estimate of SaO_2 and displays a plethysmographic waveform with a heart rate. The monitoring of hemoglobin saturation is possible by pulse oximetry because tissue is transparent to light in the near-infrared spectrum, which allows the distinct absorption spectra of chromophores such as oxyhemoglobin (HbO_2) and DeoxyHb to be viewed (Fig. 11.3). Pulse oximetry is based on the Beer-Lambert law, which states that absorption of light of a given wavelength is proportional to the concentration of the light-absorbing substance (chromophore) and the light path length.[8,9] Pulse oximetry is based on two principles: (1) spectrophotometry—HbO_2 and reduced DeoxyHb have different absorption spectra at different wavelengths of light (red and near infrared) and (2) photoplethysmography—the amount of light absorbed by blood in the tissue changes with the arterial pulse (see Fig. 11.3). The pulse oximeter probe consists of two light-emitting diodes and a photodetector that are positioned facing each other with the light passing intermittently at very high frequency through the interposed tissue. Saturation is estimated from the relative absorption of the two wavelengths during pulsatile flow (because of arterial blood—referred to as AC by convention) versus nonpulsatile flow (venous and tissue absorption—referred to as DC): $SpO_2 = f(AC_{red}/DC_{red})/(AC_{infrared}/DC_{infrared})$, where f is the calibration constant.

The calibration algorithm for pulse oximetry is generated by subjecting healthy volunteers to varying inspired oxygen concentrations and correlating the arterial gas SaO_2 with the ratio of absorption (shown in the previous formula) over a range of saturation values.[10] Because it is unethical to expose healthy

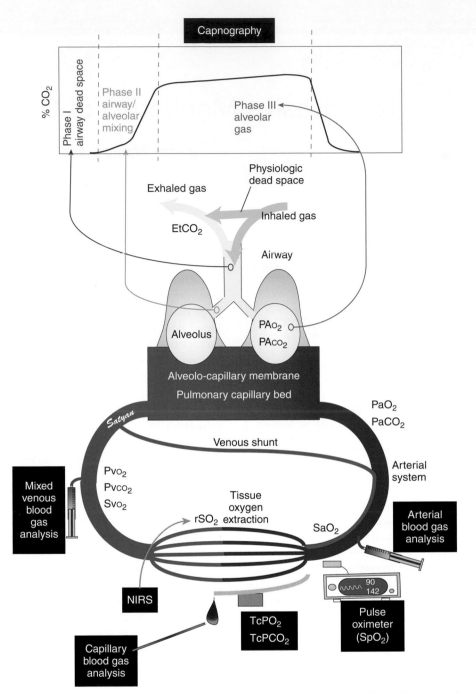

Fig. 11.1 Invasive and noninvasive assessment of gas exchange in neonates. Gas exchange in the lung occurs at the alveolocapillary membrane. Oxygen and CO_2 diffuse from and to the alveolus. The alveolar tension of CO_2 and O_2 (P_ACO_2 and P_AO_2) is in equilibration with pulmonary blood. During exhalation, the initial part of exhaled gas (phase I) is predominantly from the airway and has minimal CO_2. During phase II, a mixture of airway and alveolar gas is exhaled, resulting in an increase in CO_2. During phase III, alveolar gas is exhaled and the end-tidal CO_2 ($EtCO_2$) evaluated by capnography. The physiologic dead space "dilutes" exhaled gas, and increased dead space increases the difference between P_ACO_2 and $EtCO_2$. Arterial blood gas analysis is the gold standard invasive assessment of gas exchange and measures partial pressure of arterial oxygen, CO_2, and arterial oxygen saturation (PaO_2, $PaCO_2$, and SaO_2). Increasing venous shunt (because of pulmonary hypertension, congenital heart disease, or ventilation-perfusion mismatch) can decrease PaO_2. A pulse oximeter measures oxygen saturation (SpO_2) and is a reliable estimate of SaO_2. Transcutaneous sensors heat the cutaneous capillary bed and measure CO_2 and O_2 tension ($TcPCO_2$ and $TcPO_2$). A capillary blood sample obtained after warming the heel ("arterialized" sample) is commonly used in neonates. Near-infrared spectroscopy ($NIRS$) can measure tissue (regional) oxygen saturation (rSO_2). Mixed venous blood gas analysis provides partial pressure of CO_2 and O_2 and oxygen saturation ($PvCO_2$, PvO_2, and SvO_2).

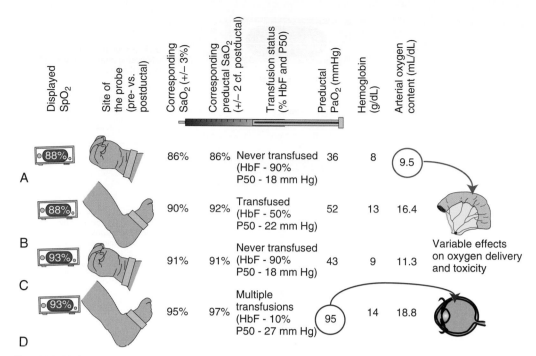

Fig. 11.2 Variables that influence oxygen delivery (based on arterial oxygen content) and oxygen toxicity (based on PaO_2). The variation in arterial oxygen content compared with pulse oximetry based on factors such as site of probe placement, hemoglobin type, and content is illustrated. Each row represents an infant with a specific combination of variables. The oxygen content can vary twofold with a 5% difference in displayed oxygen saturation (SpO_2) on the pulse oximeter, and an infant with a lower SpO_2 (88%) can actually have a higher oxygen content than one with a higher SpO_2 (93%). Infant A has a preductal SpO_2 of 88%, which can correspond to an arterial oxygen saturation (SaO_2) of 85% to 91% in approximately two-thirds of subjects ($\pm$3% variation with pulse oximeters). If the corresponding preductal SaO_2 is assumed to be 86% and she has never received a transfusion, her hemoglobin F (HbF) concentration is around 90%. The corresponding preductal PaO_2 is 36 mm Hg. If this infant has a hemoglobin (Hb) concentration of 8 g/dL, her arterial oxygen content will be approximately 9.5 mL/dL. Infant B has a postductal SpO_2 of 88%, which can correspond to an SaO_2 of 85% to 91% in approximately two-thirds of subjects. If postductal SaO_2 is assumed to be 90%, the corresponding preductal SaO_2 may be 92%. If this baby has received two transfusions, her HbF concentration is approximately 50% and the corresponding preductal PaO_2 is 52 mm Hg. If this infant's Hb concentration is 13 g/dL, her arterial oxygen content will be approximately 16.4 mL/dL. Infant C, who has never been transfused with blood and has a preductal SpO_2 of 93% and a PaO_2 of 43 mm Hg, is at significantly reduced risk of oxygen toxicity compared with infant B despite a higher displayed SpO_2. Infant D has the same displayed SpO_2 as infant C (93%). However, his pulse oximeter is located on his left foot (postductal), and he has received blood transfusions. His PaO_2 is considerably higher (95 mm Hg) compared with infant C (43 mm Hg), placing him at risk for oxygen toxicity. A higher Hb concentration results in higher arterial oxygen content.

volunteers to hazardously low saturations, readings below 75% are based on data extrapolated from calibration values obtained between 100% and 75%. Values obtained by pulse oximetry are within $\pm$2% to 3% of the true SaO_2 value between 70% and 100%. Recently, "Blue" sensors (Masimo, Irvine, CA) calibrated for the 60% to 80% range are being used in neonates with cyanotic congenital heart disease (CHD). Harris et al. reported that these sensors have better accuracy in the 75% to 85% SpO_2 range, with 86% of the samples demonstrating less than 5% difference compared with co-oximetry (compared with only 69% of samples with <5% difference from co-oximetry values from standard pulse oximetry sensors). However, there was a further increase in differences for SaO_2 values under 75% and neonates under 3 kg were not tested.[11] A study by Kim et al. comparing standard pulse oximeters to the Masimo blue sensor in pediatric patients with CHD demonstrated lower bias for the blue sensor.[12]

Although pulse oximetry is now the standard of care in the NICU, there are no clearly established normal values in neonates. Pulse oximetry studies in normal healthy term infants and preterm infants breathing room air have shown average SpO_2 to be 97% and 95%, respectively.[13,14] However, defining a target range of SpO_2 in preterm infants on oxygen therapy or mechanical respiratory support as well as in term infants with persistent pulmonary hypertension of the newborn (PPHN) remains a topic of controversy.[15,16] A recently published study on the relationship of postmenstrual age on the threshold for risk of hypoxemia (PaO_2 <40 mm Hg), normoxemia, and hyperoxemia (PaO_2 >99 mm Hg) showed that the risk of hypoxemia and normoxemia was independent of postmenstrual age. However, the risk for severe hyperoxemia changes with postmenstrual age. The cut-off SpO_2 for hyperoxemia for infants under 33 weeks was 98%, for infants 33 to 36 weeks at 97% SpO_2, and for those more than 36 weeks at 96% SpO_2.[17]

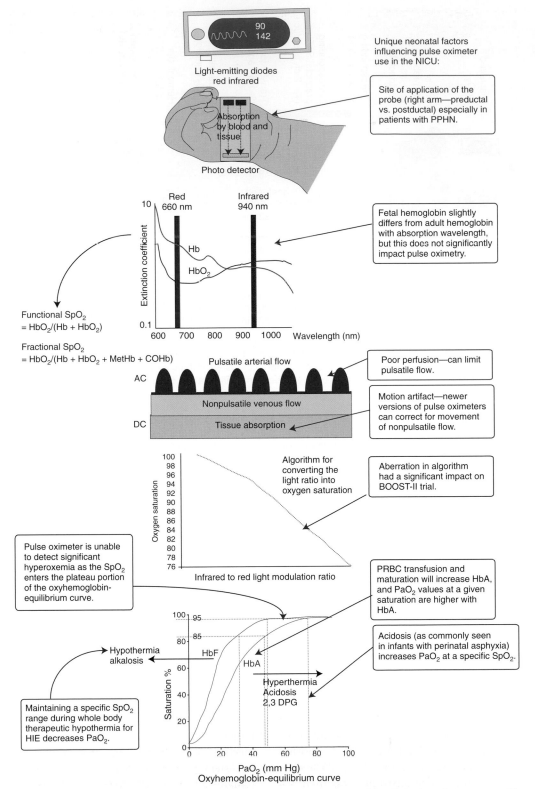

Fig. 11.3 Infographic showing the basic principles of pulse oximetry and its limitations in neonates. The pulse oximeter probe has diodes that emit light in the red and infrared spectra. After absorption of this light by pulsatile arterial blood, venous blood, and tissue, it is detected by photodetectors in the pulse oximeter probe. The extinction coefficients for deoxyhemoglobin (*Hb*) and oxyhemoglobin (*HbO₂*) are different at red and infrared spectra. The infrared-to-red light modulation ratio is converted to an SpO₂ number using an algorithm. The SpO₂ is usually within ±3% of the SaO₂. The relationship between PaO₂ and SaO₂ is the oxyhemoglobin-equilibrium curve. Limitations of pulse oximetry are shown in red boxes. *COHb*, Carboxyhemoglobin; *2,3 DPG*, diphosphoglycerate; *HbA*, adult hemoglobin; *HbF*, fetal hemoglobin; *HIE*, hypoxic–ischemic encephalopathy; *MetHb*, methemoglobin; *NICU*, neonatal intensive care unit; *PPHN*, persistent pulmonary hypertension of the newborn; *PRBC*, packed red blood cells.

A low likelihood of avoiding hypoxemia and hyperoxemia was associated with an SpO_2 target of 90% to 95% in both preterm and term infants.[18]

Indications for Pulse Oximetry

In the NICU, pulse oximetry has become the standard of care and is considered the fifth vital sign. Estimation of SpO_2 by continuous pulse oximetry is used to (1) titrate inspired oxygen concentration in infants receiving supplemental oxygen, (2) define bronchopulmonary dysplasia (BPD) with the oxygen-reduction test,[19] (3) monitor stable growing premature infants for bradycardia and desaturation spells, (4) titrate supplemental oxygen therapy during delivery room resuscitation and stabilization, (5) screen for critical CHD (CCHD) in the newborn period,[20,21] (6) monitor an infant's status during transport, (7) diagnose PPHN with ductal shunt by dual-pulse oximetry (postductal lower limb SpO_2 >5%–10% lower than right upper limb value), and (8) perform car seat testing before discharge of at-risk infants.

Delivery Room Resuscitation

With the recognition of the dangers of oxidative stress associated with hyperoxia in the immediate newborn period, the use of oxygen blenders and pulse oximetry has been recommended for resuscitation and stabilization of newborn infants in the delivery room.[22] Pulse oximetry assists in monitoring response to resuscitation (improvement in heart rate) and titration of supplemental oxygen therapy. The Neonatal Resuscitation Program (NRP) 2016 and 2021 guidelines define target saturations based on time after birth to guide optimal use of oxygen in the delivery room.[23-26] The use of pulse oximetry in the delivery room presents unique challenges. Delay in obtaining a stable tracing and readout of SpO_2 and heart rate is common. The average time to detect reliable signal on pulse oximetry has been estimated to be between 1 and 2 minutes.[24,27,28] Using the correct order of connection minimizes time to obtaining a stable signal. (1) First, connect the oximeter cable to the pulse oximeter monitor; (2) turn on the pulse oximeter monitor; (3) apply the probe to the baby; and (4) connect the probe to the oximeter cable. The average difference in time with this optimized sequence has been shown to be 7 seconds as compared with connecting the sensor to the cable first and then applying the sensor to the infant.[29] A more recent study performed in the delivery room with infants 28 weeks' or more gestation questioned this approach and suggested that applying pulse oximetry sensor to the oximeter first and then to the infant resulted in an earlier detection of a reliable signal.[30] However, with both techniques, the time from birth to obtaining a reliable signal was similar. Preductal pulse oximetry should be recorded from the right upper limb as there is a substantial pre/postductal SpO_2 difference in the immediate newborn period. The NRP guidelines for delivery room SpO_2 were created using preductal SpO_2. In addition, signal detection has been demonstrated to be faster with the pulse oximetry probe applied to the hand compared with the foot.[31] Movement, poor perfusion, difficulties with probe placement, and high ambient light can all interfere with obtaining a reliable pulse oximetry signal. Skin pigmentation is thought to slightly alter pulse oximetry reading in adults.[30] However, in newborn infants, dark skin did not appear to influence pulse oximetry.[32,33]

Limitations of Pulse Oximetry

1. Hyperoxia, hypoxia, and hypercarbia: Owing to the sigmoid shape of the oxyhemoglobin equilibration curve (see Fig. 11.3), pulse oximetry is unable to detect significant hyperoxia and is slow to detect acute hypoxemia. In infants receiving supplemental oxygen, even large changes in PaO_2 result in a small change in SpO_2 if the saturation is close to 100% (see oxygen reserve index [ORI]). Alveolar hypoventilation may also be missed in infants on supplemental oxygen monitored solely with pulse oximetry and can lead to significant hypercarbia without an appreciable change in SpO_2. Hence, patients on supplemental oxygen at risk of hyperoxia/hypoxia/hypercarbia should have intermittent PO_2 and PCO_2 measured by blood gases. Anemia (unless very severe) and polycythemia do not affect pulse oximetry readings.[34]

2. Hypoperfusion and hypothermia: Pulse oximetry relies on normal pulsatile flow for its signal and hence can be falsely low in the setting of impaired perfusion or vasoconstriction associated with hypothermia, vasopressor treatment for hypotension, tourniquet effect from blood pressure cuff, and so on.[35] When applying the sensor circumferentially to the finger, hand, or foot, it should not be applied too tightly.[36]

   Fetal hemoglobin and hypothermia shift the oxygen dissociation curve to the left. In infants with hypoxic ischemic encephalopathy (HIE) undergoing whole body therapeutic hypothermia, for a given SpO_2, the PaO_2 is significantly lower as compared with normothermia.[37] Hence, pulse oximetry and the use of uncorrected blood gas at 37° C can underestimate hypoxemia during hypothermia. Thus, during therapeutic hypothermia for HIE, frequent blood gas monitoring and maintaining temperature corrected PaO_2 between 50 and 80 mm Hg are required to prevent the risk of developing or worsening of PPHN.

3. Movement artifact: Conventional pulse oximetry is based on pulsatile flow of blood and calculates SpO_2 based on the assumption that arterial blood is the only component that moves at the site of measurement. During periods of body movement, the blood in the venous and tissue compartment also moves and interferes with the SpO_2 reading or causes a signal dropout. This can disrupt monitoring during transport or during periods of spontaneous activity. Newer pulse oximeters with signal extraction technology use adaptive filtering to separate the components of data and filter noise from the signal to limit motion artifact.[38,39]

Functional Versus Fractional Saturation

Functional saturation refers to the percentage of hemoglobin that is saturated with oxygen in relation to the amount of hemoglobin that is capable of transporting oxygen—that is, HbO_2/(HbO_2 + DeoxyHb). In contrast, fractional saturation is the percentage of oxygenated hemoglobin to the total hemoglobin, which includes variant hemoglobin molecules such as methemoglobin (MetHb) and carboxyhemoglobin (COHb) that are incapable of binding oxygen. Conventional oximeters display functional saturation and do not distinguish the variant hemoglobins from HbO_2 and provide saturation readings that are higher than the fractional saturation in patients with dyshemoglobinemias. High levels of COHb cause an increase in the SpO_2 approximately equal to the amount of COHb that is present.[40] The presence of MetHb will bias the functional SpO_2 reading toward 85%, which will result in over- or underestimation of saturation for $\%HbO_2$ values below and above 85%, respectively. In normoxic subjects, high levels of MetHb decrease the SpO_2 reading by about half of the MetHb percentage concentration.[41] New-generation oximeters are capable of detecting COHb and MetHb by using additional wavelengths of light and provide saturation readings that are more accurate in the clinical setting. When oxygen saturation determination by co-oximetry on a blood gas sample is discrepant by 5% or greater than the saturation measured by pulse oximetry, the presence of a variant hemoglobin (including fetal hemoglobin—see later) has to be considered.

Additional Considerations

Fetal hemoglobin has light absorption characteristics similar to those of adult hemoglobin and does not affect pulse oximetry readings.[42] However, one has to keep in mind its effect on the oxygen dissociation curve and tissue oxygenation at the displayed SpO_2 values (see Fig. 11.3). Indirect bilirubin has a different light absorption spectrum at 450 nm and typically will not affect SpO_2 readings.[43,44] However, interference from ambient light with phototherapy and elevated COHb with hemolysis can alter SpO_2 in neonates. Discoloration from bronze-baby syndrome (because of phototherapy in the presence of direct hyperbilirubinemia) has also been reported to interfere with pulse oximetry readings.[45]

Various indices have been derived from the data provided by oximetry and are of potential use in interpreting clinical status and guiding clinical care. These include the following:

The ORI[46]: Newer pulse oximeters use multiwavelength co-oximetry technology enabling them to monitor oxygenation in the moderate hyperoxic range, (i.e., PaO_2 between 100 and 200 mm Hg). Using this technology, it is possible to analyze arterial and venous pulsatile blood absorption changes of incident light on tissue. When supplemental oxygen delivery is progressively increased, the PaO_2 increases and as it reaches over 100 mm Hg, the SpO_2 reaches a plateau close to 100%. The venous saturation (SvO_2) continues to increase and it stabilizes around 80% as the PaO_2 reaches about 200 mm Hg. The algorithm for calculation of the ORI is based on the Fick's principle and oxygen content equations. The change in light absorption over this PaO_2 range (100–200 mm Hg) is the basis for ORI calculation. ORI is expressed as a unitless index with values ranging between 0.00 and 1.00, which indicates changes in PaO_2 in the moderate hyperoxia range. In adult patients undergoing surgery, the correlation between ORI and PaO_2 was studied.[47] At PaO_2 level less than 240 mm Hg, regression analysis showed a positive correlation with PaO_2 ($r^2 = 0.536$). At PaO_2 over 100 mm Hg, all ORI scores were more than 0.24 and at PaO_2 over 150 mm Hg, 96.6% of ORI scores were greater than 0.55. It is, however, important to bear in mind that ORI is not equivalent to PaO_2 and does not replace the need for ABG analysis. No studies to date have been published on the utility of ORI in the neonatal population.

The oxygen saturation index (OSI): The oxygenation index (OI = $FiO_2 \times 100 \times$ mean airway pressure [MAP in cm H_2O] $\div PaO_2$ [in mm Hg]) has been used to monitor the severity of hypoxemic respiratory failure (HRF) and response to treatment. Because the calculation of OI requires PaO_2 obtained by an ABG, OSI has been suggested as an alternative. Rawat et al. have shown that in newborn infants with HRF, the OSI ($FiO_2 \times 100 \times$ MAP $\div$ preductal SpO_2) correlated closely with the OI.[48] The relationship of OSI with OI in the saturation range of 70% to 99% is approximately OI = $2 \times$ OSI. The use of OSI will allow continuous assessment of the severity of HRF.[49,50]

The perfusion index (PI) is a measure derived from pulse oximetry[51] and compares the pulsatile to the nonpulsatile signal [(pulsatile signal (AC)/nonpulsatile signal (DC)) $\times$ 100] and gives an indication of the perfusion at the monitored site[52] (Fig. 11.4). The value of PI as an indicator of a patient's circulatory status is being investigated for identification of CHD (left obstructive heart disease is not typically identified on routine pulse oximetry screening for CCHD),[53] subclinical chorioamnionitis, severity of illness, and intravascular volume status.[52] The value can range from 0.02% (very weak pulse strength) to 20% (very strong pulse strength) and is influenced by stroke volume, vasoactive drugs, temperature, and vasoconstriction at the site of probe placement.[51] A study evaluating the reproducibility of PI in preterm infants less than 32 weeks' gestation in the first 48 hours of life showed a high correlation coefficient for reproducibility in the same limb. Measurements obtained in the right upper limb (preductal) were consistently higher than either lower limb.[54]

The plethysmographic variability index (PVI) is also derived from pulse oximetry. The arterial pulse volume changes during phases of the respiratory cycle, and this is more pronounced when the preload is inadequate (see Fig. 11.4). PVI measures the change in PI during a respiratory cycle and is expressed as a percentage as shown in the following equation: PVI = $[(PI_{max} - PI_{min})/PI_{max}] \times 100\%$.[55] Early studies suggest that PVI may prove helpful in assessing the hemodynamic significance of patent ductus arteriosus (PDA) in preterm infants[56] and intravascular volume status in neonatal patients.[57] A high PVI in the presence of hypotension may be an indication for a fluid bolus to increase intravascular volume.[1] Cannesson et al. showed that a PVI of more than 14% before volume expansion identified response to a fluid load in adults with a sensitivity of 81% and specificity of 100%.[58] PVI can also predict fluid responsiveness in infants undergoing congenital heart surgery, with a threshold of 13% helping to discriminate between responders and nonresponders with a sensitivity of 84% and specificity of 64%.[59]

A recent study assessing PVI at the same site of measurement and interlimb comparison in stable spontaneously breathing preterm infants between 26 and 32 weeks' gestation in the first 48 hours of life demonstrated poor reproducibility both at the

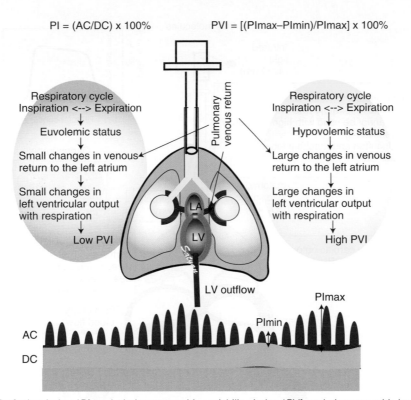

Fig. 11.4 Perfusion index (*PI*) and plethysmographic variability index (*PVI*) and changes with hypovolemia. Changes in intrathoracic pressure with respiration alter venous return to the left atrium (*LA*) and influence left ventricular (*LV*) preload and LV output and PI. These changes in LV output and PI with respiration (*PVI*) are more marked in the presence of hypovolemia and can predict response to a fluid bolus.

same site and in interlimb measurements. The presence of physiological shunts in the early neonatal period in extremely preterm infants in the study population may explain the poor reproducibility seen in this study. Further studies are needed in preterm infants to assess the clinical utility of this parameter in this patient population.[60]

Transcutaneous Oxygen Monitoring

Transcutaneous oxygen ($TcPO_2$) is occasionally used in NICUs as an alternative to arterial PaO_2 measurements in infants without arterial access but in need of continuous monitoring of PaO_2. The sensor consists of a platinum cathode and a silver reference anode. The electrode is separated from the skin surface by a thin membrane through which the oxygen diffuses. The reduction of oxygen at the platinum sensor cathode generates a current that is processed to a PO_2 readout. Studies comparing PaO_2 with $TcPO_2$ in infants show good correlation.[61] However, sensors need frequent repositioning and recalibration with ABGs, and the need for higher operating temperature is associated with a risk of thermal burns in preterm infants. With oxygenation being routinely monitored by pulse oximetry, transcutaneous monitoring of oxygen is becoming less common.

NONINVASIVE ASSESSMENT OF PARTIAL PRESSURE OF CARBON DIOXIDE

Arterial $PaCO_2$ is a reflection of the interaction of CO_2 production in the body (metabolism), transport (systemic and pulmonary

perfusion), and elimination (ventilation). Capnography provides instantaneous breath-to-breath analysis of exhaled CO_2 and has become an integral part of monitoring in the operating room. $PaCO_2$ in normal healthy infants ranges between 35 and 45 mm Hg. Cerebral blood flow is dependent on the arterial $PaCO_2$[62] and increases with hypercarbia and decreases with hypocarbia. In mechanically ventilated extremely preterm infants, fluctuations of $PaCO_2$ are common and predispose the infants to intraventricular hemorrhage (IVH), periventricular leukomalacia (PVL), and BPD.[63-65] Approaches to ventilation strategy (high frequency vs. conventional) and adjustment of ventilator settings are frequently based on $PaCO_2$. Assessment of $PaCO_2$ with intermittent ABGs can lead to unrecognized periods of hypercarbia and hypocarbia and missed opportunities for ventilator weaning. The continuous noninvasive assessment of $PaCO_2$ may be achieved using end-tidal CO_2 ($EtCO_2$) or transcutaneous CO_2 ($TcPCO_2$).

Capnography and End-Tidal Carbon Dioxide Monitoring

Capnography, the measurement of $EtCO_2$ levels in exhaled breath, is based on the principle that the CO_2 diffuses easily from the pulmonary capillary into the alveolus and rapidly equilibrates with alveolar CO_2 (P_ACO_2). The capnogram is a graphic display of the levels of CO_2 during a respiratory cycle. During inspiration, PCO_2 on the capnogram is zero as the atmospheric air contains very little CO_2. At the beginning of exhalation, the gas from the anatomic dead space is expired first and has minimal CO_2 (phase I, see Fig. 11.1). In phase II, gas

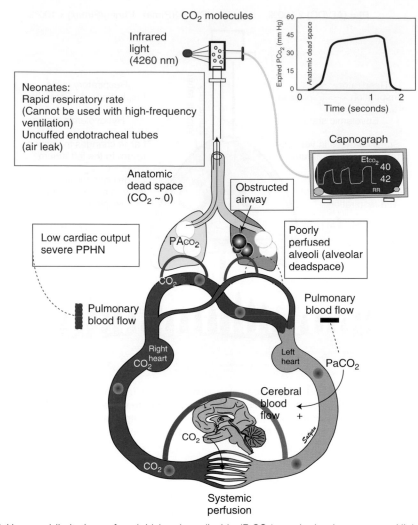

Fig. 11.5 Uses and limitations of end-tidal carbon dioxide ($EtCO_2$) monitoring in neonates. High CO_2 levels increase cerebral blood flow and decrease pulmonary blood flow. Increased dead space (anatomic and alveolar, often caused by ventilation-perfusion mismatch as shown in the left lung) contributes to inaccuracy with $EtCO_2$ monitoring. Limitations for $EtCO_2$ monitoring are shown in red boxes. *PPHN*, Persistent pulmonary hypertension of the newborn.

from the alveoli mixes with gas in the dead space, resulting in a sharp increase in the CO_2 concentration, and this reaches a peak and then plateaus as all of the expired gas is derived from the alveoli (phase III). The CO_2 level in the sampled gas is measured using infrared spectroscopy. CO_2 absorbs infrared light of a specific wavelength (4.26 μm), and this is used to calculate the amount of CO_2 in the sample (Fig. 11.5). In neonates, especially preterm, high respiratory rates and tiny tidal volumes prevent equilibration with alveolar gases limiting the utility of $EtCO_2$.

Mainstream and Sidestream Capnography

$EtCO_2$ monitors fall into two categories based on the position of the measurement device with respect to the infant's airway. In mainstream capnography, the sensor is in line with the ventilator circuit, and all the inhaled and exhaled gas passes directly over the infrared bench. In the sidestream devices, the sensor is located away from the airway, and the gas sample is continuously aspirated from the breathing circuit (via a microstream

of ~50 mL/min) and delivered to the sensor for analysis. Mainstream sensors have the advantages of faster response time and reliable single-breath capnometry measurements and are less affected by high ventilator rates. The disadvantage of mainstream capnography is that it adds respiratory dead space and can cause rebreathing of exhaled CO_2. Sidestream devices add minimal dead space and can be used for long-term monitoring; however, their accuracy is less than that of mainstream devices. At low expiratory gas flow rates, dilution of the sampled gas with the surrounding air can affect the accuracy of measurements. Sidestream measurements also tend to be less accurate in infants with high respiratory rates.

Carbon Dioxide Monitoring in the Neonatal Intensive Care Unit

Studies on capnography in the NICU have focused largely on the correlation between $EtCO_2$ and $PaCO_2$. Capnography can be used to monitor the rate, rhythm, and effectiveness of respiration (spontaneous or assisted); evaluate pulmonary and systemic perfusion and metabolism; and guide ventilator management. Kugelman et al. conducted a randomized multicenter trial in preterm ventilated infants on the use of distal end-tidal continuous capnography and demonstrated good correlation and agreement with $PaCO_2$ and improved outcomes with less time spent in unsafe $EtCO_2$ levels and decreased incidence of IVH and periventricular PVL in monitored infants.[66] Infants with HIE receiving therapeutic hypothermia have decreased metabolism, which may be reflected as a decrease in $EtCO_2$. During whole-body therapeutic hypothermia, Afzal et al. observed good correlation between $EtCO_2$ and corrected $PaCO_2$.[67] However, evaluating $EtCO_2$ alone without knowing pH or the extent of metabolic acidosis may potentially lead to erroneous respiratory management during HIE. A widening gap between $PaCO_2$ and $EtCO_2$ in a patient with lung disease indicates a mismatch between ventilation and perfusion and increasing alveolar dead space. $EtCO_2$ monitoring has been shown to be useful in cardiopulmonary resuscitation to guide the effectiveness of chest compressions and for detection of return of spontaneous circulation.[68-70]

Capnography during Neonatal Anesthesia

$EtCO_2$ monitoring is the standard of care for monitoring infants in the operating room as it provides rapid and reliable (breath by breath) assessment of the adequacy of the airway in an intubated patient. Loss of the capnogram signal or a sudden fall in $EtCO_2$ would indicate accidental extubation or plugging of the tracheal tube. Alternatively, a rapid rise in $EtCO_2$ level may indicate inadequate ventilation as commonly occurs with decreased tidal volume during surgical procedures. Examples of this include abdominal surgery, in which pressure on the diaphragm decreases tidal excursion, accidental or procedural lung collapse and migration of tracheal tube associated with patient repositioning during surgery. Changes in $EtCO_2$ are rapid and precede changes in SpO_2, and hence, capnography is able to detect airway/ventilator compromise early and may avert hypoxia and related injury.

Colorimetric Carbon Dioxide Detectors

Colorimetric CO_2 detectors are the standard of care for ensuring correct placement of tracheal tubes. A colorimetric CO_2 detector uses a modified form of litmus paper in which metacresol purple changes color depending on pH. Carbon dioxide reacts with water to form carbonic acid vapor in exhaled breath. A graded change in color from purple to yellow occurs with increasing concentration of $EtCO_2$. Lack of a color change (to yellow) after six respiratory cycles indicates esophageal intubation. False-negatives (lack of color change with correct tracheal tube placement—Fig. 11.5) may occur with (1) low cardiac output state even in the presence of severe hypercarbia or (2) impaired gas exchange in the presence of fetal lung fluid and (3) obstruction to the trachea. False-positive colorimetric CO_2 may occur with accidental contamination of the sensor with gastric acid and resuscitation drugs such as epinephrine.[71] A mnemonic for confirmation of intubation using a colorimetric capnogram is Yellow—Yes and Purple—Problem.

$EtCO_2$ in nonintubated patients can be assessed by sidestream capnography using a nasal cannula or mask. Studies by

Lopez et al. and Tai et al. have shown good correlation and minimal bias between $PaCO_2$ and $EtCO_2$ by sidestream capnography. However, in both studies, the $PaCO_2$-$EtCO_2$ gap widened in the presence of lung disease and in infants with BPD,[72,73] suggesting that $EtCO_2$ monitoring may be less reliable with the diseased lung.

Optimizing Ventilation Settings With Capnography

Volumetric capnography can assist in optimizing ventilator settings and weaning from mechanical ventilation. Hubble et al. have shown that in ventilated infants and children, capnogram-derived parameters of the ratio of physiologic dead space to tidal volume can reliably predict success of extubation.[74] Excessive positive end-expiratory pressure causes increase in the dead space and decreased pulmonary perfusion through increased intrathoracic pressure. This can be seen as a prolongation of phase I and a decline in the slope of phase II with a decrease in the volume of CO_2 eliminated through breaths per minute in the capnogram.[75]

Limitations of Capnography

Errors in estimation of $PaCO_2$ using $EtCO_2$ may occur because of ventilation-perfusion mismatch, airway obstruction as with meconium aspiration syndrome, or severe parenchymal lung disease (see Fig. 11.5). In infants with PPHN, the decreased pulmonary blood flow causes $EtCO_2$ to decrease despite elevated $PaCO_2$. Whereas impaired ventilation may elevate $EtCO_2$, a coexisting perfusion problem is likely to decrease $EtCO_2$. In infants with cyanotic CHD, decreased pulmonary blood flow and increased right-to-left shunting (e.g., during a spell in a patient with tetralogy of Fallot) cause an increase in $PaCO_2$. However, the right-to-left shunt causes a decrease in P_ACO_2 and the $EtCO_2$-$PaCO_2$ gap is widened. Rapid respiratory rates and low tidal volumes compromise the ability of sampled gas to adequately reflect alveolar gas. In preterm infants, admixture of dead space gas and fresh gas precludes a true end-tidal plateau, causing the values to underestimate the true $PaCO_2$. This is a major limitation to $EtCO_2$ monitoring in neonatology. Gas mixing proximal to the uncuffed tracheal tube because of air leaks and malfunction of the sensor that often occurs with condensation of water from the respiratory tree can also contribute to poor correlation between $PaCO_2$ and $EtCO_2$.

Transcutaneous Carbon Dioxide Monitoring

Severinghaus in 1960 first described the method for transcutaneous measurement of CO_2 in skin capillaries that are arterialized by application of heat.[76] The sensor unit consists of a glass pH electrode and a silver chloride reference electrode, a heating element, a temperature sensor, and an electrolyte reservoir (Fig. 11.6). The electrodes are separated from the surface of the skin by a membrane. When the sensor is attached to the skin, the generated heat causes local vasodilation and increases the permeability of the skin to CO_2. The CO_2 diffuses through the membrane and reacts with water to form carbonic acid, which dissociates to hydrogen and bicarbonate ions. The change in pH causes a potential difference between the electrodes. This change in pH is converted to a PCO_2 reading based on the

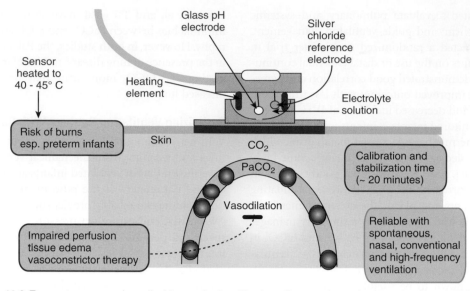

Fig. 11.6 Transcutaneous carbon dioxide monitoring. The benefits are shown in the green box, and limitations are shown in the red boxes. See text for details.

linear relationship between pH and log PCO_2. Johns et al. have shown a linear correlation of $TcPCO_2$ with $PaCO_2$ in the range of 20 to 74 mm Hg.[77] It is important to recognize that the measured value is the gas tension in the cutaneous tissue. Under stable hemodynamic conditions, these correlate closely with ABG values. As the electrodes operate at an elevated temperature, increased tissue metabolism at the site may increase the local CO_2 production. Hence, the value is corrected to the body temperature. Calibration of a $TcPCO_2$ monitor can be performed by gas calibration using mixtures of known CO_2 concentration or by using the patient's ABG sample. The in vivo calibration has been shown to align more closely with the $PaCO_2$ tension as it eliminates many of the patient-related factors that influence $TcPCO_2$ measurements. The commercially available monitors have a measurement range of $TcPCO_2$ between 0 and 200 mm Hg and accuracy within ± 4.5 mm Hg. Following application of the sensor, it takes approximately 20 minutes for stabilization and to obtain a reliable measurement of the $TcPCO_2$. Therefore, transcutaneous monitoring is used more for following $TcPCO_2$ over periods of time. In settings such as anesthesia or intubation in which a more rapid response time is needed, capnography and $EtCO_2$ monitoring may be more appropriate.

A good correlation between $TcPCO_2$ and $PaCO_2$ has been established in preterm and ill neonates.[78-80] However, a prospective study of infants of less than 28 weeks' gestation by Aliwalas et al. showed only moderate correlation.[81] A more recent study by Janaillac et al. in preterm infants showed poor correlation with a wide limit of agreement with low concordance of trends.[82] This discrepancy in results may be caused by differences in monitors, methodologies, and patient characteristics between studies. Both patient- and instrument-related factors can cause erroneous estimation of $TcPCO_2$ levels. Improper placement, trapped air bubbles, membrane, and calibration errors can lead to inaccurate readings. Despite the conflicting

results between studies, it is still possible to follow trends in change in $PaCO_2$ with transcutaneous CO_2 monitoring and may also decrease the need for repeated blood gas sampling.

There are many commercially available monitors that combine electrodes for $TcPCO_2/TcPO_2$ into a single sensor. Sensors with electrodes measuring PO_2 require a higher temperature at the site than PCO_2 sensors, and this may be a drawback of combined sensors, especially in preterm infants. Manufacturers recommend changing the position of the sensors every 4 to 12 hours, depending on the operating temperature of the electrode and the condition of the infant's skin. A comparison between transcutaneous and end-tidal CO_2 monitoring is shown in Table 11.1.

TISSUE OXYGEN SATURATION MONITORING USING NEAR-INFRARED SPECTROSCOPY

Near-infrared spectroscopy (NIRS) is an indirect assessment of tissue oxygen utilization. Oxygen delivery to the tissue is dependent on the hemoglobin content, oxygen saturation, and cardiac output. When oxygen demand exceeds the oxygen delivery, a state of oxygen debt is created, and energy is derived from the inefficient anaerobic metabolic pathway. The parameters currently in use for cardiovascular monitoring, such as blood pressure, capillary refill time, urine output, and lactate levels, lack sensitivity and specificity and are late indicators of hypoperfusion.

Franz Jobosis in 1977 first described the use of NIRS in the human brain. Much like pulse oximetry, NIRS is based on the modified Beer-Lambert law. Light of specific wavelengths is generated by light-emitting diodes and passed through the interposed tissue in an arclike configuration (Fig. 11.7). The depth of penetration of the transmitted light is proportional to the distance between the transmitting optode and the receiving optode. The reflected light is detected by the receiving optode

TABLE 11.1 Comparison of End-Tidal and Transcutaneous Monitoring of Carbon Dioxide

Capnography/End Tidal Carbon Dioxide	Transcutaneous Carbon Dioxide
Measures carbon dioxide (CO_2) in expired gas	Measures CO_2 at the cutaneous capillaries
Does not need frequent calibration	Needs frequent calibration
Responds instantaneously to change in partial pressure of carbon dioxide in alveolar gas (P_ACO_2)	Slower response to change in partial pressure of carbon dioxide ($PaCO_2$)
Reads instantaneously	Stabilization time of approximately 20 minutes before obtaining reading
Often lower than $PaCO_2$ (based on physiologic dead space)	Better correlation to $PaCO_2$
Unreliable in infants with lung disease, shunts, or ventilation-perfusion mismatch or with large leak around the tracheal tube	Unreliable in infants with impaired perfusion, acidosis, or edema or on vasoconstrictors
May increase dead space in extremely preterm infants	Risk of skin burns, need for changing sensor position to avoid thermal injury
Cannot be used with high-frequency ventilation	Can be used with any mode of ventilation: spontaneous, conventional, or high frequency
Limited use with spontaneous breathing	

and is measured and processed to estimate the amount of HbO_2 and DeoxyHb in the interposed tissue. NIRS oximetry measures a weighted average of arterial capillary and venous compartments, and a fixed ratio of venous-to-arterial blood volume is assumed, usually 70:30. There are different methodologies used by manufacturers of NIRS devices, but the most commonly used in commercially available devices is the spatially resolved spectroscopy. The following measurements are obtained through NIRS:

$$\text{Tissue (regional) oxygen saturation (rSO}_2) = SaO_2 - VO_2/DO_2,$$

where VO_2 is the oxygen consumption and DO_2 is the oxygen delivery.

$$\text{Arteriovenous oxygen saturation difference} = SpO_2 - rSO_2$$

$$\text{Fractional oxygen extraction (fOE)} = (SpO_2 - rSO_2)/SpO_2.$$

NIRS provides continuous noninvasive monitoring of the venous side of the vascular beds of various organs and provides information in real time of the balance between oxygen supply and demand. NIRS is very well suited to application in newborns and infants because of the decreased thickness of the scalp and skull and smaller amount of fat in the abdominal wall. NIRS has been applied mainly in assessing regional cerebral and

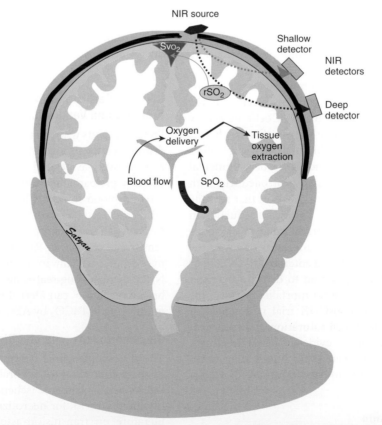

Fig. 11.7 Cerebral monitoring with near-infrared (*NIR*) spectroscopy. The light-emitting optode is placed over the scalp. Two detectors, a shallow detector and a deep detector, are placed a short distance from the emitting optode. The regional oxygen saturation (*rSO₂*) depends on oxygen delivery and tissue oxygen extraction. Low oxygen delivery or high oxygen extraction can decrease the rSO₂. *SpO₂*, Saturation by pulse oximetry; *SvO₂*, venous saturation.

splanchnic saturation in the neonatal population. There have been many studies that have demonstrated good correlation between cerebral oxygenation measured by NIRS and jugular venous oxygen saturation.[83] Cerebral oximetry has also been validated using correlation with levels of tissue adenosine triphosphate and phosphocreatine in the brain.[84] Studies of gastric tonometry (mucosal pH) have been shown to correlate with splanchnic/mesenteric rSO_2.[85]

Normal Values

In infants breathing room air, the cerebral rSO_2 is around 60% to 70% and the splanchnic rSO_2 is about 80%. The reference range of values for both term and preterm infants and changes with postnatal age have been published.[86-88] The rSO_2 also depends on the metabolic state of the tissue and is elevated in brain tissue following ischemic damage and during treatment with therapeutic hypothermia. It is decreased during increased metabolic activity, for example, during seizures, despite normal oxygen delivery. The utility of tissue oximetry at this time is in monitoring trends with determination of a baseline for each individual patient and a percentage below this baseline chosen for intervention.

Application of Near-Infrared Spectroscopy in Newborns

The clinical utility of NIRS monitoring in infants and newborns has been studied mainly in cardiac surgery. In infants undergoing surgery for CHD, low cerebral oximetry during surgery and in the postoperative period has been associated with abnormalities on neuroimaging, seizures, prolonged length of stay, need for extracorporeal membrane oxygenation, and death.[89-91]

The clinical utility of continuous brain tissue oxygen monitoring in preterm infants undergoing intensive care in the NICU has not been examined rigorously. A Cochrane review by Hyttel-Sorensen et al. to determine the benefits and harms of continuous NIRS monitoring of brain tissue oxygenation in preterm infants on mortality and neurodevelopmental outcomes identified only one randomized controlled trial with 166 preterm infants less than 28 weeks' gestation that met the eligibility criteria. Although there was a significant reduction in the cerebral oxygenation outside of normal range in the intervention group, there was no decrease in mortality or any of the morbidities (i.e., IVH, BPD, necrotizing enterocolitis [NEC], or ROP). The study, however, was powered to detect differences only in cerebral oxygenation and not for mortality or any of the listed morbidities.[92,93] The safeBoosC III trial is designed to evaluate if targeting cerebral oxygen saturation and treatment of cerebral hypoxia based on an evidence based treatment guideline will reduce death or severe brain injury at 36 weeks postmenstrual age in preterm infants less than 28 weeks' gestation at birth.[94]

Management of Hypotension

In hypotensive newborns, impaired cerebral autoregulation increases the risk of adverse neurodevelopmental outcomes. Autoregulation can be presumed to be intact when low blood pressure is not associated with a decrease in cerebral oxygenation by NIRS. In preterm neonates, NIRS can provide information on the oxygen supply and demand and guide the need for and choice of inotropes/vasopressors as well as the response to use of therapies.[95,96]

Resuscitation and Stabilization in the Delivery Room

Several studies have evaluated the rSO_2 changes in the immediate newborn period in both term and preterm infants. In the Neu-Prem trial, the infants who developed high-grade IVH were noted to have significantly lower cerebral oxygen tissue saturation from 8 to 10 minutes of life.[97] Binder-Heschl et al., in a retrospective analysis of four prospective observational studies of cerebral tissue oxygen saturation monitoring using NIRS in preterm infants who needed respiratory support in the delivery room, have shown that infants with SpO_2 less than 80% at 5 minutes of life had significantly lower rSO_2 than infants with SpO_2 of 80% or more.[98] However, it is not known if interventions to restore rSO_2 to the normal range will prevent these adverse outcomes. The COSGOD III multicenter randomized trial is designed to investigate if targeting cerebral oxygen saturations using specified clinical treatment guidelines in the first 15 minutes of life will improve survival without cerebral injury in infants under 32 weeks' gestation.[99]

Patent Ductus Arteriosus

Impairment of cerebral blood flow and oxygenation because of diastolic runoff occurs in hemodynamically significant PDA. Changes in rSO_2 and fOE by NIRS in combination with echocardiography may be used to monitor the status of the ductus arteriosus and response to pharmacological treatment for PDA.[100-102]

Cerebral Perfusion With Changes in Mean Airway Pressure and Ventilation

Preterm infants who are mechanically ventilated for respiratory distress syndrome are at high risk for IVH. Increased intrathoracic pressure associated with high mean airway pressure may decrease preload and cardiac output and cause impairment of cerebral blood flow.[103] Changes in cerebral rSO_2 and fOE by NIRS can lead to early recognition and timely intervention to prevent related complications. Cerebral blood flow is very sensitive to changes in $PaCO_2$, and rapid fluctuations in $PaCO_2$ may occur especially in infants on high-frequency ventilation. NIRS, by providing real-time information on changes in cerebral oxygenation, can alert the clinician of the need for closer monitoring of $PaCO_2$ by ABG in these infants.

Mesenteric Ischemia and Risk of Necrotizing Enterocolitis

The cerebrosplanchnic oxygenation ratio (CSOR) is the ratio of splanchnic rSO_2 to cerebral rSO_2. Values less than 0.75 are indicative of splanchnic ischemia. Low CSOR values may identify infants at risk for necrotizing enterocolitis.[104,105] A body of literature on transfusion-associated necrotizing enterocolitis and mesenteric blood flow and oxygenation during transfusion of packed red blood cells and changes associated with feeding is emerging in neonatology.[106-108]

Limitations of Near-Infrared Spectroscopy

NIRS is still an emerging technology that requires further study before adoption into practice. Limited published data on normal values based on the site of application, intervention thresholds, and impact on long-term outcomes of monitored infants justify the reluctance among practitioners toward adopting this technology. The cost of these probes and the space required to apply them on the head and abdomen have limited their use among extremely preterm infants. Further, there is wide intra- and interpatient variability in rSO_2 values, with a coefficient of variation for absolute baseline values of approximately 10%. The reading obtained is site specific and does not exclude abnormalities in other areas of the brain or other organ being monitored. To be able to obtain reliable readings, nursing and medical staff require training and experience in the correct placement and fixation of optodes and shielding from ambient light. The response to an abnormal reading should include, in addition to clinical assessment, evaluation of gas exchange, oxygen transport, hemodynamics, and regional perfusion. However, there is active ongoing research that should inform clinicians about the exact utility and indications for the use of NIRS in NICU patients in the future.

CONCLUSION

Timely, reliable, easy-to-use, comprehensive, and accurate monitoring is absolutely essential for the management of a critically ill neonate. Significant progress has been made in neonatology largely through advances in respiratory care. Survival of extremely preterm infants has improved, but morbidity remains high among survivors. Innovations in microprocessor technology and miniaturization of devices have made it possible to apply technology developed for monitoring and treatment of adults to NICU patients. In the NICU, noninvasive monitoring can decrease, but does not completely replace, the need for invasive blood gas monitoring. Noninvasive monitoring of respiratory and cardiovascular interactions has been possible through pulse oximeters, capnographs, transcutaneous monitors, and NIRS. Modern respiratory monitors offer the capability to monitor and quantify changes in respiratory mechanics and carbon dioxide elimination continuously and noninvasively using volumetric capnography. As neonatal providers, we are challenged to apply these innovations by defining the normal for our patient population and formulating interventions to rectify the abnormal. The dynamic physiology of the neonate results in rapid changes.[109] Noninvasive monitors must be capable of detecting these changes instantly so that the neonatal provider may respond promptly. Advances in our ability to monitor noninvasively should lead to better patient care, less iatrogenic blood loss, improved patient safety, and decreased need for and duration of mechanical ventilation. The cost-effectiveness and impact of these advances on clinical outcomes require validation with rigorous controlled studies. Interpretation of data from continuous noninvasive monitoring can complement clinical observations, leading to rapid diagnosis and intervention to stabilize and improve the outcomes of critically ill neonates.

A complete reference list is available at https://expertconsult. inkling.com/.

KEY REFERENCES

3. SUPPORT CWA, Finer NN, Walsh MC, et al: Target ranges of oxygen saturation in extremely preterm infants. N Engl J Med 362(21):1959–1969, 2010.

5. BOOST II: Australia and United Kingdom Collaborative Groups: Outcomes of two trials of oxygen-saturation targets in preterm infants. N Engl J Med 374(8):749–760, 2016.

6. Schmidt B, Whyte RK, Asztalos EV, et al: Effects of targeting higher vs lower arterial oxygen saturations on death or disability in extremely preterm infants: a randomized clinical trial. JAMA 309(20):2111–2120, 2013.

15. Lakshminrusimha S, Manja V, Mathew B, et al: Oxygen targeting in preterm infants: a physiological interpretation. J Perinatol 35(1):8–15, 2015.

22. Wyckoff MH, Wyllie J, Aziz K, et al: Neonatal Life Support: 2020 international consensus on cardiopulmonary resuscitation and emergency cardiovascular care science with treatment recommendations. Circulation 142(16_suppl_1):S185–S221, 2020.

48. Rawat M, Chandrasekharan PK, Williams A, et al: Oxygen saturation Index and severity of hypoxic respiratory failure. Neonatology 107(3):161–166, 2015.

66. Kugelman A, Golan A, Riskin A, et al: Impact of continuous capnography in ventilated neonates: a randomized, multicenter study. J Pediatr 168:56–61 e2, 2016.

93. Hyttel-Sorensen S, Greisen G, Als-Nielsen B, et al: Cerebral near-infrared spectroscopy monitoring for prevention of brain injury in very preterm infants. Cochrane Database Syst Rev 9: CD011506, 2017.

94. Hansen ML, Pellicer A, Gluud C, et al: Cerebral near-infrared spectroscopy monitoring versus treatment as usual for extremely preterm infants: a protocol for the SafeBoosC randomised clinical phase III trial. Trials 20(1):811, 2019.

12

Pulmonary Function and Graphics

Georg Schmölzer, MD, PhD and Helmut Hummler, MD, MBA

KEY POINTS

- Routine evaluation of bedside ventilator graphics in intubated patients can help clinicians assess a patient's respiratory physiology and pathophysiology, make management decisions about ventilator settings and use of respiratory medications, and follow a patient's course and response to treatment.
- The three most commonly used signals, usually displayed concurrently on the ventilator screen, are pressure, airflow, and volume measured using flow sensors that are pneumotachometers or hot-wire anemometers.
- There is no standardization of the techniques of measurement of pulmonary graphics and mechanics, or of the display formats across ventilators from different manufacturers. Therefore, clinicians should learn to interpret the screens of ventilators used in their institution, how exactly the measurements are obtained and analyzed, and sources of potential inaccuracy, such as a large leak around the endotracheal tube.
- Clinicians should learn to recognize patterns in ventilator graphics that are associated with specific diseases and pathophysiologic changes, and also those that indicate specific types of patient-ventilator interactions. These patterns are described in detail later, within the body of the chapter.
- Measured data, calculations, and graphic displays represent only a simplified assessment of the respiratory system as a whole and do not indicate regional variations in lung function, a particular problem with nonhomogenous lung disease. Therefore, the information obtained from pulmonary graphics and monitoring should be supplemented by the information obtained from history, clinical examination, laboratory tests (including blood gas values), and chest imaging.

INTRODUCTION

For adequate treatment of neonatal respiratory diseases, a clear understanding of pulmonary physiology is needed, which is influenced by maturity and other factors including changes in respiratory physiology during transition from the intrauterine to the extrauterine environment. Furthermore, a clear understanding of the pathophysiology of specific diseases affecting neonatal wellbeing and the effect of respiratory support is needed. Traditional monitoring of the respiratory and cardiovascular condition of neonates has focused on vital signs (i.e., respiratory rate, heart rate, or blood pressure) and blood gas exchange as these are relatively easy to assess. More recently available neonatal ventilators allow measurement and display of waveforms and loops (i.e., airway pressure [P_{aw}], airflow, tidal volume (V_T), end-tidal CO_2 [$ETCO_2$]), numerical values, real-time analysis of pulmonary function parameters, and trend monitoring, which help the clinician at bedside to choose the best ventilator mode and adjust ventilator settings.

The respiratory system interacts closely with the cardiovascular system. Therefore, more recently available methods to assess hemodynamics, such as continuous monitoring of cardiac output, tissue oxygen saturation, along with intermittent functional echocardiography, are important to assess the neonate with respiratory failure.[1,2] Adjustments of ventilator settings and treatments such as surfactant replacement therapy or the use of respiratory and/or cardiovascular drugs can be assessed using pulmonary function and hemodynamic monitoring, allowing a more comprehensive treatment of adverse conditions even in the most immature neonates.

Processing of the information available from more sophisticated respiratory and hemodynamic monitoring requires a profound understanding of the techniques used, correct interpretation of the information, and its integration into treatments based on applied pathophysiology and evidence from scientific studies if available.

Unfortunately, equipment, data processing, and analysis for pulmonary graphic monitoring have not been standardized. There is a diversity of devices, displays, and data analysis algorithms available, which may be confusing when the caregiver is exposed to different devices. However, one of the key advances in respiratory care has been the universal introduction of graphic display of respiratory signals, such as P_{aw}, airflow, and V_T in recent years. Although axis direction and scaling and the direction of loops vary between devices, they all follow the same principles and allow pattern recognition after some education and training.

In this chapter, we discuss the clinical use and limitations of pulmonary function and graphic monitoring for the daily management of neonates requiring respiratory monitoring and support. Our focus is on rather simple monitoring of respiratory parameters and a few diagnostic utilities, which are now almost universally available in devices for mechanical ventilation. We would like to emphasize that interpretation of clinical signs, along with the findings of (repeated) clinical examinations, continues to be the mainstay of excellent respiratory care.

TECHNICAL ASPECTS

Techniques for measurement of pulmonary graphics and mechanics have not been standardized and thus differ when comparing different devices. This relates to sensor techniques and display of graphics. However, pattern recognition based on experience and training allows making conclusions. The three most commonly used signals are pressure, airflow, and volume. Most pulmonary function devices or ventilators allow displaying all three signals at the same time. Signals can be used to display loops, which may help to identify altered pulmonary mechanics.

Airflow Measurement

Most commonly, flow sensors incorporated in ventilator devices for neonatal patients are usually pneumotachometers or hot-wire anemometers. Pneumotachometers are normally placed between the Y-piece of the ventilator and the endotracheal tube (Fig. 12.1). Inside the sensor are tubular or lamellar structures, which ensure laminar flow and create a small resistance to measure the pressure difference along this (small) resistor. This pressure difference is then measured using a differential pressure transducer connecting to small proximal and distal pressure lines. The pressure is higher on the proximal side (close to the Y-piece) during inspiration (Fig. 12.1A), whereas it is higher on the distal side (close to the endotracheal tube) during expiration (Fig. 12.1B) during expiration. The pressure is proportional to flow. The pneumotachometer needs to be designed for the range of gas flow expected in the population of interest. A flow sensor adds to dead space, which might cause CO_2 retention. However, effective alveolar ventilation and adequate CO_2 exhalation might still occur even with large instrumental dead space, which probably is as a result of some CO_2 washout by endotracheal leaks and gas transport other than

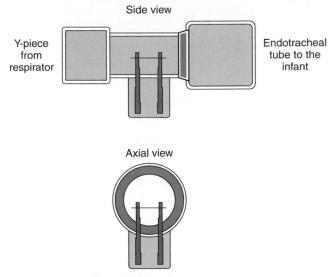

Fig. 12.2 Hot-wire anemometer.

simple in and out movement of gas volumes.[3,4] Pneumotachometers are extremely sensitive even with small flows but may be affected by humidity and secretions.

Hot-wire anemometers use a hot wire placed within the sensor with airflow changing the temperature of the wire which influences the electric current through the wire (Fig. 12.2). With more sophisticated design, the direction and magnitude of flow can be measured, although a certain minimal flow is needed to detect the direction. Hot-wire anemometers are less sensitive to safely detect very small flows and direction of flow and their measurement characteristics depend on gas humidity. However, on the other hand, sensors are less prone to gas humidity and water rain-out. With both devices, air flow/signal characteristics are often not linear and are influenced by the FiO_2,[5,6] requiring electronic calibration. Accuracy is acceptable for clinical circumstances. The devices have been designed smaller in recent years to reduce the imposed dead space.

Air flow should be measured distally and close to the patient (between the Y-piece of the ventilator and the endotracheal tube) as compressible volume will affect at least the measured inspired volume if flow is measured close to the ventilator or within the inspiratory limb. Flow sensors are usually calibrated on setup of the ventilator automatically, including calibration of zero-flow condition in pneumotachometers. It is important that bedside clinical personnel checks regularly the graphic displays including measured values for plausibility and the circuit and pressure lines of pneumotachometers for water rain-out, which can affect measurements. Especially water in pressure lines of pneumotachometers can grossly shift the zero line and affect the magnitude of the measured flow (Fig. 12.3). If this problem is being recognized, the sensor and the connecting pressure lines need to be "decontaminated" from water rainout.

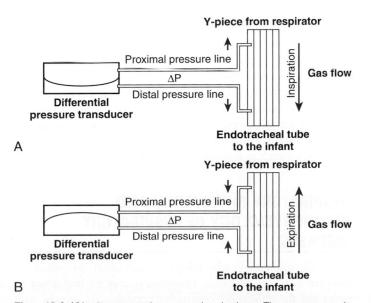

Fig. 12.1 (A) Pneumotachometer—inspiration. The pressure is higher on the proximal side (close to the Y-piece) during inspiration. **(B)** Pneumotachometer—expiration. The pressure is lower on the proximal side (close to the Y-piece) during expiration.

Pressure Measurement

P_{aw} monitoring is crucial to confirm the right pressure to be applied and to serve as a time reference of mechanical inflations to interpret flow and volume waves. P_{aw} is an important reference

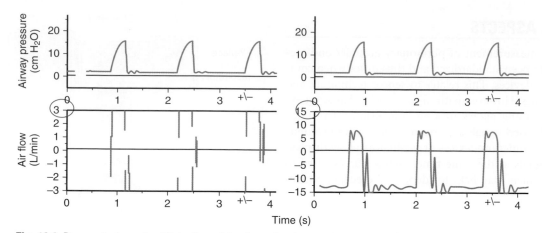

Fig. 12.3 Pneumotachometer. Distortion of the flow signal secondary to water in pressure lines. Only after increasing the flow scale, it is recognized that the measured flow is inappropriately high and the zero line during expiration is shifted to a large negative value. (Courtesy Dr. Andreas Schulze, Munich, Germany.)

signal to differentiate between spontaneous breaths and mechanical inflations. Together with airflow/volume, P_{aw} provides important information to optimize ventilator settings and for basic pulmonary function measurements (see later). The pressure needed to drive gas into the lung needs to overcome the elastic, resistive, and inertial forces of the respiratory system. For conventional mechanical inflations, the driving pressure (ΔP) is the difference between the peak (inflation) pressure (PIP) and positive end expiratory pressure (PEEP) ($\Delta P = PIP - PEEP$).

For more sophisticated pulmonary function measurements, the pressure in the pleural space is needed to get information on spontaneous respiratory activity and to separate the mechanical characteristics of the lung from the chest wall. Chest tubes (if in place for pleural drainage) or esophageal sensors or fluid-filled catheters can be used.[7-9] Although esophageal pressure measurements are useful for certain research settings, peristalsis, secretions, and positioning may affect measurements of esophageal pressure, which limit the accuracy and applicability of this technique for routine monitoring in clinical circumstances.[10]

End Tidal CO$_2$ Measurement

Measurement of exhaled CO_2 is used commonly in adult and pediatric intensive care and operating room settings[11] and is used to rapidly confirm endotracheal tube placement after intubation in patients, including neonates in the delivery room.[12,13] Mainstream and side-stream techniques have been described, and measurements somewhat reflect alveolar PCO_2 especially if the V_T is large and there is no significant lung disease. Mainstream devices add to anatomical dead space, and side-stream devices usually add none or very little dead space but may deliver a delayed signal and may affect correct flow measurements.

Considering a technically correct signal, an increase in gap between arterial CO_2 and ETCO$_2$ in a neonate with lung disease indicates increased ventilation/perfusion mismatch (i.e., increased dead space ventilation). Capnography has physiological and technical limitations, especially in very low birth weight (VLBW) and extremely low birth weight infants with the small V_Ts exhaled in this population, and cannot be used during high-frequency ventilation. In patients with more severe lung disease, the technique usually underestimates arterial values and thus limits accuracy, especially in diseases with different compartments leading to inconclusive plateau formation during expiration or with severely impaired ventilation/perfusion mismatch.[14-16] However, capnography may be very useful to follow trends in PCO_2 and help to limit invasive monitoring with blood gases.

Volume Measurement

V_T is technically obtained by integration of airflow and mathematically represents the area under the flow curve. Inspiratory and expiratory V_T measurements may differ slightly because of different fractions of gases during inspiration and expiration (FO$_2$, FCO$_2$), but more importantly secondary to leaks around the endotracheal tube or elsewhere within the respiratory system (i.e., in the presence of pulmonary air leaks), where inspiratory V_T is larger than expiratory. All modern ventilators allow V_T display, either in absolute or in weight-corrected graphs and numbers. Leaks around the endotracheal tube may affect V_T measurements, as discussed later.

Tidal volumes of healthy, spontaneously breathing preterm and term neonates early after birth and during the first weeks/months of life are approximately 5 to 8 mL/kg.[17-20] Spontaneously breathing smaller preterm infants tend to have a somewhat higher respiratory rate, which may exceed 100 breaths/min with lung disease such as respiratory distress syndrome (RDS).

RESPIRATORY PHYSIOLOGY AND PATHOPHYSIOLOGY OF RESPIRATORY DISEASES

Neonatal respiratory physiology is discussed in detail in Chapter 2 in this textbook. However, it may be important to point out the differences comparing spontaneous breaths with mechanical inflations. The main driving force for spontaneous breathing is provided by the diaphragm along with some activity of intercostal and other respiratory muscles expanding the

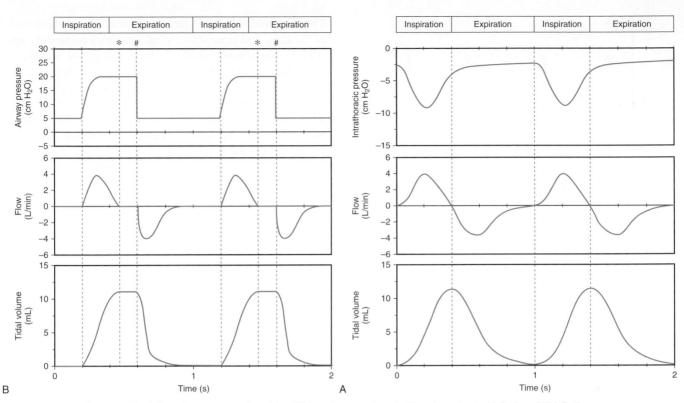

Fig. 12.4 Physiology. Spontaneous breathing (60 breaths per minute) **(A)** and mechanical inflations (60 inflations per minute), inspiratory time 0.4 seconds **(B)** * and #, see text.

thoracic cavity, decreasing intrathoracic pressure to create a gradient between the intrathoracic and ambient pressure leading to inspiratory airflow (Fig. 12.4A). Inspiration ends at the time flow returns to zero (Fig. 12.4A). In the absence of spontaneous respiratory activity, the pressure gradient to overcome elastic and resistive forces is usually provided by positive pressure to the airway (Fig. 12.4B). It is important to remember that the Hering-Breuer reflex is very active in neonates,[21,22] often resulting in temporary apnea with relaxation of the respiratory muscles. Once the lung is filled by a mechanical inflation to the desired V_T with a given peak pressure, airflow returns to and remains at zero (*)—unless there is a leak—for the remaining inspiratory time (T_{insp}) as chosen by the operator and inspiration is "on hold" until P_{aw} is returned to PEEP level (#, see Fig. 12.4B).

The mathematical relationship of these respiratory forces was discovered in the early 1900s by Fritz Rohrer but was ignored until the 1940s.[23] He described this relationship with the equation $P = P_e + P_r + P_i$ where P_e is the elastic, P_r the resistive, and P_i the inertial pressure. Elastic, resistive, and inertial forces of the respiratory system must be counterbalanced by this inspiratory driving force. The inertial forces (P_i) are usually very small because of the small specific gravity of gases and the pressure used to overcome elastic forces (P_e) is a function of pulmonary and chest wall elastance or its reverse (1/compliance). The pressure used to create air flow is the resistive pressure (P_r). It follows that at times of zero flow, all pressure is related to elastic forces. P_i can usually be neglected because of its minor influence with gas ventilation. This is a simplified description of forces in a one-compartment lung model and its implications may be limited in the presence of lung disease.

DISPLAY OF RESPIRATORY SIGNALS

Airway Pressure

Peak Inflation Pressure, Positive End Expiratory Pressure, Continuous Positive Airway Pressure

P_{aw} monitoring is helpful not only to confirm the set pressures delivered by the ventilator (PIP, PEEP, or continuous positive airway pressure [CPAP]), but also more importantly, it serves as a timely reference signal to interpret flow and V_T signals. In clinical circumstances, intrathoracic pressure measurements are usually not available, and the absence of any P_{aw} changes along with airflow present would usually indicate that the breath is of spontaneous origin. Flow/volume changes associated with an increase in airway P_{aw} would usually indicate that they are caused by mechanical inflations, although a spontaneous effort contributing to the delivered V_T may be present as well. Fig. 12.5 shows P_{aw} and V_T traces caused by spontaneous breaths (↓) along with larger flow changes associated with mechanical inflations (Δ) during synchronized intermittent mandatory ventilation (SIMV).

Mean Airway Pressure: Five Different Ways to Change MAP During Conventional Ventilation: Change in Peak Inflation Pressure, Positive End Expiratory Pressure, Inspiratory Time, Inspiratory Slope, and Rate

Mean airway pressure (MAP) is a function of PEEP, PIP, T_{insp}, and rate of mechanical inflations and flow, which influence the slope of the pressure wave form during inspiration.[24] In settings of alveolar lung disease, an increase in MAP usually improves oxygenation. Fig. 12.6 shows the five possibilities to increase

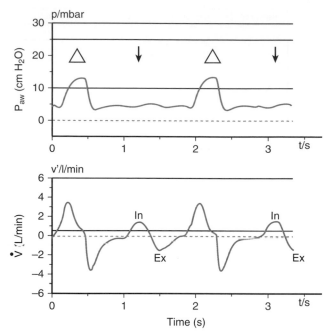

Fig. 12.5 Airway pressure (P_{aw}) and flow during synchronized intermittent mandatory ventilation (SIMV) in a preterm infant. There are two spontaneous breaths (↓) with smaller peak flows and no increase in P_{aw} and two mechanical inflations (Δ) with larger peak flows. *In/Ex*, Inspiration/expiration. (Courtesy Dr. Andreas Schulze, Munich, Germany).

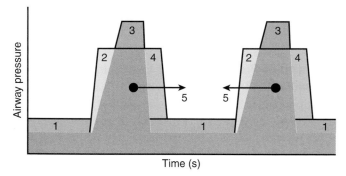

Fig. 12.6 Five options to increase mean airway pressure. Increase in positive end expiratory pressure (1), steeper slope (2), increased peak inflation pressure (3), longer inspiratory time (4), higher rate (5).

MAP during conventional ventilation (change in PEEP, PIP, T_{insp}, rate, and inspiratory slope). It was shown in neonates with severe lung disease that each of the described interventions improved oxygenation in proportion to the respective increase in MAP.[25] In clinical circumstances, it is important to consider that the described interventions have their own influence on alveolar ventilation and, thus, on CO_2 removal. Most often, PEEP is manipulated to influence MAP and oxygenation.

Effect of Inspiratory and Expiratory Time on Tidal Volume: Effect of the Time Constant on Flow and Volume

For mechanical inflations, a certain T_{insp} is needed to allow equilibrium of the delivered PIP with the alveolar pressure.

The time needed is dependent on the mechanical characteristics of the lung. The time constant of a patient's respiratory system is a measure of how quickly the lungs can inflate or deflate (see Physiological Principles, Chapter 2). The time constant (K_t) is defined as the product of lung compliance (C) and airway resistance (R) ($K_t = C \times R$). One time constant is defined as the time it takes the lung to empty 63% of the inhaled V_T. After three time constants, approximately 95% of the V_T is exhaled. For a normal full-term neonate (3 kg body weight) with a compliance of 0.005 L/cm H_2O (5 mL/cm H_2O = 1.7 mL/kg/H_2O) and a resistance of 30 cm H_2O/L/second, one time constant is 0.15 seconds and three time constants approximate to 0.45 seconds.

Fig. 12.7 shows the P_{aw}, flow, and V_T of a full-term infant with healthy lungs with normal compliance and resistance exposed to mechanical inflations with pressure limited ventilation. The PIP/PEEP is 10/3 cm H_2O. In Fig. 12.7A, the T_{insp} is adjusted to a low value for this patient (0.3 seconds) and inspiratory flow abruptly returns to zero (arrow) without allowing complete inflation, resulting in a V_T of approximately 21 mL. Prolongation of T_{insp} to 0.45 seconds allows airflow to decrease to zero (arrow), resulting in a larger V_T (24 mL) using the same PIP (Fig. 12.7B). It is important to distinguish this condition from a condition with endotracheal tube leak where inspiratory flow remains above zero until the end of the mechanical inflation owing to leak flow (see later, Fig. 12.9).

Whereas in the acute phase of RDS, a longer T_{insp} increases MAP in poorly aerated lungs and thus may improve oxygenation, babies often breathe spontaneously with a high respiratory rate when lung compliance has improved. In this phase, monitoring of the airflow trace allows seeing if the chosen T_{insp} is inappropriately long. Flow cycling to terminate the mechanical inflation is helpful during this phase (see "Cycling Off the Mechanical Inflation (Flow Cycling)" later).

Fig. 12.8 shows the P_{aw}, flow, and V_T of an infant with bronchopulmonary dysplasia (BPD) on mechanical ventilation (PIP/PEEP is 20/6 cm H_2O) with a prolonged K_t (secondary to increased resistance) resulting in expiratory flow not returning to zero before the next mechanical inflation occurs (Fig. 12.8A). Lowering the ventilator rate from 40 inflations to 30 inflations per minute allowed for complete exhalation and increased the exhaled V_T with otherwise the same settings (Fig. 12.8B). Minute ventilation decreased from 40/min × 21 mL = 840 mL/min to 30/min × 25 mL = 750 mL, because of the lower rate, which may not even affect PCO_2, as dead space ventilation usually decreases with a lower rate and a larger V_T. Another possible intervention for the described situation may be to consider increasing PEEP, which may distend the airways and reduce expiratory resistance. Whatever intervention is chosen, its effects can be followed immediately by observing airflow after the intervention.

Incomplete exhalation results in air trapping, which may not be detected clinically unless severe, but which can be easily detected if the airflow trace is observed carefully. In infants with BPD, resistance is often elevated, but compliance is often only moderately decreased secondary to distended lung units and airways, resulting in a prolonged time constant. Close observation of the P_{aw}, flow, and V_T curves allows adjustment of the inspiratory and expiratory time for optimal adjustment.

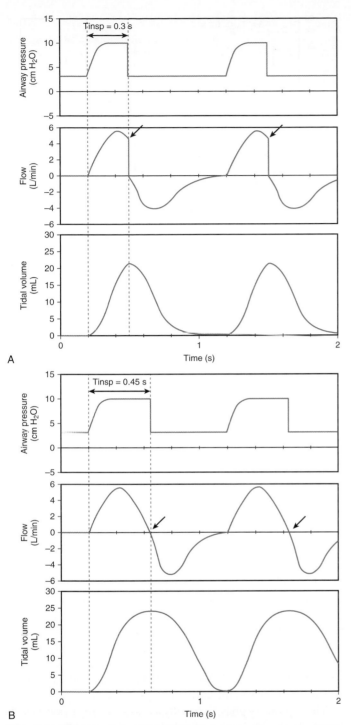

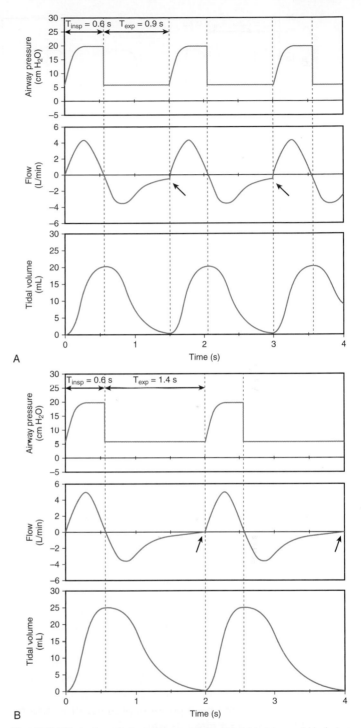

Fig. 12.7 Effect of inspiratory time on delivered tidal volume during pressure-limited mechanical inflation. Full-term infant with normal lung mechanics. **(A)** Inspiratory time (T_{insp}) 0.3 seconds. Inspiratory flow abruptly returns to zero (*arrows*) without allowing for a complete inflation (tidal volume [V_T] ≈ 21 mL). **(B)** T_{insp} 0.45 seconds. Inspiratory flow is allowed to decrease to zero (*arrows*), resulting in a larger V_T using the same peak inflation pressure (V_T ≈ 24 mL).

Fig. 12.8 Effect of expiratory time on delivered tidal volume (V_T) during pressure-limited mechanical inflation. Ex-preterm infant with bronchopulmonary dysplasia. **(A)** Inspiratory time (T_{insp}) 0.6 seconds, expiratory time (T_{exp}) 0.9 seconds. Expiratory flow does not reach zero before the next mechanical inflation (*arrow*) → incomplete exhalation. Note: V_T ≈ 21 mL. **(B)** T_{insp} 0.6 seconds, T_{exp} 1.4 seconds. Expiratory flow now reaches zero before the next mechanical inflation (*arrow*) → complete exhalation. Note: V_T ≈ 25 mL.

The clinical implication is that with (almost) normal compliance, enough time should be provided for pressure equilibration, whereas with a low compliance (such as in RDS or pneumonia), the time needed to deliver the breath is much shorter, especially if resistance is not or only minimally affected. In fact, high ventilatory rates or even high-frequency ventilation may be appropriate in these settings to limit V_T and, thus, lung injury.

As mentioned before, the inspiratory flow does not return to zero if T_{insp} is chosen too short for the given time constant. Prolonging T_{insp} would allow the inspiratory flow to return to

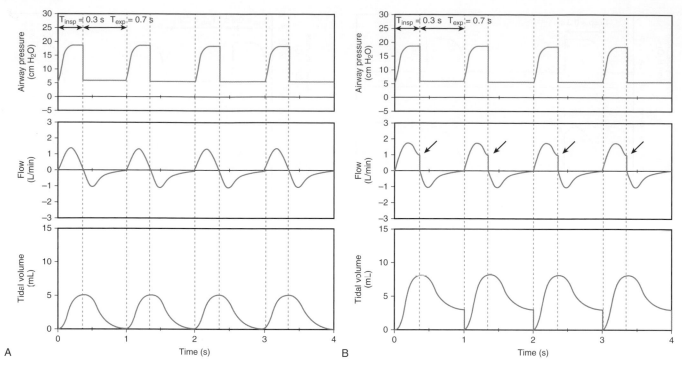

Fig. 12.9 Effect of endotracheal tube leak on flow and tidal volume (V_T) traces during pressure-limited mechanical inflation. Preterm infant with respiratory distress syndrome. **(A)** Inspiratory time (T_{insp}) 0.3 seconds, expiratory time (T_{exp}) 0.7 seconds, no leak. Inspiratory flow reaches zero before the end of the mechanical inflation. Note: V_T trace returns to 0 mL before the next inflation. **(B)** T_{insp} 0.3 seconds, T_{exp} 0.7 seconds, leak (35%). Inspiratory flow does not reach zero before the next mechanical inflation (*arrows*). Note: V_T trace does not return to 0 mL during exhalation. It is electronically zeroed before the next inflation.

zero unless the condition is caused by an air leak, which is very common in intubated neonates as most clinicians do not use cuffed tubes. Fig. 12.9A shows traces from a preterm infant with RDS without leak. Fig. 12.9B shows the same case with a small leak (calculated leak = $V_{Tinsp} - V_{Texp}/V_{Tinsp} =$ approximately 35%). During expiration, the V_T trace does not return to zero until the next mechanical inflation when the ventilator zeroes the V_T signal to avoid "runaway" of the V_T trace. In Fig. 12.9C, the T_{insp} is prolonged from 0.3 to 0.5 seconds, resulting in a longer duration of inspiratory leak flow, thus contributing to a larger leak (now ~50%). In Fig. 12.9D, gentle compression of the larynx (same ventilator settings as in Fig. 12.9C) eliminated the leak and confirmed the condition to be caused by endotracheal tube leak. Endotracheal tube leaks are often variable and factors such as tube and head position, presence of secretions, and the PIP chosen may affect its size.

It is important to recognize very large leaks (>50%–80%) as volume-targeted ventilator modes, such as volume guarantee, may not function appropriately with large leaks. If the leak is present during PEEP level, there may be an expiratory leak resulting in exhaled volume being lost into the leak, resulting in falsely low expiratory V_T measurements. Pressure-limited modes may compensate for large leaks better in this situation.

Measurement of Airflow

During spontaneous breathing, peak airflow is usually during mid-inspiration (Fig. 12.4A). Peak airflow is dependent on the patient's size (weight), the pathophysiology of the respiratory disease, and the delivered V_T during the chosen T_{insp}. Typically, inspiratory airflow is highest at mid-inspiration, whereas expiratory airflow peaks early during expiration (Fig. 12.4A).

During mechanical ventilation, the flow provided by the ventilator circuit should be much larger than the peak inspiratory flow passing through the patient's airways. In the past, circuit flow had to be selected by the operator during pressure-limited ventilation and was usually adjusted at a flow rate higher than the peak inspiratory airflow to avoid loss of pressure in the system. Modern ventilators adjust the flow automatically within a few milliseconds to achieve the desired pressure or flow profile, which usually is set by the operator. During volume-controlled ventilation, inspiratory flow accelerates to a fixed peak level, which remains constant until the V_T is delivered.

The expiratory phase is usually assessed during passive exhalation. At the beginning of exhalation, flow rapidly increases until expiratory peak flow, followed by a decelerating expiratory flow driven by the difference between alveolar pressure and P_{aw} until it reaches pressure equilibrium and zero flow (Fig. 12.4B). Rapid active exhalation on command (as used in adults and older children) cannot be used in neonates for obvious reasons. Standardized testing using rapid thoraco-abdominal compression technique can be used[26] but is quite cumbersome for daily clinical use in the neonatal intensive care unit (NICU) and probably not safe in small preterm infants at risk for IVH. Forced deflation techniques using thoracoabdominal compression or negative pressure applied to the airway has been used in intubated infants for pulmonary function testing in research, but not in clinical settings.[27-29]

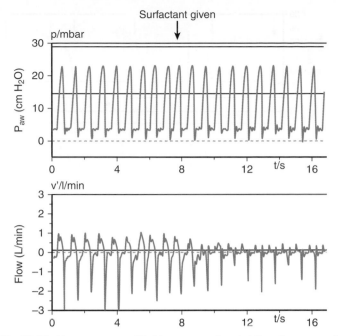

Fig. 12.10 Airway pressure (P_{aw}) (upper panel) and airflow (lower panel) in a compressed recording (16 seconds) during sudden partial airway obstruction caused by tracheal application of surfactant. Note: despite unchanged PIP, peak inspiratory and expiratory flow decreased suddenly after surfactant application. (Courtesy Dr. Andreas Schulze, Munich, Germany.)

Following P_{aw}, airflow, and V_T monitoring on the ventilator allows recognizing changes over time, i.e., a decrease in airflow caused by sudden partial airway obstruction by secretions or temporarily by surfactant administered in the airways (Fig. 12.10) or, afterward, when V_T may increase during pressure-limited ventilation once compliance improves.

Changes in lung compliance may be recognized by following flow and volume traces closely. In severe RDS with low lung compliance, the peak inspiratory and expiratory flow will be lower with a given driving pressure (PIP – PEEP) than in babies with less severe lung disease. Surfactant replacement therapy may change this within seconds/minutes, resulting in larger peak flows and V_Ts. This information is very useful for adjustment of ventilator settings (usually pressure). Volume-targeted modes will take care of the necessary weaning steps automatically.

Recognizing Spontaneous Respiratory Efforts

In research and clinical settings, esophageal pressure can be used as surrogate of pleural and, thus, intrathoracic pressure to detect negative pressure created by respiratory muscles during spontaneous inspiration[9] and has been used in term[7] and preterm[8] neonates. However, this technique has its limitations and is not applicable for widespread clinical routine monitoring.[9,10] However, the airflow and V_T traces can provide valuable information as a flow deviation from zero along with a change in V_T in the absence of a change in P_{aw} is usually related to a spontaneous breath (see Fig. 12.11B).

Checking for Synchronization

Synchronization of ventilator inflations to spontaneous efforts has many beneficial effects, including improved weaning, less

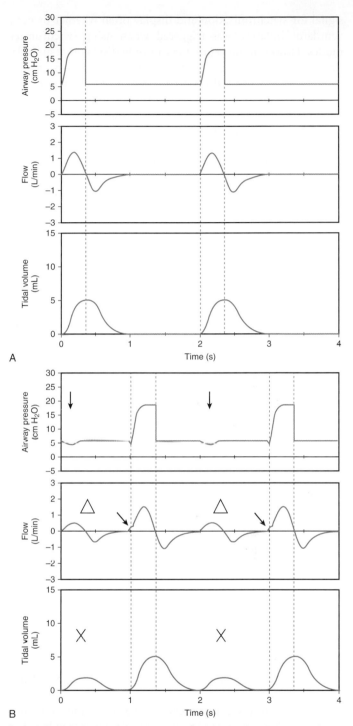

A

B

Fig. 12.11 Checking for synchronization: regular intermittent mandatory ventilation (IMV) vs synchronized IMV (SIMV). **(A)** Regular IMV (rate 30/min, T_{imp} 0.3 seconds). Note: there is no evidence for spontaneous respiratory activity. **(B)** SIMV (rate 30/min, inspiratory time 0.3 seconds). Note: presence of spontaneous breathing (60/min) as indicated by a small decrease in airway pressure (↓) and small inspiratory and expiratory flows (Δ), resulting in a small tidal volume (×) between mechanical inflations. There is a small increase in inspiratory flow before mechanical inflations "kick in" and accelerate flow further (*gray arrows*).

blood pressure fluctuations, less need for sedation, and a larger and more consistent V_T as the spontaneous negative intrathoracic inflation pressure induced by a spontaneous breath is synchronized to the positive P_{aw} imposed by the mechanical inflation.[30-33] Most ventilators for use in neonates use the flow signal for synchronization and display often whether or not a ventilator inflation was triggered when using synchronized modes. However, the ventilator can only display that an inflation was initiated once the trigger threshold has been met, whether or not this reflects a true patient effort or not. Artifacts may result in autotrigger, and trigger failure does occur,[34] and breath detection may be erroneous and thus trigger failure or autotrigger can occur even if the ventilator "claims" that the mechanical inflation has been initiated by the patient. In the absence of pleural pressure monitoring, flow and P_{aw} are nowadays available for routine monitoring in ventilators and are extremely valuable to check for correct synchronization as shown in Figs. 12.11 and 12.12. Spontaneous breaths may be identified at the P_{aw} trace and by identifying flow excursions (Fig. 12.11B). Flow and V_T excursions as seen in Fig. 12.11B in the absence of mechanical inflations (no rise in P_{aw}) refer to spontaneous breaths. If there is a P_{aw} excursion, observing a small negative dip in P_{aw} and/or small positive flow before the ventilator "kicks in" strongly suggests that this mechanical inflation is initiated by the baby and thus a correct synchronized inflation. The size of this small positive flow is dependent on the trigger delay, the baby's effort, and the threshold for synchronization selected by the clinician.

After changing from SIMV to assist-control (AC), each patient effort, as indicated by the small negative dip in P_{aw} and/or small positive flow before the ventilator "kicks in," strongly suggests that all inflations are now synchronized inflations (Fig. 12.12). Sometimes, the negative P_{aw} dips and positive flow changes before the mechanical inflations are very small and difficult to detect visually, especially if the solution of the graphical display of the ventilator or monitoring device is limited. A very uniform timing pattern of the inflations as assessed in the P_{aw}, airflow and V_T traces raises the suspicion of autotrigger, as there is usually some variability in the duration of spontaneous breaths. Another simple way to find out whether there is autotrigger during AC would be to switch for a few seconds to CPAP to observe if the patient continues to breathe. If the patient has no respirations at all, autotrigger or a high backup rate as chosen by the caretaker caused the observed breathing pattern.

Cycling Off the Mechanical Inflation (Flow Cycling)

Many ventilators can adjust the duration of the delivered mechanical inflation (T_{insp}) to flow criteria to synchronize initiation of exhalation. If this feature is chosen, the end of the mechanical inflation is then determined by flow criteria rather than based on timing (flow-cycled vs time-cycled). The trigger threshold for cycling off the inflation is often called "termination sensitivity threshold," "inspiratory time sensitivity," or "expiratory trigger sensitivity." This threshold represents the percentage of peak inspiratory flow at which the ventilator cycles from inspiration to exhalation. Depending on the device used, this threshold is often adjustable anywhere between 5% and 90%. Increasing this threshold results in a shorter T_{insp}, whereas decreasing it would result in longer T_{insp}. Using this feature avoids unnecessary "inspiratory hold" after full V_T delivery to the lung, which may elicit the Hering-Breuer reflex and result in a short apnea until the next spontaneous breathing effort begins. The advantages of using this feature include a more "natural" breathing pattern (less

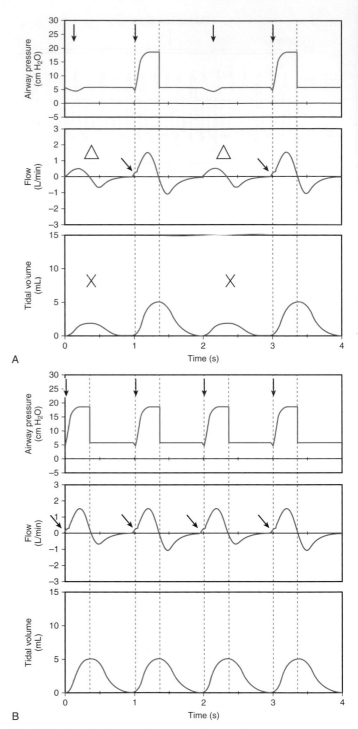

Fig. 12.12 Checking for synchronization. Synchronized intermittent mandatory ventilation (SIMV) vs assist-control (AC). **(A)** SIMV (rate 30/min, inspiratory time [T_{insp}] 0.3 seconds). Note: presence of spontaneous breathing (60/min) as indicated by a small decrease in airway pressure (P_{aw}) (↓) and small inspiratory and expiratory flows (Δ), resulting in a small tidal volume (×) between mechanical inflations. There is a small increase in inspiratory flow before mechanical inflations "kick in" and accelerate flow further (*gray arrows*). **(B)** A/C (T_{insp} 0.3 seconds). Note: spontaneous breathing as indicated by a small decrease in P_{aw} (↓) and a small increase in inspiratory flow before mechanical inflations "kick in" and accelerate flow further (*gray arrows*). Each effort is triggering a mechanical inflation resulting in a rate of 60/min.

disruption of the spontaneous breathing pattern) and prevention of air-trapping as longer T_{exp} can be provided, especially if the infant uses higher respiratory rates. However, as flow cycling shortens T_{insp}, this may result in a lower MAP, if a higher breathing rate does not compensate for the decrease in MAP. During flow cycling, there is always time cycling in the background and the inflation will be terminated by whichever criteria are met first. In case of larger leaks, flow cycling may not work as inspiratory leak flow may not decrease below the threshold chosen for cycling off (Fig. 12.13).

Measurement of Volume

Tidal Volume—Minute Ventilation

The effect of using volume-targeted ventilation can be assessed by following the V_T trace closely. Changing from pressure-limited ventilation to volume-guarantee ventilation, for example, will reduce fluctuations in V_T but increase fluctuations in P_{aw} and vice versa once switched back to pressure-limited modes.

Minute ventilation is the sum of volume delivered to the respiratory system during 1 minute. During conventional ventilation, it is calculated as minute ventilation $= V_T \times$ respiratory rate. Typical minute ventilation for term infants is approximately 240 to 360 mL/kg/min. Preterm infants ventilate with smaller V_T values and a higher rate than full-term infants, especially if they suffer from RDS. This strategy limits work of breathing with a less compliant lung with RDS and helps to maintain functional residual capacity (FRC). However, this strategy may increase dead space ventilation and decrease alveolar minute ventilation, which determines arterial PCO_2.

Tidal Volume—Effect of Endotracheal Tube Leaks

In the presence of an inspiratory endotracheal tube leak, the inspiratory is larger than the expiratory V_T, as the endotracheal tube leak usually opens with the larger inflation pressure only, but not with PEEP. Whereas the inspiratory V_T is falsely high, the exhaled V_T is considered to come out of the lung and thus is the closest approximation of delivered V_T to the lung. Therefore, ventilator adjustments to target a certain V_T should always be made based on exhaled (expiratory) rather than inspiratory V_T. In a graphic display, the volume trace is usually zeroed before the next breath to avoid runaway of the volume trace (Fig. 12.9B–C). Furthermore, in the presence of a significant leak, the pressure-volume loop fails to close (see later, Fig. 12.17).

However, if the leak is large, there may be almost no negative or only positive airflow even during the expiratory phase (Fig. 12.14). In this situation, exhaled air from the lung may bypass the flow sensor through the leak and the measured exhaled V_T may be zero or grossly underestimate true V_T. Gentle compression on the larynx may decrease or eliminate the leak and help to correct measurements at least temporarily (Fig. 12.9D).

Effect of Mechanical Characteristics of the Respiratory System on Tidal Volume

The measured V_T should always be interpreted within the context of ventilator settings (especially PEEP) and the pathophysiology of the underlying lung disease. There is a consensus

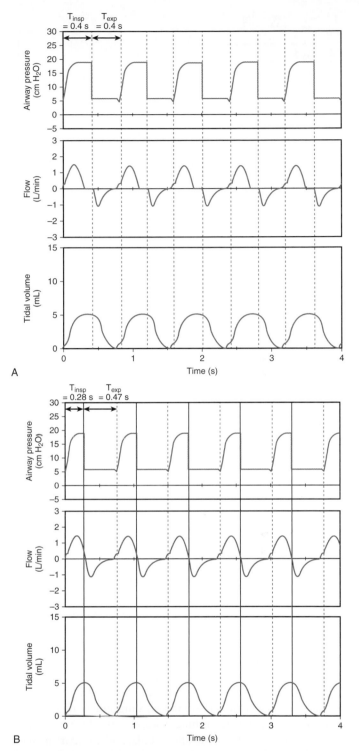

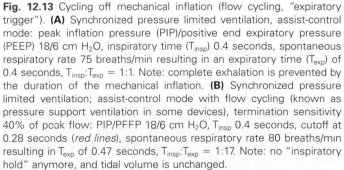

Fig. 12.13 Cycling off mechanical inflation (flow cycling, "expiratory trigger"). **(A)** Synchronized pressure limited ventilation, assist-control mode: peak inflation pressure (PIP)/positive end expiratory pressure (PEEP) 18/6 cm H_2O, inspiratory time (T_{insp}) 0.4 seconds, spontaneous respiratory rate 75 breaths/min resulting in an expiratory time (T_{exp}) of 0.4 seconds, $T_{insp}:T_{exp} = 1:1$. Note: complete exhalation is prevented by the duration of the mechanical inflation. **(B)** Synchronized pressure limited ventilation; assist-control mode with flow cycling (known as pressure support ventilation in some devices), termination sensitivity 40% of peak flow: PIP/PFFP 18/6 cm H_2O, T_{insp} 0.4 seconds, cutoff at 0.28 seconds (*red lines*), spontaneous respiratory rate 80 breaths/min resulting in T_{exp} of 0.47 seconds, $T_{insp}:T_{exp} = 1:17$. Note: no "inspiratory hold" anymore, and tidal volume is unchanged.

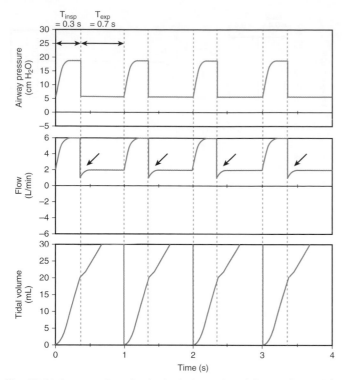

Fig. 12.14 Large endotracheal tube leak causing airflow to be positive during inspiration and expiration. Settings: inspiratory time 0.3 seconds, expiratory time 0.7 seconds, leak (100%). Airflow during inspiration is excessive and remains positive during the expiratory phase (arrows) resulting in the "runaway" of the tidal volume (V_T) trace. V_T is exhaled exclusively into the leak. V_T monitoring is not possible during this condition. Dislocation of the endotracheal tube needs to be considered. It is electronically zeroed before the next inflation.

to use a V_T of 4–6 mL/kg to avoid/limit volutrauma during mechanical ventilation.[35-37] However, if the lung is at the upper end of the pressure-volume curve because of excessive PEEP, the 4- to 6-mL/kg V_T will excessively distend the lung, resulting again in volutrauma (see later, Fig. 12.20). Conversely, if the lung resides at the lower end of the pressure-volume curve because of an inadequately low PEEP, a V_T of 4 to 6 mL/kg will allow portions of the lung to collapse and remain atelectatic. If 50% of lung volume is atelectatic, the "normal" V_T will be distributed among aerated parts of the lung to result in cycling alveolar (over)distension as if ventilated with a V_T = 8–12 mL/kg, causing both atelectotrauma and lung injury in ventilated areas. In nonhomogeneous lung disease, it may be very difficult or even impossible to aerate and ventilate all compartments in an ideal way. Monitoring pulmonary graphics can help to limit lung damage on both ends of the disease.

DISPLAY OF PULMONARY GRAPHICS USING LOOPS

Currently, there is no standardized display of the configuration of inspiratory and expiratory limbs in graphic loops. Therefore, graphic loops can vary according to the manufacturers' design and to personal preferences in setup. Some devices draw the loops clockwise, others counterclockwise. The user needs to be

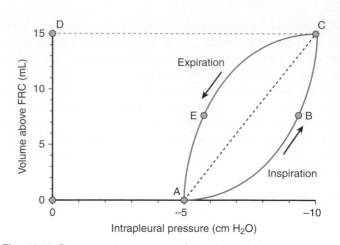

Fig. 12.15 Pressure-volume curve of the lung *during spontaneous breathing.* Inspiration starts at (*A*) and ends at (*C*). Expiration starts at (*C*) and ends at (*A*). The area *ABCD0A* represents the work of breathing to overcome elastic forces (*ACD0A*) + airway and tissue resistive forces (*ABCA*). The slope *AC* represents lung compliance.

familiar with the display to avoid incorrect interpretation of the information.

Pressure-Volume Loops

Display of pressure and volume in one graph provides information on both signals throughout the breathing cycle and can give some information on mechanical properties as shown in Fig. 12.15 in the spontaneously breathing infant without respiratory support. The loop represents one single breath. The fact that the loop during expiration does not follow the inspiration path is mainly related to resistive forces. The area ACD0A represents the total work of breathing to overcome elastic forces (ACD0A) + airway and tissue resistive forces (ABCA) during inspiration. During any point between A and C, parts of the pressure are used to compensate for elastic and resistive forces. However, points A (end-expiration) and C (end-inspiration) refer to time points with zero flow, indicating that the pressure working on the lung is used to compensate for elastic forces only, as there are no resistive forces during zero flow. The slope AC represents lung compliance. Expiration is usually passive and some of the energy stored in elastic tissue of the lung at the end of inspiration is used to overcome airway and tissue resistance during expiration (ACEA). Both a higher breathing rate and a higher airflow (widening the loop) increase the resistive work of breathing.

If the same patient is apneic and undergoes mechanical ventilation, the driving force to inflate the lung is now positive and relates to the difference of PIP – PEEP. Fig. 12.16 shows the pressure-volume curve of the lung during a mechanical inflation without simultaneous spontaneous effort. Inspiration starts at PEEP level (A) and ends at PIP (C). Expiration starts at (C) and ends at (A). When cycling to expiration during mechanical ventilation, P_{aw} usually drops quite fast to PEEP level, resulting in the expiratory part of the pressure-volume loop to be steeper than the inspiratory part (C-E-A). If pleural pressure would be measured and transpulmonary pressure ($P_{transpulmonary} = P_{aw} - P_{pleural}$) would be used as the

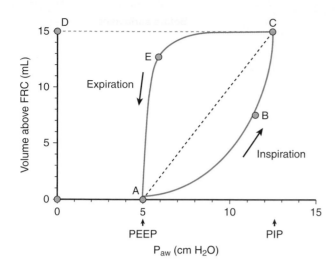

Fig. 12.16 Pressure-volume curve of the lung *during a mechanical inflation without simultaneous spontaneous effort.* Inflation starts at positive end expiratory pressure (*PEEP*) level (*A*) and ends at peak inflation pressure (*PIP*) (*C*). Expiration starts at (*C*), with a rapid drop in airway pressure to PEEP level (*E*) and ends at (*A*). Area *ABCD0A* refers to work of breathing to overcome elastic (*ACD0A*) + airway and tissue resistive forces (*ABCA*). The slope *AC* represents respiratory compliance. P_{aw}, Airway pressure; *FRC*, functional residual capacity.

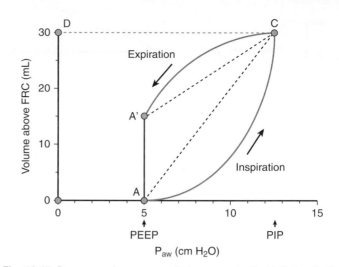

Fig. 12.17 Pressure-volume curve *during a mechanical inflation in the presence of a 50% leak.* Inspiration starts at positive end expiratory pressure (*PEEP*) level (*A*) and ends at with peak inflation pressure (*PIP*) (C). Expiration starts at (*C*) and ends at (*A'*). The volume signal ends above zero at position A' and is usually electronically zeroed before the next breath. The slope *A'C* (⋯) is a more accurate estimate of compliance than AC (⋯). P_{aw}, Airway pressure; *FRC*, functional residual capacity.

driving force for the pressure-volume loop, it would look slimmer and similar to Fig. 12.15. Again, the area ABCD0A represents the work of breathing to overcome elastic forces (ACD0A) + airway and tissue resistive forces (ABCA). As some of the pressure is needed to expand the chest wall, the slope AC represents respiratory compliance rather than lung compliance. However, unless there is a restrictive condition of the chest wall (such as severe edema), the error is not very large, as chest wall compliance is usually much higher than lung compliance in the neonatal age, especially in preterm infants with RDS.[38] More importantly, it is important to remember that in clinical circumstances, only P_{aw}, but not intrathoracic (intrapleural) pressure, is measured and any additional inspiratory spontaneous effort leads to overestimation of compliance. However, in the absence of spontaneous effort, the pressure-volume relationship—based on P_{aw} and volume measurements—allows measuring respiratory compliance at the measured PEEP, which determines the position on the overall pressure-volume curve of the lung (see later and Fig. 12.19).

If the increase in volume is smaller per pressure-unit, the pressure-volume curve becomes flatter and the calculated compliance will be lower, indicating restrictive lung disease, such as in RDS or pneumonia. Treatment of RDS with surfactant will usually show a higher volume per pressure-unit indicating improving compliance, unless the PEEP is chosen too high, causing overdistension (Fig. 12.19).

In the presence of endotracheal tube leaks, V_{Texp} is smaller than V_{Tinsp}. Therefore, the pressure-volume loop does not close at end-expiration. The volume signal ends above zero at position A' (see Fig. 12.17) and is usually electronically zeroed before the next breath (see Fig. 12.17). Using the slope AC would overestimate compliance as it would include the volume disposed into the leak. Therefore, V_{Texp} is actually the delivered V_T to the lung

and the slope A'C is a more accurate estimate of compliance than the slope AC. If the leak is very large, there may be loss of volume even during expiration and calculation becomes very inaccurate.

Note: when the inspiratory flow does not reach zero before the end of inspiration, there are two possibilities:

- T_{insp} too short. In this case, the pressure-volume loop closes (i.e., inspiratory and expiratory V_Ts are similar).
- There is an endotracheal tube leak (i.e., with leak opening during mechanical inflation as a result of the PIP distending the trachea): in this case, the pressure-volume loop fails to close, and V_{Tinsp} is larger than V_{Texp} (Fig. 12.17). Gentle compression on the larynx may decrease or eliminate the leak and help to temporarily correct measurements.

For the patient with alveolar lung disease (i.e., RDS), it is important to remember that mechanical characteristics and pressure-volume relationship are different when the lung is collapsed as compared to a situation when lung volume is recruited. More pressure is needed to recruit lung volume than to maintain the recruited lung volume. This so-called hysteresis is important to consider, as mechanical ventilation with a low distending pressure leads to repetitive closure and reopening of alveoli (atelectotrauma), even when using a small V_T. Using high distending pressure may result in overdistension, causing baro-/volutrauma with increased alveolar-capillary permeability. Both conditions may promote translocation of proinflammatory mediators into the systemic circulation and may cause distal organ injury.[39,40]

The pressure-volume relationship of a lung with alveolar disease is shown in Fig. 12.18. As P_{aw} is increased (inflation limb), air is moved and lung recruitment occurs when passing the "lower inflection point." Above the "upper inflection point," the lung becomes more and more overdistended. As P_{aw} is decreased (deflation limb), less P_{aw} is needed to maintain the

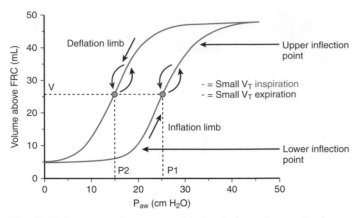

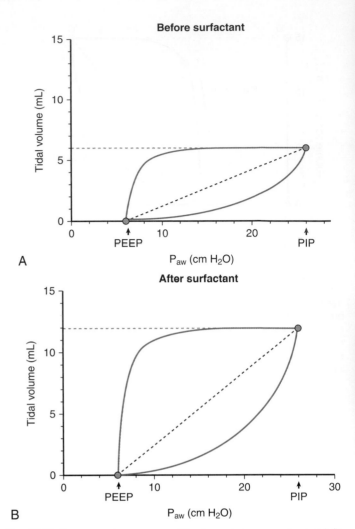

Fig. 12.18 Pressure-volume curve with alveolar lung disease. As airway pressure (P_{aw}) is increased (inflation limb), lung recruitment occurs when passing the "lower inflection point." Above the "upper inflection point," the lung becomes more and more overdistended. As P_{aw} is decreased (deflation limb), less P_{aw} is needed to maintain the same lung volume (V). Note: small tidal volumes (V_T) are provided at approximately mid–functional residual capacity (P1 and P2). There is marked hysteresis (P2 < P1).

Fig. 12.19 Pressure-volume curve of the lung *during a mechanical inflation without simultaneous spontaneous effort* in a preterm infant (birth weight of 1.2 kg) with respiratory distress syndrome before **(A)** and after **(B)** surfactant replacement therapy. Note: the tidal volume delivered doubled and compliance (*red dotted line*) improved accordingly. P_{aw}, Airway pressure; *PEEP*, positive end expiratory pressure; *PIP*, peak inflation pressure.

same lung volume (V). Note: small V_Ts are provided at approximately mid-FRC (P1 and P2). There is marked hysteresis (P2 < P1). Providing small tidal ventilation both (a) below the lower inflection point and (b) above the upper inflection point may result in lung injury (atelectotrauma vs baro-/volutrauma) secondary to (1) cyclic opening and closure and (2) overstretching of alveolar unit.[39,40]

Clinicians have successfully used the so-called "open lung concept" using recruitment maneuvers to recruit lung volume with increasing MAP during high-frequency oscillatory ventilation (HFOV) for a short period of time, followed by a decrease in PEEP/MAP thereafter to ventilate on the deflation limb, aiming for the steep portion of the pressure-volume curve (Fig. 12.18).[41]

The pressure-volume curve, along with calculation of compliance, can be used to follow the mechanical characteristics of neonates with restrictive lung disease, such as RDS or pneumonia. Fig. 12.19A–B shows the pressure-volume relationship before and after surfactant replacement therapy in an infant undergoing pressure-limited ventilation. While using the same PIP, the V_T was much larger after the surfactant was delivered and compliance improved accordingly. If volume-targeted ventilation is used in the same condition, V_T would remain constant and PIP would be reduced accordingly (automated weaning).[36]

As mentioned, it is very important to remind the user that in the absence of pleural pressure measurements, only mechanical inflations (without significant spontaneous effort) should be used to calculate compliance and that this measurement refers to respiratory compliance, which is mainly driven by lung compliance in neonates, especially in preterm infants (see earlier).

In Fig. 12.20, the role of FRC on the slope of the pressure-volume curve is shown in an infant with RDS with alveolar lung disease. There is a marked nonlinearity of volume changes in relation to P_{aw} changes, and the position on the pressure-volume curve where spontaneous or mechanical ventilation is operating is of crucial importance. A V_T of approximately 6 mL is delivered

with low/normal/high FRC resulting in large/small/large pressure changes. Compliance is shown in red lines and is higher with a normal FRC than with a low/high FRC.

The pressure-volume relationship of "the lung" is an oversimplification of a usually much more complex condition as alveolar lung disease is often very heterogeneous. In RDS, well-aerated lung areas may coexist with overdistended areas (often in nondependent regions) and/or atelectatic areas (often in dependent regions). Different lung regions may in fact have different pressure-volume relationships. Therefore, choosing a certain PEEP during conventional ventilation (or MAP during HFOV) may not serve all different areas and is always a compromise.

The pressure-volume loop may be helpful to identify appropriate PEEP and PIP to avoid overdistension and recurrent atelectasis. Overdistension may be suspected by pattern recognition when observing the pressure-volume loop, which is distorted in the upper part to a "banana-shaped" or "penguin beak" configuration. This may be formally analyzed by comparing compliance based on the last 20% of the V_T as compared

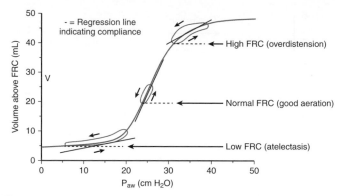

Fig. 12.20 Pressure-volume curve with alveolar lung disease—role of functional residual capacity (*FRC*). A tidal volume of approximately 6 mL is delivered with low/normal/high FRC, resulting in large/small/large pressure changes. Compliance (*red lines*) during normal FRC is higher than during low/high FRC. P_{aw}, Airway pressure.

with the overall breath (Fig. 12.21) as described by Fisher et al.[42] When this so-called C20 was compared with the overall compliance (C), the calculated C20/C ratio was significantly decreased in those patients with pressure-volume loop evidence of overdistention. When the pressure-volume loop was clearly showing signs for overdistention, C20/C values were less than 0.8.[42] The clinical implication is that the pressure-volume loop may be visually inspected and/or C20/C may be calculated to decrease PIP if there is evidence for overdistention in the loop, or when C20/C is below 0.8. It should be recognized that low C20/C may be caused not only by excessive tidal volume, but also by inadequate lung volume recruitment resulting in the tidal volume being delivered into a reduced lung volume due to atelectasis. In the former case, PIP or PEEP reduction is appropriate (depending on radiographic appearance and tidal volume); in the latter, PEEP needs to be increased to better recruit lung volume. Introducing graphic display of waveforms and loops for monitoring pulmonary mechanics in VLBW infants was associated with a lower rate of acute air leaks and IVH as compared with a historic control group from the same institution.[43]

Recurrent atelectasis during exhalation may occur if the selected PEEP is too low in an infant with alveolar lung disease. A high pressure is needed to recruit lung volume early during every inflation, resulting in a rise in P_{aw} without moving much volume at all (Fig. 12.22A–B). The left panel (A) shows a pressure-volume loop with low FRC because of atelectasis. Despite a rise in P_{aw}, there is very little air moving during early inspiration as long as P_{aw} is below opening pressure (A). During expiration, there is a rapid decrease in pressure, which is primarily related to the instantaneous reduction from PIP to PEEP. However, at PEEP level, derecruitment of lung volume occurs. After PEEP is increased, volume is increasing during tidal breathing as soon as P_{aw} increases (B). V_T is larger using the same differential pressure (PIP–PEEP), indicating successful recruitment of FRC.

Flow-Volume Loops

The flow-volume loop displays the change in airflow in relation to the change in volume. Usually, volume is displayed on the *x* axis, and airflow (in and out) on the *y* axis. Because of lack of standardization, some manufacturers place inspiration

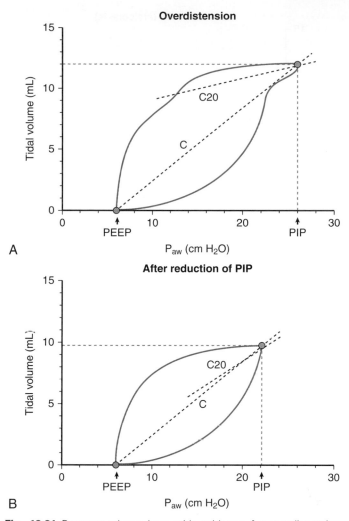

Fig. 12.21 Pressure-volume loop with evidence for overdistension. Graph A shows evidence for overdistension with flattening of the last part of the loop. After reduction of PIP flattening of the pressure-volume loop has (almost) disappeared. **(A)** Overdistension. **(B)** After reduction of PIP. *OP$_{aw}$*, Airway pressure; *PEEP*, positive end expiratory pressure; *PIP*, peak inflation pressure.

downward and expiration upward (counterclockwise loop) or vice versa. Inspiratory flow accelerates with increasing V_T to decelerate and become zero at full inspiration.

Fig. 12.23 shows the normal condition in a term neonate (A) and the decreased airflow occurring during mid- and end-expiration (increased resistance) in a BPD case (B). Increased resistance during inspiration or expiration can be displayed over the range of V_T and usually shows a lower airflow over the range of V_T where resistance is most affected. If there is a fixed increase in resistance, both limbs of the loop are affected and result in a "box-type" flow-volume loop (Fig. 12.25). In the healthy newborn, peak inspiratory flow is usually higher than peak expiratory flow because the total cross-section of the tracheo-bronchial tree is larger, and thus, resistance is lower during inspiration as compared with expiration. This is related to lung tissue distension because of the more negative intrathoracic pressure during spontaneous inspiration and/or to the higher P_{aw} during mechanical inflation.

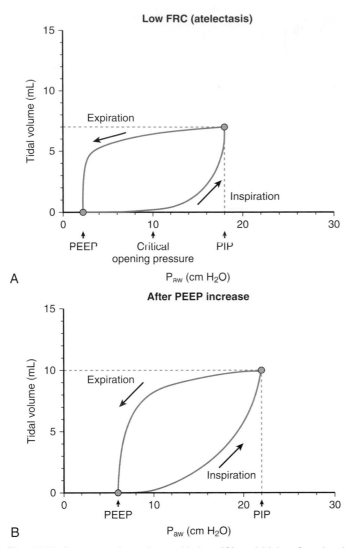

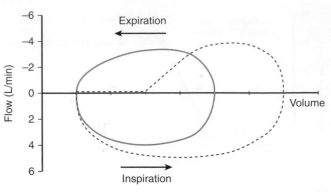

Fig. 12.24 Tidal flow-volume loops from a normal term neonate without an endotracheal tube leak (*solid blue line*) and with a 33% endotracheal tube leak (*dotted red line*). In this condition, the expiratory limb does not close with the beginning of the inspiratory loop.

Fig. 12.22 Pressure-volume loop with low **(A)** and higher functional residual capacity (FRC) **(B)**. Graph A shows an airway pressure (P_{aw}) rise without moving much air during early inspiration. After positive end expiratory pressure (*PEEP*) is increased, volume is increasing as soon as P_{aw} increases **(B)**. Tidal volume is larger using the same differential pressure (peak inflation pressure [*PIP*] – PEEP), indicating recruitment of FRC. **(A)** Low FRC (atelectasis). **(B)** After PEEP increase.

"Noise" in the flow trace as well as in the flow-volume loop may be attributed to humidity and secretions. Other reasons for significant airway obstruction may be copious secretions (improves with suctioning), a kinked endotracheal tube (improves with repositioning of the tube), or obstructive airway disease, such as in infectious bronchial inflammation, meconium aspiration syndrome, or anatomic obstruction (tracheal or bronchial stenosis). In cases with bronchial constriction, resistance may be increased primarily during expiration and may decrease following inhalation of bronchodilators. This can be followed by observing the increased expiratory flow in the flow trace or in the flow-volume loop before/after treatment.

In the presence of leaks, V_{Texp} is smaller than V_{Tinsp}. Therefore, the expiratory flow-volume loop will not meet the inspiration loop at the starting point (i.e., it does not close at end-expiration). Usually, the flow signal is electronically zeroed immediately before the next breath (Fig. 12.24). Observing either pressure-volume or flow-volume loops during manipulations to decrease leaks will provide immediate feedback on whether or not the intervention was successful.

Display of airflow over volume is useful to recognize flow limitations and may help to differentiate between underlying diseases for flow limitation. In Fig. 12.25, different tidal flow-volume loops illustrate various manifestations of flow limitation. Especially loop E is frequently observed in preterm infants with severe BPD.

PULMONARY MECHANICS

Lung Compliance

The compliance of the lung is represented by the slope of the $\Delta V/\Delta P$ curve, which is somewhat linear for a normal V_T in the midportion of the curve. Lungs with restrictive disease (such as RDS or pneumonia) are stiffer and have a lower compliance. Compliance is determined by elasticity of tissues and by alveolar surface tension. Total respiratory compliance (chest + lungs) is the V_T/change in driving pressure. In patients on mechanical ventilation, the driving pressure is equal to the difference between the PIP and the PEEP. Reference values for normal neonates, for preterm neonates with respiratory failure, and

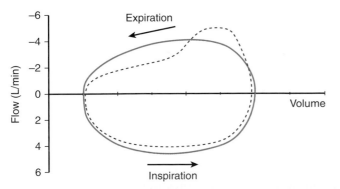

Fig. 12.23 Tidal flow-volume loops from a normal term neonate (*solid blue line*) and from an ex-preterm infant with high expiratory resistance (bronchopulmonary dysplasia) resulting in flow limitation occurring after partial expiration (*dotted red line*).

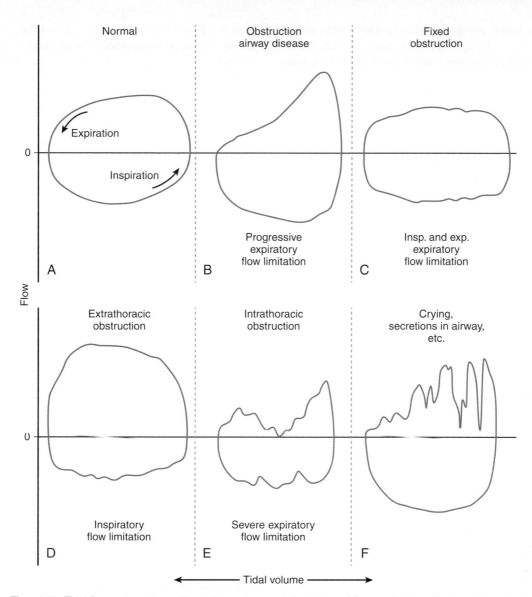

Fig. 12.25 Tidal flow-volume loops illustrating various manifestations of flow limitation. **(A)** Normal loop. **(B)** "Ski-slope" loop with expiratory flow limitation as observed in infants with expiratory flow limitation, such as in babies with bronchopulmonary dysplasia. **(C)** Extrathoracic airway obstruction with inspiratory and expiratory airflow limitation as seen in babies with subglottic stenosis or with a narrow endotracheal tube. **(D)** Intrathoracic inspiratory airflow limitation as seen in babies with intraluminal tracheal obstruction. **(E)** Unstable airways causing expiratory flow limitation, such as in tracheo-bronchomalacia. **(F)** Erratic airflow limitation, as seen with airway secretions.

after surfactant treatment are available in the literature.[17,18,44] Furthermore, sequential changes in pulmonary mechanics during the first 8 weeks of life in extremely preterm infants with respiratory failure showed that pulmonary compliance was lowest at 2 weeks of age and an average increase of 0.1 mL/cm H_2O/kg per week.[45] Typical "normal" compliance values in healthy neonates are in the range of 1.5 to 2 mL/cm H_2O/kg.

Comparing the respiratory compliance using end-inspiratory occlusions to elicit the Hering-Breuer reflex to analyze subsequent exhalations with conventional dynamic lung compliance using esophageal manometry showed good correlation without a significant difference in preterm infants, whereas in more mature neonates, respiratory compliance was approximately 80% of dynamic compliance and resistance was 24% higher,[46] which is expected as their chest wall is stiffer than the highly compliant chest wall in preterm infants.[38]

Clinical Implications

Changes in compliance can be suspected on a standard graphic display of P_{aw}, airflow, and V_T, when there is a change in peak flow and V_T during unchanged pressure-limited ventilation such as after surfactant replacement therapy. During volume-targeted ventilation, "automated weaning" of pressure may occur in the same situation. Using the pressure-volume loop, this change is easily visible and allows calculating the change in compliance. Many devices offer trend monitoring where P_{aw}, airflow, V_T, or calculated values such as compliance may be displayed in a compressed scale to show changes over minutes/hours. Obviously, this provides objective documentation of changes in certain parameters and/or measurements over time, which often is more accurate than oral/written information from healthcare professionals. Recorded data can be added to electronic medical records, which may be extremely valuable for case discussions later and for teaching and support quality management.

If after surfactant replacement therapy oxygenation improves, but V_T and compliance remain low, the PEEP used may have already shifted tidal breathing to the higher part of the now changed pressure-volume curve of the overall lung, leading to overdistension. Visualizing the pressure-volume loop of tidal breathing may allow recognizing overdistension (Fig. 12.21). Monitoring C20/C in preterm infants has been reported to be helpful to diagnose overdistension and to subsequently adjust ventilator settings (decrease in PEEP).[42]

Resistive Properties

Whenever air is moved in the respiratory system, there are resistive forces. At times of zero flow, the pressure needed to maintain the condition is related entirely to compensation of elastic forces. Motion at surfaces and within breathing media causes friction and loss of energy and requires forces to compensate for this so-called resistance. The resistances involved include frictional resistance to airflow, tissue resistance, and inertial forces. Lung resistance is predominantly (80%) attributed to frictional resistance to inspiratory and expiratory airflow in the larger airways. Tissue resistance (19%) and inertial forces (1%) also influence lung resistance but are more difficult to measure. Airflow requires a driving pressure resulting from changes in P_{aw} and/or alveolar pressure. When alveolar pressure is less than atmospheric pressure (during spontaneous inspiration), air flows into the lung. When alveolar pressure is greater than atmospheric pressure, air flows out of the lung. By definition, resistance to airflow is equal to the resistive component of driving pressure divided by airflow: resistance = pressure/flow.

To measure airway resistance, the differential between alveolar pressure and atmospheric pressure is used as the driving pressure. Under normal tidal breathing conditions, there is a linear relationship between airflow and driving pressure over a certain range of values. The slope of the flow versus pressure curve changes as the airways narrow, indicating that the patient with airway obstruction has a greater resistance to airflow. The resistance to airflow is greatly dependent on the size of the airway lumen, as indicated by the Poiseuille law: The resistive pressure (ΔP) required to achieve a given *flow* for a gas of viscosity (η) and flowing through a rigid and smooth cylindrical tube of specific length (L) and radius (r) is given as follows:

$$\Delta P = 8 \times \eta \times L \times flow/\pi r^4$$

According to this relationship, resistance to airflow increases by a power of 4 with any decrease in airway radius. Because the newborn airway lumen is approximately half that of the adult, the neonatal airway resistance is about 16-fold that of the adult. Normal airway resistance in a term newborn is approximately 20 to 40 cm H_2O/L/sec, which is much higher than in adults (1–2 cm H_2O/L/sec). In babies with obstructive airway disease, the expiratory component of resistive work of breathing is increased. Nearly 80% of the total resistance to airflow occurs in large airways up to about the fourth to fifth generation of bronchial branching. The patient usually has large airway disease when resistance to airflow is increased. Because the smaller airways contribute a small proportion of total airway resistance, they are sometimes known as the "silent zone" of the lung in which airway obstruction can occur without being readily detected. Unlike babies with RDS, babies with BPD (because of the associated airway barotrauma) have higher values of airway resistance with an associated increased resistive work of breathing.

Clinical Implications

Inspiratory peak flow usually happens during mid-inspiration and expiratory peak flow is observed during early expiration (Figs. 12.23 and 12.25). Fig. 12.25 shows typical flow-volume traces with different causes of inspiratory and expiratory flow limitation. Severe flow limitation is frequently observed in infants with severe tracheo-/bronchomalacia, particularly in growing extremely immature preterm babies developing severe BPD or in infants after tracheal or esophageal surgery. Active exhalation during crying increases intrathoracic pressure, which may promote airway collapse, exaggerating expiratory flow limitation by constriction of the tracheobronchial structures. CPAP/PEEP may provide airway splinting and alleviate increased expiratory flow resistance.[47,48] Flow-volume loops can be used to titrate CPAP/PEEP, but forced expiratory flow testing seems to be superior to mid-expiratory tidal flow measurements in assessing the best CPAP/PEEP to improve expiratory flow limitation.[47] However, the latter technique is more difficult to apply in (preterm) neonates in the NICU.

END TIDAL CO$_2$ CURVE

The ETCO$_2$ waveform consists of five parts: (1) inflation; (2) at the start of expiration, the exhaled air is a combination of dead space and alveolar gases and consists of a rapid S-shaped upswing on the tracing; (33) exhalation of mostly CO$_2$-rich gas from the alveoli (alveolar plateau); (4) end-tidal point, which represents the maximum exhaled CO$_2$; and (5) start of next inflation with a rapid decrease of CO$_2$ to baseline or zero.

Hypocarbia and/or hypercarbia have been implicated as causative factors for periventricular leukomalacia, intraventricular hemorrhage, or chronic lung disease. Fluctuations in partial pressure of arterial carbon dioxide (PaCO$_2$) are associated with worse neurodevelopmental outcomes. The gold standard of monitoring PaCO$_2$ is arterial blood gas analysis; however, this is expensive, leads to blood loss and iatrogenic anemia, causes procedural pain, and only provided a snapshot at the time of sampling. Similarly, indwelling arterial catheters or percutaneous arterial sampling are associated with digital ischemia, arterial spasm, or infection. Therefore, alternative methods to measure CO$_2$ are needed.

ETCO$_2$ is noninvasive and continuously measured with a fast response time to changes in arterial CO$_2$ levels. ETCO$_2$ is determined by alveolar ventilation, pulmonary perfusion, cardiac output, and CO_2 production. In neonatal medicine, $ETCO_2$ is mainly used during conventional mechanical ventilation in the NICU and more recently also during neonatal resuscitation in the delivery room.[49] There were concerns about the overall correlation between $ETCO_2$ and $PaCO_2$; however, recent studies reported that mainstream $ETCO_2$ monitoring is useful and accurate in neonatal patients.

ROLE OF PULMONARY GRAPHICS IN DAILY VENTILATOR MANAGEMENT—OPTIMIZING VENTILATOR SETTINGS

Optimizing Peak Inflation Pressure

Given the lower rate of morbidity, many clinicians prefer volume-targeted modes of ventilation.[35,37] However, in patients with larger leaks, the functionality of volume-targeted modes may be affected and often pressure-limited ventilation is used. During pressure-limited ventilation, PIP is usually managed to achieve a V_T of 4 to 6 mL/kg. The pressure-volume curve may help to adjust PIP and to avoid overdistension.

Optimizing Positive End Expiratory Pressure

In intubated infants, glottis function as a crucial mechanism to maintain and protect FRC is grossly impaired and the neonatal lung tends to develop atelectasis and thus require the use of PEEP. Choosing the optimal PEEP is often controversial and may change over time. Among RDS patients, surfactant responders will need less PEEP as compared with nonresponders. If distending pressures are chosen too high, there is a higher risk for air leaks and hemodynamics may be impaired because of increased intrathoracic pressure. If PEEP is chosen too low, there is a higher risk of atelectotrauma because of cyclic opening and closure of alveoli. The pressure-volume loop may be helpful to ensure that there is not a high opening pressure needed to move air during inspiration (Fig. 12.22), which indicates positioning of tidal breathing on the lower part of the pressure-volume curve. To avoid overdistension, closed observation of gas exchange along with the pressure-volume loop to follow compliance and visual appearance of overdistension should be carried out (Fig. 12.21).

Optimizing Inspiratory and Expiratory Flow by Adjusting Inspiratory and Expiratory Time

Depending on the time constant, use of a short T_{insp} may not allow pressure equilibrium between P_{aw} and alveolar pressure, resulting in incomplete inspiration (Fig. 12.7). Whereas in lungs with a short time constant (i.e., RDS) pressure equilibrium can be achieved with a short T_{insp} and T_{exp} and allows using a small V_T along with high rates to avoid lung injury, improving compliance after surfactant replacement therapy may increase the time constant and may require increasing T_{insp} and/or T_{exp} and, thus, a lower ventilator rate. Similarly, in cases with increased resistance, and thus a longer time constant (i.e., with meconium aspiration syndrome or with BPD), T_{exp} may need to be adjusted to higher values to avoid air trapping. Following closely the airflow trace allows adjusting T_{insp} and T_{exp} appropriately.

Optimizing Tidal Volume

Most clinicians limit V_T in neonates with lung disease to 4 to 6 mL/kg to avoid baro-/volutrauma. However, experimental and clinical data suggest that the use of an even smaller V_T (3 mL/kg) during conventional ventilation may result in lung injury owing to atelectasis.[50,51] However, one must emphasize that poor lung recruitment may lead to baro-/volutrauma if the "normal" V_T is distributed among the aerated part of the lung. If the lung has not been recruited adequately and only 50% of lung units participate in ventilation, that proportion will in fact receive a V_T of 8 to 12 mL/kg (double V_T)! The pressure-volume loop can help the clinician to select the best PEEP and V_T.

Optimizing Synchrony

Currently available neonatal ventilators have very sensitive devices for synchronized ventilator modes (SIMV, AC, pressure-support). However, artifacts may trigger mechanical inflations, humidity may cause dysfunction, and the trigger threshold may need to be adjusted appropriately to avoid autotrigger or trigger failure. Further, flow synchronization to cycle off the mechanical ventilation improves expiratory synchrony and may provide more patient comfort and require less sedation and paralysis. Close observation of P_{aw} and airflow traces is extremely helpful to check the proper function of synchronization.[34]

Optimizing Oxygen Exposure

High FiO_2 is causing free radical injury, which may damage not only the lung but also other organs including the brain.[52,53] The most efficient way to keep the FiO_2 low is to maintain uniform aeration and the FRC in the midportion of the pressure-volume curve. In other words, pulmonary shunts caused by atelectasis should be treated with MAP, whereas extrapulmonary right-to-left shunts causing hypoxemia should be treated with other interventions, such as nitric oxide if appropriate, and not with inappropriately high FiO_2.

Optimizing Gas Exchange—Permissive Hypercapnia

There is no clinical reason to induce hyperventilation and to lower the $PaCO_2$ below 40 mm Hg in neonates with lung disease. To limit baro-/volutrauma, normo- or mild hypercapnia has been suggested to avoid lung injury. Based on the available evidence aiming for mild hypercapnia ($PaCO_2$ 40–55 mm Hg), early after birth seems to be appropriate and safe without any risk for an increased risk for IVH.[53-56] In developing chronic lung disease or established BPD, most clinicians increase the PCO_2 target to higher values after the first days/weeks of life.[54]

Determining the Relative Contribution of Spontaneous Breaths Versus Mechanical Inflations to Minute Ventilation

Comparing the airflow and V_T of spontaneous breaths with mechanical inflations during SIMV can give an estimate on the relative contribution to minute ventilation (Fig. 12.5 and Fig. 12.11B).

Special Circumstances

RDS causes a restrictive lung disease with short time constants, which can be managed with high ventilator rates or with high-frequency ventilation. Surfactant replacement therapy may cause significant changes in lung mechanics and shifts of tidal breathing in relation to the position of the pressure-volume curve. Careful assessment of P_{aw}, airflow, and V_T traces and the pressure-volume curve helps to identify changes in lung mechanics and to detect evidence for low lung volume/atelectasis or overdistension. The aim is to ensure that tidal breathing happens in the midportion of the pressure-volume curve.

Meconium aspiration syndrome is caused by inflammation within the airways and may cause severe obstructive lung disease with significant increase in airway resistance, in airway blockage leading to emphysema, and/or atelectasis (if the respective airway is blocked completely). The disease is often nonhomogeneous with areas of atelectasis and overinflation next to each other, which explains the high risk for air leaks. Furthermore, meconium inactivates surfactant and may thus cause an acute respiratory distress syndrome like restrictive lung disease, which may be managed with higher rates or high-frequency ventilation and/or surfactant replacement therapy. Close observation of basic pulmonary graphics and function measurements can help to distinguish between these different entities and help to adjust ventilator settings based on the flow trace, or surfactant treatment.

Congenital diaphragmatic hernia is often associated with lung hypoplasia, which should be managed very carefully with low PEEP to avoid overexpansion of the hypoplastic lungs and minimal PIP consistent with acceptable gas exchange to avoid baro-/volutrauma.[57]

PITFALLS OF GRAPHICS MONITORING— TROUBLESHOOTING

Immediately after surfactant administration, airway obstruction occurs in up to 95% infants, which is displayed as partial or complete cessation of gas flow (Fig. 12.10). Further complications include inappropriate changes in ventilator pressures, decrease in V_T, changes in compliance and resistance, oxygen desaturation, and bradycardia. Close observation of basic graphic monitoring along with oxygen saturation with temporary increase in driving pressure based on the findings is helpful to avoid these complications.

One major limitation of graphics monitoring is related to the fact that lung diseases in neonates are often nonhomogeneous and it remains very difficult and often impossible to induce uniform inflation. Therefore, measured data and calculations deliver certainly a simplified picture of a more complicated pathophysiology. Leaks contribute to inaccurate measurements but sometimes may be minimized by temporary gentle compression of the larynx area for a short time to obtain useful and accurate measurements. Distensible airways may cause a high dead space ventilation and a high ratio of dead space to V_T and may cause overestimation of lung compliance and a high dead space ventilation requiring larger V_Ts than expected.

Excessive humidity and wrong calibration may cause false readings. One common mistake is to simply calculate compliance and resistance values based on measured P_{aw}, airflow, and V_T in infants undergoing mechanical ventilation without considering additive (negative) pressure exerted on the lung by spontaneous efforts. Without taking esophageal pressure into the equation, compliance will be overestimated and resistance will be falsely low. However, during apnea or muscle paralysis, P_{aw} can be used as a good surrogate driving pressure to calculate these parameters of the respiratory system.

Respiratory function monitors display waveforms and data to aid the clinician but does not provide interpretation of the signals or a diagnosis. The information given by pulmonary graphics and monitoring is only one piece in the puzzle to explain a given disease and should be always interpreted in the context of other information, such as the history, clinical, and laboratory findings including gas exchange parameters, chest x-rays and other information.

Inexperience and lack of knowledge about the displayed waveforms may lead to misinterpretation of the signals. Anyone using pulmonary graphics must be trained to interpret wave forms and numerical values. Furthermore, inexperienced users might divert their focus away from the baby to the monitor screen. Following trend data is often more useful than (over) interpretation of single measurements.

EVIDENCE FOR THE USE OF RESPIRATORY FUNCTION MONITORING TO IMPROVE NEONATAL OUTCOME

Mechanical ventilation for critically ill neonates was introduced in the 1960s and became rapidly standard of care for infants with respiratory failure. Evidence for its use is more based on common reasoning than on good evidence based on clinical trials. The available randomized trials on mechanical ventilation for newborn infants with respiratory failure caused by pulmonary disease were published in 1967 to 1970 and showed a lower risk for mortality (relative risk, 0.86, 95% confidence interval [CI], 0.74–1.00; risk difference, −0.10, 95% CI, −0.20 to −0.01; Nnumber needed to treat, 10, 95% CI, 5–100). This was entirely based on studied infants with a birth weight of more than 2000 g because there was no difference in outcome in infants with a lower birth weight.[58] However, we continue to use mechanical ventilation in all neonates based on common sense.

Respiratory function monitoring to reduce mortality and morbidity has not been studied in neonates in randomized clinical trials, neither in the delivery room[59] nor afterward during NICU care. The use of respiratory function monitoring in clinical practice is almost exclusively based on physiological reasoning. It helps the caretaker to understand the pathophysiology of the underlying disease and to make decisions for respiratory care. Some years ago, Dr. Vinod K. Bhutani concluded in his review on clinical applications of pulmonary function and graphics, that "pulmonary function testing in conjunction with clinical, radiological, and blood gas monitoring changed neonatal ventilation from good judgement to informed judgement."[60] We would like to add that knowledge of pulmonary function monitoring and graphics improves understanding of the physiology and pathophysiology of neonatal respiratory diseases, which is extremely important for the clinical team.

More recently, an expert panel of the American Thoracic Society/European Respiratory Society concluded that respiratory function measurements can provide useful information to guide management on (1) assessing the physiologic nature and progression of the disease, (2) optimizing respiratory support and minimizing ventilator-associated lung injury, (3) assessing the effect of therapeutic interventions, and (4) assessing readiness to wean from respiratory support.[29] Newer techniques such as forced deflations to measure flow limitation during exhalation, forced oscillation technique to measure compliance and resistance, nitrogen washout or helium dilution techniques to measure FRC, inert gas washout to assess inhomogeneity, electrical impedance tomography to assess air distribution, and occlusion pressure techniques to assess respiratory muscle strength are available and have been studied in technical and validation studies. They are very valuable techniques for research settings but—in the absence of randomized trials to assess the effect of these techniques on clinical outcomes—are too expensive and/or not ready for daily clinical care.[29]

Pulmonary function and graphics add to our understanding of respiratory physiology if the staff is trained adequately, as well as to the pathophysiology of the diseases of individual patients. This permits continuous surveillance of the respiratory condition and readjustment of ventilator settings according to the individual needs of patients, which may add to patient safety.[61] However, this remains to be proven in larger clinical trials.

ACKNOWLEDGMENTS

The authors acknowledge the contributions of Drs. Donald Morely Null Jr. and Gautham K. Suresh, previous authors of this chapter.

KEY REFERENCES

6. Verbeek C, van Zanten HA, van Vonderen JJ, et al: Accuracy of currently available neonatal respiratory function monitors for neonatal resuscitation. Eur J Pediatr 175:1065–1070, 2016.
11. Ortega R, Connor C, Kim S, et al: Monitoring ventilation with capnography. N Engl J Med 367:e27, 2012.
13. Hawkes GA, Kelleher J, Ryan CA, et al: A review of carbon dioxide monitoring in preterm newborns in the delivery room. Resuscitation 85:1315–1319, 2014.
19. Gaultier C: Lung volumes in neonates and infants. Eur Respir J Suppl 4:130S–134S, 1989.
22. Greenough A, Morley C, Davis J: Interaction of spontaneous respiration with artificial ventilation in preterm babies. J Pediatr 103:769–773, 1983.
26. Lum S, Hülskamp G, Merkus P, et al: Lung function tests in neonates and infants with chronic lung disease: forced expiratory maneuvers. Pediatr Pulmonol 41:199–214, 2006.
36. Klingenberg C, Wheeler KI, Davis PG, et al: A practical guide to neonatal volume guarantee ventilation. J Perinatol 31:575–585, 2011.
37. Klingenberg C, Wheeler KI, McCallion N, et al: Volume-targeted versus pressure-limited ventilation in neonates. Cochrane Database Syst Rev 10:CD003666, 2017.
60. Bhutani VK: Clinical applications of pulmonary function and graphics. Semin Neonatol 7:391–399, 2002.
61. Sinha SK, Nicks JJ, Donn SM: Graphic analysis of pulmonary mechanics in neonates receiving assisted ventilation. Arch Dis Child Fetal Neonatal Ed 75:F213–F218, 1996.

13

Airway Evaluation: Bronchoscopy, Laryngoscopy, and Tracheal Aspirates

Clarice Clemmens, Erik B. Hysinger, and Joseph Piccione

KEY POINTS

- Airway pathology is common in infants requiring mechanical ventilation.
- In experienced hands, airway evaluation can be performed and well tolerated, even in the most critically ill mechanically ventilated infants.
- Direct rigid telescope microlaryngoscopy and rigid bronchoscopy can be used for both diagnostic and therapeutic purposes.
- Lower respiratory tract infections are common in mechanically ventilated infants and bronchoalveolar lavage can help guide diagnosis and treatment.
- Although tracheal aspirates can also be used to identify microorganisms, culture results are poorly correlated with those obtained during bronchoalveolar lavage.

INTRODUCTION

Over the past few decades, instruments available for examining the airway have evolved to become increasingly smaller while providing better optical resolution. It is now possible to directly evaluate the airway of even the smallest premature infants. The optimal approach to airway evaluation depends upon the indication for the procedure, the risk of adverse effects, and the magnitude of potential benefit. This chapter will assist those caring for critically ill neonates in determining which diagnostic modalities will obtain the most relevant information while minimizing risk to the patient.

FLEXIBLE NASOPHARYNGOLARYNGOSCOPY IN THE NEONATE

Indications

Flexible laryngoscopy is used as a diagnostic tool to assess pathology at or superior to the glottis. This procedure may be performed at the bedside during wakefulness or sleep. It is noninvasive, with relatively low risk to the patient as sedation is not necessary.

Flexible laryngoscopy is valuable for narrowing the differential diagnosis in infants with noisy breathing. The evaluation begins at the nares and proceeds through the nasal turbinates to the choana. Because neonates are obligate nasal breathers, severe nasal obstruction can lead to significant respiratory distress with cyclical cyanosis and feeding difficulties. Narrowing

of the pyriform aperture, known as congenital nasal pyriform aperture stenosis (CNPAS), is a rare cause of severe nasal obstruction in the neonate. Choanal atresia is a congenital anomaly representing complete obstruction of the nasal airway, with an incidence of 1 in 10,000 live births.[1] Infants typically experience severe respiratory distress, especially when it is bilateral (50% of cases). It can be bony or membranous or have features of both.[2]

After passing through the nasopharynx, the oropharynx and larynx can be examined. Obstruction at the level of the supraglottic or glottic structures results in inspiratory stridor. The most common cause of stridor in infants is laryngomalacia, which in severe cases presents with dyspnea, feeding difficulties, failure to thrive, dysphagia, and obstructive sleep apnea. It is the result of a congenital abnormality of the laryngeal cartilage or its supportive muscle tone resulting in dynamic collapse of the supraglottic structures during inspiration. Severity initially worsens with growth, but in most cases, it resolves between 6 and 18 months of age.[3] Treatment of laryngomalacia is dependent upon the severity of symptoms. Those with mild to moderate laryngomalacia may be managed by observation. Medical therapies can improve symptoms in those with concurrent gastroesophageal reflux disease (GERD). Surgical management with supraglottoplasty can resolve the associated respiratory and feeding problems.[4]

Vocal cord paralysis (VCP) is the second most common laryngeal anomaly identified in neonates. Unilateral VCP often results from iatrogenic injury during cardiothoracic surgery or ligation of a patent ductus arteriosus. It may also be idiopathic or result from neurologic disorders. Iatrogenic unilateral VCP frequently resolves with time, and regular follow-up with repeated endoscopic examinations is recommended before considering surgical interventions.[5,6] Bilateral VCP is less common, usually congenital and associated with other anomalies in 50% of cases.[7] It presents at birth with respiratory compromise and either inspiratory or biphasic stridor. Infants with unilateral VCP typically have a hoarse cry, whereas those with bilateral VCP vocalize well.

Flexible laryngoscopy is also helpful in differentiating the etiology of hoarse cry in neonates. Hoarse cry may develop following endotracheal intubation as a consequence of glottic edema or granulomata. In the majority of cases, these problems resolve spontaneously or with management of coincident GERD.

Risks, Contraindications, and Limitations

Flexible laryngoscopy, when performed correctly, is a relatively low-risk procedure. Risks include vasovagal reactions resulting in bradycardia and laryngospasm. They generally resolve with the removal of the laryngoscope. Maintaining a superior location of the scope and avoiding contact with the glottic structures help prevent laryngospasm. Coagulopathies are considered a relative contraindication, as the risk of mucosal bleeding from the nose must be weighed against the anticipated benefit of the procedure. The presence of an endotracheal tube substantially limits the value of this procedure. Although the nasal airway can still be visualized well, useful information about the larynx is rarely obtained.

Equipment

The necessary equipment required for flexible nasopharyngolaryngoscopy (NPL) includes only a light source and the scope itself. At our institution, the 2.2-mm flexible NPL is used most often in neonates. Use of "antifog" solutions or alcohol swabs minimizes condensation on the objective lens of the scope and improve visualization.

DIRECT MICROLARYNGOSCOPY AND RIGID BRONCHOSCOPY IN THE NEONATE

Indications

Direct rigid telescope microlaryngoscopy and rigid bronchoscopy (ML&B) can be useful as a diagnostic and therapeutic tool for upper airway and subglottic pathology (Fig. 13.1). In contrast to bedside flexible laryngoscopy, general anesthesia is required. Evaluation with ML&B should be considered when a need for surgical intervention is determined based on findings during NPL or when better visualization of the airway is required.

If vocal cord immobility has been established, arytenoid mobility should be assessed by palpation during microlaryngoscopy to determine if the cord mobility is impaired as a result of recurrent laryngeal nerve pathology or arytenoid fixation resulting from fibrosis or atresia of the posterior glottis. In cases of severe laryngomalacia (Fig. 13.2), ML&B can be used to perform cold surgical or laser supraglottoplasty.

Laryngeal webs, cysts, clefts, and laryngoceles are rare congenital anomalies of the larynx that are difficult to visualize on bedside examination. Laryngeal webs are caused by incomplete recanalization of the laryngotracheal tube during the third month of gestation.[8] Laryngoceles are air-filled dilations of the laryngeal saccule that communicate with the laryngeal ventricle, whereas saccular cysts are fluid-filled dilations of the saccule that do not communicate with the airway. Rigid microlaryngoscopy is also used in the diagnosis and treatment of submucosal lesions, such as venolymphatic malformations. Laryngeal and subglottic infantile hemangiomas may cause progressive, biphasic stridor within the first few months of life. They are sometimes associated with cutaneous hemangiomas and often respond well to chronic propranolol therapy, which is used until the growth phase has subsided and involution has occurred.[9]

Laryngeal clefts are rare anomalies that often present with stridor and aspiration. A type I laryngeal cleft is confined to the interarytenoid space; a type II cleft extends through part of the cricoid; a type III cleft extends completely through the cricoid; and a type IV cleft extends beyond the cricoid into the trachea.[10]

When the etiology for noisy breathing in the neonate is not apparent based on NPL examination, it is important to visualize

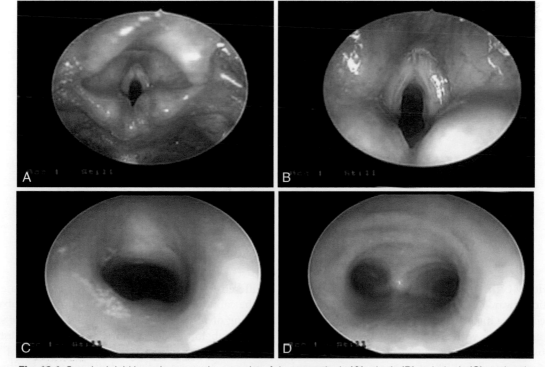

Fig. 13.1 Standard rigid bronchoscopy photographs of the supraglottis **(A)**, glottis **(B)**, subglottis **(C)**, and main stem bronchi **(D)**.

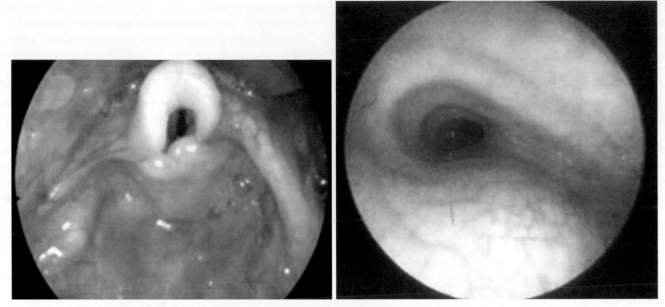

Fig. 13.2 Left, Laryngomalacia: omega-shaped epiglottis with arytenoid prolapse. Right, Tracheomalacia: collapse of the trachea.

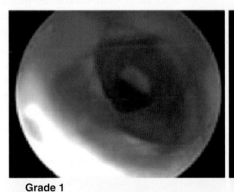

Grade 1
Stenosis 0%-50%

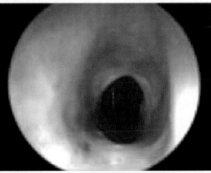

Grade 2
Stenosis 51%-70%

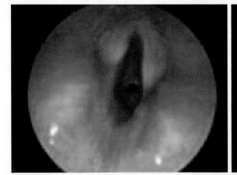

Grade 3
Stenosis 71%-99%

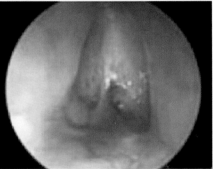

Grade 4
Stenosis 100%

Fig. 13.3 Examples of subglottic stenosis.

the subglottis with ML&B. Subglottic cysts can cause obstruction of the subglottic airway, resulting in stridor. They are almost always associated with a history of endotracheal intubation and often occur in association with subglottic stenosis (Fig. 13.3). Subglottic stenosis is an important cause of stridor in neonates. In most cases, it is acquired, but 5% of cases represent congenital forms of this condition.[11] It should be considered in the differential diagnosis when an age-appropriate endotracheal tube cannot be passed during attempts at intubation or in the setting of recurrent croup. Acquired subglottic stenosis results when subglottic edema associated with the presence of an endotracheal tube impairs capillary perfusion of the subglottic mucosa. Necrosis and chondritis ensue and a fibrocartilaginous scar is formed.[12] Risks are increased with larger endotracheal tubes, prolonged intubation, repeat or traumatic intubations, and infection.

The severity of subglottic stenosis is graded using the Cotton-Meyer grading system. A stenosis is grade 1 when 0% to 50% of the lumen is obstructed; grade 2, with 51% to 70% obstruction; grade 3, with 71% to 99% obstruction; and grade 4, when the airway lumen is completely obstructed.[13] Based on the etiology, grade, and thickness of the obstruction, various surgical techniques have been developed for the management of subglottic stenosis, including laryngotracheal reconstruction with costal cartilage grafting, cricoid split, and cricotracheal resection. In neonates with severe stenosis, a tracheostomy may be required until definitive surgical management can be performed.

Another important cause of stridor in the neonate is congenital tracheal stenosis owing to complete cartilaginous tracheal rings. In these infants, the membranous posterior wall of the trachea is replaced by cartilage. The number of rings varies and the diameter tends to narrow with each subsequent ring, giving a funneled appearance on radiographic images.[14] The airway of a neonate with complete tracheal rings is tenuous and must be treated with caution because of risk of obstructive mucus plugs and limited options for endotracheal intubation. Irritation of the mucosa in the stenotic segment by rigid bronchoscopy or an endotracheal tube can result in airway edema and exacerbate airflow obstruction in the trachea.

Tracheoesophageal fistulae (TEF) are well visualized with rigid bronchoscopy. A TEF results from failed closure of the tracheoesophageal septum during embryologic development. There are five types of TEF, the most common of which is associated with proximal esophageal atresia and the distal esophagus arises from the lower trachea or carina. Some degree of associated tracheomalacia is inherent to this disorder.[15]

Risks, Contraindications, and Limitations

The requirement of general anesthesia for ML&B makes it a higher-risk procedure than NPL; however, the risk of serious complications remains low. Common adverse events include cough, oxyhemoglobin desaturation, hypoventilation, and laryngospasm. Bleeding and damage to the lips, gums, and maxillary alveolus are uncommon when appropriate precautions are taken.

Equipment

The procedure requires a light source; rigid laryngoscope, telescope, or microscope; and a suspension arm if interventions are to be performed. Laryngoscopes are available in a variety of lengths, diameters, and angles. Selection is based upon surgeon preference, indications for the procedure, and which interventions need to be performed (Fig. 13.4).

The setup should also include "antifog" solutions for the telescope and a topical anesthetic (1%–2% lidocaine) to prevent laryngospasm. Care must be taken to avoid lidocaine toxicity in neonatal populations. The maximum safe dose of lidocaine (without epinephrine) is 4 mg/kg.

FIBEROPTIC FLEXIBLE BRONCHOSCOPY

Indications

Flexible bronchoscopy may be considered for both diagnostic and therapeutic purposes. A comparison with ML&B is summarized in Table 13.1. One of the most common indications for flexible bronchoscopy is sampling the contents of the airways and alveoli by obtaining bronchoalveolar lavage (BAL) fluid. Another important role of flexible bronchoscopy is to assist endotracheal intubation in neonates with difficult airway access. The bronchoscope may be inserted through an endotracheal tube and after navigating through the airway to a suitable position; the tube is advanced into place along the shaft of the bronchoscope.[16]

Infants with artificial airways (endotracheal intubation/ tracheostomy) may require inspection of the tube lumen when obstruction is suspected or positioning needs to be optimized.[17] When the tube diameter is sufficient to accommodate a bronchoscope with an internal suction channel, mucus plugs[18] and blood clots can be evacuated from the airway (see later). Similarly, in those with persistent or recurrent chest radiographic opacities, flexible bronchoscopy can help differentiate among anatomical, infectious, hemorrhagic, and mechanical etiologies. An important anatomical consideration for infants with recurrent or persistent right upper lobe opacities is the possibility of a tracheal bronchus, in which the right upper lobe bronchus originates from the distal trachea. A seemingly appropriate placement of the endotracheal tube can occlude the right upper lobe orifice, resulting in localized atelectasis when this common anatomic variant is present.[19]

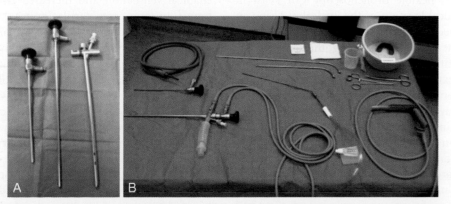

Fig. 13.4 Bronchoscopy setup. **(A)** Ventilating bronchoscope setup. **(B)** Complete rigid bronchoscopy setup. (Courtesy Joanne Stow, CRNP.)

TABLE 13.1 Flexible Bronchoscopy in Comparison with Direct Rigid Telescope Microlaryngoscopy and Rigid Bronchoscopy

Indication	Rigid Instruments	Flexible Instruments
Stridor	May alter airway dynamics	Preferred
Persistent wheeze (not responsive, or poorly responsive, to bronchodilator therapy)		Preferred, especially to evaluate distal airway structure and dynamics
Atelectasis (persistent, recurrent, or massive)	May be needed to remove airway obstruction (e.g., foreign body)	
Localized hyperinflation		Preferred
Pneumonia		Preferred (much better to obtain BAL specimens)
• Recurrent		
• Persistent		
• Patients unable to produce sputum		
• Atypical or in unusual circumstances (e.g., immunocompromised patients)		
Hemoptysis	May be best if there is brisk bleeding	Preferred to evaluate distal airways
Foreign body aspiration	Mandatory for removal of foreign bodies	May be useful to examine for possibility of foreign body; rarely useful for removal
• Known		
• Suspected		
Cough (persistent)		Preferred
Suspected aspiration	Preferred to evaluate posterior larynx and cervical trachea	• Preferred to obtain BAL
		• Combined use of both instruments very useful
Evaluation of patients with tracheostomies	Preferred to evaluate posterior larynx and subglottic space	Preferred to evaluate tube position and airway dynamics
Suspected mass or tumor	Preferred for laryngeal or tracheal lesions	Preferred for lesions in distal airways
Suspected airway anomalies		
Complications of artificial airways		

BAL, Bronchoalveolar lavage.

When recurrent opacities are observed in varied locations and aspiration of gastroesophageal refluxate is suspected, flexible bronchoscopy can be performed to identify TEF. The more common distal-type TEF is easily seen at the posterior wall of the carina, whereas the H-type TEF is located more proximally in the trachea beneath a mound of mucosa on the posterior tracheal wall.[20] In the case of known or suspected pulmonary hemorrhage, flexible bronchoscopy can be used to evacuate clots from the lower airways and identify mucosal and endoluminal sources of bleeding. This may be particularly useful in neonates requiring extracorporeal membrane oxygenation (ECMO).

In children with persistent pneumothoraces or suspected bronchopleural fistulae, flexible bronchoscopy can assist in identifying the anatomical location of the air leak.[21] Using an inflatable balloon-tipped catheter advanced sequentially into each bronchial segment in the affected lung, the source of air leak will become evident when the chest tube output ceases.

When attempts at extubation fail in association with noisy breathing (stridor, stertor, or wheezing), flexible fiberoptic evaluation of the airway is critical to uncovering the etiology. Techniques for evaluating obstruction in the upper airway are described in the section on flexible laryngoscopy; however, as lower airway obstruction commonly occurs concomitant with these abnormalities, careful inspection from nose to bronchi may be prudent. Evaluation of dynamic obstruction in the airway requires the presence of spontaneous respiratory effort and careful modulation of the level of sedation.[22] The presence and severity of airway pathology are likely to be masked by positive pressure ventilation, inadequate respiratory effort, or the stenting effect of an endotracheal tube.

Tracheomalacia and bronchomalacia are the most commonly identified pathologies of the intrathoracic airway in infants and can be present in up 50% of infants in select populations.[23] Tracheomalacia and bronchomalacia result from inherent weakness in the airway cartilage, reduced large airway smooth muscle tone, or both.[24] During exhalation, the diameter of the airway lumen can be reduced owing to transmural pressure differences. The collapse of the airway lumen can result in more than a 300% increase in respiratory work. Consequently, infants with tracheomalacia may have longer need for mechanical ventilation and increased risk of needing tracheostomy.[23] In some cases, cartilaginous weakness is further exacerbated by compression from the heart and great vessels. Vascular compression may result from a right-sided or double aortic arch, pulmonary artery sling, aberrant innominate artery, or anomalous subclavian artery. If pulsatile tracheal compression is noted during bronchoscopy, further vascular imaging may be warranted. Symptoms of tracheomalacia typically include homophonous wheezing, barking quality cough, and hypoxemic spells resulting from end-expiratory airway collapse. Treatment options range from supportive care (supplemental oxygen and continuous positive airway pressure [CPAP]) and medical therapies (inhaled ipratropium bromide and bethanechol)[25-27] in moderate cases to surgical intervention (tracheostomy, aortopexy, or tracheopexy) in severe cases.[28] In some children, inhaled beta-agonists may exacerbate symptoms; however, co-existing small airways bronchial constriction is common in these infants, and the potential benefit of inhaled bronchodilators may greatly exceed the risk.

Risks, Contraindications, and Limitations

Flexible bronchoscopy can be safe and well tolerated even in critically ill neonates with chronic respiratory failure,[29,30] provided that a skilled and experienced team is available to perform the procedure, administer sedation with careful hemodynamic monitoring, and provide adequate respiratory support. Clear and effective communication between team members is of utmost importance because a stable situation can quickly deteriorate in neonates with minimal cardiorespiratory reserve. Situational awareness is critical, and failure to recognize impending problems can result in resuscitation delay and poor outcomes. Resuscitation equipment and medications should be readily available.

Mild hypoxemia is the most common complication during the procedure; severe hypoxemia and bradycardia occur in <5% of patients and are transient.[31] Other complications include fever, cough, hypoventilation, and in spontaneously breathing infants, laryngospasm.[32] Fever is observed in approximately 25% of cases when BAL is performed. It is typically low grade (<102° F), develops within 12 hours, and resolves within 24 hours. Persistent fever should warrant consideration of infectious etiologies. Cough and laryngospasm can be mitigated by topical anesthesia such as lidocaine, sedation, and neuromuscular blockade (when dynamic examination is not indicated). Hypoxemia and hypoventilation may develop as a consequence of anesthesia, bronchospasm, and obstruction of the airway lumen by the bronchoscope. In mechanically ventilated infants, positive airway pressures may need to be increased to accommodate for the increased resistance attributable to the presence of the bronchoscope in the endotracheal or tracheostomy tubes; however, care must be taken to ensure complete exhalation and avoid generating auto positive end expiratory pressure.[33] Likewise, higher fractions of inspired oxygen administered during the procedure will also reduce the risk of hypoxemia. Serious complications such as bleeding and pneumothorax are rare.

Often, the most serious complications of flexible bronchoscopy are the result of cognitive errors. Clinically significant diagnostic findings may be quite subtle and misinterpretation could delay appropriate treatment or lead to more invasive interventions without benefit to the patient. Another type of error is the failure to perform a bronchoscopy when results of the procedure can lead to significant therapeutic benefit. A careful assessment of the probability and magnitude of potential risks and benefits should be considered in the context of the team's experience and abilities. An experienced bronchoscopist can be a critical asset for an advanced neonatal critical care program.

Equipment

Flexible bronchoscopes are available from several manufacturers in a variety of sizes. They may be inserted via an endotracheal tube or laryngeal mask airway in the mechanically ventilated neonate or through the nares when a better assessment of airway dynamics in desired and mechanical ventilation is not required. Flexible bronchoscopes require a light source, which transmits light through thin glass fibers to the tip of the instrument. An objective lens in the tip transmits the image back to the eyepiece or into a video processor for viewing on the monitor. Recording devices can be used and allow for review of the procedure findings at a later time (Fig. 13.5).

The 2.2-mm external diameter bronchofiberscope allows airway evaluation in neonates of virtually any size or gestational age but lacks a channel for suction or saline administration needed to perform BAL. It can be accommodated through tracheostomy and endotracheal tubes of 2.5 mm or larger. The 2.7- and 2.8-mm bronchoscopes contain a 1.2-mm suction channel. They can be used to assist endotracheal intubation in tubes as small as 3.0 mm; however, the ventilator circuit connector must be removed from the endotracheal first. A 3.5-mm tube is required to allow for adequate ventilation and maneuverability during diagnostic and therapeutic bronchoscopy. They are also available as a hybrid bronchofibervideoscope with which a magnified video image can be displayed on a monitor. The standard bronchofiberscope requires direct visualization via an eyepiece. A camera adapter can be attached to the eyepiece and displayed on a monitor; however, the clarity and brightness of the image are reduced.

A lever positioned on the bronchoscope handle allows the user to flex or extend the tip of the bronchoscope when navigating the airway. Bronchoscopes with suction capability offer a suction valve and biopsy/injection port for instrumentation

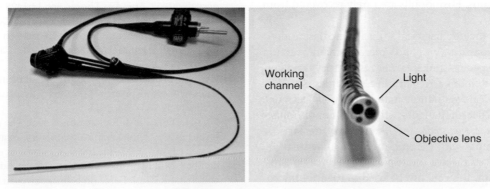

Fig. 13.5 Flexible bronchoscope.

and lavage. Supplemental oxygen can be insufflated via the suction valve to maintain oxyhemoglobin saturation and clear airway secretions when flexible bronchoscopy is performed via a transnasal approach. This is particularly helpful during transnasal flexible fiberoptic intubation; however, care must be taken to avoid insufflation distal to carina because of risk of pneumothorax. Biopsy forceps and brushes can prove useful for obtaining diagnostic samples as well as aid in the evacuation of mucus plugs and clots from the airway.

At the conclusion of the procedure, careful handling and cleaning of the bronchoscope will reduce the risk of infection via contamination in future patients and ensure longevity of the equipment.

BRONCHOALVEOLAR LAVAGE AND TRACHEAL ASPIRATES

BAL refers to the sampling of airway and alveolar spaces by washing a segment or subsegment of the lung with saline and recovering the contents of the epithelial fluid lining (EFL).[34] It is best performed with bronchoscopic guidance in which the tip of the bronchoscope is wedged into the desired location. This effectively isolates the region to be lavaged and reduces spill over into other parts of the lung. Simple tracheal aspirates and nonbronchoscopic lavage can be performed by blindly inserting a catheter via the endotracheal tube. These options may be useful for obtaining cultures but are more likely to sample the contents of the large airways as opposed to the EFL.

Factors to be considered in selecting the location for BAL include physical examination findings, chest radiography, endoscopic findings, and the relative ease or difficulty in fluid recovery. The right middle lobe and lingula provide the greatest potential yield of fluid return due their anterior position in the supine patient. Lavage volumes of 5- to 20-mL aliquots of body temperature saline are usually sufficient. A sterile collection container is attached to the suction valve of the bronchoscope and the sample can be distributed into additional containers for a variety of laboratory analyses.

The BAL fluid will contain both cellular and noncellular elements. Cytological analysis can be useful in determining the presence of infection. Whereas macrophages typically represent more than 90% of the alveolar white blood cell count, an abundance of neutrophils suggests the presence of bacterial infection. Lymphocyte predominance may prompt further evaluation for fungal or viral infections. Eosinophils are rarely recovered from the BAL fluid.

Microbial studies include bacterial, fungal, acid-fast and viral cultures, immunoassays, viral polymerase chain reaction tests, and organism-specific stains. Lower respiratory tract cultures from BAL are often of particular interest in infants requiring chronic mechanical ventilation and identify at least one organism in up to 70% of patients with bronchopulmonary dysplasia. *Pseudomonas*, *Klebsiella*, and *Enterobacter* are particularly common in infants with chronic mechanical ventilation, and many patients can have multiple isolated organisms. Although tracheal aspirates can also be used to identify microorganisms, culture results are poorly correlated with those

obtained during BAL.[31] Gomori methenamine silver stain can detect pneumocystis and fungal infection, whereas acid-fast stains identify tuberculous and nontuberculous mycobacterial infection. Other special stains can be used in the case of suspected pulmonary hemorrhage or chronic pulmonary aspiration. Iron stains can identify hemosiderin-laden macrophages, which are found in abundance approximately 72 hours following a pulmonary bleed. The lipid-laden macrophage index can be calculated as a marker for chronic aspiration. Unfortunately, this procedure is relatively time-intensive and limited by a degree of subjectivity in its interpretation. Published reports demonstrate a wide range of sensitivity and specificity.[35] Pepsin content is another potential marker of chronic aspiration; however, evidence to support this is still limited at this time.[36]

SUMMARY

Flexible and rigid endoscopic examination of the neonatal airway provides valuable diagnostic information and can be safely performed in even the smallest neonates. Identifying the most appropriate diagnostic modalities requires understanding the strengths and limitations of each approach. This will allow the neonatal care team to communicate effectively with collaborating otolaryngology and pulmonary specialists and deliver the highest standard of care.

SUGGESTED READINGS

3. Holinger LD: Etiology of stridor in the neonate, infant and child. Ann Otol Rhinol Laryngol 89:397–400, 1980.

4. Holinger LD, Konior RJ: Surgical management of severe laryngomalacia. Laryngoscope 99:136–142, 1989.

12. Hawkins DB: Pathogenesis of subglottic stenosis from endotracheal intubation. Ann Otol Rhinol Laryngol 96:116–117, 1987.

13. Myer CM 3rd, O'Connor DM, Cotton RT: Proposed grading system for subglottic stenosis based on endotracheal tube sizes. Ann Otol Rhinol Laryngol 103:319–323, 1994.

16. Midulla F, de Blic J, Barbato A, et al: Flexible endoscopy of paediatric airways. Eur Respir J 22:698–708, 2003.

22. Wood RE: Pediatric bronchoscopy in the 21st century: challenges and opportunities. Pediatr Pulmonol Suppl 18:130, 1999.

23. Hysinger EB, Friedman NL, Padula M, et al: Tracheobronchomalacia is associated with increased morbidity in bronchopulmonary dysplasia. Ann Am Thorac Soc 14:1428–1435, 2017.

28. Shieh HF, Smithers CJ, Hamilton TE, et al: Descending aortopexy and posterior tracheopexy for severe tracheomalacia and left mainstem bronchomalacia. Semin Thorac Cardiovasc Surg 31:479–485, 2018.

31. Hysinger E, Friedman N, Jensen E, et al: Bronchoscopy in neonates with severe bronchopulmonary dysplasia in the NICU. J Perinatol 39:263–268, 2018.

33. Hsia D, DiBlasi RM, Richardson P, et al: The effects of flexible bronchoscopy on mechanical ventilation in a pediatric lung model. Chest 135:33–40, 2009.

34. de Blic J, Midulla F, Barbato A, et al: Bronchoalveolar lavage in children. ERS Task Force on bronchoalveolar lavage in children. European Respiratory Society. Eur Respir J 15:217–231, 2000.

14

Delivery Room Stabilization and Respiratory Support

Louise S Owen, Gary Weiner, and Peter G Davis

KEY POINTS

- The majority of infants transition to extrauterine life unassisted, but the need for assistance cannot always be predicted. All settings where births occur should have staff trained in newborn resuscitation immediately available. Providers should receive regular practical and team-based resuscitation training.
- Best stabilization practice includes delayed cord clamping, stimulation and drying/wrapping, good thermal management, and no routine suctioning for those born through meconium-stained liquor.
- For infants born in poor condition, positive pressure ventilation should be initiated without delay, initially in 21% oxygen for term and near-term infants and with titrated supplemental oxygen for preterm infants, and including positive end expiratory pressure where possible. Monitoring using pulse oximetry and electrocardiography is recommended.
- Regardless of the device used to deliver positive pressure ventilation, peak pressures should commence at 20 to 30 cm H_2O. A rising heart rate is a good sign of effective ventilation. For infants who remain hypoxic or bradycardic or who have no respiratory effort, endotracheal intubation or insertion of a laryngeal mask airway should be considered.
- Very preterm infants should be delivered where adequate resources and trained personnel are available. No guidelines advise resuscitation of infants below 22 weeks' gestation. Survival before 25 weeks' gestation is increasing but remains below 50%; however, rates of serious morbidity in extremely preterm survivors have remained static.

INTRODUCTION

Rapid and complex physiological changes occur around the time of birth. The keys to a successful transition are the clearance of lung fluid and the establishment of a functional residual capacity (FRC). These changes are accompanied by an increase in pulmonary blood flow and the onset of regular respiration. Most infants achieve the transition unaided, but 15% need help to establish spontaneous breathing in the first minutes of life; 10% will respond to drying and stimulation, 3% will commence breathing after positive pressure ventilation, 2% will be intubated, and 0.1% receive chest compression and/or drug therapy.[1] Successful aeration of the lungs can reduce the need for more extensive resuscitation and should be the focus of initial resuscitative efforts. Therefore, ensuring that clinicians acquire and maintain the skills necessary to deliver effective respiratory support is vital.

Intrapartum-related neonatal death and neonatal encephalopathy impose a substantial burden worldwide, particularly in resource-limited settings.[2] The International Liaison Committee on Resuscitation (ILCOR) evaluates and synthesizes the available evidence, producing updated guidelines every 5 years, most recently in 2015.[1] From these guidelines, national resuscitation councils (such as the Neonatal Resuscitation Program [NRP™] Steering Committee in the United States) formulate recommendations suitable for application their own countries.

This chapter will outline the important developments in the assessment and management of babies in the first minutes of life.

PHYSIOLOGY OF TRANSITION, ASPHYXIA, AND RESUSCITATION

Physiology of Normal Transition

At birth, the first spontaneous breath generates a large negative pressure, up to −100 cm of water (cm H_2O),[3] inflating the lungs and driving lung fluid distally into the interstitial tissues. Studies of the initiation of respiration in healthy term infants from more than 50 years ago,[3] and more recently data from preterm infants,[4] demonstrate that the first breaths have a short, deep inspiration, followed by a prolonged phase of chest muscle contraction with a closed[3] (expiratory braking) or partially closed (crying) glottis,[4] then finally a small-volume, short expiration. These breaths push back the air-liquid interface; more volume is inspired than expired and the FRC is established.[5]

As the lungs aerate, pulmonary vascular resistance falls and blood flow through the ductus arteriosus changes from right-to-left to become left-to-right. Pulmonary venous return then starts to provide ventricular preload. Within three breaths, carbon dioxide (CO_2) starts to be exhaled, increasing to levels of around 50 mm of mercury (~67 kilopascals) after 1 minute.[6]

If the umbilical cord is cut immediately after birth, before lung aeration, cardiac output falls because left ventricular preload is still dependent on umbilical blood flow. Then, as pulmonary blood flow rises, cardiac output increases, followed by an increase in heart rate and blood pressure.[7,8] Newborn term and preterm infants not requiring resuscitation and undergoing immediate cord clamping typically have a heart rate under 100 beats per minute at 1 minute of age, rising quickly to more than 160 beats per minute by 3 minutes.[9] Therefore, delaying cord clamping until after lung aeration may stabilize preload and cardiac output, and reduce potential swings in arterial pressures and blood flows, leading to a more stable circulatory transition.[7,10]

Physiology of Asphyxia

Many pre- and peripartum events can reduce the supply of oxygenated blood to the fetus, resulting in varying degrees of fetal hypoxia-ischemia. Classic studies of acute total hypoxia-ischemia (asphyxia) in animal models have guided our understanding of neonatal asphyxia. The physiological changes and their response to resuscitation are shown in Fig. 14.1.

At the onset of hypoxia, breathing movements become deep and rapid. As the level of consciousness falls, respiratory efforts stop. This is the period of primary apnea, during which heart rate falls to around 100 beats per minute and blood pressure transiently rises before falling. Because left ventricular preload continues to come from umbilical blood flow before lung aeration, early clamping of the umbilical cord in an infant who has

unaerated lungs, and who therefore does not have any pulmonary venous return, may exacerbate hypoxia by reducing preload and cardiac output,[7] contributing to bradycardia.

As cardiac output falls, there is an increase in noncerebral vascular resistance, redirecting remaining cardiac output to the brain to maintain cerebral blood flow and maximize cerebral oxygen delivery. Spinal reflexes, no longer inhibited by higher (conscious) brain activity, trigger the classic diving reflex: respiratory efforts recommence as slow, deep, effortful gasps. This period lasts for several minutes while heart rate, blood pressure, and oxygen levels fall and carbon dioxide, lactate, and acidosis increase. Hypoxia and acidosis increase vasoconstriction of the pulmonary vasculature, resulting in reduced pulmonary blood flow, lower left atrial pressure, increased right-to-left shunting, and exacerbation of hypoxia. Animal studies show that, eventually, all respiratory efforts cease (terminal or secondary apnea), the myocardium fails, cardiac output and blood pressure drop,[11] and without intervention, the animal dies. In human infants, this sequence may last up to 20 minutes after the onset of hypoxia.[12]

However, animal models have focused on acute total asphyxia, whereas asphyxia in newborn infants may be intermittent, subacute, or chronic. The varying types of asphyxia make it difficult to translate the knowledge gained from animal models to the different pathophysiologies seen in newborn infants.

Physiology of Resuscitation

The primary aims of resuscitation are to sustain life while preventing brain injury. In the newborn setting, the focus is on lung aeration, to reduce pulmonary vascular resistance and increase pulmonary blood flow. This results in more oxygenated blood flowing through the coronary arteries to reperfuse the myocardium and an increased cardiac output. Newborn resuscitation guidelines focus primarily on good ventilatory support to achieve these goals. Even partial lung aeration will significantly increase pulmonary blood flow.[13]

Infants presenting in primary apnea can go on to make a successful transition through gasping reflexes; however, at birth, it is not possible to be sure of the duration of compromise, nor whether the presenting apnea is primary or terminal. The earlier in the asphyxial process that resuscitation is started, the more likely it is to be successful. Animal studies demonstrate that resuscitative efforts are more likely to be successful during primary apnea, and the longer the delay in initiating resuscitation after the last gasp, the longer the time to spontaneous breathing. For every 1-minute delay, the time to first spontaneous breath extends by around 2 minutes, and the time to onset of regular respiration extends by around 4 minutes.[14] The decision whether to intervene at birth is complicated by the fact that healthy babies may not take their first breath for more than 30 seconds,[15] and if decisions to intervene are made too early, unnecessary interventions may be applied. However, if decisions are delayed, there may be further cardiorespiratory compromise. In considering whether to intervene, it is helpful to remember that an infant who has good tone is unlikely to be severely hypoxic, and the key sign of an infant's condition in the minutes after birth, and response during stabilization, is the heart rate.

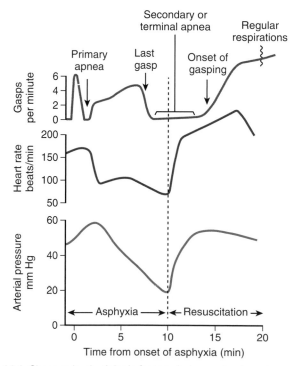

Fig. 14.1 Changes in physiologic factors during asphyxia and resuscitation in newborn rhesus monkeys. (Modified from Adamsons K Jr, Behrman R, Dawes G, et al: The treatment of acidosis with alkali and glucose during asphyxia in foetal rhesus monkeys. J Physiol 169:679, 1963; Dawes GS: Foetal and Neonatal Physiology. Chicago, Year Book Medical Publishers, 1968. By permission of Elsevier, Inc.)

ANTICIPATION AND PREPARATION FOR RESUSCITATION

The need for respiratory support and other interventions immediately after birth is a relatively frequent emergency.[16,17] The probability that term and late preterm newborns will require some assistance to establish spontaneous respirations increases in the presence of known risk factors. The best outcome is achieved when there is a skilled, organized, and efficient response from a highly effective team. Ensuring such a response requires effective team behaviors including comprehensive training, deliberate practice, anticipation, and careful preparation.

Training

All health providers working with newborns should complete a standardized neonatal resuscitation training course. Examples include the NRP developed by the American Academy of Pediatrics (AAP) and American Heart Association and the European Resuscitation Council's Newborn Life Support course. These programs focus on the cognitive, technical, and teamwork skills required to resuscitate a newborn in the hospital. Other courses teach critical skills for births occurring in limited-resource settings[18] and outside the typical delivery room (DR) setting.[19] By simulating both common and unusual neonatal emergencies, providers can identify weaknesses in their skills and develop proficiency.[20-26] Although a participant's knowledge and skills improve after a resuscitation course, both have been demonstrated to decay rapidly over time.[27,28] Without deliberate practice, providers are unlikely to acquire and maintain competence with infrequently used technical skills such as tracheal intubation and emergency vascular access. Even basic assisted ventilation skills have been shown to decay within months of course completion.[28] The ideal frequency of training has not been established; however, several studies have shown that brief practice with short intertraining intervals (low-intensity, high-frequency) may improve skill acquisition and retention.[24,29-32]

Teamwork

A complex neonatal resuscitation requires health providers to precisely execute multiple assessments and interventions within minutes of birth. Although each individual may have mastered the skills to resuscitate a newborn, optimal performance in the high-intensity setting of a neonatal resuscitation will not be achieved without effective teamwork. Poor teamwork and communication are the most common causes of potentially preventable deaths in the DR.[33] Simply assembling a team of expert health providers does not ensure that they will work efficiently together.

High-performance resuscitation teams precisely execute structured protocols that allow them to recognize important patterns, share information efficiently, and trigger the appropriate response. Each team member's roles and responsibilities are well defined before the resuscitation begins. The team is directed by an identified leader who gives clear direction, delegates responsibilities, and maintains awareness of the overall clinical situation without becoming distracted by individual procedures. During a critical event, when many human factors

can lead to confusion and delays, experienced leadership is particularly important. Training that includes multidisciplinary, high-fidelity simulation with structured communication has been shown to improve teamwork skills and the outcome of resuscitation.[21,23,34]

Anticipation

Anticipating the need for neonatal resuscitation allows a fully prepared team to be present and ready to begin lifesaving procedures without delay. Before every birth, neonatal healthcare providers should review the pregnancy history with the obstetric care team to determine which personnel should attend the birth. Using a comprehensive list of antepartum and intrapartum risk factors, Aziz et al.[35,36] demonstrated that approximately 80% of newborns who required resuscitation at a single tertiary perinatal center could be identified before birth (Table 14.1). When risk factors were stratified into moderate- and high-risk categories, positive pressure ventilation was required in 16% of moderate-risk births and 47% of high-risk births. In a logistic regression model, requiring positive pressure ventilation after birth was associated with maternal hypertension, oligohydramnios, maternal infection, preterm multiple pregnancy, opiates received during labor, meconium-stained fluid, breech presentation, abnormal fetal heart rate patterns, delivery at 34 to 35 weeks' gestation, emergency cesarean birth, and shoulder dystocia. However, the individual risk factors had limited discriminatory power and identified many births where no intervention was needed. To avoid missing a newborn who required resuscitation, the resuscitation team attended approximately two-thirds of all births.

Despite the use of a risk stratification system, the need for positive pressure ventilation will not always be predicted. Among births with no identified risk factor, Aziz et al. found that 7% of newborns received positive pressure ventilation.[36] In a large tertiary academic hospital, Niles et al. reported that 33% of newborns who received positive pressure ventilation

TABLE 14.1 Risk Factors for Neonatal Resuscitation	
Antepartum Risk Factors	**Intrapartum Risk Factors**
Preterm birth at less than 36 weeks' gestational age	Abnormal fetal heart rate pattern (category II or III)
Intrauterine growth restriction	Prolapsed cord
Polyhydramnios	Placenta previa
Oligohydramnios	Placental abruption
Maternal diabetes	Meconium-stained fluid
Maternal hypertension	Shoulder dystocia
Major fetal anomaly or hydrops	Breech or transverse presentation
Maternal infection	Vacuum or forceps birth
Chorioamnionitis	Emergency cesarean birth
	Opiates received in labor
	General anesthesia

Adapted from Aziz K: Ante- and intra-partum factors that predict increased need for neonatal resuscitation. Resuscitation 79: 444–452, 2008.

after a vaginal birth were not preidentified and the resuscitation team was alerted after delivery.[37] These data highlight the importance of having adequate personnel available at every birth.

Can risk factors predict the need for complex procedures such as endotracheal intubation, chest compressions, and emergency vascular access that require a team with advanced skills in the DR? In a prospective, multicenter study evaluating term and late-preterm births, Berazategui et al. developed a risk calculator to predict the need for advanced resuscitation.[38] The final model included 10 antepartum and intrapartum variables (birth at 34–37 weeks, intrauterine growth restriction, gestational diabetes, meconium-stained fluid, forceps or vacuum delivery, clinical chorioamnionitis, fetal bradycardia, placental abruption, general anesthesia, and emergency cesarean birth). Although the calculator showed a moderate degree of discrimination (area under the receiving operating characteristic curve = 0.85), it failed to identify almost 25% of newborns who required advanced resuscitation (sensitivity of 75%).

Preparation

After evaluating the perinatal risk factors, the necessary personnel should be assembled. The number and qualifications of the health providers will vary depending upon the specific circumstances. Every birth should be attended by at least one qualified health provider whose only job is to manage the newborn.[39] At a minimum, this person must be proficient at newborn assessment, the initial steps of newborn care, and positive pressure ventilation. A rapid and reliable method of calling for additional help is imperative. If risk factors are identified, at least two qualified providers should be present at the time of birth. Regardless of the setting, every hospital that delivers newborns should have a team proficient in all resuscitation skills immediately available if a complex resuscitation is required. The full team should be present at the time of birth if the need for a complex resuscitation is anticipated. If the newborn has cardio-respiratory collapse, multiple procedures will need to be completed without delay.

If there is time before delivery, a preresuscitation briefing or "Time Out" should be performed to review the clinical situation, identify a team leader, plan the response and possible contingencies, delegate roles and responsibilities, and prepare the necessary equipment (Box 14.1 and Box 14.2). The equipment required to initiate positive pressure ventilation should be checked and ready for immediate use at every birth. All equipment necessary to

---

BOX 14.1   The Preresuscitation "Time Out"

Introduce team members
Review maternal history and risk factors
Identify team leader
Review anticipated clinical scenarios
Describe the planned response and contingencies
Delegate roles and responsibilities
Prepare supplies and equipment
Are special consultants or equipment needed?
"If any team member identifies concerns or safety issues, alert the team leader immediately"

BOX 14.2   Neonatal Resuscitation Supplies and Equipment

Basic supplies
Radiant warmer with servo control sensor
Warm towels/blankets
Clock with second hand
Stethoscope
Pulse oximeter, sensor and sensor cover
Electronic cardiac monitor and leads
Gloves and gowns

Suction equipment
Bulb syringe
Mechanical suction
Suction catheters (5–6 French [F], 8–12 F)
8F feeding tube and 20-mL syringe
Meconium aspirator

Positive pressure ventilation equipment
Resuscitation bag or T-piece and mask
Compressed air and oxygen
Oxygen blender and flow-meter tubing

Intubation equipment
Laryngoscope (size 00, 0, and 1)
Tracheal tubes (internal diameter 2.5, 3.0, 3.5, 4.0)
Stylet
Measuring tape
Tape or securing device
Scissors
CO_2 detector
Laryngeal mask or other supraglottic device

Medications
Epinephrine (0.1 mg/mL)
Normal saline (50–250 mL bag)
Syringes (1 mL, 3 mL, 20–60 mL)

Umbilical vessel catheterization kit
Sterile gloves
Antiseptic solution
Umbilical tie
Small clamp (hemostat)
Forceps
Scalpel
Umbilical catheters (single lumen), 3.5 F or 5 F
Three-way stopcock
Syringes (3–5 mL)
Intraosseous needle (18 gauge or 15 mm)

For very preterm
Food grade plastic wrap or bag
Exothermic mattress

For thoracentesis and paracentesis
Antiseptic solution
18- or 20-gauge percutaneous catheter-over-needle device
Three-way stopcock
20–60 mL syringe

---

perform a complex resuscitation should be readily available if needed and prepared for immediate use if a complex resuscitation is anticipated. Using a standardized prebirth checklist helps to ensure adequate preparation, improves communication and teamwork, supports quality assurance data collection, and facilitates postresuscitation debriefing.[40-42]

CLINICAL ASSESSMENT, APGAR SCORE, SATURATION, AND HEART RATE MONITORING

Clinical Evaluation

Initial assessment of the newborn baby must be rapid and accurate to identify babies who need resuscitation and to evaluate the effectiveness of interventions.

The Apgar score was first published in 1953 and represents an important landmark in the care of newly born infants. It marked the author's reaction to the scant attention paid to newborns in the DR at that time; "nine months observation of the mother surely warrants one minute's observation of the baby."[43] For many decades, the score (Table 14.2) and its five

TABLE 14.2 The Apgar Score

Sign	SCORE		
	0	1	2
Heart rate	Absent	Slow (<100 beats per minute)	>100 beats per minute
Respirations	Absent	Slow, irregular	Good, crying
Muscle tone	Limp	Some flexion	Active motion
Reflex irritability	No response	Grimace	Cough, sneeze, cry
Color	Blue or pale	Pink body, blue extremities	Completely pink

components have been used "as a basis for discussion and comparison of the results of obstetric practices, types of maternal pain relief and the effects of resuscitation."[44] Conventionally, scores are assigned at 1 and 5 minutes of life, although it has been acknowledged that assessment and intervention may be required before 1 minute. The precision and accuracy of the component signs have recently been evaluated. Observers disagree about the presence or absence of cyanosis, and the correlation between color and oxygen saturations is poor.[45] Assessment of color no longer forms part of the ILCOR guidelines for resuscitation. Heart rate determined by auscultation of the chest or palpation of the cord has long been considered critical in monitoring the need for and effectiveness of resuscitation. However, both methods of clinical measurement are inconsistent and systematically underestimate heart rate by approximately 15 to 20 beats per minute relative to measurement by electrocardiogram.[46] Assessment of respiration is also difficult. Although no studies have evaluated spontaneously breathing infants, assessment of chest rise in those being ventilated indicates that observers differ substantially in their perceptions of chest rise and there is considerable disparity between clinical assessment and objective tidal volume measurements.[47] Not surprisingly, studies of the precision and accuracy of the Apgar score have shown that experienced observers differ considerably in their assessments.[48] Hence, clinicians need to be aware of the limitations of clinical signs obtained in the DR.

Pulse Oximetry and Electrocardiograph

Pulse oximetry has been used for decades to safely administer oxygen to infants in the intensive care unit. Advances in technology have enabled reliable readings of both oxygen saturation and heart rate to be obtained within the first 90 seconds of life.[49] Continuous display, particularly of heart rate, means that resuscitation can be continued without interruption for intermittent auscultation. The sensor should be attached to the right hand or wrist to measure preductal saturations. Normal ranges of saturation measurements[50] and heart rate[51] have been defined by monitoring healthy term infants. However, these infants were managed with immediate cord clamping. Oxygen saturation levels are higher in the first 10 minutes after birth in infants undergoing delayed cord clamping (DCC).[52] Electrocardiography (ECG) provides an alternative method of measuring heart rate in the DR. It provides data quicker than the pulse oximeter[53,54] and is now the recommended method of obtaining

an accurate measurement immediately after birth. Both methods require further evaluation to determine whether their use improves outcomes for at-risk infants.

ECG is not without problems. Pulseless electrical activity during neonatal resuscitation has been described in a case series. The presence of an ECG signal can falsely reassure clinicians and cause a delay in initiating advanced resuscitation of an infant with little or no cardiac output.[55] Johnson et al. conducted a systematic review identifying and comparing techniques of assessing heart rate in the DR.[56] They concluded that ECG was the fastest and most reliable method of HR measurement at birth but suggested that it should not be used alone. Other methods including digital stethoscopes, photoplethysmography, and piezoelectric transducers were found to be promising but required further assessment during neonatal resuscitation before use in practice.

INTERVENTION BASICS: CORD CLAMPING, WARMTH, POSITION, SUCTION, STIMULATION

The basic steps of newborn care include management of umbilical cord, ensuring adequate warmth, positioning the baby's head and neck so that the airway is open, clearing the airway of secretions if necessary, and providing gentle stimulation.

Management of the Umbilical Cord

There is good evidence to support DCC for at least 1 minute in term and near-term infants; delaying clamping increases infant blood volume and hemoglobin[57] and has a beneficial effect on neurodevelopmental outcome at 12 months of age.[58] Animal studies have demonstrated that initiation of breathing before umbilical cord clamping stabilizes cardiovascular transition[59] and there is increasing support for "physiologically based cord clamping" (PBCC), rather than timed-based clamping.[60] Meanwhile, DCC is now recommended for infants who do not require immediate resuscitation at birth.[1] DCC is more complicated in very preterm infants and is discussed in the Special Cases section of this chapter. Umbilical cord "milking" (UCM) is a technique in which a section of the umbilical cord is compressed and emptied toward the infant, sometimes repeatedly. The technique appears feasible even in infants depressed at birth[61] and is similarly effective in placental blood transfusion in term and near-term infants as DCC.[62,63] However, the technique focuses on the benefits of placental blood transfusion rather than stabilization of cardiorespiratory transition. There are some concerns that UCM may cause wide fluctuations in blood pressure and cerebral blood flow in very preterm infants,[64] especially those who have not initiated breathing; see the Special Cases section of this chapter.

Warmth

Newborns lose heat and rapidly and become hypothermic unless adequate attention to thermal regulation is provided. Hypothermia after birth is associated with increased mortality and morbidities, including respiratory distress, late-onset sepsis, metabolic acidosis, and hypoglycemia. The DR should be appropriately warm and free from draughts. Immediately after birth, a vigorous term newborn may be placed on the mother's chest or abdomen and covered with a warm, dry blanket. Warmth will be maintained by drying the newborn's skin and maintaining direct skin-to-skin contact with the mother. A nonvigorous newborn should be placed on a warm, dry blanket under a prewarmed radiant heat source, the skin dried and the wet linen removed. The baby should remain uncovered to allow visualization and effective radiant warming. Newly born infants, without evidence of hypoxic injury, should have their temperature maintained between 36.5° C and 37.5° C. If the baby remains under the radiant warmer for more than a few minutes, a servo-controlled temperature sensor should be used to adjust the radiant warmer's output and avoid overheating.

Very preterm newborns will require additional interventions to prevent hypothermia, which are discussed later in this chapter.

Position

The infants should be placed supine with the head and neck in a neutral or slightly extended position. This has been called the "sniffing" position (Fig. 14.2). This position opens the baby's airway, aligns the posterior pharynx and trachea, and allows unrestricted air movement. Excessive flexion or extension of the baby's neck may cause airway obstruction.[65] If the baby has a prominent occiput, it may be helpful to place a small towel or blanket roll under the baby's shoulders to lift the shoulders and straighten the neck.

Suction

If the newborn is vigorous after birth, a soft cloth or towel may be used to gently wipe the baby's face, mouth, and nose. Among vigorous newborns, there is no benefit to routine oropharyngeal, nasopharyngeal, or gastric suction and this practice may interfere with pulmonary transition and the initiation of feeding.[66-69] Gentle oral and nasal suction should be reserved for babies who are having difficulty breathing or who have secretions obstructing their airway and for those who require positive pressure ventilation. Prolonged, vigorous, or deep pharyngeal suction should be avoided because it may cause bradycardia and traumatize tissues.

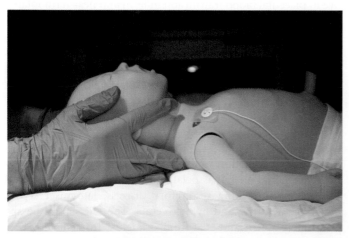

Fig. 14.2 The "sniffing" position.

Meconium-Stained Amniotic Fluid

The approach to babies born through meconium-stained amniotic fluid has evolved over recent years. Large, multicenter, randomized trials have shown no benefit from routine intrapartum oropharyngeal suction, or from tracheal suction of the vigorous newborn.[70,71] Previous treatment guidelines from the ILCOR recommended selective tracheal intubation and suction for nonvigorous newborns in an attempt to prevent meconium aspiration syndrome.[72] These recommendations were largely based on nonrandomized observational studies completed in the 1970s.[73,74] Because of the lack of supportive evidence, potential delays in providing ventilation, and the risk of complications associated with tracheal intubation, the ILCOR (2015),[1] American Heart Association (2015),[75] and the NRP's *Textbook of Neonatal Resuscitation* (7th edition, 2016)[39] stopped recommending routine tracheal suction for nonvigorous newborns. A recent meta-analysis of four randomized controlled trials (RCTs) enrolling 581 nonvigorous newborns delivered through meconium-stained fluid and one observational study including 231 newborns found that laryngoscopy and tracheal suction, compared with immediate resuscitation, did not reduce the incidence of meconium aspiration syndrome, hypoxic ischemic encephalopathy, or survival.[76] There is insufficient evidence to support routine intubation and tracheal suction of nonvigorous newborns delivered through meconium-stained fluid and the most updated ILCOR consensus on science suggests against this practice.[77] A large, multicenter randomized trial enrolling nonvigorous newborns is needed to inform this guideline, but organizing this trial presents tremendous logistical challenges.

Stimulation

Most newborns, including preterm newborns, breathe spontaneously within the first 30 seconds after birth.[78,79] Tactile stimulation for nonbreathing newborns is a practice that has been recommended in varying methods for over 100 years.[80] Although few studies have rigorously evaluated this intervention, it has been recommended in international guidelines based on experience and expert opinion.[75,81-83] Stimulating an apneic newborn seems to be common sense. Human fetuses respond to vibro-acoustic and tactile stimulation in utero with an increase in heart rate, movement, and crying.[84,85] Rats instinctively stimulate their newborns to breathe by biting, licking, and pushing on the pup's chest.[86] However, recent observational studies in both high- and low-resource settings have shown that tactile stimulation after birth is performed inconsistently, often delayed, and likely has a limited effect on bradycardia or hypoxemia.[87-89] It is unclear how effective tactile stimulation is for initiating breathing and preventing the need for positive pressure ventilation. Estimates range from 9% to 50%.[78,87,89,90] The interpretation of these observational studies is limited by variations in the timing of stimulation, the definition of a positive response, and the lack of an unstimulated control group.

Stimulation is often omitted from the immediate care of preterm newborns.[90] This may occur because the baby is wrapped in polyethylene plastic and not being dried or because the resuscitation team is focused on providing respiratory support quickly after birth. In a randomized trial enrolling preterm newborns (27–32 weeks' gestation), mandatory repetitive stimulation every 10 seconds alternating with 10 seconds of rest during the first 4 minutes compared with standard stimulation provided only as needed did not improve respiratory minute volume or decrease the need for positive pressure ventilation.[91]

The process of positioning and drying the newborn may provide sufficient stimulation to initiate spontaneous respirations. If the newborn is apneic, brief additional stimulation by drying or rubbing the baby's back or chest may be effective,[90] but caution must be exercised to avoid aggressive stimulation and cutaneous injury.[92] If an apneic newborn does not initiate spontaneous respirations within 1 minute after birth, positive pressure ventilation is indicated. Continued tactile stimulation alone is unlikely to be helpful and only delays appropriate interventions.

OXYGEN

Oxygen is perhaps the most widely used drug in neonatology but until recently remained poorly evaluated. An appreciation of its life-sustaining properties is now balanced by an understanding of its potential toxicity, even from a relatively short period of resuscitation. ILCOR guidelines on the use of oxygen for the resuscitation of term and late-preterm infants were updated in 2019[93] based on a systematic review undertaken in 2018.[94] This review identified five RCTs and five quasi-randomized trials enrolling a total of 2164 patients. The certainty of the evidence was graded as low for short-term outcomes and very low for neurodevelopmental outcomes. The recommendations of the updated guidelines remain unchanged; that is, the initial use of 21% oxygen is reasonable when providing respiratory support to term and late-preterm newborns (>35 weeks' gestation). Starting resuscitation with 100% oxygen is associated with excess mortality.[93]

The establishment of a normal range for term babies provides targets for clinicians, but the optimal increments and timing of changes remain uncertain. It is vital that operators continue to ensure adequate ventilation throughout the resuscitation and are not distracted by making frequent adjustments to oxygen concentrations. No human data exist, and animal data do not demonstrate any difference in outcomes between resuscitation in air versus oxygen whilst receiving chest compressions;[95] however, ILCOR guidelines recommend the use of 100% oxygen whenever cardiac compressions are provided. The use of oxygen in the preterm infant may have a different risk/benefit profile and recommendations are detailed in the Special Cases section of this chapter.

VENTILATION

Any newborn infant who does not initiate regular respiration, or who fails to respond to initial measures of drying, wrapping, and gentle stimulation should be given positive pressure support. This is typically first applied noninvasively using a face mask or nasal prong(s) and a pressure generating device. If the infant is making inadequate respiratory effort, continuous positive airway pressure (CPAP) may be sufficient to aid lung inflation, to establish FRC and to regularize breathing.[96] An infant who has no respiratory effort, or is bradycardic (heart rate <100 beats per minute), or remains hypoxic despite CPAP support should be given positive pressure inflations, ideally with positive end expiratory pressure (PEEP).[97] The aim of positive pressure ventilation is to provide effective ventilation and gas exchange, without causing lung injury, which can occur within a few large volume positive pressure inflations (volutrauma).[98-100] Actions to prevent lung injury include avoiding large tidal volumes and facilitating formation and maintenance of FRC.

Observation of the first breaths in well term infants suggests that prolonged (sustained) initial inflations may be advantageous;[4,15] this idea is supported by studies of sustained inflation in preterm animal models that show rapid lung inflation without overexpansion, immediate development of appropriate FRC, and uniformly aerated lungs[101] without serious side effects.[102] Randomized trials of sustained inflations at birth in preterm infants have produced mixed results.[103-107] This may be because the effect of sustained inflations in newborns varies with spontaneous breathing, opening and closing of the glottis,[108] and face mask leak, compared with controlled sustained inflation delivery via endotracheal tube (ETT) in animal studies.[109] Consequently, sustained inflations have been included in some resuscitation guidelines, whereas others recommend against their use.[1] Two recent reviews have evaluated the published trials, reaching similar conclusions, that there is no evidence of benefit[110] nor evidence to support routine use.[111] The Cochrane review[111] also highlights that the largest clinical trial addressing this topic was stopped early[107] because of a higher mortality rate in the sustained inflation group.

The ideal target volumes for positive pressure ventilation of term and preterm infants after birth have not been established; animal studies demonstrate that initial high tidal volumes are detrimental.[112] Recent data have shown that in spontaneously breathing term infants, expired tidal volumes rise after birth to plateau at an average of 5 to 6 mL/kg by the third minute of life,[113] but that some very high volumes breaths approaching 20 mL/kg are seen. Keeping tidal volumes under 8 mL/kg seems reasonable,[114] but delivered volumes are difficult to measure with standard DR equipment and are consequently rarely targeted or measured at birth. Clinicians still rely on setting a peak pressure and observing clinical signs as a proxy for "appropriate" volume delivery. Guidelines suggest that peak pressures should begin in the range of 20 to 30 cm H_2O[1] and these have been shown to produce adequate tidal volumes.[115] Infants without any respiratory effort may require higher peak pressures initially, which should be reduced as the lungs aerate and become more compliant.[116] The actual delivered volume will vary because of many factors; spontaneous breathing effort, lung compliance, laryngeal closure, facemask leak, obstruction at the mouth and nose, and the resuscitation device used. The result is that delivered tidal volumes vary widely and can be much higher than those generated during spontaneous breathing.[117] A rising heart rate is a good sign that effective ventilation is being delivered and is preferable to using achievement of peak pressure or assessing chest rise, neither of which is reliable.[47,118]

Although use of PEEP in the DR is not strongly supported by clinical evidence, it is a well-established technique with convincing animal data to support its use in establishing FRC, whether or not a sustained inflation is given.[101,119] A "standard" level of PEEP is unlikely to suit all infants. ILCOR does not specify which PEEP levels to use, and the levels recommended by resuscitation councils vary. The American NRP suggests 5 to 7 cm H_2O,[120] the Australian Resuscitation Council suggests 5 cm H_2O,[121] and the British Resuscitation Council recommends 4 to 5 cm H_2O.[122] European guidelines advise using PEEP of at least 6 cm H_2O.[123] The reported typically used level of PEEP in the DR is 5 cm H_2O,[124] but infants who have not fully established FRC are likely to benefit from higher PEEP.[125] A single PEEP level from birth until NICU admission may not be optimal; recent data from a study where escalating PEEP according to cardiorespiratory response was used were promising,[126] and a large study to investigate this is underway.[127]

Continuous ventilation, at a rate of 40 to 60 per minute, is recommended (unless chest compressions are being given concurrently); this matches the typical respiratory rate of healthy newborns. The optimal duration of each inflation is uncertain. Current guidelines suggest that matching the spontaneous inspiratory time of newborn infants (~0.3 seconds) is reasonable.[128] Set gas flow will vary with the pressure device being used. When using a T-piece, operators should be aware that PEEP and tidal volume may vary with changes to set flow. Manufacturer recommendations regarding flow should be followed.[129,130]

If chest wall movement is poor or absent and heart rate does not improve during mask ventilation, corrective steps need to be taken. These include repositioning of the head to ensure neutral position and reapplication of the mask to reduce leak and nasal obstruction. Other measures to consider include increasing the applied peak pressure, opening the mouth, suctioning secretions, and holding the mask on the face with two hands.[120]

Once heart rate exceeds 100 beats per minute and spontaneous breathing is established, positive pressure ventilation can be stopped; CPAP should be continued in premature infants. Positive pressure ventilation must continue if spontaneous respiration is inadequate, or if the heart rate remains less than 100 beats per minute. Endotracheal intubation should be considered for infants who do not develop adequate respiratory effort or who remain bradycardic and/or hypoxic in spite of adequate mask ventilation. Options for the management of preterm infants who require ongoing respiratory support include intubation and surfactant administration in the DR or initial CPAP support with rescue intubation and surfactant treatment only if required.[1,131]

PRESSURE SOURCES

In resource-limited settings, there may be no device available to generate positive pressure support. Mouth-to-mouth resuscitation can be used, but it carries the risk of infection. Mouth-to-mask[132] or mouth-to-tube[133] ventilation may be viable options and carry somewhat lower risks of infection.[134] Worldwide, many devices are available for generating positive pressure in the DR (Fig. 14.3).

The choice of device may be made based on cost, availability of a gas supply, desire to deliver sustained inflations, PEEP and CPAP, operator experience, or personal preference (Table 14.3).

Self-inflating bags (SIBs) reexpand after compression. They are the only devices that can be used without a gas supply and may be the most useful in limited-resource settings. Several types and sizes of SIB exist; the smallest size, around 240 mL, is for newborns. The peak pressure delivered by an SIB depends on how hard and fast the bag is squeezed. Although SIBs usually incorporate a valve to limit the maximum delivered pressure, it can be inadvertently or manually overridden to deliver higher pressures. Pressures greater than100 cm H_2O have been reported, resulting in excessive tidal volumes.[135] It is difficult to

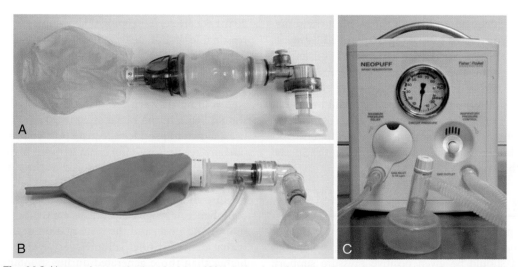

Fig. 14.3 Neonatal resuscitation devices. **(A)** A 240-mL self-inflating bag with an oxygen reservoir attached (Laerdel Medical, Stavanger, Norway). **(B)** A flow-inflating bag or anesthetic bag (Parker Health Care Pty, Mitcham, Australia). **(C)** A T-piece pressure-limited device (Neopuff Infant Resuscitator; Fisher & Paykel, New Zealand).

TABLE 14.3 Comparison of Attributes Across the Range of Positive Pressure-Generating Devices

Device	Self-Inflating Bag	Flow-Inflating Bag	T-Piece	Ventilator
Can function without gas supply	✓	–	–	–
Achieves accurate, consistent peak pressure	–	–	✓	✓
Measures delivered peak pressure	–	–	✓	✓
Potential to deliver sustained inflation	–	Possible with experience	✓	–
Delivers PEEP	Possible with PEEP valve	Possible with PEEP valve	✓	✓
Delivers CPAP	–	–	✓	✓
Delivered pressures are independent of gas flow	✓	✓	–	✓
Measures delivered tidal volume	–	–	–	Possible with some ventilators

CPAP, Continuous positive airway pressure; PEEP, positive end expiratory pressure.

give consistent peak pressures with an SIB,[136] even when using a manometer, although recent "upright" designs deliver more consistent tidal volumes than traditional devices.[137] If a PEEP valve is attached, some PEEP can be generated, but again, this is inconsistent,[138] and PEEP is lower at slower inflation rates.[138,139] SIBs cannot deliver CPAP or sustained inflations[140] and therefore may not be the optimal device for stabilizing preterm infants. SIBs entrain room air during reexpansion but can still deliver up to 70% inspired oxygen when used without a reservoir bag.[141]

A flow-inflating bag (FIB) needs a continuous gas supply to inflate the bag. Like the SIB, delivered pressure and volume depend on how hard the bag is squeezed. A pressure-limiting valve can be attached, and a manometer is recommended to increase consistency of peak pressure delivery.[142,143] PEEP can be generated by controlling the rate of gas flow from the back of the bag, although this requires experience; many operators find the FIB more difficult to use than the SIB.[144] Experienced FIB users can deliver sustained inflations with an FIB, but the delivered pressure fluctuates.[140] It is very difficult to deliver reliable CPAP using an FIB.

A T-piece device is flow controlled and pressure limited; it also requires a continuous gas supply to operate. Gas flow through an expiratory valve is used to generate PEEP. Peak pressure is achieved by occluding the port in the expiratory valve with a finger. Inflation time depends on how long the port is occluded. T-pieces are easy to use and are preferred by both experienced and inexperienced operators.[143] T-pieces deliver more accurate and consistent peak and PEEP pressures than other devices, resulting in more stable tidal volume delivery,[145] including with new operators.[146] However, operators are less responsive to changing lung compliance than when using other devices.[147] The T-piece effectively delivers CPAP while the port is open,[145] and occlusion of the port efficiently delivers sustained inflations of any duration or pressure.[140] Therefore, T-pieces may be the optimal device for providing respiratory support for preterm infants at birth.[143] A 2018 study of almost 1500 infants under 34 weeks' gestation showed higher rate of survival to hospital discharge without major morbidities when a T-piece was used.[148] If either a T-piece device or an FIB is used, there must be a back-up SIB for use in the event of failure of the compressed gas source.

Lastly, infants can also be stabilized using a ventilator. Ventilators can provide accurate delivery of peak and PEEP pressures, sustained inflations, CPAP, synchronization, and tidal volume measurement.[149] Alternative techniques, where pressure sources with their own specific interfaces, such as nasal high flow therapy delivered via nasal cannulae, are discussed in the section later.

INTERFACES

Positive pressure ventilation is most often delivered via a face mask that covers both the mouth and nose. These can be attached to an SIB, FIB, T-piece, or ventilator. Although the principles of face mask ventilation are simple, good technique is essential. To achieve effective stable tidal volumes, a good seal must be achieved between the mask and face. Without a good seal, there will be substantial leak around the mask and inadequate ventilation will ensue. In an effort to prevent mask leak, excessive force may be applied, distorting the nose and obstructing the airway.[150,151] Masks are available in many sizes and shapes. The most commonly used masks are round and have cushioned rims. Choosing the correct mask size is important. The mask should extend from the chin tip to the nasal bridge without encroaching upon the eyes. For a single operator, the "two-point top hold" provides the most stable mask application without distortion.[152] The mask should be rolled up from the chin, rather than directly placed onto the face. A finger positioned on the baby's chin tip may be used to align the lower edge of the mask, which can then be rolled gently upward (Fig. 14.4).[153] Difficulties with mask technique, plus the observation that simply the pressure exerted by the facemask can induce reflex apnea via the trigeminal cardiac reflex,[154] have led to investigation of alternative interfaces. A nasal tube, made by cutting down a 3- to 4-cm piece of ETT placed inside the nostril, has been used and studied. Two randomized trials compared this interface with a face mask and found no important differences in efficacy.[155,156] However, in a trial enrolling more than 600 babies, Capasso et al. found that infants resuscitated with short binasal prongs were less likely to require endotracheal intubation or chest compressions, although there were no differences in Apgar scores or mortality rates.[157]

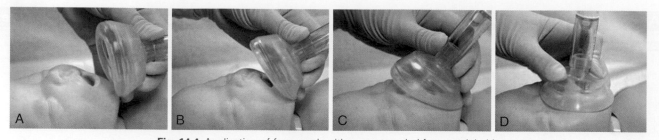

Fig. 14.4 Application of face mask with recommended face mask hold.

ENDOTRACHEAL INTUBATION

Indications for intubation after birth vary depending on gestational age, respiratory effort, response to noninvasive ventilation, and the skill and experience of the resuscitator. International resuscitation guidelines suggest intubation be considered at several stages:[1] if the heart rate is less than 100 beats per minute after 30 seconds of effective positive pressure ventilation, if the infant continues to be apneic despite adequate mask ventilation, if mask ventilation is prolonged or ineffective, or if there are congenital anomalies affecting transition, for example, diaphragmatic hernia. Infants without a detectable heartbeat should be intubated and ventilated as soon as possible; the endotracheal route of adrenaline administration may be needed before intravenous access being established. Neonatal intubation is a difficult skill to acquire and maintain. Uncuffed, uniform-diameter, radio-opaque tubes of 2.5 to 4.0 mm internal diameter are used. The narrow subglottic section of the neonatal trachea means that there is a risk of tracheal tissue damage when cuffed ETTs are used. Because of the focus on noninvasive respiratory support in preterm infants from birth, and the move away from routine suctioning below the cords for term infants born through meconium-stained liquor, fewer newborns are intubated and skills are declining. Trainees have fewer opportunities to learn[158] and are successful in less than half of intubation attempts,[159] compared with 85% success rates by experienced operators. Trainees take longer to perform intubations, frequently longer than the recommended 30 seconds, with consequent clinical deterioration in the infant.[159] Success rates are improved when trainees use videolaryngoscopy under senior supervision.[160,161]

INTUBATION EQUIPMENT AND PROCEDURE

Equipment for endotracheal intubation should be readily available wherever infants may be born. The required items are outlined in Box 14.3. The infant should be placed supine in a neutral position, avoiding both flexion and hyperextension of the neck, which makes the glottis hard to visualize.

The tip of the laryngoscope should be advanced over the tongue, either to the vallecula or over the top of the epiglottis, and elevated (not rotated) to reveal the vocal cords (Fig. 14.5). The laryngoscope should remain midline and support the tongue toward the left of the mouth, leaving sufficient space to see the larynx while passing the ETT. If the laryngoscope

---

BOX 14.3 Recommended Equipment and Supplies for Endotracheal Intubation

Positive pressure delivery device (self-inflating bag/flow inflating bag with manometer and positive end expiratory pressure valve if possible, or T-piece device)
Air/oxygen supply with flow meter and blender
Neonatal cushioned, round facemasks in range of sizes
Pulse oximeter (attached to right hand/wrist)
Laryngoscope(s) with straight blades, Miller sizes 00, 0, and 1
Uncuffed, uniform diameter, radio-opaque, endotracheal tubes, with a standard curve, depth marked, in sizes 2.5-, 3.0-, 3.5-, and 4.0-mm internal diameter
Stylet (optional)
Magill forceps (for nasal intubation)
Neonatal stethoscope
Colorimetric carbon dioxide detector
Suction equipment and suction catheters (5-, 6-, 8-, and 10-French size)
Equipment to secure the endotracheal tube in place (adhesive tape/ties/hat)

---

is advanced too far, the larynx will not be visible. Gentle external cricoid pressure may help to bring the anterior larynx into view.

Initially, the ETT should be inserted to the level of the vocal cord marker on the ETT. At this depth, the tube is expected to be above the carina; however, the marker position varies by manufacturer and should not be used as the primary method of determining the insertion distance. Previous recommendations suggested an insertion depth measured from the ETT tip to the infant's upper lip, estimated by adding 6.0 cm to the infant's weight (kg). This formula tends to overestimate the insertion depth and may inadvertently insert the tube into the infant's right mainstem bronchus, especially in extremely low-birth-weight infants. Other methods of estimating the insertion depth have been validated in term and preterm newborns; updated estimates based on the baby's weight or gestational age have been shown to be accurate (Table 14.4),[162] as is measuring the distance (cm) between the newborn's nasal septum and ear tragus (nasal-tragus length [NTL]). The tube is inserted the distance NTL + 1 cm, with the appropriate centimeter mark located at the infant's upper lip.[163] The ultimate goal is to place the ETT in the midtrachea, aligning the tip of the ETT between the first and second thoracic vertebrae.

A stylet can be used for ETT insertion; however, there is no evidence that this improves the rate of successful intubation.[164]

Properly Positioned in Vallecula

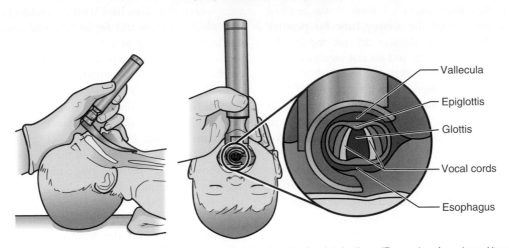

Fig. 14.5 Proper placement of laryngoscope and landmarks for intubation. (From the American Heart Association/American Academy of Pediatrics: Textbook of Neonatal Resuscitation. Dallas, American Heart Association, 2006, pp. 5–13. Reproduced with permission.)

Weight (g)	Gestation (weeks)	Endotracheal Tube Size Internal Diameter (mm)	Insertion Depth "Tip-to-Lip" Oral Endotracheal Tube (cm)
500–600	23–24	2.5	5.5
700–800	25–26	2.5	6.0
900–1000	27–29	2.5/3.0	6.5
1100–1400	30–32	3.0	7.0
1500–1800	33–34	3.0	7.5
1900–2400	35–37	3.0/3.5	8.0
2500–3100	38–40	3.5	8.5
3200–4200	41–43	3.5/4.0	9.0

TABLE 14.4 Guidelines for Endotracheal Tube Size

(Modified from Kempley ST, Moreiras JW, Petrone FL: Endotracheal tube length for neonatal intubation. Resuscitation 77(3):369–373, 2008.)

The stylet must not protrude beyond the tip of the ETT, as this can result in tracheal damage. It is also easy to inadvertently dislodge a correctly placed ETT when removing a stylet. Magill's forceps are often required to advance the ETT through the vocal cords during nasal intubation.

The placement of the ETT must always be verified; the best clinical indicator is a rapid increase in heart rate. Correct placement can be assessed by observing the tube passing through the vocal cords, auscultating air entry in both axillae, observing condensation inside the ETT during expiration and observing chest rise during positive pressure inflations. However, these signs can be misleading and the use of an end-tidal CO_2 detector on the ETT connector is recommended.[1] The depth of ETT tube insertion should then always be assessed with chest radiography.

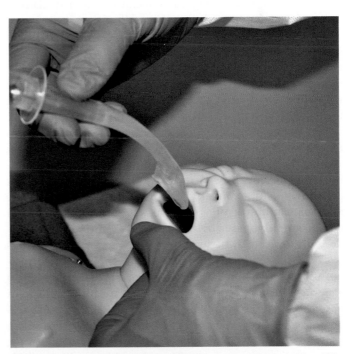

Fig. 14.6 A laryngeal mask airway (iGel, Intersurgical, Berkshire, UK).

LARYNGEAL MASK AIRWAY

Supraglottic devices, such as a laryngeal mask airway (LMA), are effective alternatives to face-mask and ETT ventilation. The LMA is a small elliptical mask attached to an airway tube (Fig. 14.6). The mask has either a soft gel or inflatable rim. The device is inserted into the baby's mouth with the operator's index finger and advanced along the palate into the posterior pharynx, and the mask is positioned over the laryngeal inlet. After insertion, the soft gel conforms to the of the tissue surrounding the larynx, or the rim is inflated, creating a seal over the glottis. A resuscitation bag or a T-piece is attached to a standard 15-mm connector on the airway tube for positive pressure ventilation. Supraglottic devices do not require the operator to visualize the vocal cords and do not require instruments for insertion. Their major limitation is the lack of small sizes. Most size 1 LMAs are designed for infants greater than 2000 g. Although successful insertion has been reported in smaller babies,[165,166] it may not be possible to use an LMA in infants smaller than approximately 1250 g, or about 29 weeks' gestational age.

In a metaanalysis of five randomized trials, the LMA was found to be an effective alternative to either bag-mask ventilation (five studies) or endotracheal intubation (three studies).[167] Use of an LMA compared with a bag-mask device was associated with a decreased need for endotracheal intubation and a shorter duration of positive pressure ventilation. No differences were found between endotracheal intubation and LMA insertion; however, the success with endotracheal intubation in the included studies was higher than typically reported. The time required for laryngeal mask insertion was short, the first attempt success rate was high, and operators required relatively little training to acquire the insertion skill.

Several studies have investigated the use of an LMA for surfactant administration in preterm newborns. In a metaanalysis of five randomized trials, surfactant administered through an LMA decreased the need for intubation compared with either continued CPAP or surfactant administered using the INSURE (INtubation-SURfactant-Extubation) approach.[168]

The most commonly reported use for LMAs during neonatal resuscitation has been as a rescue airway when face-mask ventilation and endotracheal intubation were both unsuccessful. This includes newborns with orofacial anomalies that prevent operators from achieving an effective seal with a face mask or that obstruct the upper airway. Because the operator does not need to visualize the vocal cords during LMA insertion, the device may be successful when an obstruction interferes with laryngoscopy.[169] Published examples include newborns with a small mandible or large tongue complicating a wide variety of congenital syndromes.[170] In addition, the LMA has been used to secure the airway during helicopter and ambulance transport when laryngoscopy for intubation is not feasible.[171,172] An LMA may provide a life-saving airway during an unanticipated emergency. They should be readily available in every birth setting and clinicians should become proficient in their use.

MONITORING

As noted previously, effective ventilation is the key to successful resuscitation. This means delivering a tidal volume that is sufficient to achieve adequate gas exchange, but not so much as to cause lung damage. As few as six large inflations can cause severe lung injury in a preterm lamb model of resuscitation.[98] Leak around the face mask and obstruction to gas flow may lead to reduced tidal volumes, which may result in an unsuccessful resuscitation. Clinical assessment of lung inflation based on

chest rise during ventilation is imprecise and inaccurate.[47] For many years, clinicians have used ventilators in the intensive care unit which measure and display flow and volume of gas entering and leaving the lung. Stand-alone respiratory function monitors are available to perform similar functions in the DR. A recording of effective face mask ventilation is shown in Fig. 14.7. This technology enables clinicians to detect ineffective ventilation because of excessive mask leak (Fig. 14.8) or airway obstruction (Fig. 14.9) and then adjust mask position or inspiratory pressure to obtain optimal tidal volumes (Fig. 14.10). A small pilot randomized trial demonstrated the feasibility of this approach and showed that operators responded to the information provided by the monitor and reduced mask leak and excessive tidal volumes.[173] A recent RCT investigating the use of respiratory monitoring in the DR for extremely preterm infants has recently been completed and the results are awaited.[174] Respiratory monitoring is not yet widely available and more data are required before the technology is widely adopted. Nevertheless, this technology has potential for improving training in mask ventilation as well as providing valuable information during resuscitation of high-risk infants.

A simple alternative to respiratory function monitoring is provided by colorimetric carbon dioxide detectors. Leone and colleagues describe the use of these devices to demonstrate airway patency during mask ventilation.[175] Blank et al. demonstrated further proof of concept by showing that color change preceded improvement in heart rate and oxygen saturations.[176] This technique has considerable potential, particularly in resource-limited settings.

CHEST COMPRESSIONS

Approximately 1 per 1000 term and late preterm newborns receive chest compressions in the DR.[16] Most newborns requiring resuscitation have primary respiratory failure and only require effective positive pressure ventilation to recover. If gas exchange is impaired over a prolonged period of time, progressive hypoxemia and acidosis may deplete myocardial energy stores and depress myocardial function to the point that assisted ventilation alone will not be sufficient. In this setting, chest compressions may be required to augment circulation and allow the myocardium to recover. By directly compressing the heart between the sternum and vertebral column or causing phasic changes in the intrathoracic pressure, chest compressions increase the diastolic pressure gradient between and ascending aorta and coronary sinus, resulting in increased coronary artery blood flow.[177]

Recommendations for chest compressions during neonatal resuscitation are based on expert opinion because the guidelines have been informed almost exclusively from human observational studies and physiologic studies in animal models. Current guidelines recommend initiating chest compressions if the newborn's heart rate remains less than 60 beats per minute after at least 30 seconds of effective positive pressure ventilation.[1] To optimize the efficiency of positive pressure ventilation, an ETT should be placed if possible before initiating compressions.

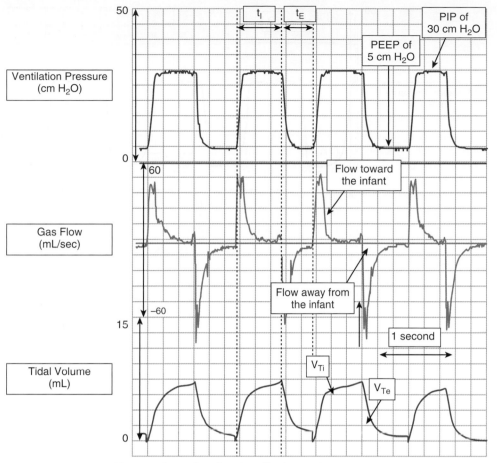

Fig. 14.7 Recording showing effective mask ventilation.

Chest compressions are performed using two thumbs centered on the middle of the sternum, over the lower third of the chest, with the hands and fingers encircling the chest (Fig. 14.11). Compressions should be given with sufficient force to depress the sternum approximately one-third of the anterior-posterior diameter of the chest.[178,179] Once an ETT is secured, the individual providing ventilations may move to the side of the bed and allow the compressor to stand at the head of the bed. This position allows the operator to continue two-thumb compressions while permitting access to the baby's umbilicus for another team member to insert a catheter for medication administration.

After intubation, adult and pediatric cardiopulmonary resuscitation is performed with continuous chest compressions and a low rate of asynchronous ventilations. Unlike adults where the cause of cardiac arrest is most often a primary arrhythmia, neonatal bradycardia and cardiac arrest are most often caused by hypoxia and metabolic acidosis. It is therefore important to provide effective ventilation and adequate oxygen delivery during neonatal chest compressions to improve the chance for myocardial recovery. The currently recommended compression method synchronizes compressions with inflations.[1] Three rapid compressions are followed by a short pause to interpose one inflation, yielding a total of 90 compressions and 30 inflations each minute. Manikin models indicate that this 3:1 compression-to-ventilation (C:V) ratio results in better compression depth and ventilation dynamics than the 15:2 C:V ratio recommended for adults and older children.[180,181] Animal studies comparing alternative C:V ratios and continuous chest compressions with asynchronous inflations have found no difference in return of spontaneous circulation (ROSC) or survival.[182-185] Studies in asphyxiated piglets and a pilot randomized trial enrolling preterm infants have suggested that using sustained inflations (20–30 seconds duration) to maintain lung inflation combined with continuous chest compressions (90–120 compressions per minute) may improve minute ventilation and shorten the time to ROSC.[186-188] A multicenter randomized trial investigating this alternative method is planned (SURV1VE-NCT02858583).[189]

Although the ideal oxygen concentration for ventilation during chest compressions is not known, current guidelines recommend ventilating with 100% oxygen until the heart rate exceeds 60 beats per minute and a reliable pulse oximetry reading can be obtained.[1] This recommendation is based on expert opinion and reflects an attempt to balance the potential harms from inadequate oxygen delivery during chest compressions and excessive exposure to oxygen. In addition, pulse oximeters

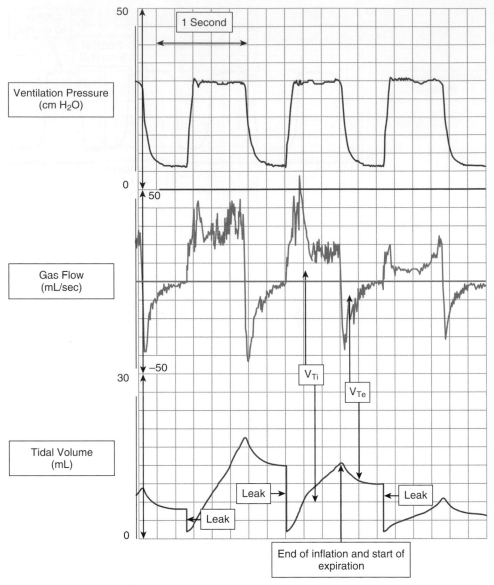

Fig. 14.8 Recording showing excessive mask leak.

may not reliably assess oxygenation during cardiovascular collapse. There are no published human studies comparing different oxygen concentrations during neonatal chest compressions. Animal studies using lamb and piglet models of asphyxia-induced cardiac arrest have shown that systemic oxygenation and oxygen delivery to the brain are very low during chest compressions with either 21% or 100% oxygen.[190,191] No differences have been found in time to ROSC, survival, or measurements of inflammatory mediators and oxidative stress.[95,192] However, animals receiving 100% oxygen during compressions have increased carotid blood flow and hyperoxia after ROSC that could increase the risk of reperfusion injury.[190] Although it may be reasonable to use 100% oxygen during chest compressions, the inhaled oxygen concentration should be adjusted to achieve a physiologic oxygen saturation target once circulation has been restored.

In an effort to limit interruptions that may decrease coronary artery perfusion, chest compressions should be continued for 60 seconds before pausing to check the heart rate response.[1] Physical examination methods of determining the baby's heart rate are inaccurate and a pulse oximeter may not achieve a reliable signal during cardiovascular collapse. An electrocardiogram provides a more accurate and continuous measure of the newborn's heart rate and is recommended during chest compressions.[53,54,193,194] Other methods of monitoring the return of circulation during compressions have been investigated. During asystole, blood is not flowing to the lungs and carbon dioxide is not exhaled. Once circulation is restored, carbon dioxide is carried to the lungs and exhaled. Studies performed in animal models have shown that detecting the return of exhaled carbon dioxide (14–32 mm Hg) by continuous capnography during compressions correlates with ROSC.[195,196]

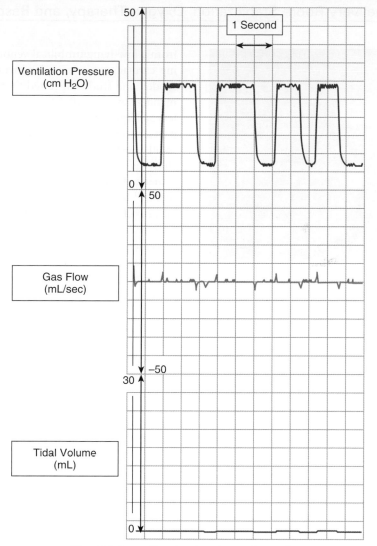

Fig. 14.9 Recording showing airway obstruction.

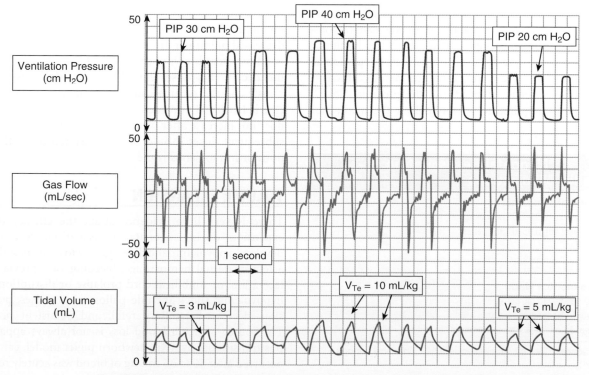

Fig. 14.10 Adjustment of peak inspiratory pressure to attain effective tidal volume.

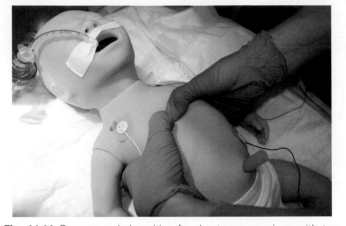

Fig. 14.11 Recommended position for chest compressions with two thumbs centered on the middle of the sternum, over the lower third of the chest, with the hands and fingers encircling the chest.

EPINEPHRINE

Epinephrine is the only medication included on the neonatal resuscitation algorithm and it is rarely needed.[197] It is an endogenous catecholamine that constricts vascular smooth muscle by stimulating alpha-adrenergic receptors. The resulting increase in systemic vascular resistance increases coronary artery perfusion pressure and enhances the efficacy of chest compressions. In addition, epinephrine increases the rate and strength of cardiac contractions by stimulating myocardial beta-adrenergic receptors.

Epinephrine is recommended if the newborn's heart rate remains less than 60 beats per minute after 30 seconds of effective ventilation, preferably through an ETT, followed by an additional 60 seconds of ventilation coordinated with chest compressions.[1] The recommended dose is 0.01 to 0.03 mg/kg (0.1 to 0.3 mL/kg using a 0.1 mg/1 mL solution) administered rapidly into the central venous circulation (Box 14.4).[75] If an adequate response is not achieved, the dose may be repeated every 3 to 5 minutes.

Medications rapidly reach the central venous circulation after administration into a low-lying umbilical venous catheter[198] or an intraosseous needle inserted into the proximal tibia.[199] The flush volume required to reliably deliver the medication

BOX 14.4 Neonatal Resuscitation: Emergency Medications

Epinephrine (0.1 mg/mL)
- UVC or IO needle: 0.01–0.03 mg per kg
- ETT (less effective): 0.05–0.1 mg per kg
- Infuse rapidly
- Repeat every 3–5 minutes

Normal saline (0.9 NaCl)
- UVC or IO needle: 10 mL per kg
- Infuse over 5–10 minutes
- May repeat 10 mL/kg if inadequate response

ETT, Endotracheal tube; *IO*, intraosseous; *UVC*, umbilical venous catheter.

from a low-lying umbilical venous catheter into the heart during cardiac arrest is under investigation. In a newborn lamb model, one study suggested that the volume currently recommended by the NRP (0.5–1.0 mL)[39] is insufficient and may leave a large portion of the medication in the umbilical vein and portal venous system.[200] Although experienced providers commonly use the umbilical vein for emergency access, a simulation study using a neonatal manikin found that umbilical venous catheter insertion took longer than intraosseous needle placement.[201] Intraosseous needles are commonly used by prehospital providers and in pediatric emergency departments. There are case reports of local complications from intraosseous needle placement;[202,203] however, they should be available with standard neonatal resuscitation supplies and neonatal health providers should be trained how to insert them. Peripheral veins are not recommended for emergency medication administration during resuscitation because cannulation is unlikely to be successful in the setting of cardiovascular collapse and drug delivery to the central circulation is likely to be impaired. Delays in epinephrine administration can be prevented by anticipation, preparation, and training. If risk factors for severe neonatal depression are identified, such as persistent fetal bradycardia, epinephrine and the equipment for emergency vascular access should be prepared before the baby is born.

While vascular access is being secured, some clinicians may choose to administer one dose of epinephrine through the ETT. Although endotracheal administration is an option, neonatal animal and human studies indicate that epinephrine absorption is delayed[198,204] and may be less effective in comparison with the intravenous route.[197,205] In a retrospective study, only 20% (6/30) of newborns achieved ROSC after an initial dose of endotracheal epinephrine (0.03–0.05 mg/kg).[205] Among newborns who did not respond to the endotracheal dose but received a subsequent intravenous dose, most (21/24) were successfully resuscitated.[205] This may reflect unique physiology in the newborn, including fluid-filled lungs and decreased pulmonary blood flow. If endotracheal epinephrine is administered, a higher dose (0.05–0.1 mg/kg) is recommended.[75] This dose should not be administered intravenously and the syringe containing the higher dose should be clearly labeled "Endotracheal use only". If the baby's heart rate does not increase after one dose of endotracheal epinephrine, subsequent doses should be administered using the intravenous or intraosseous route.

VOLUME EXPANSION

There is very little evidence about the efficacy of volume expansion during neonatal resuscitation. Newborns may develop hypovolemic shock secondary to acute blood loss from a fetal-maternal hemorrhage, bleeding vasa previa, placental laceration, or umbilical cord prolapse or disruption. Signs of hypovolemic shock include pallor, weak pulses, poor perfusion, decreased capillary refill, and persistent bradycardia. The source of acute blood loss is not always apparent. In a posttransitional hypoxic newborn piglet model, cardiac arrest occurred after 30 to 35 mL/kg of blood was acutely removed.[206]

Despite blood loss, nearly 25% of animals did not require volume expansion because they achieved ROSC with ventilation, chest compressions and epinephrine. Animals who received volume expansion with either isotonic saline or blood achieved ROSC after only 10% to 15% of the volume lost was returned. There was no difference in ROSC or time to achieve ROSC between animals randomized to receive saline or blood.

Volume expansion is currently recommended if the baby does not respond to epinephrine and has clinical signs of hypovolemic shock or risk factors that suggest the possibility of unrecognized blood loss. Routine volume expansion is not indicated in the absence of hypovolemia because it may worsen pulmonary edema without beneficial effects.[207] Normal saline is a readily available isotonic crystalloid solution and it is the most commonly recommended volume expander. The initial dose of normal saline for hypovolemic shock is 10 mL/kg infused over 5 to 10 minutes (Box 14.4).[39] If the baby does not improve, an additional 10 mL/kg may be infused. In unusual circumstances, additional volume expansion may be considered; however, caution should be used to avoid infusing excessive volume and increasing demands on the newborn's heart. Emergency, noncross-matched, type-O, Rhesus (Rh)-negative packed red blood cells should be available and considered for the acute replacement of large volume blood loss.

SPECIAL CASES

Preterm Neonates

Preterm infants, particularly those born less than 32 weeks' gestation, should be delivered in settings with adequate physical resources and trained personnel available. In a recent meta-analysis, DCC in extremely preterm infants has been shown to reduce mortality compared with immediate cord clamping.[208] ILCOR now recommends that DCC should be facilitated in preterm infants unless immediate resuscitation is required after birth. Research is underway to evaluate the practicality, safety, and utility of providing respiratory support to those who require it, before cord clamping.[209] Already, this technique has demonstrated reduced bradycardia and hypoxia in very preterm infants resuscitated with an intact cord.[209] The technique may allow providers to support placental transfusion without delaying resuscitative efforts in this vulnerable population. Meanwhile, there is evidence that UCM in the extremely preterm population may induce fluctuations in blood pressure and cerebral blood flow,[64] resulting in higher risk of intraventricular hemorrhage.[210] Two recent systematic reviews have reported that cord milking improved mean blood pressure and reduced need for blood transfusions but did not improve other clinical outcomes.[211,212]

Maintenance of normal body temperature is vital. Very preterm infants are particularly vulnerable to hypothermia owing to their large surface area–to–mass ratio and thin epidermis. Plastic bags and wraps are effective in maintaining temperature[213] and are standard of care for infants less than 28 weeks' gestational age. ILCOR recommends that infants be placed in plastic bags or wraps without prior drying and managed under a radiant warmer.[1] Temperatures need to be regularly measured

and hyperthermia avoided as it is associated with increased risk of adverse outcomes. Maintenance of DR temperatures of at least 26° C (~79° F) is also recommended. If respiratory support is required, it may be beneficial to use warmed and humidified gases, to limit evaporative heat loss.[214]

Recommendations regarding the optimal method of respiratory support have changed in recent years. Whereas some preterm infants are in poor condition at birth and require immediate resuscitation, the majority cry and breathe spontaneously[79] and require support through transition rather than immediate intubation. Following a series of multicenter randomized trials,[215-217] ILCOR and the AAP[218] now recommend that preterm infants with respiratory distress after birth should be managed with CPAP rather than intubation. If intubation is required, surfactant should be administered, and the ETT removed as soon as possible. With the increasing use of less-invasive surfactant techniques in NICUs, clinicians have trialed the technique in the DR.[219] If intermittent positive pressure is required during the first minutes of life, PEEP is likely to be beneficial in facilitating rapid aeration of the lungs and should be used if available.[1] The ideal concentration of oxygen to begin resuscitation and the optimal targets of oxygen saturations remain to be determined for preterm infants. Investigators have noted that in preterm infants, commencing resuscitation with air leads to saturations that fall below the recommended range.[220,221] A small RCT noted that a higher initial supplemental oxygen concentration is associated be better respiratory drive and a shorter period of mask ventilation than 21% oxygen.[222] However the question of whether it is better to start in higher (≥40%) or lower (<40%) oxygen remains unclear[223] and is the subject of ongoing studies.[224] For infants less than 35 weeks' gestation, it seems reasonable to begin resuscitation with 21% to 30% oxygen and adjust the concentration to maintain saturations in the range measured in healthy term infants.[93] Aiming for saturations of 80% by 5 minutes after birth may reduce the risk of later intraventricular hemorrhage.[225]

Congenital Diaphragmatic Hernia

Congenital diaphragmatic hernia (CDH) is a defect of the diaphragm, most commonly on the left side, which allows the abdominal viscera to herniate into the fetal chest. Compression from the herniated contents disturbs development of the lungs and pulmonary vasculature, causing varying degrees of pulmonary hypoplasia and pulmonary hypertension. Despite advances in care, most newborns with CDH develop severe respiratory failure with cardiovascular dysfunction shortly after birth and the mortality risk remains high.

Whenever possible, the birth should occur at a high-risk center with an experienced, coordinated team capable of offering advanced resuscitation, cardiorespiratory care, and neonatal surgery. Birth outside of a high-risk center has been associated with a higher risk of mortality.[226,227]

Before birth, the resuscitation team should prepare a comprehensive management plan because the use of a standardized protocol has been shown to decrease CDH mortality.[228,229]

Newborns with CDH often experience hypoxemia and acidosis during fetal-to-neonatal transition. Delaying cord clamping until the lungs have been aerated may improve cardiopulmonary transition and decrease the severity of pulmonary hypertension. By allowing pulmonary vascular resistance to decrease before removing the placental circulation, pulmonary venous return is allowed to maintain left ventricular preload and cardiac output when the cord is clamped. Improving the transition from fetal to neonatal circulation may prevent the cycle of events triggered by acidosis and hypoxia that ultimately results in severe pulmonary hypertension.[230] This concept was supported by a lamb CDH model where PBCC resulted in a marked increase in pulmonary blood flow during the first minutes after birth.[231] Two small pilot studies have demonstrated that it is feasible to perform intubation and stabilization in newborns with a CDH and an intact umbilical cord.[232,233] A larger randomized trial in the Netherlands is investigating this approach (NCT04373902).

The goal of DR management is to achieve an acceptable preductal oxygen saturation without causing lung injury from high ventilating pressure, excessive tidal volume, and oxygen toxicity. Consensus guidelines have been published by the CDH Euro Consortium and the Canadian CDH Collaborative.[234,235] Positive pressure ventilation with a face mask should be avoided to prevent gaseous distention of the herniated abdominal contents and increased lung compression. Although some infants predicted to have good lung development based on antenatal testing may be allowed a trial of spontaneous breathing,[234] current guidelines support immediate intubation after birth and ventilation with low peak pressure (<25 cm H_2O).[234,235] A T-piece resuscitator or mechanical ventilator may be preferred during initial stabilization and transport to avoid inadvertent high inspiratory pressure.[235] Although 100% oxygen is commonly used to initiate respiratory support, the ideal oxygen concentration has not been established.[236] Current guidelines recommend maintaining preductal oxygen saturation above 80% to 85% but not greater than 95%, postductal saturation over 70%, arterial pH greater than 7.2–7.25, and arterial PCO_2 45 to 60 mm Hg.[234,235] During the first 2 hours of life, the CDH Euro Consortium suggests that a lower preductal saturation (70%) may be acceptable if the baby is gradually improving, ventilation is adequate, and organ perfusion is maintained.[234] A nasogastric tube with intermittent or continuous suction should be inserted promptly to decompress the abdominal contents. An umbilical or radial artery catheter should be placed for continuous blood pressure monitoring and blood gas sampling. An umbilical venous catheter is helpful for fluid and medication administration; however, the catheter may not advance properly if the liver is herniated into the chest. Volume expansion and inotropic support may be required to maintain normal blood pressure for gestational age.

Fetal Hydrops

Fetal hydrops is defined as the presence of two or more abnormal fluid collections in the fetus and usually presents as generalized subcutaneous edema with abdominal ascites, pleural, or pericardial effusions. Nonimmune hydrops fetalis (NIHF) is the most common type and specifically refers to cases not caused by red cell alloimmunization.[237] The most common associated diagnoses are structural heart defects, abnormalities in heart rate, twin-to-twin transfusion, congenital anomalies such as pulmonary masses, lymphatic vessel dysplasia and obstruction, chromosomal abnormalities, congenital viral infections, and congenital anemia.[237,238] In many cases, the etiology of NIHF remains unknown.

Birth should be planned in a high-risk center with the capability to resuscitate critically ill newborns.[237] Ultrasonography performed just before birth may be helpful to identify the location of fluid collections and plan interventions. If there is a large pleural effusion or significant ascites, the obstetric provider may remove fluid before delivery. The DR resuscitation team should anticipate complex problems including restricted ventilation from pleural effusions and ascites, pulmonary hypoplasia, pulmonary edema, surfactant deficiency, pulmonary hypertension, severe anemia, intravascular volume depletion, and myocardial dysfunction.[239] Sufficient personnel with proficiency in endotracheal intubation, emergency vascular access, thoracentesis, and paracentesis should be present in the DR. Multiple procedures may be required in a short period of time and specific roles should be delegated in advance. The equipment to perform these procedures should be prepared before birth and ready for immediate use.

After birth, respiratory distress should be expected. The resuscitation team should be prepared to promptly intubate the trachea and provide positive pressure ventilation. Tracheal intubation may be difficult if there is soft tissue edema or a neck mass. If the abdomen is distended and interfering with ventilation, paracentesis should be performed. Only enough fluid to permit diaphragmatic excursion and effective ventilation should be removed. If pleural effusions interfere with ventilation, thoracentesis may be required in the DR. Less commonly, emergency pericardiocentesis must be performed to relieve cardiac tamponade. If the baby is born preterm, surfactant administration may be helpful. Once the airway has been secured and ventilation has been established, umbilical arterial and venous catheters should be inserted to monitor arterial blood pressure, obtain blood samples, and infuse fluids. Despite marked edema, the newborn may have intravascular volume depletion, and careful volume expansion with isotonic saline or packed red blood cells may be needed. Hypoglycemia, metabolic acidosis, and hypothermia are common problems and should be anticipated. If severe anemia is present, an isovolemic partial volume exchange transfusion with type-O, Rh-negative packed red blood cells cross-matched against the mother may be required to avoid volume overload.

ETHICS

Deciding Whether to Commence Resuscitation

Noninitiation of resuscitation at birth can be ethically acceptable under certain circumstances. Families with fetuses known to be affected by anencephaly, confirmed trisomy 13 or 18, or severe brain, cardiac, lung, or renal malformations may opt not to offer intensive care support at birth. For infants at very low gestational age, the decision of whether to initiate intensive care is complex. Initiation of resuscitation in the DR does not mandate continued provision of intensive care. Parents should be informed that a decision made before birth to initiate resuscitation can and may need to be altered, depending upon the infant's response to resuscitation and their subsequent progress. Redirection of care toward palliation is considered ethically equivalent to noninitiation of support.

International guidelines have provided some consistency in the development of gestational age–based guidelines on resuscitation,[240] but large variation in recommendations still exists.[241] Initiation of resuscitation is nearly always indicated where there is a high survival rate and acceptable morbidity. Typically, this includes babies with gestational age of 25 weeks or more. No published guidelines advise initiation of resuscitation for infants born before 22 weeks' gestation. Between these two time points, there is a gray zone, where the wishes of parents, the experience and beliefs of clinicians, and local policy and guidelines will influence whether resuscitation is offered, advised, or given.[242] Some countries, and centers within countries, offer resuscitation to infants born at 22 weeks' gestation as standard, others practice selective resuscitation, and some recommend no resuscitation at less than 23 or 24 weeks' gestation.[243] A recent framework from the British Association of Perinatal Medicine on the management of extreme preterm birth uses gestational age, sex, plurality, fetal growth, use of antenatal corticosteroids, and hospital setting to guide management decisions for babies born between 22 and 25 weeks' gestation.[244] When there is uncertainty surrounding the gestational age, an infant's birth weight may be used as a guide, with survival known to be significantly lower below 400 g.[245] A therapeutic trial may be an option; however, it should be noted that clinicians are very poor at predicting which infants will do well in the long-term on the basis of their appearance at birth.[246]

The gestational age recommendations for active resuscitation are based on the poor outcomes associated with extreme preterm birth, but determining outcome for extremely low gestational age infants is challenging. It is a self-fulfilling prophecy that if resuscitation is not offered at certain gestations, then survival will be very low. A 2017 metaanalysis[247] reported that from 47 studies, survival of infants born at 22 weeks' gestation was 9%, whereas in Japan, where initiation of intensive care support at 22 weeks has occurred for many years, 37% of 22-week infants survived to hospital discharge in 2013.[248] Subsequently, reports have emerged of other sites with encouraging outcomes, from Sweden, where more than 50% of 22-week infants survived,[249] and from Iowa, United States, where 70% of 22-week infants survived and where more than half of survivors had mild or no neurodisability at 18 to 22 months corrected age.[250] In contrast, in the French EPIPAGE study from 2011, where resuscitation at 22 and 23 weeks was not recommended, less than 1% of infants under 24 weeks' gestation survived to discharge.[251] Although survival below 25 weeks has increased over the past decades,[252] rates of serious morbidity have either remained static or increased,[253,254] meaning that the number of preterm survivors with or at risk of later health problems has increased. For infants born at 22 to 25 weeks, overall mortality is still 50% or more; rates of surviving minimally or unimpaired are less than 20% for those born below 25 weeks' gestation, but less than 5% for those

born at 22 and 23 weeks' gestation.[255] Poor neurodevelopmental outcome is often cited as a reason for noninitiation of resuscitation, as is poor long-term quality of life. However, quality of life is subjective; physical or intellectual impairment does not necessarily equate to poor quality of life. Teenage children born extremely preterm rate their life quality similarly to term-born teenagers,[256] with a majority of adults healthy, living productive lives.[257]

Deciding Whether to Stop Resuscitation

It is reasonable to avoid prolonged resuscitation if the outcome is likely to be death or survival with severe disability. Therefore, clinicians have sought to determine how much intervention, and for how long, is appropriate. Data from the late 1990s showed that two-thirds of term infants who received epinephrine in the DR survived, and almost three-quarters of survivors who were assessed at 1 year had no neurological deficit.[258] However, for those under 29 weeks' gestation, survival was 30%, and within this group, 78% ultimately died or had neurodevelopmental disability. The American Heart Association registry reported survival after DR cardiopulmonary resuscitation of infants born across all gestational age groups between 2004 and 2016.[259] They found that 83% of infants more than 36 weeks' gestation survived to discharge, decreasing with lower gestational age, to 25% survival for those at 22 to 24 weeks' gestation.

Several studies have evaluated outcomes of very preterm infants who have received intensive resuscitation at birth in infants. In two very preterm cohorts, 6% to 7% of infants received chest compressions and/or epinephrine.[260,261] Perhaps unsurprisingly, mortality, intraventricular hemorrhage, and neurodisability are all significantly higher in infants who receive extensive resuscitation (cardiopulmonary resuscitation and/or epinephrine) in the DR, compared with those who do not.[262,263] Some studies have seen the largest differences in mortality between those receiving and those not receiving intensive DR resuscitation in the extremely preterm, less than 1000 g infants,[261] whereas other studies have seen wider differences in outcome in babies less preterm, at 1000 to 1500 g[264] and 28 to 31 weeks' gestation.[265]

A report in 1991 showed that of a cohort of infants of various gestational ages, with an Apgar score of 0 at 10 minutes of life ($n = 58$), 98% died and the single survivor had poor neurological outcome. These results led to the recommendation that resuscitation should be stopped if there is no ROSC at 10 minutes of life. A recent report, including term and preterm infants with an Apgar score of zero at 10 minutes, found survival was 61% for those more than 36 weeks' gestation, falling to 35% for those under 32 weeks' gestation.[266]

However, studies of term and near-term infants born in the era of neuroprotective hypothermia have been more encouraging. They have reported better survival,[267] and lower rates of death/severe neurodevelopmental disability, of 73% to 76%,[268,269] inferring that almost a quarter survive without major neurodevelopmental sequelae. These data may influence recommendations for resuscitation duration in the future, but currently, the ILCOR guidelines conclude that discontinuation of resuscitation may be justified after "10 minutes of continuous and adequate resuscitative efforts of an infant with no heartbeat and no respiratory effort."[1]

POSTRESUSCITATION CARE

Examination/Monitoring

Infants who required resuscitation after birth have an increased risk of multiple organ injury. These complications may be anticipated and promptly addressed by careful assessment and appropriate monitoring. Even newborns who required only brief (<1 minute) positive pressure ventilation after birth have a higher risk of short-term respiratory and neurologic complications and should have postresuscitation monitoring.[270] The nature and duration of monitoring are dependent upon the newborn's condition and identifiable risk factors.

A thorough examination should be performed to identify anomalies that may have contributed to cardiorespiratory compromise after birth and any evidence of trauma from the birth or resuscitation procedures. The newborn should be evaluated for signs of ongoing respiratory distress such as retractions, nasal flaring, or grunting. The chest should be auscultated to assess the presence of bilateral breath sounds. Asymmetric breath sounds may be a sign of pneumothorax. If cyanosis is apparent when the baby is quiet and resolves with crying, ensure that both nares are patent. The abdomen should be examined for evidence of trauma, distention, masses, or unusual flattening ("scaphoid"). If the baby required prolonged resuscitation, a standardized neurologic examination including alertness, pupillary response, sucking, tone, and reflexes should be completed to rule out encephalopathy.

Vital signs should be monitored frequently during postresuscitation care. Term and late preterm babies who received either CPAP or positive pressure ventilation have an increased risk of pneumothoraces (2%–5%) and ongoing respiratory distress requiring assisted ventilation (5%–16%).[270-272] Delayed transition increases the risk of persistent pulmonary hypertension and caregivers should be attentive to signs of worsening hypoxemia. Chest radiography and arterial blood gases may be indicated to inform treatment decisions. Hypotension may occur because of hypovolemia, peripheral vasodilation, myocardial dysfunction, or sepsis. Routine volume expansion without evidence of hypovolemia, however, is not recommended and may contribute to worsening respiratory distress.[207] Babies who required significant resuscitation may require pharmacologic agents to support their blood pressure. Hypotension, hypoxia, and acidosis can decrease renal blood flow and cause renal failure associated with acute tubular necrosis. Babies who required significant resuscitation should have their urine output, body weight, and serum electrolyte levels checked frequently. Perinatal stress increases glucose consumption and may causes hypoglycemia. Milk feeds may be delayed because of clinical instability and intravenous fluids may be required to maintain the blood glucose in the normal range. Blood glucose levels should be checked at regular intervals until milk feeds are established and the infant is able to maintain a normal glucose level. Newborns with hypotension, hypoxemia, and acidosis may develop apnea and seizures associated with hypoxic ischemic encephalopathy.

Therapeutic Hypothermia for Hypoxic Ischemic Encephalopathy

Death and long-term neurodevelopmental sequelae are the most important consequences of peripartum hypoxia. Neuronal death following a severe insult occurs in two phases.[273] Immediate primary neuronal death because of primary energy failure is followed by a latent period of at least 6 hours. A secondary, delayed neuronal death phase ensues during which a substantial proportion of cell loss occurs. The 6-hour "therapeutic window" allows amelioration of injury through brain cooling by rescuing cells from apoptotic death and reducing cerebral metabolic rate. The Cochrane review on this topic found 11 randomized trials, which recruited 1505 term and late preterm infants with evidence of peripartum asphyxia. Infants typically had Apgar scores of 5 or less at 10 minutes, required ventilation at 10 minutes or had cord or arterial pH under 7.1 within 1 hour of birth, and had evidence of encephalopathy.[274] Infants treated with either whole-body or selective head cooling were compared with standard treatment. Cooling reduced the risk of death or neurodevelopmental disability to 18 months of age (relative risk, 0.75 [0.68–0.83]; number needed to treat, 7 [5–10]). Both whole-body and selective head cooling are effective and both moderately and severely encephalopathic patients appear to benefit from cooling. The benefits of cooling outweighed the short-term adverse effects of sinus bradycardia and thrombocytopenia. Therapeutic cooling should be undertaken according to protocols similar to those used in the randomized trials and in settings with sufficient resources in terms of both staff and equipment. Infants who undergo therapeutic hypothermia should be followed up throughout childhood to identify and support those with neurodevelopmental impairment. Although the improved outcomes seen following therapeutic hypothermia are maintained into later childhood,[275] almost half of newborns with moderate to severe encephalopathy die or survive with adverse neurodevelopment.[274]

A complete reference list is available at https://expertconsult. inkling.com/.

KEY REFERENCES

1. Perlman JM, Wyllie J, Kattwinkel J, et al: Part 7: neonatal resuscitation: 2015 international consensus on cardiopulmonary resuscitation and emergency cardiovascular care science with treatment recommendations (reprint). Pediatrics 136(suppl 2): S120–S166, 2015.
77. Strand ML, Lee HC, Kawakami MD, et al: Tracheal suctioning of meconium at birth for non-vigorous infants; a systematic review and meta-analysis. International Liaison Committee on Resuscitation (ILCOR) Neonatal Life Support Task Force CoSTR, 2019. https://costr. ilcor.org/document/tracheal-suctioning-of-meconium-at-birth-for-non-vigorous-infants-a-systematic-review-and-meta-analysis-nls-865.
82. Helping Babies Breathe. 2020. https://www.aap.org/en-us/advocacy-and-policy/aap-health-initiatives/helping-babies-survive/Pages/ Helping-Babies-Breathe.aspx. Accessed May 23, 2020.

93. Escobedo MB, Aziz K, Kapadia VS, et al: 2019 American Heart Association focused update on neonatal resuscitation: an update to the American Heart Association guidelines for cardiopulmonary resuscitation and emergency cardiovascular care. Pediatrics 145(1), 2020.

110. Foglia EE, Te Pas AB, Kirpalani H, et al: Sustained inflation vs standard resuscitation for preterm infants: a systematic review and meta-analysis. JAMA Pediatr e195897, 2020.

123. Sweet DG, Carnielli V, Greisen G, et al: European consensus guidelines on the management of respiratory distress syndrome—2019 update. Neonatology 115(4):432–450, 2019.

208. Fogarty M, Osborn DA, Askie L, et al: Delayed vs early umbilical cord clamping for preterm infants: a systematic review and meta-analysis. American J Obstet Gynecol 218(1):1–18, 2018.

213. McCall EM, Alderdice F, Halliday HL, et al: Interventions to prevent hypothermia at birth in preterm and/or low birthweight infants. Cochrane Database Syst Rev (3):CD004210, 2010.

223. Lui K, Jones LJ, Foster JP, et al: Lower versus higher oxygen concentrations titrated to target oxygen saturations during resuscitation of preterm infants at birth. Cochrane Database Syst Rev 5:CD010239, 2018.

241. Guillen U, Weiss EM, Munson D, et al: Guidelines for the management of extremely premature deliveries: a systematic review. Pediatrics 136(2):343–350, 2015.

250. Watkins PL, Dagle JM, Bell EF, et al: Outcomes at 18 to 22 months of corrected age for infants born at 22 to 25 weeks of gestation in a center practicing active management. J Pediatr 217:52–58 e1, 2020.

257. Saigal S, Morrison K, Schmidt LA: Health, wealth and achievements of former very premature infants in adult life. Semin Fetal Neonatal Med 101107, 2020.

274. Jacobs SE, Berg M, Hunt R, et al: Cooling for newborns with hypoxic ischaemic encephalopathy. Cochrane Database Syst Rev (1):CD003311, 2013.

15

Exogenous Surfactant Therapy

K. Suresh Gautham and Roger F. Soll

KEY POINTS

- Mammalian surfactant obtained by lung lavage consists of 80% phospholipids, 8% neutral lipids, and 12% protein. There are four unique surfactant-associated apoproteins: SP-A, SP-B, SP-C, and SP-D.
- Three types of exogenous surfactant are available: (1) surfactant derived from animal sources, (2) synthetic surfactant without protein components, and (3) synthetic surfactant with protein components.
- In preterm infants with respiratory distress syndrome, administration of exogenous surfactant therapy reduces mortality and pulmonary air leaks.
- Infants with respiratory distress syndrome should be given rescue surfactant early in the course of the disease, when the FiO_2 requirements exceed 0.30 or 0.40.
- Animal-derived surfactants have greater benefits than synthetic surfactants in the treatment of respiratory distress syndrome.
- Less invasive surfactant administration using a thin catheter without endotracheal intubation or positive pressure is emerging as the preferred method to administer surfactant, with the other reasonable option being the INSURE (intubate-surfactant-extubated to continuous positive airway pressure [CPAP]) method.
- Surfactant therapy has been used in infants with other pulmonary conditions leading to hypoxic respiratory failure, but its benefits and risks in these conditions are, in general, poorly studied.

The development of exogenous surfactant therapy in the early 1990s was a historic advance in neonatology that led to significant reductions in neonatal mortality.[1-3] Exogenous surfactant therapy is now routinely used in the management of respiratory distress syndrome (RDS) in preterm infants and increasingly in other neonatal respiratory disorders such as meconium aspiration syndrome (MAS). This chapter provides an evidence-based overview of the use of exogenous surfactant therapy in neonatal respiratory disorders.

HISTORY

The development of effective surfactant preparations was the culmination of a series of investigations by pioneers of surfactant research, who described the existence and composition of surfactant, the role of surfactant in lowering surface tension, and the role of surfactant in maintaining alveolar stability.[4,5] A landmark in our understanding of RDS was the demonstration of surfactant deficiency in the lungs of infants dying of extreme prematurity or hyaline membrane disease.[6] Although the introduction of surface-active substances into the lung was suggested as early as 1947,[7] the initial attempts to provide exogenous surfactant therapy for immature lungs were unsuccessful.[8,9] These were followed several years later by successful attempts in animals[10] and then in human neonates.[11] After these initial efforts, numerous animal experiments and human clinical trials were conducted to study the efficacy of surfactant therapy, the relative efficacies of different surfactant preparations, the optimal timing of administration, the optimal dosage, and other aspects of exogenous surfactant therapy. The history and evolution of surfactant therapy have been reviewed in detail by several authors.[12-17]

SURFACTANT FUNCTION, COMPOSITION, AND METABOLISM

The function, composition, secretion, and metabolism of mammalian surfactant have been reviewed by several authors[18-20] and are summarized here.

Function

Pulmonary alveoli, where gas exchange occurs, are bubble shaped and have a high degree of curvature. The surface tension of the moist inner surface is as a result of the attraction between the molecules in the alveolar fluid and tends to make the alveoli contract. Unchecked, this tendency would result in lung collapse. Surfactant greatly reduces the surface tension on the inner surface of the alveoli, thus preventing the alveoli from collapsing during expiration.

Composition

An accurate determination of the composition of pulmonary surfactant is difficult. To obtain surfactant for analysis, one must either wash out lungs (with the possible limitation of leaving important components behind) or extract surfactant from minced lungs (with the possible problem of adding cellular contaminants). Mammalian surfactant obtained by lung lavage consists of 80% phospholipids, 8% neutral lipids, and 12% protein. The predominant class of phospholipid (nearly 60%) is dipalmitoyl phosphatidylcholine (DPPC), with lesser amounts of unsaturated phosphatidylcholine compounds (25%), phosphatidylglycerol (15%), and phosphatidylinositol. Of all the constituents of surfactant, DPPC alone has the appropriate properties to reduce alveolar surface tension. However, DPPC alone is a poor surfactant because it adsorbs very slowly to air–liquid interfaces. Surfactant proteins or other lipids facilitate its adsorption.

Approximately half the protein in surfactant consists of contaminating protein from the plasma or lung tissue.[20] The remaining proteins include four unique surfactant-associated apoproteins: SP-A, SP-B, SP-C, and SP-D. SP-A and SP-D are hydrophilic proteins and belong to a subgroup of mammalian lectins called *collectins*. They may play important roles in the defense against inhaled pathogens, and SP-A may have a regulatory function in the formation of the monolayer that lowers the surface tension.[18] SP-B and SP-C are hydrophobic proteins and are required to enhance spreading of phospholipid in the airspaces. SP-B promotes phospholipid adsorption and induces the insertion of phospholipids into the monolayer, thus enhancing the formation of a stable surface film.[18] SP-C enhances phospholipid adsorption, stimulates the insertion of phospholipids out of the subphase into the air–liquid interface, and may increase the resistance of surfactant to inhibition by serum proteins or by edema fluid.[18,19]

Secretion and Metabolism

Surfactant is produced in the type II cells of the alveoli (Fig. 15.1). It is assembled and stored in the lamellar bodies, which consist of concentric or parallel lamellae, predominantly composed of phospholipid bilayers. Lamellar bodies are extruded into the fluid layer lining the alveoli by exocytosis and form structures known as *tubular myelin*. Tubular myelin consists of long stacked tubes composed mainly of phospholipid bilayers, the corners of which appear fused, resulting in a lattice-like appearance on cross section. Tubular myelin is thought to be the major source of the monolayer surface film lining the air–liquid interface in the alveoli, in which the hydrophobic fatty acyl groups of the phospholipids extend into the air, whereas the hydrophilic polar head groups bind water.[21] This surfactant monolayer lowers the surface tension at the air–liquid interface by replacing water at the surface.[21] The phospholipid from the monolayer eventually reenters the type II cells through endocytosis and forms multivesicular bodies. These multivesicular bodies are either "recycled" by rapid incorporation into the lamellar bodies or degraded in lysosomes. Of note, all critical components of surfactant (DPPC, phosphatidylglycerol, SP-A, SP-B, and SP-C) are recycled.[20]

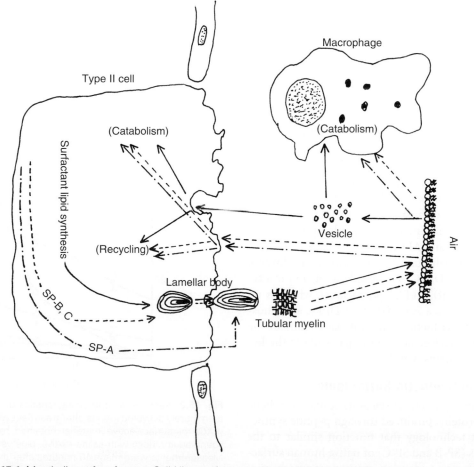

Fig. 15.1 Metabolism of surfactant. *Solid line,* surfactant + liquid; *dashed and dotted line,* SP-A; *dashed line,* SP-B, SP-C. (From Jobe AH, Ikegami M: Clin Perinatol 28:655, 2001.)

TYPES OF SURFACTANT

Three types of exogenous surfactant are available: (1) surfactant derived from animal sources, (2) synthetic surfactant without protein components, and (3) synthetic surfactant with protein components.

Animal-Derived Surfactants

Current commercially made animal-derived surfactants are obtained from either bovine or porcine lungs. Beractant (Survanta) and surfactant TA (Surfacten) are lipid extracts of bovine lung mince with added DPPC, tripalmitoylglycerol, and palmitic acid. Calf lung surfactant extract (calfactant, Infasurf), SF-RI 1 (Alveofact), and bovine lipid extract surfactant (BLES) are bovine lung washes subjected to chloroform–methanol extraction. Poractant (Curosurf) is a porcine lung mince that has been subjected to chloroform–methanol extraction and further purified by liquid–gel chromatography. It consists of approximately 99% polar lipids (mainly phospholipids) and 1% hydrophobic, low-molecular-weight proteins (SP-B and SP-C).[22] All the animal-derived surfactants contain SP-B and SP-C, but the lung mince extracts (Survanta and Curosurf) contain less than 10% of the SP-B that is found in the lung-wash extracts (Infasurf, Alveofact, and BLES).[23] The purification procedure including extraction with organic solvents removes the hydrophilic proteins SP-A and SP-D, leaving a material containing only lipids and small amounts of hydrophobic proteins. Poractant, which is further purified by liquid–gel chromatography, contains only polar lipids and about 1% hydrophobic proteins (SP-B and SP-C in an approximate molar ratio of 1:2).[24] None of the commercial preparations contain SP-A.[23] A surfactant obtained from human amniotic fluid was originally tested in clinical trials[25,26] but is not used as of this writing.

Synthetic Surfactants Without Protein Components

The original exogenous products tested in the 1960s were synthetic surfactants composed solely of DPPC, which by itself cannot perform all the functions required of pulmonary surfactant. Current synthetic surfactants without protein are mixtures of a variety of surface-active phospholipids (principally DPPC) and spreading agents to facilitate surface adsorption. These products include Exosurf and ALEC (artificial lung-expanding compound). Colfosceril palmitate, hexadecanol, and tyloxapol (Exosurf) consist of 85% DPPC, 9% hexadecanol, and 6% tyloxapol (a spreading agent). ALEC (pumactant), which is no longer manufactured,[27] was a 7:3 mixture of DPPC and phosphatidylglycerol. These synthetic surfactants lack many of the components of animal-derived surfactant, particularly the hydrophobic surfactant proteins B and C.

Protein-Containing Synthetic Surfactants

The protein-containing synthetic surfactants contain synthetic phospholipids and proteins produced through peptide synthesis and recombinant technology that function similar to the hydrophobic proteins (SP-B and SP-C) of native human surfactant. Research is in progress to develop component protein analogues of the hydrophilic proteins SP-A and SP-D as well.

Of the surfactants containing SP-B analogues, the best studied is lucinactant (Surfaxin), which contains a mimic of SP-B called *sinapultide* or *KL4 peptide*. KL4 is a 21-residue peptide consisting of repeated units of four hydrophobic leucine (L) residues, bound by basic polar lysine (K) residues arranged in the following order: KLLLLKLLLLKLLLLKLLLLK. This structure mimics the repeating pattern of hydrophobic and hydrophilic residues in the C-terminal part of SP-B and stabilizes the phospholipid layer by interactions with the lipid heads and the acyl chains.[28] In lucinactant, sinapultide is combined with DPPC, palmitoyl-oleoyl-phosphatidylglycerol, and palmitic acid.[28,29] Other synthetic surfactants containing SP-B and SP-C analogues have also been tested in animal studies.[30-32]

Of the surfactants containing SP-C analogues, recombinant SP-C (rSP-C) surfactant or lusupultide (Venticute) has been studied in vitro and in animals and has shown efficacy. It contains rSP-C combined with DPPC, palmitoyloleoylphosphatidylglycerol, palmitic acid, and calcium chloride.[33,34] rSP-C is similar to the 34-amino-acid human SP-C sequence, except that it contains cysteine (in place of phenylalanine) in positions 4 and 5 and contains isoleucine (instead of methionine) in position 32.

ACUTE PULMONARY AND CARDIAC EFFECTS OF SURFACTANT THERAPY

Immediate Pulmonary Effects of Surfactant Therapy

In animal models of RDS, administration of exogenous surfactant results in improved lung function (Fig. 15.2)[35] and improved alveolar expansion (Fig. 15.3).[36] Several studies in human neonates have shown that the administration of exogenous

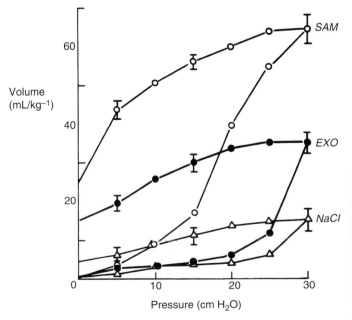

Fig. 15.2 Pressure–volume characteristics of lungs from 10 matched prematurely delivered rabbits after treatment with saline (*NaCl*), Exosurf (*EXO*), or surface-active material obtained by lavaging the lungs of young adult rabbits with saline (*SAM*), plus ventilation for 30 minutes. Measurements were made 10 minutes after the animals died and their lungs were allowed to degas spontaneously. (From Tooley WH, Clements JA, Muramatsu K, et al: Am Rev Respir Dis 136:651, 1987.)

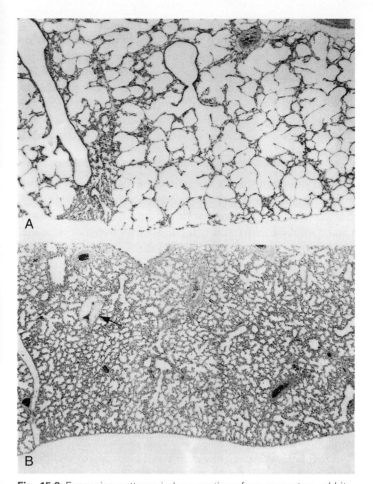

Fig. 15.3 Expansion patterns in lung sections from premature rabbits. **(A)** Well-expanded area in surfactant-treated fetus. The rounded appearance of the aerated alveoli contrasts with the pattern in panel B and with the wedge of unexpanded parenchyma (lower left). **(B)** "Unexpanded" lung in control fetus that did not receive surfactant. The configuration of the alveoli reflects the fluid-filled state. Note abundant interstitial fluid around a pulmonary vein (*arrow*) (hematoxylin and eosin, original magnification ×27). (From Robertson B, Enhorning G: Lab Invest 31:54, 1974.)

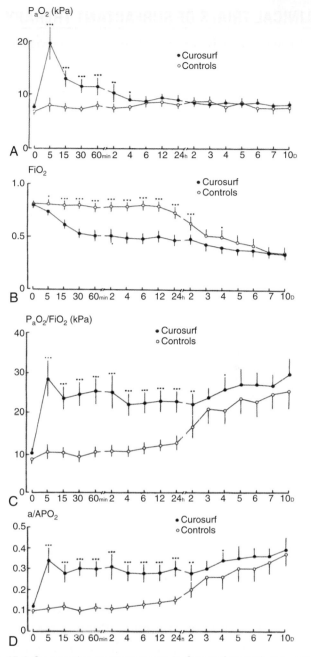

Fig. 15.4 Oxygenation measurements in Curosurf-treated and control infants at various intervals after randomization. **(A)** Partial pressure of oxygen. **(B)** Fraction of inspired oxygen. **(C)** Ratio of partial pressure of oxygen to fraction of inspired oxygen. **(D)** Arterio-alveolar oxygen ratio. Results are mean values and 95% confidence intervals. If confidence intervals are overlapping, bars are shown on only one side of the data point. Note that the time scale is not linear. Conversion factor: 1 kPa = 7.52 mm Hg. $*P < .05$; $**P < .01$; $***P < .001$. (From Collaborative European Multicenter Study Group. Pediatrics 82:683, 1988[13].)

surfactant therapy leads to rapid improvement in oxygenation and a decrease in the degree of support provided by mechanical ventilation (Fig. 15.4).[37] These rapid changes are accompanied by an increase in the functional residual capacity and are followed by a slower and variable increase in lung compliance.[38-40] A decrease in pulmonary ventilation–perfusion mismatch has also been reported.[41-43]

Immediate Effects on Pulmonary Circulation

The effect of surfactant treatment on the pulmonary circulation is unclear. In three studies, pulmonary blood flow was unchanged with surfactant therapy.[44-46] In contrast, others have reported a decrease in pulmonary artery pressure or an increase in pulmonary artery flow with surfactant therapy,[47-50] as well as an increase in the ductal flow velocity from the systemic to the pulmonary circuit.[49] It is uncertain whether these changes in pulmonary circulation are related to ventilation practices, blood gas status, or the surfactant treatment itself.[51]

Radiographic Changes

In addition to these physiologic changes, treatment with exogenous surfactant also results in radiologic improvement, with chest radiographs after treatment often (but not always) showing a decrease in the signs of RDS. This clearing of the lungs can be uniform, patchy, or asymmetric, sometimes with disproportionate improvement of radiologic changes in the right lung.[52-56]

CLINICAL TRIALS OF SURFACTANT THERAPY

Surfactant therapy is one of the best-studied interventions in neonatology and has been subjected to numerous randomized controlled trials comparing various treatment strategies. The findings from these trials, many of which are included in multiple systematic reviews in the Cochrane Database of Systematic Reviews, are summarized in the following sections. The results of meta-analyses are presented as the "typical" or "pooled" estimates of relative risk (RR) and absolute risk difference (ARD), with 95% confidence intervals (CIs).

Surfactant Therapy Compared With Placebo or No Therapy

Many of the early trials in the late 1980s and early 1990s studied the effects of surfactant therapy compared with placebo or no therapy. Some of these trials studied the effects of prophylactic administration of surfactant to preterm infants at risk for developing RDS (prophylactic or prevention trials). Others studied the effects of treatment with surfactant in preterm infants with clinical and/or radiologic features of RDS (rescue or treatment trials). Some of these studies used animal-derived surfactant and others used synthetic surfactant. Systematic reviews of these trials[57-60] show that, compared with placebo or no therapy, surfactant treatment or prophylaxis (with either animal-derived or synthetic surfactant) decreases the risk of pneumothorax and of mortality. Estimates from the meta-analyses indicate that there is a 30% to 65% relative reduction in the risk of pneumothorax and up to a 40% relative reduction in the risk of mortality. There were no consistent effects on other clinical outcomes such as chronic lung disease, patent ductus arteriosus, and intraventricular hemorrhage.

Further evidence of the benefits of surfactant therapy is derived from studies demonstrating decreased mortality and morbidity in very low birth weight infants after the introduction of surfactant therapy into practice.[1,3,61,62]

Prophylactic Surfactant Administration Compared With Post-Birth Stabilization on Continuous Positive Airway Pressure and Selective Surfactant Administration

The rationale for prophylactic administration of surfactant was the observation that in animal studies, a more uniform and homogeneous distribution of surfactant is achieved when it is administered into a fluid-filled lung[63,64] and by the belief that administration of surfactant into a previously unventilated or minimally ventilated lung will diminish acute lung injury. Even brief (15–30 minutes) periods of mechanical ventilation before surfactant administration have been shown, in animal models, to cause acute lung injury resulting in alveolar-capillary damage, leakage of proteinaceous fluid into the alveolar space, and release of inflammatory mediators,[65-67] and to decrease the subsequent response to surfactant replacement.[68,69] Surfactant-deficient animals who receive assisted ventilation develop necrosis and desquamation of the bronchiolar epithelium as early as 5 minutes after onset of ventilation.[70] Prophylactic surfactant

has been administered after intubating the infant immediately after birth ("before the first breath"). However, administration after initial resuscitation and confirmation of endotracheal tube position were found in a randomized trial to be equivalent or superior to immediate administration.[71] A systematic review[72] included 11 randomized controlled trials that compared prophylactic surfactant administration to selective surfactant treatment, that is, treatment of established RDS. All these trials used animal-derived surfactant. The selective treatment group had two categories of infants—those who were routinely stabilized on nasal continuous positive airway pressure (CPAP) immediately after birth and received surfactant if CPAP "failed" (more recent, larger studies with a high rate of maternal antenatal steroid administration) and those who were not stabilized on CPAP and received surfactant treatment at anywhere from 1.5 to 7.4 hours of age (older studies with a low rate of maternal steroid administration). A meta-analysis of studies without routine application of CPAP in controls demonstrated benefits with the use of prophylactic surfactant—a decrease in the risk of air leak and neonatal mortality. However, the analyses of studies that allowed for routine stabilization on CPAP demonstrated a decrease in the risk of chronic lung disease or death in infants stabilized on CPAP. When all studies were evaluated together, no benefits of prophylactic surfactant could be demonstrated. Furthermore, infants receiving prophylactic surfactant had a higher incidence of bronchopulmonary dysplasia (BPD) or death than did infants stabilized on CPAP (RR, 1.12; 95% CI, 1.02–1.24). Therefore, in extremely preterm infants, the early use of CPAP with subsequent selective surfactant administration is the preferred management immediately after birth.[73] Infants managed with CPAP should be monitored closely after birth, and those who show evidence of progressive respiratory failure from RDS should be intubated and given surfactant treatment early without delay. Administration of surfactant should preferably be followed by rapid extubation, and prolonged ventilation should be avoided.

In preterm infants who do not receive prophylaxis, early surfactant treatment of those with signs and symptoms of RDS is preferred. Six randomized controlled trials, including the largest randomized trial conducted in neonatology (the OSIRIS trial), have evaluated early versus delayed selective surfactant administration. The results of these trials are summarized in a systematic review.[74] Of note, this is a comparison of what to do once an infant is intubated and not a decision about when to intubate for surfactant treatment. In these trials, early administration of surfactant consisted of administration of the first dose within the first 30 minutes to 2 hours of life. Two of the trials used synthetic surfactant (Exosurf Neonatal) and four used animal-derived surfactant preparations. The meta-analyses demonstrate significant benefits to early treatment of intubated infants with RDS: reductions in the risk of neonatal mortality (typical RR, 0.84; 95% CI, 0.74–0.95; typical risk difference [RD], −0.04; 95% CI, −0.06 to −0.01), chronic lung disease (typical RR, 0.69; 95% CI, 0.55–0.86; typical RD, −0.04; 95% CI, −0.06 to −0.01), and chronic lung disease or death at 36 weeks (typical RR, 0.83; 95% CI, 0.75–0.91; typical RD, −0.06; 95% CI, −0.09 to −0.03). Intubated infants randomized to early selective surfactant administration also demonstrated a decreased risk of acute lung injury, including a decreased risk of pneumothorax (typical RR, 0.69; 95% CI, 0.59–0.82; typical RD, −0.05; 95% CI, −0.08 to −0.03), pulmonary interstitial emphysema (typical RR, 0.60; 95% CI, 0.41–0.89; typical RD, −0.06; 95% CI, −0.10 to −0.02), and overall air-leak syndromes (typical RR, 0.61; 95% CI, 0.48–0.78; typical RD, −0.18; 95% CI, −0.26 to −0.09). A trend toward risk reduction for BPD or death at 28 days was also evident (typical RR, 0.94; 95% CI, 0.88–1.00; typical RD, −0.04; 95% CI, −0.07 to −0.00). No differences in other complications of RDS or prematurity were noted. Therefore, preterm infants who do not receive prophylactic surfactant and exhibit the signs and symptoms of RDS should receive the first dose of surfactant as early as possible. Outborn infants are at highest risk of delayed administration. Tertiary referral units accepting outborn infants should attempt to develop systems to ensure that surfactant is administered as early as possible to these infants, either by the transporting team or, if appropriate, by the referring hospital. In inborn infants, delays in the administration of surfactant occur if other admission procedures such as line placement, radiographs, and nursing procedures are allowed to take precedence over surfactant dosing soon after birth. Surfactant administration should be given priority over other admission procedures.

Early Surfactant Administration Followed Immediately by Extubation to Nasal Continuous Positive Airway Pressure

When surfactant therapy was first used, infants were maintained on mechanical ventilation after surfactant administration, ventilator support was gradually weaned as the pulmonary status improved, and the infant was extubated from low ventilator settings. This approach has been compared with a strategy of surfactant administration followed immediately (within 1 hour) by extubation to nasal CPAP (nCPAP) to prevent ventilator-induced lung injury (VILI) that can result from even brief periods of mechanical ventilation.[75,76] This approach has been called the INSURE technique (intubate, surfactant, extubate to CPAP). Six randomized trials, all of which were trials of rescue surfactant administration, have compared the INSURE approach in spontaneously breathing infants with signs of RDS to later, selective administration of surfactant in infants with respiratory insufficiency related to RDS, followed by continued mechanical ventilation and extubation from low respiratory support. These trials are summarized in a systematic review.[77] Most of these studies included infants with a gestation of 35 weeks or less and a birth weight of 2500 g or less. The meta-analysis in this review showed that compared with the traditional management strategy of gradual weaning, the INSURE approach reduced the need for mechanical ventilation (typical RR, 0.67; 95% CI, 0.57–0.79), air-leak syndromes (typical RR, 0.52; 95% CI, 0.28–0.96), and BPD (oxygen at 28 days; typical RR, 0.51; 95% CI, 0.26–0.99). A lower threshold for treatment at study entry (FiO$_2$ less than 0.45) resulted in a lower incidence of air leak (typical RR, 0.46; 95% CI, 0.23–0.93) and BPD

(typical RR, 0.43; 95% CI, 0.20–0.92). A higher treatment threshold (FiO$_2$ >0.45) at study entry was associated with a higher incidence of patent ductus arteriosus requiring treatment (typical RR, 2.15; 95% CI, 1.09–4.13). Since this systematic review, two large randomized controlled trials have been published. In a randomized trial by the Colombian Neonatal Research Network,[78] 279 infants of 27 to 31 weeks' gestation with RDS who were randomly assigned within the first hour of life to intubation, very early surfactant, extubation, and nCPAP required less ventilation and had a lower incidence of mortality and air leaks (pneumothorax and pulmonary interstitial emphysema) than infants assigned to nasal continuous airway pressure alone. In a large trial using the INSURE technique, the Vermont Oxford Network[79] randomized 648 infants to prophylactic surfactant followed by a period of mechanical ventilation (PS), prophylactic surfactant with rapid extubation to bubble nCPAP (ISX), or initial management with bubble nCPAP and selective surfactant treatment (nCPAP). Compared with the PS group, the RR of BPD or death was 0.78 (95% CI, 0.59–1.03) for the ISX group and 0.83 (95% CI, 0.64–1.09) for the nCPAP group. There were no statistically significant differences in mortality or other complications of prematurity. In the nCPAP group, 48% were managed without intubation and ventilation, and 54% without surfactant treatment. These data suggest that spontaneously breathing preterm infants who show early signs of RDS should be given surfactant at a low threshold, after which they can be quickly extubated and placed on nCPAP to reduce VILI.

Targeted Surfactant Therapy

Several studies have addressed the use of rapid bedside tests such as the click test, lamellar body count, or stable microbubble test on a tracheal aspirate or a gastric aspirate specimen.[80-82] Such tests can potentially supplement the use of clinical criteria in selecting preterm infants whose likelihood of RDS is high enough to merit surfactant therapy and perhaps avoid needless intubations and, in those already intubated, needless surfactant therapy. However, it is unclear whether the logistic challenges of performing these tests are worth the additional refinements in decision making. In expert hands, the use of lung ultrasound can also help identify infants who require surfactant therapy.[83]

Single Versus Multiple Surfactant Doses

Many of the initial trials of surfactant therapy tested a single dose of surfactant. However, surfactant may become rapidly metabolized, and functional inactivation of surfactant can result from the action of soluble proteins and other factors in the small airways and alveoli.[20] The ability to administer repeat or subsequent doses of surfactant is thought to be useful in overcoming such inactivation. The results of two randomized controlled trials that compared multiple dosing regimens to single-dose regimens of animal-derived surfactant extract for treatment of established RDS have been evaluated in a systematic review.[84] In one study,[85] after the initial dose of BLES, infants assigned to the multiple-dose group could receive up to three additional doses of surfactant during the first 72 hours of life if they had a respiratory deterioration, provided they had shown a positive response to the first dose and a pneumothorax had been eliminated as the cause of the respiratory deterioration. In the other study,[86] infants in the multiple-dose group received additional doses of poractant at 12 and 24 hours after the initial dose if they still needed supplemental oxygen and mechanical ventilation. Approximately 70% of the infants randomized to the multiple-dose regimen received multiple doses.

The meta-analysis supports a decreased risk of pneumothorax associated with multiple-dose surfactant therapy (typical RR, 0.51; 95% CI, 0.30–0.88; typical ARD, 0.09; 95% CI, 0.15–0.02). There was also a trend toward decreased mortality (typical RR, 0.63; 95% CI, 0.39–1.02; typical ARD, 0.07; 95% CI, 0.14–0.00). No differences were detected in other clinical outcomes. No complications associated with multiple-dose treatment were reported in these trials. In a third study, in which synthetic surfactant was used in a prophylactic manner, the use of two doses of surfactant in addition to the prophylactic dose led to a decrease in mortality, respiratory support, necrotizing enterocolitis, and other outcomes compared with a single prophylactic dose.[87] In the OSIRIS trial, which used synthetic surfactant, a two-dose treatment schedule was found to be equivalent to a treatment schedule permitting up to four doses of surfactant.[88]

Criteria for Repeat Doses of Surfactant

The use of a higher threshold for retreatment with surfactant appears to be as effective as a low threshold and can result in significant savings in costs of the drug. The criteria for administration of repeat doses of surfactant have been investigated in two studies, both of which used animal-derived surfactant. In one study,[89] the retreatment criteria compared were an increase in the fraction of inspired oxygen by 0.1 over the lowest baseline value (standard retreatment) versus a sustained increase of just 0.01 (liberal retreatment). There were no differences in complications of prematurity or duration of respiratory support. However, short-term benefits in oxygen requirement and degree of ventilator support were noted in the liberal retreatment group.

In another study,[90] retreatment at a low threshold (FiO_2 >30%, still requiring endotracheal intubation) was compared with retreatment at a high threshold (FiO_2 >40%, mean airway pressure >7 cm H_2O). Again, there were minor short-term benefits to using a low threshold with no differences in major clinical outcomes. However, in a subgroup of infants with RDS complicated by perinatal compromise or infection, infants in the high-threshold group had a trend toward higher mortality than the low-threshold group. Based on current evidence, it appears appropriate to use persistent or worsening signs of RDS as criteria for retreatment with surfactant. A low threshold for repeat dosing should be used for infants with RDS who have perinatal depression or infection.

METHODS OF ADMINISTRATION OF SURFACTANT

A theoretical model for the transport of exogenous surfactant through the airways has been proposed,[91] consisting of four distinct mechanisms: (1) the instilled bolus may create a liquid

plug that occludes the large airways but is forced peripherally during mechanical ventilation; (2) the bolus creates a deposited film on the airway walls, either from the liquid plug transport or from direct coating, that drains under the influence of gravity through the first few airway generations; (3) in smaller airways, surfactant species form a surface layer that spreads because of surface-tension gradients, that is, Marangoni flows; and (4) the surfactant finally reaches the alveolar compartment, where it is cleared according to first-order kinetics.

Administration Through Catheter, Side Port, or Suction Valve

According to the manufacturers' recommendations, beractant and poractant should be administered through a catheter inserted into the endotracheal tube; colfosceril should be administered through a side-port adapter attached to the endotracheal tube, and calf lung surfactant extract can be administered either through a catheter or through a side-port adapter. Other methods of administration of surfactant have been tested in randomized trials. In one randomized trial, the administration of beractant through a catheter inserted through a neonatal suction valve without detachment of the neonate from the ventilator was compared with the administration of the dose (with detachment from the ventilator) in two aliquots through a catheter and to the standard technique of administration of the dose in four aliquots through a catheter.[92] Administration through the suction valve led to less dosing-related oxygen desaturation but more reflux of beractant than the two-aliquot catheter technique. In another study,[93] the administration of poractant as a bolus was compared in a randomized trial to administration via a catheter introduced through a side hole in the tracheal tube adaptor without changing the infant's position or interrupting ventilation. The numbers of episodes of hypoxia and/or bradycardia, as well as other outcomes, were similar in both groups. A slight and transient increase in $PaCO_2$ was observed in the side-hole group.

Administration Through Dual-Lumen Endotracheal Tube

The administration of poractant through a dual-lumen endotracheal tube without a change in position or interruption of mechanical ventilation was compared with bolus instillation in a randomized trial.[94] The dual-lumen group had fewer episodes of dosing-related hypoxia, a smaller decrease in heart rate and oxygen saturation, and a shorter total time in increased supplemental oxygen than the bolus group. The dual-lumen method has also been compared with the side-port method of administration of colfosceril in a randomized trial.[95] No difference was found between the two methods in dosing-related hypoxemia.

Administration Through a Laryngeal Mask Airway

Surfactant administration through a laryngeal mask airway (LMA) is noninvasive, avoids endotracheal intubation, and potentially avoids the complications associated with intubation. It has been reported in a series of eight preterm infants (mean birth weight 1700 g) with RDS managed with nCPAP.[96] The mean arterial-to-alveolar oxygen tension ratio improved significantly after the treatment, and no complications were reported. Moreover, although the smallest infant in this study was 880 g, the use of the currently available LMA is recommended only for babies above 1500 g. A randomized controlled trial of 26 infants resulted in reduction of FiO_2 in the first 12 hours after surfactant administration, but later, no significant difference was found in subsequent need for mechanical ventilation or BPD. However, this study reported several adverse events with the use of LMA.[97] Another randomized trial of 61 patients found that surfactant administration through an LMA reduced the proportion of preterm infants with moderate RDS who required mechanical ventilation compared with standard endotracheal administration following intubation with premedication. The efficacy of surfactant in decreasing RDS severity was similar with both methods.[98] Another randomized trial of 70 infants used i-gel for surfactant administration.[99] i-gel is a laryngeal device modeled on the LMA. The study resulted in significantly higher a-APO_2 after treatment with i-gel compared with INSURE in controls. Thus, although there is accumulating evidence for the administration of surfactant through an LMA or similar device, further research is required to establish the efficacy and risk-versus-benefit ratio of these methods.

Nasopharyngeal Administration of Surfactant

Another noninvasive method of surfactant administration is instillation of surfactant into the nasopharynx during or immediately after delivery and before the first breath. Such instillation is thought to cause the surfactant to be aspirated into the fluid-filled airway as an air–fluid interface is established. A case series[100] of 23 preterm infants of 27 to 30 weeks' gestation receiving such intrapartum nasopharyngeal instillation of surfactant followed by placement on CPAP immediately after birth (mask CPAP initially followed by nCPAP) demonstrated the feasibility of such administration. However, more evidence is required to prove the efficacy of this approach before it can be used or recommended.

Thin Catheter Endotracheal Administration (Less Invasive Surfactant Administration)

Instead of an endotracheal tube, this method uses a thin catheter that is inserted into the trachea while the patient is spontaneously breathing on CPAP, and surfactant is administered through this thin tube, after which it is removed. Three main methods of less invasive surfactant administration (LISA) have been described in randomized controlled trials. All used catheters have a smaller external diameter (1.33–1.7 mm) than that of a standard endotracheal tube. In the Cologne method, the surfactant was administered through a 4-Fr feeding tube inserted 1.5 cm below the vocal cords under direct laryngoscopy with the aid of Magill forceps after premedication with atropine. In the Take Care method, a shortened 5-Fr feeding tube without Magill forceps and premedication was used. In the minimally invasive surfactant therapy (MIST) method, a 16-gauge vascular catheter (Angiocath, BD, Sandy, UT) without premedication was used. An in vitro study comparing different catheters in a mannequin model showed that stiff catheter insertion is quicker and easier compared with flexible catheters.

The adverse events associated with thin catheter insertion include coughing, gagging, desaturation, bradycardia, and surfactant reflux. The success rate for insertion of the catheter on the first attempt has been reported to be between 72% and 95% in randomized control trials. The stiffer and straight catheter is an attractive option for US, Canadian, and Australian centers, where oral intubation is the preferred practice and use of Magill forceps is uncommon. Two custom-made stiff catheters specifically designed for LISA have been manufactured but are currently not available in the United States.

A Cochrane systematic review of LISA[101] included 16 studies that compared surfactant administration via a thin catheter with surfactant administration through an endotracheal tube with early extubation (INSURE technique) or with delayed extubation, or with continuation of CPAP and rescue surfactant administration at prespecified criteria, or compared different strategies of surfactant administration via thin catheter. Meta-analyses of 14 studies in which LISA was compared with endotracheal administration of surfactant as a control demonstrated a significant decrease in risk of the composite outcome of death or BPD at 36 weeks' postmenstrual age (PMA) (risk ratio [RR], 0.59; 95% CI, 0.48–0.73; RD, −0.11; 95% CI, −0.15 to −0.07; number needed to treat for an additional beneficial outcome [NNTB], 9; 95% CI, 7–16), the need for intubation within 72 hours (RR, 0.63; 95% CI, 0.54–0.74; RD, −0.14; 95% CI, −0.18 to −0.09; NNTB, 8; 95% CI, 6–12), severe intraventricular hemorrhage (RR, 0.63; 95% CI, 0.42–0.96; RD, −0.04; 95% CI, −0.08 to −0.00; NNTB, 22; 95% CI, 12–193), death during first hospitalization (RR, 0.63; 95% CI, 0.47–0.84; RD, −0.02; 95% CI, −0.10 to 0.06; NNTB, 20; 95% CI, 12–58), and BPD among survivors (RR, 0.57; 95% CI, 0.45–0.74; RD, −0.08; 95% CI, −0.11 to −0.04; NNTB, 13; 95% CI, 9–24). There was no significant difference in risk of air leak requiring drainage (RR, 0.58; 95% CI, 0.33–1.02; RD, −0.03; 95% CI, −0.05 to 0.00). The publication of the results of a large randomized multicenter trial (OPTIMIST-A) that compared catheter administration of surfactant to sham administration is pending at the time of writing.

A consensus-based guideline on LISA[102] recommends that while many infants can be managed without requiring additional sedation/analgesia during LISA, fentanyl along with atropine may be considered. It also emphasizes that parents should be provided with sufficient information about medication side effects and involved in treatment discussions. A quality improvement report describing the safe and successful introduction of LISA into a neonatal intensive care unit[103] provides a good description of a structured and systematic way of implementing this practice.

Other Methods

In one randomized clinical trial,[104] the slow infusion of colfosceril using a microinfusion syringe pump over 10 to 20 minutes was compared with manual instillation over 2 minutes. Pump administration resulted in fewer infants with loss of chest wall movement during dosing as well as a smaller increase in peak inspiratory pressure than with hand administration. However, in animals, slow infusion of surfactant into the endotracheal tube results in nonhomogeneous distribution of surfactant in the lung.[105,106] Therefore, currently, bolus administration of surfactant is preferred. Other methods of administration, such as nebulization or aerosolization[107-110] and in utero administration to the human fetus,[111,112] have also been reported. In one randomized trial, compared with a standard administration method, the administration of calfactant by nebulization decreased the rate of intubation from 50% to 25% ($P < .0001$), with a number needed to treat of 5 to prevent one intubation. However, respiratory support at days 3, 7, and 28 was not different in the two groups of infants.[113] This study had a high risk of bias because of its design, and a significant proportion of enrolled infants were more than 28 weeks' gestation. These methods require further clinical testing and require specialized nebulization equipment.

Chest Position During Administration of Surfactant

In a study in rabbits, pulmonary distribution of intratracheally instilled surfactant was largely determined by gravity, and changing the chest position after instillation did not result in any redistribution of the surfactant. Therefore, for neonates receiving surfactant, keeping the chest in the horizontal position may result in the most even distribution of the surfactant in the two lungs.[114]

Summary of Administration Methods

In summary, based on available evidence, surfactant should be administered in the standard method of aliquots instilled into an endotracheal tube. There is evidence to suggest that the administration of surfactant using a dual-lumen endotracheal tube or through a catheter passed through a suction valve is effective and may cause less dosing-related adverse events than standard methods. The side-port method of administration and the catheter method of administration through the endotracheal tube appear to be equivalent. Less invasive surfactant administration is a promising method to improve the outcome of extremely preterm infants. More studies are required before firm conclusions can be drawn about the optimal method of administration of surfactant and whether the optimal method is different for different types of surfactant.

CHOICE OF SURFACTANT PRODUCT

Comparison of Animal-Derived Surfactant Extract Versus Protein-Free Synthetic Surfactant for the Prevention and Treatment of Respiratory Distress Syndrome

Although both synthetic and animal-derived surfactants are effective, their compositions differ. Animal-derived surfactant extracts contain surfactant-specific proteins that aid in surfactant adsorption and resist surfactant inactivation. Fifteen randomized trials have compared the effects of animal-derived and protein-free synthetic surfactants in the treatment or prevention of RDS. More than 5000 infants were studied in these trials. A systematic review of these trials is available.[115]

Compared with synthetic surfactant without protein, treatment with animal-derived surfactant extracts resulted in a significant reduction in the risk of pneumothorax (typical RR, 0.65; 95% CI, 0.55–0.77; typical ARD, −0.04; 95% CI, −0.06 to −0.02) and the risk of mortality (typical RR, 0.89; 95% CI, 0.79–0.99; typical ARD, −0.02; 95% CI, −0.04 to 0.00). Animal-derived surfactant extract is associated with an increase in the risk of necrotizing enterocolitis (typical RR, 1.38; 95% CI, 1.08–1.76; typical ARD, 0.02; 95% CI, 0.01–0.04) and borderline significant increase in the risk of intraventricular hemorrhage (typical RR, 1.07; 95% CI, 0.99–1.15; typical ARD, 0.02; 95% CI, 0.00–0.05), but no increase in grade 3 or 4 intraventricular hemorrhage (typical RR, 1.08; 95% CI, 0.91–1.27; typical ARD, 0.01; 95% CI, −0.01 to 0.03). The meta-analysis also supports a marginal decrease in the risk of BPD or mortality associated with the use of animal-derived surfactant preparations (typical RR, 0.95; 95% CI, 0.91–1.00; typical ARD, −0.03; 95% CI, −0.06 to 0.00).

In addition to these benefits, animal-derived surfactants have a more rapid onset of action, allowing ventilator settings and inspired oxygen concentrations to be lowered more quickly than with synthetic surfactant.[116-120] A comparison of physical properties and the results of animal studies also suggest that animal-derived surfactants have advantages over protein-free synthetic surfactants.[121] These properties are attributed to the presence of the surfactant proteins SP-B and SP-C in certain animal-derived surfactants.[122]

The use of animal-derived surfactant preparations should be favored in most clinical situations because their use results in greater clinical benefits than synthetic surfactants.

Comparison of Protein-Containing Synthetic Surfactant Versus Animal-Derived Surfactant Extract for the Prevention and Treatment of Respiratory Distress Syndrome

Clinical trials have compared the effects of synthetic surfactants containing peptides to those of animal-derived surfactant preparations. These synthetic surfactants do not have the theoretical concerns associated with animal-derived surfactants, namely, transmission of microorganisms, exposure to animal proteins and inflammatory mediators, susceptibility to inactivation, and inconsistent content. Lucinactant, the synthetic surfactant containing an analogue of SP-B, sinapultide, has been compared with beractant in the Safety and Effectiveness of Lucinactant Versus Exosurf in a Clinical Trial (SELECT) of RDS in premature infants, a multicenter, masked randomized trial of surfactant prophylaxis in infants of 24 to 32 weeks' gestation.[123] Lucinactant was also compared with poractant in Surfaxin therapy against RDS in a multicenter randomized trial (STAR) of surfactant prophylaxis in infants of 24 to 28 weeks' gestation that was structured as a noninferiority trial.[124] A meta-analysis of these two studies[125] found no significant differences in outcomes between lucinactant and the compared animal-derived surfactant in mortality at 36 weeks' PMA (typical RR, 0.81; 95% CI, 0.64–1.03), chronic lung disease at 36 weeks' PMA (typical RR, 0.99; 95% CI, 0.84–1.18), the composite outcome of mortality or chronic lung disease at 36 weeks' PMA (typical RR, 0.96; 95% CI, 0.82–1.12), or other respiratory outcomes. A decreased risk of necrotizing enterocolitis, a secondary outcome, was noted in infants receiving lucinactant (typical RR, 0.60; 95% CI, 0.42–0.86; typical RD, −0.06; 95% CI, −0.10 to −0.01).

However, both trials of lucinactant described previously had multiple methodologic problems[126] that undermined their validity, and there is no clear evidence of the equivalence or superiority of lucinactant over any animal-derived surfactant product.[127] In March 2012, the US Food and Drug Administration approved lucinactant for use in the United States. The drawbacks of the lucinactant preparation were its high viscosity at room temperature and a gel formulation, which required heating, mixing, and subsequent cooling to body temperature before administration. Also, the dose-equivalent volume was approximately 2.5 times that of poractant alfa. Lucinactant was withdrawn from the European market in 2006, and production was completely stopped by the US manufacturer in 2015. It is currently under development as an aerosolized surfactant.

Another protein-containing synthetic surfactant, lusupultide, which contains rSP-C, has only been tried in adults with acute RDS (ARDS). It was not found to have significant clinical benefits in these patients and was not commercialized. An additional synthetic surfactant enriched with SP-B and SP-C protein analogues (CHF5633) has also been tested in human trials that demonstrated the feasibility of administration, but had inconclusive results.[128] Further research is required to elucidate the role of newer surfactants in the prevention or treatment of RDS.

Comparison of Protein-Containing Synthetic Surfactant Versus Protein-Free Synthetic Surfactant for the Prevention and Treatment of Respiratory Distress Syndrome

In the SELECT trial,[124] the randomized trial of lucinactant, in which lucinactant was compared with beractant, lucinactant was also compared with colfosceril. Infants who received protein-containing synthetic surfactant compared with protein-free synthetic surfactant did not demonstrate significantly different risks of mortality at 36 weeks' PMA (RR, 0.89; 95% CI, 0.71–1.11), chronic lung disease at 36 weeks' PMA (RR, 0.89; 95% CI, 0.78–1.03), or the combined outcome of mortality or chronic lung disease at 36 weeks' PMA (RR, 0.88; 95% CI, 0.77–1.01). Regarding the secondary outcome of RDS at 24 hours of age, a decrease in the incidence was demonstrated in the group that received lucinactant (RR, 0.83; 95% CI, 0.72–0.95).[129]

Comparison of Different Types of Bovine Surfactants

Two prevention studies and seven treatment studies compared bovine lung lavage surfactant extract to modified bovine minced lung surfactant extract. The meta-analysis[130] of the prevention trials, representing high-quality evidence, found no significant difference in death or chronic lung disease (typical RR, 1.02; 95% CI, 0.89–1.17; typical RD, 0.01; 95% CI, −0.05 to 0.06). Analysis of the treatment trials also found no significant differences between these two types of bovine surfactants in

death or chronic lung disease (typical RR, 0.95; 95% CI, 0.86–1.06; typical RD, −0.02; 95% CI, −0.06 to 0.02, high-quality evidence).

Comparison of Porcine and Bovine Surfactants

Nine treatment studies compared modified bovine minced lung surfactant extract with porcine minced lung surfactant extract. A meta-analysis of these studies[130] found a significant increase in mortality before hospital discharge (typical RR, 1.44; 95% CI, 1.04–2.00; typical RD, 0.05; 95% CI, 0.01–0.10) in patients treated with modified bovine surfactant extract compared with porcine minced lung surfactant extract. Other outcome parameters like death or oxygen requirement at 36 weeks' PMA (typical RR, 1.30; 95% CI, 1.04–1.64; typical RD, 0.11; 95% CI, 0.02–0.20), receiving more than one dose of surfactant (typical RR, 1.57; 95% CI, 1.29–1.92; typical RD, 0.14; 95% CI, 0.08–0.20), and patent ductus arteriosus requiring treatment (typical RR, 1.86; 95% CI, 1.28–2.70; typical RD, 0.28; 95% CI, 0.13–0.43) also favored treatment with porcine minced lung surfactant. The dose of beractant was uniformly 100 mg/kg across all five studies. When only studies that used a 100 mg/kg dose of poractant were considered, the reduction in mortality before discharge and risk of death or oxygen requirement at 36 weeks' PMA were not statistically significant. It is uncertain that the statistical difference between the two types of surfactants was related to the source of extraction (porcine vs bovine) or to the higher initial dose of porcine surfactant.

ADVERSE EFFECTS OF SURFACTANT THERAPY

Transient hypoxia and bradycardia can occur as a result of acute airway obstruction immediately after surfactant instillation.[92,131] Other acute adverse effects of surfactant administration include reflux of surfactant into the pharynx from the endotracheal tube, increase in transcutaneous carbon dioxide tension, tachycardia, gagging, and mucous plugging of the endotracheal tube. These complications of surfactant administration generally respond to a slower rate of surfactant administration or to an increase in the airway pressure or FiO_2 during administration. Rapid improvement in oxygenation after surfactant administration necessitates close monitoring and appropriate reduction of ventilatory parameters.

Several authors have reported a transient decrease in blood pressure,[132-134] a transient decrease in cerebral blood flow velocity,[135-137] a transient decrease in cerebral oxyhemoglobin concentration,[137] and a transient decrease in cerebral activity on amplitude-integrated electroencephalography[132] immediately after surfactant administration. The electroencephalogram (EEG) depression observed after surfactant instillation is not caused by cerebral ischemia,[138] and the EEG suppression is not directly related to alterations in blood gases or systemic circulation.[139] The clinical significance of these findings is uncertain. One study[140] reported an increase in the incidence of intraventricular hemorrhage, and a case report documents a temporal association between the development of intraventricular hemorrhage and the administration of surfactant TA to improve respiratory failure caused by pulmonary hemorrhage.[141] However, the meta-analyses of multiple trials do not show an increase in the risk of intraventricular hemorrhage with surfactant therapy compared with placebo.[57-60]

There is a well-described increase in the risk of pulmonary hemorrhage with surfactant therapy.[142,143] Although trials in which animal-derived surfactants were used reported a higher incidence (5%–6%) of pulmonary hemorrhage than trials of synthetic surfactant (1%–3%), direct comparison of the two types of surfactants demonstrates no difference in the risk of pulmonary hemorrhage. The overall incidence of pulmonary hemorrhage was low, and the absolute magnitude of the increased risk is small.[142] However, moderate and severe pulmonary hemorrhage is associated with an increased risk of death and short-term morbidity. It is not associated with increased long-term morbidity.[144] The occurrence of pulmonary hemorrhage may be related to the presence of a hemodynamically significant patent ductus arteriosus.[145,146] Seppanen studied the association of neonatal complications with the Doppler-derived aortopulmonary pressure gradient (APPG) across the ductus arteriosus, which reflects pulmonary artery pressure during the first day of life. Infants in whom the APPG decreased after birth had a lower frequency of patent ductus arteriosus and pulmonary hemorrhage[147] than those whose APPG remained low. Another mechanism for pulmonary hemorrhage may be a direct cytotoxicity, which has been demonstrated in in vitro studies and appears to be different for different surfactants and different dosages.[148]

When surfactant initially became available for clinical testing, there was concern that the introduction of foreign proteins from animal-based lung surfactants into the lungs of preterm infants could lead to immunologic responses. Two studies did not find antibodies specific to surfactant protein in the sera of preterm infants treated with bovine surfactant.[149,150] In other studies, immune complexes or antibodies to the protein in exogenous porcine, bovine, or human surfactant have been identified in the sera of neonates with RDS. However, similar immune complexes or antibodies were also noted in control infants who did not receive surfactant. Positive enzyme-linked immunosorbent assay values with regard to SP-A, and IgM against SP-A and SP-B and C, were more frequently found in the control group than in the surfactant-treated group in sera from neonates at 1 week of age.[147,151,152] This occurrence was less frequent in surfactant-treated neonates, suggesting that surfactant treatment reduces leakage of these proteins in the circulation.[151]

With animal-derived surfactants, there is a theoretical risk of the transmission of infectious agents, including bovine spongiform encephalitis, with surfactants derived from bovine sources and other viral infections in swine. Organic solvent processing of phospholipids, terminal sterilization techniques, and screening of animal sources have been used to minimize this risk.

ECONOMIC ASPECTS OF SURFACTANT THERAPY

With the introduction of surfactant therapy, there was concern that the increased number of survivors and a possible increase in the length of hospital stay would lead to an increase in the overall cost of neonatal care.[153] These increased costs can be offset to a variable extent by the fact that surfactant therapy can lead to lower hospital charges,[154] reduce the costs or charges per survivor of neonatal intensive care,[3,155,156] and reduce the charges for infants who ultimately die.[3] In an economic analysis for a hypothetic cohort of infants weighing 700 to 1350 g and treated with synthetic surfactant, based on the results of a randomized controlled trial,[157] the total hospital charges through 1-year adjusted age were similar to those for a comparable cohort of infants receiving air placebo, despite the fact that more babies in the synthetic surfactant cohort survived and thus required prolonged hospital care during their first year of life. The incremental cost per survivor estimated in this study was $1585 (in 1995 dollars).

In 1990, the cost per quality-adjusted life year (QALY) with surfactant therapy was estimated in one study to be $1500[158] and in another study to be £710.[159] From a societal perspective, the cost-effectiveness of surfactant therapy is more favorable than that of health care interventions such as renal transplantation, coronary bypass surgery, and dialysis.[159] In a geographically defined, population-based study from Australia, cost effectiveness and cost-utility ratios in presurfactant and postsurfactant periods were compared for 500- to 999-g birth weight infants. When costs incurred during the primary hospitalization were considered, both of these ratios were lower (i.e., economically better) in the postsurfactant era than in the presurfactant era (presurfactant vs postsurfactant, $7040 vs $4040 per life year gained; $6700 vs $5360 per QALY). Both ratios fell with increasing birth weight. With costs for long-term care of severely disabled children added, both cost ratios were higher in the postsurfactant era.

FACTORS AFFECTING THE RESPONSE TO SURFACTANT THERAPY

Several factors have been reported by various authors to be associated with a poor response to surfactant therapy, either in terms of immediate pulmonary response or in terms of later morbidity and mortality. These factors include high total fluid and colloid intake in the first days of life;[160] a low mean airway pressure relative to the FiO_2;[160] the presence of an additional pulmonary disorder such as infection;[161] perinatal asphyxia, infection, or other complications of prematurity;[162] and high fraction of inspired oxygen requirement at entry (had a negative impact on a-APO_2 6 and 24 hours after treatment), lower birth weight, male sex, outborn status, perinatal asphyxia, and high airway pressure requirement at entry.[163] Low birth weight, low Apgar scores, and initial disease severity were associated with an increased mortality.[164]

A high pulmonary resistance before therapy was associated with a poor response to therapy at 24 and 48 hours.[165] In addition, the immediate response to surfactant therapy itself has been reported to be a significant prognostic indicator for mortality and morbidity.[166] In animal studies, poor response to surfactant has been associated with delayed administration[64] and the leakage of proteinaceous fluid into the alveolar spaces. Within some multicenter trials, significant differences in outcomes of surfactant-treated infants have been noted between participating hospitals,[163,164] suggesting that variations in patient care practices have an important influence on the outcomes of surfactant-treated infants.

As noted earlier, observational studies have demonstrated a decrease in mortality and morbidity for such infants after the introduction of surfactant therapy. However, racial differences in this decline in mortality have been reported. In one study, the overall neonatal mortality for Black very low birth weight (VLBW) infants did not change after the introduction of surfactant therapy,[62] and in another study, declines in neonatal mortality risks caused by RDS and all respiratory causes were greater for non-Hispanic White VLBW infants than for Black VLBW infants.[167] Although such racial differences have been noted at a population level, the role of racial factors in the response pattern of individual infants with RDS to exogenous surfactant therapy is unknown.

LONG-TERM OUTCOMES AFTER SURFACTANT THERAPY

Long-term outcomes after surfactant therapy have been well studied for synthetic surfactant. Follow-up studies of long-term outcomes after animal-derived surfactant therapy have consisted of small numbers of patients, with a variable proportion of survivors being tested. For both synthetic and animal-derived surfactant, the long-term outcomes reported consist of outcomes predominantly in the first 3 years of life, with very few reports of outcomes at school age or higher. Given these limitations, the evidence suggests that not only do more infants survive from surfactant therapy, but also they are at no selective disadvantage for neurodevelopmental sequelae because of the surfactant therapy. Most comparisons of long-term outcomes have been between infants treated with surfactant and placebo. There are few or no comparisons of long-term outcomes between infants treated with different types of surfactant or different regimens of the same surfactant. The following sections mainly address comparisons between infants treated with surfactant and placebo.

Neurodevelopmental Outcomes

No significant differences have been reported in the long-term neurodevelopmental outcomes of infants treated with surfactant compared with those treated with placebo, either with synthetic surfactant[87,168,169] or with animal-derived surfactant.[170-174]

Long-Term Respiratory Outcomes

Compared with infants treated with placebo, infants treated with surfactant in the neonatal period have been reported either to have improved[175-177] or to have equivalent[178-180] results on pulmonary function testing. Some studies have reported a lower frequency of subsequent clinical respiratory disorders in surfactant-treated infants compared with placebo,[181,182] whereas others have reported no difference[147,168,170,175] or a trend toward an increase in allergic manifestations.[174]

Physical Growth

No significant differences have been reported in weight or height outcomes between surfactant-treated and placebo-treated infants on follow-up.[147,169,174-176,182]

Outcomes of Prophylactic Versus Rescue Treatment Strategies

Two studies compared the long-term outcomes of infants treated with prophylactic surfactant to those treated with a "rescue" strategy. In one, there were no differences at school age in neurodevelopmental outcome or in the results of pulmonary function testing between the two groups, although infants who had received prophylactic surfactant showed fewer clinical pulmonary problems than those who received rescue treatment.[183] In another study in which there was significant loss of infants to follow-up (and therefore a high likelihood of attrition bias), the mean scores on the Bayley scales of infant development at 12 months' adjusted age were higher in the rescue group than in the prophylactic group.[181]

EXOGENOUS SURFACTANT THERAPY FOR CONDITIONS OTHER THAN RESPIRATORY DISTRESS SYNDROME

Exogenous surfactant therapy has been attempted in a variety of neonatal respiratory disorders other than RDS, with variable quality of evidence and variable efficacy.[184]

Meconium Aspiration Syndrome

In vitro studies[185,186] and animal studies[187,188] have demonstrated that meconium inhibits surfactant function and is likely to be partially responsible for alveolar collapse in MAS. Components of meconium that may contribute to altered surfactant function include cholesterol, free fatty acids, bile salts, bilirubin, and proteolytic enzymes.[185-187]

In uncontrolled studies of human infants with MAS, improved oxygenation has been reported with exogenous surfactant therapy.[189-191] A randomized trial in infants of greater than 34 weeks' gestation with severe respiratory failure on extracorporeal membrane oxygenation (ECMO) (including infants with MAS) showed that infants treated with beractant had improved lung function, a shorter duration of ECMO, and fewer complications after ECMO.[192]

Four randomized trials[193-196] have studied the effects of animal-derived surfactant in term infants with MAS and are included in a systematic review. In these trials, surfactant therapy was administered as a continuous infusion over 20 minutes[194] or as a bolus. A systematic review and meta-analysis of these four trials[197] showed a decreased need for ECMO with surfactant therapy (typical RR, 0.64; 95% CI, 0.46–0.91; typical ARD, -0.17; 95% CI, -0.30 to -0.04). One trial reported a reduction in the length of hospital stay (mean difference, 8 days; 95% CI, -14 to -3 days). There were no statistically significant effects on mortality (typical RR, 0.98; 95% CI, 0.41–2.39; typical RD, 0.00; 95% CI, -0.05 to 0.05) or other outcomes (duration of assisted ventilation, duration of supplemental oxygen, pneumothorax, pulmonary interstitial emphysema, air leaks, chronic lung disease, need for oxygen at discharge, or intraventricular hemorrhage).

In summary, infants with severe MAS are likely to benefit from treatment with animal-derived surfactants. Multiple doses are usually required in such infants. Only animal-derived surfactants have been tested in human clinical trials in this setting, and the efficacy of synthetic surfactants is unknown. Each dose should be administered cautiously, with close cardiac, respiratory, and oxygen saturation monitoring, because surfactant can aggravate preexisting airway obstruction from meconium, and transient oxygen desaturation and endotracheal tube obstruction have been reported with bolus administration in nearly one-third of infants.[193]

Investigators have also attempted to treat MAS by lavaging the airways with diluted surfactant solutions to wash out residual meconium.[198] This approach to surfactant treatment requires further study before it can be recommended.

Acute Respiratory Distress Syndrome

Surfactant dysfunction is well described in acute lung injury.[199] Therefore, surfactant replacement has been proposed as a treatment for patients with acute lung injury and ARDS, which, although more common in adults and older children, can occur in term neonates.[200,201] Exogenous surfactant therapy has been attempted in ARDS in adults, but the results of clinical trials have not been promising.[202] There are scant randomized trials of exogenous surfactant therapy specifically for ARDS in neonates,[203] but in older children with acute respiratory failure, surfactant use decreased mortality and duration of ventilation.[204,205] Extrapolating from these pediatric studies, and based on the pathophysiologic, clinical, and radiologic similarities between RDS and ARDS, term infants with clinical and radiologic features of ARDS (severe respiratory failure with pulmonary opacification and air bronchograms on chest radiographs) are often treated with exogenous surfactant.[206] A consensus statement from the European Society for Pediatric and Neonatal Intensive Care (ESPNIC) based on a review of existing literature (that found significant flaws in existing studies) recommended targeted research enrolling infants meeting current definitions of neonatal ARDS and considering the more recent knowledge on ARDS pathobiology[207] (DeLuca 2021, PMID: 33618742).

Other Conditions

There are reports (anecdotal or case series) of the use of exogenous surfactant therapy in human infants for the management of pulmonary hemorrhage[208,209] and neonatal pneumonia.[189,210-212] However, the efficacy of surfactant in these conditions is uncertain, and its routine use in these conditions cannot be recommended. Surfactant therapy for infants with congenital diaphragmatic hernia (CDH) has also been attempted[213-219] but actually resulted in worse outcomes, and routine surfactant administration in CDH therefore is not recommended.

CONCLUSION

Exogenous surfactant therapy has been a significant advance in the management of preterm infants with RDS and has become established as a standard part of the management of such infants. Both animal-derived and synthetic surfactants lead to clinical improvement and decreased mortality, with animal-derived surfactants having advantages over synthetic surfactants. Infants with RDS who are spontaneously breathing should be initially stabilized on CPAP of at least 6 cm H_2O via mask or nasal prongs. In infants requiring surfactant therapy, earlier treatment (before 2 hours) has benefits over later treatment. Less invasive surfactant administration without endotracheal intubation and positive pressure is emerging as the preferred way to administer surfactant. The use of multiple doses of surfactant as needed is superior to the use of a single dose, and the use of a higher threshold for retreatment appears to be as effective as a low threshold. The adverse effects of surfactant therapy are infrequent and usually not serious; long term follow-up of infants treated with surfactant in the neonatal period is reassuring. Research on synthetic surfactants is ongoing. Further research is required on the optimal use of surfactant in conjunction with other respiratory interventions. Optimal respiratory outcomes in infants with RDS require attention to not just exogenous surfactant therapy but also to administration of antenatal steroids in mothers at risk for preterm delivery, management in the delivery room immediately after birth, oxygen therapy, and modalities of respiratory support.[220]

A complete reference list is available at https://expertconsult.inkling.com/.

KEY REFERENCES

16. Halliday HL: History of surfactant from 1980. Biol Neonate 87(4):317–322, 2005.
59. Seger N, Soll R: Animal derived surfactant extract for treatment of respiratory distress syndrome. Cochrane Database Syst Rev (Online) (2):CD007836, 2009.
62. Hamvas A, Wise PH, Yang RK, et al.: The influence of the wider use of surfactant therapy on neonatal mortality among blacks and whites. N Engl J Med 334(25):1635–1640, 1996.
74. Bahadue FL, Soll R: Early versus delayed selective surfactant treatment for neonatal respiratory distress syndrome. Cochrane Database Syst Rev (Online) 11:CD001456, 2012.
101. Abdel-Latif ME, Davis PG, Wheeler KI, et al: Surfactant therapy via thin catheter in preterm infants with or at risk of respiratory distress syndrome. Cochrane Database Syst Rev 5(5):CD011672, 2021.
102. Reynolds P, Bustani P, Darby C, et al: Less-invasive surfactant administration for neonatal respiratory distress syndrome: a consensus guideline. Neonatology 118(5):586–592, 2021.
130. Singh N, Halliday HL, Stevens TP, et al: Comparison of animal-derived surfactants for the prevention and treatment of respiratory distress syndrome in preterm infants. Cochrane Database Syst Rev (Online) 12:CD010249, 2015.
142. Raju TN, Langenberg P: Pulmonary hemorrhage and exogenous surfactant therapy: a metaanalysis [see comments]. J Pediatr 123(4):603–610, 1993.
197. El Shahed AI, Dargaville PA, Ohlsson A, et al: Surfactant for meconium aspiration syndrome in term and late preterm infants. Cochrane Database Syst Rev (Online) 12:CD002054, 2014.
220. Sweet DG, Carnielli V, Greisen G, et al: European consensus guidelines on the management of respiratory distress syndrome—2019 update. Neonatology 115(4):432–450, 2019.

16

Oxygen Therapy

Maximo Vento

KEY POINTS

- Aerobic metabolism, in the presence of oxygen, renders essential for growth and development of multicellular organisms. However, excessive oxygen supplementation leads to the formation of reactive oxygen species, which are highly damaging for cell components such as lipids, proteins, and nucleic acids. Mass spectrometry methods have been developed to measure biomarkers of oxidative stress and damage in controlled clinical studies.
- With the initiation of airborne breathing oxygen saturation as measured by preductal pulse oximetry, SpO_2 rapidly increases to reach values of 85% at 5 minutes after birth. Thereafter, SpO_2 slowly increases to reach 90% to 95% at 10 minutes.
- Term infants with asphyxia should be initially ventilated with an inspired fraction of oxygen (FiO_2) of 0.21 (room air). FiO_2 should be titrated according to the infant's response assessed by heart rate and SpO_2.
- Preterm infants, especially very preterm (<28 weeks' gestation), should be ventilated in the delivery room with an initial FiO_2 of 0.3. FiO_2 should be then titrated aiming to reach a preductal SpO_2 of 85% at 5 minutes after birth. Delays in reaching this target saturation significantly increase the risk of death and/or intraventricular hemorrhage.
- Preterm infants should be kept within an SpO_2 range of 90% to 95% during their neonatal intensive care unit stay if they are receiving oxygen supplementation therapy. Prolonged periods of intermittent hypoxia (SpO_2 <80%) cause neurodevelopmental delay and should be avoided. Automatic loop devices to keep SpO_2 within preestablished limits have become a promising tool to avoid damage caused either by hyperoxia or hypoxia.
- Babies with severe respiratory insufficiency may need oxygen supplementation at home to maintain an adequate growth and development. Strict protocols and implication of parents and primary care pediatricians are essential to avoid complications.

HISTORY OF THE USE OF OXYGEN IN CLINICAL MEDICINE

Although anecdotal information indicates that oxygen was already known by the Chinese in the thirteenth century, our present knowledge of its chemical and biological characteristics and its clinical application derives from the discoveries made almost simultaneously by C.W. Scheele (Sweden), Joseph Priestley (Britain), and Antoine-Laurent de Lavoisier (France). By heating mercury oxide, silver carbonate, magnesium nitrate, and potassium nitrate, they all produced the same gas previously known as phlogiston and that later was identified as a source of life because it allowed the survival of a mouse in a sealed jar, whereas without addition of this gas, the mouse would die. Moreover, Priestley showed that plants were capable of producing it, and thus, he opened the path for further studies on photosynthesis. The name oxygen comes from the Greek words oxys (acrid) and gene (something that produces something), meaning a substance that produces acids. Still today, in German, oxygen is known as Sauerstoff, or acidic substance.[1]

Oxygen was first used in neonatology in the eighteenth century for the resuscitation of newborn infants. At the beginning of the twentieth century, oxygen was infused in the umbilical vessels of asphyxiated infants or directly given into the pharynx or via a gastric catheter.[2] In the 1930s, oxygen started to be used liberally in the treatment of preterm infants suffering respiratory distress. With the ongoing use of oxygen, clinical scientists started to describe its positive and negative effects undoubtedly associated with its restricted or liberal use in the treatment of neonatal patients. Oxygen, when liberally used, was identified as the agent that caused what was initially called retrolental fibroplasia (RLF), characterized by the formation of a thick membrane in the retrolental space that resulted in damage and detachment of the retina and frequently blindness. This severe ophthalmologic condition had already caused blindness in about 10,000 infants in the early 1950s. Randomized trials performed in 1954 to 1956 clearly showed that the liberal use of oxygen was a major cause of RLF. It is important to note that at that time, the level of oxygenation of the patients could be monitored only by observing respiratory rate, heart rate (HR), and/or color. Beginning in the 1960s, objective oxygen monitoring, such as blood gas analysis, transcutaneous oxygen monitoring, and later on pulse oximetry, was incorporated into the routine of care of preterm infants, allowing a more precise means of supervising oxygen status and supplementation.

The establishment of a causative relationship between excessive oxygen and RLF unfortunately pushed the pendulum to the opposite extreme, and oxygen was drastically limited even in the most severe cases of respiratory distress. Prolonged and extreme hypoxemia resulted in an exponential increase in cerebral palsy and mortality from respiratory failure; thus, for every baby saved from RLF, 16 died of respiratory insufficiency.

Since 1995, experimental and clinical research has exponentially increased our knowledge of oxygen metabolism and its toxic consequences in the neonatal period. The front line of neonatal research is directed especially at three different stages during the perinatal period when oxygen is most frequently needed: (1) the fetal-to-neonatal transition and postnatal adaptation—that is, the need for oxygen in the delivery room; (2) the oxygen saturation target ranges when oxygen is supplemented in the neonatal intensive care unit (NICU); and (3) the need for oxygen at home after hospital discharge of patients with chronic conditions.[3,4]

This chapter is meant to provide a comprehensive approach to the relevant basic, metabolic, and clinical aspects related to oxygen therapy in the newborn period.

BASIC PRINCIPLES OF OXYGEN PHYSIOLOGY

Aerobic Metabolism

Oxygen (O_2) is one of the most abundant elements in nature; the second most abundant component of breathing air, constituting 21% of its composition; and probably the most widely used drug in neonatology.[5] The presence of oxygen will allow the complete combustion of glucose, amino acids, and free fatty acids in a highly efficient process that produces approximately 20 times more energy than anaerobic combustion. This process takes place within the mitochondria, which act as the energy factories of the cell (Fig. 16.1). Substrates are metabolized into acetyl coenzyme A, which enters the tricarboxylic acid cycle (Krebs cycle) where energy in the form of highly energized electrons is liberated and transported by specific proteins (NADH, NADPH, FADH) to the electron transport chain (ETC) located in the inner mitochondrial membrane. Electrons, considered reducing equivalents, provide the energy necessary to maintain the electrochemical gradient that drives adenosine triphosphate (ATP) synthesis. Components of the ETC pump protons across the inner mitochondrial membrane against an electrochemical gradient, and the protons are taken in again by ATP synthase. In this process, energy is recovered and employed to transform adenosine diphosphate into ATP. Electrons are captured by oxygen, thus permitting the formation of water and avoiding electron leakage and formation of free radicals; thus, each molecule of dioxygen will be completely reduced by four electrons.[6] Metabolic substrates used to provide energy are highly organ specific; thus, the central nervous system and erythrocytes almost exclusively depend on glucose, whereas cardiac contraction uses energy provided from the combustion mainly of free fatty acids.[7] Oxidative phosphorylation provides most of the ATP needed by the body and is especially relevant in aerobic-dependent tissues known as oxyregulators, such as brain. These organs cannot adapt for even short periods of time in the absence of oxygen without undergoing necrosis and/or apoptosis.[8]

Reactive Oxygen Species, Redox Regulation, and Antioxidant Enzymes

The term reactive oxygen species (ROS) refers to a series of molecules derived from incomplete reduction of molecular dioxygen

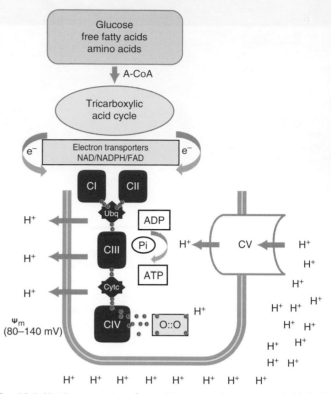

Fig. 16.1 Nutrients are transformed into acetyl coenzyme A (*A-CoA*), which is metabolized in the inner mitochondrial space along the tricarboxylic acid cycle. During this process, energized electrons are liberated and transported to the electron transport chain, creating a mitochondrial transmembrane potential (Ψm). Energy is used to first extrude protons (H^+) that are thereafter taken in again by adenosine triphosphate (*ATP*) synthase, and liberated energy is employed to resynthesize ATP from adenosine diphosphate (*ADP*). Oxygen will be reduced with four electrons. This process is known as *oxidative phosphorylation*. *FAD*, Flavin adenine dinucleotide; *NAD*, nicotine adenine dinucleotide; *NADPH*, nicotine adenine dinucleotide phosphorylated.

(Fig. 16.2). Even under physiologic conditions, a small percentage of electrons will "leak," causing a "partial" reduction of oxygen (oxygen with fewer than four electrons). The incomplete reduction of oxygen with one electron elicits the production of anion superoxide ($\cdot O_2-$), [$\cdot O_2-$] with the addition of two electrons will lead to the generation of hydrogen peroxide (H_2O_2), and with a third electron, the highly reactive hydroxyl radical (OH) will be produced.[9] ROS are also relevant in the regulation of nitric oxide (NO) metabolism and availability and therefore indirectly have an important influence on airway and vascular reactivity. Hence, when superoxide anion binds to NO, peroxynitrite ($ONOO-$) will be produced. Peroxynitrite is a highly reactive nitrogen species but also influences vascular reactivity in such areas as the lung, where its production can lead to increased vasoconstriction, causing pulmonary hypertension.[10] The production of ROS under physiologic and also pathologic conditions is highly dependent on the concentration of oxygen in the tissue. ROS are produced in hypoxic and hyperoxic situations and especially when the oxygen concentration fluctuates from hyperoxia to hypoxia and vice versa. ROS can be extremely aggressive when acting as free radicals, causing direct structural and/or functional damage and/or interfering with essential redox-regulatory elements. In other

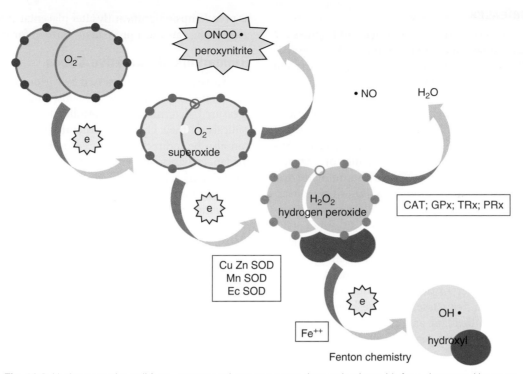

Fig. 16.2 Under normal conditions, oxygen undergoes a tetravalent reduction with four electrons. However, under certain circumstances, oxygen is reduced stepwise by one electron at a time. This leads to the formation of reactive oxygen species, some of which are free radicals (e.g., superoxide anion from monovalent reduction and hydroxyl radical from trivalent reduction), whereas others are not (hydrogen peroxide from divalent reduction). Hydrogen peroxide acts as a signaling molecule. Hydroxyl radical formation is enhanced in the presence of transition metals such as iron, copper, and manganese by the so-called Fenton chemistry. The antioxidant system neutralizes the chemical reactivity of free radicals. *CAT*, Catalase; *GPx*, glutathione peroxidase; *PRx*, peroxiredoxin; *SOD*, superoxide dismutase; *TRx*, thioredoxin.

circumstances, ROS can be relatively stable and act as signaling molecules in physiologic processes.[11]

The term free radical refers to any molecule capable of independent existence with one or more unpaired electrons in the outer shell (e.g., anion superoxide, hydroxyl radical). Free radicals form covalent bonds to share one electron with other molecules; however, the resulting molecule easily decomposes, leading to the formation of toxic products. Free radicals may also react with nonradical molecules in typical chain reactions, causing damage to DNA, proteins, and lipids or promoting the formation of adducts with DNA. Under very stressful conditions (ischemia-reperfusion, inflammation, or hyperoxia), damage caused by free radicals can lead to cell death by necrosis or apoptosis or marked cellular dysfunction.[12] In addition to mitochondrial respiration, ROS are produced also by the cytochrome P450 monooxygenase system, xanthine oxidoreductase, NO synthases, heme oxygenases (HOs), and other enzymes involved in inflammatory processes. Moreover, in the presence of transition metals such as iron, copper, zinc, and manganese, the generation of ROS can be exponentially increased.[8]

ROS also have a relevant role in cell physiology. At low/moderate concentrations, especially those ROS that are not free radicals (e.g., hydrogen peroxide) elicit an ample array of cellular responses acting as signaling molecules. Thus, ROS-mediated actions can be protective against ROS-induced oxidative stress and reestablish or maintain redox homeostasis. One of the most important roles of ROS is the regulation of NO production, the oxidative burst produced as a response to infectious agents by phagocytic NAD(P)H oxidase, or acting as sensing elements for regulating tissue oxygen needs, cell adhesion, immune responses, or induced apoptosis.[13]

Redox Regulation

The concept of oxidative stress as a global imbalance affecting the entire economy no longer adequately explains redox biology. Central sulfur-disulfide couples, which include reduced and oxidized glutathione (GSH/GSSG), cysteine/cystine, and reduced and oxidized thioredoxin, function as reducing counterparts of H_2O_2 and other oxidants in controlling the redox state of oxidizable thiols in proteins. These sulfur switches in which hydrogen peroxide has a relevant role are used for cell signaling, protein structure, protein trafficking, and regulation of enzyme, transporter, receptor, and transcription factor activity. Redox mechanisms control proinflammatory and profibrotic signaling, cell proliferation, apoptosis, and a range of other biologic processes by modifying the protein structure without involving oxidative structural or functional changes. This concept differs from previous thinking in which the importance of free radical mechanisms and macromolecular damage as an underlying mechanism was overemphasized.[14]

Antioxidant Defenses

The redox balance at various sites in our organism requires the intervention of antioxidant defenses to counterbalance the generation of ROS. These mechanisms include both enzymatic and nonenzymatic processes. Antioxidant enzymes, through catalytic reactions, remove ROS and protect proteins through the use of chaperones, transition metal-containing proteins (transferrin, ferritin, ceruloplasmin), and low-molecular-weight compounds that function as oxidizing or reducing agents. Superoxide dismutases (SODs) constitute a family of enzymes located in the cytoplasm (Cu/Zn SOD), in the mitochondria (Mn/Cu SOD), or extracellularly (Zn/Cu SOD), which convert or dismutate superoxide anions to H_2O_2. Catalases and glutathione peroxidases (GPx) convert H_2O_2 into H_2O and O_2. GPx couples H_2O_2 reduction to water with the oxidation of GSH to GSSG. GSSG is again reduced to GSH by the activity of the pentose shunt. Other systems that detoxify hydrogen peroxide in mitochondria and other organelles include glutaredoxin, thioredoxin, thioredoxin reductase, and the peroxiredoxins. Other enzymes with antioxidant and signaling functions are HOs (HO-1 and HO-2). HO-1 removes heme, a prooxidant, and generates biliverdin, an antioxidant-releasing iron, and carbon monoxide. Finally, nonenzymatic antioxidants such as GSH, vitamin C, vitamin E, and β-carotene also function to protect cells from the damaging effects of ROS.[9] The ontogeny of enzymatic antioxidant expression progresses gradually during gestation. Compared with full-term infants, preterm infants have immature antioxidant defenses, which are more susceptible to ROS-associated conditions derived from hypoxia-reoxygenation, inflammation, or infection. In addition, transplacental passage of antioxidants also occurs late in gestation. In assays performed in human abortus materials, it has been shown that antioxidant enzyme activities in response to oxidant insults increase with advancing gestation. As a consequence, conditions occurring during pregnancy such as preeclampsia significantly alter placental antioxidant enzyme expression, causing a prooxidant burden for the fetus.[15]

Biomarkers of Oxidative Stress

Oxidative stress can be assessed by various means. Direct damage to molecules such as proteins, lipids, and DNA can be measured, determining the results of the interaction with free radicals on their chemical structure. However, oxidative stress can also be indirectly measured by increased activity of antioxidant enzymes or increment in the concentration of oxidized antioxidants such as the GSH/GSSG ratio. In clinical research, determination of the concentration derived from free radical aggregation in biofluids such as blood, plasma, serum, urine, or cerebrospinal fluid has gained popularity. Table 16.1 summarizes the most widely employed biomarkers of oxidative stress. The GSH/GSSG ratio is a comprehensive indicator of redox status and can be determined in whole blood. Lipid peroxidation is determined by measuring malondialdehyde in blood or urine. However, isoprostanes, reflecting noncyclooxygenase oxidation of arachidonic acid, are now widely employed because they are very stable and not influenced by diet, parenteral nutrition, or gestational age (GA). The preferred method is liquid chromatography coupled to mass spectrometry. Isofurans, which reflect the oxidation of arachidonic acid under hyperoxic conditions, have been very satisfactorily employed in neonatal studies involving the use of oxygen. Other similar biomarkers are neuroprostanes and neurofurans. Neurofurans reflect the oxidation of docosahexaenoic acid specifically present in the brain and therefore may reflect damage caused by oxidative stress to brain tissue.16 Recently, biomarkers of oxidative damage to adrenic acid, a principal component of cerebral white matter, have been incorporated into the armamentarium of biomarkers. Oxidation of adrenic acid leads to the formation of Di-homo-isoprostanes and Di-homo-isofurans, both of which are highly selective indicators of damage to

---

TABLE 16.1   Main Oxidative Biomarkers Used in the Clinical Setting and Human Research and the Most Reliable Techniques to Measure Them

Biomarker	Target Molecule	Biologic Effect	Biofluid Determination	Analytical Method
Glutathione (GSH/GSSG ratio)	Antioxidants	General redox status	Total blood	LC-MS/MS
MDA	Lipids	PUFA peroxidation	Plasma	HPLC (UV detection)
HNE	Lipids	PUFA peroxidation	Plasma	HPLC
o-Tyrosine (o-Tyr/Phe ratio)	Proteins	Tyrosine hydroxylation	Urine	LC-MS/MS
m-Tyrosine (m-Tyr/Phe ratio)	Proteins	Tyrosine hydroxylation	Urine	LC-MS/MS
3N2-tyrosine	Proteins	Tyrosine nitration	Urine	LC-MS/MS
8OHdG (8OHdG/2dG ratio)	Lipids	AA peroxidation	Urine/plasma	LC-MS/MS
F2-IsoPs	Lipids	AA peroxidation	Urine/plasma	GC-MS/MS; LC-MS/MS
D2/F2-IsoPs	Lipids	AA peroxidation	Urine/plasma	GC-MS/MS; LC-MS/MS
IsoFs	Lipids	AA peroxidation	Urine/plasma	GC-MS/MS; LC-MS/MS
NeuPs	Lipids	DHA peroxidation	Urine/plasma	GC-MS/MS; LC-MS/MS
NeuFs	Lipids	DHA peroxidation	Urine/plasma	GC-MS/MS; LC-MS/MS

AA, Arachidonic acid; *DHA*, docosahexaenoic acid; *8OHdG*, 8-hydroxy-2′-deoxyguanosine; *GC*, gas chromatography; *GSH*, reduced glutathione; *GSSG*, oxidized glutathione; *HNE*, 4-hydroxy-2-nonenal; *HPLC*, high-performance liquid chromatography; *IsoFs*, isofurans; *IsoPs*, isoprostanes; *LC*, liquid chromatography; *MDA*, malondialdehyde; *MS/MS*, tandem mass spectrometry; *m-Tyr*, *meta*-tyrosine; *NeuFs*, neurofurans; *NeuPs*, neuroprostanes; *PUFA*, polyunsaturated fatty acid; *o-Tyr*, ortho-tyrosine; *3N2-tyrosine*, 3-nitrotyrosine; *2dG*, 2′-deoxyguanosine; *UV*, ultraviolet.

cerebral white matter by free radicals.[17] Damage to proteins can be assessed by mass spectrometry determining *ortho-* or *meta-*tyrosine, which reflects the oxidation of circulating phenylalanine in a nonphysiologic metabolic pathway. Finally, determining the oxidation of the guanidine bases in urine or plasma assesses DNA damage, reflecting oxidation of the cell nucleus. There are many other biomarkers (RNA, glycoproteins, exhaled compounds, etc.) under evaluation, but these are still applicable only in more basic research.[16]

Oxygen-Sensing Mechanisms and Physiologic Response

The following is a brief description of oxygen and hypoxia-inducible factor (HIF-1) interaction and erythropoietin (EPO) expression. Oxygen homeostasis is critical for the survival and function of cells and organisms. On one hand, oxygen in excess (hyperoxia) inevitably causes an excessive production of ROS, causing cell damage. On the other hand, the complete absence of oxygen (anoxia) is lethal. Physiologic systems are therefore adapted to achieve the proper equilibrium between oxygen demand and availability to ensure correct cellular functioning. A number of redox-sensitive transcription factors such as HIF-1, cyclic adenosine monophosphate response element-binding protein, nuclear factor κB, activator protein 1, and p53 regulate gene expression in response to changes in the concentration of ROS.[18]

Variations in oxygen concentration in the body elicit two types of responses. During acute hypoxia, pulmonary vasoconstriction and carotid body neurosecretion dependent on increased intracellular calcium levels mediated by ROS are essential for survival. If hypoxia is prolonged, activation of the HIF transcription factors will be triggered.[19] The oxygen level in utero at the time of implantation is around 15 to 20 mm Hg and remains at this low level until the end of the first trimester, providing an adequate environment (reductive) for fetal and placental development.[20-22] Angiogenesis is stimulated by low oxygen concentrations in tissue through transcriptional and posttranscriptional regulation of growth factors such as vascular endothelial growth factor (VEGF), EPO, placental growth factor, and angiopoietins 1 and 2.[18] The master regulator of the cell's adaptive response to hypoxia is HIF-1, a heterodimeric transcription factor comprising HIF-1α and HIF-1β subunits. HIF-1α protein is continuously synthesized; however, if the O_2 concentration in tissue is normal or high, it will undergo proteasomal degradation. Under conditions below the specific critical oxygen threshold, HIF-1α protein will be stabilized and will bind to the hypoxia-responsive element of DNA and elicit the expression of numerous genes (Fig. 16.3). HIF-1β is constitutively present in the cell nucleus. Activated genes, and especially VEGF and EPO, are meant to enhance O_2 delivery to tissues.[22]

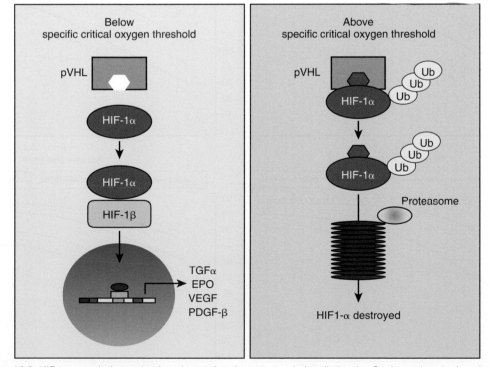

Fig. 16.3 HIF-1α protein is predominantly regulated posttranscriptionally by the O_2-dependent hydroxylation of two proline residues by the prolyl-hydroxylase enzymes, leading to ubiquitination and proteasomal degradation. HIF-1α is stabilized when the concentrations of oxygen are below the specific critical oxygen threshold, thus accumulating in the hypoxic cell. When oxygen overcomes metabolic needs, HIF-1α binds to the von Hippel-Lindau *(pVHL)* protein, which recruits a ubiquitin *(Ub)* ligase that targets *HIF-1α* for proteasomal degradation. *HIF-1β* is constitutively present in the cell nucleus. *EPO,* Erythropoietin; *HIF-1α,* hypoxia-inducible factor 1α; *PDGF-β,* platelet-derived growth factor β; *TGFα,* transforming growth factor α; *VEGF,* vascular endothelial growth factor. (Modified from Vento M, Teramo K: Evaluating the fetus at risk for cardiopulmonary compromise. Semin Fetal Neonatal Med 8(6):324–329, 2013.)

OXYGEN IN THE FETAL-TO-NEONATAL TRANSITION AND POSTNATAL ADAPTATION

Fetal-to-Neonatal Transition

The fetal arterial partial pressure of oxygen (PaO_2) is 25 to 35 mm Hg (3.5–4.5 kPa), reaching even lower values of 17 to 19 mm Hg (2.2–2.5 kPa) in the pulmonary circulation.[23] Although apparently isolated by the fetal membranes, the fetus is highly susceptible to changes in the mother's oxygenation status. Therefore, maternal hypoxia and/or hyperoxia will rapidly induce changes in the oxygen metabolism of the fetus. Hence, maternal hyperoxia induced by oxygen supplementation during anesthesia will cause an oxidative stress in the fetus with increased concentrations of malondialdehyde and F2-isoprostanes in the cord blood.[24] With the initiation of air respiration and the cardiopulmonary circulatory changes that characterize postnatal adaptation after cord clamping, PaO_2 will rise to approximately 65 to 75 mm Hg in the first 5 to 10 minutes after birth in the healthy full-term infant. Increased oxygen availability will cause physiologic oxidative stress and trigger specific gene expression to ensure postnatal adaptation. Term newborn infants reach stable arterial oxygen saturation (SpO_2) values around 85% to 90% by 5 minutes after birth. However, some healthy normal newborn infants need even more time, especially if they are born by cesarean section. Remarkably, preterm infants, especially extremely preterm, those with GAs 28 weeks or less, need almost 10 minutes to reach preductal SpO_2 of around 85%. Postnatal oxygenation is highly dependent on GA, type of delivery, and whether the baby is breathing spontaneously or requires some type of respiratory support.[4]

Arterial Oxygen Saturation Nomogram

By collecting data prospectively using preductal pulse oximetry with identical methodology in 468 newly born infants with GAs ranging from 25 to 42 weeks who did not receive oxygen at birth, it was possible to build an oxygen saturation nomogram reflecting the first 10 minutes after birth. The data were represented in a smoothed graph that included mean and ±3 standard deviations of preductal SpO_2 minute by minute for the first 10 minutes after birth. Data collected by Dawson and coworkers in term and preterm infants are shown in Fig. 16.4A–D. As of this writing, Dawson's oxygen saturation nomogram represents the best estimate of the physiologic oxygenation that occurs in normal term or well-adapted preterm infants in the first minutes after birth.[25]

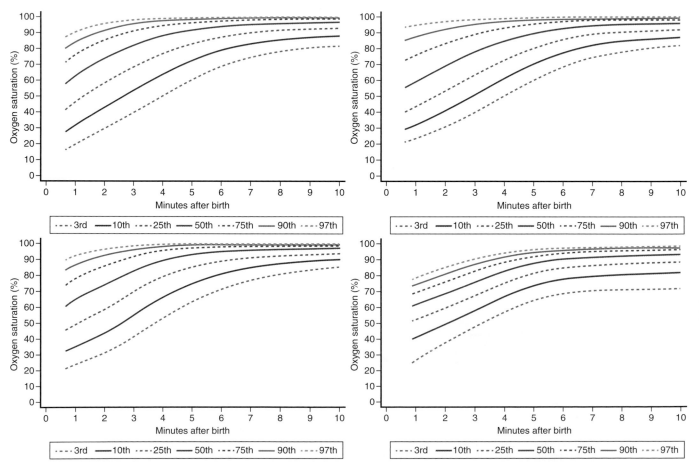

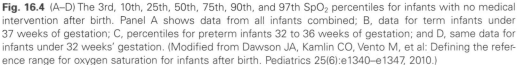

Fig. 16.4 (A–D) The 3rd, 10th, 25th, 50th, 75th, 90th, and 97th SpO_2 percentiles for infants with no medical intervention after birth. Panel A shows data from all infants combined; B, data for term infants under 37 weeks of gestation; C, percentiles for preterm infants 32 to 36 weeks of gestation; and D, same data for infants under 32 weeks' gestation. (Modified from Dawson JA, Kamlin CO, Vento M, et al: Defining the reference range for oxygen saturation for infants after birth. Pediatrics 25(6):e1340–e1347, 2010.)

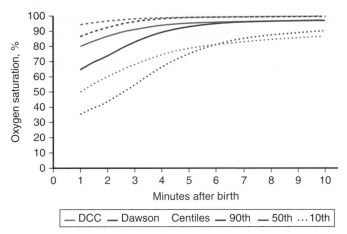

Fig. 16.5 Comparison of the 10th, 50th and 90th percentiles for SpO₂ measured with preductal PO between Dawson's reference range[30] and term newborn babies born by vaginal delivery not needing resuscitation after birth and delayed cord clamping for ≥60 seconds reproduced according to Padilla-Sánchez et al. *DCC*, DCC = delayed cord clamping. (From Padilla-Sánchez C, Baixauli-Alacreu S, Cañada-Martínez AJ, et al: Delayed vs. immediate cord clamping changes oxygen saturation and heart rate patterns in the first minutes after birth. J Pediatr 227:149–156, 2020.)

In the last decade, delaying cord clamping for at least 1 minute after birth in term and preterm babies has been recommended by international guidelines.[26,27] Patent cord allows a substantial volume of blood to be transferred from the placenta to the newly born infant's circulation, contributing to increasing the right ventricular preload and enhancing pulmonary blood flow and hemodynamic stability.[28] Recently, reference ranges for term infants, born by vaginal delivery allowed cord patency for more than 1 minute, and not needing resuscitation or oxygen at birth have been constructed. Minute-by-minute data for HR and preductal oxygen saturation (SpO₂) were retrieved during the first 10 minutes after fetal expulsion. Significantly higher values for SpO₂ for the 10th, 50th, and 90th centiles compared with Dawson's reference range for the first 5 minutes and for HR for the first 1–2 minutes after birth were reported.[25,29] Hence, in healthy infants born by vaginal delivery and with delayed cord clamping more than 60 seconds, higher SpO₂ and HR were achieved in the first 5 minutes after birth compared with term neonates born with immediate cord clamping (Fig. 16.5).[29]

OXYGEN SATURATION IN PRETERM INFANTS WITH POSITIVE PRESSURE VENTILATION AND AIR

Continuous positive airway pressure (CPAP) applied immediately after birth with a pressure of 5 to 6 cm H₂O facilitates the achievement of a functional residual capacity (FRC) in preterm babies immediately, thereby improving oxygenation and decreasing work of breathing.[30] Very preterm babies with GAs 28 weeks or less receiving CPAP and inspiratory fraction of oxygen (FiO₂) of 0.21 achieved stable preductal SpO₂ values significantly earlier than babies of similar GAs who were breathing spontaneously without CPAP. It was intriguing that female premature infants

achieved saturation targets significantly more rapidly than males.[31] These data indicate that the use of CPAP facilitates lung volume recruitment and the establishment of an adequate FRC, which in turn reduces the need for supplemental oxygen during postnatal stabilization, consistent with numerous experimental studies that have shown the benefit of positive end expiratory pressure in the fetal-to-neonatal transition.[32,33]

Oxygen Administration in the Delivery Room

The use of room air (21% oxygen) in the resuscitation of asphyxiated term newborn infants reduces the time needed to achieve a spontaneous respiration, improves Apgar score at 1 minute, reduces the oxygen load and oxidative stress, reduces damage to the heart and kidney, and most importantly, significantly reduces mortality compared to the initial use of 100% oxygen.[34] International guidelines in 2015 have recommended the use of air as the initial gas mixture for the depressed neonate. Moreover, both pulse oximetry monitoring of SpO₂ and titration of the FiO₂ to avoid hyperoxic or hypoxic damage are also encouraged.[26,27,35]

Initial FiO2 for preterm infants in the delivery room remains a matter of debate. No reference ranges are available to guide neonatologists how to start and how to titrate FiO₂ during postnatal stabilization. In a recent Cochrane review, the use of lower (<40%) versus higher (>40%) oxygen concentrations to achieve targeted saturations during resuscitation of very preterm infants after birth was compared. No differences in relevant outcomes such as mortality, bronchopulmonary dysplasia (BPD), combined outcome of death or BPD, retinopathy of prematurity (ROP), intra/periventricular hemorrhage (IPVH), or necrotizing enterocolitis (NEC) when using an initial FiO₂ of less than 40% vs more than 40% were found.[36] In addition, the most recent and largest systematic review with metaanalysis including 10 studies and 5607 preterm infants under 35 weeks' gestation performed by Welsford et al.[37] also failed to show differences between babies receiving higher (>50%) and babies receiving lower (<50%) initial FiO₂ in the delivery room. However, the authors pointed out that the majority of newborns 32 weeks' gestation or less would require oxygen supplementation upon stabilization.[37] The use of lower initial FiO₂ could have the advantage of reducing the oxygen load received during initial stabilization and thus reduce oxidative stress. In two studies, initiation of resuscitation with very high initial FiO₂ (90% or 100%) with subsequent titration resulted in increased oxidant stress and BPD incidence compared to starting with 21% or 30%.[38,39] In contrast, no differences in clinical outcomes or biomarkers of oxidative stress were found when an initial FiO₂ of 30% was compared with 60% or 65%.[40,41] However, recent observations in extremely premature infants (<28 weeks' gestation) have raised doubts about the optimal strategy to supplement these vulnerable patients with oxygen in the first minutes after birth. The Targeted Oxygenation in the Resuscitation of Premature Infants (TORPIDO) study randomized infants under 32 weeks' GA to air or 100% oxygen.[42] In a post hoc analysis, infants under 28 weeks' GA had a relative increased risk for mortality of almost four-fold if initially started with air compared with 100% O₂ (risk ratio [RR], 3.9; 95% confidence interval

[CI], 1.1–13.4).[42] Oei et al., seeking an explanation for the results of the TORPIDO trial, performed a systematic review of the outcomes of infants ≤28 + 6 weeks' gestation randomized to resuscitation with low (≤0.3) versus high (≥0.6) FiO_2 at delivery. They did not find differences in the overall risk of death or other common preterm morbidities, including BPD, NEC, ROP, patent ductus arteriosus, and intraventricular hemorrhage, after resuscitation is initiated at delivery with lower or higher FiO_2.[43] The key for resolving this conundrum resides in the achievement of saturations of at least 80% to 85% in the first 5 minutes after birth independently of the initial FiO_2, GA, gender, or type of delivery. Reaching adequate oxygenation and avoiding episodes of bradycardia in the first 5 minutes after birth seem essential to enhance postnatal stability and avoid death or serious complications such as IVH.[44] Hence, Oei et al. analyzed data from 768 infants under 32 weeks' GA enrolled in eight randomized controlled trials (RCTs) initially resuscitated with higher (≥0.6) or lower (≤0.3) initial FiO_2. Those babies who, independent from the initial FiO_2, did not reach a SpO_2 of 80% within 5 minutes after birth had higher mortality, more severe IVH, and poorer neurodevelopmental outcome than those who reached this level.[45] Until further studies shed light on this important issue, both experts and consensus guidelines recommend to initiate resuscitation of infants 28 to 31 weeks with an initial FiO_2 of 0.21 to 0.30 guiding oxygen titration up and down with the use of pulse oximetry aiming to achieve SpO_2 of 80% to 85% and HR over 100 beats per minute within 5 minutes.[46,47]

The use of pulse oximetry has become an essential tool in the delivery room. Preductal pulse oximetry reflects oxygenation of blood going to the brain and therefore is preferred during postnatal stabilization. Reliable preductal readings within 1 to 2 minutes of birth can be rapidly obtained with adequate training. Data are rapidly displayed if these steps are followed: (1) turn on the oximeter, (2) apply the sensor to the infant's right hand or wrist, (3) connect the sensor to the oximeter cable, and (4) shield the sensor from light. By attaching the sensor to the baby before connecting the oximeter cable to the monitor, the response time to reliable readings is shortened. Once reliable readings of the pulse oximeter are achieved and the baby is being ventilated, FiO_2 should be titrated against pulse oximeter readings of the HR and saturation. The air/oxygen blender should be adjusted accordingly to avoid hyperoxia and hypoxia. Hence, if SpO_2 is below the 10th percentile, then FiO_2 should be increased in 10% increments every 30 seconds until SpO_2 reaches its 10th to 50th percentile, always avoiding going above the 90th percentile of SpO_2.[30] These recommendations are based on experts' opinions; there is no evidence-based information as of this writing regarding the best way of adjusting the oxygen concentration according to the pulse oximeter readings. The American Heart Association has defined the target ranges for 1, 2, 3, 4, 5, and 10 minutes after birth at 60% to 65%, 65% to 70%, 70% to 75%, 75% to 80%, 80% to 85%, and 85% to 90%, respectively.[26] Hence, until sufficiently powered studies are available, our aim should be to reduce the oxygen load during resuscitation in the first minutes of life, trying to adjust SpO_2 to the reference charts, which at present are our best estimate of the best oxygenation targets in preterm infants. It should be underscored that delayed cord clamping may introduce substantial changes in the reference ranges and, consequently, in the target saturations in the first minutes after birth.

OXYGEN DURING NEONATAL CARE IN THE NEONATAL INTENSIVE CARE UNIT

The establishment of optimal oxygen saturation targets for preterm infants needing oxygen supplementation in the NICU remains elusive. Preterm infants are very sensitive to hyperoxia, which may lead to lung and retinal damage and also to hypoxia, which may cause increased mortality, NEC, or white matter injury.[5] The lung of the extremely preterm infant has a tendency to suffer oxidative stress and inflammation because it lacks an adequately developed antioxidant defense system, is structurally and functionally immature, and frequently requires mechanical ventilation and supplemental oxygen. Additionally, the lungs are prone to infection and are exposed to increased circulating free iron.[48,49] A connection between oxygen, oxidative stress, mechanical ventilation, and genetic factors and later appearance of BPD has been substantiated in various studies.[50] Thus, preterm neonates who later developed BPD exhibited elevated concentrations in blood and tracheal aspirates of carbonyl adducts, which represent by-products of the attack of oxygen free radicals upon structural and functional proteins of the lung.[51-53] Similarly, elevated plasma isofurans immediately after birth with higher oxygen load and F2α-isoprostanes in the first week after birth have also been associated with later development of BPD and periventricular leukomalacia, indicating an important role for oxidative injury.[39,40,54] In addition to the acute and direct effects of free radicals upon the lung tissue, evidence reveals that specific oxygen species such as hydroperoxides may act as signaling molecules inducing the expression of transcription factors that may alter cell growth, differentiation, chemotaxis, inflammatory response, and/or apoptosis.[55]

Exposure to elevated oxygen concentration leads to the release of specific mediators such as VEGF and angiopoietin 2 capable of disrupting the alveolar-capillary membrane and thus causing pulmonary edema and subsequent lung injury. Other cytokines are also released from lung cells and attract inflammatory cells to the lung. These inflammatory cells, as well as hyperoxia per se, release ROS, which can initiate the mitochondrial-dependent cell death pathway.[56]

A series of RCTs has tried to assess the optimal SpO_2 range for preterm infants needing oxygen supplementation after postnatal stabilization. In the Benefits of Oxygen Saturation Targeting (BOOST) I trial, the effect of higher (95%–98%) versus lower (91%–94%) targeted saturations for babies of less than 30 weeks' gestation was compared. The use of higher SpO_2 limits was associated with an increased length of oxygen therapy, increased incidence of chronic lung disease, and increased frequency of babies discharged on home oxygen therapy, whereas it did not improve neurodevelopment or somatic growth.[57] In another RCT (STOP-ROP, or Supplemental Therapeutic Oxygen for Prethreshold Retinopathy of Prematurity), a group of preterm infants with prethreshold ROP was randomized to SpO_2 limits set between 89% and 94% or between 95% and 99% for a minimum of 2 weeks. The beneficial effect of higher SpO_2 on the evolution of eye disease was minimal, whereas the negative effects such as prolonged hospitalization, respiratory morbidity, and prolonged need for oxygen supplementation were significantly higher.[58]

Five multicenter, international, masked RCTs, the NeOProM studies, have been conducted. These trials enrolled nearly 5000 extremely low birth weight (ELBW) infants of under 28 weeks' gestation and sought to identify the optimal saturation target while following almost identical designs to allow for subsequent individual-level patient metaanalysis. All of these studies compared low-target SpO_2 (85%–89%) with high-target (91%–95%).[59] The Surfactant, Positive Pressure, and Oxygenation Randomized Trial (SUPPORT) trial confirmed that surviving ELBW infants randomly assigned to lower SpO_2 target ranges (85%–89%) had a lower risk of ROP (8.6% vs. 17.9%; $P < .01$) than those in the higher target group (91%–95%). However, unexpectedly, a significantly increased mortality was present in the low saturation group (19.9% vs. 16.2%; $P < .04$).[60] In addition, the BOOST II trial performed in the United Kingdom, Australia, and New Zealand showed similar results, with higher ROP in babies maintained in the high saturation range and higher mortality in babies kept in the low saturation range.[61] In contrast, the Canadian Oxygen Trial, using a primary outcome that was a composite of death, gross motor disability, cognitive or language delay, severe hearing loss, or bilateral blindness at a corrected age of 18 months, with secondary outcomes of ROP and brain injury, did not find significant differences in death or disability in babies in the lower compared with the higher saturation range.[62] In a metaanalysis that included all the NeOProM studies, with a total of approximately 5000 babies, it was concluded that when targeting SpO_2 in the lower range there was an increased risk of mortality (RR, 1.41; 95% CI, 1.14–1.74) and NEC (RR, 1.25; 95% CI, 1.05–1.49). However, in the lower saturation range, there was a significantly decreased risk of ROP (RR, 0.74; 95% CI, 0.59–0.92). The authors of this metaanalysis concluded that SpO_2 targets of 90% to 95% for babies born at less than 28 weeks' gestation needing supplemental oxygen were recommended until 36 weeks' postmenstrual age.[63] In a more recent metaanalysis using Cochrane Review methodology, the same five NeoProm trials were analyzed. When an aligned definition of major disability was used, there was no significant difference in the composite primary outcome of death or major disability in extremely preterm infants when targeting a lower (SpO_2 85%–89%) versus a higher (SpO_2 91%–95%) oxygen saturation range (typical RR, 1.04; 95% CI, 0.98–1.10; typical RD, 0.02; 95% CI, –0.01 to 0.05). However, compared with a higher target range, a lower target range significantly increased the incidence of death at 19 to 24 months corrected age and NEC. Targeting the lower range significantly decreased the incidence of ROP requiring treatment. No differences for blindness, hearing loss, cerebral palsy, or other important neonatal morbidities were noted.[64] Moreover, in a prospectively planned metaanalysis of individual participant data that included the NeoProm patients, results confirmed the previous Cochrane Review by Askie et al.[64] Hence, a lower SpO_2 target range was associated with a higher risk of death and NEC, but lower risk of ROP treatment.[65]

Although all of these trials had an impeccable design, some concerns especially from a technical perspective raised doubts about the practical applicability of their conclusions. It is relevant to know that the accuracy of the reading of the pulse oximeters employed was 2.9%. Thus, if the displayed SpO_2 is 88%, true saturation may be in the 85% to 91% range in 68% of observations and in the 82% to 94% range in 95% of observations.[66] In addition, the algorithm used in these trials resulted from the fusion of a high- and a low-range algorithm. The effect of this dual curve was that the SpO_2 values in the region of 87% to 90% (at the junction of the lower and higher algorithm curves) were shifted upward. Readings were therefore factitiously elevated around 2% in the proximity of saturations in the 90% range.[67] Given the relatively small separation in the mean SpO_2 between the high and the low target groups, these technical considerations make interpretation of the data challenging, and the optimal saturation range for extremely preterm infants needing oxygen supplementation remains elusive. It is likely that there is no fixed SpO_2 range or oxygen supply that safely satisfies the metabolic demands of all infants born at different GAs. Moreover, even for a given GA, postnatal age is also a relevant factor to be taken into consideration when establishing oxygen saturation limits. Although SpO_2 is relatively easily measured, it is not a direct reflection of tissue oxygen delivery. In addition to oxyhemoglobin saturation, oxygen delivery at the tissue level is affected by oxygen carrying capacity (hemoglobin level) and circulation and may more directly reflect the organism's oxygen sufficiency or excess. Finally, it is important to note that the findings of these trials may be largely related to our limited ability to maintain the SpO_2 within the target ranges during routine care. The exposure to extreme levels of SpO_2 may be more strongly related to the observed outcomes than the target ranges. In these trials, the actual SpO_2 levels did not exactly match the target ranges, and the exposure to extremely high or low SpO_2 ranges may have differed between the target ranges. In daily practice, during routine care, SpO_2 levels above the target range are frequently tolerated to reduce hypoxemia, but this practice increases the exposure to high SpO_2. Conversely, targeting lower SpO_2 ranges to avoid hyperoxemia can increase exposure to very low SpO_2 levels. Tolerance of high SpO_2 to avert hypoxemia spells or targeting low SpO_2 ranges to avoid hyperoxemia may not be necessary if the maintenance of the intended range of SpO_2 could be improved and exposure to extreme high or low SpO_2 minimized.

Until further evidence is available, keeping preterm babies within a range from 90% to 95% seems a reasonable approach. Minimizing fluctuation in SpO_2 would be desirable because alternating hypoxia and hyperoxia is known to be a proinflammatory stimulus. To that effect, there is a great deal of interest in improving oxygen saturation targeting by automatic control of FiO_2 (see Chapter 21).

EVOLVING OXYGEN NEEDS IN THE FIRST WEEKS OF LIFE AND NEW METABOLIC INDICES

Saugstad et al. suggested that it would be possible to differentiate between two periods with different oxygen limits.[68] Very preterm infants below 32 weeks' postmenstrual age would benefit from lower SpO_2 limits (e.g., 85%–95%) in a phase of rapid vascular growth and extreme sensitivity to free radical damage owing to an immature antioxidant defense system. During this stage, the use of higher oxygen limits would lead to oxidative stress and inflammation in the lung, intestine, or brain, leading to BPD, NEC, or IPVH. However, older neonates (>32 weeks' postmenstrual age) with a more mature antioxidant system and a tendency toward hyperproliferation of the vascular bed of the retina owing to a relative hypoxia of the retinal tissue would benefit from higher SpO_2 ranges (95%–97%). The latter approach, while based on sound physiologic principles, has not been conclusively established.[68] Hence, in the immediate postnatal period and independent of GA, the target saturation during the fetal-to-neonatal transition until postnatal stabilization is completed should be 90%. However, based on the findings of the SUPPORT and BOOST II trials, during the NICU stay, keeping the baby within a range of 90% to 95% seems adequate and safe. However, any attempt to maintain oxygen saturation in a narrow range must be balanced with alarm fatigue, as bedside caregivers must respond to the fluctuations of saturation levels in individual babies. Because there is very likely to be substantial individual variation in the susceptibility to oxidative injury, it would be useful to have at our disposal functional and noninvasive biomarkers, which would allow clinicians to monitor cell aerobic metabolism and evaluate the response to intervention. Traditional biomarkers of hypoxemia such as lactic acid do not significantly correlate with intensity but especially with the duration of hypoxia. Apparently, glycine/branched-chain amino acid or alanine/branched-chain amino acid ratios are far better predictors of duration of hypoxia. In addition, when metabolites from the Krebs cycle such as succinate and propionyl-l-carnitine were also taken into consideration, the correlation with the duration of cell hypoxia was further increased.[69] In a piglet model of hypoxic ischemic encephalopathy, Kuligowski et al. proposed a metabolite score calculated based on the relative intensities of choline, 6,8-dihydroxypurine and hypoxanthine that showed maximum correlation with hypoxia time. This combination of metabolites was compared to the performance of lactate, which is currently considered the gold standard. In the immediate posthypoxic insult period, both lactate and the metabolite score performed similar to lactate. However, after 2 hours of the insult, the metabolite score performed significantly better and provided an enhanced predictive capacity.[70] As of this writing, studies are being done on the levels of growth factors, such as insulin-like growth factor and VEGF, and metabolite ratios, which might be used at the bedside in the future to enable the clinician to have reliable information relative to cell oxygenation, which could ensure oxygen sufficiency and avert the initiation of retinal vascular proliferation.[68,69]

GOING HOME ON OXYGEN

Chronic lung disease and prolonged oxygen needs after discharge among extremely preterm infants (≤28 weeks' gestation) are a matter of clinical concern. In a 2013 study of 48,877 newborn infants of 23 to 43 weeks' gestation discharged from the NICUs of 228 hospitals in the United States, rates of BPD varied by GA, from 37% in extremely preterm infants to 0.7% in term infants. Of this cohort, 1286 infants (2.6%) were discharged on home oxygen, and 722 (56%) of the infants discharged on home oxygen were extremely preterm. Hence, GA was by far the most significant risk factor for needing home oxygen; however, other relevant factors were small-for-gestational-age infants, congenital anomalies, need for mechanical ventilation or for FiO_2 over 40% in the first 72 hours after birth, and patent ductus arteriosus.[71] The goal of home oxygen therapy is to prevent the effects of chronic hypoxemia, which include pulmonary vasoconstriction and pulmonary vascular remodeling leading to pulmonary hypertension, bronchial constriction leading to airway obstruction, and changes in growth of the ocular vasculature. Improved oxygenation may lead to improved lung growth and repair, better nutritional status, and somatic growth.[72,73] It is relevant to note that although BPD is a predictor of poor developmental outcome, those patients with severe BPD who were discharged home on oxygen did not score worse in neurodevelopmental tests than did patients with BPD who did not need home oxygen supplementation.[74] The decision about sending a baby home with oxygen is not an easy one. Before discharge, the baby has to fulfill a series of requirements or criteria, which are common to most institutions (Box 16.1). As a safety measure, oxygen reduction tests can be performed before discharge. The purpose of the oxygen reduction test is to see the nadir of SpO_2 reached in room air after supplemental oxygen has been discontinued. In most units, a minimum SpO_2 of greater than 80% should be maintained in air for 30 minutes before discharge, and after discharge, clinical signs such as respiratory rate and growth combined with continuous overnight oximetry (or polysomnography) are monitored. Interestingly, oxygen supplementation after hospital discharge may have some advantages in babies with BPD. DeMauro and colleagues compared medical and developmental outcomes over the first 2 years of life in

---

BOX 16.1 **Criteria Followed at Our Institution for Decision Making on Sending a Preterm Infant Home on Oxygen**

A. Corrected age over 34 weeks' gestation
B. Able to maintain body temperature (axillary 37.0° C) in an open crib
C. Effective bottle/breast feeding without fatigue or cardiorespiratory compromise
D. Adequate weight gain in the week before discharge (10–15 g/kg/day)
E. Physiologically mature
F. Stable cardiorespiratory function with continuous SpO2 monitoring values within the established range (90%–95%) in the previous 12 to 24 hours
G. No apnea of prematurity (no need for caffeine treatment)
H. No active medical condition needing hospital treatment
I. Appropriately immunized
J. Metabolic screening performed
K. Basic family training (use of the pulse oximeter, basic resuscitation maneuvers) and attachment to an emergency department and outpatient clinic follow-up program
L. Acceptance by the family

extremely preterm infants with BPD who were discharged on supplemental oxygen via nasal cannula with outcome infants with a similar severity but discharged breathing in room air. Oxygen supplementation was associated with marginally improved growth and increased resource; however, they were more likely to be rehospitalized for respiratory illness and to use respiratory medications and equipment. Rates of neurodevelopmental impairment were similar between groups.[75]

OXYGEN SATURATION RECOMMENDATIONS

We would suggest that preterm babies should reach an SpO_2 of 90% to 95% in the delivery room at around 5 to 15 minutes after birth depending on GA, type of delivery, gender, and response to stabilization maneuvers. Once in the NICU and until the baby reaches 36 weeks' postmenstrual age, the range of SpO_2 should be 90% to 95% according to the most recent publications at the time of writing. If BPD and/or pulmonary hypertension are concomitantly present, a median SpO_2 of 94% should be allowed, meaning that most of the time, the baby will be around 95% to 97% saturation. Finally, pulse oximetry should be monitored at home and periodically retrieved for prolonged periods of 8 to 12 hours. During these monitoring periods, the SpO_2 range should be 95% to 97% most of the time. If pulmonary hypertension is under control and the patient is growing, weaning from oxygen should be considered.

KEY REFERENCES

3. Saugstad OD, Sejersted Y, Solberg R, et al: Oxygenation of the newborn: a molecular approach. Neonatology 101(4):315–325, 2012.
5. Vento M, Escobar J, Cernada M, et al: The use and misuse of oxygen during the neonatal period. Clin Perinatol 39:165–176, 2012.
11. Semenza GL: Regulation of oxygen homeostasis by hypoxia-inducible factor 1. Physiology (Bethesda) 24:97–106, 2008.
22. Semenza GL: Hypoxia-inducible factors in physiology and medicine. Cell 148:399–408, 2012.
25. Dawson JA, Kamlin CO, Vento M, et al: Defining the reference range for oxygen saturation for infants after birth. Pediatrics 125:e1340–e1347, 2010.
26. Wyckoff MH, Aziz K, Escobedo MB, et al: Part 13. Neonatal resuscitation. 2015 American Heart Association guidelines update for cardiopulmonary resuscitation and emergency cardiovascular care. Circulation 132:S543–S560, 2015.
34. Saugstad OD, Ramji S, Soll RF, et al: Resuscitation of newborn infants with 21% or 100% oxygen: an updated systematic meta-analysis. Neonatology 94:176–182, 2008.
36. Lui K, Jones LJ, Foster JP, et al: Lower versus higher oxygen concentrations titrated to target oxygen saturations during resuscitation of preterm infants at birth. Cochrane Database Syst Rev 5(5):CD010239, 2018.
43. Oei JL, Vento M, Rabi Y, et al: Higher or lower oxygen for delivery room resuscitation of preterm infants below 28 completed weeks gestation: a meta-analysis. Arch Dis Child Fetal Neonatal Ed 102:F24–F30, 2017.
65. Askie LM, Darlow BA, Finer N, et al: Association between oxygen saturation targeting and death or disability in extremely preterm infants in the neonatal oxygenation prospective meta-analysis collaboration. *JAMA* 319:2190–2201, 2018.

17

Respiratory Gas Conditioning

Andreas Schulze

PHYSIOLOGY AND PATHOPHYSIOLOGY

The inner surface of the upper respiratory tract serves two major functions: (1) inspiratory gas conditioning (i.e., warming and humidification), and (2) mucus clearance. To accomplish these interrelated tasks, the inner airway wall consists of three layers: (1) a basal epithelial layer with ciliated cells, mucus-producing goblet cells, and cells that have a capacity to secret or absorb water; (2) an aqueous (sol) layer; and (3) a luminal viscous gel layer carrying mucous particles that can encapsulate inhaled foreign particles, infectious agents, cell debris, and other compounds. The depth of the aqueous layer is tightly regulated under normal circumstances. This provides an adequate environment for the ciliae to beat and reach up into the gel layer, which is a prerequisite for the mechanisms of the ciliary escalator to work effectively.[1,2]

Breathing is associated with a net heat and water loss unless the respiratory gas is artificially preconditioned to core body temperature and saturated with water vapor (body temperature pressure saturated [BTPS] gas). Ambient air is cooler and contains less water. It gains heat and moisture while travelling through the upper airway during inspiration. During expiration, the nasal and pharyngeal mucosa is rewarmed but remains below core body temperature. Therefore, water is then condensed back to the upper airway lining. This countercurrent heat and moisture exchange function of the upper airway preserves heat and water. However, losses will still occur as long as the expired air temperature stays above inspiratory air temperature. The greater the difference in temperature, the larger is the respiratory water loss.

The location along the airway at which the inspired gas reaches body temperature and full saturation is called the isothermic saturation boundary (ISB). During normal breathing, it is located at about the mid-trachea to main bronchi level, but it may move downward with a deep and fast breathing pattern or in disease. This knowledge is derived from measurements in adults.[3] Such data are unavailable for term or preterm human infants.

Dehydration of the mucosa may lead to progressive airway dysfunction with decreased cilia beat frequency, inspissated secretions, airway occlusion, atelectasis, epithelial cell damage, ulceration, and ultimately, necrotizing tracheobronchitis.[4-6] Systemic and long-term effects such as respiratory infections, sepsis, and chronic lung disease have been reported.[7] The extend and potential reversibility of such injuries depend on exposure time and magnitude of the moisture depletion.[8,9]

Conversely, excessive heat exposure of the respiratory epithelium that results in thermal injury and/or delivery of excess water to the airway even with flooding of alveoli may develop as a result of humidifier malfunction or misuse. This, however, is unlikely to occur with modern humidifiers given the internationally imposed technical regulations and standards for manufacturing these devices.[10]

Basics of the Physical Relationships Among Temperature, Water Vapor, and Energy Content of Gases

Three different states of water are encountered during patient care: liquid water, aerosol, and water vapor. Aerosol is a distribution of small droplets of water in air that can be obtained by nebulization. Both the liquid form and an aerosol can adsorb or dissolve particles and thereby transmit infectious diseases. In contrast, water vapor is an invisible molecular distribution of water in a gas, unable to carry infectious agents. In this state, water exerts a gaseous pressure that amounts to a partial pressure of water of 47 mm Hg when air is fully saturated with water vapor at 37° C. This corresponds to a water vapor mass of 44 mg of water per liter of gas.

The term "absolute humidity" (AH) is defined as the amount of water vapor (in milligrams) per gas volume (in liters) at a given temperature. "Relative humidity" (RH) is the actual water vapor content of the gas volume (in milligrams) relative to the water vapor content (in milligrams) of this same gas volume at saturation at the same temperature. There is a fixed relationship among AH, RH, and temperature (Fig. 17.1).

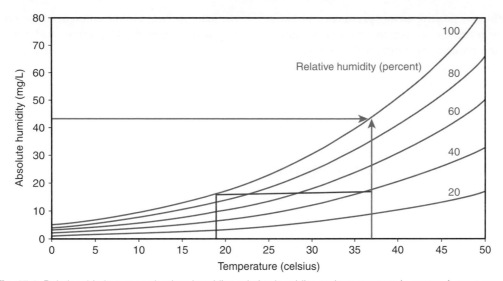

Fig. 17.1 Relationship between absolute humidity, relative humidity, and temperature in gases. A gas accommodates 44 mgH$_2$O/L at 37° C and 100% relative humidity (body temperature pressure saturated gas, *arrows*). A cold passover or bubble-through humidifier can deliver a maximum of less than 20 mgH$_2$O/L with its water reservoir at room temperature (*purple line*). This gas will have about 40% relative humidity if it is dry heated to core body temperature; that is, the respiratory tract needs to vaporize more than another 20 mgH$_2$O/L to condition it to the alveolar gas composition.

Air takes up energy when nebulized water, or liquid water, is converted into water vapor. Conversely, heat is generated in the process of rainout of water vapor (condensation). Hence, there are two components to the total energy content of air: a sensible and a latent heat content. The air temperature solely reflects the former, whereas the water vapor mass reflects the latter energy component. It is important to understand that changing the air temperature alone without changes in water vapor mass constitutes a small change in total energy content compared with changing the humidity of the gas. The difference may approach an order of magnitude. Therefore, warming of frigid inspiratory air does little cooling to the upper airway lining compared with the amount of heat loss that incurs when this air is particularly dry. Conversely, if air is inhaled at 39° C without being fully saturated with water vapor, it will quickly cool to core body temperature without significant heating of the airway lining. The following illustrates this issue quantitatively in an example: If air is saturated with water vapor at 37° C in a humidifier chamber and subsequently dry heated to 39° C in a heated breathing circuit, this dry heating adds almost no energy to the gas: it contains 143 J/g at 37° C, 100% RH versus 145 J/g at 39° C, 90% RH. If, however, air enters the airway at much higher than core body temperature and full saturation, there may be a risk of thermal injury to the respiratory epithelium.

STANDARDS ON HUMIDIFICATION OF MEDICAL GASES FOR USE WITH ARTIFICIAL RESPIRATORY SUPPORT MODALITIES

It is important to recognize that medical-grade gases from gas cylinders or hospital pipeline systems have virtually no water content at room temperature and thus require conditioning before entering the patient's airway especially when the normal upper airway pathways are bypassed in intubated patients. The need for warming and humidification of inspired gases during neonatal mechanical ventilation was recognized more than 50 years ago. It was common practice at this time to change the endotracheal tube once or twice daily to prevent plugging of the tip of the tube and associated serious complications from dry tracheobronchial secretions.[11] The optimum level of respiratory gas conditioning has been debated since. Standards on minimum required levels of inspired gas humidity during artificially supported respiration have been published in the United Kingdom (33 mgH$_2$O/L)[12] and in the United States (30 mgH$_2$O/L).[13] More recently, the International Organization for Standardization (ISO) specified requirements for respiratory humidifying devices.[14] According to this document, 33 mgH$_2$O/L is the minimum required level of humidification at the patient connection port during invasive ventilation with the upper airway bypassed. For noninvasive ventilation, this minimum level was defined at 12 mgH$_2$O/L. Specifications for the neonatal age group in general or for specific neonatal respiratory support modalities have not been issued.

The ISO acknowledges, however, that it is rational to avoid any additional requirement of heating and humidification of inspired gas by a compromised airway. Such additional challenge of the airway is generally present if the inspired gas is less humid and colder than the alveolar air. This implies supplying breathing gases with a humidity as close to 44 mgH$_2$O/L as possible at body temperature.[15]

Although the upper airway is anatomically not "bypassed" by nasal cannula, the airway surface may still dry out when high flow rates (high-flow nasal cannula [HFNC] therapy) are applied using inadequately humidified gas because the nasal cavity and pharynx are continuously purged. With the application of nasal prongs during continuous positive airway pressure or noninvasive ventilation, this entire airway region will also be flushed unidirectionally in the presence of mouth leaks, and flow rates will increase with higher airway pressures.[16,17]

In addition, striving for the "alveolar" level of inspiratory gas conditioning during resuscitation in the delivery room in extremely low-birth-weight infants may reduce evaporative respiratory heat loss and thereby contribute to avoid hypothermia.[18]

PROCEDURES AND DEVICES FOR RESPIRATORY GAS CONDITIONING

Cold Passover, Bubble-Through, and Heated Water Humidifiers for use With Nasal Cannula Therapy

Cold passover or bubble-through humidification can be used for low-flow (<2 L/min) supplemental oxygen therapy in infants with chronic lung disease. Provided the incoming gas flow does not cool down the water reservoir below room temperature, moisture up to a maximum of about 18 mgH$_2$O/L will be added (saturation at 20° C; see Fig. 17.1). During low flow, small-bore nasal cannula therapy, room air is additionally entrained from the environment during inspiration as peak flow rates of spontaneous inspirations exceed the cannula flow rate. This is different from HFNC therapy when the provided flow rates match or exceed peak flow rates of spontaneous inspiration, and a positive pressure develops in the nasal and pharyngeal cavities. During mouth-open states, the positive airway pressure generates a unidirectional flow that precludes any heat and moisture exchange functioning of the nose and pharynx. Prolonged and repeated purging of the nasopharyngeal cavity may dry the epithelial surface if the gas is underhumidified. To avoid this and to improve the general comfort with HFNC therapy, cannula sets have been made available that intend to provide heated air and oxygen mixtures with a humidity level close to alveolar air.[19-22]

Heated Humidifiers With Heated Wire Tubing Circuitry

The cold and dry respiratory gas flow from an air-oxygen blender leaves the ventilator and passes through an unheated tube into the humidifier's water-vaporizing chamber. The amount of water vaporized inside the chamber depends on water temperature, water surface, and the gas flow rate. At 37° C water temperature, the gas may be loaded with a maximum of 44 mg/L of water vapor (fully saturated, 100% RH). The vapor load, however, may be lower if the gas flow rate is high relative to the vaporizing capacity of the chamber. The water in the chamber is manually or automatically refilled from a reservoir to maintain the water level inside the chamber. The gas mixture is then commonly dry-heated above 37° C by a heated wire inside the inspiratory limb of the circuitry. Dry-heating the gas to about 39° C on its way through the inspiratory limb of the tubing circuit does not involve a risk of thermal injury to the infant because increasing gas temperature alone involves only a small gain in energy compared with raising the temperature and adding water vapor. There are different ventilator tubing circuit configurations on the market. They vary with respect to (1) position and number of temperature probes (at humidification chamber outlet, at entry into the incubator, at circuit Y), (2) extension of the heater coil inside the inspiratory limb (only the segment outside the incubator, or throughout the inspiratory limb up to the circuit Y), and (3) degree of insulation of the tubing circuit from the environmental temperature. These variables influence the overall performance of the system.[23]

It is important to understand that rainout in the inspiratory limb of the circuit does not indicate proper humidification; rather it indicates a detrimental moisture loss. Condensation of water vapor shows that the gas temperature must have decreased to or below the dew point. A critical loss of temperature and humidity may easily set in along unheated segments of the circuitry. This is promoted by the large outer surface area of small diameter tubing (particularly when corrugated), by drafts around the tubing (air-conditioned rooms), and by a low room temperature. The decrease in temperature will be larger with smaller circuit gas flow rates because of the longer contact time. Insulating unheated segments of the inspiratory circuit may partly obviate these problems.[23,24] However, the maximum heat output of any heated wire circuit may not be sufficient to meet target gas temperatures under extremes of room and incubator temperatures. For safety reasons, manufacturing standards impose an upper limit to the power output of circuit heater coils. There has been a warning that covering heated wire circuits with drapes or other material for insulation may involve a risk of melting or charring of circuit components.

Condensation and accumulation of liquid water may occur inside the Y adapter, inside an unheated pneumotach probe at the Y adapter, and within a lengthy, uncut neonatal endotracheal tube because of a relevant temperature drop with low incubator temperatures.[24,25] Again, this phenomenon does not necessarily mean that humidifier and circuit provide excessive levels of humidity. To the contrary, it may be a sign of appropriate function of the humidifier chamber and should not lead the clinician into reducing water chamber temperature rather than take insulation measures.

Rainout should also be avoided for reasons other than moisture depletion: condensate becomes easily contaminated, may be flushed down the endotracheal tube with risks of airway obstruction and nosocomial pneumonia, and may disturb the functions of the ventilator.

Heat and Moisture Exchangers ("Artificial Noses")

Heat and moisture exchangers (HMEs) recover part of the heat and moisture contained in the expired air for subsequent release during inspiration. A sponge material inside the clear plastic housing absorbs heat and condenses water vapor during expiration. Hydrophobic HMEs use water-repelling condenser elements. Condensers in hygroscopic HMEs employ salts such as $CaCl_2$, $MgCl_2$, and LiCl. Some brands of HMEs combine both types of condensers; others are additionally coated with bacteriostatic substances and equipped with bacterial or viral filters (HME filters [HMEFs]). Filters are expected to prevent viruses or bacteria from reaching the lung from the environment. "Active" HMEs use a heated water source to enhance the moisturizing performance or use chemical reactions with exhaled CO_2 to release additional heat.

HMEs may be an alternative to heated humidifiers for short-term applications like transport for several reasons, such as simplification of the ventilator circuit, passive operation without requirement of external energy and water sources, no ventilator circuit condensate, low risk of circuit contamination, and low expense.

However, depending on their actual water load and other variables, HMEs add a variable resistance and a dead space to the circuit.[26] A risk of airway occlusion from clogging with secretions or from a dislodgement of the HME's internal components[27] is reported for infants even during short-term application. Also, an expiratory air leak will impair or abrogate the barrier effect against moisture loss.[28,29]

Small HMEs for neonatal applications are commercially available, but data on their use are sparse.[30,31] A pediatric HME maintained an average inspiratory humidity greater than 30 mg/L in a clinical study involving neonates for a test period of 6 hours.[32] Other clinical studies on pediatric and neonatal application confirmed the ability of HMEs to conserve heat and to provide humidity levels that are appropriate for short-term conventional mechanical ventilation.[33-35] The safety and effectiveness of HME for long-term mechanical ventilation are controversial in adults.[36-38] It has not been shown conclusively in neonates. In 30 preterm infants with a birth weight greater than 900 g who required invasive ventilation, HMEs were exclusively used with no detectable differences in outcome compared with a group randomized to conventional heat vaporizers.[39] Bench studies on high-frequency oscillatory ventilation in a neonatal lung model showed that a neonatal HME was able to provide more than 35 mg/L of mean humidity at the proximal end of the endotracheal tube adapter. The HME dampened the oscillatory pressure amplitude less than a neonatal endotracheal tube of 3.5 mm internal diameter.[40]

There is no evidence from studies in adults that HMEs reduce the incidence of ventilator-associated pneumonia (VAP) compared with the use of active humidifiers with heated circuits.[41]

HMEs must not be used in conjunction with heated humidifiers, nebulizers, or metered dose inhalers. This may cause a hazardous increase in device resistance and/or wash off the hygroscopic coating.[42,43]

Device performance has improved during recent years and further advances can be expected to facilitate neonatal short-term applications, for example, during transport.

Aerosol Application

Aerosol water particles that range in size from about 1 to 10 μm may deposit in the airway by impaction (larger particles) or sedimentation (smaller particles). Sedimentation occurs as a gravitational effect when airflow velocity declines in the smaller airways. An aerosol cannot contribute to respiratory gas conditioning downstream to the ISB because the gas is already fully saturated. For this same reason, aerosol water particles cannot be eliminated in this airway region through evaporation and

exhalation. They will therefore become a water burden on the mucosa, which needs to be absorbed by the airway epithelium to maintain an appropriate periciliary fluid depth. An increase in depth of the airway lining's fluid aqueous layer may make it impossible for the cilia to reach the mucous layer and thus may impair mucus transport. Furthermore, if the aerosol deposition rate exceeds absorption capacity, this may lead to increased airway resistance[44,45] and possibly narrowing or occlusion of small airways. Severe systemic overhydration subsequent to ultrasound aerosol therapy has been described in a term newborn infant[46] and similar occurrences were reported in adults.[47]

If an aerosol stream meets the airway proximal to the ISB, the particulate water can theoretically contribute to the gas conditioning process by evaporation before and after deposition. The droplets, however, contain sensible heat only and the mucosa needs to supply most of the latent heat for vaporization. This will cool the airway. If the inspiratory gas is supplied through the endotracheal tube at core body temperature and close to full saturation, the ISB is located near the tip of the endotracheal tube. In such a situation, any aerosol may contribute little if at all to appropriate gas conditioning.

Water or normal saline nebulization therefore appears to offer no significant benefit for inspiratory gas conditioning and may entail a risk of overhumidification.[10]

Irrigation of the Airway

It has been common clinical practice to instill small amounts of water, normal saline solution, or a normal saline dilution of sodium bicarbonate into the endotracheal tube before suctioning procedures in the belief that this provides moisture, loosens tenacious secretions, and facilitates their removal. Suggested amounts of fluid to be used in infants vary widely from 0.1 mL/kg to 0.5 mL/kg. It has been shown, however, that this fluid is not uniformly distributed within the bronchial tree. It enters preferentially dependent regions of the lung.[48] More than 80% of the instillate may remain inside the airway after suctioning and will probably later be absorbed or removed by the mucociliary system.[49] There is no evidence that this practice is beneficial under conditions of appropriate warming and humidification of respiratory gases.[50] Instillation of bulk fluid in patients on mechanical ventilation, however, has an adverse effect on their oxygen status.[51-53] Moreover, instillation of saline into the endotracheal tube may increase the risk of VAP, presumably by washing bacteria from a colonized endotracheal tube deeper into the lungs. Consequently, avoidance of this practice has become a standard part of many neonatal VAP prevention bundles.

ESTIMATION AND MEASUREMENT OF THE EFFICIENCY OF RESPIRATORY GAS CONDITIONING DEVICE BRANDS

Direct, precise measurement of the humidity in inspired air is a demanding engineering challenge. To date, no "gold standard" for hygrometric measurements has been defined for the evaluation of clinically used devices. Scientific studies used complex

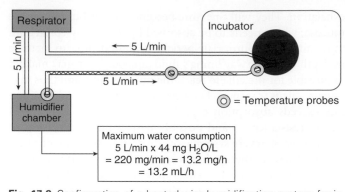

Fig. 17.2 Configuration of a heated-wire humidification system for infants on invasive or noninvasive mechanical ventilation. The ventilator's air/oxygen blender delivers a cold and dry gas mixture to the heated humidification chamber. The gas can accommodate a maximum of 44 mgH$_2$O/L if the humidification chamber warms the water to 37° C. The user sets a target temperature to be reached at the endotracheal tube adaptor. This temperature is commonly set at or above 37° C. A heated wire inside the inspiratory limb of the circuit maintains or slightly raises the gas temperature to avoid moisture depletion because of rainout. This dry heating adds little energy to the gas. It therefore cools down rapidly to body temperature near the airway entrance. The water consumption rate of a humidifier chamber required to reach a target respiratory gas humidity can be calculated from the circuit flow rate. Observation of this water consumption rate can be employed as a simple test of the efficiency of a humidifier.

techniques such as psychrometry,[35] capacitive hygrometers, or dew point hygrometers[54]—all of which appear unsuitable for use in clinical routine care settings.

Recording the water consumption of the humidifier chamber over time is a simple and clinically useful test to check for sufficient vaporization. Because most infant ventilators use a continuous constant circuit flow or a circuit flow rate range of known size, the absolute and RH delivered at the humidification chamber outlet can be calculated from the humidifier's water consumption rate (Fig. 17.2). This principle for estimation of inspired gas humidity can also be applied for cold passover and bubble-through humidification. It is applicable to HFNC therapy, invasive and noninvasive ventilation.

Different brands of HMEs may vary widely in their performance characteristics. In a large-scale bench study, some HMEs' moisture output deviated considerably from manufacturer data.[55] The ISO 9360 standard[56] recommends the gravimetric method for HME performance evaluation, but this technique can also not be used with patients nor for comparisons with heated humidifiers. Indirect clinical measures such as the occurrence of nosocomial pneumonia, number of endotracheal tube occlusions, frequency of required tracheal suctioning, and instillations do not reliably reflect an HME's effectiveness.[57] However, visual evaluation of the amount of moisture in the adapter segment between the endotracheal tube and the HME was found to closely correlate with objective measurements of the delivered humidity.[58]

Clinicians should be aware that the humidity output of humidifiers may change with a ventilator's flow rate range, settings, ambient temperature, and gas inlet temperature. Therefore, manufacturers need to disclose these conditions when humidity output levels are presented in user manuals.

KEY REFERENCES

1. Williams R, Rankin N, Smith T, et al: Relationship between the humidity and temperature of inspired gas and the function of the airway mucosa. Crit Care Med 24:1920–1929, 1996.
2. Schulze A: Respiratory gas conditioning in infants with an artificial airway. Semin Neonatol 7:369–377, 2002.
4. Pillow JJ, Hillman NH, Polglase GR, et al: Oxygen, temperature and humidity of inspired gases and their influences on airway and lung tissue in near-term lambs. Intensive Care Med 35: 2157–2163, 2009.
18. te Pas AB, Lopriore E, Dito I, et al: Humidified and heated air during stabilization at birth improves temperature in preterm infants. Pediatrics 125:e1427–e1232, 2010.
23. Todd DA, Boyd J, Lloyd J, et al: Inspired gas humidity during mechanical ventilation: effects of humidification chamber, airway temperature probe position and environmental conditions. J Paediatr Child Health 37:489–494, 2001.
30. Kelly M, Gillies D, Todd DA, et al: Heated humidification versus heat and moisture exchangers for ventilated adults and children. Cochrane Database Syst Rev Issue 4. Art. No.: CD004711, 2010.
31. Gillies D, Todd DA, Foster JP, et al: Heat and moisture exchangers versus heated humidifiers for mechanically ventilated adults and children. Cochrane Database Syst Rev Issue 9. Art. No.: CD004711, 2017.
35. Fassassi M, Michel F, Thomachot L, et al: Airway humidification with a heat and moisture exchanger in mechanically ventilated neonates. Intensive Care Med 33:336–343, 2007.

18

Noninvasive Respiratory Support

Brett J. Manley, Peter G. Davis, Bradley A. Yoder, and Louise S. Owen

---

KEY POINTS

- Early continuous positive airway pressure (CPAP) confers a small benefit over endotracheal intubation for initial management of extremely preterm infants, reducing the rate of the combined outcome of death or bronchopulmonary dysplasia.
- Preliminary evidence suggests that minimally invasive surfactant therapy provided to infants with respiratory distress syndrome on CPAP is safe and effective.
- Synchronized nasal intermittent positive pressure ventilation is a useful method of augmenting the benefits of CPAP, particularly as postextubation respiratory support.
- High-frequency nasal ventilation is a promising therapy, but more research is required before it is widely applied.
- Nasal high flow (nHF) is less effective than CPAP as primary support for preterm infants but is an appropriate therapy for moderately preterm infants with signs of mild to moderate respiratory distress.
- nHF is an alternative to CPAP as postextubation respiratory support, although caution is recommended in extremely preterm infants.

INTRODUCTION

History of Noninvasive Respiratory Support

The beginning of the modern era of neonatal intensive care may be defined by the introduction of invasive mechanical ventilation (MV) via an endotracheal tube (ETT). Previously, respiratory support was provided in the form of supplemental oxygen delivered directly into an incubator or via an oxygen hood. Supplemental oxygen alone saved lives but proved insufficient for infants with moderate to severe lung disease or poor respiratory drive. Initial attempts to ventilate immature newborn infants using equipment and techniques appropriate for older patients were largely unsuccessful. In response to unacceptably high mortality rates, Gregory et al. pioneered the use of continuous positive airway pressure (CPAP), although infants in their initial case series were predominantly managed with CPAP delivered using an ETT.[1] Other interfaces, including mono- and binasal prongs and nasal masks, were subsequently developed to provide genuinely noninvasive respiratory support. However, subsequent improvements in both the equipment and techniques used to deliver MV, along with the uptake of treatment with exogenous surfactant, predominantly delivered via an ETT, led to a decrease in popularity of noninvasive support. Some units persisted with a strategy of minimizing lung damage through the aggressive use of CPAP, and in one of the most influential observational studies in neonatology, Avery and colleagues showed that this approach was associated with lower rates of bronchopulmonary dysplasia (BPD) than MV.[2] However, widespread use of noninvasive support, particularly as primary therapy for preterm infants with respiratory distress syndrome (RDS), did not occur until a series of multicenter randomized controlled trials (RCTs) in the early 2000s demonstrated the feasibility and safety of this approach.[3-6] The simplicity and low cost of noninvasive support modes have led to its uptake around the world, including settings where both personnel and equipment are limited.

What Are the Clinical Indications and How Does Noninvasive Respiratory Support Help?

Respiratory Distress Syndrome

RDS is characterized by immature lung development and inadequate surfactant production. Predominantly a disorder affecting preterm infants, it leads to widespread lung atelectasis and difficulty establishing and maintaining residual volume. The tendency toward lung collapse is exacerbated by increased compliance of the chest wall and relative muscle hypotonia.[7] The cycle of atelectasis and reexpansion leads to inflammation and leakage of protein exudate into alveoli, which in turn inactivates surfactant.[8] By preventing alveolar collapse at the end of expiration, noninvasive support preserves whatever surfactant is present, allowing maintenance of functional residual capacity (FRC), reducing ventilation-perfusion mismatch, and enhancing oxygenation.[9] The alternative mode of support, MV via an ETT, ensures a clear upper airway and relieves the infant of much of the work of breathing. The ETT also provides the traditional route of administration for replacement surfactant therapy. However, it is associated with many unwanted adverse effects. The presence of an ETT in contact with the fragile mucosa may lead to upper airway trauma with the risk of progression to subglottic stenosis. Likewise, in the relatively immunocompromised newborn infant, MV increases the risk of pulmonary and systemic infections. Insertion of the ETT is associated with physiological instability, and ongoing ventilation is associated with volutrauma (overdistension of the lungs) and atelectotrauma (repetitive opening and closing of lung units), leading to acute and chronic lung injury. For these reasons, noninvasive respiratory support is the preferred mode of initial support for spontaneously breathing infants, with intubation and MV reserved for those infants who develop respiratory failure.

Apnea of Prematurity

Apnea of prematurity is considered a developmental disorder related to immaturity of the brain's respiratory center. The airway of newborn infants, especially those born preterm, is highly compliant and prone to collapse. This includes the pharynx, the trachea, major bronchi, and the small airways. Pressure delivered to the upper airway acts to keep these passages open and, in doing so, reduces airway resistance and the work of breathing.[10] The tendency of the upper airways to collapse, in conjunction with poor respiratory drive, particularly in very preterm infants, leads to apnea. Currently, the combination of noninvasive support and the respiratory stimulant caffeine represents standard therapy for preterm infants at risk of apnea.

Postextubation Care

Prolonged MV increases the risk of BPD, sepsis, neurological injury, and retinopathy of prematurity. Clinicians try to extubate preterm infants as quickly as possible to reduce these risks. However, extubation is often unsuccessful and about two-thirds of infants born less than 29 weeks' gestation require reintubation.[11] Loss of lung volume following removal of the ETT and cessation of tidal ventilation often leads to instability, particularly in the first hours to days following extubation. Noninvasive support provides distending pressure to maintain alveolar and airway patency and reduces obstruction, work of breathing, and apnea.

An Overview of Equipment Used to Provide Noninvasive Respiratory Support

Interfaces

After unsuccessful trials of pressure chambers and face masks, nasal interfaces (prongs, masks and cannulae) have become the most frequently used interfaces for noninvasive support. Excellent nursing care is required to maintain optimal nasal interface positioning and to avoid nasal trauma.

Pressure Generators

All pressure generators incorporate appropriate gas blending, heating, and humidification as per international standards. CPAP can be generated by mechanical ventilators, but the use of such sophisticated and expensive devices may limit accessibility. Low-cost alternatives for CPAP delivery that do not require a power source, such as "bubble" CPAP, have made noninvasive support accessible and affordable in resource-limited settings,[12,13] where it has been shown to be effective.[14]

Efforts to improve the effectiveness of CPAP include superimposing intermittent higher pressures, delivered by a mechanical ventilator or specialized device. These devices vary in pressures generated and the ability to synchronize with the infant's spontaneous breathing patterns. Delivery of CPAP augmented by noninvasive high-frequency oscillations via the nasal interface is another promising method of augmenting the action of CPAP, which also requires specialist equipment.

CONTINUOUS POSITIVE AIRWAY PRESSURE

Indications for Continuous Positive Airway Pressure Support

Nasal CPAP has most commonly been used to support breathing in preterm infants; it has become increasingly popular since the 1990s. CPAP is also used in the treatment of apnea of prematurity and for many other respiratory conditions in term and preterm infants.

Continuous Positive Airway Pressure Support for Preterm Infants from Birth

Trials from as early as the 1970s, supported by a Cochrane review,[15] demonstrated that continuous distending pressure was effective in reducing mortality in preterm infants. By the mid to late 1990s, CPAP had become the mainstay of early treatment of RDS for very preterm infants. However, extremely preterm infants, born less than 28 weeks' gestation, were almost always managed with initial intubation, MV, and surfactant treatment.

Between 1993 and 2001, a series of observational studies from the United States and Scandinavia were published demonstrating that extremely preterm infants could be managed with CPAP from birth, reducing intubation and BPD rates without increasing mortality or morbidity.[16-19] Following these publications, CPAP gained more credibility as a first-line treatment for extremely preterm infants.[20,21] Subsequently, several large RCTs were completed that compared CPAP with intubation at birth. The first of these was published in 2008,[4] and although it showed no difference in the primary outcome of death or BPD at 36 weeks' corrected gestation, there was a trend toward a lower rate of the combined outcome in the CPAP group (34% vs. 39%). Less than half of the CPAP-treated group required intubation, although a higher rate of pneumothorax was seen in this group.[4] Another of the trials also showed no difference in the primary outcome of death or BPD[3] but reported that there was no difference in death or neurodevelopmental impairment at 18 to 22 months' corrected age between groups[22] and less respiratory morbidity in the CPAP group.[23] Individually, these trials showed little differences in outcomes between groups, but they did establish that CPAP from birth was a safe and effective alternative to routine intubation for surfactant delivery. These trials have now been the subject of meta-analyses,[24] and they have formed part of a Cochrane review[25] concluding that when compared with MV, prophylactic CPAP reduces the need for intubation and surfactant treatment, while reducing death and BPD. This evidence has been incorporated into international guidelines that recommend the practice of initiating CPAP from birth wherever possible.[26,27] Attention has now turned to the best way to support infants who are managed with early CPAP but who also need treatment with exogenous surfactant.

Continuous Positive Airway Pressure Support for Preterm Infants Postextubation

As part of the modern philosophy to minimize the time preterm infants receive invasive support, attempts are made to extubate these infants quickly. However, unlike their term-born counterparts, who typically recover quickly from early postnatal respiratory disorders, preterm infants have ongoing respiratory support requirements. They have ongoing lung disease,[28] thoraco-abdominal asynchrony,[29] apnea,[30] and poor muscle stamina and excessively compliant chest wall, resulting in progressive atelectasis.[31] A Cochrane review of trials randomizing preterm infants to CPAP or head box oxygen postextubation showed less requirement for escalation of support in those extubated to CPAP (of at least 5 cm H$_2$O) than in those managed with supplemental oxygen alone (relative risk [RR], 0.62; 95% confidence interval [CI], 0.51–0.76; number needed to treat, six infants).[32] No difference in the rate of reintubation or BPD was seen; however, many infants in the supplemental oxygen group received "rescue" CPAP. Postextubation CPAP support is now standard practice in the preterm population.[26] Despite this, around half of extremely preterm infants will require reintubation following their first extubation attempt,[33] even when validated tests have been applied to predict success. Predicting success is challenging, but factors associated with higher success rates include higher gestational age, lower peak oxygen requirements in the first 24 hours, lower carbon dioxide levels, and higher pH with less need for supplemental oxygen before extubation.[33,34]

Continuous Positive Airway Pressure Support for Apnea of Prematurity

Although there are sound physiological reasons supporting the use of CPAP to treat apnea, there is limited direct clinical evidence of benefit. CPAP can alter the Hering-Brauer reflex,[35] stimulate laryngeal mechanoreceptors,[36] and suppress the intercostal phrenic inhibitory reflex to support inspiration.[37] CPAP has been shown to reduce mixed and obstructive apneas,[38] shorten central apneas, and reduce apnea-associated desaturation.[39] However, the only RCT examining CPAP versus methylxanthine therapy was carried out almost 40 years ago, in just 32 very preterm infants.[40] A CPAP pressure of 2 to 3 cm H$_2$O was compared with theophylline treatment, which was found to be more effective in reducing prolonged apneas and preventing escalation to intubation. This was the only study included in the subsequent Cochrane review[41] in 2001. No further studies have evaluated CPAP for the treatment of apnea in preterm infants in a RCT.

Continuous Positive Airway Pressure Support for Other Conditions

Given the well-established physiological benefits of CPAP, it has been used to treat many other respiratory conditions. These include transient tachypnea of the newborn,[42] meconium aspiration syndrome,[43] pulmonary hypertension,[44] pulmonary hemorrhage,[45] cardiac failure with pulmonary edema,[46] respiratory infections such as congenital pneumonia,[47] and bronchiolitis.[48] CPAP supports infants following thoracic and cardiac surgery, those with hypoventilation syndromes, and infants with obstructive conditions such as laryngo- or tracheomalacia.[49,50]

CPAP is accessible and easy to apply in many settings; however, infants treated with CPAP are cared for in newborn nurseries, separated from their mothers. They may also be treated

with intravenous fluids and antibiotics and may have reduced opportunities to breast feed. Therefore, it is important to ensure that CPAP is used appropriately and that newborn term and late preterm infants with tachypnea or grunting are carefully observed and given the opportunity to complete their transition independently, before making a decision to commence CPAP.

Contraindications to Continuous Positive Airway Pressure Support

There are few true contraindications to CPAP;[51] however, it may not be the optimal choice for infants with poor respiratory drive and frequent apnea or for those with progressive respiratory acidosis. CPAP can be more challenging to successfully apply in infants with a cleft lip and palate and infants with other facial anomalies, and it may not be possible to use it in infants with choanal atresia. Some conditions are exacerbated by the use of CPAP and it should be avoided in these infants. These conditions include anomalies in which the addition of gas into the gastrointestinal tract compromises ventilation or gastrointestinal integrity: congenital diaphragmatic hernia, tracheoesophageal fistula, and gastroschisis, as well as acute gastrointestinal events such as spontaneous intestinal perforation or necrotizing enterocolitis.

Continuous Positive Airway Pressure Devices and Interfaces

Ventilator-Generated Continuous Positive Airway Pressure

During ventilator-generated CPAP, a continuous set gas flow is directed past and into the infant's nose via the chosen interface. The ventilator expiratory assembly employs various methods to maintain a set pressure within the circuit that is applied to the infant.

Bubble Continuous Positive Airway Pressure

A second form of continuous-flow CPAP is "bubble" CPAP. Although it was originally described in 1914,[52] commercially available devices only become widely available in the last 20 years. Bubble CPAP uses an underwater seal at the distal end of the expiratory limb of the breathing circuit to generate circuit pressure. Tubing is inserted to a specific underwater depth to obtain the desired circuit pressure. Typically, markings on the tubing indicate the insertion depth to achieve a given circuit pressure (Fig. 18.1).

The generated pressure varies slightly with the set gas flow; very high gas flows can generate pressure higher than the level indicated by the depth markings with some systems.[53,54] As gas leaves the underwater expiratory tubing (by bubbling out), small pressure oscillations are generated within the circuit. The amplitude of these oscillations varies with the system used and with the vigor of the bubbling. Some of these pressure oscillations may reach the chest, potentially supporting gas exchange.[55,56] The amount of oscillation transfer varies between systems[56] and may be minimal in some systems and under some conditions.[53] One mode of bubble CPAP, known as "Seattle-PAP", has altered the orientation of the expiratory limb of the circuit upward to 135 degrees. Early data showed that this

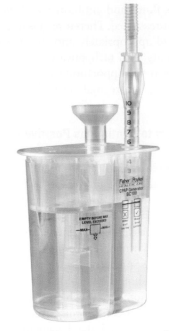

Fig. 18.1 Continuous positive airway pressure (CPAP) circuit with underwater seal, set to deliver 6 cm of water (Bubble CPAP, Fisher & Paykel Healthcare, Auckland, New Zealand).

modification improved arterial oxygen and significantly reduced work of breathing.[57] However, these advantages have not been shown to reduce CPAP failure rates or any other morbidity in preterm infants.[58] Studies have attempted to determine whether the pressure oscillations of bubble CPAP translate into advantages in respiratory physiology that may improve outcome; a study in preterm infants examined whether the amplitude of the bubbling had any effect on short-term outcome and reported that whether bubbling was minimal or vigorous did not affect gas exchange.[59] Bubble CPAP systems neither routinely monitor delivered pressure nor provide pressure-relief valves or alarms, which differs from other CPAP delivery devices. Dislodging of the nasal interface, inadvertent high or low set gas flow, and condensation in the expiratory limb can result in CPAP levels different from those desired.[60] There are several commercially available bubble CPAP systems, many of which

have been modified from the original design. Unrestricted modifications have the capacity to alter the mechanics of the device and may increase the imposed work of breathing.[61]

Variable-Flow Continuous Positive Airway Pressure

The alternative to continuous-flow CPAP is variable-flow CPAP, where alterations to the gas flow result in changes in the delivered pressure. Two distinct modes of variable-flow CPAP are readily available. The original Infant Flow mechanism (SiPAP, Vyaire Medical Inc., Mettawa, IL, USA) uses a dedicated flow driver, circuit, and prongs. Gas flow is driven through the inspiratory limb of the circuit. A short, narrower, expiratory limb exhausts gases, generating pressure. The short expiratory limb is angled in such a way that during expiration, the inspiratory gas flow is also directed out the expiratory limb (Fig. 18.2) using the Coandă effect (termed "fluidic flip"). This potentially reduces expiratory resistance and work of breathing.[62] Residual gas pressure is provided by the constant gas flow, enabling stable CPAP delivery throughout the respiratory cycle. Comparable systems with similar functionality have become available.[63]

Benveniste Gas-Jet Valve Continuous Positive Airway Pressure

The second mode of variable-flow CPAP is generated using a Benveniste gas-jet valve. This valve was first described in the 1960s;[64] it uses the Venturi effect to entrain and pressurize gas between two metal tubes connected by a metal ring. One end of the tubing is connected to the humidified, blended gas supply, and the other, to the patient interface. Increasing the applied gas flow increases the delivered pressure, delivered pressure is not monitored, and there are no blow-off valves or alarms to avoid delivery of excessive pressure.

Comparison of Continuous Positive Airway Pressure Devices

There are no large-scale RCTs investigating the differences between CPAP delivery devices. Several small studies exist, but there is little convincing evidence to support or refute one form over another, a conclusion reached by the 2008 Cochrane review.[65] A recent systematic review of bubble CPAP versus other CPAP delivery modes included 19 studies. The authors

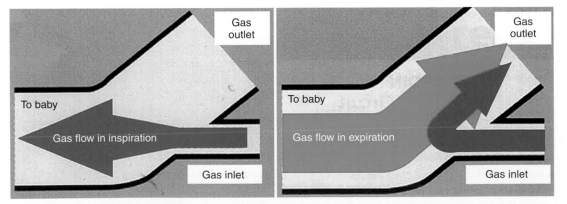

Fig. 18.2 A diagram demonstrating the fluidic flip mechanism of variable-flow continuous positive airway pressure.

report that there was no difference in mortality or BPD between modes and that there was less CPAP failure within 7 days with bubble CPAP (RR, 0.75; 95% CI, 0.57–0.98), but more nasal injury with bubble CPAP than other modes (RR, 2.04; 95% CI, 1.33–3.14).[66]

Comparisons have previously been complicated by the use of different nasal interfaces; however, direct comparisons have been made between ventilator and bubble CPAP, between ventilator and variable-flow (Infant Flow) CPAP, and between bubble and ventilator CPAP.

Ventilator Continuous Positive Airway Pressure Versus Variable-Flow (Infant Flow) Continuous Positive Airway Pressure

There is some evidence that variable-flow CPAP imposes less work of breathing than ventilator CPAP,[62,67,68] with one study measuring 75% less work.[67] Other studies have reported better lung recruitment,[69] increased tidal volume,[70] improved thoraco-abdominal synchrony,[71] and more stable airway pressures[62,67,70] with variable-flow devices. However other comparisons have failed to find any differences in clinically important outcomes including respiratory rate, heart rate, blood pressure, comfort levels,[72] or rates of extubation failure[73] when compared with ventilator CPAP.

Ventilator Continuous Positive Airway Pressure Versus Bubble Continuous Positive Airway Pressure

Comparisons between ventilator and bubble CPAP have also shown conflicting results. In vitro studies have shown that bubble CPAP pressures vary more than may be appreciated (as pressures are not typically recorded during bubble CPAP delivery), and this variation can be more than the small variations seen in ventilator-generated CPAP.[53] However, another in vitro model, albeit without leak, found that lung recruitment was better with bubble CPAP than with ventilator CPAP.[74] In a preterm lamb study, bubble CPAP delivered via an ETT resulted in improved oxygenation and better carbon dioxide clearance than ventilator-generated CPAP,[75] as well as decreased markers of lung injury. A small clinical study that compared ventilator with bubble CPAP in recovering preterm infants found lower respiratory rates in the bubble CPAP group, but no difference in blood gases.[55]

Variable-Flow Continuous Positive Airway Pressure Versus Bubble Continuous Positive Airway Pressure

A few studies in preterm infants have compared short-term outcomes between variable-flow CPAP and bubble CPAP. A small crossover study reported that work of breathing and thoraco-abdominal synchrony were both better with variable-flow (Infant Flow) CPAP than with bubble CPAP.[76] Three RCTs have compared bubble CPAP with variable-flow CPAP (Infant Flow) in preterm infants. When used postextubation before 14 days of age, CPAP failure rate was found to be lower, with shorter postextubation support needed, in infants supported with bubble CPAP.[77] A small earlier study (n = 36) had reported that preterm infants treated with bubble CPAP had higher oxygen requirements and higher respiratory rates than

those managed with variable-flow (Infant Flow) devices; however, different nasal interfaces were used between groups in this study, potentially confounding the results.[78] The most recent study (n = 40) found no differences between infants treated with either variable-flow or bubble CPAP devices.[79] One RCT has compared bubble CPAP with variable-flow Benveniste-valve jet CPAP[80] in preterm infants. A total of 170 preterm infants received one intervention as initial respiratory support. CPAP failure rates and all other studied outcomes were not different between groups.

Continuous Positive Airway Pressure Interfaces

Originally, CPAP was delivered using ETTs, various head chambers, and face-covering masks. These interfaces either increased the work of breathing, were uncomfortable for the infant, caused pressure injuries, or limited movement of and access to the infant; consequently, they are no longer used. Infants are obligate nose breathers; therefore, modern CPAP interfaces have focused on the nose. Although this route avoids unnecessary noxious stimuli to the mouth and keeps the mouth free for oral care and nonnutritive sucking, it also allows the mouth to open, potentially limiting the benefits of pressurized gas entering the nose. Clinicians may attempt to limit pressure loss through the mouth by using a pacifier or a strap under the infant's chin, although there is minimal evidence that this is safe and effective. Downward pressure on the palate from nasally applied CPAP can be sufficient to press the palate against the tongue, providing a natural barrier to some of the pressure loss from the mouth. Modern neonatal CPAP uses a variety of nasal interfaces (Fig. 18.3). Nasal prongs are very common; these may be binasal or mononasal, short (<15 mm) or long (up to 90 mm), wide bore or narrow. Prongs vary in material, length,

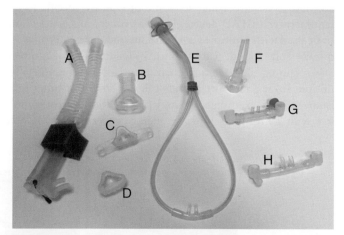

Fig. 18.3 Examples of continuous positive airway pressure interfaces include nasal masks: (A) Flexitrunk with short binasal prongs (Fisher & Paykel Healthcare, Auckland, New Zealand), (B) Stephan EasyFlow mask (Stephan, Gackenback, Germany), (C) nasal mask (Medical Innovations, Puchheim, Germany), (D) nasal mask (Fisher & Paykel Healthcare, Auckland, New Zealand), (E) RAM nasal cannulae (RAM, Neotech Products, Valencia, CA, USA), (F) nasopharyngeal prongs (Binasal Airway, Neotech Products, Valencia, CA, USA), (G) short binasal prongs (Inca Prong, SLE, Surrey, UK), (H) short binasal prongs (Hudson Prongs, Teleflex Medical, Durham, NC, USA).

and diameter; these aspects affect the resistance to flow and therefore the pressure delivered to the upper airway. Nasal masks are readily available and are increasingly frequently used.

Mononasal Prongs, Cut-Down Endotracheal Tubes, and Binasal Nasopharyngeal Prongs

Longer nasal prongs, where the tip sits in the nasopharynx, whether single or binasal, impose an increased work of breathing. A single nasopharyngeal prong is typically an ETT that may have been shortened, and then inserted via one nostril into the nasopharynx. Commercially available binasal nasopharyngeal prongs exist (Fig. 18.3F) and can be of narrower bore than a cut-down ETT, further increasing respiratory load and reducing the transmitted pressure.[81] Use of these interfaces is less common since the Cochrane review in 2008, which concluded that short binasal prongs are more effective.[65] However a recent RCT by Hochwald et al.[82] compared longer, narrower prongs to short binasal prongs or masks while providing nasal intermittent positive pressure ventilation (NIPPV, discussed later) to 166 preterm infants: the longer, narrower prongs were noninferior by the trial definition for the primary outcome of intubation within 72 hours and resulted in less severe nasal trauma.

Cut-down ETTs may be a useful alternative to ideal CPAP interface options under certain circumstances, such as when using standard nasal masks or prongs are inadequate (e.g., for an infant with a cleft lip). However, it is important to be aware that the relatively narrow bore and increased length contribute to greater resistance and more loss of pressure transmitted to the airways, which can be as much as 4 cm of water pressure;[81] additionally, transmitted pressure can be lost via the contralateral nostril.

Short Binasal Prongs

Short binasal prongs are commonly used to deliver nasal CPAP and many types are available. Some prongs are specific to the manufacturer's CPAP device, whereas others are generic and can be used with multiple CPAP circuits and devices. Prongs are typically soft, round, 6 to 15 mm in length, and of uniform cross-sectional shape along their length. Most brands offer multiple sizes, and some brands offer a variety of interprong distances. Two examples of nasal prongs that are commonly used with continuous-flow, ventilator-generated, and bubble

CPAP include Hudson prongs (Hudson Respiratory Care, Inc., Arlington Heights, IL, USA) (Fig. 18.3H) and Inca prongs (Ackrad Laboratories, Inc., Cranford, NJ, USA) (Fig. 18.3G). Both these types of prongs are placed across the face, over the moustache area, with the CPAP circuit running up each side of the face and secured using a CPAP hat and strapping (Fig. 18.4A). An example of an alternative is the midline Flexitrunk CPAP system (Fisher & Paykel Healthcare, Auckland, New Zealand), where the CPAP circuit is secured to a hat and passed over the center of the forehead, over the bridge of the nose, into the nostrils (Fig. 18.3A, B). The nasal prongs (or mask) used with the Infant Flow SiPAP (Care Fusion, San Diego, CA, USA) also use a midline position (Fig. 18.4C).

Future Nasal Prong Development

Nasal prongs are a well-established interface, but they are not perfect. It can be challenging for clinicians to determine the optimal prong fit to create a seal at the nares, without blanching and damaging the surrounding skin. Prongs are round, but the nares are triangular and the internal shape of the nostrils is variable. These issues make the design of comfortable, well-fitting prongs more challenging. In addition, infants with different ethnic backgrounds have different face and nasal shapes that mean that current CPAP prong systems may be more suited to infants from some regions of the world than others. Future designs of nasal prongs should consider the true shape and size of infants' nostrils internally and externally, as well as accommodate variations in face and nose shape and size. With the advent of rapid three-dimensional printing, it may be possible in the future to design individualized prongs for babies that can be changed as the infant grows.

Nasal Masks

Nasal masks are a relatively recent innovation. As with nasal prongs, there are several commercially available brands. Typically, these masks are triangular in shape and can be fitted to either midline or cross-face CPAP circuits. The masks are small and soft and sit over the bridge of the nose and onto the philtrum (Fig. 18.3B–D). Nasal masks are much smaller than the round face masks used to deliver positive pressure ventilation, such as in the delivery room. Nasal masks have been used as an alternative to short binasal prongs, in an attempt to increase

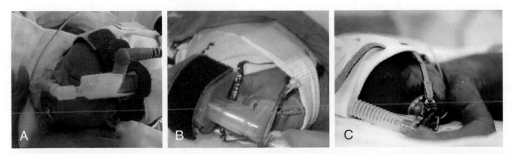

Fig. 18.4 (A) Short binasal prongs (Hudson prong, Teleflex Medical, Durham, NC, USA) demonstrating "cross-face" continuous positive airway pressure (CPAP). **(B)** Midline CPAP (Flexitrunk system, Fisher & Paykel Healthcare, Auckland, New Zealand). **(C)** Infant flow nasal mask CPAP (CareFusion, Becton, Dickinson and Company, Franklin Lakes, NJ, USA).

infant comfort and reduce nasal trauma, while providing equivalent CPAP support. Some units cycle between masks and binasal prongs to avoid serious nasal trauma. As very small mask sizes are available, masks can be used in infants who are too small for the smallest sized nasal prongs. As with nasal prongs, it is essential to strike a balance between maintaining a good nasal seal to maintain CPAP pressure and overly tight application that increases the risk of nasal trauma.

Nasal Cannulae

Nasal cannulae were originally used to deliver low-flow supplemental oxygen, typically using flows of 0.5 L/min or lower. Nasal cannulae are also used to deliver nasal high flow (nHF) therapy (Fig. 18.5), where heated, humidified gases are delivered at flows of 2 to 8 L/min. Subsequently, products have been developed to deliver CPAP via nasal cannulae. CPAP circuits using nasal cannulae do not have an expiratory limb and are therefore designed to be fitted while leaving part of the nares unfilled, creating an intentional leak, in an effort to avoid uncontrolled high-pressure delivery.

Cannulae are of much narrower cross-sectional area than nasal prongs, and the adjoining circuits used are also typically of smaller diameters than standard CPAP circuits. This can make it more challenging to adequately heat and humidify gases to the point of delivery and can potentially reduce the transmission of the applied pressure. One commercially available example of cannulae for CPAP use is the RAM Nasal Cannula (Neotech, Valencia, CA, USA) (Fig. 18.3E). This product has short, stiff, binasal cannulae with larger-bore tubing than standard low-flow oxygen or nHF circuits. The device has gained acceptance in some parts of the United States to provide CPAP[83] (and in some cases NIPPV) because it is quicker and easier to apply and secure than standard CPAP. However, the long segment of narrow tubing between the circuit connection and the interface creates substantial resistance. This leads to a considerable drop in pressure from the circuit to the patient interface, especially with the smallest size cannula and when there is a large leak at the nares.[84] This is of particular concern as there is no pressure monitoring system intrinsic to the device, meaning that the clinician would

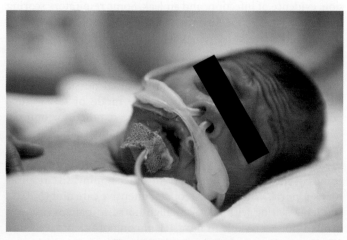

Fig. 18.5 Nasal high flow.

be unaware that a lower pressure than desired was being delivered. Higher CPAP pressures than those required when short binasal prongs are used may be needed to achieve the same level of support when nasal cannulae are used.[85]

Comparison Between Nasal Interfaces

Few comparative data exist to guide clinicians in choosing one type of nasal interface over another. Those that have been done have often been confounded by use of different CPAP delivery devices. Where evidence is lacking, individual centers should focus on developing expertise in the use of one device to optimize its benefits and minimize adverse effects.

Comparison Between Nasal Prong Types

De Paoli et al.[81] compared the pressure drop for five different CPAP prong types of various sizes, at various gas flows. They reported a wide variation in pressure drop between devices, which may account for clinically important differences in outcomes in studies comparing nasal interfaces. A meta-analysis of studies comparing short binasal prongs with single nasal or nasopharyngeal prongs found that use of short binasal prongs prevented more reintubations (RR, 0.59; 95% CI, 0.41–0.85; number needed to treat, five infants).[65]

Comparison Between Nasal Masks and Nasal Prongs

There have now been multiple RCTs exploring the relative effectiveness of nasal masks compared with nasal prongs. There have also been several systematic reviews, the most recent of which included 11 studies.[86] This review concluded that nasal mask CPAP reduced the rate of intubation (RR, 0.72; 95% CI, 0.58–0.90), reduced the need for surfactant (RR, 0.85; 95% CI, 0.74–0.97), and reduced the rate of BPD (RR, 0.47; 95% CI, 0.23–0.95) compared with nasal prong CPAP. The authors also reported a slightly longer CPAP duration during nasal mask CPAP (mean difference, 1.78 days; 95% CI, 1.67–1.89).

Comparison Between Standard Interfaces and Nasal Cannulae

In a bench-top study, Green et al. demonstrated that nasal masks showed the lowest resistance and smallest pressure drop across the interface. Short binasal prongs had very variable levels of resistance, with Infant Flow prongs showing the least pressure loss. Nasal cannulae (RAM cannulae) showed the largest pressure loss across the device.[87] In 12 preterm infants, Singh et al. measured pharyngeal pressure during CPAP delivered via nasal cannulae (RAM) and short binasal prongs (Hudson). They reported a significantly different pressure loss between set and delivered pressures (2.5 cm H_2O with nasal cannulae, RAM) compared with no pressure drop with short binasal (Hudson) prongs.[88] Similarly, Sharma studied 30 preterm infants, comparing delivered CPAP pressures using three devices (nasal mask, binasal prongs, and nasal cannulae).[89] Measured oropharyngeal pressures were below the set CPAP level with all three interfaces. The largest pressure drop was seen with the nasal cannulae (RAM) cannula, and the smallest was measured with the use of the nasal mask. Clinicians should be cautious in applying a cannula interface to deliver CPAP, as there is marked attenuation of the desired pressure delivered to the infant.

Optimal Continuous Positive Airway Pressure

Determining the optimal CPAP to treat infants is challenging. The optimal distending pressure will vary between infants and will vary throughout an infant's course. High pressures may be needed to achieve lung inflation and clear lung fluid in the delivery room. Variable, intermediate pressures may be required to support preterm infants with respiratory distress who have atelectasis and poor lung compliance. Lower pressures may be required later in an infant's course, during recovery, and to manage apnea. The aim is to find the ideal pressure to adequately oxygenate and ventilate each individual infant at each timepoint, avoiding both atelectasis and overdistension. Ascertaining such an ideal pressure is hampered by the lack of easy-to-use, reliable bedside tools. Clinicians have traditionally relied on clinical assessment (respiratory rate and effort), oxygen requirement (as a proxy for ventilation/perfusion matching), and chest radiography (as a substitute for lung inflation) to judge whether more or less support is required. More recently, electrical impedance tomography has been used to visualize lung inflation in preterm infants at the bedside.[90] The technique shows promise but is not yet a simple, real-time, clinically accessible modality.[91]

Animal studies have shown that the alveolar-arterial gradient falls as pressure is increased from 0 to 8 cm H_2O.[92] This is supported by data from preterm infants demonstrating increasing FRC and tidal volume, decreasing respiratory rate, and improved thoracoabdominal synchrony over a similar CPAP pressure range.[93] There is likely to be an upper limit to safe CPAP, although this level will change throughout an infant's course. Excessive CPAP pressure can result in overexpansion, which in turn can result in air leak,[4] decreased venous return,[94] and reduced ventilation.[95]

We know that clinicians typically commence CPAP pressures in the region of 5–6 cm H_2O, with many allowing an increase up to 8 cm H_2O and some up to 10 cm H_2O.[96-98] However, a short period of time at higher pressure can lead to a sustained improvement in aeration. A study of preterm infants demonstrated that the lung volume gained when moving from a CPAP of 5 to 6 cm H_2O to 10 cm H_2O was maintained in the majority when the CPAP was decreased to 8 cm H_2O.[90] There are limited data in regard to optimal CPAP pressures to use postextubation in preterm infants. The one published RCT reported that in 93 infants, extubation failure was lower in those treated with CPAP pressures of 7 to 9 cm H_2O, compared with those treated using 4 to 6 cm H_2O (RR, 0.60; 95% CI, 0.35–1.00; number needed to treat, five infants).[99] A trial enrolling extremely preterm infants is currently underway, comparing postextubation CPAP pressures of 6 to 8 cm H_2O with 9 to 11 cm H_2O (Trial Registration ACTRN12618001638224). Regardless of the chosen pressure, it may be difficult to consistently deliver it as there is considerable pressure loss across CPAP interfaces,[81] some of which may not be appreciated or quantified, as well as further pressure loss via leak at the upper airway from the mouth and nose.[100] Whatever level is initially set, infants who require increasing oxygen concentration or who have increasing respiratory effort likely require more support, whereas those with decreasing oxygen needs and who are breathing comfortably likely have improving lung compliance and may tolerate reduced levels of support.

Supportive Care During Continuous Positive Airway Pressure

Although local management strategies vary, there are some overarching philosophies that should be applied when caring for infants on CPAP. There is good evidence that active preterm infants requiring respiratory assistance should be stabilized using CPAP in the delivery room[24] and continue to receive this support during transfer to the newborn nursery. More mature preterm (and term) infants who do not initially require CPAP may subsequently develop signs of respiratory distress and require support. The optimal mode of initial noninvasive support in older preterm infants is discussed later in this chapter.

Infants supported with CPAP require meticulous nursing care. Nasal prongs that are too large or too small risk nasal injury or prong dislodgement. Close observation is especially important when there are no inbuilt alarm systems to alert the clinician to either obstruction or loss of delivered pressure. Nasal prongs are designed to entirely fill the nares without blanching the surrounding tissue. Nasal masks should fit comfortably over the bridge of the nose and rest on the philtrum without encroaching on the upper lip, and nasal cannulae should fill about half the nares, leaving a clear leak. Careful attention must be paid to the infant's position, both in terms of maintaining a neutral airway and in regard to their developmental needs. These details are especially important as infants are now treated with CPAP for many weeks, even months, and longer treatment times increase the risk of nasal injury.[101] Infants typically have an orogastric tube placed in an attempt to "vent" the stomach and prevent bowel distension, which is a common problem with CPAP; however, there is little evidence that this is useful.

Infants supported with CPAP should undergo continuous cardiorespiratory monitoring including peripheral oxygen saturations or transcutaneous measurements. Arterial or capillary blood gas analysis should drive assessment of ventilation, and a baseline chest x-ray should be performed to assess lung expansion, evidence of infection, and air leak. Some respiratory scoring tools exist, such as the Silverman-Anderson respiratory severity score, which have good reliability in determining the need for additional support.[102]

Centers with highly successful CPAP programs attribute their success to a team approach, dedicated nursing care and consistent management using a single mode of CPAP support.[103] Given the highly specialized care required for optimal CPAP support described above, nurse-to-patient ratios, specific training of bedside nursing staff or respiratory therapists, and the overall clinical acuity on the unit may contribute to outcomes of infants receiving CPAP or other noninvasive respiratory supports. Whereas the neonatal intensive care unit (NICU) is often a setting with relatively high nurse-to-patient ratios, it is often not achievable to have 1:1 nursing of infants receiving CPAP or other noninvasive respiratory supports, which may not be optimal.[104] There are other examples of how the health outcomes of infants and families in NICUs may be jeopardized when nursing care is suboptimal.[105,106]

Administration of Surfactant to Infants on Continuous Positive Airway Pressure

Surfactant is one of the most studied treatments in neonatology. It is now 40 years since the first trials of surfactant. At that time, ventilation via an ETT was the standard treatment for very preterm infants, antenatal corticosteroids were given to a minority of eligible mothers, and rates of neonatal mortality and morbidity were much higher than today. Then, and until recently, surfactant was administered via the ETT with a subsequent period of MV. However, in the last decade or so, alternative "less invasive" techniques for surfactant instillation without an ETT have been described.

Oropharyngeal, Nebulized, and Laryngeal Mask Airway Surfactant Administration

Several methods of surfactant administration without endotracheal catheterization have been proposed. Pharyngeal instillation before delivery of the shoulders is feasible,[107] but as yet untested in large RCTs, although a trial of oropharyngeal surfactant at birth is underway.[108]

Aerosolized administration, an attractive option as it is truly "noninvasive," has been unsuccessful in the past because of inefficient aerosol devices. Newer nebulizers may be more efficient and reliable: a trial by Minocchieri et al.[109] found that surfactant delivered using a customized vibrating membrane nebulizer (eFlow neonatal nebulizer system, PARI Pharma, Starnberg, Germany) reduced the requirement for intubation within 72 hours, although the benefit seemed to be limited to more mature preterm infants. Further trials of surfactant nebulization are ongoing, although technical challenges remain in delivering the surfactant efficiently.

Surfactant has also been administered by supraglottic airway, also called laryngeal mask airway (LMA) (Fig. 18.6). A recent systematic review and meta-analysis[110] that included five RCTs showed LMA surfactant administration was associated with a reduction in MV in comparison with both continued CPAP (RR, 0.57; 95%, CI, 0.38–0.85) and surfactant administration via an ETT (RR, 0.43; 95% CI, 0.31–0.61). However, the authors caution that these findings are based on a limited number of infants in studies of varying designs and qualities and recommended that LMA surfactant administration be limited to clinical trials. The size of currently available LMAs limits their use to larger and more mature preterm infants,[111] and LMA surfactant delivery has not been reported in infants weighing <1000 g.[110]

Less Invasive Surfactant Administration and Minimally Invasive Surfactant Treatment: Surfactant Administration via Thin Catheter

The most extensively studied "less invasive" surfactant administration techniques are LISA (less invasive surfactant administration) and MIST (minimally invasive surfactant treatment). These are similar procedures during which infants on CPAP

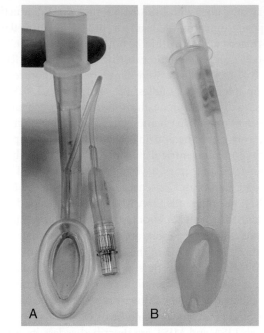

Fig. 18.6 Laryngeal mask airways. **(A)** Ambu Inc., Linthicum, MD, USA, shown with the rim inflated, and **(B)** iGel LMA, Intersurgical, Berkshire, UK.

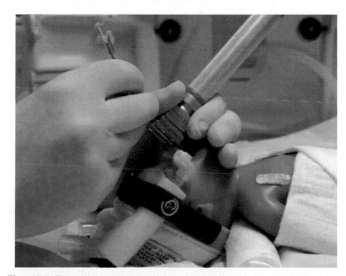

Fig. 18.7 The minimally invasive surfactant treatment procedure in a preterm infant who is spontaneously breathing on continuous positive airway pressure.

spontaneously breathe during the administration of surfactant via a feeding tube or thin catheter inserted through the vocal cords into the trachea under direct laryngoscopy, with or without premedication (Fig. 18.7).

Following promising observational studies suggesting improved short-term outcomes, LISA/MIST techniques have been further evaluated in RCTs[112-119] and meta-analyses.[120,121] These RCTs, including a total of more than 1200 preterm infants, are all unblinded and vary by the technique, the mode of noninvasive respiratory support used, the comparator, and study population. A meta-analysis by Aldana-Aguirre et al. in 2017 (which does not include the more recently published RCTs) reported improved respiratory outcomes with LISA/MIST, including a reduction in the composite outcome of death or BPD (RR, 0.75; 95% CI, 0.59–0.94), need for MV within 72 hours of birth (RR, 0.71; 95% CI, 0.53–0.96), and MV anytime during the admission (RR, 0.66; 95% CI, 0.47–0.93). There were fewer pneumothoraces in the LISA group infants (five studies; RR, 0.61; 95% CI, 0.37–1.02). There was no difference in death or in important neonatal morbidities such as pulmonary hemorrhage, patent ductus arteriosus requiring treatment, necrotizing enterocolitis, retinopathy of prematurity, or intraventricular hemorrhage. It must be noted that longer-term outcomes have not been reported. The 2019 update to the European Consensus Guidelines on the Management of RDS recommends LISA/MIST as the preferred method of surfactant treatment for spontaneously breathing infants receiving CPAP support.[26] Results are currently awaited of the largest (and only blinded) RCT of the MIST procedure, the international OPTIMIST-A trial.[122] It is enrolling preterm infants born 25 to 28 completed weeks' gestation, administering surfactant via a thin vascular catheter (the "Hobart method"), and has the important primary outcome of death or BPD.

Although LISA and MIST are described as less invasive than intubation with an ETT, these techniques still require laryngoscopy. They have attracted debate as to whether pharmacological analgesia should be routine, and if so, which drug(s) are safe and effective. Several medications have been proposed or tested (including propofol, fentanyl, ketamine and remifentanil), but none fits the ideal safety and efficacy profile required, and long-term outcomes from their use have not yet been reported.[123] Analgesic medications may be sedating, and spontaneous respiration is critical to the success of these procedures. Desaturation and bradycardia are known complications of tracheal catheterization,[124-127] which can be significantly reduced by administering atropine before the procedure, as shown in several studies.[128,129]

When Has Treatment With Continuous Positive Airway Pressure "Failed?"

Clinicians strive to avoid MV and limit its duration by using noninvasive supports such as CPAP; however, it is still important to recognize the need for surfactant administration and/or MV in preterm infants, lest they become more unstable or suffer the complications of respiratory failure. Despite this clinical scenario being very common in neonatal units around the world, there remains no universally accepted definition of "CPAP failure." The failure criteria used in trials of CPAP in the delivery room in extremely preterm infants vary: in the COIN trial,[4] these were a fraction of inspired oxygen (FiO_2) greater than 0.6 or pH over 7.25 with partial pressure of carbon dioxide ($PaCO_2$) under 60 mm Hg, or more than one apnea per hour requiring stimulation; in the SUPPORT trial,[3] these were FiO_2 over 0.50, $PaCO_2$ more than 65 mm Hg, or hemodynamic instability.

It can be difficult to determine the optimal CPAP pressure for an individual infant, although the FiO_2 required to maintain peripheral oxygen saturation targets is important, and investigations such as chest x-ray or lung ultrasound (to determine the severity of lung pathology and assess inflation), blood gas analysis, or transcutaneous carbon dioxide monitoring (to detect respiratory failure) may be useful adjuncts. Point-of-care

lung ultrasound is increasingly used to make clinical decisions around escalation of care in preterm infants with RDS, with a recent systematic review of six studies (total 485 infants) finding a higher lung ultrasound score accurately predicted the need for surfactant or MV.[130] Lung ultrasound has the added potential advantage of avoiding radiation if used in place of chest x-ray.[131] Some units have adopted respiratory scoring tools, such as the Silverman-Anderson score[132] or newer variants, to guide clinical management.

In general, in preterm infants with RDS, CPAP failure is usually based clinically on an increasing or persistently high FiO_2 above a prespecified upper limit despite maximal CPAP: typically an FiO_2 greater than 0.30 in preterm infants.[133] In many centers, the maximum set CPAP pressure is 8 cm H_2O or less, but some centers may be comfortable to increase the set pressure to more than 10 cm H_2O, especially in infants already treated with surfactant.[97-99] The substantial pressure drop documented for the RAM cannula should be taken into account when determining the appropriate pressure limit to use with CPAP.[84,85] However, particularly in the most immature infants, an increasing oxygen requirement from RDS is not the only factor, and apnea or acidosis may be a reason to escalate respiratory support. Studies suggest that lower gestational age, more severe radiographic lung disease, and escalating FiO_2 are key markers for preterm infants in whom CPAP is more likely to fail.[20,133] Whatever threshold for CPAP treatment failure is applied, it is important that remediable causes are sought and treated before progressing to endotracheal intubation. These include ensuring optimal prong size (filling the nares without blanching the surrounding tissue), avoiding prong dislodgement, optimal airway positioning, and measures to reduce leak.

Complications of Continuous Positive Airway Pressure

Aside from issues with maintaining the prongs in place with an adequate seal, which are important considerations, CPAP use in preterm infants has been associated with complications, most relatively minor, but some that are more severe and result in significant morbidity.

Gaseous Intestinal Distension

A usually minor but frequently seen complication is gaseous distension of the intestine presenting as abdominal distension, or "CPAP belly," owing to both direct passage of delivered gas into the esophagus and the infant swallowing additional gas. In severe cases, there may be pressure on the diaphragm from this distension, worsening the respiratory status of the infant. Placement of an orogastric tube should be routine during CPAP and indeed with other modes of respiratory support. Some of the more important complications are discussed later.

Pneumothorax or Other Air Leak

Pneumothorax is a well-recognized, sometimes severe complication of CPAP, and clinicians need to be proficient at diagnosing and treating this condition. In preterm infants, the risk of pneumothorax seems to be mainly limited to surfactant-deficient infants receiving CPAP for treatment of RDS in the first days of life and is much less common during CPAP as postextubation/surfactant support.[32,134] Early treatment with surfactant appears to substantially reduce the risk of pneumothorax and other air leaks.

In the COIN trial,[4] there were significantly more pneumothoraces in the CPAP group than in the ventilated group (9% vs. 3%, respectively), raising concerns about the use of early nasal CPAP. In the Colombian Neonatal Network study, the group managed with early surfactant therapy had fewer pneumothoraces compared with the group managed with nasal CPAP alone (2% vs. 9%).[135] Conversely, the SUPPORT trial found no difference in the rate of pneumothoraces between early CPAP and early MV.[3] An RCT of early CPAP compared with supplemental oxygen therapy alone for more mature newborn infants with respiratory distress born in Australian nontertiary centers by Buckmaster et al. found an almost threefold higher rate of pneumothorax in the CPAP group: 9% versus 3%.[136] Two recent RCTs comparing noninvasive respiratory supports for newborn infants who had not yet received surfactant treatment in tertiary NICUs[137] and nontertiary centers[138] had pneumothorax rates in the CPAP groups of 2% and 8%, respectively.

Nasal Skin Trauma

The use of binasal prongs to deliver nasal CPAP in very preterm infants is associated with pressure-related nasal trauma ranging from mild erythema to severe injury requiring surgery.[139] A recent systematic review by Imbulana et al. of CPAP-related nasal trauma found the condition was common (reported ranges from 20% to 100%), with very preterm infants born less than 30 weeks' gestation and those requiring longer duration of CPAP most at risk.[140] However, some centers with extensive experience in using nasal CPAP in preterm infants report much lower rates, which they attribute to their careful management and nursing skill.

The systematic review found that strategies shown to reduce nasal trauma in preterm infants include the use of nasal barrier dressings (three studies, $n = 345$; RR, 0.27; 95% CI, 0.13–0.55), using nHF therapy as an alternative to CPAP (eight studies, $n = 1640$; RR, 0.46; 95% CI, 0.37–0.57), and using a nasal mask rather than binasal prongs (four studies, $n = 476$; RR, 0.70; 95% CI, 0.51–0.94).[140] Subsequent to this review, there has been an additional single-center RCT performed of a hydrocolloid nasal barrier dressing during CPAP in 108 very preterm infants born under 30 weeks' gestation and/or with birth weight under 1250 g.[141] Infants in the nasal barrier group had a significantly lower rate of nasal injury compared with the no barrier group, although the injuries described were mainly mild.

In units with high rates of CPAP-related injury it seems reasonable to use hydrocolloid nasal dressings. Otherwise, it is important to be meticulous with appropriate positioning of the nasal prongs, with frequent examination by bedside staff to identify infants at risk of injury. Some units alternate use of nasal prongs with nasal masks in an attempt to minimize nasal injury.

Continuous Positive Airway Pressure Weaning

It is important to minimize exposure of preterm infants to respiratory support and oxygen supplementation. Practice around weaning from CPAP varies greatly around the world, and the optimal method of CPAP weaning remains uncertain. Proposed weaning methods include the cessation of CPAP when certain clinical criteria are met, "cycling" CPAP on and off with a gradual increase in the time off CPAP (with or without supplemental oxygen or nHF [discussed later] when off CPAP), a gradual reduction of set CPAP pressure followed by cessation, or a combination of these methods. Several RCTs with differing methodologies have compared these strategies.

In a Danish multicenter RCT by Jensen et al.,[142] sudden cessation of CPAP was compared with pressure weaning (gradual reduction in pressure before cessation) in infants born under 32 weeks' gestation, with 354 infants completing the trial. Although in a subgroup of infants born less than 28 weeks of gestation, more were successfully weaned from CPAP during the first attempt in the pressure wean group compared with the sudden discontinuation group (risk difference, 31%; 95% CI, 13%–50%), there was no overall difference in the duration of CPAP or supplemental oxygen. Rastogi et al.[143] undertook a pilot RCT comparing sudden and gradual weaning methods in 56 preterm infants born under 33 weeks' gestation and found no difference in the rate of success of initial weaning, the postmenstrual age at which infants were weaned off CPAP, or the length of hospital admission between the two methods.

An Australian multicenter RCT enrolled 177 very preterm infants born under 30 weeks' gestation[144] who were stable on CPAP, and then randomly allocated them to one of three CPAP weaning strategies: (1) sudden cessation of CPAP with a view to remain off; (2) cycling on and off CPAP with incremental increases in time off CPAP; and (3) cycling on and off CPAP with incremental increases in time off CPAP, but with infants supported by nasal cannula with gas flow 0.5 L/min during periods off CPAP. In contrast to the findings of the earlier studies, this study found that sudden cessation (method 1) significantly reduced the time to wean from CPAP (mean ± SD, 11.3 ± 0.8 days) compared with methods 2 and 3 (16.8 ± 1.0 days and 19.4 ± 1.3 days respectively) and reduced CPAP duration (24.4 ± 0.1, 38.6 ± 0.1, and 30.5 ± 0.1, respectively). In addition, sudden cessation was associated with shorter duration of supplemental oxygen and hospital admission and a reduction in the diagnosis of BPD.

Several RCTs have assessed the role of nHF, a support mode discussed in a later section, in weaning preterm infants from nasal CPAP, with conflicting results at least partially explained by their methodology and sample sizes. Three trials[146-148] found that nHF use contributed to shorter time on CPAP without reducing the overall duration of noninvasive support, one trial found that the use of nHF 2 L/min to wean from CPAP resulted in more days on oxygen and respiratory support,[148] and another found that nHF 2 L/min significantly reduced the duration of supplemental oxygen and hospital stay but did not increase successful weaning from CPAP.[149]

NASAL VENTILATION

Nasal ventilation is the noninvasive application of an additional positive airway pressure above the baseline nasal CPAP at some added rate. The most common terms to denote this approach to noninvasive respiratory support include NIPPV, noninvasive ventilation (NIV), and nasal intermittent mandatory ventilation (NIMV). In this section, we will use the acronym NIPPV when describing noninvasive nasal ventilation. The additional airway pressure can be synchronized (sNIPPV) or nonsynchronized (nsNIPPV) with an infant's spontaneous breaths.

Historically, the first publication on neonatal NIPPV appears to be that by Donald and Lord in 1953 employing a face mask interface.[150] Over a decade later, the first reports on successful application of NIPPV via face mask interface were published by Helmrath et al. and Llewellyn and colleagues.[151,152] Owing to a variety of clinical concerns and technical issues with prolonged face mask application in preterm infants, devices were developed and studied to apply positive pressure noninvasively via the nares and nasopharynx.[153-155] Subsequently, Moretti and colleagues published one of the first reports incorporating NIPPV via nasal prongs.[156] In the 40 years since, a wide range of devices and approaches to NIPPV have been studied.

Physiologic Mechanisms

The physiologic effects of NIPPV are generally the same as for nasal CPAP. The primary goal is to improve end-expiratory lung volume via the application of positive end-expiratory pressure. Improved FRC is accompanied by decreased intrapulmonary shunt, improved compliance, and reduced work of breathing. Studies in preterm infants show a "dose-dependent" effect of CPAP on tidal volume, end-expiratory lung volume, and oxygenation.[69,93,157] Additionally, there is evidence for lower respiratory rate and work of breathing.[69,93,157] Reduction in apnea has also been reported as a benefit from NIPPV, although meta-analyses do not suggest convincing evidence for this effect and note that additional studies are needed.[41,158]

A key physiologic question in comparing NIPPV with CPAP is, what are the effects of the imposed nasal pressures provided by the delivery device? Specifically, does the added pressure augment pressure and volume delivery to the lung to improve gas exchange? The answer to this question remains unclear but the evidence is summarized here:

1. Pressure delivery: Most studies suggest limited and variable additional pressure delivery during NIPPV pressure changes, even when synchronized with spontaneous breaths.[160-163] Additionally, during episodes of central or obstructive apnea, none (or very little) of the NIPPV delivered pressure is transmitted beyond the glottis.[159,160,162]
2. Volume delivery: Given that pressure delivery during NIPPV support appears limited, it is not surprising that these studies also found no or minimal augmentation of tidal volumes, with or without synchronization.[9,157,159-162] Again, during episodes of apnea, limited to no volume delivery is measurable, even with synchronization.
3. Gas exchange: Although studies by Ali et al. and Chang et al. suggest that measures of gas exchange (minute ventilation, FiO_2, peripheral oxygen saturation, and transcutaneous $PaCO_2$) are no different between preterm infants managed on CPAP and those on either sNIPPV or nsNIPPV, they do demonstrate improvement in measures for work of breathing.[9,161]

On the other hand, Huang and colleagues showed that sNIPPV, compared with nsNIPPV, had more effective gas exchange in preterm infants when applied in the immediate/early postextubation period.[163]

A key difference between any form of NIPPV and CPAP is the intermittent delivery of added positive pressure to the nasopharyngeal-glottic region. During spontaneous breathing, there is a well-synchronized neural interplay that optimizes the flow of inspired gas from outside the body into the gas exchange regions. This includes activation of glottal dilator muscles in synchrony with activation of the diaphragm. The likely physiologic benefit is reduced resistance to flow during inspiration. CPAP alone does not appear to alter glottal dilator muscle activation during inspiration.[164] The introduction of NIPPV pressures significantly changes the inspiratory dynamics of the glottic region; there is both an inhibition of the normal glottic dilator muscle activity as well as an increase in glottic constrictor muscle activity.[164,165] The net effect of this change in glottic muscle activation is a narrowing of the glottis and limitation in lung ventilation.[164,166] Interestingly, neither sNIPPV nor noninvasive high-frequency nasal ventilation (HFNV, discussed later) induces this glottic constrictor muscle activity.[167,168] These findings suggest that, at least from a physiologic perspective, some approaches to NIPPV may be less noxious and more supportive than others.

Clinical Trials
Nasal Intermittent Positive Pressure Ventilation

The first randomized clinical trials comparing NIPPV with other modes of noninvasive support for the respiratory management of neonates were performed over 20 years ago.[169-172] Over the ensuing two decades, there have been numerous additional trials, with several recent meta-analyses related to the overall efficacy and safety of NIPPV in neonates (Table 18.1).[173-177]

The general consensus from meta-analyses is that, compared with all other noninvasive approaches, NIPPV significantly lowers the risk for intubation and MV. This effect is found when NIPPV is used as primary therapy for respiratory distress, as well as for postextubation support. When analyzed by synchronization (sNIPPV versus nsNIPPV), a benefit from synchronization is not consistently found when the approach is for primary therapy of RDS. However, there appears to be a strong signal favoring sNIPPV versus nsNIPPV, as well as all other noninvasive modes, when used for postextubation support of preterm infants.[174,175] Although there is a strong suggestion for reduced rates of intubation and MV, studies have not demonstrated an NIPPV benefit for mortality, BPD, or the combined outcome of death or BPD. Synchronization may have a positive signal for these outcomes, but the studies are limited.[173-176] It is important to point out the overall low quality of studies included in these meta-analyses. Additionally, the majority of studies are of fairly small size and there is a wide range of approaches to each of the noninvasive modes studied.

The results of Kirpalani et al.'s trial[178] comparing NIPPV with CPAP dominate any meta-analyses of NIPPV. This large, pragmatic, multicenter, randomized trial conducted between 2007 and 2011 hypothesized that NIPPV would reduce the risk

TABLE 18.1 Summary of Recent Meta-analyses for Nasal Intermittent Positive Pressure Ventilation

Author Intervention	Lemyre	Ramaswamy	Isayama
NIPPV vs. nasal CPAP Failure ETT/MV BPD	Primary therapy 0.65 (0.51–0.82) 10 trials, 1060 pts 0.78 (0.64–0.94) 9 trials, 950 pts 0.78 (0.58–1.06) 9 trials, 899 pts No signal effect for sNIPPV vs. nsNIPPV	Primary therapy 0.56 (0.44–0.71) 13 trials, 1508 pts 0.60 (0.44–0.77) 13 trials, 1514 pts 0.75 (0.48–1.09) 6 trials, 855 pts No signal effect for sNIPPV vs. nsNIPPV	Primary therapy Did not analyze for failure or ETT/MV Multiple interventions: LISA, INSURE, NIPPV, nasal CPAP LISA consistently had lowest rates for BPD, death, or combined outcome
NIPPV vs. nasal CPAP Failure ETT/MV BPD	Postextubation 0.70 (0.60–0.80) 10 trials, 1431 pts 0.76 (0.65–0.88) 8 trials, 1301 pts 0.95 (0.59–1.55) 6 trials, 1140 pts	Postextubation Compared nCPAP to sNIPPV, nsNIPPV, nHF, and HFNV sNIPPV consistently showed lowest rates for ETT/MV and BPD vs. all other modes	Did not include postextubation studies

Data are presented as relative risk (95% confidence interval).
BPD, Bronchopulmonary dysplasia; *CPAP*, continuous positive airway pressure; *ETT*, endotracheal tube; *HFNV*, high-frequency nasal ventilation; *INSURE*, INtubation-SURfactant-Extubation technique; *LISA*, less invasive surfactant administration; *MV*, mechanical ventilation; *nHF*, nasal high flow; *s/nsNIPPV*, synchronized/nonsynchronized nasal intermittent positive pressure ventilation.

of BPD in extremely low birth weight infants (<30 weeks' gestation and <1000 g birth weight) by minimizing the duration of endotracheal intubation. This trial enrolled 1009 infants and differs from smaller studies in that it recruited a heterogeneous study population and permitted a variety of devices to deliver NIPPV, including some that delivered sNIPPV. There was no difference in the composite primary outcome of death or BPD: NIPPV 38.4% versus CPAP 36.7% (adjusted odds ratio, 1.09; 95% CI, 0.83–1.43; $P = .56$).

The mechanism(s) for the apparent benefit of NIPPV remain unclear. Several studies have noted that NIPPV does not typically provide additional pressure or volume support, and this is particularly so during periods of apnea.[159-161,179] One consistently proposed effect may be related to the fact that NIPPV is consistently applied with higher overall mean distending pressure than comparative modes, specifically CPAP.[174,180,181] The evidence to support the improved efficacy of higher versus lower CPAP pressures is limited.[99] Clinical trials are underway to help address the question whether NIPPV has greater efficacy than CPAP when comparable mean distending pressures are employed.

Synchronized Nasal Intermittent Positive Pressure Ventilation

Physiologically, sNIPPV makes sense. Animal studies show normalized glottic muscle activation with a synchronized approach compared with nsNIPPV.[164,167] Several studies suggest improved tidal volume, oxygenation, and work of breathing during sNIPPV support.[161,170,179] However, not all studies agree. The study by Chang et al. compared nasal CPAP, nsNIPPV, and sNIPPV in otherwise stable preterm infants and found no benefit during sNIPPV for tidal volume and minute ventilation or measures of gas exchange.[161] However, they (and others)

measured a significant reduction in work of breathing during sNIPPV. Although perhaps not as important for larger preterm infants, lower respiratory effort may enhance the ability of very preterm infants to tolerate noninvasive support.

There are a variety of approaches and devices that can support sNIPPV (Table 18.2). The approaches included synchronization with abdominal respiratory movements, flow synchronization, and synchronization with electrical activity of the diaphragm (Edi). The early trials assessing sNIPPV predominantly used an abdominal sensor called the Graseby capsule (Graseby Medical, UK) interfaced with the Infrasonics Infant Star 950 ventilator (Infrasonics Inc., San Diego, CA, USA).[169,171,172] This capsule can be interfaced with other devices, but clinical trials have not been done.[160] Promising results for sNIPPV have been reported by Ding et al. for a different abdominal sensor interfaced with the Comen NV8 neonatal ventilator (Shenzhen Comen Medical Instruments Co., Ltd., China), as well as by Moretti, Gizzi, and colleagues using flow synchronization via the Giulia V3 neonatal ventilator (Ginevri srl, Italy).[180,182-184] All of these sensors appear to have relatively rapid response time and high rates of trigger efficacy and can adjust to variable degrees of system leak. None of these devices are approved for use with NIPPV in the United States. Ideally, future investigations will be done to gain approval for more sNIPPV devices.

A promising approach to sNIPPV is neurally adjusted ventilatory assist, or NAVA, termed NIV-NAVA when used to for noninvasive respiratory support. NAVA synchronizes respiratory support (assist) via the electrical activity of the diaphragm (EAdi). The EAdi signal, obtained via miniaturized electrodes embedded on a specially developed naso-orogastric tube, is a measure of the central nervous system respiratory drive. The specialized catheter has been developed to work with the Servo ventilator (Maquet Critical Care AB, Sweden) and is approved

TABLE 18.2 **Potential Devices for Synchronized Approach to Nasal Intermittent Positive Pressure Ventilation**

Device	Comen NV8	Giulia V3	InfantStar 950	Servo-*i*
Manufacturer and country	Comen Medical China	GINERVI Italy	No longer made	Maquet Sweden
FDA approved	No	No	Yes	Yes
Synchronization mechanism	Abdominal sensor	Flow sensor	Abdominal Graseby capsule	Diaphragm electrical activity
Response time	Not reported	~64 milliseconds	~26 milliseconds	<20 milliseconds
Leak compensation	Yes, ~25%	Yes	Yes	Yes
Trigger efficacy	Not reported	>90%	>85%	>95%
Clinical trials	Ding	Morretti Gizzi	Friedlich Barrington Khalaf	Kallio Yagui Makker

FDA, U.S. Food and Drug Administration.

in many countries, including the United States. Employing the EAdi signal for synchronization eliminates concerns raised about approaches using either abdominal movement, or flow-based approaches to synchronization. One apparently unique aspect of the NAVA approach is that the level of assistance delivered is proportional to the diaphragmatic signal and NAVA level; thus, assisted respiratory support can be adjusted to provide more or less support for the patient as needed. As it is based on the neural-EAdi signal, NAVA provides rapid response time and excellent ventilatory synchrony. As with all other approaches to synchronization, NIV-NAVA is only possible when the infant has a reasonably stable respiratory drive and thus may not be an option with severe central or obstructive apnea, with oversedation, or when an effective EAdi signal cannot be generated.

There are numerous observational studies reporting the potential for NIV-NAVA to safely support sNIPPV in preterm infants.[185-187] Several small randomized trials comparing NIV-NAVA with CPAP have been reported.[188-190] Although the results are mixed, these small studies support possible benefits of using NIV-NAVA for sNIPPV. Large multicenter randomized trials targeting high-risk populations and assessing important long-term respiratory outcomes are needed. Such trials should attempt to employ similar mean airway pressures in all study groups and should include comparisons of NIV-NAVA with other synchronized NIPPV modes and with CPAP at equivalent mean pressures.

HIGH-FREQUENCY NASAL VENTILATION

HFNV can be described as any noninvasive approach in which high-frequency pressure changes are added via any device, to provide high-frequency modulations to flow. These modulations can be oscillatory, interruptive, or pulsatile in design. Potential noninvasive interfaces can include standard nasal prongs, a nasal mask, a nasopharyngeal tube, or even a nasal cannula. In many ways, the path incorporating use of HFNV within the NICU mirrors that for nHF (discussed later); use escalated over several years before any randomized trials were actually performed and before a definitive benefit has been shown.

Mechanisms of Gas Exchange

Multiple factors are likely to determine the effectiveness of gas exchange during HFNV (Fig. 18.8). Most of these factors are interactive, although interface resistance likely has the largest functional influence. To date, no single device has demonstrable superiority. One variable that has not been well studied is the role for added conventional pressure changes during HFNV (i.e., combining NIPPV with HFNV). With the exception of the SensorMedics 3110A (CareFusion, San Diego, CA, USA), most other high-frequency ventilators available across the world have

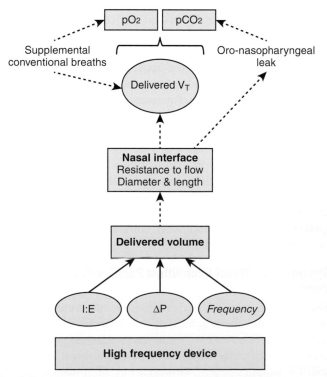

Fig. 18.8 Interactive factors contributing to delivered tidal volume and effectiveness of gas exchange during noninvasive high-frequency nasal ventilation. *I:E,* Inspiratory to expiratory ratio; *ΔP,* pressure amplitude; *PCO₂,* partial pressure of carbon dioxide; *PO₂,* partial pressure of oxygen; *V$_T$,* tidal volume.

TABLE 18.3 Potential Factors Determining the Efficacy and Safety of High-Frequency Nasal Ventilation

Variable	Comments
Ventilator	A variety of "drivers" are possible; not all have been studied
	Majority are not currently FDA approved
	SensorMedics, VDR-4, Life Pulse Jet, medinCNO, Leoni Plus, Stephanie/Sophie, SLE 5000, Fabian
Frequency	Unclear the role for active v passive expiration
	Optimum f unclear; bench studies suggest <10 Hz
	Most studies used 10 Hz, with range 6–14 Hz
Inspiratory time	Longer I:E increases V_T delivery; studies vary, 1:1 to 1:3
	Recommend maximum on-time for jet
Amplitude/P	Increased $\Delta P \rightarrow$ larger V_T
	Markedly limited by interface resistance, leak
	Most recommend adjusting to get upper chest vibration
	Unclear effect; leak may play a larger role for ventilation
Nasal interface	Standard binasal CPAP prongs or mask
	Single nasopharyngeal tube
	Nasal cannula
Conventional breaths	Not all devices can incorporate added conventional breaths
	Studied in animal models, but not described in neonatal reports

Device manufacturers: FDA approved: 3100A (Carefusion, San Diego, CA, USA), VDR4/Bronchotron (Percussionaire, Sandpoint, ID, USA), and Life Pulse Jet (Bunnell Inc., Salt Lake City, UT, USA). Non–FDA approved: Drager VN500/Babylog 8000 (Draeger Medical, Lubeck, Germany), medinCNO (medin Medical Innovations GmbH, Olching, Germany), Leoni Plus (Heinen+Lowenstein, Bad Ems, Germany), and Sophie (Fritz Stephan-GmbH, Gackenbach, Germany). *FDA*, U.S. Food and Drug Administration; *I:E*, inspiratory:expiratory ratio; ΔP, oscillatory pressure amplitude; V_T, tidal volume.

this as a potential option (Table 18.3). The dynamics of gas exchange during HFNV remain less clear than during invasive high-frequency oscillatory ventilation (HFOV).[74] Laboratory evidence demonstrates substantial loss of pressure and volume across the noninvasive interface during HFNV in both test lungs[191-193] and animal studies.[194] Tidal volume appears to be affected by the same factors that control tidal volume during invasive HFOV: amplitude, inspiratory time, and frequency.[191,192] However, ventilatory efficiency appears to be much more impacted by the nasal interface during noninvasive support than the ETT during MV, likely related to differences in resistance and leak. Bench studies show that nasal prongs with larger internal diameters (i.e., lower resistance) allow larger tidal volume delivery,[192] whereas nasal masks allow very minimal pressure or volume delivery[193] (Fig. 18.8). Mukerji et al. performed bench testing to assess the effect of high-frequency oscillatory rate on carbon dioxide removal and found markedly more removal from a test lung at all HFNV rates compared with conventional NIPPV, with optimal removal at a frequency of 8 Hz.[195] Although most studies have used ventilators specifically manufactured for the purpose of high-frequency ventilation, even a very simplified system employing an in-line solenoid valve to provide high-frequency flow interruptions during the application of

CPAP or nHF can enhance carbon dioxide clearance.[196,197] Studies also show, however, that incorporating at least a moderate leak during HFNV enhances this process.[198] This finding, akin to that shown with nHF (discussed later) where increased leak also supports enhanced carbon dioxide clearance,[199] suggests that some element of nasopharyngeal dead space "washout" may play a role in how HFNV supports gas exchange. As described later, clinical trials have employed a variety of devices and settings, but studies have not yet begun to investigate the optimal settings for HFNV by device or interface.

As noted in the NIPPV section, there is a different response of the laryngo-pharyngeal musculature during various modes of noninvasive support. During normal spontaneous breathing, laryngeal muscles act in synchrony to open the upper airway during inspiration, decreasing resistance and easing the flow of gas through the glottis. This synchrony persists during CPAP support, as well as with sNIPPV (including NIV-NAVA) but is markedly altered during nsNIPPV.[164,167] Similar to CPAP and sNIPPV, HFNV has also been shown to support the normal synchrony of laryngeal muscle activation.[168]

Clinical Trials

Van der Hoeven et al. first reported the use of HFNV as a noninvasive technique over 20 years ago.[200] Several additional small, retrospective reports followed, but it was not until recently that randomized trials were published. Table 18.4 shows the study characteristics and findings for five recently completed randomized trials enrolling a total of 513 babies.[201-205] There are wide ranges in the gestational ages among the studies, as well as differences in timing of the intervention and the approaches to HFNV support. Additionally, not all studies attempted to employ equivalent mean airway pressures between the HFNV and CPAP groups. Recognizing the differences in study design, most studies suggested a statistical difference in the subsequent use of MV. The sole study not reporting this difference, by Mukerji et al., enrolled the fewest patients at the lowest gestational age. Two studies reported significantly lower carbon dioxide values in the HFNV group, although the relative clinical benefit of this difference is unclear.[203,205] Because of the generally high gestational age across these studies, no differences were seen in rates for BPD or survival, nor for duration of oxygen support or hospitalization. Limited data from two recently published meta-analyses related to the evidence base for HFNV are also shown in Table 18.4.[206,207] The apparent benefit from HFNV compared with CPAP was an overall reduction in risk for MV of about 50%. Given the methodological differences and issues with these trials, it is clear that adequately powered multicenter trials with relevant primary clinical outcomes are needed before we can better determine the efficacy and safety of HFNV in the management of high-risk preterm infants. At least one such study is planned to compare HFNV with nsNIPPV and CPAP.[208] However, there are methodological concerns because of important between-group differences in starting and maximum allowed mean airway pressure.

None of the clinical studies published to date has incorporated NIPPV-style pressure changes during HFNV support. This approach has been used in animal studies investigating

TABLE 18.4   High-Frequency Nasal Ventilation: Demographics, Nasal Interface, Ventilator Driver and Settings, and Effects for Published Randomized Trials and Meta-analyses

	Mukerji	Zhu	Chen	Iranpour	Malakian
No. infants	39	76	206	68	124
GA (weeks)	~26	28–34	<37	30–36	28–34
Timing	Failing CPAP	Post-INSURE	Post-extubation	Primary RDS	Primary RDS
Control	Nasal CPAP	Nasal CPAP	Nasal CPAP	Nasal CPAP	Nasal CPAP
Paw (cm H_2O)	Same	Same	Different	Different	Same
	8–10	6	10 vs. 6	8 vs. 6–7	4–8
HFNV driver	Drager vn500	medinCNO	SLE5000	Fabian	medinCNO
HFNV settings	6–14 Hz	10 Hz	8–12 Hz	10 Hz	5 Hz
	8–10 cm H_2O	6 cm H_2O	8–10 cm H_2O	8 cm H_2O	4–8 cmH_2O
	Variable ΔP	Variable ΔP	Variable ΔP	Variable ΔP	Variable ΔP
Comments	HFNV vs. CPAP	HFMV vs. CPAP	HFNV vs. CPAP	HFNV vs. CPAP	HFNV vs. CPAP
	MV: 31% vs. 23%	MV: 24% vs. 56%[a]	MV: 17% vs. 36%[a]	MV: 0% vs. 12%[a]	MV: 7% vs. 14%
	BPD: 83% vs. 74%	BPD: 8% vs. 13%	BPD: 3% vs. 6%	BPD: 15% vs. 6%	BPD: None
	"Fail": 38% vs. 65%		pCO2: 50 vs. 57a		Hours NIV: 37% vs. 50[a]
Meta-analysis		No. Studies (No. Patients)	Mechanical Ventilation	Change in PCO2 (mm Hg)	
Li		8 (463)	0.50 (0.36–0.70)	−4.6 (−1.3 to −7.9)	
Shehedah		5 (275)	0.43 (0.25–0.75)	−3.8 (−0.4 to −7.3)	

[a]$P < .05$.

BPD, Bronchopulmonary dysplasia; *cm H_2O,* centimeters of water; *CPAP,* continuous positive airway pressure; *GA,* gestational age; *INSURE,* INtubation-SURfactant-Extubation technique; *MV,* mechanical ventilation; *NIV,* noninvasive ventilation; *ΔP,* oscillatory pressure amplitude; *Paw,* mean airway pressure; *PCO2,* partial pressure of carbon dioxide; *RDS,* respiratory distress syndrome.

HFNV as support for preterm lambs with RDS.[194,209] Although the published studies only reported HFNV support with the Percussionaire VDR4 high-frequency device (Percussionaire Corp., Sandpoint, ID, USA), the lamb model has also been supported by HFNV using the Dräger VN500 (Drägerwerk AG and Co. KGaA, Lübeck, Germany) and the Bunnell Life Pulse Jet ventilators (Bunnell Inc., Salt Lake City, UT, USA). Intermittent conventional NIPPV pressure changes might augment tidal volume delivery and improve FRC and gas exchange. Clearly, such an approach requires rigorous clinical trials before possible incorporation into clinical practice. Concerns have been raised over the potential for adverse effects from HFNV related to lowered relative humidity and temperature.[210] Relative loss of airway humidification over extended periods of time could lead to issues with epithelial injury and/or inspissated/thickened secretions throughout the respiratory system. Given the relatively high flow rates that may be employed during HFNV, additional concerns related to excessive gastrointestinal gas flow should also be considered for safety monitoring in future trials.

Future Directions

Numerous aspects related to HFNV need to be better studied and clarified, including comparisons of high-frequency "drivers," determining optimal frequencies and inspiratory times, the relative benefit of different interfaces and leaks, the potential role (if any) for NIPPV-style pressure changes during HFNV, and ease of user interface. The primary reason for promoting any mode of noninvasive respiratory support, including HFNV, rather than invasive MV is to potentially minimize injury to the immature lung, to improve lung growth, and possibly redirect the preterm lung back toward more normal development pathways. Long-term

studies, out to adolescence, will be required to effectively determine how well, or even if, we can achieve these goals. Such studies will require a long-term investment in time, money, and effort.

NASAL HIGH FLOW

CPAP is the mainstay of noninvasive respiratory support for newborn infants, although it has some potential disadvantages: nasal injury, bulky interfaces, and need for highly trained nursing staff to provide effective CPAP. In recent years, nHF, a simpler alternative to CPAP, has rapidly increased in popularity (Fig. 18.5). Somewhat confusingly, nHF is known by other names or acronyms around the world and in the literature, including high-flow nasal cannula (HFNC) or even (noting that all noninvasive respiratory supports should be, and routinely are, heated and humidified) heated, humidified HFNC (HHHFNC). HFNC/HHHFNC appears to reference the interface rather than the therapy applied via that interface and we prefer and will use nHF throughout this chapter.

nHF uses smaller binasal prongs (cannulae) than CPAP, with a simpler interface, and delivers heated, humidified gas at flows of more than 1 L/min, although in clinical practice and clinical trials, the flow is typically set at 2 to 8 L/min. Parents and nursing staff report a preference for nHF over CPAP, particularly in more stable infants;[211,212] the simpler nHF interface is perceived to be easier to use and more comfortable for infants than CPAP[211-213]; and it has been shown to result in lower rates of nasal skin trauma.[140] The most commonly used commercial nHF devices are the Optiflow Junior (Fisher & Paykel, Auckland, New Zealand) and the Precision Flow (Vapotherm Inc., Exeter, NH, USA) (Fig. 18.9). Although one or other device is

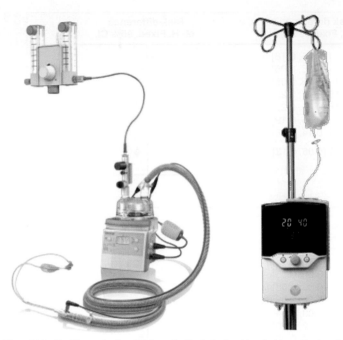

Fig. 18.9 Optiflow Junior (Fisher & Paykel, Auckland, New Zealand) (left) and the Precision Flow (Vapotherm Inc., Exeter, NH, USA) (right).

preferred in different units, only one small trial has compared their efficacy in preterm infants, as postextubation support, and found no difference.[214]

The mechanisms of action of nHF include heating and humidification of the gases, reduction in work of breathing, and the application of continuous (although variable and not set) distending pressure to the airways.[215] Washout of the nasopharyngeal dead space and subsequent carbon dioxide removal may also be important.[216,217] In contrast to CPAP, where the clinician sets the applied distending pressure, nHF requires gas flow rather than pressure to be selected. However, nHF does generate some distending pressure, probably similar to or below pressures commonly set during CPAP. The delivered pressure increases with increasing gas flow[218-221] and is higher in smaller infants[218,219] and with smaller leaks at the nares. Unlike a CPAP circuit that has an inspiratory and expiratory limb, nHF only has an inspiratory limb and relies either on gas escaping around the cannula and through the mouth or on an inbuilt pressure relief valve as included in some circuits. Thus, care must be taken to avoid a tight fit in the nostrils to avoid the potential of excessive pressure buildup.

Clinical Trials in Preterm Infants
Primary (Early) Respiratory Support

Since a 2016 Cochrane review,[222] there have been five new RCTs[137,138,223-225] and one updated RCT.[226] For an updated pooled analysis of the outcomes of treatment failure within 72 hours and MV within 72 hours, we excluded unpublished data and also the trial by Shin et al.[225] because the timeframe for these outcomes was not reported, leaving seven trials with a total of 1833 preterm infants that could be included (Fig. 18.10). When interpreting the results of these trials and the results of a meta-analysis, it is important to note that the studies differ in the devices used to deliver

nHF, the set gas flows, and the set CPAP pressures. Some studies allowed the use of "rescue" CPAP in the event of nHF treatment failure,[137,138,223,225] potentially preventing the need for MV, and similarly some allowed the use of biphasic positive airway pressure in infants in whom CPAP failed.[225,226] Three studies allowed surfactant administration via the INSURE (Intubation, Surfactant, Extubation) technique without this being deemed treatment failure.[224,226,227] There were no extremely preterm infants born under 28 weeks' gestation enrolled in any of the included studies.

The use of nHF as primary respiratory support after birth, when compared with CPAP, resulted in a higher rate of treatment failure within 72 hours (risk difference, 0.10; 95% CI, 0.06–0.13) (Fig. 18.10). Significant heterogeneity is evident between included trials. There was no difference in the rate of MV within 72 hours (risk difference, 0.01; 95% CI, -0.01 to 0.04; $P = .33$), possibly because of the use of "rescue" CPAP for infants in whom nHF failed in some trials. In other updated meta-analyses, there was no difference in the risk of death (RR, 1.10; 95% CI, 0.53–2.27; eight studies, 1900 infants) or BPD (RR, 1.14; 95% CI, 0.74–1.76; nine studies, 1987 infants). nHFs use reduced the rate of nasal trauma (RR, 0.49; 95% CI, 0.36–0.68; seven studies, 1286 infants) but resulted in a slightly longer duration of respiratory support (mean difference, 0.7 days; 95% CI, 0.4–1.0; six studies, 1429 infants). There was no difference in the rate of pneumothorax. The two largest studies that compared nHF with CPAP as primary support in newborn infants[137,138] undertook secondary analyses of their trial data to determine predictors of nHF success as early support to help guide clinicians.[228,229] In both, nHF treatment failure was moderately predicted by a lower gestational age and higher prerandomization oxygen requirement.

Three trials (total 272 preterm infants) compared nHF with NIPPV as early respiratory support,[224,230,231] and pooled analysis shows no difference in the rates of death, BPD, MV, or treatment failure. Infants randomized to nHF had a lower rate of nasal trauma, compared with NIPPV (RR, 0.21; 95% CI, 0.09–0.47).

In summary, nHF is associated with a higher rate of treatment failure when used as primary respiratory support for preterm infants, compared with CPAP. There is no difference in the rate of MV, likely owing to the use of "rescue" CPAP in several trials for patients in whom nHF failed. The rate of nasal trauma is lower with the use of nHF. Factors such as the approach to surfactant administration, availability of CPAP, and the severity of RDS may be important: it may be prudent to choose CPAP for more immature infants and infants with a higher supplemental oxygen requirement, especially given no RCTs of nHF as early support have included extremely preterm infants. However, clinicians highly experienced with the use of nHF have shown that it can be used successfully as early support for preterm infants without the use of CPAP backup.[232]

Postextubation/Surfactant Respiratory Support

Since a 2016 Cochrane review,[222] there have been another two published RCTs.[233,234] For an updated pooled analysis of the outcomes of treatment failure within 7 days and reintubation within 7 days, we included eight trials with a total of 1039 preterm infants. Most studies compared nHF with CPAP as

Study or subgroup	Nasal HF Events	Nasal HF Total	CPAP Events	CPAP Total	Weight	Risk difference M–H, Fixed, 95% CI
Farhat 2018	15	54	14	53	5.8%	0.01 [–0.15, 0.18]
Iranpour 2011	0	35	0	35	3.8%	0.00 [–0.05, 0.05]
Lavizzari 2016	17	158	15	158	17.3%	0.01 [–0.05, 0.08]
Manley 2019	49	185	22	194	20.7%	0.15 [0.07, 0.23]
Murki 2018	37	133	13	139	14.8%	0.18 [0.09, 0.27]
Roberts 2016	71	278	38	286	30.8%	0.12 [0.06, 0.19]
Yoder 2013	6	58	9	67	6.8%	–0.03 [–0.14, 0.08]
Total (95% CI)		**901**		**932**	**100.0%**	**0.10 [0.06, 0.13]**
Total events	195		111			

Heterogeneity: $Chi^2 = 30.60$, df = 6 (P < 0.0001); $I^2 = 80\%$
Test for overall effect: Z = 5.69 (P < 0.00001)

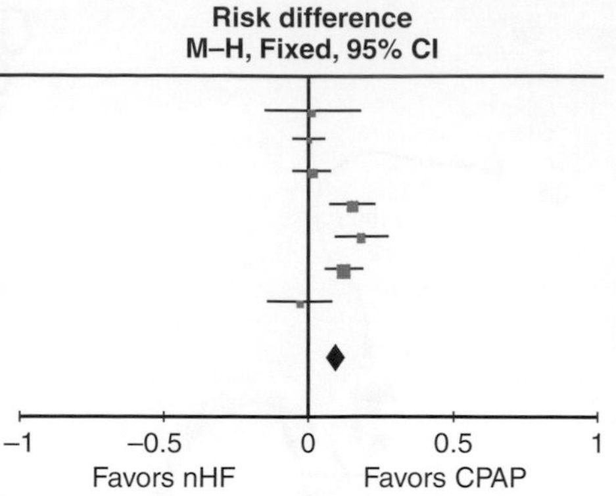

A

Study or subgroup	Nasal HF Events	Nasal HF Total	CPAP Events	CPAP Total	Weight	Risk difference M–H, Fixed, 95% CI
Farhat 2018	15	54	14	53	5.8%	0.01 [–0.15, 0.18]
Iranpour 2011	0	35	0	35	3.8%	0.00 [–0.05, 0.05]
Lavizzari 2016	17	158	15	158	17.3%	0.01 [–0.05, 0.08]
Manley 2019	17	185	14	194	20.7%	0.02 [–0.04, 0.08]
Murki 2018	8	133	11	139	14.8%	–0.02 [–0.08, 0.04]
Roberts 2016	43	278	33	286	30.8%	0.04 [–0.02, 0.10]
Yoder 2013	6	58	9	67	6.8%	–0.03 [–0.14, 0.08]
Total (95% CI)		**901**		**932**	**100.0%**	**0.01 [–0.01, 0.04]**
Total events	106		96			

Heterogeneity: $Chi^2 = 2.84$, df = 6 (P = 0.83); $I^2 = 0\%$
Test for overall effect: Z = 0.98 (P = 0.33)

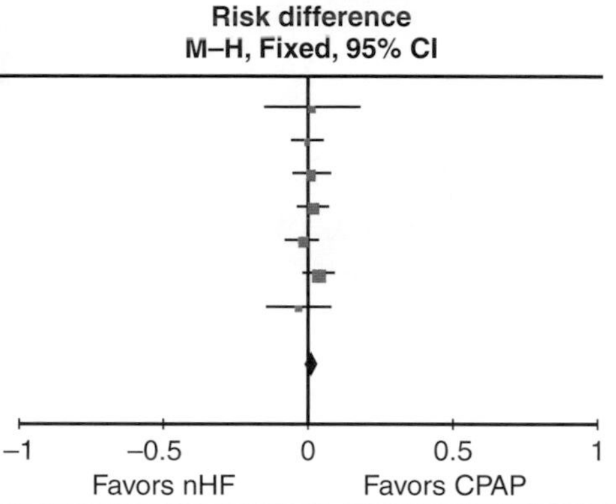

B

Fig. 18.10 Nasal high flow (*HF*) versus continuous positive airway pressure (*CPAP*) as early respiratory support for preterm infants. **(A)** Treatment failure within 72 hours. **(B)** Mechanical ventilation within 72 hours. *95% CI*, 95% Confidence interval.

postextubation support (to prevent extubation failure), whereas two studied nHF as support after surfactant administration via the INSURE technique.[234,235] Several of these trials permitted the use of rescue CPAP before reintubation in the event of nHF treatment failure. The largest study of postextubation nHF reported that 48% of infants in whom nHF treatment failed were successfully treated with rescue CPAP and avoided reintubation for at least 7 days.[134]

Fig. 18.11 shows the pooled analysis of nHF versus CPAP as postextubation/surfactant support in preterm infants for the outcomes of treatment failure and MV. nHF as postextubation/postsurfactant support, when compared with CPAP, resulted in a higher rate of treatment failure within 7 days, although the difference did not reach statistical significance (RR, 1.23; 95% CI, 0.98–1.54; eight trials, 1039 infants). There was no difference in the rate of MV (reintubation) within 7 days (RR, 1.01; 95% CI, 0.77–1.32; eight trials, 1037 infants). There was evidence of moderate heterogeneity between the studies for these analyses. Again, when interpreting the results of these studies and the results of the meta-analysis, it is important to note that the studies differ in the devices used for delivering nHF and the set gas flows and CPAP pressures.

Two RCTs included extremely preterm infants born under 28 weeks' gestation following extubation. Collins et al.[236] reported no statistically significant difference in extubation failure between the nHF and CPAP groups in extremely preterm infants: 37% versus 52%. Although there was no statistically significant difference between treatment groups, the study by Manley et al.,[134] which included the largest number of extremely preterm infants, reported a very high nHF treatment failure rate (81%) in infants born less than 26 weeks' gestation, and the authors advised caution in using nHF for these infants. None of these trials reported a difference in the mortality or BPD between groups, and the 2016 Cochrane review[222] also found no difference in these important outcomes.

The 2016 Cochrane review found that the use of nHF as postextubation support significantly reduces nasal trauma compared with CPAP (four studies, 645 infants; RR, 0.64; 95% CI, 0.51–0.79). Subsequently, Soonsawad et al.[233] also found a significant reduction in nasal trauma with nHF (17% vs. 44%); Kadivar et al.[234] reported no nasal trauma in either group. The Cochrane review also reported a reduction in pneumothoraces with nHF use, but this was not statistically significant (five studies, 896 infants; RR, 0.35; 95% CI, 0.11–1.06). Subsequently, Kadivar et al.[234] reported difference in the rate of pneumothorax, and Soonsawad et al.[233] reported no pneumothoraces in either group.

In summary, nHF has similar efficacy to CPAP as respiratory support after extubation/surfactant in preterm infants, although caution is recommended using nHF in this role in extremely preterm infants as there is a paucity of data in this high-risk population. nHF use reduces the risk of nasal trauma and may reduce the rate of pneumothorax after extubation/surfactant.

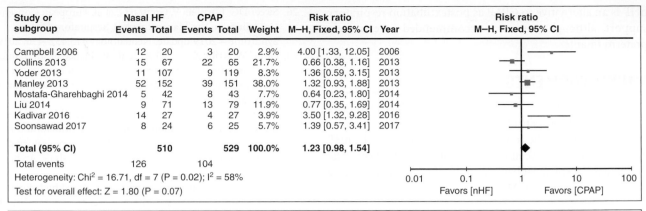

Fig. 18.11 Nasal high flow (*HF*) versus continuous positive airway pressure (*CPAP*) as postextubation/surfactant respiratory support for preterm infants. **(A)** Treatment failure within 7 days. **(B)** Reintubation within 7 days. *95% CI*, 95% Confidence interval.

Future Directions

nHF is a relatively new mode of respiratory support in neonatology that is still undergoing investigation, and potential new applications have been proposed. Because it is quick and easy to apply, nHF could be useful as a method of stabilization for preterm infants in the delivery room. To date, this use of nHF has only been reported in a small case series of infants born less than 30 weeks' gestation in a center experienced with nHF use in very preterm infants.[237] Most infants were successfully stabilized with nHF and transferred to the NICU, where they received ongoing nHF support, although the most immature infants still mainly required endotracheal intubation soon after birth.

Another potential use of nHF is during endotracheal intubation of neonates. Neonatal intubation is a technically challenging procedure, and with changing practices, neonatal trainees have fewer opportunities to gain proficiency in this procedure. Also, neonates are vulnerable to physiological instability and clinical deterioration during intubation. Applying nHF during apnea has been found to prolong the time to desaturation after induction of anesthesia in children,[238] a technique known as transnasal humidified rapid insufflation ventilatory exchange (THRIVE). Applying the simple nHF interface (and providing supplemental oxygen if required) during neonatal intubation may improve stability and potentially prolong the safe procedure duration; an RCT of this intervention is currently underway (ACTRN12618001498280).

CONCLUSION

A growing body of evidence confirms the safety and efficacy of noninvasive respiratory support for a variety of indications including initial management of RDS and postextubation care. CPAP is the most widely used form, but alternatives have been developed to increase the effectiveness and usability of the technique. In summary:

- Early CPAP confers a small benefit over endotracheal intubation for initial management of extremely preterm infants, reducing the rate of the combined outcome of death or BPD.
- Bubble CPAP systems are simple and inexpensive and appear to be as effective as alternative pressure generators.
- Nasal masks and short binasal prongs are suitable interfaces for CPAP delivery.
- Preliminary evidence suggests that minimally invasive surfactant therapy provided to infants with RDS on CPAP is safe and effective.
- NIPPV, when synchronized with the infant's own efforts, is a useful method of augmenting the benefits of CPAP, particularly in the postextubation scenario.
- HFNV is a promising therapy, but more research is required before it is widely applied.
- nHF, although less effective than CPAP as primary support, is an appropriate therapy for moderately preterm infants with signs of mild to moderate respiratory distress, especially when rescue CPAP is available.

- nHF is an alternative to CPAP as postextubation respiratory support, although caution is recommended in extremely preterm infants.

ACKNOWLEDGMENTS

The authors wish to thank Dr. Kate Hodgson (The Royal Women's Hospital and The University of Melbourne, Melbourne, Australia) for her assistance with the content and data analysis for the nHF section of this chapter. We also thank Professor Peter Dargaville (Royal Hobart Hospital, Hobart, Australia) for providing a figure for the section on LISA and MIST.

KEY REFERENCES

4. Morley CJ, Davis PG, Doyle LW, et al: Nasal CPAP or intubation at birth for very preterm infants. N Engl J Med 358:700–708, 2008.

11. Ferguson KN, Roberts CT, Manley BJ, et al: Interventions to improve rates of successful extubation in preterm infants: a systematic review and meta-analysis. JAMA Pediatr 171: 165–174, 2017.

24. Schmolzer GM, Kumar M, Pichler G, et al: Non-invasive versus invasive respiratory support in preterm infants at birth: systematic review and meta-analysis. BMJ Clin Res Ed 347:f5980, 2013.

26. Sweet DG, Carnielli V, Greisen G, et al: European Consensus Guidelines on the Management of Respiratory Distress Syndrome—2019 update. Neonatology 115:432–450, 2019.

113. Gopel W, Kribs A, Ziegler A, et al: Avoidance of mechanical ventilation by surfactant treatment of spontaneously breathing preterm infants (AMV): an open-label, randomised, controlled trial. Lancet 378:1627–1634, 2011.

121. Aldana-Aguirre JC, Pinto M, Featherstone RM, et al: Less invasive surfactant administration versus intubation for surfactant delivery in preterm infants with respiratory distress syndrome: a systematic review and meta-analysis. Arch Dis Child Fetal Neonatal Ed 102:F17–F23, 2017.

138. Roberts CT, Owen LS, Manley BJ, et al: Nasal high-flow therapy for primary respiratory support in preterm infants. N Engl J Med 375:1142–1151, 2016.

174. Lemyre B, Laughon M, Bose C, et al: Early nasal intermittent positive pressure ventilation (NIPPV) versus early nasal continuous positive airway pressure (NCPAP) for preterm infants. Cochrane Database Syst Rev 12:CD005384, 2016.

175. Lemyre B, Davis PG, De Paoli AG, et al: Nasal intermittent positive pressure ventilation (NIPPV) versus nasal continuous positive airway pressure (NCPAP) for preterm neonates after extubation. Cochrane Database Syst Rev 2:CD003212, 2017.

179. Kirpalani H, Millar D, Lemyre B, et al: A trial comparing noninvasive ventilation strategies in preterm infants. N Engl J Med 369:611–620, 2013.

19

Overview of Assisted Ventilation

Martin Keszler

KEY POINTS

- Mechanical ventilation is a complex intervention increasingly reserved for the most immature and sickest infants. Although it may be life-saving, it is associated with many possible adverse effects and requires a thorough understanding of respiratory physiology and a familiarity with the operating principles of ventilators.
- Optimal outcomes can be achieved only if appropriate strategies are used that effectively address the patient's specific pathophysiology.
- Unit protocols and guidelines are useful, but individualized patient care ultimately requires a careful choice of modalities and frequent assessments of the patient's response to ventilator settings.

INTRODUCTION

Effective mechanical ventilation of newborn infants is a relatively late phenomenon in the care of newborn infants, having evolved within the lifetime of many practitioners active today. The death in 1963 of the late preterm son of President Kennedy from respiratory failure is a stark reminder of how inadequate respiratory care was in the early days of our specialty. Today, few babies die as a result of primary respiratory failure; early mortality is more often from complications of extreme prematurity and from infection. However, although mechanical ventilation has greatly reduced mortality from pulmonary causes, morbidity, including bronchopulmonary dysplasia, remains high.

As discussed in Chapter 18, avoidance of mechanical ventilation may be the best way of avoiding ventilator-induced lung injury. With increased use of antenatal steroids and improved delivery room stabilization approaches, most moderately preterm and many very preterm infants are able to be supported noninvasively. Although a substantial proportion of extremely low gestational age neonates (ELGANs) continue to require mechanical ventilation, the proportion of infants treated without mechanical ventilation appears to be increasing. Almost 90% of extremely low-birth-weight (ELBW) infants cared for in Neonatal Research Network centers during the early years of this century were treated with mechanical ventilation during the first day of life, and 95% of survivors were invasively ventilated at some point during their hospital stay.[1] In the Surfactant, Positive Pressure, and Oxygenation Randomized Trial (SUPPORT), published in 2010, 83% of the ELBW infants initially assigned to noninvasive support received endotracheal

intubation and mechanical ventilation at some point during their newborn intensive care unit (NICU) stay.[2] Unpublished data from the Neonatal Research Network indicate that in 2018, 56% of infants below 29 weeks or 1000 g were intubated in the delivery room, with 75% being mechanically ventilated at least briefly in the first 3 days of life. Similarly, 55% of the 23 to 26 weeks' gestational age infants in the Sustained Aeration of Infants Lungs (SAIL) trial required intubation in the delivery room and 51% were receiving mechanical ventilation on day 3 of life.[3] Thus, invasive ventilation remains largely reserved for the relatively small number of the most immature infants or those affected by a variety of pregnancy and perinatal complications. Because fewer infants now receive mechanical ventilation, there is a decreased level of experience for trainees and practitioners. Infants who receive mechanical ventilation today tend to be smaller, sicker, and more immature than those ventilated in an earlier era and may remain ventilator dependent for extended periods, sometimes for reasons not related to their lung disease. The spectrum of lung disease that neonatologists treat has expanded into more chronic conditions that we are less accustomed to treating. Furthermore, today's patients may be uniquely susceptible to lung injury because of the very early stages of lung development at which they are born.

All these issues make it important to optimize the way mechanical ventilation is managed so that preventable mortality and morbidity can be avoided. Some degree of lung injury is probably inevitable in mechanically ventilated ELGANs, even with optimal respiratory support. However, the wide range of the rate of bronchopulmonary dysplasia (BPD) in the individual NICUs within the National Institute of Child Health and Human Development Neonatal Research Network and the Vermont-Oxford Network suggests that mechanical ventilation may be a potentially modifiable risk factor.[4] Although the evidence to guide respiratory support strategies remains incomplete, the potentially best practices and the rationale for them will be outlined in this and subsequent chapters. The focus of this chapter is conventional mechanical ventilation. High-frequency ventilation is discussed in detail in Chapter 24.

UNIQUE CHALLENGES IN MECHANICAL VENTILATION OF NEWBORN INFANTS

Individuals involved in the care of critically ill newborn infants should be keenly aware that newborns are not simply small children, any more than children are simply small adults. Sophisticated microprocessor-based ventilators with advanced features enabling effective synchronized ventilation are now widely available. However, better technology alone will not improve outcomes. Unless used with care and with optimal ventilation strategies that are appropriate for the specific condition being treated, these machines cannot materially impact outcomes. To optimally use the complex devices at our disposal, we need to be aware of the many unique aspects of a newborn infant's respiratory physiology. These are reviewed in detail in Chapter 2, but key aspects that directly affect the provision of invasive mechanical ventilation are summarized here.

Lung Mechanics

Small infants with poorly compliant lungs have very short time constants and normally have rapid respiratory rates with very short inspiratory times to match their lung mechanics. They have limited muscle strength and a very compliant chest wall, so they struggle to develop adequate inspiratory flow or pressure. This situation imposes great technological challenges on device design, especially in terms of triggering ventilator inflations in synchrony with the onset of inspiratory effort, inflation termination, and tidal volume (V_T) measurement. Suboptimal ventilator design for neonatal applications may lead to excessive trigger delay with asynchrony, failure to trigger or flow-terminate inflation, and errors in V_T measurement or delivery. These technological challenges have largely been overcome in modern ventilators but remain a problem in some older devices still in use.

Uncuffed Endotracheal Tubes

Uncuffed endotracheal tubes (ETTs) have traditionally been used in newborn infants, because of concern about pressure necrosis of the tracheal mucosa from inflated cuffs. The small size of the tubes also makes inflatable cuffs difficult to incorporate without compromising lumen size. For this reason, some degree of gas leak around the ETT is present in most infants. Despite lack of contemporary supporting evidence, some practitioners believe that it is important to have an audible leak around the tube to ensure that the fit is not too tight. Unfortunately, substantial leak makes V_T estimation increasingly inaccurate, an issue that has become more relevant with increasing use of volume targeted ventilation. Moreover, increasing leak around the ETT develops over time in infants who require prolonged ventilation, because the immature structures of the larynx and trachea progressively dilate from the cyclic stretch of thousands of inflations per day. A ventilator rate of 50 per minute stretches the trachea 3000 times per hour or 72,000 times per day! Leak is greater during inflation, because the pressure gradient driving the leak is greater and because the trachea distends with peak inflation pressure (PIP). Therefore, it is important to measure both inspiratory and expiratory V_T, with the latter more closely approximating the volume of gas that had entered the lungs. The leak varies from moment to moment because the ETT is inserted only a short distance beyond the larynx and thus the leak will change with any change in the infant's head position and movement of the ETT up and down within the trachea. Because of these difficulties, a reconsideration of the prohibition of cuffed tubes has been proposed[5] but subsequently rendered unnecessary by technological advances that make it possible to accurately estimate the true V_T even with a large endotracheal leak.

Measurement of Tidal Volume

The importance of very accurate V_T measurement in any sort of volume-controlled/volume-targeted ventilation of extremely small infants is self-evident, considering that infants weighing 400 to 1000 g require V_T in the range of 2 to 5 mL. Unfortunately, most so-called universal ventilators designed primarily for adult patients but capable of supporting the full range of patients from newborns to adults measure flow and calculate V_T at the output of the flow control valve within the ventilator rather than at the input to the patient (i.e., the airway opening). This approach is convenient and avoids extra wires and the added instrumental dead space of a flow sensor. However, in neonates, this remote placement of flow measurement introduces a high degree of inaccuracy of the V_T data. When the V_T is measured at the ventilator end of the circuit, the value does not account for compression of gas in the circuit, distention of the circuit, or leak around the ETT and is subject to inaccuracies related to approximate corrections for heat and humidification of the cold dry air from the control valve. The loss of delivered V_T in the circuit is proportional to the compliance of the ventilator circuit and humidifier (and the compressibility of the volume of gas they contain), relative to the compliance of the patient's lungs. In large patients with a cuffed ETT, the volume measured at the ventilator correlates reasonably well (using appropriate corrections) with the actual V_T entering the lungs. In tiny infants whose lungs are very small and noncompliant, the loss of volume to the circuit is proportionally much larger and not easily corrected, especially in the presence of significant ETT leak.

BASIC VENTILATOR MODE CLASSIFICATION

To understand how ventilators work, the clinician should focus on how the specific modes work and on understanding the sometimes complex interactions between an awake, breathing infant, and the particular mode on the specific device in use. This is made more difficult by the confusing terminology used by device manufacturers intent on differentiating their device from the rest. Consequently, ventilation modes with identical names may function differently on various devices and essentially identical modes often bear different names on competing devices, making communication among users of different devices increasingly difficult.

A basic classification of modes is presented here. A more sophisticated approach is described in Chapter 27. A mode of ventilation describes a pattern of interaction between a patient and a ventilator. A ventilator cycle consists of a positive flow phase (inflation) and a negative flow phase (expiration) defined in terms of the flow-time curve (Fig. 19.1). The easiest way to think of ventilator modes is to consider three points: What triggers the ventilator to deliver an inflation, how is pressure and gas flow controlled during the ventilator cycle, and finally, how is the inflation terminated (Fig. 19.2).[6] The term "inflation" is preferred

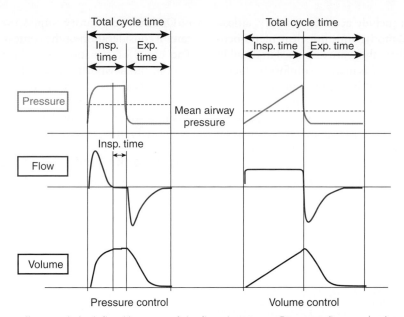

Fig. 19.1 A ventilator cycle is defined in terms of the flow-time curve. Pressure, flow, and volume curves are depicted as displayed on ventilator interface. Important timing parameters related to ventilator settings are labeled. With pressure-controlled ventilation (*left panel*), pressure is the primary control variable. When the circuit is pressurized, gas flows into the lungs until pressure equilibrates and gas flow ceases. If pressure equilibrates before inspiratory time is reached, there will be an inspiratory hold, followed by exhalation. The tidal volume (V_T) is a function of inflation pressure and lung compliance. With volume-controlled ventilation, volume is the primary variable. Constant flow is delivered into the circuit until the set V_T is reached, at which time exhalation occurs. Pressure rises passively in inverse proportion to lung compliance. Mean airway pressure and lung volume are higher with pressure-controlled ventilation, at equal V_I and inspiratory time, because the bulk of flow occurs early in the inspiratory phase of pressure controlled ventilation.

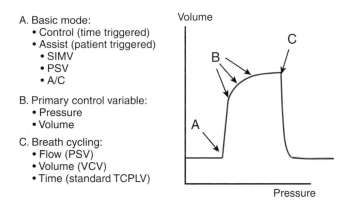

A. Basic mode:
  • Control (time triggered)
  • Assist (patient triggered)
    • SIMV
    • PSV
    • A/C

B. Primary control variable:
  • Pressure
  • Volume

C. Breath cycling:
  • Flow (PSV)
  • Volume (VCV)
  • Time (standard TCPLV)

Fig. 19.2 Basic classification of ventilation modes is best understood by considering what initiates an inflation (*point A*), how pressure and flow are regulated during inflation (*point B*), and finally, what causes the ventilator to terminate the inflation (*point C*). *AC,* Assist control ventilation; *PSV,* pressure support ventilation; *SIMV,* synchronized intermittent mandatory ventilation; *TCPLV,* time-cycled, pressure-limited ventilation; *VCV,* volume-controlled ventilation.

over "breath" to avoid confusion between ventilator and patient-generated gas flow. We have argued that ventilators do not breathe. Only living things breathe; therefore, ventilators do not deliver breaths, they deliver inflations.[7]

Ventilator inflation may be triggered by a timing mechanism independent of any patient effort (referred to as controlled ventilation) or by some sort of trigger mechanism allowing the

patient to initiate the ventilator inflation. The various forms of synchronized or assisted ventilation make it possible to maximally use the patient's own respiratory effort, preserving respiratory muscle training, reducing ventilator dependence and hemodynamic impairment. A detailed discussion of basic modes of synchronized modes of ventilation can be found in Chapter 20.

Gas flow during the ventilator cycle may be regulated by pressure (pressure-controlled [PC] ventilation) or by volume (volume-controlled [VC] ventilation). An approach unique to neonatal ventilation is PC ventilation with volume targeting, an approach that combines the advantage of both basic modes of gas flow regulation. The advantages and disadvantages of pressure vs volume as the primary control variable are discussed in detail in Chapter 22.

In the VC mode of ventilation, inflation is terminated when the set V_T is delivered. In PC modes, inflation may be terminated when a preset inflation time has been reached (time-cycled) or when gas flow during inflation drops to a set percentage of peak flow (flow cycled).

INITIATION OF MECHANICAL VENTILATION

Indications for Mechanical Ventilation

The goal of mechanical ventilation is to maintain acceptable gas exchange with a minimum of adverse effects and to wean from invasive support at the earliest opportunity. Adverse effects of positive pressure ventilation include acute lung injury, airleak syndrome, airway damage, hemodynamic impairment, nosocomial infection, and brain injury; these are discussed in detail in Chapters 39 and 43. Secondary goals include comfort (reducing asynchrony), reducing the work of breathing, and minimizing oxygen consumption. Because of the wide range of clinical conditions, weights, and gestational ages of neonatal patients, no simple formula exists to define indications for intubation and mechanical ventilation. In general, reasonable indications include inadequate or absent respiratory effort, clinical signs of impending respiratory failure, a high and rising partial pressure of carbon dioxide (PCO_2) level, persistent high oxygen requirement (fraction of inspired oxygen [FiO_2] >0.40–0.60), and excessive work of breathing despite optimized noninvasive support (Table 19.1).

Optimal respiratory support of the neonate requires a careful consideration of the context in which it is being applied. The range of situations in which mechanical ventilation is used in the newborn infant is broad, with a variety of pathophysiological disturbances. Table 19.2 provides a list of the common situations in which mechanical ventilation is used and includes some key considerations regarding ventilator modes and initial settings for each situation.

Choosing the Ventilator Mode

The clinician's choice of ventilator modes may be limited by the equipment available in his or her NICU. Although most modern ventilators are capable of providing the basic modes of synchronized ventilation, there are a variety of hybrid modes and combinations that may be unique to each device, as discussed earlier and reviewed in detail in Chapter 27. Ventilators designed primarily for adult/pediatric patients, but capable of also supporting neonates (so-called universal ventilators), have a greater variety of modes including volume-controlled ventilation. Some of these modes have never been evaluated in newborn infants. Therefore, when ventilating newborns with these devices, the clinician must be aware of the pitfalls of applying various "adult" or novel modes to this unique population. Unlike the specialty neonatal ventilators, pressure support ventilation on these devices does not have a continuous backup rate and thus requires a reliable respiratory effort, seldom present in preterm infants. Universal ventilators are not designed with uncuffed ETTs in mind and thus cope less well with ETT leaks in terms of triggering and V_T measurement. Volume-controlled ventilation controls the volume delivered into the proximal (ventilator) end of the circuit (known as V_{del}), not the V_T entering the patient's lungs. Because of compression of gas and stretching of the circuit, as well as a variable leak around uncuffed ETTs, there is only a very indirect relationship between V_{del} and the volume of gas that enters the patient's lungs. For this reason, PC ventilation (commonly referred to as time-cycled, pressure-limited ventilation in the neonatal literature) became the initial standard ventilation mode in the NICU, more recently with modifications that allow volume-targeting. Despite decades of routine use, controversy persists regarding

TABLE 19.1 Suggested Indications for Mechanical Ventilation

Category	Specific Findings or Values
Inadequate/absent respiratory effort	Absent, weak, or intermittent spontaneous effort
	Frequent (>6 events/hour) or severe apnea requiring PPV
Excessive work of breathing (relative)	Marked retractions, severe tachypnea, >90–100/min
High oxygen requirement	FiO_2 >0.40–0.60; labile SpO_2 if PPHN is suspected
Severe respiratory acidosis	pH <7.2 and not improving, PCO_2 >65 on days 0–3, >70 beyond day 3
Moderate or severe respiratory distress *and* contraindications for noninvasive support	Intestinal obstruction; intestinal perforation; recent gastrointestinal surgery; ileus; CDH
Postoperative period	Residual effect of anesthetic agents; fresh abdominal incision; need for continued muscle relaxation (e.g., fresh tracheostomy)

CDH, Congenital diaphragmatic hernia; *FiO2*, fraction of inspired oxygen; *PCO2*, partial pressure of carbon dioxide; *PPHN*, persistent pulmonary hypertension; *PPV*, positive pressure ventilation; *SpO2*, oxygen saturation.

TABLE 19.2 Common Situations When Mechanical Ventilation is Employed and Key Considerations in Choosing Support

Situation	Example	Predominant Pathophysiologic Disturbance	Suggested PEEP	V_T Range[a]	Considerations Regarding Ventilator Mode and Settings
Apnea					
	• Preterm infant with apnea of prematurity	Poor respiratory drive, relatively normal lung function	4–5 cm H_2O	4–5 mL/kg	Should need only minimal ventilator support. Lungs often relatively compliant, care must be taken to avoid lung injury, excessive V_T
	• Preterm infant with RDS apnea because of impending respiratory failure	Support should address the underlying RDS (see later)			Same as for RDS (see later)

TABLE 19.2 **Common Situations When Mechanical Ventilation is Employed and Key Considerations in Choosing Support—cont'd**

Situation	Example	Predominant Pathophysiologic Disturbance	Suggested PEEP	V_T Range[a]	Considerations Regarding Ventilator Mode and Settings
Lung Disease					
Diffuse alveolar disease	• Preterm infant with RDS	Low lung compliance, compliant chest wall, microatelectasis, ventilation:perfusion mismatch, very prone to ventilator-associated lung injury	6–8 cm H_2O, transiently may be higher	4–5 mL/kg	Recruitment using PEEP with CMV or MAP increments with HFOV. Short T_I and fast rate well tolerated. Optimizing lung inflation and avoiding volutrauma are key considerations
	• Term or preterm infant with hemorrhagic pulmonary edema	Poor lung compliance, surfactant inactivation, pulmonary edema, fluid in the airways	8–10 cm H_2O during acute event	4–6 mL/kg	Acutely increase PEEP and PIP to tamponade edema fluid. Recruitment using PEEP increments and fixed V_T may be helpful. Longer T_I needed to help recruitment
Obstructive and/or heterogeneous disease	• Term infant with meconium aspiration syndrome	High airway resistance, low compliance, heterogeneous inflation, prolonged time constants. With thin meconium, surfactant inactivation predominates and mimics diffuse alveolar disease	4–6 cm H_2O	5–6 mL/kg	Potential for overdistention of relatively normal lung regions. Need for lower ventilator rate to avoid air trapping. Higher V_I/kg is needed owing to increased alveolar dead space. When surfactant dysfunction predominates, treat like RDS
Pulmonary hypoplasia	• Preterm infant born after prolonged oligohydramnios • Term infant with congenital diaphragmatic hernia	Low lung compliance related to small total lung volume. Prone to overdistention, air leak, and pulmonary hypertension	4–6 cm H_2O	4–5 mL/kg	Avoid high V_T/PIP, avoid overexpansion. Consider high-frequency ventilation if PIP >25 cm H_2O or if there is refractory hypoxic respiratory failure
Air leak	• Preterm infant with pulmonary interstitial emphysema • Pneumothorax	Compression of normal airspaces by interstitial gas, poor compliance, and high airway resistance Continued leak of gas into the pleural space	4–6 cm H_2O	4–5 mL/kg	Accept higher partial pressure of carbon dioxide (PCO_2), avoid large V_T, maintain lung volume with moderate PEEP. Low PEEP leads to atelectasis, resulting in need for higher PIP. Selective single bronchus intubation if unilateral. High-frequency ventilation (especially HFJV) is preferable
Persistent pulmonary hypertension (PPHN)	• PPHN with parenchymal lung disease	Reduced pulmonary blood flow secondary to increased pulmonary vascular resistance superimposed on underlying lung disease	6–8 cm H_2O	4–6 mL/kg	V_T and PEEP requirements depend on associated parenchymal disease. Optimize lung inflation, correct acidosis, avoid overexpansion, avoid lung injury
Pulmonary arterial hypertension	• PPHN with normal lung parenchyma	Reduced pulmonary blood flow secondary to increased pulmonary vascular resistance. Pulmonary vascular remodeling	4–5 cm H_2O	4–5 mL/kg	Avoid overexpansion, excessive V_T. Avoid increasing airway pressure to improve oxygenation. Early use of iNO may be beneficial
	• Severe chronic lung disease (BPD)	Reduced pulmonary vascular bed, pulmonary vascular remodeling, increased pulmonary vasoreactivity	6–8 cm H_2O	6–8 mL/kg	Optimize treatment of BPD, maintain high oxygen saturation (SpO_2). Consider long-term pulmonary vasodilator therapy
Severe chronic lung disease (BPD)	• Former preterm infant with established chronic lung disease	Multicompartmental lung with regions of low compliance and increased resistance, poorly supported airways prone to collapse. Decreased alveolarization with less gas-exchanging surface and fewer pulmonary capillaries. Increased pulmonary vascular resistance	8–10 cm H_2O, sometimes higher	6–10 mL/kg, sometimes higher	Slow rate, longer T_I and T_E to allow ventilation of the diseased lung regions with long time constants. Sufficient PEEP is needed to prevent expiratory flow limitation at low lung volumes. Larger V_T is needed because of increased alveolar and anatomic dead space

Continued

TABLE 19.2   Common Situations When Mechanical Ventilation is Employed and Key Considerations in Choosing Support—cont'd

Situation	Example	Predominant Pathophysiologic Disturbance	Suggested PEEP	V_T Range[a]	Considerations Regarding Ventilator Mode and Settings
Cardiac Disease					
Left to right shunts	• Preterm infant with patent ductus arteriosus • Term infant with large ventricular septal defect	Pulmonary overcirculation with decreased lung compliance from pulmonary engorgement and edema	5–8 cm H_2O	5–6 mL/kg	High PEEP mitigates left to right shunt. Increasing carbon dioxide (CO_2) can help limit blood flow to some degree
Vulnerable pulmonary circulation	• Pulmonary atresia with duct-dependent pulmonary circulation • Hypoplastic left heart syndrome, post Norwood operation	Pulmonary blood flow highly variable and under the influence of intra-alveolar pressure	3–5 cm H_2O	4–6 mL/kg	Lung overdistention with high pressure settings will impede pulmonary blood flow. Manipulation of PCO_2 can help to control pulmonary blood flow: lower CO_2 to encourage blood flow, increase CO_2 to restrict blood flow
Neuromuscular Disease					
	• Term infant with myopathy	Poor muscle strength, low FRC and V_T secondary to compromised respiratory muscle function	3–5 cm H_2O	4–5 mL/kg	Pressure support for each spontaneous breath is optimal
Airway Obstruction					
Large airway obstruction	• Tracheobronchomalacia	Increased airway obstruction with crying or increased respiratory effort because of airway collapse	6–10 cm H_2O	4–6 mL/kg	Titrate PEEP upward until obstruction is relieved by splinting airway open
Small airway obstruction	• Former preterm infant with BPD	Inflammation, secretions, smooth muscle hypertrophy lead to mostly fixed airway obstruction. There may be a variable bronchospastic component. Prolongation of T_E and gas trapping. Expiratory flow limitation at low lung volumes	6–8 cm H_2O, sometimes higher	4–6 mL/kg	Slower rate, longer T_I and T_E to accommodate long time constants. Titrate PEEP upward until obstruction is relieved by splinting airway open. Antiinflammatory agents and bronchodilators may be of some value
Postoperative Support					
General aspects	• Any infant with a painful surgical incision	Suppression of respiratory drive because of sedation. Limitation of respiratory excursion because of pain	4–6 cm H_2O	4–5 mL/kg	Heavy sedation may predispose to atelectasis by suppressing sighs. Adequate set rate needed as the infant may not breathe above set rate or trigger adequately (40/min term, 50/min preterm)
Abdominal surgery	• Term infant with gastroschisis repair • Preterm infant s/p laparotomy for necrotizing enterocolitis	Raised intra-abdominal pressure and diaphragmatic splinting	6–8 cm H_2O	4–5 mL/kg	High PEEP needed to maintain EELV and recruitment but may compromise venous return if lung compliance is normal. Adequate V_T may be difficult to achieve without very high PIP. HFOV or HFJV preferred

[a]V_T refers to exhaled tidal volume measured at the airway opening. V_T need is also affected by patient size. Very small infants need a larger V_T/kg. V_T may be controlled directly when using volume-targeted ventilation modes or be a target value achieved by adjusting PIP when using pressure-controlled modes.

BPD, Bronchopulmonary dysplasia; *CMV*, conventional mechanical ventilation; *EELV*, end-expiratory lung volume; *FRC*, functional residual capacity; *HFOV*, high-frequency oscillatory ventilation; *HFJV*, high-frequency jet ventilation; *iNO*, inhaled nitric oxide; *MAP*, mean airway pressure; *PEEP*, positive end-expiratory pressure; *PIP*, peak inflation pressure; *PPHN*, persistent pulmonary hypertension of the newborn; *RDS*, respiratory distress syndrome; *s/p*, status post; *T_I*, inflation time; *T_E*, expiratory time; *V_T*, tidal volume.

the relative merits of the commonly used modes of synchronized ventilation, discussed in detail in Chapter 20.

Initial Settings for Pressure Controlled Ventilation

Immediately after intubation, a period of manual ventilation using a portable ventilation device is usually required until the ETT is secured, nasogastric tube inserted, and the baby properly positioned for ventilation. If intubation occurred in the delivery suite, bolus surfactant may be given at this time and some distance of in-house transport may be needed until initiation of mechanical ventilation. Use of adequate positive end-expiratory pressure (PEEP) is strongly recommended during this period. If the manual ventilation device does not allow for delivery of PEEP (e.g., self-inflating bag), the infant should be connected to the ventilator as quickly as possible.

The initial ventilator settings should consider the gestational age, underlying pulmonary pathology, and the clinical response to settings used during ventilation with a portable device. There should be a logical approach to choosing ventilator settings and an immediate assessment of their effectiveness, guided by a combination of careful clinical evaluation, observation of waveforms, and other displayed parameters on the ventilator screen and early evaluation of arterial blood gases. PEEP level is a key determinant of end-expiratory lung volume (EELV) and therefore of adequacy of oxygenation. An initial level of 5 to 7 cm H_2O is a reasonable starting point for most infants, with titration upward if FiO_2 remains above 0.30. Adequate PEEP is a key factor in lung protective ventilator strategies. PEEP optimization schemes and approaches to lung-protective ventilation strategies are discussed in detail in Chapter 21.

The key considerations to guide PEEP setting are as follows: (1) There is no universal PEEP setting that is appropriate for all patients and all lung diseases. Even for an individual patient, the PEEP requirement evolves over time. Mandating a standard PEEP level for reasons of simplicity misses opportunities to manage respiratory support optimally and according to sound physiological reasoning. Suggested ranges for PEEP are given in Table 19.2, but these should be considered in the context of the individual circumstances, with further adjustment according to the physiological response and the course of the disease. See also Chapter 25 for a discussion of the appropriate settings for various lung pathologies. The PEEP setting should be reevaluated whenever there is an alteration to pulmonary mechanics, for example, after surfactant administration. (2) Very low PEEP (<4 cm H_2O) is inappropriate in the diseased lung, predisposing the infant to low EELV, poor oxygenation, impaired pulmonary mechanics, greater turnover of surfactant, and a risk of greater lung injury. (3) Conversely, a PEEP level that is set too high (or becomes too high when PEEP is not reduced as lung compliance improves) leads to overdistention of the lung, incomplete exhalation with hypercapnia, increased pulmonary vascular resistance, and impairment of venous return with decreased cardiac output. (4) PEEP is not, by itself, a recruitment tool; PEEP increments will not recruit the lung optimally without an adequate inflating pressure that must reach the critical opening pressure to reinflate nonaerated lung units. Once the lung is recruited, it becomes more compliant and the

PEEP and PIP must then be reduced to avoid overventilation and lung injury.

Choice of the inflation time (T_I) should be based on the time constant of the infant's respiratory system (how quickly gas gets in and out; see Chapter 2 for a detailed explanation of the concept of time constant). It should be set at around 0.4 to 0.5 seconds for term infants and 0.25 to 0.35 seconds for a preterm infant and quickly adjusted if needed based on the analysis of the flow-time curve displayed on most modern neonatal ventilators. T_I should be long enough to allow completion of inspiratory flow before the ventilator cycles off but should avoid a long inspiratory hold that increases patient-ventilator asynchrony and risk of airleak. For flow-cycled modes (e.g., pressure support or volume support), the T_I set value is really the upper limit that comes into play only if flow cycling fails to occur; it should be set long enough to permit flow cycling to occur. In some devices, the inflation termination criterion is adjustable by the user (typically at 10%–25% of peak flow); in neonatal ventilators with effective leak compensation, this value is fixed at 15%. Setting PIP should be guided by a visual appreciation of a just adequate chest rise, audible breath sounds, and preferably the measured exhaled V_T, which should range between 4 and 6 mL/kg, depending on the patient size, age, and diagnosis (except in severe established BPD, which requires substantially larger V_T). There is no optimal PIP for all infants and the PIP required to achieve adequate V_T is not a function of the size of the infant. Very small infants may have very poor lung compliance and transiently need quite high PIP. The reason larger infants often need higher PIP compared with the ELBW infant is that they cope better with the increased load imposed by lung disease and thus develop signs of respiratory failure at a point of more severe disease than tiny infants. Peak pressure by itself is not injurious to the lungs without generating an excessive V_T (see Chapter 22). Finally, expiratory time (T_E) (determined by direct setting or indirectly by preset ventilator rate) is adjusted to achieve a sufficient level of support to reduce work of breathing and produce adequate minute ventilation, a value also usually available on the ventilator display. Care must be taken to ensure that the expiratory time is sufficient to allow for complete exhalation and avoid inadvertent PEEP as verified by inspection of the flow waveform. Depending on the ventilator mode, the ventilator rate may be a minimum value, with the actual rate determined by the infant as in assist-control (AC) or pressure support ventilation (PSV) or may directly determine the actual ventilator cycling frequency in an apneic infant or with synchronized intermittent mandatory ventilation (SIMV). Please see Chapter 20 for further discussion of various modes of synchronized ventilation.

Assessment After Starting Ventilation

A thorough clinical evaluation after initiation of ventilation is essential, recognizing that further adjustments to ventilator settings may be indicated after evaluating the patient's response to the initial choices (Table 19.3). Relying solely on blood gas measurement potentially exposes the patient to a period of suboptimal support, something that can usually be discerned

TABLE 19.3   Clinical Evaluation After Initiation of Mechanical Ventilation

Observation	• Color and activity
	• Patient-ventilator interaction
	• Triggering
	• Autocycling
	• Chest rise and diaphragmatic excursion
	• Work of breathing
	• Respiratory rate
	• Circulation
	• Gastric distention
Auscultation	• Breath sounds to all lung areas
	• Adequacy of air entry
	• Symmetry of air entry
	• Adventitial sounds
	• Large airway sounds
	• Endotracheal tube leak
	• Obstruction on carina
	• Heart sounds
Ventilator monitor display	• Exhaled tidal volume of
	• Mechanical inflations
	• Spontaneous breaths (if applicable)
	• Spontaneous respiratory rate/is infant breathing above set rate?
	• Working (measured) peak inspiratory pressure (if applicable)
	• Percentage leak
	• Flow-time curve—evidence of sufficient inspiratory and expiratory time
	• Excessive inspiratory hold
	• Evidence of triggering/autocycling

clinically and corrected before obtaining a blood gas. Careful note of the rate of spontaneous breathing and the effectiveness of triggering should be made as the infant recovers from the intubation and the effects of any sedative and muscle relaxant drugs used during the procedure. Adequacy and symmetry of breath sounds and exhaled V_T should be evaluated. FiO_2 should be coming down with adequate support, and if it remains high, an increase in PEEP (and perhaps PIP) should be seriously considered.

Observation of the chest rise and abdominal motion gives a rough estimate of the adequacy of V_T, although this clinical skill requires some time to master, and often underestimates the actual V_T.[8] For this reason, the chest rise should be only just perceptible—a large, easily seen chest rise indicates excessive V_T. Auscultation of both sides of the chest is essential to detect mainstem bronchus intubation, atelectasis, or pneumothorax. Low pitched sounds may indicate a large ETT leak or partial tube obstruction against the carina. Listening over the larynx or the open mouth will help confirm the source of the upper airway noise. Slight tension on the ETT may confirm ETT position as the source of the noise. Persistent increased work of breathing may reflect inadequate V_T, inadequate minute ventilation, or tube obstruction or malposition, which must be corrected promptly. In the immediate postintubation period, respiratory system compliance may be transiently decreased because of

gastric distention, especially after prolonged face mask ventilation, or because of atelectasis resulting from interruption of distending pressure during the procedure. Venting of the stomach with an adequately sized nasogastric tube should be routine to avoid gastric distention.

A key component of the clinical assessment after initiating ventilation is a careful appraisal of the data available on the ventilator display. In actively breathing infants, the displayed values will fluctuate; therefore, observations should be made over a number of cycles. The exhaled V_T for a set PIP, or, conversely, the PIP required to deliver a set V_T should be evaluated and adjustments made if necessary. In a volume targeted mode, the PIP limit may need to be increased if the desired V_T cannot be delivered.

An estimate of minute ventilation can be made using the product of measured V_T and respiratory rate before the first PCO_2 reading is obtained. A value of 200 to 300 mL/kg/min usually indicates adequate ventilation. Prompt assessment of the flow waveform is essential to detect insufficient T_E, which is recognized by failure of the expiratory flow to return to zero before the next inflation. For expiratory flow to still be occurring at the end of the inflation cycle, there must still be a pressure gradient between the trachea and the ventilator circuit (i.e., inadvertent, also known as dynamic PEEP), which can impair ventilation as well as hemodynamics and thus must be avoided. A detailed discussion of ventilator waveforms is available in Chapter 12. Avoidance of inadvertent PEEP can be difficult when an infant has a rapid spontaneous breathing rate and each breath is being supported by the ventilator. Tachypnea is sometimes because of pain or agitation, which should be recognized and treated if present, but more commonly reflects inadequate ventilator support. Increasing PEEP and/or PIP will typically achieve more adequate support and allow the infant's respiratory rate to return to more physiologic values, thus allowing adequate T_E.

Trigger sensitivity may need to be adjusted to optimize patient-ventilator interaction. In general, the trigger threshold should be as low as possible without causing auto-triggering (inadvertent initiation of inflation without patient effort), because a higher trigger threshold is associated with increased work of breathing and longer trigger delay. If a patient remains tachypneic despite apparently good support, an attempt should be made to confirm whether the ventilator is auto-triggering. The latter situation is more likely when there is a significant ETT leak,[9] or with condensed water collecting in the ventilator tubing, and can lead to hyperventilation and air-trapping, especially in modes that support every spontaneous breath (AC and PSV). Specialized neonatal ventilators, such as the Dräger VN 500, have effective leak compensation and are much less susceptible to auto-triggering owing to ETT leak, but may still be affected by water in the circuit. Insertion of water traps at the lowest point of the expiratory limb of the ventilator circuit can mitigate this problem. The use of heated patient circuits and modern ventilator circuits with a semipermeable expiratory limb, which effectively eliminates water condensation (Evaqua™, Fisher and Paykel, Auckland, New Zealand), has virtually eliminated autotriggering. Therefore, when using specialty neonatal ventilators with effective leak compensation and these circuits, the trigger sensitivity should normally remain at the most sensitive value (i.e., lowest) with no concern about auto-triggering.

A chest radiograph should always be performed to confirm the position of the ETT, evaluate the lung parenchyma, and assess lung inflation. Because radiographs are theoretically taken at peak inflation, the apparent lung volume reflects end-inspiratory lung volume (EELV + V_T), and thus, the chest radiograph is not very helpful for titrating PEEP. Moreover, chest radiographs are often not taken at peak inflation and thus are not always reliable indicators of lung inflation. Adequacy of PEEP is better determined on the basis of oxygen requirement, because PEEP is the key determinant of ventilation/perfusion matching.

The need for further sedation/analgesia should be assessed. Muscle relaxation is rarely indicated in the era of effective synchronized ventilation. Narcotic analgesia should be used judiciously, if at all. Evidence from a large, randomized trial indicates that although morphine administration relieves pain in ventilated neonates, it may result in more feeding intolerance, increase the risk of adverse neurological outcomes, and prolong the duration of ventilation.[10] When an infant is "fighting the ventilator," it is tempting to prescribe sedation. However, it must be clearly understood that this sign typically means that support is inadequate, even if gas exchange as measured by a blood gas is satisfactory. When gas exchange is inadequate, sedation will only mask the clinical signs of inadequate support. The infant is, in fact, struggling to breathe and the blood gas is not bad because the infant is fighting the ventilator, the infant is fighting the ventilator because the blood gas is bad! Finding the optimal level of support along with physical means of comfort will allow most infants to settle down without pharmacotherapy.

Subsequent Ventilator Adjustments

The therapeutic goals of mechanical ventilation include adequate oxygenation, sufficient alveolar minute ventilation to achieve an acceptable range of pH and PCO_2, avoidance of air-hunger, and reduction in the work of breathing.

Oxygenation

In the absence of right-to-left shunting through fetal channels, oxygenation is a reflection of ventilation/perfusion matching and is most effectively addressed by manipulation of the EELV, commonly referred to as functional residual capacity. The most effective way of optimizing EELV during conventional ventilation and high-frequency jet ventilation is adjustment in PEEP. With high-frequency oscillatory ventilation (HFOV), direct adjustments in mean airway pressure (MAP) are used to optimize lung volume and ventilation:perfusion matching. Increases in PIP also increase MAP and thus can improve oxygenation, but excessive PIP may lead to excessive V_T and volutrauma and thus should not be used primarily to control oxygenation, unless V_T is inadequate.[11] Prolonging the inspiratory time will also increase MAP but may lead to active exhalation against the inspiratory hold with a variety of potential adverse consequences. Adequate end-expiratory pressure is critical in maintaining end-expiratory alveolar stability, more uniform lung inflation, and

reducing volutrauma, as discussed in detail in Chapter 21. Increased PIP without adequate PEEP is likely to overdistend already expanded lung units and increase lung injury.

There is no easy direct way of visualizing lung volume. Chest radiographs are of limited value in assessing lung inflation/EELV,[12] and more precise techniques, such as electrical impedance tomography, remain research tools at this time.[13] Under most circumstances, the best assessment of EELV is the oxygen requirement. Oxygenation-guided lung volume recruitment strategies have been described with both HFOV[14] and conventional ventilation.[15] The approach with conventional ventilation is to increase PEEP in increments of 0.5 to 1 cm H_2O until FiO_2 is under 0.30 or until there is no further improvement in oxygenation for two consecutive steps. This is probably best accomplished while keeping V_T stable with volume-targeted ventilation, thus increasing PIP in the process, which will serve to ensure that the critical opening pressure is reached to recruit atelectatic portions of the lungs. Whereas an attempt at lung volume recruitment is indicated in most neonates with significant oxygen requirements, it must be recognized that not all causes of hypoxemia are caused by atelectasis. If the hypoxemia is the result of diffuse severe pneumonia or right to left shunting through fetal channels, lung volume recruitment may not be feasible or helpful. However, low lung volume and/or severe lung disease in and of themselves will increase pulmonary vascular resistance. If an echocardiogram indicates elevated pulmonary arterial pressure and the lungs are diffusely opacified, lung recruitment should still be attempted and will often mitigate the pulmonary hypertension when lung volume is improved. Optimizing lung volume is not only important in improving oxygenation and thus reducing oxygen toxicity from lung exposure to high FiO_2 but is also a critical component of lung-protective ventilation strategies.[16] Please see also Chapter 16 for a discussion of target PaO_2 and SpO_2 ranges and Chapter 21 for a discussion of lung-protective ventilation strategies.

Ventilation/Carbon Dioxide Elimination

Ventilation (i.e., carbon dioxide [CO_2] elimination), is primarily determined by alveolar minute ventilation, which maintains the partial pressure gradient between blood and alveolar gas. Alveolar minute ventilation is the product of respiratory rate and the difference between V_T and dead space volume. Increasing either rate or V_T will increase alveolar minute ventilation, but increasing V_T has a greater impact than increasing rate, because of the effect of dead space. If we assume dead space to be 2 mL and we are ventilating with a V_T of 4 mL, the alveolar V_T is 2 mL. Increasing V_T by 1 mL to 5 mL, a 25% increase, will increase alveolar V_T from 2 to 3 mL and thus increase alveolar minute ventilation by 50%. Note that the minute ventilation displayed on the ventilator screen does not account for alveolar or anatomical/instrumental dead space, which may be substantial in some circumstances. The benefit of improved ventilation with larger V_T must be weighed against the potential for volutrauma. However, rapid shallow breathing, such as may occur with an insufficient PIP or low SIMV rate without adequate PS, leads to high dead space to V_T ratio and reduced alveolar ventilation with increased work of breathing. The V_T therefore needs to be sufficiently large to overcome dead space. Mainstream end-tidal CO_2 monitors should be avoided in the small preterm infants because of the added dead space and the ETT should always be cut to the shortest length compatible with good fixation and positioning. The flow sensor that is essential to measure V_T and to provide synchronized ventilation also adds some dead space but is essential for state-of-the-art care. Although the effect of dead space is real, it has been demonstrated that some of the dead space is effectively bypassed in small infants ventilated through narrow ETTs.[17,18]

MONITORING AND DOCUMENTATION DURING MECHANICAL VENTILATION

Infants receiving mechanical ventilation are critically ill and are receiving life support. Thus, they require intensive monitoring and careful documentation of physiologic and ventilatory parameters. All mechanically ventilated infants should have, at a minimum, continuous cardiorespiratory monitoring, continuous pulse oximetry (SpO_2), and intermittent blood pressure and temperature monitoring. An indwelling arterial catheter for continuous monitoring of blood pressure and periodic arterial blood gas sampling is highly desirable in the unstable and critically ill infant and helpful during the acute phase of invasive respiratory support of all infants. Continuous transcutaneous PCO_2 monitoring is desirable when using PC ventilation or high-frequency ventilation and less necessary when volume-targeted ventilation is used. Mainstream end-tidal CO_2 monitoring adds significantly to the instrumental dead space and is often inaccurate in small infants whose rapid respiratory rates do not allow for an end-tidal plateau to be reached. Side-stream capnography avoids the dead space issue but affects V_T measurement and is also adversely affected by the rapid respiratory rate with absence of an end-expiratory plateau in small infants. Thus, transcutaneous monitoring is preferred in most ventilated neonates when continuous monitoring of carbon dioxide is desirable (see also Chapter 11).

Ventilation settings and measured variables should be recorded at regular intervals. Most modern ventilators provide the ability to trend key variables over time, allowing the user to see the evolution of the disease process and patient-ventilator interactions at a glance. The specific variables to be recorded depend on the mode that is in use but should include ventilator set and measured pressures, set and observed ventilator rate, exhaled V_T (and the target V_T, if using volume-targeted ventilation), and the percentage of leak. To be accurate, V_T must be measured at the airway opening, not at the ventilator end of the circuit. The humidifier temperature should be regularly checked and recorded. Most modern ventilators also provide continuous display of waveforms and/or tidal ventilation loops, and these can be very helpful in fine-tuning ventilator settings, as described in this and other chapters in this text. Most modern ventilators allow for screen capture of waveforms, which can be a useful tool for teaching and for subsequent evaluation/consultation when something unusual or unexplained appears to be happening.

VENTILATION PROTOCOLS

Mechanical ventilation is one of the most common therapies in the NICU and is associated with substantial morbidity and mortality. Mechanical ventilation is a complex and highly specialized area of neonatology, made more complicated by the availability of many different modes, techniques, and devices. Yet, the management of infants receiving mechanical ventilation remains largely dependent on individual preferences and an individual's training, rather than scientific evidence. Thus, it comes as no surprise that mechanical ventilation has been identified as one of the major risk factors for iatrogenic errors in the NICU.[19] Although the preceding considerations argue in favor of developing ventilation protocols for management of mechanically ventilated infants,[20] there is a danger of oversimplifying a very complex procedure and failing to provide optimal support for individual patients. For this reason, because establishing a common and standard basic approach to mechanical ventilation is important, such unit protocols must take into account the need to tailor ventilation strategies to the underlying pathophysiology and its evolution over time and allow for reassessment of the strategy/settings based on the patient's response to the initially chosen ventilation approach. Nonetheless, available evidence indicates that having a unit protocol improves outcomes with the existence of a protocol being more impactful than the specific details of that protocol. Table 19.2 provides a brief outline of the approach to various clinical scenarios when mechanical ventilation may be employed. A detailed discussion of common neonatal respiratory conditions and approaches to mechanical ventilation best suited for these patients in provided in Chapter 25. It is hoped that the information provided in this book will provide a sound basis for establishing such unit-based protocols.

KEY REFERENCES

4. Ambalavanan N, Walsh M, Bobashev G, et al: Intercenter differences in bronchopulmonary dysplasia or death among very low birth weight infants. Pediatrics 127(1):e106–e116, 2011.

8. Schmolzer GM, Kamlin OC, O'Donnell CP, et al: Assessment of tidal volume and gas leak during mask ventilation of preterm infants in the delivery room. Arch Dis Child Fetal Neonatal Ed 95(6):F393–F397, 2010.

9. Bernstein G, Knodel E, Heldt GP: Airway leak size in neonates and autocycling of three flow-triggered ventilators. Crit Care Med 23(10):1739–1744, 1995.

10. Anand KJ, Hall RW, Desai N, et al: Effects of morphine analgesia in ventilated preterm neonates: primary outcomes from the NEOPAIN randomised trial. Lancet 363(9422):1673–1682, 2004.

15. Castoldi F, Daniele I, Fontana P, et al: Lung recruitment maneuver during volume guarantee ventilation of preterm infants with acute respiratory distress syndrome. Am J Perinatol 28(7):521–528, 2011.

16. van Kaam AH, Rimensberger PC: Lung-protective ventilation strategies in neonatology: what do we know—what do we need to know? Crit Care Med 35(3):925–931, 2007.

17. Nassabeh-Montazami S, Abubakar KM, Keszler M: The impact of instrumental dead-space in volume-targeted ventilation of the extremely low birth weight (ELBW) infant. Pediatr Pulmonol 44(2):128–133, 2009.

18. Keszler M, Montaner MB, Abubakar K: Effective ventilation at conventional rates with tidal volume below instrumental dead space: a bench study. Arch Dis Child Fetal Neonatal Ed 97(3):F188-F192, 2012.

19. Snijders C, van Lingen RA, van der Schaaf TW, et al: Incidents associated with mechanical ventilation and intravascular catheters in neonatal intensive care: exploration of the causes, severity and methods for prevention. Arch Dis Child Fetal Neonatal Ed 96(2):F121–F126, 2011.

20. Sant'Anna GM, Keszler M: Developing a neonatal unit ventilation protocol for the preterm baby. Early Hum Dev 88(12):925–929, 2012.

20

Basic Modes of Synchronized Ventilation

Martin Keszler and Mark C. Mammel

INTRODUCTION

The standard mode of ventilation used in newborn infants before the availability of synchronized ventilation was known as intermittent mandatory ventilation (IMV). This pressure-controlled, time-cycled mode of ventilation provides a set number of "mandatory" mechanical inflations. The patient continues to breathe spontaneously, using the fresh gas flow available in the ventilator circuit. However, without synchronization of the infant's spontaneous effort, the irregular respiratory pattern of a newborn baby leads to frequent asynchrony between the infant and the ventilator, sometimes resulting in a ventilator inflation that occurs just as the infant is exhaling (Fig. 20.1).[1] High airway pressure, pneumothorax, poor oxygenation, and large fluctuations in intracranial pressures leading to increased risk of intraventricular hemorrhage were observed with such asynchrony.[2,3] In the past, heavy sedation or muscle paralysis was often necessary to prevent the baby from "fighting the ventilator."[2-4] These interventions resulted in greater dependence on respiratory support, lack of respiratory muscle training, generalized edema, impaired gut motility, and inability to assess the infant's neurologic status. The advantages of synchronizing the infant's spontaneous effort with the ventilator cycle, rather than using muscle relaxants, are intuitively obvious and supported by a number of short-term physiologic studies and small randomized clinical trials demonstrating improved gas exchange and other benefits of synchronized ventilation (Box 20.1).[5-10] Unfortunately, the two largest randomized trials of synchronized ventilation failed to clearly demonstrate benefits of synchronization, but they were conducted many years ago using outdated technology (pressure trigger) and had other methodologic issues.[11,12] A Cochrane metaanalysis demonstrated shorter duration of mechanical ventilation with synchronized vs nonsynchronized ventilation, but no effect on other important outcomes.[13] The

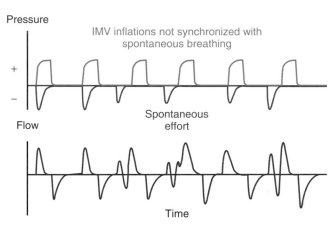

Fig. 20.1 Pressure and flow waveforms indicating lack of synchrony between ventilator inflations and a patient's spontaneous effort. Positive pressure inflations are shown in *teal* above the baseline and patient's spontaneous effort is shown as negative pressure deflection in *purple*. Note the consequences of asynchrony with disorganized flow, which will lead to highly variable tidal volume. *IMV*, Intermittent mandatory ventilation.

BOX 20.1 Benefits of Triggering/Synchronization

- Elimination of asynchrony
- Greater patient comfort
- Improved gas exchange
- Decreased need for sedation
- Avoidance of muscle paralysis
- Reduction of airway pressures
- Decreased work of breathing
- Decreased risk of baro/volutrauma
- Decreased risk of intraventricular hemorrhage
- Better respiratory muscle training
- Faster weaning from mechanical ventilation

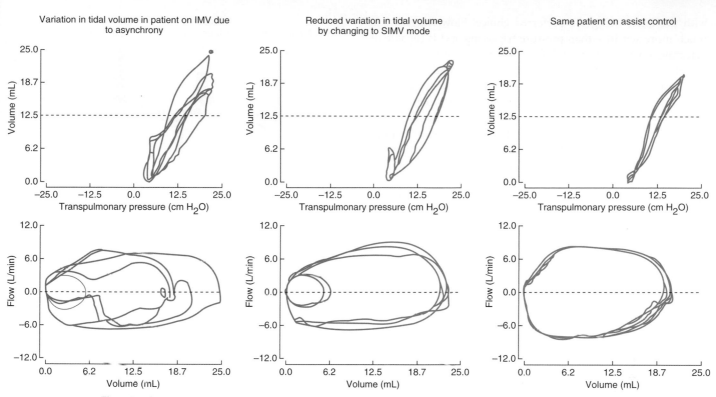

Fig. 20.2 Pressure-volume (*upper panel*) and flow-volume (*lower panel*) loops during nonsynchronized intermittent mandatory ventilation (*IMV*), synchronized IMV (*SIMV*), and assist control (*AC*) ventilation in a single patient. Note the large and random variation in the loops with IMV, the more consistent loops but with a large difference between spontaneous breaths and mechanical inflations with SIMV and the consistent superimposable loops with AC.

effect of synchronizing the ventilator inflations with the patient's own effort is illustrated in Fig. 20.2. This chapter focuses on the commonly used modes of synchronized ventilation. Less widely used modes are discussed in Chapter 23 on Special Ventilation Techniques, and a detailed discussion of ventilator nomenclature is available in Chapter 27.

TRIGGER TECHNOLOGY

Availability of effective synchronized ventilation for neonatal applications lagged considerably behind its use in adults because of the technological challenges occasioned by the small size, weak respiratory effort, and short time constants of preterm

infants. The ideal triggering device for newborn ventilation must be sensitive enough to be activated by a small preterm infant and at the same time must also be relatively immune from autotriggering. A very rapid response time to match the short inspiratory times and rapid respiratory rates of small premature infants is also critically important. An additional challenge is the ubiquitous leak of gas around uncuffed endotracheal tubes (ETTs). The types of triggering devices used in clinical care and their relative advantages are listed in Table 20.1. Flow triggering using a flow sensor at the airway opening has proven to be the best method that is currently widely available.[14,15] Either a variable orifice differential pressure transducer (pneumotachometer) or a hot wire anemometer may be used for flow detection,

TABLE 20.1 Available Trigger Technologies With Their Advantages and Shortcomings

Method/Technology	Advantages	Disadvantages
Airway pressure/pressure transducer	Simple, no added dead-space	Lacks sensitivity, causes long trigger delay, high WOB. No tidal volume (V_T) measurement.
Airflow/hot wire anemometer or pneumotachograph	Good sensitivity, rapid response, provides V_T measurement	Added dead space, prone to autotriggering with ETT leak.
Thoracic impedance/EKG leads	No added dead space	Affected by placement, poor electrode adhesion. No V_T measurement.
Abdominal motion/aplanation transducer (Graseby capsule)	Rapid response, no added dead space	Susceptible to artifact with incorrect position. Affected by change in patient position. Limited availability. No V_T measurement.
Electrical activity of the diaphragm (EADi)/transesophageal electromyography	No added dead-space, very rapid response, not affected by leak—ideal for NIV	Costly, somewhat invasive. Limited availability. No V_T measurement.

ETT, Endotracheal tube; *NIV*, noninvasive ventilation; *WOB*, work of breathing.

with the latter being the preferred choice. Flow triggering is much more sensitive than pressure triggering and is capable of detecting a patient effort with flow as low as 0.2 mL/min.

An attractive synchronization technology currently only available on the Maquet Servo ventilators (Maquet, Wayne, NJ) uses the electrical activity of the diaphragm (EADi), detected by transesophageal electromyography, to trigger ventilator inflation. This approach is attractive because it has the shortest trigger delay and is not affected by ETT leakage, thus being particularly suitable for noninvasive synchronized ventilation.[16-18] However, it cannot currently be used independent of the neurally adjusted ventilatory assist (NAVA) mode, which has not yet been adequately evaluated in small preterm infants with immature respiratory control and is not available on other devices.

Although flow triggering is the best widely available method of synchronization, it is not without limitations. The interposition of the flow sensor adds 0.6 to as much as 1.2 mL of instrumental dead space to the ventilator circuit (depending on the device and manufacturer), a volume that becomes a larger proportion of the tidal volume (V_T) as the size of the patient decreases.[19] The second limitation is its susceptibility to autotriggering in the presence of a leak around the ETT.[20] A substantial leakage flow during the expiratory phase may be erroneously interpreted by the ventilator as an inspiratory effort, potentially resulting in an excessively rapid ventilator rate, hypocapnia, or air-trapping. Autotriggering is potentially more of a problem with ventilation modes that support every patient breath and should be suspected when the ventilator rate is more than 70 per minute with no evidence of patient inspiratory effort. Autotriggering can also occur when there is water in the ventilator circuit that causes pressure and flow fluctuation in the circuit. Removing water from the circuit should immediately resolve the problem if that was the culprit. Most modern ventilators display the magnitude of the endotracheal leak—thus, a quick check of that value will usually suggest the cause. If in doubt, the simplest way to verify that tachypnea is caused by autotriggering is to briefly switch the ventilator to continuous positive airway pressure (CPAP) or low rate synchronized IMV (SIMV) mode. If autotriggering was occurring, the patient's respiratory rate will immediately drop and may fall to zero for a few minutes because the induced respiratory alkalosis suppressed the infant's respiratory drive. When autotriggering is recognized, it can be mitigated by making the trigger less sensitive. Unfortunately, the size of the leak can change quite rapidly, requiring constant vigilance and frequent adjustment. Furthermore, when the trigger sensitivity is decreased, increased patient effort is needed to trigger inflation and the trigger delay increases, both of which are highly undesirable (Fig. 20.3). Most devices now allow a fixed amount of leak compensation to mitigate this problem, but a fixed compensation level does not account for the variability of the leak. Some specialty neonatal ventilators employ effective leak compensation technology (Leak Adaptation) that derives the instantaneous leak flow throughout the ventilator cycle and mathematically subtracts this flow from the raw measurement (Fig. 20.4). This approach eliminates ETT leak-related autotriggering, but the device may still be affected by water in the circuit. Water traps placed at the lowest point in the

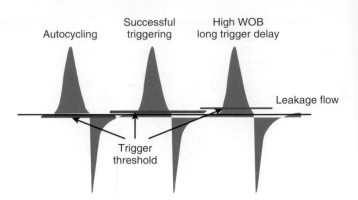

Fig. 20.3 Impact of leakage flow on flow triggering. When leakage flow exceeds trigger threshold, autotriggering will occur (first ventilator cycle on the left). With a trigger sensitivity just above the leakage flow, there is rapid response time and no autotriggering (second cycle in the middle). This is the ideal situation, but because leakage flow varies, autotriggering can recur when the sensitivity is too close to the leakage flow. The danger of autotriggering can be eliminated by substantially increasing the trigger threshold (making the trigger less sensitive), but this results in increased trigger delay and requires increased effort to trigger the ventilator (third cycle on the right). *WOB*, Work of breathing.

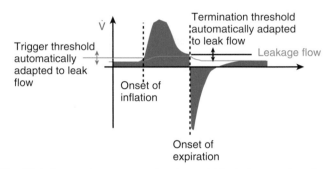

Fig. 20.4 Automatic compensation for variable leak around endotracheal tube as implemented on Dräger Babylog 8000+ and VN 500. The magnitude of leakage flow is derived throughout the ventilator cycle based on measured pressure and the impedance of the leakage flow and electronically subtracted from measured flow. This approach allows the trigger sensitivity to remain at the most sensitive value without danger of autotriggering with leaks of up to 70%. The same leak compensation concept is also applied to inflation termination in pressure support ventilation, which is addressed later in the text. The termination criterion is fixed at 15% of peak flow and reliable flow cycling will occur even in the face of 70% to 80% leak without premature inflation termination when the leak decreases. This is known as Leak Adaptation.

ventilator circuit are helpful but offer an imperfect solution. The use of ventilator circuits with semipermeable expiratory limb that eliminates water condensation (Evaqua™, Fisher and Paykel, Auckland, New Zealand) has virtually eliminated autotriggering, allowing trigger sensitivity to remain at the most sensitive value and preserving the rapid response time and minimal work to trigger inflation.

PATIENT-VENTILATOR INTERACTIONS WITH SYNCHRONIZED VENTILATION

The key concept in minimizing the need for invasive respiratory support is to avoid heavy sedation and muscle paralysis and to

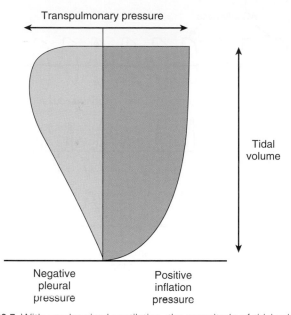

Fig. 20.5 With synchronized ventilation, the magnitude of tidal volume on the vertical axis is the result of the combined effort of ventilator and patient. The transpulmonary pressure on the horizontal axis is the sum of the positive inflation pressure from the ventilator (to the right in *blue*) and the negative pressure generated by the patient's inspiratory effort (on the left in *yellow*). Ventilator graphics and calculated compliance and resistance values do not include the patient's spontaneous effort.

maximally use the patient's spontaneous respiratory effort. Although allowing the patient to breathe spontaneously during mechanical ventilation has clear advantages as described earlier, it leads to considerable challenges for the clinician, who needs to appreciate the complex interaction between the awake, spontaneously breathing infant and the various modes of synchronized ventilation.[21] A key concept in understanding these interactions is an appreciation of the additive nature of the patient inspiratory effort and the positive pressure generated by the ventilator. As illustrated in Fig. 20.5, the V_T entering the infant's lungs is driven by the transpulmonary pressure, the sum of the negative inspiratory effort of the infant, and the positive inflation pressure from the ventilator. Because in a preterm infant, the spontaneous effort is often sporadic and always highly variable, the resulting transpulmonary pressure and V_T inevitably vary considerably from breath to breath. The following paragraphs will describe the way an infant's spontaneous respiratory pattern interacts with the common ventilator modes.

SYNCHRONIZED INTERMITTENT MANDATORY VENTILATION

SIMV provides a preset number of inflations as with standard IMV, but these are synchronized with the infant's spontaneous respiratory effort, if present. SIMV may be pressure or volume controlled (PC-SIMV or VC-SIMV) but in neonatal applications, it is usually pressure controlled and time-cycled. To prevent mandatory inflations during expiration, there is a brief

refractory period after each cycle, so that triggering can only occur within a trigger window. If no spontaneous effort is detected during a trigger window, a mandatory inflation will be given. Spontaneous breaths in excess of the set ventilator rate are not supported. This is not a major problem with a relatively rapid ventilation rate typically used in the acute phase of the disease but results in uneven tidal volumes and high work of breathing during weaning, especially in very small infants who must breathe through a narrow ETT. As discussed in Chapter 2, resistance to flow is inversely proportional to the fourth power of the radius, making it hard for tiny infants to breathe effectively through the small ETT. The high ETT resistance, coupled with limited muscle strength and mechanical disadvantage of the infant's excessively compliant chest wall, results in ineffective spontaneous breathing with a high dead space:V_T ratio. Because anatomical and instrumental dead space is fixed, small breaths that largely rebreathe dead space gas will contribute minimally to effective alveolar ventilation (alveolar ventilation – minute ventilation – dead space ventilation). To maintain adequate alveolar minute ventilation, a relatively large V_T, typically around 6 mL/kg, is thus required with the limited number of ventilator inflations (Fig. 20.6). From a practical standpoint, an additional disadvantage of SIMV is that the operator must adjust both rate and pressure (V_T) to wean the infant from respiratory support. Whereas many find these adjustments reassuring because they keep the clinician involved in the weaning process, in fact the infant is both faster and better able to self-adjust respiratory rate and volume needed for tidal breaths.

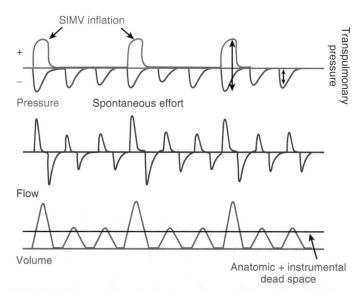

Fig. 20.6 Pressure, flow, and volume scalar waveforms during synchronized intermittent mandatory ventilation (*SIMV*). Drawn in *purple* is the spontaneous respiratory effort of the patient, which is not displayed on the ventilator screen, but which contributes to the transpulmonary pressure (*vertical arrow in top panel*) and, thus, size of the tidal volume. Note the large difference in tidal volume (V_T) between unsupported spontaneous breaths and ventilator inflations. In a small infant with high endotracheal tube resistance and weak respiratory effort, the V_T barely exceeds anatomical and instrumental dead space leading to inefficient rapid shallow breathing.

Assist Control

Assist control (AC) is a synchronized mode that supports every spontaneous breath that is sufficient to trigger ventilator inflation (this is the "assist" part) and provides a minimum rate of ventilator inflations in case of apnea (the "control" part). In various parts of the world, the mode is sometimes referred to as synchronized intermittent positive pressure ventilation or patient-triggered ventilation. AC is a time-cycled mode that can be pressure or volume controlled, but in neonatal applications, it is typically pressure controlled. Because every spontaneous breath is supported, AC provides more uniform V_T delivery and lower work of breathing than SIMV (Fig. 20.7). An inspiratory time is set, which may produce an inspiration that is either too long or too short, a problem that is avoided with the use of flow cycling (see later). The clinician sets a ventilator rate for mandatory "backup" inflations that provide a minimum ventilator rate in case of apnea and the inflations can only be triggered within the trigger window. The backup rate should be set just below the infant's spontaneous rate, usually at 30 to 40 inflations per minute depending on the baby's size, to allow the infant to trigger the ventilator. The goal is to have the infant and the ventilator work together, resulting in lower ventilator pressure. Excessively high backup rate will result in an increased number of untriggered inflations when the ventilator backup rate kicks in before the infant has a chance to breathe (Fig. 20.8).[22] A backup rate that is too low will result in excessive fluctuations in minute ventilation and oxygen saturations during periods of apnea. Because the infant controls the inflation rate, gradual withdrawal of support is accomplished by lowering the peak inflation pressure (PIP) (V_T), rather than ventilator rate. In fact, the ventilator rate should never need adjustment once the baby is generating spontaneous respiratory effort. In this fashion, the amount of support provided to each breath is decreased, allowing the infant to gradually take over the work of breathing. This slightly less intuitive weaning strategy, along with some

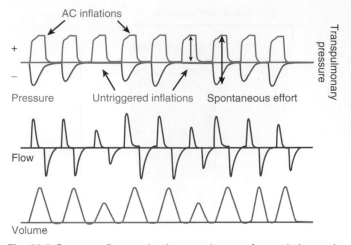

Fig. 20.8 Pressure, flow, and volume scalar waveforms during assist control (*AC*) with a backup rate that is too high. Drawn in *purple* is the spontaneous respiratory effort of the patient, which is not displayed on the ventilator screen. Note the occasional untriggered ventilator inflations that result in a smaller transpulmonary pressure when the ventilator cycles before the infant breathes.

long-held misconceptions addressed later in this chapter, appears to be the reasons for the apparent reluctance of some practitioners to adopt this mode.

Pressure support ventilation

A variety of modes are referred to as pressure support ventilation (PSV), a situation that greatly complicates communication. As implemented on specialty neonatal ventilators, PSV is a flow-cycled and pressure-controlled mode that supports every spontaneous breath just like AC, with the only difference being flow-cycling. On some devices, this mode is referred to as "flow-cycled AC." Flow cycling means that the inflation is terminated when inspiratory flow declines to a preset threshold, usually around 15 % of peak flow (Fig. 20.9). Flow cycling eliminates the inspiratory hold (prolonged inflation time [T_I] that keeps the lungs at peak inflation) and thus presumably provides more optimal synchrony. Eliminating the inspiratory hold should limit fluctuations in intrathoracic and intracranial pressure that occur when an infant attempts to exhale against the high positive pressure during inspiratory hold. The time needed for the lungs to fill and the flow to decline to the termination threshold is a function of the patient's inspiratory effort and the time constants of the patient's respiratory system. Thus, PSV automatically adjusts inflation time to be appropriate to the changing lung mechanics of the patient. The reader should recognize that changing from basic time-cycled AC to PSV usually results in a shorter T_I and, thus, lower mean airway pressure and therefore may lead to atelectasis, unless adequate positive end expiratory pressure (PEEP) is used to maintain mean airway pressure (Fig. 20.10). As with triggering, a substantial leak around the ETT may affect flow cycling. When leakage flow is greater than the threshold for inflation termination (known also as termination criteria), flow cycling will not occur (Fig. 20.11). For this reason, the user must still set a T_I limit, which should be about 50% longer than the baseline spontaneous inspiratory time, to allow the infant an opportunity to receive a longer inflation

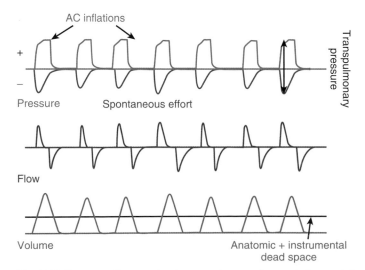

Fig. 20.7 Pressure, flow, and volume scalar waveforms during assist control (*AC*). Drawn in *purple* is the spontaneous respiratory effort of the patient, which is not displayed on the ventilator screen. Note the relatively uniform transpulmonary pressure and tidal volume when each patient breath is supported by a ventilator inflation.

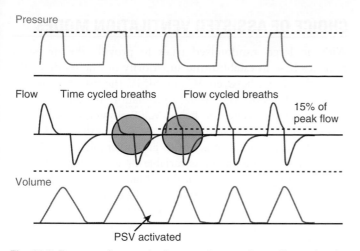

Fig. 20.9 Pressure, flow, and volume scalar waveforms illustrating the concept of flow-cycling. The left half of the tracing shows time-cycling with a fixed inspiratory time that results in a pressure plateau, also known as inspiratory hold. The pressure has equilibrated and there is no further inspiratory flow during the latter phase of the cycle. On the right side of the tracing, flow-cycling has been activated. The ventilator now cycles into exhalation when flow drops to 15% of peak flow. Flow-cycling results in a shorter inflation time (top tracing) and allows the infant to exhale as soon as inspiratory flow is nearly completed. This is a more natural breathing pattern and eliminates active exhalation against the inspiratory hold. *PSV*, Pressure support ventilation.

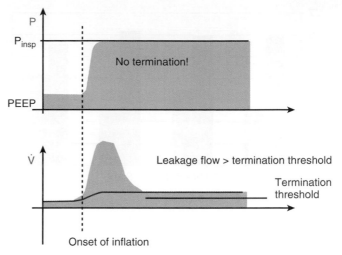

Fig. 20.11 Possible consequence of large leak around endotracheal tube on flow cycling. When the leakage flow is greater than the termination threshold, flow cycling would not occur. For this reason, manual setting of maximum inflation time is required. Manual adjustment of the termination criteria is necessary on some ventilators; others have an automatic leak adaptation (see Fig. 20.4). *PEEP*, Positive end-expiratory pressure.

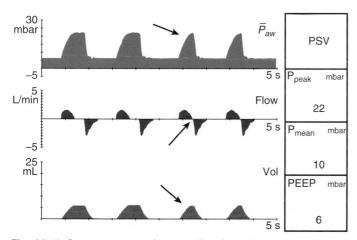

Fig. 20.10 Screen capture of a transition from time-cycling to flow-cycling. The time that flow-cycling was activated is indicated by the *black arrows*. Note that the gap between inspiratory and expiratory flow disappears (*middle panel*). Also note the shorter inflation time, which results in a drop in mean airway pressure and could lead to atelectasis if positive end-expiratory pressure (*PEEP*) was not adjusted to maintain adequate distending pressure. *PSV*, Pressure support ventilation.

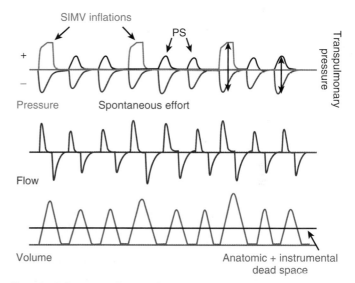

Fig. 20.12 Pressure, flow, and volume scalar waveforms during synchronized intermittent mandatory ventilation (*SIMV*) with pressure support (*PS*). Drawn in *purple* is the spontaneous respiratory effort of the patient, which is not displayed on the ventilator screen. Note that the addition of PS to spontaneous effort now increases the transpulmonary pressure and tidal volume, allowing the tidal volume to reach a more adequate value that results in less tachypnea and a more efficient breathing pattern.

time when he or she takes a longer, deeper spontaneous breath (i.e., a sigh). Because of the risk of failure to flow-cycle because of ETT leak, some devices allow the user to manually set the termination criteria (i.e., the percentage of peak flow that will terminate inflation) up to as much as 25% to 50% of peak flow. The problem once more is that ETT leaks are highly variable and when the leak decreases, terminating an inflation at 50% of peak flow can result in rather short inflation times and an uncomfortable breathing pattern. The need for such manual adjustment is obviated by the

effective leak compensation known as leak adapted pressure support on the Dräger ventilators, which automatically compensates for leakage flow and maintains effective inflation termination even in the face of very large ETT leak (Fig. 20.4).

Similar to AC, a backup rate will maintain a minimum inflation rate. In most devices, PSV can also be used to support spontaneous breathing between low-rate SIMV, to overcome the problems associated with inadequate spontaneous respiratory effort, and high ETT resistance (Fig. 20.12). Adding PSV

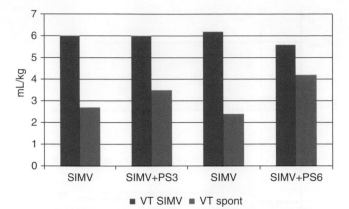

Fig. 20.13 The effect of the addition of pressure support (*PS*) during synchronized intermittent mandatory ventilation (*SIMV*) on tidal volume (*V_T*). Figure drawn based on data from Osorio et al.[25] Note that in these small infants in the recovery phase of respiratory distress syndrome on SIMV without PS, the spontaneous V_T was at or below the typical anatomical and instrumental dead space of 3 mL/kg (*blue bar*), whereas the ventilator inflations were about 6 mL/kg (*purple bar*). The addition of 3 cm H_2O of PS increased the spontaneous V_T slightly (second set of bars). Upon return to baseline of SIMV alone, the spontaneous V_T again becomes inadequate (third set of bars). The addition of 6 cm H_2O of PS increased the spontaneous V_T to a reasonable physiologic value, allowing the V_T of the ventilator inflations to come down slightly (last set of bars). The PS setting for individual patients should be guided by the V_T that it achieves, with 4 mL/kg being a reasonable goal.

to SIMV has been shown to decrease work of breathing,[23] increase minute ventilation and reduce tachypnea,[24] increase the V_T of spontaneous breaths (Fig. 20.13),[25] and to lead to more rapid weaning from mechanical ventilation.[26] PSV can also be used as a fully spontaneous mode, which lacks a backup rate and depends instead on an "apnea ventilation" setting that kicks in after a user-preset period of apnea. When used to support spontaneous breaths between SIMV or with CPAP, PSV does not come with a backup mandatory rate, so a reliable spontaneous respiratory effort is required. When used with SIMV, PSV can be thought of as a pressure boost given for each spontaneous breath that helps overcome the resistance of the ETT and augments the infant often inadequate spontaneous V_T. Although this approach is effective, it adds complexity and does not appear to have any advantage over either PSV used alone (or AC with appropriate settings), as long as atelectasis is avoided by avoiding sedation and using adequate level of PEEP to compensate for the lower MAP. In addition, using PSV typically results in different populations of supported breaths, some with higher V_T (the SIMV inflations) and some with lower (pressure-supported spontaneous breaths). Because in this application PSV is a pressure-controlled mode, and not volume targeted, it can distract the clinician from patient needs.

Withdrawal of support for PSV as a primary mode is accomplished in the same way as for AC. When used in conjunction with SIMV, there is no consensus and no data to determine the best way to wean. Both the SIMV inflation rate and PIP, as well as the PSV support level, need to be lowered at some point, again adding a level of unnecessary complexity.

CHOICE OF ASSISTED VENTILATION MODES

With no large, randomized trials to provide the necessary evidence base to establish the superiority of one mode or the other, the choice between AC and SIMV, the two most widely used modalities of synchronized ventilation, remains a matter of personal preference or habit. Valid physiologic considerations and short-term studies, however, suggest that modes that support every spontaneous breath are preferable in small preterm infants. Smaller and less variable V_T, less tachypnea, more rapid weaning from mechanical ventilation, and smaller fluctuations in blood pressure have been documented many years ago with AC, when compared with SIMV.[8,27,28] Despite indications that SIMV does not provide optimal support in extremely low gestational age newborns with small ETTs, SIMV remains the most widely used modality, especially during weaning from mechanical ventilation,[29-31] based on the widely accepted but not evidence-based belief that both rate and pressure must be weaned before extubation.[8,32] Preference for the lower inflation rate of SIMV appears to be based on the superficially plausible assumption that fewer ventilator inflations are inherently less damaging. However, this concept ignores the fact that the slower ventilator rate is accomplished at the expense of a larger V_T, a variable that is clearly more injurious than a higher ventilator rate. The emphasis on slower ventilator rate is also contradicted by available evidence from both animal and human studies.[33,34] Many clinicians also mistakenly believe that assisting every breath prevents respiratory muscle training. This concern reflects a lack of understanding of the complex patient-ventilator interaction during assisted ventilation. As illustrated earlier in Fig. 20.5, the V_T produced during synchronized ventilation is driven by the sum of the negative inspiratory pressure generated by the infant and the positive inflation pressure delivered by the ventilator. This transpulmonary pressure, together with the compliance of the respiratory system, determines the resulting V_T. During weaning, as the ventilator inflation pressure is decreased, the infant progressively takes over a greater proportion of the work of breathing with effective training of the respiratory muscles. As weaning progresses, the inflation pressure is decreased to the point when it only overcomes the added resistance of the ETT and circuit, at which point the infant can be extubated to noninvasive support. Table 20.2 summarizes the key aspects of the common pressure-controlled synchronized modes.

GUIDELINES FOR CLINICAL APPLICATION

As discussed previously, initial ventilator settings are a function of the nature and severity of the disease process and the age and size of the patient, refined subsequently by an immediate assessment of how the patient is responding to these initial settings. A general approach to respiratory support of infants under various conditions is outlined in Chapter 19, and disease-specific ventilation strategies are discussed in greater detail in Chapter 25. Here, we will briefly discuss general aspects of how the various synchronized modes may be implemented in the neonatal intensive care unit.

TABLE 20.2 **Key Characteristics of the Common Modes of Synchronized Ventilation in Pressure-Controlled Mode**

	Intermittent Mandatory Ventilation	Synchronized Intermittent Mandatory Ventilation	Synchronized Intermittent Mandatory Ventilation + Pressure Support	Assist Control	Pressure Support Ventilation
Trigger	None	Set no. of breaths	Every breath but different support	Every breath	Every breath
Cycling	Time	Time	Time/flow	Time	Flow
Ventilator rate	Set by user	Set by user	Set by user + PS rate driven by baby	Driven by baby (+backup rate)	Driven by baby (+backup rate)
Tidal volume	Variable	Variable	Less variable but two patterns	Relatively stable	Relatively stable
Work of breathing	High	High/depends on rate	Variably decreased, depends on PS level	Lowest	Lowest
Weaning	Decrease rate and PIP	Decrease rate and PIP	Decrease SIMV rate and PIP, continue PS	Decrease PIP, leave rate same	Decrease PIP, leave rate same

PIP, Peak inflation pressure; *PS*, pressure support; *SIMV*, synchronized intermittent mandatory ventilation.

Synchronized Intermittent Mandatory Ventilation

As explained previously, SIMV without pressure support should be avoided in small preterm infants when the inflation rate is under 30, but it is a reasonable choice in larger infants who are able to generate adequate spontaneous V_T. The variables that require user input include PEEP, PIP when using in pressure-control mode, or V_T target when using in a volume-targeted mode, and inflation time. Ventilator rate is set indirectly by adjusting expiratory time or directly by setting the rate, depending on the specific ventilator. Care should be taken to choose PIP that results in an appropriate V_T and to adjust it as needed when lung mechanics change. Generally, a volume targeted mode should be employed (see Chapter 22). Adequacy of the V_T of spontaneous breaths should be assessed, and if these are 3 mL/kg or less and/or the infant remains tachypneic, an increase in ventilator rate, addition of pressure support or change to AC mode should be seriously considered. Reduction of support is accomplished by reducing inflation pressure and rate. Ventilator rate should not be reduced below 15 inflations per minute before extubation to avoid excessive work of breathing. Although not optimal for small infants, SIMV is the preferred mode for older ventilator-dependent infants with established severe BPD (see also Chapters 25 and 36).

Assist Control

AC is a mode that allows the patient to control the ventilator rate but provides a minimum number of inflations in case of inadequate or absent respiratory support. The backup rate can be thought of as a safety net that is designed to avoid large fluctuations in minute ventilation in preterm infants with sporadic respiratory effort. Small preterm infants with respiratory distress syndrome (RDS) have relatively short time constants and their breathing rate is typically in the 50s and 60s. Thus, a backup rate of 40 per minute is reasonably close to their own rate but not so high that it would interfere with the infant's ability to trigger the ventilator. A backup rate that is too low (e.g., 25–30) would result in excessive fluctuations in minute ventilation during periods of apnea that lead to fluctuations in partial pressure of arterial carbon dioxide ($PaCO_2$) and oxygen saturation (SpO_2), both of which are undesirable. Because their normal respiratory

rate is lower, a slower backup rate of around 35 is appropriate in full-term infants. PIP, PEEP, and T_I are the other variables under user control. As mentioned previously, AC can be a pressure-controlled or volume-controlled mode. Pressure-controlled AC may be used with or without volume targeting. When used without volume targeting, the PIP should be carefully chosen to achieve appropriate V_T and adjusted as necessary in response to changing lung mechanics. This requires near-constant monitoring of measured V_T during ventilation. This need for manual adjustment is obviated by the use of volume targeting, which is preferred. As with all modes of support, adequate blood gas values alone do not guarantee adequacy of respiratory support. If the infant remains tachypneic after a period of adjustment to the new settings (respiratory rate >70), the reason for the tachypnea should be sought. Autocycling should be ruled out if marked unexplained tachypnea is observed, especially when no apparent respiratory effort is noted. Any condensed water in the ventilator circuit should be drained and evidence of a large leak around ETT should be excluded. If confirmed to be intrinsic to the baby, tachypnea usually indicates inadequate V_T, discomfort or an effort to maintain FRC when PEEP level is insufficient. If tachypnea persists after adjusting PIP to achieve adequate V_T, ensuring optimal patient positioning and verifying that the ETT is not pushing on the infant's upper gum (a common cause of discomfort), a trial of higher PEEP should be considered, especially when the oxygen requirement is greater than 30%. It should be remembered that AC itself does not cause tachypnea, but because the ventilator rate is driven by the infant's own respiratory rate, AC makes it more obvious to the observer. Moderate tachypnea with a slightly low $PaCO_2$ is often seen in infants with a metabolic acidosis, of any etiology. Typically, the pH is not alkalotic and the tachypnea in fact reflects the infant's respiratory compensation for the base deficit that may be the result of perinatal events, low renal threshold for bicarbonate or intolerance of large amount of protein in the parenteral nutrition in the first days of life in very immature infants. Changing to SIMV may make the clinician happy by allowing the $PaCO_2$ to rise to what may be seen as a more desirable partial pressure of carbon dioxide (PCO_2) level, but this will change little else, because it is pH, not $PaCO_2$, that is the primary driver of the infant's respiratory effort. Any increase in $PaCO_2$ which may occur results from less effective support provided by SIMV and increases the work of breathing for the baby.

As long as the infant has a reasonably sustained respiratory effort, lowering the backup rate will not affect the overall level of support; weaning from mechanical ventilation is instead achieved primarily by lowering inflation pressure, as well as PEEP and fraction of inspired oxygen (FiO_2).

Pressure Support Ventilation

When used in conjunction with SIMV, the PSV support is set as "X" cm H_2O above PEEP (e.g., PS of 8 cm H_2O). There is no backup rate. The choice of the level of support should be guided by the goal of achieving an adequate V_T of at least 3.5 to 4 mL/kg for the spontaneous supported breaths. Six cm H_2O may be a reasonable starting level but should be titrated upward if needed. The goal is to augment the inadequate respiratory effort of the infant and ensure that spontaneous breathing actually contributes to effective alveolar ventilation. Adequacy of pressure support should be confirmed by adequacy of spontaneous V_T and resolution of tachypnea. PSV becomes more important as the SIMV rate is progressively lowered. There is no evidence base on which to base weaning during SIMV + PS, but keeping in mind the goals of the PS, it seems reasonable to lower SIMV rate until it is low enough to consider extubation (typically 15/min) and adjust PS to maintain just adequate V_T during the weaning process. Infants can typically be extubated when they are able to maintain good oxygenation and are generating adequate V_T with PS of 6 to 8 cm H_2O.

When used as a primary mode, the PIP and PEEP are set as with AC (i.e., PIP/PEEP). PSV theoretically results in more optimal synchronization than AC and so should probably be the preferred mode in most situations. The exception would be extremely small infants with RDS during the first few days of life who have such extremely short time constants that the T_I with PSV would be under 0.2 seconds. Such a short T_I may contribute to tachypnea and limits the time for intrapulmonary gas distribution. We therefore avoid PSV in infants less than 800 g during the first 3 to 4 days of life. It should be kept in mind that the shorter T_I of PSV results in relatively low mean airway pressure and may lead to atelectasis unless adequate PEEP is employed—typically 6 to 8 cm H_2O. If switching from AC to PSV, the simple approach is to make note of the mean airway pressure on AC and then adjust the PEEP to return to the same value after PSV is activated. If an infant remains ventilated beyond a week of life, care must be taken to ensure that the T_I limit is adjusted as needed to allow flow cycling to occur, because airway resistance will be increasing and therefore the time constants are now more prolonged with the spontaneous T_I now potentially exceeding the set limit.

CONCLUSION

Synchronized mechanical ventilation modes represent a significant advance in respiratory support of newborn infants. Despite the limited evidence base from published literature, their benefits are generally accepted. Although debate continues regarding the specific choice of synchronized modes, there is strong rationale for using modes that support every patient spontaneous effort in very small infants.[35] Specific details of clinical application should be based on disease-specific strategies and on the advantages and limitations of specific ventilators at the disposal of the clinician. A good understanding of the underlying physiologic principles and the particular capabilities of the available device are critical for providing optimal respiratory support in critically ill newborn infants.

KEY REFERENCES

3. Perlman JM, Goodman S, Kreusser KL, et al: Reduction in intraventricular hemorrhage by elimination of fluctuating cerebral blood-flow velocity in preterm infants with respiratory distress syndrome. N Engl J Med 312(21):1353–1357, 1985.

5. Cleary JP, Bernstein G, Mannino FL, et al: Improved oxygenation during synchronized intermittent mandatory ventilation in neonates with respiratory distress syndrome: a randomized, crossover study. J Pediatr 126(3):407–411, 1995.

13. Greenough A, Dimitriou G, Prendergast M, et al: Synchronized mechanical ventilation for respiratory support in newborn infants. Cochrane Database Syst Rev (1):CD000456, 2008.

20. Bernstein G, Knodel E, Heldt GP: Airway leak size in neonates and autocycling of three flow-triggered ventilators. Crit Care Med 23(10):1739–1744, 1995.

21. Keszler M: Update on mechanical ventilatory strategies. NeoReviews 14(5):e237–e251, 2013.

23. Patel DS, Rafferty GF, Lee S, et al: Work of breathing during SIMV with and without pressure support. Arch Dis Child 94(6): 434–436, 2009.

24. Gupta S, Sinha SK, Donn SM: The effect of two levels of pressure support ventilation on tidal volume delivery and minute ventilation in preterm infants. Arch Dis Child Fetal Neonatal Ed 94(2):F80–F83, 2009.

26. Reyes ZC, Claure N, Tauscher MK, et al: Randomized, controlled trial comparing synchronized intermittent mandatory ventilation and synchronized intermittent mandatory ventilation plus pressure support in preterm infants. Pediatrics 118(4):1409–1417, 2006.

30. van Kaam AH, Rimensberger PC, Borensztajn D, et al: Ventilation practices in the neonatal intensive care unit: a cross-sectional study. J Pediatr 157(5):767–771 e761–763, 2010.

35. Keszler M: Time to abandon your comfort zone? Pediatr Crit Care Med 21:495–496, 2020.

21

Principles of Lung-Protective Ventilation

Anton H. van Kaam

INTRODUCTION

Respiratory failure is a common and serious clinical condition in newborn infants that is associated with an increased risk of neonatal morbidity and mortality.[1-3] Although respiratory failure occurs in both term and preterm infants, it is especially common in the latter group. Despite the fact that many of the very low birth weight infants can initially be managed on noninvasive respiratory support, such as nasal continuous positive airway pressure, historically, almost 70% of them have needed to be supported by invasive mechanical ventilation at some point during their admission.[4] Unfortunately, in its goal to correct gas exchange, mechanical ventilation often results in secondary lung damage, also referred to as ventilator-induced lung injury (VILI).[5] VILI is considered one of the major risk factors for the development of chronic pulmonary morbidity in newborn infants, that is, bronchopulmonary dysplasia (BPD).[6] Studies in both animal models and humans have provided valuable insight into the mechanisms of VILI, and this knowledge has been used to develop so-called lung-protective ventilation strategies, aiming to minimize the risk of (respiratory) morbidity and mortality. This chapter will summarize the basic principles of VILI and the basic concepts of lung-protective ventilation strategies.

NEONATAL RESPIRATORY FAILURE

As noted previously, preterm infants are most at risk of respiratory failure. This is to a large extent explained by the fact that their lungs are both structurally and biochemically immature. This is reflected by surfactant deficiency (neonatal respiratory distress syndrome [RDS]), which results in an increase in elastic recoil forces of the lung owing to the higher surface tension at the alveolar/saccular air–liquid interface and a concomitant reduction in lung compliance. In addition, the end-expiratory lung volume (EELV) or functional residual capacity is reduced and unstable, because the excessively high compliance of the chest wall of the preterm infant is unable to counteract the increased recoil forces. A low EELV will lead to a further reduction in lung compliance, an increase in airway resistance, and an increase in work of breathing. Furthermore, collapse of saccules will increase intrapulmonary right-to-left shunting, leading to (severe) hypoxia and to uneven distribution of tidal volume. These physiologic concepts are also applicable to term infants although the immaturity of the respiratory system is much less compared with the preterm infant and the surfactant dysfunction is not caused by surfactant deficiency but surfactant inactivation (meconium aspiration syndrome [MAS] or pneumonia) or loss of type 2 cell function (e.g., status post asphyxia neonatorum). Understanding these physiologic concepts is essential when designing and applying so-called lung-protective ventilation strategies.

VENTILATOR-INDUCED LUNG INJURY

Although BPD is considered a multifactorial disease, VILI remains an important determinant in its pathophysiology. Animal studies conducted since 1974 have greatly improved our knowledge about the mechanisms of VILI. These studies have identified the most important risk factors for VILI and its pulmonary and systemic consequences.

Risk Factors for Ventilator-Induced Lung Injury
Volutrauma

In 1974, Webb and Tierney showed that the application of high peak inflation pressures during conventional mechanical ventilation resulted in alveolar and perivascular edema, leading to deteriorating lung mechanics and, ultimately, death in healthy rats.[7] Additional experiments showed that application of high peak inflation pressures will damage the lung only if the thorax can freely expand and volume can enter the lungs. Preventing this expansion by thoracic strapping (low volume, high pressure) will protect the lung against VILI.[8] These results clearly indicate that the volume entering the lungs (volutrauma) and not the pressure applied to the lungs causes VILI. The importance of volutrauma in the development of VILI has also been confirmed in preterm animal models.[9]

Volutrauma is often thought to be equivalent to high tidal volume ventilation. Although this is true in most cases, it is important to realize that even low tidal volumes can induce volutrauma. First of all and explained in more detail in the next paragraph, low tidal volumes provided at the airway opening can result in regional overdistention if part of the lung is atelectatic. Second, if low tidal volumes are superimposed on a high EELV, the end-inspiratory lung volume can still exceed total lung capacity and result in volutrauma.[10]

Atelectrauma

As previously discussed, neonatal respiratory failure is often accompanied by surfactant deficiency or inhibition, resulting in collapse of small airways and alveoli/saccules (atelectasis). Owing to the heterogeneous nature of lung disease and gravitational effects on the lung, the distribution and behavior of unstable lung units differ at the regional level. Roughly three zones can be identified (Fig. 21.1): (1) alveoli that remain open during the entire ventilatory cycle, (2) alveoli that are recruitable during the inspiration phase but collapse during expiration, and (3) alveoli that remain collapsed during the entire ventilatory cycle.[11] Alveoli in zone 2 will be subjected to repetitive opening and collapse during conventional (tidal) ventilation. Animal experiments in both adult and preterm models have shown that the repetitive tidal recruitment and collapse are injurious to the lung.[12,13] Because alveoli in zone 3 do not participate in tidal ventilation, the tidal volume administered to the lung during conventional ventilation is redistributed to the alveoli in the other two zones. This may increase the risk of regional overdistention (volutrauma) and subsequent VILI.[14]

Oxygen Toxicity

Ventilation with high fractions of inspiratory oxygen concentrations can result in excessive production of oxygen radicals, overwhelming the normal antioxidant-detoxifying capacity of the cell and leading to VILI.[15] Both animal and human studies have indicated that prematurity impairs the ability to increase antioxidant enzymes in response to hyperoxia, making this group of patients extremely vulnerable to oxidative stress often present after preterm birth.[16,17] Low EELV results in high oxygen requirement because of poor ventilation/perfusion matching and intrapulmonary right-to-left shunt, thus contributing to oxidative stress.

Pulmonary and Systemic Consequences of Ventilator-Induced Lung Injury
Structural Injury

Volutrauma can cause direct structural injury to the alveolar-capillary unit. The coexistence of atelectatic and open alveoli may further increase this risk owing to so-called shear forces that exceed transpulmonary pressures.[18] Finally, hyperoxia can have a direct cytotoxic effect on alveolar endothelial and epithelial cells. This loss of structural integrity will increase endothelial and epithelial permeability, leading to pulmonary edema and hemorrhage.[15,19]

Biotrauma

In vitro studies have shown that cyclic stretch of alveolar epithelial cells and alveolar macrophages stimulates the production of proinflammatory cytokines such as tumor necrosis factor α and interleukin-8 (IL-8).[20,21] Ex vivo and in vivo animal studies showed that volutrauma, atelectrauma, and especially the combination of these risk factors result in a significant inflammatory response in the lung.[22-24] Pulmonary inflammation is further upregulated by hyperoxia, which stimulates neutrophil migration into the alveoli and enhances proinflammatory cytokine response of alveolar macrophages.[19,25,26]

One of the changes induced by the production of proinflammatory mediators like IL-8 is the recruitment of polymorphonuclear (PMN) white blood cells in the lung.[27,28] PMN cells can inflict tissue damage through the release of proteases, the production of reactive oxygen species, and the release of cytokines.[29] The importance of PMN cells in the development of VILI has been shown by Kawano et al., who found little evidence of VILI in rabbits depleted of granulocytes before initiation of injurious conventional ventilation.[30]

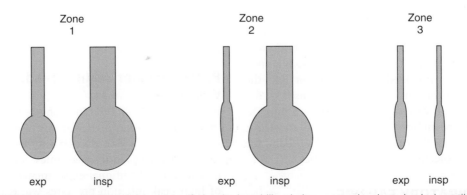

Fig. 21.1 Schematic drawing of the zones of alveolar instability during conventional mechanical ventilation. Zone 1: alveoli that remain open during the entire ventilatory cycle. Zone 2: alveoli that are recruitable during the inspiration phase but collapse during expiration. Zone 3: alveoli that remain collapsed during the entire ventilatory cycle. *exp*, Expiration phase; *insp*, inspiration phase.

In addition to upregulation of local inflammation in the lung, there is now also evidence from both experimental and human data that injurious ventilation will also lead to a decompartmentalization of inflammatory mediators into the systemic circulation, possibly leading to multiple organ failure.[22,31-33]

Surfactant Dysfunction

Although surfactant dysfunction is often already present at the start of invasive respiratory support, conventional mechanical ventilation may further compromise its function.

As previously mentioned, VILI is often accompanied by an increased permeability of both the endothelial and the epithelial barriers, promoting an influx of plasma proteins into the alveolar space.[34,35] It has been shown that these proteins result in a dose-dependent inhibition of surfactant.[36]

Studies investigating the alveolar metabolism of pulmonary surfactant have shown that surfactant exists in different subfractions. The two major subfractions of surfactant obtained from lung lavage material are large aggregates (LAs) and small aggregates (SAs).[37] LA surfactant is able to lower alveolar surface tension, but SA surfactant is not surface active and is the metabolic product of the LA fraction.[38] Animal experiments have shown that the conversion from LA to SA surfactant is increased when high tidal volumes are applied during ventilation of the injured lung.[39,40] The increased conversion of surfactant has also been documented in newborn and adult patients with acute lung injury.[41,42]

Animal experiments have shown that ventilation can enhance the secretion of endogenous surfactant by the type 2 cells.[43,44] This surfactant can subsequently be squeezed out of the alveolar space into the small airways as a result of compression of the surfactant film when the surface of the alveolus becomes smaller. Ex vivo experiments in rat lungs showed that this movement of surfactant into the airways is directly related to the tidal volume and inversely related to the end-expiratory pressure.[45] Hyperoxia results in both inactivation and decreased synthesis of pulmonary surfactant, resulting in a deterioration of lung mechanics.[46]

Lung Development

Experimental studies in preterm animal models have shown that mechanical ventilation and hyperoxia are able to arrest the normal alveolarization process during lung development.[47-50] This arrest in lung development is considered one of the histologic hallmarks of the "new" BPD and highlights the link between mechanical ventilation, VILI, and the development of BPD.[6]

Susceptibility of Newborn Lungs to Ventilator-Induced Lung Injury

Animal experiments have shown that the magnitude of VILI is highly dependent on the condition of the lung at the start of mechanical ventilation. Exposing the preterm lungs antenatally to intra-amniotic endotoxin before starting mechanical ventilation after birth results in a more pronounced inflammatory response compared with subjecting the lungs to either of these insults alone.[51] The same is true when exposing the lungs to postnatal inflammation by systemic injection of endotoxin.[52]

These experiments strongly suggest that the inflammatory status of the lungs is an important mediator in the effect of mechanical ventilation on lung injury. In addition to inflammation, the surfactant status of the lungs also seems to be an important mediator of VILI. Applying high-pressure ventilation to surfactant-deficient lungs results in more VILI compared with similar ventilation given to surfactant-sufficient lungs.[53]

These experimental results suggest that preterm lungs are highly susceptible to VILI, as antenatal inflammation (chorioamnionitis), postnatal inflammation (sepsis, pneumonia), and surfactant deficiency (RDS) are often present in the preterm population and are reasons for starting invasive mechanical ventilation.[54]

Studies in preterm animal models also suggest that just a few injurious inflations administered immediately after birth are sufficient to trigger the cascade of VILI.[9,55]

LUNG-PROTECTIVE VENTILATION: BASIC PRINCIPLES

The basic goal of lung-protective ventilation is to establish an acceptable level of gas exchange while minimizing VILI as much as possible. Based on the experimental data on the pathogenesis of VILI, the cornerstones of a lung-protective ventilation strategy are (1) minimizing end-inspiratory (alveolar) overdistention (volutrauma) and (2) optimizing EELV by reversing atelectasis (recruitment) and stabilizing lung units throughout the ventilatory cycle (avoiding atelectrauma). Applying such a strategy will often improve oxygenation and allow for a reduction in the fraction of inspired oxygen (less oxygen toxicity). A lung-protective ventilation strategy based on these principles is often referred to as an optimal lung volume strategy or open lung ventilation strategy.[56]

Minimizing Volutrauma

Minimizing volutrauma has mainly been associated with reducing tidal volume during mechanical ventilation. Indeed, animal studies have shown that reducing alveolar overdistention by limiting tidal volumes during mechanical ventilation will attenuate VILI.[8,9,23,55,57] However, it is important to realize that it is equally important to distribute the tidal volume evenly into optimally inflated and adequately recruited lungs; small tidal volumes can still result in (regional) volutrauma if superimposed on a relatively high EELV or administered during heterogeneous lung disease with significant atelectasis.[10,14]

Minimizing Atelectrauma

It is essential to realize that in a diseased lung, the reduction of atelectasis is based on two principles. First, already collapsed alveoli/saccules need to be reopened or recruited by applying sufficient inflation pressure. Second, after recruitment, sufficient (end-expiratory) airway pressure should be applied to stabilize the lung volume and prevent subsequent collapse during expiration. Fig. 21.2 shows the pressure-volume (P/V) relationship of an individual alveolus. Staub and colleagues proposed that the behavior of alveoli is quantal in nature.[58] After reaching a critical opening pressure, the collapsed alveolus pops open, immediately

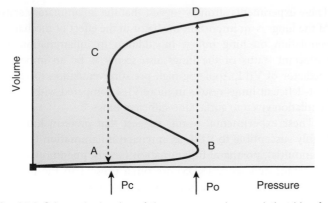

Fig. 21.2 Schematic drawing of the pressure-volume relationship of a single alveolus during inspiration and expiration (*solid line*). At the start of the inflation (*A*), the alveolus is collapsed. At point *B*, the pressure increase has reached the critical opening pressure (*Po*), leading to an immediate volume increase (*dashed line*) as the alveolus is recruited (*D*). As the pressure is slowly decreased, there is little volume loss until the critical closing pressure (*Pc*) is reached at point *C*. The alveolus immediately collapses to point *A*. Note that Pc is lower than Po owing to the law of LaPlace.

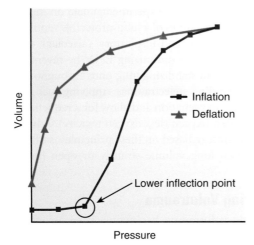

Fig. 21.3 Pressure-volume relationship of the lung showing the inflation (*red line*) and the deflation limb (*green line*). Note the clear difference in lung volume between the limbs at identical pressures (*hysteresis*).

resulting in a large volume (radius) increase. As follows from the law of LaPlace, which states that the pressure (P) necessary to keep a spherical structure opened is two times the surface tension (γ) divided by the radius (r), the critical closing pressure of the alveolus will be lower than the opening pressure.

The P/V curve of the entire lung, as shown in Fig. 21.3, will be the cumulative relationship of all alveoli/saccules of the lung, each with a different severity of lung disease and thus a different opening and closing pressure. The inflation limb of the P/V curve shows the changes in lung volume during incremental airway pressures and usually contains a so-called lower inflection point above which lung volume suddenly increases in a linear fashion. As lung volume approaches total lung capacity (TLC), the inflation limb flattens off. The deflation limb represents the changes in lung volume

during decremental airway pressure steps starting at TLC. Again, as explained by the law of LaPlace, lung volume is initially maintained as pressures are lowered but eventually decreases owing to progressive alveolar collapse as the distending pressure drops below the critical closing pressure. The clear difference in lung volume at identical airway pressures between the inflation and the deflation limb of the P/V relationship is called lung hysteresis. Studies in newborn infants have shown that lung hysteresis is present in preterm infants with RDS and term infants with more heterogeneous causes of lung disease.[59-61]

It was initially assumed that lung recruitment occurred primarily around the lower inflection point of the P/V curve. However, observations in adults and newborn infants have indicated that recruitment occurs along the entire inflation limb of the P/V curve.[60,62] Although sometimes stated differently, the inflation pressures or volumes, and not positive end-expiratory pressure (PEEP), are responsible for alveolar recruitment during conventional ventilation. PEEP is an expiratory phenomenon, and its main purpose is to stabilize the previously opened alveoli and thereby prevent subsequent collapse during expiration. Failing to recruit the lungs before or concomitant with increasing PEEP will not prevent VILI.[13,63] On the other hand, recruiting the lungs but applying insufficient PEEP to prevent subsequent collapse will augment rather than reduce lung injury.[64]

It was also believed that the optimal PEEP levels preventing alveolar collapse should be above the lower inflection point of the P/V curve.[65] However, experimental and human data have shown that the critical closing pressure of the lungs is not related to the lower inflection point.[66,67]

Both mathematical models and animal experiments have shown that adequate recruitment of collapsed alveoli, followed by optimal stabilization with adequate levels of PEEP, will place ventilation on the deflation limb of the P/V curve.[68,69] This position will improve compliance and reduce VILI compared with ventilation on, or close to, the inflation limb of the P/V curve.[63,69]

Because most underlying lung diseases causing neonatal respiratory failure are heterogeneous in nature, regional overdistention of relatively healthy lung parts has been a major concern during recruitment. Although this concern seems valid, there is little evidence that recruitment maneuvers actually damage the lungs if accompanied by sufficient PEEP. More importantly, to date most experiments have indicated that derecruitment is more injurious than recruitment.[70,71]

One of the difficulties of practical implementation of lung recruitment is the lack of tools that can assess changes in EELV in ventilated newborn infants at the bedside. Although often used in clinical practice, chest radiography provides only general information on lung aeration at one point in time and does not seem to correlate well with actual lung volumes.[72] This may in part be caused by suboptimal technique in terms of centering of the film and the difficulty in timing exposure at a particular point in the respiratory cycle at rapid respiratory rates. Tracer gas washout techniques can be used to measure changes in EELV, but they do not provide continuous information and are not applicable during high-frequency ventilation.[73] Respiratory

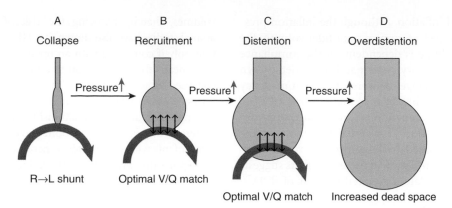

Fig. 21.4 Basic principle of oxygenation-guided recruitment illustrated by one alveolar-capillary unit. **(A)** Collapsed but perfused alveolus with no uptake of oxygen in the bloodstream. Blood returns to the left atrium in a hypoxic state. This is called intrapulmonary right-to-left shunting. **(B)** The increased airway pressure exceeds the critical opening pressure of the alveolus, resulting in opening of the alveolus, a (rapid) volume increase, and an uptake of oxygen owing to the optimal ventilation/perfusion match. This process is called recruitment. **(C)** A further increase in pressure will distend the already open alveolus, resulting in an increase in volume but no change in the optimal ventilation/perfusion match. This process is called distention. **(D)** A further increase in pressure will result in overdistention of the alveolus, resulting in absent perfusion owing to compression of the alveolar blood vessels. This will result in an increase in (alveolar) dead space and rising partial pressure of carbon dioxide.

inductive plethysmography has been successfully used in newborn infants to measure changes in EELV and to reconstruct the P/V relationship of the lung.[61] However, its application is hampered by signal instability over time, especially in unsedated nonmuscle-relaxed infants.[74] Another disadvantage that applies to all of the aforementioned techniques is the inability to differentiate between lung volume changes caused by alveolar recruitment (which is the aim of volume optimization) and those caused by alveolar distention (of already open alveoli). A more recent imaging technique called electrical impedance tomography does provide regional information on changes in lung aeration and has been successfully used in (preterm) infants.[60,74] However, the hardware, software, and patient interface of this technique need to be improved before it can be used in daily clinical practice.

Owing to these limitations of the currently available monitoring tools, most clinicians use oxygenation as an indirect tool to measure changes in lung volume at the bedside. The basic principle is illustrated in Fig. 21.4. In a collapsed alveolus, blood flowing through the alveolar-capillary unit will not be able to take up oxygen before returning to the left atrium. This is called intrapulmonary right-to-left shunting, which results in hypoxemia. If the alveolus is recruited with sufficient airway pressure, gas exchange will be restored at the alveolar level, resulting in an improvement of the ventilation/perfusion ratio, reflected by improved oxygenation. Increasing the airway pressure further will increase the volume of the alveolus (distention) but will not affect the ventilation/perfusion ratio. In the case of overdistention, the capillaries will be compressed, resulting in increased alveolar dead space and hypercarbia. The same concepts also apply when reducing the airway pressure once the alveolus is recruited. This means that oxygenation is able to differentiate between volume changes based on alveolar recruitment and distention.

LUNG-PROTECTIVE VENTILATION: CONVENTIONAL MECHANICAL VENTILATION

Conventional mechanical ventilation is the most frequently used modality in newborn infants.[54] It is a broad term for various modalities that all use the concept of tidal ventilation. In this section, we will focus on the various elements of lung protection during conventional mechanical ventilation without going into the specifics of the available conventional ventilation modes. For these details, the reader is referred to other chapters in this textbook.

Low Tidal Volume Ventilation

Based on the experimental evidence that higher tidal volumes can lead to VILI, experts have advocated targeting a tidal volume between 4 and 7 mL/kg during conventional mechanical ventilation in (preterm) infants. The evidence to support this recommendation, however, is limited. As of this writing, there are no large randomized controlled trials comparing higher and lower tidal volumes and their impact on clinically relevant outcomes, such as BPD. A small clinical trial comparing a tidal volume of 3 mL/kg with 5 mL/kg in preterm infants with RDS showed an increased inflammatory response in the tracheal aspirates of infants treated with 3 mL/kg.[75] This study seems to suggest that tidal volumes below 4 mL/kg, combined with a relatively low PEEP of 3 to 4 cm H_2O, may cause lung injury, probably because of alveolar collapse. Other studies have indicated that the optimal tidal volume in terms of gas exchange is probably not a fixed number but instead a dynamic parameter that changes over time.[76]

Tidal Volume Stabilization

Pressure-limited ventilation, the most widely used mode in neonatology, delivers a preset inflation pressure above PEEP during each mechanical inflation. Although the inflation pressure is initially set to target an appropriate tidal volume, the actual delivered tidal volume is dependent on the compliance and resistance of the respiratory system and the patient's own effort. As these variables change, delivered tidal volumes may become too high or too low, thereby increasing the risk of VILI. Applying volume-targeted ventilation will result in a more stable tidal volume and less VILI.[77,78] A systematic review of the (small) randomized controlled trials comparing volume-targeted to pressure-limited ventilation in preterm infants suggests that this approach also translates into a reduced risk of BPD.[79]

Permissive Hypercarbia

In an attempt to reduce tidal volume as much as possible, some clinicians accept higher carbon dioxide levels during mechanical ventilation, a strategy also referred to as permissive hypercarbia. Despite the fact that experimental evidence suggests a protective effect on the lungs, studies in ventilated preterm infants did not show a clear benefit in terms of BPD-free survival.[80,81]

Open Lung Ventilation

As previously mentioned, an open lung ventilation strategy aims to optimize lung volume by recruiting and stabilizing unstable lung units and by ventilating the lungs with low tidal volumes. Animal studies have shown that such an open lung ventilation strategy is feasible during positive-pressure ventilation (PPV) using relatively high peak inflation pressures and PEEP to, respectively, recruit and stabilize the lung.[82,83] Open lung PPV improves gas exchange and attenuates VILI compared with more conventional ventilation strategies. These beneficial effects are similar during open lung PPV and open lung high-frequency ventilation, suggesting that the open lung ventilation strategy is probably more important than the ventilation mode.

Despite these promising animal data, studies on open lung PPV in human infants are limited. As of this writing, only one study has assessed the short-term benefits of open lung PPV in preterm infants with RDS. This study reported better oxygenation and shorter oxygen dependency.[84]

Several studies explored the short-term effects of various levels of PEEP without a recruitment procedure during conventional mechanical ventilation in preterm infants. Higher levels of PEEP improved functional residual capacity and oxygenation but also resulted in a reduction in lung compliance and higher carbon dioxide levels.[85-87] These findings may reflect failure to achieve lung recruitment before increasing PEEP. Unfortunately, the effects on markers of VILI or the incidence of BPD were not reported. Another study explored the effects of a higher versus a lower PEEP in term infants on extracorporeal membrane oxygenation and showed that lung function was better preserved by using higher PEEP levels, resulting in a more rapid recovery.[88]

LUNG-PROTECTIVE VENTILATION: HIGH-FREQUENCY VENTILATION

In neonatology, high-frequency ventilation (HFV) has been the ventilation mode associated most with lung-protective ventilation. This is probably because HFV, by design, applies very small tidal

volumes, thereby reducing the risk of volutrauma. However, animal studies have also shown that HFV will provide lung protection only if combined with an open lung ventilation strategy.[89,90] This means that, in addition to applying the small tidal volumes, collapsed lung units need to be recruited and stabilized with the lowest possible airway pressure. This will place ventilation on the deflation limb of the P/V relationship, taking advantage of the lung hysteresis that is present in both preterm infants with RDS and term infants with more heterogeneous causes of lung disease.[60,61]

Reports on oxygenation-guided lung recruitment during (primary) HFV are limited to preterm infants with RDS. Fig. 21.5 shows the basic scheme of this ventilation strategy. Changes in oxygenation are monitored at the bedside using pulse oximetry (oxygen saturation [SpO_2]). Assuming that alveolar/saccular collapse resulting in intrapulmonary right-to-left shunt is the main cause of hypoxemia, reversing atelectasis will allow for normal oxygenation with minimal or no supplemental oxygen. For this reason, most clinicians will define an optimally recruited lung as needing a fraction of inspired oxygen (FiO_2) less than or equal to 0.25 to 0.30 to maintain SpO_2 within the appropriate target. To minimize the risk of overdistention, the continuous distending pressure (CDP) during HFV is usually set between 6 and 8 cm H_2O at the start of the recruitment procedure. The FiO_2 is adjusted in such a way that the SpO_2 is within the target range. If the FiO_2 is over 0.30, the lung volume is considered as not being optimal, and the CDP is increased in steps of 2 cm H_2O every 2 to 3 minutes. If lung units are recruited, oxygenation will improve, allowing for a stepwise reduction in FiO_2 (5% to 10%

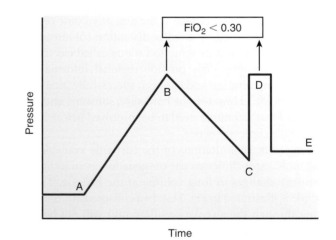

Fig. 21.5 Schematic representation using oxygenation to optimize lung volume in preterm infants with respiratory distress syndrome. At the start (A), airway pressure is low and fraction of inspired oxygen (FiO_2) is high, indicating a high degree of atelectasis and intrapulmonary shunt. Over time, airway pressures are increased stepwise, resulting in alveolar recruitment, a reduction in intrapulmonary shunt, and improvement in oxygenation. The last will allow a stepwise reduction in FiO_2, thus preventing hyperoxia. Airway pressures are increased until FiO_2 is below 0.30 or oxygenation no longer improves (B). The pressure level at point B is called the opening pressure. Airway pressures are reduced stepwise until oxygen saturation starts to deteriorate, indicating alveolar collapse (C). This pressure level is called the closing pressure. After reopening collapsed alveoli with the known opening pressure (D), airway pressure is set 2 cm H_2O above the closing pressure to ensure a stabilization of lung volume (E).

each step). The CDP is increased stepwise until the FiO_2 is under 0.30 or oxygenation does not improve during three consecutive pressure steps. At that point, referred to as opening pressure, the lung is considered as being optimally recruited. It is essential at this point to reduce the distending pressure because the pressure needed to keep the lungs open will be lower than the opening pressure (law of LaPlace, lung hysteresis). Using a fixed FiO_2, the CDP is decreased stepwise (2 cm H_2O every 2–3 minutes) until SpO_2 deteriorates, indicative of alveolar/saccular collapse. The corresponding pressure is called the closing pressure. Next, the CDP is increased to the opening pressure for several minutes and then decreased to 2 cm H_2O above the closing pressure. The corresponding pressure is called the optimal CDP.

In addition to oxygenation, changes in (transcutaneous) partial pressure of carbon dioxide (PCO_2) can also assist the clinician in lung recruitment.[91] PCO_2 will change depending on the position of ventilation on the inflation and deflation limbs of the P/V relationship. A rise in PCO_2 when determining the opening pressure is an indication that the lung is almost fully recruited because ventilation is moving up the flat part of the inflation limb.

Administering exogenous surfactant will improve both EELV and its stability at lower pressures.[92] This means that following surfactant treatment, the CDP can usually be significantly lowered. A prospective cohort study in preterm infants with RDS subjected to primary HFV provided useful and practical information on this open lung ventilation strategy during HFV.[93] It showed that the mean opening pressure before surfactant treatment was 20 cm H_2O. Optimal recruitment resulting in an FiO_2 under 0.30 was feasible in 90% of the infants. It is important to emphasize that the strategy as described uses an individual and dynamic approach. The pressures applied to the lungs are different for each individual patient depending on the severity of lung disease. This is probably the most important reason that the incidence of adverse effects of lung recruitment, such as hemodynamic instability and air leaks, is relatively low.

It is also important to acknowledge that oxygenation is an indirect tool for guiding lung recruitment. In case hypoxemia is also caused by extrapulmonary right-to-left shunt owing to persistent pulmonary hypertension or the presence of alveolar debris (pneumonia) impairing normal diffusion in the alveolar-capillary unit, oxygenation is no longer a reliable marker of lung volume. Clinicians should be aware of this drawback.

Although the basic concepts of open lung HFV are also applicable to other causes of respiratory failure, there are some important differences compared with preterm infants with RDS. First, lung disease in older preterm infants or term infants with respiratory failure is much more heterogeneous in nature compared with RDS.[94] Studies have indicated that the time constants of the lungs—that is, the time it takes collapsed lung units to open up or to close after a change in airway pressure—are much longer compared with infants with RDS.[73,95] Furthermore, the heterogeneous nature of lung disease often results in higher optimal pressures and concomitant FiO_2 compared with infants with RDS. Finally, lung disease in more mature infants is often accompanied by persistent pulmonary hypertension and, as previously mentioned, this complicates the process of oxygenation-guided lung recruitment during HFV.

The strategy described earlier is applicable in lung disease accompanied by alveolar/saccular collapse. HFV can also be lung protective during lung disease not characterized by atelectasis, such as lung hypoplasia associated with prolonged premature rupture of membranes and congenital diaphragmatic hernia. However, in these cases, it is usually not necessary to apply a recruitment procedure. The optimal lung volume can be maintained with relatively low CDPs. Lung protection is focused on preventing alveolar/saccular overdistention by clearing carbon dioxide with relatively small tidal volumes.

Most randomized studies of HFV have been done in preterm infants with RDS. A systematic review of all randomized controlled trials comparing HFV to conventional mechanical ventilation shows, at most, a modest reduction in BPD in favor of HFV.[96] However, this effect is weakened by the heterogeneity between trials. Differences in the characteristics of the included patients, supportive therapies, and ventilation strategy used during both HFV and CMV probably account for this heterogeneity. Studies that failed to use or achieve an optimal lung volume strategy did not show any benefit of HFV. Based on the two largest randomized controlled trials, it has been suggested that HFV used with the optimal lung volume strategy might be superior to conventional mechanical ventilation in preterm infants with more severe RDS if consistently used during every ventilation period during hospitalization.[97,98]

As of this writing, only one randomized controlled trial has compared HFV with conventional mechanical ventilation in term infants who were candidates for extracorporeal membrane oxygenation, mostly because of MAS.[99] This study showed that high-frequency oscillatory ventilation (HFOV) was an effective mode of ventilation especially when conventional mechanical ventilation failed. However, mortality and significant long-term morbidity did not differ between the groups. This may have been influenced by the relatively advanced age at randomization (40 hours) and the high crossover rate in each treatment arm (>50%). Another randomized controlled trial investigating the use of HFOV and/or inhaled nitric oxide also showed improved oxygenation when switching from conventional ventilation to HFOV in the treatment of MAS.[100] Furthermore, combining inhaled nitric oxide with HFOV was superior compared with combination with conventional mechanical ventilation.

The use of HFV in lung hypoplasia has been reported in human case reports and case series. Most of these reports described improved survival after adopting HFV in the management of congenital diaphragmatic hernia mostly compared with historical controls.[101,102] Reports that showed no benefit from HFV often used this ventilation mode as a rescue therapy, applying it to those patients who failed (high-pressure) conventional mechanical ventilation, thus subjecting their lungs to volutrauma for a considerable period of time.[103,104] As of this writing, only one randomized controlled trial compared HFV with CMV in infants with congenital diaphragmatic hernia, reporting no benefit on the combined outcome death or BPD.[105] Patients treated with CMV were ventilated for fewer days; less often needed extracorporeal membrane oxygenation support, inhaled nitric oxide, and sildenafil; and had a shorter duration of vasoactive drugs as compared with infants treated with HFV.

Despite the fact that congenital diaphragmatic hernia is not a recruitable lung disease, this study did adopt a recruitment procedure in the HFV ventilation protocol. This may explain the lack of benefit and the adverse hemodynamic effects.

LUNG-PROTECTIVE VENTILATION: WEANING AND EXTUBATION

Although a lung-protective ventilation strategy can attenuate lung injury, it can never totally prevent it. For this reason, infants should be weaned from invasive support as soon as possible and transferred back to noninvasive modes of respiratory support. Prolonging mechanical ventilation for more than a few days will already increase the risk of BPD.[3] Furthermore, (protracted) mechanical ventilation has also been associated with an increased risk of adverse neurodevelopmental outcome in preterm infants.[2]

Studies have shown that noninvasive support modes such as continuous positive airway pressure and nasal intermittent PPV will increase the chance of successfully transitioning preterm infants from invasive to noninvasive support.[106,107] This is probably the most important reason protracted ventilation is nowadays less common in preterm infants.

IMPLICATIONS FOR PRACTICE AND RESEARCH

The goal during mechanical ventilation of newborn infants should be to establish adequate gas exchange while minimizing VILI as much as possible. Animal studies suggest that the ventilation strategy is probably more important than the ventilation mode when trying to achieve this goal. Such a lung-protective ventilation strategy should reduce both alveolar/saccular overdistention (volutrauma) and collapse (atelectrauma). When using conventional mechanical ventilation, clinicians should probably aim for a tidal volume between 4 and 7 mL/kg and reduce fluctuations as much as possible by choosing a volume-targeted ventilation mode. In addition, sufficient PEEP should be used to stabilize lung volume at the end of expiration, using oxygenation as an indicator of lung volume. A good alternative for conventional ventilation is HFV. This mode uses very small tidal volumes, thereby reducing the risk of volutrauma. However, HFV will provide optimal lung protection only if combined with an optimal lung volume or open lung ventilation strategy. Again, oxygenation can serve as an indirect monitoring tool for EELV. Finally, patients who require invasive mechanical ventilation should be extubated as soon as possible, limiting the duration of ventilation and the subsequent lung injury as much as possible.

Although invasive mechanical ventilation has been used in newborn infants for almost 50 years, there are still several unresolved issues that need to be addressed in future studies. First, the optimal tidal volume during conventional mechanical ventilation needs to be established in a randomized controlled trial comparing a higher to a lower tidal volume in specific patient populations. Second, the beneficial effects of volume-targeted ventilation reported in a meta-analysis summarizing several small trials need to be confirmed in a large randomized trial. Third, future studies need to confirm the presumed beneficial effect of lung recruitment and stabilization (open lung strategy) during conventional mechanical ventilation. Finally, more direct tools for measuring (changes in) lung volume, such as electrical impedance tomography, are urgently needed. These tools need to be optimized for clinical use and their impact on clinically relevant outcomes tested.

A complete reference list is available at https://expertconsult.inkling.com/.

KEY REFERENCES

5. Dreyfuss D, Saumon G: Ventilator-induced lung injury: lessons from experimental studies. Am J Respir Crit Care Med 157: 294–323, 1998.
54. van Kaam AH, Rimensberger PC, Borensztajn D, et al: Ventilation practices in the neonatal intensive care unit: a cross-sectional study. J Pediatr 157:767–771 e761–e763, 2010.
55. Bjorklund LJ, Ingimarsson J, Curstedt T, et al: Manual ventilation with a few large breaths at birth compromises the therapeutic effect of subsequent surfactant replacement in immature lambs. Pediatr Res 42:348–355, 1997.
56. van Kaam AH, Rimensberger PC: Lung-protective ventilation strategies in neonatology: what do we know—what do we need to know? Crit Care Med 35:925–931, 2007.
60. Miedema M, de Jongh FH, Frerichs I, et al: Changes in lung volume and ventilation during lung recruitment in high-frequency ventilated preterm infants with respiratory distress syndrome. J Pediatr 159:199–205, e192, 2011.
61. Tingay DG, Mills JF, Morley CJ, et al: The deflation limb of the pressure-volume relationship in infants during high-frequency ventilation. Am J Respir Crit Care Med 173:414–420, 2006.
63. Rimensberger PC, Pristine G, Mullen BM, et al: Lung recruitment during small tidal volume ventilation allows minimal positive end-expiratory pressure without augmenting lung injury. Crit Care Med 27:1940–1945, 1999.
77. Keszler M, Abubakar K: Volume guarantee: stability of tidal volume and incidence of hypocarbia. Pediatr Pulmonol 38:240–245, 2004.
79. Klingenberg C, Wheeler K, McCallion N, et al.: Volume-targeted versus pressure-limited ventilation in the neonate. Cochrane Database Syst Rev 10:CD003666, 2017.
81. Thome UH, Genzel-Boroviczeny O, Bohnhorst B, et al.: Permissive hypercapnia in extremely low birthweight infants (PHELBI): a randomised controlled multicentre trial. Lancet Respir Med 3:534–543, 2015.
82. van Kaam AH, de Jaegere A, Haitsma JJ, et al: Positive pressure ventilation with the open lung concept optimizes gas exchange and reduces ventilator-induced lung injury in newborn piglets. Pediatr Res 53:245–253, 2003.
89. McCulloch PR, Forkert PG, Froese AB: Lung volume maintenance prevents lung injury during high frequency oscillatory ventilation in surfactant-deficient rabbits. Am Rev Respir Dis 137:1185–1192, 1988.
93. De Jaegere A, van Veenendaal MB, Michiels A, et al: Lung recruitment using oxygenation during open lung high-frequency ventilation in preterm infants. Am J Respir Crit Care Med 174: 639–645, 2006.
96. Cools F, Offringa M, Askie LM: Elective high frequency oscillatory ventilation versus conventional ventilation for acute pulmonary dysfunction in preterm infants. Cochrane Database Syst Rev CD000104, 2015.

22

Volume-Targeted Ventilation

Martin Keszler, MD and Kabir Abubakar, MBBS

KEY POINTS

- Pressure-controlled ventilation has been the standard approach to mechanical ventilation of newborn infants but can cause excessive tidal volume delivery and inadvertent hyperventilation when lung compliance improves. As a result, volume-targeted ventilation is increasingly used to avoid volutrauma and the dangers of respiratory alkalosis.
- Neonatal volume-targeted ventilation is pressure-controlled ventilation with automatic adjustment of inflation pressure to maintain a user-selected target tidal volume. Newer devices deal more effectively with problems related to leak around uncuffed endotracheal tubes and measure tidal volume more accurately using a flow sensor at the airway opening.
- Selection of the tidal volume appropriate for the specific patient and underlying condition is key to success. One size does NOT fit all. Use of volume-targeted ventilation results in more complex patient–ventilator interactions, making clinical assessment of the patient and ventilator waveforms essential tools in assessing appropriateness of ventilator settings.

As described in Chapter 19, two fundamentally different approaches to positive pressure ventilation are possible. In pressure-controlled (PC) ventilation, the primary control variable governing gas delivery to the lungs is inflation pressure, while the tidal volume delivered to the lungs is the dependent variable that changes if the baby breathes more forcefully and/or lung compliance and resistance change. In volume-controlled ventilation (VCV), tidal volume delivery into the ventilator circuit is directly controlled and pressure becomes the dependent variable, changing as necessary to compensate for the baby breathing and to overcome resistive and elastic forces of the lungs (Fig. 22.1).

Pressure-controlled, time-cycled, continuous-flow ventilation has been the standard of care in neonatal ventilation for more than 30 years because early attempts at VCV in small preterm neonates were unsuccessful with the devices available at the time. The perceived advantages of PC ventilation are the ability to directly control the inflation pressure and time, and to ventilate despite large leaks around the uncuffed endotracheal tubes (ETTs) used with neonates. Preoccupation with high inflation pressure as the chief culprit in ventilator-associated lung injury (VALI) and airleak has led to a deeply ingrained "barophobia" that has persisted despite mounting evidence that pressure by itself, without generating excessively large tidal volume, is not the main cause of lung injury.

RATIONALE FOR TIDAL VOLUME-TARGETED VENTILATION

Preclinical studies clearly demonstrate that tidal volume, rather than inflation pressure, is the critical determinant of ventilator-induced lung injury. Dreyfuss and colleagues demonstrated, as early as 1988, that severe acute lung injury occurred in animals ventilated with large tidal volume, regardless of whether that volume was generated by a high or low inflation pressure[1]. On the other hand, animals whose chest wall and diaphragmatic excursion were limited by external binding experienced much less lung damage despite being exposed to the same high inflation pressure[2,3]. This and other similar studies clearly show that pressure by itself, without correspondingly high tidal volume, is not injurious to the lungs, although it could be injurious to immature airways.

An equally compelling reason for tidal volume-targeted ventilation (VTV) is the extensive body of evidence documenting that both hypercapnia and hypocapnia are associated with neonatal brain injury[4-8]. Despite increasing awareness of its adverse consequences, inadvertent hyperventilation remains a common problem with pressure-limited ventilation, especially early in the clinical course when the baby starts breathing, lung compliance changes rapidly in response to clearing of lung fluid, surfactant administration, and optimization of lung volume. Luyt et al. demonstrated that 31% of ventilated infants had at least one blood gas with $PaCO_2$ less than 25 torr during the first day of life, whether they were ventilated with patient-triggered ventilation or unsynchronized intermittent mandatory ventilation[9].

Although there are important differences in how volume targeting is achieved with various ventilators, the primary benefit of VTV probably rests in the ability to regulate and maintain an appropriate tidal volume (V_T), regardless of how that goal is achieved. When V_T is the primary control variable, inflation pressure will fall as lung compliance and patient inspiratory effort improve, resulting in real-time weaning of pressure, in contrast to intermittent manual lowering of pressure in response to blood gases. Real-time lowering of pressure avoids excessive V_T and achieves a shorter duration of mechanical ventilation. The inflation pressure will also rise if, for some reason, the set tidal volume is not delivered. Two recent meta-analyses that included a combination of several different modalities of volume-controlled and VTV documented a number

Volume vs Pressure Ventilation

Volume Control	Pressure Control
- Controls the set flow rate	- Controls the set pressure
- Cycles when set volume is delivered	- Cycles by time or flow
- Pressure rises passively	- Volume depends on compliance

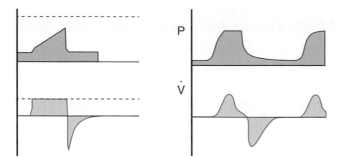

Fig. 22.1 Key differences between volume-controlled (VC) and pressure-controlled (PC) ventilation. Volume delivered into the ventilator circuit is the primary control variable in VC. Circuit pressure rises passively and reaches its peak just before exhalation. The device generates whatever pressure is needed to deliver the set volume. Inflation pressure is the primary control variable in PC ventilation. Delivered volume is proportional to inflation pressure and compliance of the respiratory system; therefore, the tidal volume will vary with changes in respiratory mechanics.

of advantages of volume-controlled or targeted ventilation, compared with pressure controlled ventilation; these included a significant decrease in the combined outcome of death or BPD, lower rate of pneumothorax, less hypocapnia, decreased risk of severe intraventricular hemorrhage/periventricular leukomalacia, and significantly shorter duration of mechanical ventilation (Table 22.1).[10,11] These results are very encouraging, but some limitations should be recognized. Included studies were quite small and used a variety of different modalities, and many of the key outcomes reported in the meta-analysis were not prospectively collected or defined. In some of the studies, other

variables beyond volume vs pressure targeting also differed. The studies focused on short-term physiologic outcomes, rather than BPD, as a primary outcome. Except for one follow-up study based on parental questionnaire, no long-term pulmonary or developmental outcomes have been reported.

VOLUME-CONTROLLED VERSUS VOLUME-TARGETED VENTILATION

Volume-controlled, also known as volume-cycled, ventilators deliver a constant, preset V_T into the ventilator circuit with each inflation. In theory, these ventilators allow the operator to select V_T and respiratory rate and therefore directly control minute ventilation. Pressure rises passively, in inverse proportion to lung compliance, as the tidal volume is delivered, reaching its peak just before the ventilator cycles off, allowing little time for intrapulmonary gas distribution. The ventilator delivers the set V_T into the circuit, generating whatever pressure is necessary to overcome lung compliance and airway resistance, up to a set safety pop-off, typically set at a pressure of 40 cm H_2O or greater. A maximum inflation time is also set as an additional safety measure. The ventilator cycles into expiration when the preset V_T has been delivered, or when the maximum inflation time has elapsed. The latter ensures that with very poor lung compliance, the ventilator does not generate a very prolonged inflation in an attempt to deliver a set V_T that cannot be reached at the pressure pop-off value.

The major limitation of VCV is that what is controlled is the volume injected into the ventilator circuit, not the V_T that enters the patient's lungs. This limitation is based on the fact that the tidal volume is measured at the ventilator end of the circuit and does not account for compression of gas in the circuit and humidifier or distention of the compliant circuit.[12] In large patients with cuffed ETTs, this loss is insignificant and easily compensated, but such is not the case in small preterm infants, whose lungs are only a fraction of the total volume of the circuit (Fig. 22.2). Most modern ventilators have provisions to compensate for circuit compliance/gas compression, but this ability

---

TABLE 22.1 Documented Benefits of Volume-Targeted Ventilation

	Relative Risk or Mean Difference	95% Confidence Interval	Number Needed to Benefit (95% CI)
Death at BPD at 36 weeks	0.75	0.53 to 1.07	NA
BPD at 36 weeks PMA	0.73	0.59 to 0.89[a]	8 (5–20)
Grade 3–4 IVH	0.53	0.37 to 0.77[a]	11 (7–25)
PVL ± severe IVH	0.53	0.27 to 0.80[a]	11 (7–33)
Pneumothorax	0.52	0.31 to 0.87[a]	20 (11–100)
Hypocapnia	0.49	0.33 to 0.72[a]	3 (2–5)
Days of MV	−1.35	−1.83 to −0.86[a]	

Sixteen parallel studies with 977 infants + four crossover studies were included.
[a]Statistically significant benefit of volume-targeted ventilation.
BPD, Bronchopulmonary dysplasia; *CI,* confidence interval; *IVH,* intraventricular hemorrhage; *MV,* mechanical ventilation; *PVL,* periventricular leukomalacia.
(Data from Klingenberg C, Wheeler KI, McCallion N, et al: Volume-targeted versus pressure-limited ventilation in neonates. Cochrane Database Syst Rev 10:CD003666, 2017.)

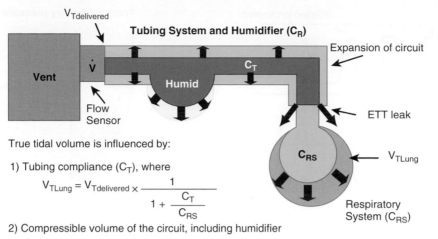

$V_{Tdelivered}$

Tubing System and Humidifier (C_R)

Expansion of circuit

Vent

$\dot{V}$

C_T

Humid

Flow
Sensor

ETT leak

C_{RS}

V_{TLung}

True tidal volume is influenced by:

1) Tubing compliance (C_T), where

$$V_{TLung} = V_{Tdelivered} \times \dfrac{1}{1 + \dfrac{C_T}{C_{RS}}}$$

2) Compressible volume of the circuit, including humidifier

3) Magnitude of ETT leak

Respiratory
System (C_{RS})

Fig. 22.2 Functional limitation of volume-controlled ventilation in newborn infants. Volume-controlled ventilation regulates the volume of gas delivered into the proximal end of the ventilator circuit ($V_{Tdelivered}$). The volume of gas entering the lungs (V_{TLung}) is affected by three factors: (1) tubing compliance (C_T), (2) compressible volume of the circuit and humidifier, and (3) magnitude of the leak around an uncuffed endotracheal tube. In newborn infants, the volume of the lungs is only a fraction of the circuit/humidifier volume and often poorly compliant. Thus, the loss of volume to compression of gas in the circuit and to stretching of the compliant circuit is very substantial. Variable leak around endotracheal tubes makes compensation very challenging. *ETT,* Endotracheal tube.

breaks down with the ubiquitous and highly variable leak around uncuffed ETTs used in newborn infants. These limitations can be overcome to a degree by using a separate flow sensor at the airway opening to monitor exhaled tidal volume. This will allow the user to manually adjust the set tidal volume (also known as V_{del}) to achieve the desired exhaled tidal volume. Unfortunately, the ETT leak is usually variable, and thus, frequent monitoring and adjustment may be necessary. An alternate approach to VCV is to rely on clinical assessment of adequacy of chest rise and breath sounds to set the V_{del}, which typically needs to be set at 10 to 12 mL/kg, to achieve effective tidal volume of 4 to 5 mL/kg, and to make subsequent adjustments based on blood gas measurement. Despite these limitations, VCV has been shown to be feasible even in small preterm infants when a flow sensor at the airway opening is used.[13]

NEONATAL TIDAL VOLUME-TARGETED VENTILATION

In contrast to traditional VCV, VTV modalities are modifications of PC ventilation designed to deliver a target tidal volume by real-time microprocessor-directed adjustments of inflation pressure. Some devices regulate tidal volume delivery based on flow measurement during inflation and others during exhalation. Each approach has advantages and disadvantages—leak is greater during inflation and thus exhaled tidal volume more closely approximates true tidal volume. Use of exhaled tidal volume results in regulation of the peak pressure based on the previous ventilator cycle, whereas using inflation volume makes same-cycle control possible, but it is then not possible to compensate for ETT leak in real time. If the inflation volume were 10 mL and the ETT leak 50%, then the baby would only be

getting a tidal volume of 5 mL. When a large ETT leak is present, even the exhaled tidal volume underestimates true volume and inspiratory measurement will overestimate the true tidal volume that enters the lungs. On balance, the use of exhaled V_T offers the best balance of safety and effectiveness. In recent years, newer modalities of VTV have increasingly come to closely resemble volume guarantee (VG) ventilation, which focuses on expired tidal volume, as described below.

VOLUME GUARANTEE

VG is an option available on the Draeger Babylog 8000+; the VN 500, 600, and 800 (Draeger Medical, Lubeck, Germany); and the Leoni Plus (Heinen + Löwenstein GmbH, Bad Ems, Germany; not available in the United States). More recently, a version of VG has been implemented on the Avea ventilator (Vyaire, Mettawa, IL). VG may be combined with any of the basic ventilator modes, including controlled mechanical ventilation (CMV), assist control (AC), synchronized intermittent mandatory ventilation (SIMV), or pressure support ventilation (PSV). It is a volume-targeted, time- or flow-cycled, pressure-limited form of ventilation. The operator chooses a target V_T and a pressure limit up to which the ventilator operating pressure (working pressure) may be adjusted. The microprocessor compares the exhaled V_T of the previous inflation and adjusts the working pressure up or down to target the set V_T (Fig. 22.3A and B). The algorithm limits the pressure increment from one inflation to the next to a percentage of the amount needed to reach the target V_T to avoid excessive oscillations, up to a maximum increase of 3 cm H_2O. Consequently, with rapid, large changes in compliance or patient inspiratory effort, several cycles are needed to reach target V_T. If the ventilator is unable to reach the target V_T

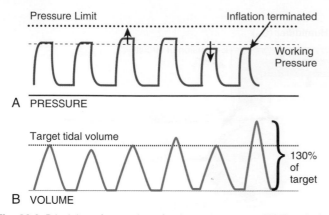

A PRESSURE

B VOLUME

Fig. 22.3 Principles of operation of volume guarantee. **(A)** The device compares the measured expired tidal volume to the target volume and automatically regulates the PIP (peak inflation pressure, working pressure) within preset limits (as low as end-expiratory pressure to as high as the set pressure limit) to achieve the tidal volume that is set by the user. **(B)** This figure illustrates that regulation of PIP is in response to *exhaled* tidal volume of the previous inflation to decrease error because of endotracheal tube leak. The PIP increase from one cycle to the next is limited to avoid overshoot and undesirable oscillations. If tidal volume exceeds 130% of target, inflation will be terminated at that point (a secondary safety volume-limit function).

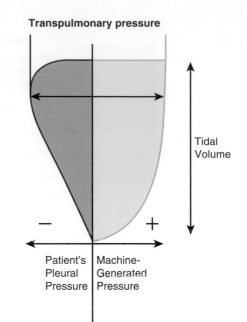

Fig. 22.4 In an awake, breathing infant, the tidal volume that enters the lungs is generated by the transpulmonary pressure, the sum of the negative intrathoracic pressure generated by the infant's spontaneous respiratory effort and the positive inflation pressure generated by the ventilator. Because the respiratory effort of a preterm infant is variable and inconsistent, the infant's contribution to the transpulmonary pressure is variable thus resulting in a variable tidal volume.

with the set inflation pressure limit, a "low tidal volume" alarm will sound, alerting the operator that an assessment is needed. The VG modality, as implemented on the Draeger Babylog 8000+ and VN500, 600, and 800 ventilators, which are designed specifically for newborn infants, employs separate controls for triggered and untriggered inflations. This is an important feature when ventilating spontaneously breathing preterm infants whose respiratory effort is intermittent and highly variable, because, as with all forms of synchronized ventilation, the tidal volume is determined by a combination of the positive pressure from the ventilator and the negative intrapleural pressure resulting from the spontaneous effort of the infant (Fig. 22.4). Consequently, VG leads to a more stable tidal volume than would be seen in similar modalities that use a single control algorithm (Fig. 22.5). The impact of VG with the dual control algorithm compared to simple PC ventilation is seen in Fig. 22.6. A secondary safety feature designed to prevent delivery of excessively large inflations terminates an inflation on the same cycle if the tidal volume target is exceeded by more than 30% based on inspiratory volume measurement (corrected for leakage). In an awake, actively breathing infant, the variable patient contribution to transpulmonary pressure is always perturbing the equilibrium, causing the V_T to fluctuate around the target V_T. Thus, the term volume "guarantee" is arguably a misnomer. However, there is good evidence that a completely constant V_T leads to atelectasis over time; thus, a physiologic variability of V_T is actually desirable.[14]

The VG modality, as implemented on a Draeger ventilator, has been studied more thoroughly than other modes of VTV and has been shown to reduce the incidence of hypocapnia and the number of excessively large tidal volumes.[15] Specific clinical guidelines for VG have been published and are also provided

later and in Tables 22.2 and 22.3.[16,17] VG has been shown to be more effective when used with AC than with SIMV, likely because all inflations are subject to volume targeting.[18]

The choice of appropriate V_T (see later) depends on infant size, pulmonary diagnosis, and basic synchronization mode. It is critical to appreciate that one size DOES NOT fit all when it comes to neonatal tidal volume settings. The smallest infants require a slightly larger V_T/kg owing to the proportionally larger fixed dead space of the flow sensor.[20] Infants with pulmonary conditions that lead to increased alveolar dead space (e.g., meconium aspiration syndrome or bronchopulmonary dysplasia) also require relatively larger V_T.[21,29] Depending on the set rate, SIMV may require a larger V_T than AC to deliver the same alveolar minute ventilation, because fewer breaths are supported and volume targeted. As the underlying pulmonary pathology evolves, the V_T target that provides optimal support will also change.

Some older devices, including the Babylog 8000+, which is no longer produced but still in occasional use, regulate the peak pressure for the current inflation based on the uncorrected exhaled V_T of the previous inflation. This measurement begins to progressively underestimate the true V_T with increasing ETT leak.[30] In that situation, the ventilator will increase inflation pressure in an attempt to reach the target, but because it is now working with falsely low exhaled V_T values, the resulting VT is actually larger than the target, potentially resulting in inadvertent hypocapnia when the ETT leak exceeds about 40% (Fig. 22.7). Progressively larger ETT leak commonly occurs if a preterm infant remains intubated for >2 weeks, because of

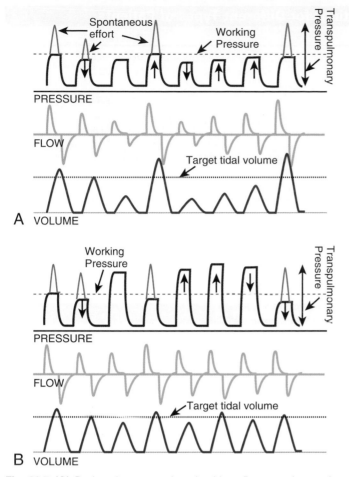

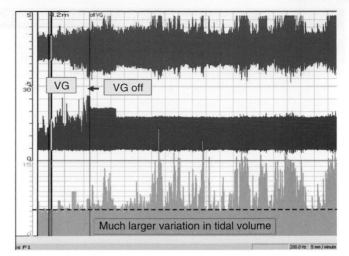

Fig. 22.6 The impact of VG with dual control algorithm vs PC ventilation. Flow is displayed in the *upper panel*, pressure in the *middle panel*, and V_T in the *lower panel*. Relatively stable V_T is seen in the first part of the recording, while PIP is highly variable. After VG is turned off, PIP becomes fixed (after it is manually lowered in two steps), while V_T begins to fluctuate from inflation to inflation, because now we see the impact of a fixed PIP on top of a highly variable and sometimes absent spontaneous effort of the baby. *PC*, Pressure-controlled; *PIP*, peak inflation pressure; *VG*, volume guarantee.

Fig. 22.5 (A) Basic volume-targeting algorithm. Because the respiratory effort of a preterm infant is variable and inconsistent, the infant's contribution to the transpulmonary pressure is variable, thus resulting in a variable tidal volume. In this figure, the infant's own inspiratory effort is drawn in *blue*, superimposed on the ventilator pressure. This contribution is not measured or displayed by the ventilator. When an actively breathing infant who was contributing substantially to the transpulmonary pressure fails to take a breath before the next ventilator cycle, there will be a large drop in delivered tidal volume. The ventilator adjusts the working pressure based on the tidal volume of the previous cycle, but the infant again resumes her breathing, resulting in large fluctuations in tidal volume. Because of the limited increment in working pressure from breath to breath, it takes several cycles to reach the target tidal volume when the infant remains apneic. **(B)** The volume guarantee modality as implemented on Draeger devices has a separate control algorithm to regulate triggered and untriggered inflations. The microprocessor will use the working pressure for the previous cycle of the same type (triggered or untriggered) as a starting point for the adjustment. Consequently, the transpulmonary pressure remains more stable, resulting in more stable tidal volume delivery.

stretching of the trachea and larynx (acquired tracheomegaly),[31] and may require reintubation with a larger ETT, or reversion to PC ventilation because reliable measurement of V_T is no longer possible with such a large leak. With the VN 500, 600, and 800 ventilators, this problem has largely been eliminated. These ventilators, being specifically designed for newborn infants, employ an effective leak compensation algorithm (Fig. 22.8). We recommend that the leak compensation feature

be selected in the ventilator default setting to minimize measurement error caused by ETT leakage. The ability to compensate effectively for leaks of up to 75% to 80% is a remarkable technological advance on the VN series ventilators that makes VG feasible and safe in virtually all infants.

An obvious advantage of VG is that weaning occurs automatically, in real time, and requires fewer blood gas measurements. With stable minute ventilation ensured by VG along with noninvasive pulse oximetry monitoring, fewer invasive blood gas measurements are needed once the appropriate settings are confirmed. This effective self-weaning mechanism appears to be counterintuitive to some practitioners who are accustomed to manual adjustments of ventilator settings. As a consequence, there is sometimes inappropriate lowering of target V_T in an effort to wean the patient off the ventilator. It should be clearly understood that the physiologic V_T required by the patient does not decrease (over time it may actually increase); what goes down is the pressure required to achieve that V_T because of improved compliance of the respiratory system and the infant breathing more effectively. Decreasing V_T target below the patient's physiologic need will increase the work of breathing[32] and may delay successful extubation.

SUGGESTED CLINICAL GUIDELINES (SEE ALSO TABLE 22.3)

These guidelines are based on research and extensive clinical experience of the authors based on the VG modality on the Draeger devices. Although the principles described in this section generally apply to all modalities of VTV, there may be some device-related differences that may require slightly different approaches.

TABLE 22.2 Suggested Initial Tidal Volume Settings for Different Types of Patients

Condition	Initial V_T	Rationale	Reference
Term, late preterm, normal lungs	4–4.5 ml/kg	Baseline	Dawson et al.[19]
Preterm RDS 1250–2500 g	4–4.5 mL/kg	Low alveolar dead space	Dawson et al.[19]
Preterm RDS 700–1249 g	4.5–5 mL/kg	Dead space of the flow sensor	Nassabeh-Montazami et al.[20]
Preterm RDS <700 g	5.5–6 mL/kg	Dead space of the flow sensor	Nassabeh-Montazami et al.[20]
Preterm evolving BPD, 3 weeks old	5.5–6.5 mL/kg	Increased anatomical and alveolar dead space	Keszler et al.[21]
Term MAS with classic CXR[a]	5.5–6 mL/kg	Increased alveolar dead space	Sharma et al.[22]
Term MAS with whiteout CXR	4.5–5 mL/kg	Alveolar dead space less of a problem	Keszler[23]
Term CDH	4–4.5 mL/kg	Normal CO_2 production requires normal alveolar minute ventilation	Sharma et al.[24]
Established severe BPD	7–12 mL/kg	Greatly increased alveolar and anatomical dead space; lower respiratory rate because of long time constants needs larger V_T	Abman et al.[25]

[a]Classic CXR in MAS shows heterogeneous inflation and air trapping.

BPD, Bronchopulmonary dysplasia; *CDH,* congenital diaphragmatic hernia; *CXR,* chest radiograph; *MAS,* meconium aspiration syndrome; *RDS,* respiratory distress syndrome; V_T, tidal volume.

TABLE 22.3 Clinical Guidelines for Volume-Targeted Ventilation

Initiation of Volume-Targeted Ventilation

Recommendation	Rationale
• Implement VTV as soon as ventilation is started.	• Compliance and respiratory effort change rapidly soon after birth.
• Choose the basic mode of synchronized ventilation: PC-AC or PC-PSV is preferred.	• These ventilator modes result in more stable V_T and lower WOB.
• If using SIMV + PSV, be aware that only SIMV inflations are volume targeted.	• The PSV pressure is a set value, not subject to volume targeting.
• Select a backup rate about 10/min below spontaneous breathing rate: 30/min for term, 40/min for preterm infants.	• Backup rate is a safety net for apnea. If too low, there will be more fluctuation in $PaCO_2$ and minute ventilation; if too close to the spontaneous rate, there will be more untriggered inflations.[26]
• Select PEEP appropriate to the infant's diagnosis, current condition, and FiO_2.	• Because VG uses the lowest possible PIP, adequate PEEP is essential to maintain FRC.
• Ensure that flow sensor is calibrated and functioning properly.	• Accurate V_T measurement is essential for VTV.
• Select target expired V_T (see Table 22.2).	• V_T is now the primary control variable.
• Set PIP limit 3–5 cm H_2O above expected PIP need.	• To allow adjustment of working pressure both up and down.
• If V_T target is not met, ensure that the ET tube is in good position, then increase PIP limit if needed.	• ETT obstructed on carina would cause high PIP; ETT in the right bronchus would cause high PIP and volutrauma.
• Confirm adequacy of support by observing chest rise, auscultating breath sounds and monitoring SPO_2 and obtaining blood gas.	• Recommended V_T targets are population averages; individual patients may need higher or lower V_T.
• If converting from PC to VTV, match the V_T generated by PC mode if $PaCO_2$ was satisfactory and increase PIP limit by 3–5 cm H_2O.	• Changing primary control variable does not affect the relationship of compliance, PIP, and V_T. Allow PIP to float both up and down as needed. Average PIP will be equal to or less than on PC.

Subsequent Adjustment

• Once the range of working PIP is known, set the PIP limit 25%–30% above the upper end of the range.	• Important safety feature to alert provider to changes in support.
• Record and present on rounds range of working (measured) PIP as well as PIP limit.	• PIP limit does not accurately reflect actual level of support.
• If indicated, adjust V_T in steps of ~0.5 mL/kg.	• This step leads to meaningful change
• Base V_T adjustments on both pH and $PaCO_2$; do not lower V_T target if pH is not alkalotic and accept higher PCO_2 if pH is OK.	• pH, not $PaCO_2$, is the primary control of respiratory drive. Infants compensate for a base deficit by hyperventilating.
• Lower PIP limit as needed to keep it 25%–30% above the upper end of the range of PIP.	• This maintains the early warning benefit, alerting user to changes in PIP need.
• Assess the patient's respiratory rate, comfort, oxygen requirement, and working pressure, not just blood gas. Increase V_T if necessary to achieve adequate support.	• Tachypnea and retractions indicate increased WOB. If V_T is set below the patient's physiologic need, the ventilator lowers the PIP and the infant has to work harder to maintain his or her minute ventilation.
• Always verify appropriateness of support by clinical assessment, especially if a large increase in support appears to be needed.	• Machines are fallible. Do not blindly trust any mechanical device.
• Use birth weight initially to determine V_T target and remember to adjust for weight gain if the baby remains ventilated.	• Short-term changes in weight after birth reflect fluid shifts, but once the baby begins to grow, the V_T needs to keep up with current weight.

TABLE 22.3 Clinical Guidelines for Volume-Targeted Ventilation—cont'd

Initiation of Volume-Targeted Ventilation

Weaning

- When pH is low enough to ensure respiratory drive (<7.35), weaning is automatic; do not lower target V_T to wean, unless the patient is alkalotic.
- Withhold/reduce sedation/analgesia if used.
- Do not reduce V_T below 3.5–4 mL/kg.
- Consider raising PEEP to maintain adequate distending pressure as PIP comes down.
- Avoid using SIMV without PSV; do not wean backup rate on PC-AC or PC PSV.
- Observe the graphic display to detect excessive periodic breathing or apnea.

- Physiologic V_T need does not decrease; the PIP needed to achieve it does—self-weaning.
- Avoid suppressing the respiratory drive.
- Setting the V_T below what the infant needs imposes excessive WOB.
- Automatic lowering of PIP may lead to atelectasis if PEEP is relatively low.
- As PIP comes down, the WOB is gradually shifted from ventilator to infant. The infant controls the ventilator rate.
- Inconsistent respiratory effort may set up the infant for extubation failure.

Extubation

- Consider extubation if PIP is <12–15 cm H₂O with satisfactory blood gas.
- Older infants can be extubated from higher PIP.
- Ability to sustain adequate respiratory effort can be assessed using the SBT.
- If not given earlier, caffeine should always be used before extubation of preterm infants <32 weeks.
- Distending pressure with CPAP, NIPPV, or HHHFNC should always be used for at least 24 hours post extubation.

- These pressures are low enough to ensure that the infant is able to take over.
- Older infants can generate stronger respiratory effort.
- The SBT has its limitations, but may help predict extubation readiness (see Chapter 26).
- Caffeine reduces extubation failure in preterm infants.[27]
- The use of distending airway pressure after extubation reduces the risk of extubation failure.[28]

AC, Assist control; *CPAP*, continuous positive airway pressure; *ETT*, endotracheal tube; *FRC*, functional residual capacity; *HHHFNC*, high-humidity, high-flow nasal cannula; *NIPPV*, nasal intermittent positive pressure ventilation; *PC*, pressure controlled; *PEEP*, positive end-expiratory pressure; *PIP*, peak inflation pressure; *PSV*, pressure support ventilation; *SBT*, spontaneous breathing test; *SIMV*, synchronized intermittent mandatory ventilation; *VG*, volume guarantee; *VT*, tidal volume; *VTV*, volume-targeted ventilation; *WOB*, work of breathing.

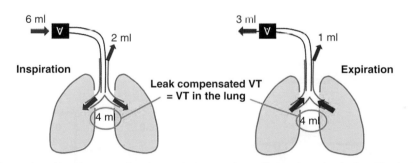

Fig. 22.7 Illustration of inspiratory and expiratory leak around uncuffed endotracheal tubes. The leak is always larger during inspiration, driven by the greater pressure gradient of peak inflation pressure. Leak also occurs during expiration, driven by the positive end-expiratory pressure. Expiratory time is typically longer than inspiratory time, allowing more time for volume loss. In this example, there is a 50% leak. Measured inspiratory V_T is 6 mL, and measured expiratory V_T is 3 mL. The actual V_T entering and exiting the patient's lungs is 4 mL. *VT*, Tidal volume.

When starting with VG as the initial mode of support, the tidal volume target should be chosen carefully, based on the infant's size and pulmonary condition (see Table 22.2). Failure to select the V_T target appropriate for the infant and failure to make subsequent adjustments based on the baby's response are the most common causes of "failure" of VTV.[33] There is now a body of literature providing normative data to guide initial V_T settings, but this information does not appear to be widely appreciated.[34] It is important to understand that the published values were based on the VG modality of VTV and may not directly apply to other devices. Moreover, these values represent population means, which, like all physiologic measurements, have substantial standard deviation, meaning that individual

patients may require larger or smaller volume. These values are a good starting point, but each patient's response to the initial settings needs to be assessed and appropriate adjustments made even before obtaining the initial blood gas measurement.

The inflation pressure limit should initially be set 3 to 5 cm H₂O above the level estimated to be sufficient to achieve that V_T. If the target V_T cannot be reached with this setting, the pressure limit may be increased modestly until the desired V_T is generated. It is important to make sure the ETT is not kinked, malpositioned in the mainstem bronchus, or obstructed on the carina, all of which can cause unexpectedly high inflation pressure. Significant volutrauma and/or air leak could result from failure to recognize single-lung intubation. If changing from PC

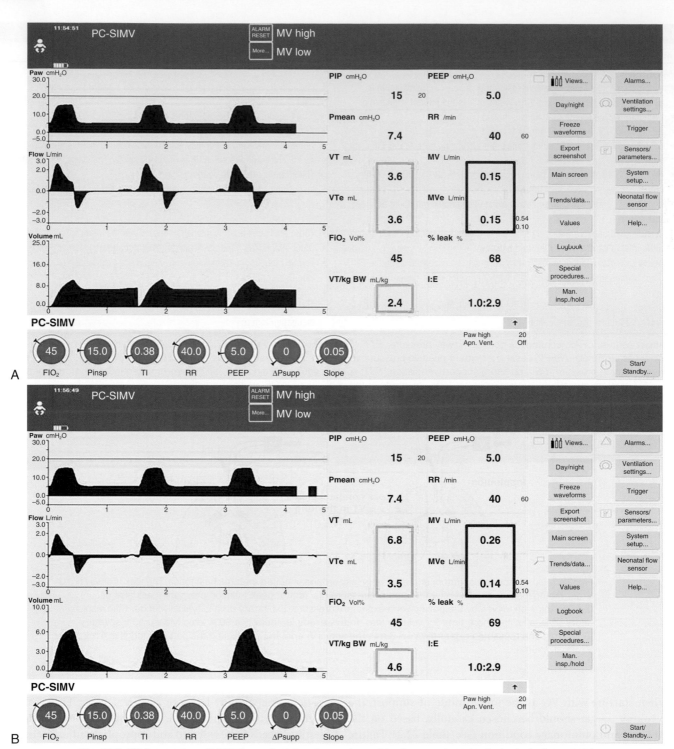

Fig. 22.8 **(A)** Screenshot of VN500 user interface in a patient with a large endotracheal tube leak. Automated Leak Compensation is **off**. The tidal volume used to adjust inflation pressure (denoted on the screen as *VT*) is the measured exhaled volume (*VTe*). Expiratory leak leads to underestimation of true V_T. Minute ventilation calculation (*MV*) is based on the measured VTe. Tidal volume per kg (*VT/kg BW*) uses VTe. Flow and volume graphics are unaltered, indicating the presence of a leak. In this example, there is a 68% leak and the measured exhaled VTe is 3.6 mL and VT/kg BW is 2.4 mL. The clinician believes that the patient is ventilated adequately with a very small V_T. **(B)** Automated leak compensation is activated. Tidal volume used to adjust inflation pressure and calculate MV is a calculated value, reflecting actual V_T reaching the lungs (denoted on the screen as *VT*). Because of the large leak, the VTe, the actual measured exhaled tidal volume, is much lower than the calculated value. VT/kg BW uses the calculated V_T. Flow and volume graphics are altered to represent the calculated V_T. With the same settings and leak magnitude as in Panel A, we see that the actual (calculated) VT is 6.8 mL, while the measured VTe, as before, is 3.5 mL. The VT/kg is 4.6 mL. The clinician knows the true V_T that is being used to ventilate the patient. In both instances, the inflation pressure and true V_T are the same. *PEEP,* Positive end-expiratory pressure; *PIP,* peak inflation pressure; *RR,* respiratory rate

in an infant whose $PaCO_2$ is in an appropriate range, it is best to match the average measured V_T of several ventilator cycles and increase pressure limit 3 to 5 cm H_2O above that used during the PC ventilation, to allow the microprocessor to adjust the working pressure up as well as down as needed. If using SIMV, be sure to use the V_T of the ventilator inflations, not the spontaneous breaths. It is advisable to keep the pressure limit 25% to 30% above the upper end of the range of current working pressure and adjusted periodically as lung compliance and the infant's breathing improves. Maintaining this relationship serves as an early warning system and a key safety feature. A persistent "low V_T" alarm indicates that there has been a change in the patient's condition or with the circuit/ETT; this should encourage a prompt evaluation of the reason for a change in respiratory system compliance, ETT position, or patient respiratory effort. Please note that with some older versions of VG, when the flow sensor is temporarily removed (such as around the time of surfactant administration or delivery of nebulized medication), if its function is affected by reflux of secretions or surfactant, the working pressure will default to the peak inflation pressure (PIP) limit. If the limit is much higher than the infant requires, a dangerously high tidal volume could be reached, and if the situation persists, hypocapnia will develop. Additionally, when the manual inflation function is used, the ventilator will use the PIP limit pressure. Therefore, it is important to keep the PIP limit sufficiently close to the working pressure to avoid volutrauma and hypocapnia. The newer Draeger VN ventilators avoid this danger by using the most recent working pressure instead of the pressure limit to continue support in the absence of a V_T signal and to deliver manual inflations. Some clinicians chose to leave the PIP limit at 40 cm H_2O, regardless of the level of working pressure. This simplifies the application of VG and minimizes alarms but defeats important safety features and inactivates the valuable early warning system. The benefits of the interactive VG system clearly outweigh the drawbacks, despite the increase in alarm frequency and some added complexity that requires more sophisticated thought process than simple PC ventilation. Use of longer alarm delay settings, appropriate pressure limit settings, avoidance of large leak around ETTs, proper positioning, and adequate physical comfort measures or sedation will minimize nuisance alarms. Please see Tables 22.2, 22.3, and 22.4 for further detail and troubleshooting tips.

Subsequent adjustments of V_T should be guided by $PaCO_2$ measurement as well as clinical observation. Increased work of breathing and tachypnea indicate a need for increased support even if the blood gas values are acceptable. Failure of the infant to breathe above the set backup rate may indicate respiratory alkalosis and a need to lower the V_T target. Other causes of prolonged apnea, such as sepsis, exhaustion, and oversedation, should be ruled out first. Several conditions indicate a need for increasing the V_T target. If the infant remains intubated for more than a few days, a modestly higher V_T is required even with permissive hypercapnia, because of increasing anatomical dead space owing to cyclic stretching of the immature upper airway by positive pressure ventilation (acquired tracheomegaly)[31] and increased alveolar dead space because of development of bronchopulmonary dysplasia, which results in more heterogeneous inflation and air-trapping.[21] The V_T target needs to be adjusted for weight gain, much as we adjust drug dosage and fluid intake. Allowing the infant to outgrow the set V_T is a common cause of respiratory deterioration and poor weight gain. Another common source of difficulty often encountered in extremely preterm infants is immature renal function that results in transient renal tubular acidosis. It is not widely appreciated that pH, not $PaCO_2$ is the primary respiratory control driver. Consequently, it is common to see inappropriate lowering of V_T target in response to a slightly low $PaCO_2$ when the pH is under 7.30 because of a substantial base deficit. In this situation, the infant's respiratory drive responding to the low pH will cause the infant to generate a spontaneous V_T greater than the set target. As described earlier, when the measured V_T is greater than target V_T, the ventilator responds by lowering the inflation pressure, sometimes all the way down to the level of PEEP (Fig. 22.9). This situation results in excessive work of breathing, decreases the mean airway pressure potentially leading to loss of lung volume, and is likely to cause fluctuations in $PaCO_2$ because the extremely preterm infant is unable to sustain this increased effort. Consequently, the infant intermittently brings down the $PaCO_2$ to normalize the pH, but when no longer able to do so, will fall back to the set V_T and backup rate, which results in rising $PaCO_2$ and falling pH. Available data suggest that hypercapnia and large fluctuations in $PaCO_2$ are a particularly high risk for severe intraventricular hemorrhage, death, and adverse neurodevelopmental outcome.[37]

During weaning, pH should be allowed to be low enough to ensure adequate respiratory drive, and if sedation is being used, it should be lightened or discontinued. V_T should normally not be weaned below 4 mL/kg to avoid shifting all the work of breathing to the infant. When V_T is set below the infant's physiologic need, the baby will spontaneously generate a tidal volume above the set value, causing the working pressure to drop all the way to PEEP with the infant essentially on a prolonged endotracheal CPAP trial and should be avoided. When the infant is able to maintain good gas exchange with low inflation pressure, extubation should be attempted.

PRESSURE-REGULATED VOLUME CONTROL

The pressure-regulated volume control (PRVC) mode on the Servo ventilators (Maquet, Solna, Sweden) is a time-cycled, pressure-limited mode that uses the V_T of the previous cycle to regulate the inflation pressure needed to achieve the desired V_T. Pressure increment is limited to 3 cm H_2O. Because pressure adjustment is based on the previous cycle, regardless of whether it was an assisted breath or an untriggered inflation, variable and/or intermittent patient respiratory effort will cause large fluctuations in tidal volume. The older Servo-i ventilator is still widely used but has now been supplanted by the Servo-n, specifically designed for newborn use, and the Servo-u, designed for both adult and neonatal use. The main limitation of the PRVC mode of the older Servo-i ventilator when used in newborn infants is the overestimation of tidal volume measured at the ventilator end of the circuit, rather than at the airway

TABLE 22.4   Troubleshooting

Problem	Possible Cause	Suggested Action

Low VT alarm—not reaching target Recurrent alarms	• Decreased compliance:
	  • Atelectasis
	  • Pneumothorax/PIE
	  • ETT in RMSB
	  • ETT obstructed on the tracheal wall or carina
	  • Abdominal distention
	  • Chest wall edema
	  • Decreased patient effort (oversedation, sepsis)
	  • Baby splinting chest and reducing delivered tidal volume
	• Increased resistance:
	  • Airway secretions
	  • Partial kinking of FTT
	  • Bronchospasm (rare)
	• PIP limit too close to working (measured) PIP
	• Alarm delay is too short
	• Large ETT leak
	• Flow sensor malfunction
	• Forced exhalation episodes
	• Interrupted exhalation
	Some infants intermittently perform expiratory braking and briefly reverse expiratory flow, thus interrupting full exhalation. The ventilator misinterprets this as a new breath and uses the exhaled volume of only the second portion of the exhalation, thus underestimating the true value of V_T.[35]
		• Evaluate breath sounds.
		• Evaluate chest rise.
		• Examine ventilator waveforms.
		• Reposition the patient and/or the ETT.
		• Assess overall condition.
		• Obtain CXR.
		• Assess the patient's level of sedation, activity.
		• Evaluate breath sounds.
		• Examine ETT, circuit.
		• Listen to the patient, examine flow waveform.
		• Observe working pressure in relation to PIP limit; the limit needs to be about 5 cm H_2O above upper end of range of working pressure to allow the ventilator to increase pressure when the baby fails to breathe.
		• Increase alarm delay for low V_T; it is not important to know a few inflations fell short of target, but we do want to know if it persists.
		• Check for ETT leak on the ventilator display. Note that when using the VN500/800 leak compensation feature, the waveforms do not visually indicate the leak, because the ventilator displays the corrected value.
		• Evaluate V_T clinically, recalibrate flow sensor as needed.
		• Recognize these by observing sudden cessation of airflow despite appropriate inflation pressure. These are preceded by a large expiratory flow and the infant is bearing down with a Valsalva maneuver. There is no effective way to abolish these short of muscle relaxation. Setting a higher PIP limit than usual mitigates their effect and achieves faster recovery.
		• Recognize these by a typical brief blip of the expiratory flow above 0 during exhalation. In most infants, these are infrequent and benign, but if more regular, may need intervention. Try increasing PEEP to obviate the need for expiratory breaking.

Ventilator is not generating any PIP	• Tubing disconnection • V_T is too low for the infant's physiologic need	• Check for leak, disconnection. • Reevaluate V_T setting. If the infant consistently generates V_T in excess of the target, the device continues to decrease PIP until it is equal to PEEP.
Ventilator is generating a low PIP, which is not increasing despite low or absent V_T	• Complete ETT obstruction. When the device senses complete ETT or circuit obstruction, the PIP drops to about half of the previous value and an alarm sounds. This is a safety feature to avoid a large overshoot of PIP once the obstruction is relieved.	• Check for ETT obstruction or kinked tubing and correct if present. ETT may be obstructed with secretions or viscous surfactant.[36]
Persistently low $PaCO_2$	• Metabolic acidosis • Agitation	• Consider pH, not just $PaCO_2$; the respiratory control center responds to pH and respiratory compensation for a base deficit is normal. • Ensure optimal positioning, comfort. Provide sedation if necessary.
Tachypnea, increased WOB	• V_T set too low • Agitation	• Insufficient support leads to tachypnea and retractions. Reassess appropriateness of V_T setting. • As earlier.

CXR, Chest x-ray; *ETT*, Endotracheal tube; *PEEP*, positive end-expiratory pressure; *PIE*, pulmonary interstitial emphysema; *PIP*, peak inflation pressure; *RMSB*, right main-stem bronchus; *VT*, tidal volume; *WOB*, work of breathing.

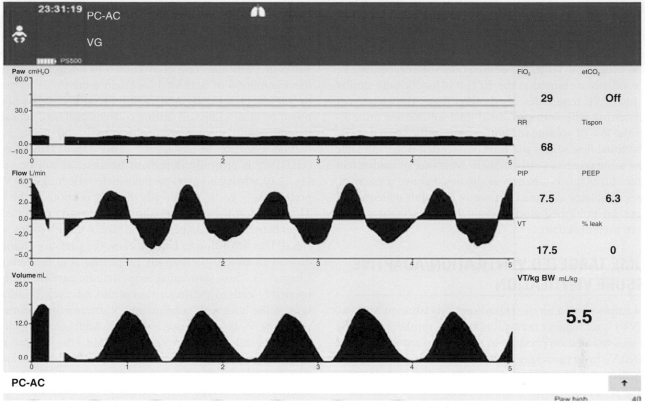

Fig. 22.9 Screenshot of the user interface showing the effect of a V_T target that is too low for this term baby with metabolic acidosis after a difficult delivery. The infant is vigorous enough to generate a strong respiratory effort and is reacting to her low pH. Note that the pressure waveform is flat, indicating that the ventilator is not generating any inflation pressure above positive end-expiratory pressure. The infant is tachypneic (respiratory rate of 68) and is generating a V_T that is larger than the set value, which for a term infant would typically be around 4 to 4.5 mL/kg.

opening. An optional flow sensor at the wye-piece allows for more accurate monitoring of tidal volume, but the servo-regulation of inflation pressure is still based on the remote flow measurement. PRVC is solely an AC mode on the Servo-i but can be either AC or SIMV with the newer Servo ventilators. Circuit compliance compensation is available to correct for compression of gas in the circuit but is ineffective when there is a leak around the ETT. The reliability of compliance compensation falls with lower infant weights and may result in wide swings of apparent V_T in tiny infants. Therefore, the compliance compensation feature is generally not used in small preterm infants. Because substantial loss of V_T to compression of gas in the circuit occurs, the set V_T must be 2 to 3 times larger than the target exhaled V_T at the airway opening. The manufacturer has corrected these major issues in the newer Servo-n and Servo-u models, which now can use the optional Wye-piece sensor to measure V_T at the airway opening and to regulate inflation pressure. Therefore, the V_T targets used with these devices and general ventilation procedures should be similar to those specified earlier for VG when the optional Wye sensor is used.

When initiating PRVC with the older Servo-i, several methods may be used for setting the target V_T. If a proximal (Wye-piece) flow sensor is available, it should be used to measure directly the exhaled V_T and adjust the set value (V_{del}) to achieve an exhaled V_T of approximately 5 mL/kg, with the same caveats for matching target V_T to the specific condition as outlined for VG. If the infant is being switched from a pressure-limited mode, a common approach is to set the target volume either (1) to match the volumes (V_{del}) generated by PC ventilation or (2) to generate inflation pressures similar to those being used in PC ventilation. If the infant is being started directly on PRVC without the optional Wye-piece flow sensor, the operator must rely on clinical assessment of chest rise and breath sounds to determine the appropriate V_{del}, keeping in mind that a substantial portion of the V_T will be lost in the circuit. Clinical assessment of the adequacy of support should supplement blood gas analysis. Similar to other VTV modalities, the pressure needed to achieve the target V_T comes down automatically as lung compliance and patient effort improve. The target V_T should not be reduced below 4 mL/kg exhaled volume at the airway opening for the same reasons as described in the previous section on VG. A randomized clinical trial of PRVC on the Servo 300 ventilator compared to pressure-limited SIMV in VLBW infants failed to show any advantage of PRVC.[38]

VOLUME VENTILATION PLUS

Volume Ventilation Plus (Puritan Bennett 840, Covidien, Mansfield, MA) is a complex mode that combines two different dual mode volume-targeted inflation types—Volume Control Plus (VC+) for delivery of mandatory inflations in A/C and SIMV and Volume Support (VS) for support of spontaneous breaths in the spontaneous ventilation mode. The ventilator adjusts inflation pressure to target the desired tidal volume. Because V_T is not routinely measured at the ETT, it is functionally similar to VC and PRVC modes described earlier. Thus, the selection of volume setting reflects the proximal tidal volume and must allow for the loss of volume to compression in the ventilator circuit. Proximal flow sensor use is recommended where available with the same targets as earlier. Again avoidance of inadvertent mainstem bronchus intubation as discussed above is essential. This is a ventilator designed primarily for adult patients and there are no published studies evaluating its clinical performance in preterm infants.

VOLUME TARGETED VENTILATION/ADAPTIVE PRESSURE VENTILATION

VTV as implemented on the Hamilton G5 (Hamilton Medical, Reno, NV) is a modality that is functionally similar to VG. The device adjusts inflation pressure in response to any deviation of measured V_T from the target value. This is a relatively new modality with no published literature on its safety and effectiveness, but it appears to have similar functionality to standard VG, and therefore, similar guidelines should be applied to its use. On the newer Hamilton C1 neo, this mode is referred to as adaptive pressure ventilation, but it appears to be essentially the same concept of inflation pressure modulation based on exhaled VT using a flow sensor at the airway opening.

TARGETED TIDAL VOLUME

Targeted tidal volume (TTV) was a modality on the SLE 4000 and 5000 neonatal ventilators (Specialised Laboratory Equipment Ltd., South Croydon, UK). These devices are not available in the United States but are widely used outside of North America. The original volume-targeted mode on the SLE 4000 was called TTV and was, in essence, a modified volume limit function. The device increased the rise time of the pressure waveform to improve the chance of effectively limiting V_T to the desired target. To avoid the risk of excessive PIP when the TTV function is turned off, the PIP automatically dropped to 5 mbar above the set PEEP and the user had to actively adjust the PIP. Reliance on inspiratory V_T measurement had the potential to lead to inadequate V_T delivery with significant leak around the ETT. The newer SLE 5000 ventilator came with an enhancement referred to as TTV plus, which made the modality function more like VG by using exhaled tidal volume measurement and actively modulating inflation pressure to target the desired V_T. A leak compensation feature has also been added. The new SLE 6000 has abandoned the terminology of TTV and now uses the term "volume-targeted ventilation." This newest iteration appears to closely mimic the basic VG approach, and therefore, the device function should be consistent with the guidelines presented in this chapter.

IMPORTANCE OF OPEN LUNG STRATEGY

The benefits of VTV cannot be fully realized unless we ensure that the V_T is evenly distributed into an "open lung." Although adequate PEEP has long been known to mitigate lung injury, the admonition of Burkhard Lachman more than 25 years ago to "OPEN THE LUNG AND KEEP IT OPEN!"[39] has been ignored by many clinicians during conventional mechanical ventilation despite a sound physiologic basis and strong experimental evidence in its favor.[40] This Open Lung Concept (OLC)[41-43] is critically important because, as can be seen in Fig 22.10, when gas enters partially atelectatic lungs, the V_T will preferentially go to the already aerated portion of the lungs. This is because the pressure required to expand the aerated lung is less than the critical opening pressure of the atelectatic alveoli (recall that according to Laplace's law, the pressure required to distend an alveolus is inversely proportional to the radius; see Chapter 2). Thus, ventilating lungs that are partially atelectatic inevitably leads to overexpansion of this relatively healthy portion of the lung with subsequent volutrauma/biotrauma even when the V_T is in the normal range. Additionally, atelectasis leads to exudation of protein-rich fluid (the hyaline membranes seen histologically) with increased surfactant inactivation and release of inflammatory mediators. Shear forces and uneven stress in areas where atelectasis and overinflation coexist add to the damage.

Consequently the open lung approach, which ensures that the V_T is distributed evenly throughout the lungs, is a fundamental component of any lung-protective ventilation strategy (see also Chapter 21 for a full discussion of lung-protective ventilation concepts).

ALARMS/TROUBLESHOOTING

VTV modes generate alarms not encountered with simple PC ventilation; these become annoying when they are excessive. The alarms are designed to provide feedback as to whether the patient is receiving the desired level of ventilator support. Significant fall in lung compliance, decreased spontaneous respiratory effort, impending accidental extubation, and forced exhalation episodes will all generate "low tidal volume" alarms. When properly used, this information should improve care in the most vulnerable infants. It is important to evaluate the cause of the alarms and correct any correctable problems. Large leak results in underestimation of delivered V_T and triggers the low V_T alarm when the device is unable to reach the target V_T at the set PIP limit. With the older Babylog 8000+ and other devices with VG modes that lack effective leak compensation, when the leak exceeds 40% to 50%, the VG mode no longer functions reliably because of inability to accurately measure V_T. This is much less of a problem with the newer VN series ventilators, which can compensate for leak of up to 75%. The alarms serve an important function and should not be ignored. If the low tidal volume alarm sounds repeatedly in the absence of excessive leak, increase the pressure limit AND INVESTIGATE THE CAUSE. Please see Table 22.4 for troubleshooting advice.

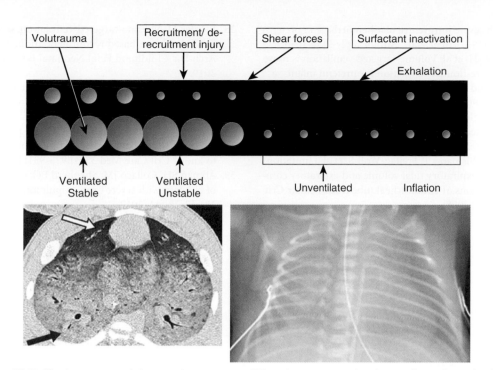

Fig. 22.10 The importance of the open lung concept. Although anteroposterior chest radiographs make the lungs of an infant with respiratory distress syndrome appear homogeneous (*right lower panel*), this is an artifact of a two-dimensional view of a three-dimensional structure. Atelectasis has a gravity-dependent distribution as illustrated on the computer tomography view in the *lower left panel*. This situation is diagrammatically represented in the *middle panel*. Ventilating lungs in the presence of extensive atelectasis result in atelectrauma. Surfactant inactivation in the atelectatic portion, shear forces at the boundary between the aerated and the unaerated lung, and damage from repeated collapse and opening of unstable alveoli all contribute to lung injury. Perhaps most importantly, the gas expanding partially atelectatic lungs will preferentially enter the already aerated portion of the lung (*white arrow*), which requires less distending pressure than the critical opening pressure of the atelectatic lungs, indicated by the *heavy black arrow* (Laplace's law; see Chapter 2). Therefore, even a normal, physiologic tidal volume entering the small proportion of open alveoli will inevitably lead to overexpansion and volutrauma.

Unnecessary alarms can be avoided by optimizing settings and alarm limits.

Use of longer alarm delay settings, appropriate pressure limit settings, avoidance of large leak around ETTs, and adequate physical comfort measures or sedation will minimize alarms.

CONCLUSION

There is now strong evidence in support of using tidal volume as the primary control variable for mechanical ventilation of newborn infants. VTV has been shown to improve a variety of important clinical outcomes, yet its penetration into clinical practice has been surprisingly slow in most parts of the world, with Canada, Australia, Scandinavia, and Italy being the exceptions. It appears that many clinicians are still unwilling to abandon their comfort zone and embrace the paradigm shift that VTV represents.[44] Availability of equipment is no longer a barrier to acceptance, at least in reasonably well-resourced parts of the world. Some form of VTV is now available on virtually all ventilators used in neonatal intensive care and the newest devices designed specifically for newborn infants now perform very well even in very small infants. However, it is important to

point out that each ventilator functions differently. It is critical that the user becomes familiar with the specific features and limitations of their particular device. The reader is referred to Chapter 27 of this book and to user manuals of their respective devices for further guidance. A ventilator is only a tool in the hands of the clinician, a tool that can be used well, or not. It is probably time to abandon the term "ventilator-induced lung injury" in favor of "physician-induced lung injury" as it is we who select the ventilator settings!

KEY REFERENCES

1. Dreyfuss D, Soler P, Basset G, et al: High inflation pressure pulmonary edema. Respective effects of high airway pressure, high tidal volume, and positive end-expiratory pressure. Am Rev Respir Dis 137(5):1159-1164, 1988.
6. Fabres J, Carlo WA, Phillips V, et al: Both extremes of arterial carbon dioxide pressure and the magnitude of fluctuations in arterial carbon dioxide pressure are associated with severe intraventricular hemorrhage in preterm infants. Pediatrics 119(2):299 305, 2007.
8. Kaiser JR: Both extremes of arterial carbon dioxide pressure and the magnitude of fluctuations in arterial carbon dioxide pressure

are associated with severe intraventricular hemorrhage in preterm infants. Pediatrics 119(5):1039, 2007. Author reply 1039-1040.

10. Peng W, Zhu H, Shi H, et al: Volume-targeted ventilation is more suitable than pressure-limited ventilation for preterm infants: a systematic review and meta-analysis. Arch Dis Childhood Fetal Neonatal Edi 2014;99(2):F158-F165.

11. Klingenberg C, Wheeler KI, McCallion N, et al: Volume-targeted versus pressure-limited ventilation in neonates. Cochrane Database Syst Rev 10:CD003666, 2017.

22. Herber-Jonat S, von Bismarck P, Freitag-Wolf S, et al: Limitation of measurements of expiratory tidal volume and expiratory compliance under conditions of endotracheal tube leaks. Pediatr Crit Care Med 9(1):69-75, 2008.

25. Keszler M: Volume-targeted ventilation: one size does not fit all. Evidence-based recommendations for successful use. Arch Dis Childhood Fetal Neonatal Ed 104(1):F108-F112, 2019.

30. Tsuchida S, Engelberts D, Peltekova V, et al: Atelectasis causes alveolar injury in nonatelectatic lung regions. Am J Respir Crit Care Med 174(3):279-289, 2006.

33. van Kaam AH, Rimensberger PC: Lung-protective ventilation strategies in neonatology: what do we know—what do we need to know? Crit Care Med 35(3):925-931, 2007.

39. Abman SH, Collaco JM, Shepherd EG, et al: Interdisciplinary care of children with severe bronchopulmonary dysplasia. J Pediatr 181:12-28 e11, 2017.

23

Special Techniques of Respiratory Support

Nelson Claure and Eduardo Bancalari

KEY POINTS

- In premature infants, arterial oxygen saturation (SpO$_2$) is not consistently maintained within the targeted range by manual adjustment of the fraction of inspired oxygen during routine clinical care.
- Automated fraction of inspired oxygen (FiO$_2$) control can improve SpO$_2$ targeting and reduce exposure to hyperoxemia, supplemental oxygen, and episodes of severe hypoxemia. The impact of extended clinical use of this technology on neonatal outcomes is still to be determined.
- Proportional assist ventilation can maintain comparable ventilation with lower pressures compared with conventional pressure-controlled modes. Further studies are needed to determine if longer-term use of this modality can improve respiratory outcome.
- Neurally adjusted ventilatory assist is effective in synchronizing the positive pressure with the infant's spontaneous inspiration and can maintain ventilation with lower pressures compared with pressure-controlled ventilation. Its impact on short- and long-term respiratory outcomes in premature infants still needs to be investigated.
- Modalities of targeted minute ventilation conduct automatic adjustments to the ventilator rate to maintain a more stable ventilation. Feasibility studies have shown that they can provide comparable gas exchange with less ventilatory support than conventional modalities. Data on neonatal outcomes are not yet available.

INTRODUCTION

The care of premature infants with respiratory failure has advanced considerably over the past decades, but a substantial proportion of very premature infants survive with some degree of respiratory, visual, and neurodevelopmental impairment. There is increasing evidence that many of these complications can be related to the use of respiratory support. This reality highlights the need for further improvement in the strategies of respiratory support used in this population. New techniques to provide respiratory support and supplemental oxygen to the premature infant have become available, but their use is not yet widespread and there is limited information on their benefits or limitations. This chapter describes some of these modalities and discusses the rationale and the evidence for the advantages and possible limitations. Standard modes of respiratory support are discussed in other chapters of this book.

AUTOMATED CONTROL OF INSPIRED OXYGEN

Most premature infants require supplemental oxygen to maintain arterial oxygen saturation (SpO$_2$) within the prescribed target range. However, it is well documented that in routine clinical care, manual adjustment of the fraction of inspired oxygen (FiO$_2$) commonly fails to keep SpO$_2$ within range. It has been reported that premature infants spend nearly a third of the time with SpO$_2$ levels above the target range because of excessive FiO$_2$.[1,2] The resulting hyperoxemia increases the risk of damage to the eye, brain, and other organs, whereas exposure to higher-than-necessary FiO$_2$ can result in oxidant damage to the lungs.[3-8] The same report showed that premature infants spend nearly a fifth of the time with SpO$_2$ below the target range.[1] This is attributed to episodes of intermittent hypoxemia that occur frequently in premature infants because of their respiratory instability. The frequency of these episodes increases with postnatal age, especially in infants with chronic lung disease.[9-12] Most episodes of hypoxemia are spontaneous,[13-15] but some are related to care procedures. The prompt response of the clinical staff can reduce the duration and severity of hypoxemia episodes. However, staff availability to perform this task is often limited. The impact of staff availability on the maintenance of SpO$_2$ within target was documented by a decline in the proportion of time with SpO$_2$ within range as the nurse-to-infant ratio decreased.[16] This was mainly because of an increased time in hyperoxemia. Also, FiO$_2$ is increased during the episodes, but the resolution of hypoxemia is not always followed by a prompt return of FiO$_2$ to baseline, which results in hyperoxemia.[17] Because episodes of hypoxemia are in part related to the basal level of SpO$_2$,[18-20] higher SpO$_2$ levels are often tolerated in an attempt to prevent their occurrence, but this practice can lead to increased exposure to hyperoxemia.[17]

These problems explain why consistent maintenance of SpO$_2$ within the prescribed target range is seldom achieved in premature infants receiving supplemental oxygen. In an attempt to solve this problem, different systems for automated closed-loop control of FiO$_2$ have been developed to assist caregivers in the maintenance of SpO$_2$ within the prescribed target range and reduce exposure to hyperoxemia and hypoxemia. These systems continuously adjust FiO$_2$, aiming at keeping SpO$_2$ within a target range set by the clinician. Fig. 23.1 shows representative recordings of SpO$_2$ and FiO$_2$ from a premature infant with frequent episodes of hypoxemia during automated FiO$_2$ control showing minimal need for manual adjustment of FiO$_2$.

Short-term clinical studies have shown that automated FiO$_2$ control systems are more effective in keeping SpO$_2$ within the target range than manual control during routine care and equal to or better than a fully dedicated nurse.[21-36] The relative efficacy of automated systems compared with conventional manual adjustment obtained in these clinical studies is shown in Table 23.1. Automated FiO$_2$ control also produced a consistent reduction in the proportion of time with SpO$_2$ above the target range compared with manual control. The proportion of time with SpO$_2$ below target was not consistently reduced by automated compared with manual FiO$_2$ control. Studies in infants with frequent hypoxemia episodes showed more episodes

of mild hypoxemia during automated control. This was likely as a result of the fact that during routine manual FiO$_2$ control, infants were kept at a higher basal SpO$_2$. These studies showed a consistent reduction in the number of more severe and prolonged episodes of hypoxemia during automated FiO$_2$ control. This is important in light of reports of significant neurodevelopmental and eye damage related to prolonged hypoxemia episodes.[37,38] These findings illustrate the fact that automated FiO$_2$ control systems do not prevent hypoxemia episodes, but their faster response can attenuate their duration and severity.

The number of manual changes in FiO$_2$ was minimal during automatic FiO$_2$ control. This suggests potential savings in staff workload and the possibility of shifting the staff effort to other areas of clinical care. SpO$_2$ alarms are among the most common events in the neonatal intensive care unit. Although not yet examined, systems for automatic FiO$_2$ control may reduce SpO$_2$ alarm fatigue during extended use. On the other hand, reduced staff attentiveness is a potential unintended consequence of automated FiO$_2$ control. An automatic increase in FiO$_2$ can mask a respiratory deterioration that would otherwise manifest as a persistently lower SpO$_2$. Hence, it is essential that automated FiO$_2$ control systems alert the clinician when there is a persistent need for a higher FiO$_2$.

Significant discrepancies can exist between the target and the actual range of SpO$_2$ during routine care. Caution is recommended when setting the range of SpO$_2$ to be targeted by automatic systems because there may be important clinical implications that become evident when SpO$_2$ is kept more consistently within such range. This is particularly important because the optimal range of SpO$_2$ for this population has not been clearly established.

In summary, short-term clinical studies showed that automated FiO$_2$ control can improve SpO$_2$ targeting and reduce exposure to hyperoxemia, supplemental oxygen, and episodes of severe hypoxemia. Whether extended clinical use of this technology can have an impact on long-term visual, respiratory, and neurodevelopmental outcomes in premature infants is still to be determined.[39]

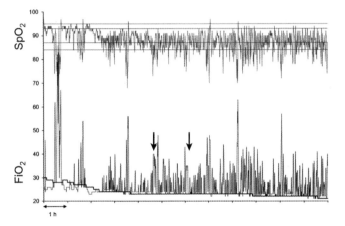

Fig. 23.1 The graph shows frequent automated fraction of inspired oxygen (*FiO$_2$*) adjustments to keep oxygen saturation (*SpO$_2$*) within the target range (*light gray horizontal lines*) in an infant with frequent hypoxemia spells. Automated adjustments reduced periods with SpO$_2$ above the target range and achieved a consistent reduction of the baseline FiO$_2$ level. Arrows show infrequent manual adjustments during 12 hours. The thicker line under FiO$_2$ shows the decreasing basal FiO$_2$ level.

TABLE 23.1	Maintenance of Oxygen Saturation Target Ranges During Manual and Closed-Loop Inspired Oxygen Control		
		% TIME WITHIN TARGET RANGE	
	Oxygen Saturation (SpO$_2$) Target Range	**Manual Fraction of Inspired Oxygen (FiO$_2$) Control**	**Closed-Loop FiO$_2$ Control**
Bhutani, 1992	94%–96%	54	81
Morozoff, 1993	90%–95%	39	50
Claure, 2001	88%–96%	66	75
Urschitz, 2004	87%–96%	82	91
Claure, 2009	88%–95%	42	58
Morozoff, 2009	90%–96%	57	73
Claure, 2011	87%–93%[a]	39	47
Waitz, 2014	88%–96%	69	76
Hallenberger, 2014	Four centers (90%–95%, 80%-92%, 83%–93%, 85%–94%)	61	72
Zapata, 2014	85%–93%	34	58
Lal, 2015	90%–95%	60	69
Van Kaam, 2015	89%–93%[a]	54	62
	91%–95%	58	62

[a]Includes periods with SpO$_2$ > target range while FiO$_2$ = 0.21.

VENTILATION TECHNIQUES THAT PROVIDE SUPPORT PROPORTIONAL TO PATIENT EFFORT

Proportional Assist Ventilation

The underlying lung disease can affect differently the mechanical properties of the infant's respiratory system. Restrictive conditions such as respiratory distress syndrome (RDS) decrease lung compliance that imposes an increased elastic load on the infant's respiratory pump. Obstructive conditions increase airway resistance and impose resistive loads. These respiratory loads lead to an increased breathing effort that is necessary to sustain ventilation. When the effort is insufficient, the patient develops hypoventilation and respiratory failure.

Proportional assist ventilation (PAV) is a modality in which the pressure generated by the ventilator increases in proportion to the volume, flow, or both, generated by the infant's inspiratory effort. The proportional gain by which the positive pressure increases in relation to the measured tidal volume (V_T) or flow is the elastic gain (volume proportional, in units of pressure per milliliter of measured volume) or resistive gain (flow proportional, in units of pressure per unit of measured flow). The simultaneous increase in ventilator pressure augments the infant's spontaneous inspiratory effort to achieve the required V_T. The proportional increase in ventilator pressure to the infant's spontaneous effort is illustrated in Fig. 23.2.

Studies in infants recovering from RDS showed that PAV produced similar ventilation with lower ventilator pressures compared with pressure-controlled modalities such as assist-control (AC) and synchronized intermittent mandatory ventilation (SIMV).[40-42] In premature infants with evolving chronic lung disease, PAV improved oxygenation compared with pressure controlled AC.[43]

During PAV, the elastic and resistive gains should be set to produce enough unloading to compensate for the disease-induced respiratory loads. An elastic gain that exceeds what is needed to compensate for the decrease in lung compliance can result in an excessive increase in pressure. A resistive gain that exceeds what is needed to overcome the increased airway resistance can induce rapid oscillations in pressure. To minimize the risk of overinflation, the peak pressure and V_T limits must be set appropriately by the clinician. It must be recognized that the underlying assumption of PAV is that the patient's respiratory drive is appropriate, and the device is simply overcoming disease-induced mechanical loads. When applied to premature infants with immature respiratory control, there is a potential for hypoventilation attributed to central apnea unless a backup rate is provided.

A clear understanding of the theory behind unloading by PAV is essential when setting the elastic or resistive gains. As compliance changes, the elastic gain must be adjusted accordingly to avoid excessive V_T and possible volutrauma when the infant becomes agitated and generates excessively large V_T, for example, with handling.

In summary, published data indicate that PAV is effective in the short term in maintaining comparable ventilation with lower pressures compared with conventional pressure-controlled modes. Further studies are needed to determine if longer-term use of this strategy can be advantageous in reducing the need for ventilatory support and improving respiratory outcome. The complexity of this modality and limited availability appear to have limited its penetration into clinical practice. As of this writing, this mode of support is unique to the Stephanie ventilator (F. Stephan GmbH Medizintechnik, Gackenbach, Germany).

Neurally Adjusted Ventilatory Assist

Neurally adjusted ventilatory assist (NAVA) is a novel modality in which the ventilator pressure is adjusted in proportion to the electrical activity of the diaphragm measured by esophageal electrodes mounted on a feeding tube. The ventilator pressure during NAVA increases in proportion to the diaphragmatic activity with a proportionality factor or gain that is set by

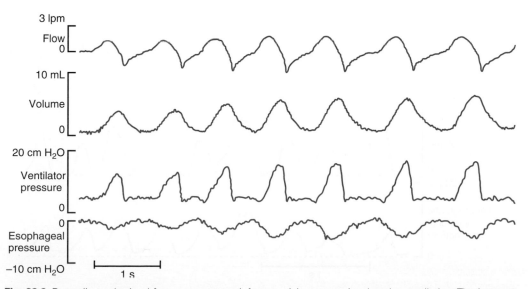

Fig. 23.2 Recordings obtained from a premature infant receiving proportional assist ventilation. The increase in positive pressure is proportional to the spontaneous inspiratory effort of the infant measured by esophageal manometry. The increase in inspiratory effort and positive pressure results in a larger tidal volume.

the clinician (in units of pressure per microvolt of electrical activity), known as the "NAVA level." When the ventilator pressure is increased simultaneously with and proportionally to the rise in the diaphragm's electrical activity, NAVA can enhance the diaphragm's ability to generate a larger V_T or maintain a similar V_T with less inspiratory effort. The increase in the ventilator pressure in proportion to the magnitude of the diaphragmatic activity is illustrated in Fig. 23.3.

Studies in premature infants have shown that NAVA is effective in synchronizing the positive pressure with the infant's spontaneous inspiration. These studies showed that NAVA maintained ventilation and gas exchange with lower airway pressures compared with pressure-controlled ventilation.[44-47] The effects of NAVA on breathing effort and ventilator pressure were relative to the specific settings of pressure or target volume used in the conventional modality. NAVA reduced diaphragmatic activity compared with pressure-controlled ventilation and provided similar V_T with smaller peak pressures.[45,46] In contrast, the activity of the diaphragm was higher during NAVA in comparison with volume-targeted ventilation, but peak airway pressure and V_T were lower.[47] In a more recent randomized trial including preterm infants with RDS, NAVA achieved comparable weaning rates from the ventilator to pressure controlled modes.[48]

Management of NAVA differs from conventional modalities because in NAVA, the support is adjusted by setting the NAVA gain. There are no normative or reference values for diaphragmatic activity in preterm infants and it cannot be assessed as an absolute value. Although it appears to be safe, little has been reported on the effects of different NAVA gains in premature infants.[49] Also, little is known about the interaction of NAVA with the infant's immature respiratory control that typically manifests as irregular and highly variable respiratory effort. Similar to PAV, the positive feedback approach that NAVA employs has the potential to result in the delivery of large V_T. Therefore, pressure and volume limits must be set at appropriate levels by the clinician. A backup mechanical support is needed to deal with periods of apnea.

NAVA is an interesting modality of respiratory support, but its impact on short- and long-term respiratory outcomes in premature infants needs to be explored further before recommending its routine use. As of this writing, this modality is available only on the Maquet Servo ventilator.

Airway Pressure Release Ventilation

Airway pressure release ventilation (APRV) is a modality used primarily in adults with acute respiratory failure as an alternative method to improve oxygenation.[50] APRV is a modality whereby a continuous high positive pressure is applied at the airway with an intermittent release phase. In APRV, the higher level positive pressure (P_{high}) is used to maintain lung volume and alveolar recruitment, and the brief release phase is expected to produce some ventilation. However, the bulk of minute ventilation must come from spontaneous respiratory effort of the patient during the application of P_{high}. This alternating pattern of low and high pressure can be thought of as extreme inspiratory to expiratory inverse ratio ventilation. It also bears some similarity to the various forms of bilevel continuous positive airway pressure (BiPAP), because of its reliance on spontaneous breathing activity. APRV is usually used as a rescue technique, and unlike BiPAP, the upper pressure level

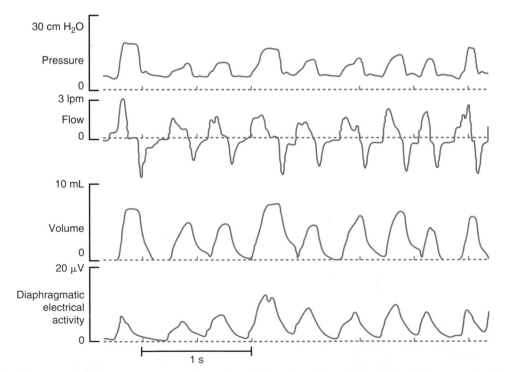

Fig. 23.3 Representative recording of a premature infant receiving neurally adjusted ventilatory assist. The increase in the ventilator pressure above positive end-expiratory pressure is proportional to the amplitude of the electrical activity of the diaphragm.

P_{high} is maintained for the majority of the respiratory cycle (T_{high}). The pressure to which the lungs are released is called P_{low}, and the release time is called T_{low}. The technique has primarily been used in adult patients with acute lung injury, in whom there may be some short-term benefits in terms of oxygenation. No clear survival advantage or reduction in complications has been demonstrated. A recent randomized trial in pediatric patients was terminated early because of increased mortality in the APRV arm.[51,52] There is insufficient evidence to assess the utility of this technique in newborn infants, with only a handful of case reports available and no controlled trials.

VENTILATION TECHNIQUES DESIGNED TO MAINTAIN MINUTE VENTILATION

Targeted Minute Ventilation

Standard modes of mechanical ventilation provide a relatively constant level of ventilatory support determined by the peak inflation pressure and ventilator rate. The level of support set by the clinician is adequate in most instances, but in infants who have fluctuations in spontaneous ventilation due to a weak respiratory pump, immature respiratory drive, or unstable respiratory mechanics, the ventilatory support is often insufficient, whereas at other times, it can be excessive. The rationale for targeted minute ventilation (TMV) is that the automatic adjustments to the ventilator rate will maintain a more stable ventilation and gas exchange and reduce the possibility of excessive ventilatory support. Modalities of TMV are based on automatic adjustments to the mandatory rate to maintain minute ventilation at or above a minimal level. When spontaneous breathing is enough to maintain minute ventilation above such level, the ventilator rate is reduced, or vice versa. Continuous adjustments to the ventilator rate during TMV are shown in Fig. 23.4.

In preterm infants recovering from RDS, TMV achieved a 50% reduction in the SIMV rate without affecting gas exchange compared with conventional SIMV.[53] This study showed that although premature infants can sustain their ventilation for significant periods of time, they frequently have periods when they need much higher ventilator rates. In a subgroup of infants with frequent spontaneous episodes of hypoxemia, TMV attenuated the hypoxemia episodes compared with SIMV. It should be noted that this technique is specifically applicable to the SIMV mode and has been compared only with SIMV. It is not known whether this approach is superior to other modes of synchronized ventilation, such as AC and pressure support ventilation as implemented on neonatal ventilators (modes that assist every spontaneous breath), or SIMV with pressure support.

Mandatory Minute Ventilation

Mandatory minute ventilation (MMV) is a modality of TMV used in the adult that has been adapted for neonates. In MMV, the minute ventilation target is maintained by the product of a constant ventilator rate of volume-targeted ventilator breaths. When minute ventilation exceeds the target level, the ventilator rate stops. MMV is generally used in combination with pressure support to assist every spontaneous breath. In late preterm infants without lung disease, MMV achieved a reduction in the mandatory rate and mean airway pressure compared with SIMV without alterations in gas exchange.[54]

Apnea Backup Ventilation

Apnea backup ventilation is a modality available in most neonatal ventilators. Spontaneous breaths are usually assisted by pressure support, but in the presence of apnea, the ventilator initiates a preset mandatory rate of mechanical inflations. Although it is available in most neonatal ventilators, its clinical benefits or disadvantages have not been evaluated.

Adaptive Backup Ventilation

Adaptive backup ventilation is a modality whereby a mandatory rate is provided during periods of apnea or during episodes of reduced SpO_2. In preterm infants recovering from RDS, this modality attenuated the frequency and severity of episodes of hypoxemia compared with the backup mandatory rate for apnea alone.[55]

The findings from short-term clinical studies evaluating various modalities of TMV showed that these modalities can better match the mechanical support to the varying ventilatory

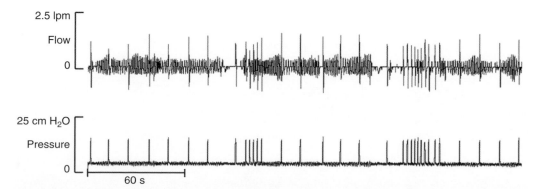

Fig. 23.4 Recordings of flow and pressure from a premature infant undergoing targeted minute ventilation. The ventilator rate is automatically reduced during periods of consistent spontaneous breathing (darker areas in flow waveform), and it is increased when spontaneous breathing decreases. (From Claure N, Bancalari E. Automated respiratory support in newborn infants. Semin Fetal Neonatal Med. 2009 Feb;14(1):35-41. doi: 10.1016/j.siny.2008.08.008. Epub 2008 Oct 1. PMID: 18829405.)

needs of premature infants. Whileed to these findings are promising, the benefits and possible shortcomings of these modalities need to be assessed in longer-term clinical trials.

Adaptive Support Ventilation

Adaptive support ventilation (ASV) is an automatic modality of ventilation used in pediatric and adult patients.[56] ASV provides a combination of adjustments to respiratory rate and V_T. For this, the ASV algorithm determines the respiratory rate based on the patient's dead space volume, desired minute ventilation, and respiratory time constant. V_T is calculated by dividing minute ventilation by the respiratory rate. The clinician can adjust the target minute ventilation depending on the patient's condition. Thereafter, ASV adjusts the ventilator peak pressure to maintain the target V_T. The set respiratory rate, V_T, and respiratory mechanics are reassessed on a breath-to-breath basis. In periods during which the spontaneous breathing rate decreases, mandatory inflations are provided to maintain the desired rate.

By adapting the respiratory rate depending on the dead space, respiratory mechanics, and consistency of the respiratory drive, ASV aims to maintain adequate minute ventilation and facilitate weaning. ASV represents a novel and sophisticated approach to the management of ventilatory support in pediatric and adult patients, but at this time there are no reports on its use in neonates.

CONCLUSION

Many of the novel respiratory support techniques discussed in this chapter are promising and address some of the limitations in conventional mechanical ventilation or oxygen administration. Although most of these novel techniques are available or may become available for clinical use in the near future, additional evidence for their safety and benefits in premature infants is necessary before they gain wider clinical application.

KEY REFERENCES

1. Hagadorn JI, Furey AM, Nghiem TH, et al: Achieved versus intended pulse oximeter saturation in infants born less than 28 weeks' gestation: the AVIOx study. Pediatrics 118(4): 1574–1582, 2006.
25. Claure N, D'Ugard C, Bancalari E: Automated adjustment of inspired oxygen in preterm infants with frequent fluctuations in oxygenation: a pilot clinical trial. J Pediatr 155(5):640–645 e1–e2, 2009.
27. Claure N, Bancalari E, D'Ugard C, et al: Multicenter crossover study of automated control of inspired oxygen in ventilated preterm infants. Pediatrics 127(1):e76–e83, 2011.
31. van Kaam AH, Hummler HD, Wilinska M, et al: Automated versus manual oxygen control with different saturation targets and modes of respiratory support in preterm infants. J Pediatr 167(3):545–550, e1–e2, 2015.
37. Di Fiore JM, Kaffashi F, Loparo K, et al: The relationship between patterns of intermittent hypoxia and retinopathy of prematurity in preterm infants. Pediatr Res 72(6):606–612, 2012.
38. Poets CF, Roberts RS, Schmidt B, et al: Association between intermittent hypoxemia or bradycardia and late death or disability in extremely preterm infants. JAMA 314(6): 595–603, 2015.
40. Schulze A, Gerhardt T, Musante G, et al: Proportional assist ventilation in low birth weight infants with acute respiratory disease: a comparison to assist/control and conventional mechanical ventilation. J Pediatr 135(3):339–344, 1999.
41. Schulze A, Rieger-Fackeldey E, Gerhardt T, et al: Randomized crossover comparison of proportional assist ventilation and patient-triggered ventilation in extremely low birth weight infants with evolving chronic lung disease. Neonatology 92(1):1–7, 2007.
44. Beck J, Reilly M, Grasselli G, et al: Patient-ventilator interaction during neurally adjusted ventilatory assist in low birth weight infants. Pediatr Res 65(6):663–668, 2009.
53. Claure N, Gerhardt T, Hummler H, et al: Computer-controlled minute ventilation in preterm infants undergoing mechanical ventilation. J Pediatr 131(6):910–913, 1997.

24

High-Frequency Ventilation

Martin Keszler, J. Jane Pillow, and Sherry E. Courtney

First described in the 1970s, high-frequency ventilation (HFV) is a form of mechanical ventilation that uses small tidal volumes (sometimes less than anatomic dead space) and very rapid ventilator rates (2.5 to 20 Hz or 150 to 1200 cycles per minute). Potential advantages of this technique over conventional mechanical ventilation (CMV) include the use of lower peak alveolar pressures, the ability to manage oxygenation and ventilation relatively independently in the recruited lung while using very small tidal volumes (V_T), and the preservation of normal lung architecture even when using high mean airway pressures (MAPs).[1-5] The ability of HFV to sufficiently oxygenate and ventilate the fragile preterm lung with peak alveolar pressures that are lower than those used with CMV, the relative ease of achieving alveolar recruitment and improving distribution of medications such as inhaled nitric oxide (iNO), makes HFV a crucial constituent of neonatal respiratory therapy. In this chapter, current HFV techniques and technology are described, and their application in the newborn with pulmonary dysfunction is discussed.

Currently, two types of HFV are commonly used: high-frequency oscillatory ventilation (HFOV), which is produced by a device that moves gas back and forth at the airway opening, resulting in limited bulk gas flow; and high-frequency jet ventilation (HFJV), which is produced by ventilators that deliver a high-velocity jet of gas directly into the airway and have passive exhalation. A third type, high-frequency flow interruption (HFFI), also known as high-frequency percussive ventilation (HFPV), is less well studied and is less commonly employed. HFFI generates pulses of fresh gas similar to HFJV and also uses passive exhalation, but unlike HFJV, it does not produce a high-velocity stream of gas.

HFV appears to enhance both the distribution and the diffusion of respiratory gases. All types of HFV shift the transition point between convective and diffusive gas transport progressively in a cephalad direction from the acinus into the larger airways. The net effect of this shift is efficient CO_2 elimination relatively independent of mean lung volume.[6]

Conventional pulmonary physiology tells us that the amount of gas available for gas exchange, the alveolar tidal volume (VA), is the product of the tidal volume (V_T) delivered into the airway minus anatomic dead space (VD): $VA = V_T - VD$. If this relationship is true, tidal volumes near anatomic VD should produce little, if any, alveolar ventilation. In an attempt to clarify the mechanisms of HFV gas exchange at V_T less than anatomic VD, Chang demonstrated that multiple modes of gas transport occur, including bulk convection, high-frequency "pendelluft" (movement of gas among alveoli with differing time constants), convective dispersion, Taylor-type dispersion, and molecular diffusion.[7] These multiple mechanisms of enhanced intrapulmonary gas mixing are common to all forms of HFV. They contribute to tidal volume having a greater impact than the impact of ventilator rate at frequencies greater than 5 Hz, with minute ventilation being roughly equal to frequency times tidal volume squared ($f \cdot V_T^2$). The practical implication of this relationship is that even small changes in V_T can result in large changes in $PaCO_2$. With HFOV, the usual direct linear relationship between ventilator rate and CO_2 elimination is no longer valid, because changes in frequency affect the delivered V_T at any given pressure amplitude. This nonlinear relationship between frequency and V_T is because the inspiratory-to-expiratory time ratio (I:E) is held constant and therefore a reduction in frequency results in a longer inspiratory time. Consequently, gas flow occurs over a longer period of time, producing a larger V_T (Fig. 24.1). As gas exchange is proportional to $f \cdot V_T^2$, any reduction in minute ventilation resulting from lower frequency is

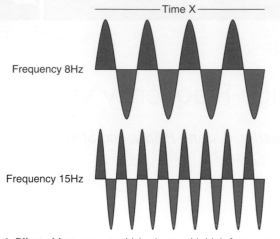

Fig. 24.1 Effect of frequency on tidal volume with high-frequency oscillatory ventilation. When the inspiratory-to-expiratory time ratio (I:E) is held constant, a reduction in frequency results in a longer inspiratory time. Consequently, gas flow occurs over a longer period of time, producing a larger V_T at any given pressure amplitude (volume = flow integrated over time, indicated by the shaded area in each cycle).

overshadowed by the impact of the larger V_T. With HFJV, the inspiratory time rather than I:E ratio is held constant, and therefore, frequency change does not impact V_T to a significant degree, unless the frequency is set too high, resulting in insufficient expiratory time and air-trapping. In that scenario, decreasing the rate will increase expiratory time and allow for complete passive exhalation.

In 2002, Slutsky and Drazen concisely summarized the gas exchange mechanisms of HFV (Fig. 24.2).[8] The theoretical explanations of gas exchange during HFV are beyond the scope of this clinical chapter. For those interested, there are a number of excellent review articles, as well as a review of physiologic principles in Chapter 2.[9-11]

TYPES OF HIGH-FREQUENCY VENTILATORS

As of this writing, only three HFV devices are approved by the US Food and Drug Administration (FDA) for clinical use in the United States. However, many HFOV devices are in use elsewhere in the world. Table 24.1 lists the commonly used HFV devices as of this writing.

High-Frequency Jet Ventilators

High-frequency jet ventilators deliver short pulses of pressurized gas directly into the upper airway through a narrow-bore cannula or jet injector. High-frequency jet ventilators are capable of maintaining ventilation over wide ranges of patient sizes and lung compliances. Jet ventilators have been tested extensively in laboratory animals and have been used clinically in neonates for over 35 years.[12-27] The Bunnell Life Pulse jet ventilator (Bunnell, Inc., Salt Lake City, UT), initially approved by the FDA in 1988, is the only jet ventilator available in the United States and Canada. As of this writing, there is limited availability of the device outside North America. The original model

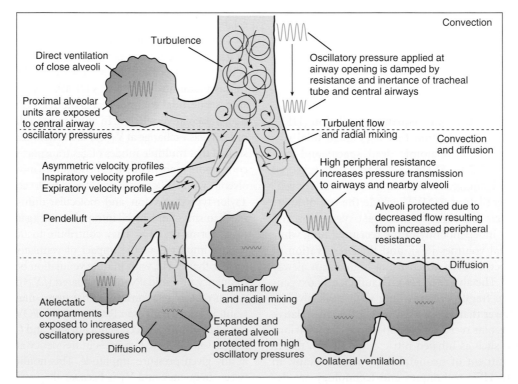

Fig. 24.2 Gas transport mechanisms and pressure damping during high-frequency ventilation. Major gas transport mechanisms include convective flow, convection and diffusion, diffusive flow, pendelluft, laminar flow with Taylor dispersion, turbulent flow, cardiogenic mixing, and perialveolar collateral ventilation. (From Pillow JJ: High-frequency oscillatory ventilation: mechanisms of gas exchange and lung mechanics. Crit Care Med. 2005 Mar; 33(3 Suppl):S135–41 as adapted from Slutsky S, Drazen JM: Ventilation with small tidal volumes. N Engl J Med 2002;347:630.)

TABLE 24.1 Classification and Key Characteristics of High-Frequency Ventilators

Ventilator	High-Frequency Ventilator Type	Conventional Ventilation + High-Frequency Ventilator	Volume Measurement	Exhalation
SensorMedics 3100A	"Piston" oscillator (=large diaphragm)	No	No	Active
Metran Humming Vue	Piston oscillator	Yes	Yes	Active
Flowline Dragonfly	Piston oscillator	No	Yes	Active
Dräger VN500, VN600, VN800	Diaphragm oscillator	Yes	Yes	Active
Fabian HFO	Diaphragm oscillator	Yes	Yes	Active
Leoni Plus	Diaphragm oscillator	Yes	Yes	Active
SLE5000, 6000	Reverse jet oscillator	Yes	Yes	Active
Stephan Stephanie and Sophie	Reciprocating valve oscillator	Yes	Yes	Active
VDR-4, IPV-2C Bronchotron	Flow interrupter	Yes	No	Passive
Bunnell Life Pulse 203, 204	Jet pulse via pinch valve	No	No	Passive

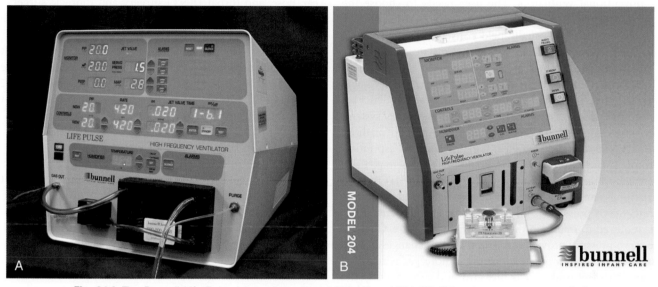

Fig. 24.3 The Bunnell Life Pulse jet ventilator Model 203 **(A)** and 204 **(B)**. This microprocessor-controlled pressure-limited time-cycled ventilator servo controls delivered airway pressure as measured at the endotracheal tube tip. Frequency range is from 240 to 660 cycles per minute. Pressure range is from 8 to 50 cm H2O. Inspiratory time is adjustable from 0.02 to 0.034 seconds. The Servo Pressure displayed on the front panel is an indirect indicator of changes in lung compliance and delivered tidal volume. The new Model 204 is smaller and lighter with enhanced user interface and updated electronics, but functionally similar to the sister device. (Courtesy Bunnell, Salt Lake City, UT.)

203 was recently replaced by the smaller and lighter model 204, but the functionality of the new device is essentially unchanged. The Bunnell device was designed specifically for infants and at the time it was the first microprocessor controlled neonatal ventilator (Fig. 24.3). This device delivers its jet pulse of heated, humidified gas into the endotracheal tube through the LifePort endotracheal tube adapter's injector port and then servo controls the driving pressure (servo pressure) of the jet pulse to maintain a constant user-preset peak pressure within the endotracheal tube. The LifePulse operates at rates from 240 to 660 cycles per minute (4–11 Hz), with the most common rates being 240 to 420 cycles per minute (4–7 Hz). The rates are less than those typically used in HFOV because exhalation during HFJV is a result of passive lung recoil. The device has negligible compressible volumes owing to the placement of the patient

box, which contains the pinch valve that controls gas flow and the airway pressure monitoring sensor near the patient. An open ventilator-patient circuit is essential, and HFJV is used in combination with a conventional ventilator to provide positive end-expiratory pressure (PEEP) and occasional sighs if needed. Tidal volume is difficult to measure but appears to be equal to or slightly greater than anatomical dead space.[28] Unpublished data from one of the authors (JJP) suggest that at equivalent pressure amplitude and inspiratory time (TI 0.02 seconds on HFJV and frequency of 15 Hz with 1:2 I:E ratio on HFOV), the V_T generated by HFJV and HFOV are similar.

In addition to V_T delivered through the jet injector, some gases surrounding the injector are pulled or entrained into the airway with each jet pulse, although this effect is minimal in small subjects.[29] The high-flow jet pulse produces a Venturi effect that creates an area of negative pressure at its periphery, entraining ambient gases into the airway. Because of high gas velocities, Venturi effects, and pressure gradients within the delivery system, pressure monitoring must occur far enough downstream from the jet injector to minimize Venturi effects.

With HFJV, CO_2 removal may be achieved at lower peak airway pressures and MAPs than with HFOV.[13,14,18,30-32] Although initially primarily used to treat air leak, HFJV is also effective in homogeneous lung disorders such as respiratory distress syndrome (RDS), provided an appropriate strategy that prioritizes optimal lung inflation is utilized. A randomized multicenter trial showed a beneficial pulmonary effect (lower rates of chronic lung disease) with the use of early HFJV over CMV in RDS.[23]

The Bunnell jet ventilator controls are similar to those used with conventional ventilators. The user needs to choose the peak inspiratory pressure (PIP), PEEP, and rate. The inspiratory time (valve on-time) is usually held constant at 0.02 seconds but can be increased modestly at lower ventilatory rates (e.g., 240–300 cycles per minute) or when needed to deliver a high PIP in sicker patients. The maximum inspiratory time possible is 0.034 seconds. The appropriate ventilator rate (frequency) is related to the time constants of the infant's respiratory system; longer time constants are seen in larger infants and in those with increased airway resistance, e.g., meconium aspiration syndrome (MAS), pulmonary interstitial emphysema (PIE), and bronchopulmonary dysplasia (BPD). As with HFOV, CO_2 elimination is controlled by the product of tidal volume squared and rate. Servo pressure is an indicator of the amount of gas that is required to maintain the peak airway pressure. Changes in the servo pressure provide important cues to changes in lung compliance; when compliance improves, more gas is required to maintain the set peak airway pressure, and consequently, the servo pressure rises to meet the need. When less gas is needed, servo pressure falls. A fall in servo pressure may occur if lung compliance deteriorates (for example because of atelectasis or pneumothorax), or when the endotracheal tube is partially obstructed. Acute changes in servo pressure should prompt an evaluation of the patient and endotracheal tube position and patency. In general, falling servo pressure is a concerning sign and increasing servo pressure is indicative of patient improvement. However, a leak in the system could also cause increasing servo pressure. Oxygenation is determined by fractional inspired oxygen (FiO_2) and MAP (labeled MAP on this device), which is primarily controlled by the level of PEEP.

HFJV appears to be uniquely effective in nonhomogeneous lung disorders in which CO_2 elimination is the major problem, such as air-leak syndromes, especially PIE,[18,31] or in diseases in which atelectasis and overdistention occur simultaneously, such as MAS.[24] In the former, the very short inspiratory time and the high-velocity jet pulse contribute to the resolution of air leak. In the latter, the ability to provide a low-rate sigh (two to five inflations per minute) assists with opening atelectatic areas. HFJV is also safe and effective when used in neonatal transport and can be used with simultaneous delivery of iNO.[25,33] There may also be a benefit of the shorter I:E ratio (longer expiratory time) during HFJV, as the pressure decrease to PEEP allows

better pulmonary blood flow compared to HFOV, where there is little variation in pressure between inspiratory/expiratory cycle phase; this feature of HFJV may offer a benefit over HFOV (particularly when high MAP is required) in terms of less impairment of venous return resulting in improved cardiac output and improved pulmonary blood flow leading to better oxygenation. During HFJV, adequate humidification is essential due to the high gas flow and is ensured by a very efficient humidification system integrated into the device. Before the implementation of this humidification system, necrotizing tracheobronchitis (NTB) was described as a complication of HFJV;[34-36] however, tracheal injury is not unique to HFJV[32,37] and is no longer an issue with current technology.

In Europe, the Monsoon jet ventilator (Acutronic Medical Systems AG, Hirzel, Switzerland) has been used primarily for ear, nose, and throat (ENT) surgery and thoracic surgery and has seen limited applications in intensive care for adult patients with severe respiratory failure and air-leak complications. The device has an integrated humidification and heating system, making it potentially suitable for extended use. It operates at frequencies of 0.2 to 10 Hz, percentage inspiratory time of 20% to 70%, PEEP 10 to 40 cmH_2O. No systematic evaluation of safety and effectiveness is available.

High-Frequency Oscillators

High-frequency oscillatory ventilators (HFOVs) have been tested extensively in animals and in humans.[1,2,5,38-56] HFOVs operate at frequencies ranging from 180 to 1200 cycles per minute (3–20 Hz) to move small volumes of gas in and out of the lungs. During HFOV, inspiration and expiration are both active (proximal airway pressures are negative during expiration). In the Vyaire (formerly SensorMedics) 3100A (Vyaire, Mettawa, IL), fresh gas flows continuously past the electromagnetically operated piston, generating the oscillations. The 3100B is a more powerful oscillator that can be used in children and adults. In both devices, a controlled-leak or low-pass filter allows gas to exit the system without dampening the high-frequency pressure swings. The balance between the inflow of fresh gas and the controlled leak through the low pass filter determines the mean airway pressure (P_{aw}) (Fig. 24.4). The amplitude of the pressure oscillations within the airway is controlled by adjusting the power applied to the piston and determines the V_T that is delivered to the lungs around a constant P_{aw}. This allows avoidance of high peak airway pressures for ventilation as well as maintenance of lung recruitment by avoidance of low end-expiratory pressures. Frequency (3–15 Hz or 180–900 cycles per minute), percentage inspiratory time (33%–50%), and power applied to the piston can be adjusted. The original SensorMedics HFO was approved for clinical use in 1990 (Fig. 24.5).

Newer HFOV devices are available in Canada, Europe, and other countries. These microprocessor-controlled devices have many important advantages. Most have the ability to generate both conventional and HFV, avoiding the cumbersome need to change machines should HFO be necessary or vice versa. Changing to a different ventilator is not merely inconvenient. The need to disconnect the patient from the ventilator circuit

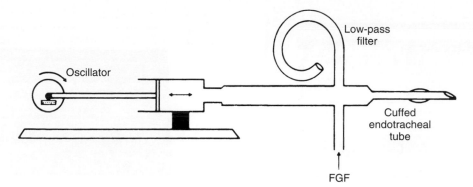

Fig. 24.4 Schematic of a piston high-frequency oscillator. A piston mechanism generates oscillating pressures. Fresh gases enter the system proximal to the endotracheal tube. Excess gas and mixed expired gases exit via a low-pass filter. *FGF*, Fresh gas flow. (From Thompson WK, Marchak BE, Froese AB, Bryan AC: High-frequency oscillation compared with standard ventilation in pulmonary injury model. J Appl Physiol. 52:543, 1982.)

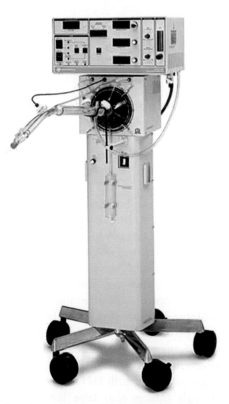

Fig. 24.5. The SensorMedics 3100A high-frequency oscillator. This electronically controlled ventilator uses a sealed piston with adjustable volume displacement to generate oscillations into the airway. Frequency is adjustable from 180 to 900 cycles per minute (3–15 Hz). Mean airway pressure can be set between 3 and 45 cm H2O; oscillatory pressure amplitude is adjustable to more than 90 cm H2O. Inspiratory time can be set from 33% to 50% of the total cycle. (Courtesy SensorMedics Corp, Yorba Linda, CA.).

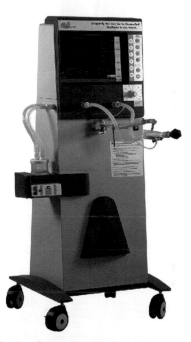

Fig. 24.6 The Flowline Dragonfly high-frequency oscillator. This piston oscillator is somewhat similar to the 3100A and only capable of delivering high-frequency ventilation via a short, rigid circuit at frequencies of 5 to 18 Hz, inspiratory time of 33% or 50% and mean airway pressure up to 40 cm H_2O. Unlike the 3100A, it is capable of measuring tidal volume and automatically maintains mean airway pressure constant when other parameters are changed. (Courtesy Flowline Healthcare Co., Kothrud Pune, Maharashtra, India.)

A variety of mechanisms provide HFOV with these ventilators, but they are all true oscillators based on the waveform they generate. They operate quietly as compared to the noisy SensorMedics and Dragonfly HFO.[57] Some of these devices are capable of frequencies up to 20 Hz. Sighs can be superimposed or interposed if necessary, to aid lung volume recruitment. Low-compliance conventional circuits are used, making handling and kangaroo care easier. These HFO ventilators include the SLE 5000 and 6000 (SLE Limited, South Croydon, UK; Fig. 24.7), the Fabian (Acutronic Medical Systems, Hirzel, Switzerland, recently acquired by Vyaire Mettawa, IL;

risks dislodging the endotracheal tube and the transient loss of distending pressure leads to derecruitment of lung volume. The exception is the Flowline Dragonfly (Pune, India; Fig. 24.6), which is based on the 3100, uses a similar patient circuit, and is capable only of HFOV. This device is no longer produced, but many are still in use in parts of Asia.

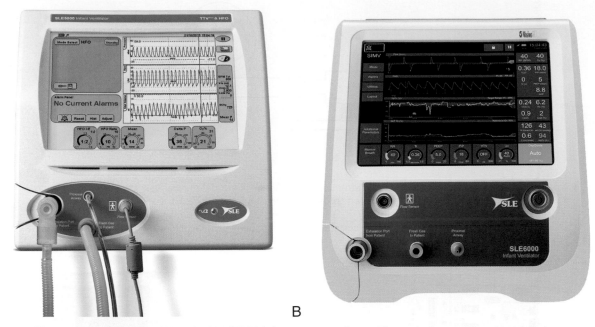

Fig. 24.7 The SLE 5000 **(A)** and 6000 **(B)** high-frequency ventilators. These devices are capable of both conventional and high-frequency ventilation with volume targeting. The oscillations are produced by a valveless mechanism involving forward- and backward-facing jets that alternately direct gas into the patient and facilitate active exhalation. Inspiratory:expiratory ratio is adjustable from 1:1 to 1:3 and frequency is adjustable up to 20 Hz. Sighs can be applied at adjustable pressure and inspiratory time. Set and measured values are displayed. (Courtesy SLE, South Croydon, UK.)

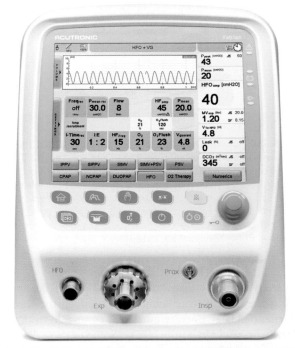

Fig. 24.8 The Fabian high-frequency oscillator. Conventional and high-frequency ventilation is available with this device, which is designed for use in patients from 300 g to 30 kg. Frequency is adjustable from 300 to 1200 cycles per minute (5–20 Hz). Amplitude is set between 5 and 100 cm H2O, and it uses automatic leak compensation with volume targeting. Mean airway pressure is adjustable between 0 and 40 cm H2O. Measured and derived respiratory parameters are displayed. (Courtesy Vyaire, Mettawa, IL.)

Fig. 24.8), the Leoni Plus (Löwenstein Medical Technology, Bad Ems, Germany; Fig. 24.9), the Stephanie and the Sophie (Stephan, Gackenbach, Germany; Fig. 24.10), the Humming Vue (Metran, Saitama, Japan; Fig. 24.11), and the VN500 and the VN600/800 (Dräger, Lubeck, Germany; Fig. 24.12). Perhaps most importantly, they can also measure and in some cases automatically control V_T by an approach analogous to conventional volume guarantee (VG) ventilation, thus decreasing the risk of inadvertent overventilation and avoiding the frequent need to change the amplitude in the face of overventilation or underventilation.

Control of gas exchange with HFOV is relatively straightforward. Although this is also true for other modes of ventilation, HFOV more clearly separates control of oxygenation and CO_2 elimination at a given level of compliance. Oxygenation is controlled by FiO_2 and $\bar{P}_{aw}$, while ventilation (CO_2 removal) is controlled by adjustment of delivered tidal volume. The latter is controlled by the pressure amplitude (ΔP) and the frequency and, to a lesser extent, by percent inspiratory time. As previously explained, a lower frequency generates a larger V_T at any given pressure amplitude and thus increases CO_2 elimination, but the increased V_T is accomplished at the expense of increased transmission of pressure to the lung. There is more interdependence between ventilation and oxygenation than has traditionally been taught. When changes in $\bar{P}_{aw}$ cause significant change in lung compliance, there is substantial impact on both oxygenation and CO_2 elimination.

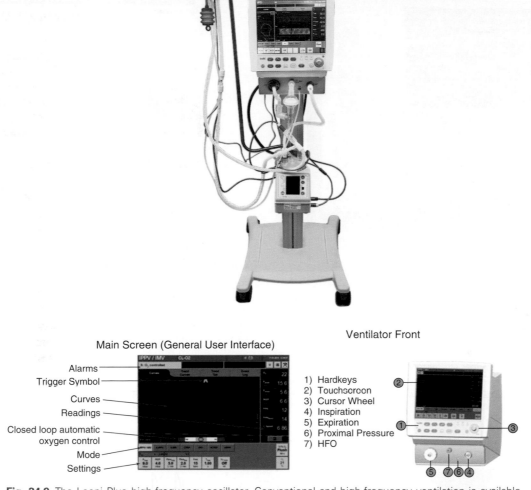

Fig. 24.9 The Leoni Plus high-frequency oscillator. Conventional and high-frequency ventilation is available with this device, which is designed for use in patients up to 30 kg. HFO frequency is adjustable from 300 to 1200 cycles per minute (5-20 Hz). Amplitude is set between 0 and 100 cm H2O, and it uses automatic leak compensation with tidal volume measurement and targeting. Mean airway pressure is adjustable between 0 and 30 cm H2O. Measured and derived respiratory parameters are displayed. (Courtesy Löwenstein Medical Technology, Bad Ems, Germany.)

As with HFJV, the site of pressure monitoring in HFOV is important. During HFOV, airway pressures usually are measured either at the proximal end of the endotracheal tube or within the ventilator itself. The amplitude of pressure oscillations is considerably damped across the endotracheal tube and further within the airways (Fig. 24.13). The clinical relevance of pressure measurements in the ventilator circuit is unclear, as they are some distance away from the patient and the relationship of intrapulmonary pressures measured during HFOV to those measured during CMV is not consistent. Depending upon the size and resonant frequency of the lung, alveolar oscillatory pressures can be the same, lower, or even higher than those measured in the trachea.[39,58,59] Similarly, with the exception of an I:E ratio of 1:1, mean pressure in the airways and the lung is lower than mean pressure recorded at the airway opening and displayed on the ventilator. The drop in MAP is flow dependent and hence depends on oscillatory frequency, I:E ratio, oscillatory power (amplitude), and tracheal diameter.[60]

High-Frequency Flow Interrupters/Percussive Ventilators

The term flow interrupter originally was used to describe a group of ventilators that were neither true oscillators nor true jets. Some had jet-type injectors but delivered their bursts of gas not directly into the airway but into the ventilator circuit some distance back from the trachea and endotracheal tube. For this reason, these machines also were called setback jets. Most of these ventilators are no longer in production. Early clinical studies yielded mixed results.[61-63]

In recent years, HFFI ventilation has experienced a modest resurgence in the form of several devices from the company of Forrest Bird, the inventor of the first neonatal ventilator, the

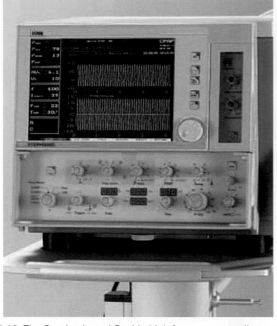

Fig. 24.10 The Stephanie and Sophie high-frequency ventilators. These ventilators provide both conventional and high-frequency ventilation. Frequency range is 5 to 15 Hz; inspiratory time can be adjusted between 33%, 40%, and 50%; mean airway pressure: up to 30 cm H_2O. At maximum amplitude, a tidal volume of 24 mL can be reached at 10 Hz using a valve system that alternately directs flow into the patient circuit and away from the patient to generate active exhalation. (Courtesy Stephan, Gackenbach, Germany.)

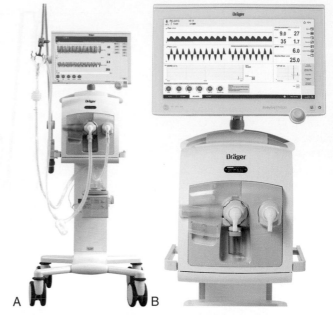

Fig. 24.12 The Dräger VN500 **(A)** and 800 **(B)** neonatal/pediatric ventilators. These ventilators provide both conventional and high-frequency ventilation using the same platform. High-frequency oscillatory ventilation is adjustable from 5 to 20 Hz with an inspiratory:expiratory ratio setting from 1:1 to 1:3. Mean airway pressure range is 5 to 50 cm H_2O, with amplitude adjustable from 5 to 90 cm H_2O. Tidal volumes and calculated index of CO_2 elimination are displayed. Volume guarantee is available for both conventional and high-frequency ventilation with a range of tidal volume from 0.2 to 40 mL. Sigh inflations are available at a rate ranging from 1 to 30 and pressure of 6 to 80 cm H_2O. There is another version of this ventilator that is functionally identical to the VN800 but has a smaller screen, known as VN600 (not pictured). (Courtesy Dräger, Lubeck, Germany.)

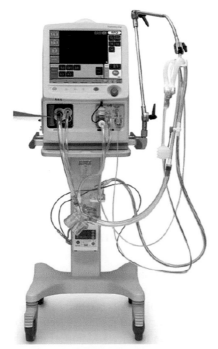

Fig. 24.11 The Metran Humming Vue is a descendent of the original Hummingbird ventilator used in the HIFI trial. It is a piston oscillator also capable of conventional ventilation. A frequency of 5 to 17 Hz is available and a 1:1 inspiratory:expiratory ratio is used. Tidal volume is measured by a proximal flow sensor. Amplitude is controlled as percentage of maximal power and superimposed conventional inflations can be applied at adjustable pressure and rate up to 120 per minute. Set and measured values are displayed. (Courtesy Metran, Saitama, Japan.)

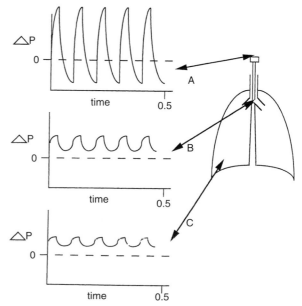

Fig. 24.13 Airway pressure drop across the airway using high-frequency oscillatory ventilation using a 33% inspiratory time. (The graph was adapted from unpublished observations using the SensorMedics 3100A.) *Curve A* is the pressure measured at the proximal endotracheal tube. *Curve B* is the pressure measured at the carina. *Curve C* is the pressure measured in the distal airways. The magnitude of drop is affected by percentage inspiratory time, size of the endotracheal tube, and amplitude. Similar attenuation of pressure swings occurs with other modalities of high-frequency ventilation.

BabyBird. The Bronchotron (Percussionaire Corp., Sandpoint, ID) is a pneumatically driven flow interrupter/percussive ventilator increasingly used during transport.[64] The Bronchotron is attractive as a transport ventilator because of its light weight, ability to function as both conventional and high-frequency ventilator, and relatively low gas consumption (Fig. 24.14A). The ventilator's internal pneumatic timer cycles high-pressure gas flow at a frequency ranging from 3 to 10 Hz. Rate and amplitude are continuously adjustable. The inspiratory time is determined by the frequency and the mechanical properties of the lungs. The high-frequency gas pulses enter a sliding piston mechanism called a Phasitron through a Venturi cavity in its central axis. The Phasitron creates pulses of gas flow by the rapid movement of a spring mechanism that balances inspiratory and expiratory pressures within preset pressures for PEEP and MAP, acting as both an inspiratory and an expiratory valve. In the inspiratory phase, the pulse of gas is augmented by entrained gas proportional to the pressure difference before and after the Venturi. During expiration, the piston springs back, opening an exhalation port, and gas is allowed to exit the patient through an adjustable resistor that provides PEEP and regulates MAP. The MAP, frequency, and flow (which adjusts the gas flow to the Phasitron and controls the pulse amplitude) are continuously adjustable.

The main limitation of the Bronchotron device is the lack of real values for the ventilator variables—all dials are marked with unit-less values of 1 to 10, but these numbers do not translate to constant values. Adjustments must be made based solely on clinical observation of chest movement and patient response. Frequency is displayed as cycles per minute (not Hz),

and MAP ($\overline{P}_{aw}$) can be measured intermittently by flipping a toggle switch and changing the phasic pressure display to an integrated mean. The phasic pressure displayed by the rapidly oscillating needle of a mechanical gauge is difficult to read. The other major concern is the bulk/weight of the Phasitron device located near the endotracheal tube that must be carefully positioned and supported to avoid inadvertent endotracheal tube kinking or dislodgment. The generally accepted safety and efficacy of the Bronchotron are not well documented; the device was "grandfathered" by the FDA, meaning that it was approved based on its "substantial equivalence" to a device in existence prior to the effective date of the law (1979). The Bronchotron and the 3100A oscillator achieved similar gas exchange when the devices were adjusted to deliver identical V_T at the same $\overline{P}_{aw}$ and frequency in saline-lavaged newborn piglets, but higher pressure amplitude was needed with the Bronchotron.

The IPV 2C is a hospital version of the Bronchotron and shares similar features and functionality (Fig. 24.14B). The VDR-4 (Percussionaire Corp., Sandpoint, ID) is a time-cycled, pressure-controlled, pneumatically driven high-frequency percussive ventilator similar to the Bronchotron but more complex and designed for hospital use (Fig. 24.14C). The device delivers gas from a pressurized source through a pneumatic timing cartridge system. The source gas is interrupted to produce a pulsatile flow, which enters the breathing circuit via the Phasitron as with its sister devices. Warmed, humidified gas is entrained to augment V_T. V_T delivery is determined by flow velocity, inspiratory duration, and supplementary gas entrainment. The VDR-4 is composed of two subsystems: conventional and high frequency. The conventional component can

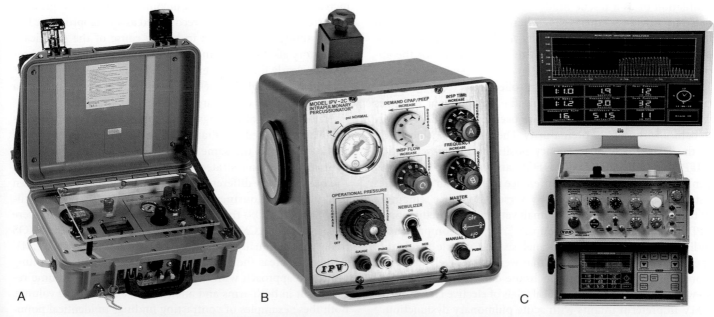

Fig. 24.14 (A) The Bronchotron transport ventilator. **(B)** The IPV-2C ventilator. **(C)** The VDR 4 percussive ventilator. These devices employ a unique valve system known as the Phasitron to direct pulses of gas into the patient's airway. The Bronchotron operates at a rate of 200 to 800 cycles per minute at a 1:1 inspiratory:expiratory ratio. The IPV 2C operates at lower rates of 60 to 330 cycles and the VDR 4 can combine conventional inflations with percussive ventilation at rates of 50 to 900 per minute and adjustable inspiratory time. (Courtesy Percussionaire Corp., Sandpoint, ID.)

deliver up to 70 inflations per minute with independent control of inflation time and pressure. The high-frequency component can deliver frequencies from 0.5 to 30 Hz, amplitudes from 0 to 100 cm H2O, and I:E from 1:1 to 1:5. The conventional and high-frequency modalities can be superimposed, and thus, a variety of conventional and high-frequency combinations can be used. Like the Bronchotron, the VDR-4 was approved by the FDA without requiring proof of safety and efficacy. The literature regarding the safety and efficacy of this device in the pediatric population is limited to a few small studies in adult and pediatric patients and a single case series of six newborn infants.[65] The device is often used in burn patients as clinicians feel it can clear the airways of patients with severe smoke inhalation better than other devices.[66] There is also interest in using this device to deliver HFV via the nasal route, as a means to provide noninvasive ventilation.[67,68]

EVIDENCE BASE FOR CLINICAL APPLICATIONS OF HIGH-FREQUENCY VENTILATION

Elective Versus Rescue High-Frequency Ventilation

HFV has been studied in animal models for over 40 years. The majority of animal data support the superiority of various forms of HFV over CMV, in terms of both short-term physiology and pressure exposure, as well as in lung pathology over days to weeks. Animal studies suggest that HFV works at lower distal oscillatory airway pressures than CMV, reduces ventilator-induced lung injury (VILI) and lung inflammatory markers, improves gas exchange in the face of air-leak syndromes, is synergistic with surfactant and nitric oxide, and decreases oxygen exposure. Unfortunately, these findings have not been consistently reproduced in the human studies of HFV versus CMV, whether looking at HFV either as an initial, elective mode of ventilation or as a rescue mode of ventilation when CMV has failed to provide adequate gas exchange. Failure to use an open lung strategy in the conventionally ventilated controls in these preclinical studies may be one of the explanations for the apparent superiority of HFV.[69]

Over a dozen randomized controlled trials (RCTs) of elective use of HFV versus CMV for the treatment of neonates with respiratory insufficiency have been performed, primarily in babies with RDS of prematurity. These studies include HFV in the forms of high-frequency positive-pressure ventilation (HFPPV), HFFI, HFJV, and HFOV, and most were unable to demonstrate any significant difference in pulmonary outcomes between babies treated with HFV versus CMV. The remainder of the studies demonstrated a small yet significant reduction in BPD in the HFV-treated groups.[23,45,49,50,53] A comprehensive individual patient data meta-analysis was unable to identify specific subgroups of patients that were more likely to benefit from HFOV.[70] In 2015, the Cochrane database provided a review and meta-analysis of clinical trials of elective HFOV versus CMV in preterm infants with acute pulmonary dysfunction.[71] The review demonstrated no evidence of effect on mortality and no substantial advantage to the preferential use of elective HFO over CMV as the initial ventilation strategy in premature babies with respiratory distress. However, in contrast to earlier

reviews, the risk ratio was shifted just enough to reach significance due to a 2014 study by Sun et al. that suggested a large reduction in the combined outcome of death or BPD.[72] The authors of the Cochrane review concluded that the overall conclusion was weakened by the inconsistency of benefit across studies. A reduction in the rate of retinopathy of prematurity was also noted as a possible benefit of HFOV.

A number of efforts have been made to identify factors that may explain the heterogeneity in the outcomes of HFOV trials. In general, an "optimal lung volume" strategy with HFOV, early use of HFOV (<6 hours), I:E of 1:2, extubation to continuous positive airway pressure rather than a trial of CMV, and lack of lung-protective strategies in the CMV groups were associated with the trials that demonstrated a reduction in chronic lung disease in the HFOV groups. Piston oscillator use also appeared to be associated with better outcomes, but it is impossible to disentangle this characteristic from the other factors, which likely are more important. The nature of the pressure and flow waveform that the lungs are exposed to, rather than the mechanism by which the waveform is produced, is what ultimately matters.

A metaregression analysis performed by Bollen and colleagues[73] demonstrated that variation in ventilation strategies in both the HFV and the CMV groups most likely explains the observed differences in outcomes. This analysis did not support the widely held beliefs that early initiation of HFOV and the use of piston oscillators are associated with better HFOV outcomes.

The Cochrane database also reviewed the elective use of HFJV versus CMV and from the three studies reviewed concluded that there may be a decreased risk of BPD in the elective HFJV groups.[74] However, the authors raised questions about these apparent positive findings because of significant heterogeneity among the studies and the fact that one study showed increased adverse neurologic outcomes in the HFJV group.[75] That study used what is now recognized as an inappropriate low PEEP strategy that appears to be the cause of the significant respiratory alkalosis seen in the HFJV group, which was subsequently clearly linked to periventricular leukomalacia (PVL).[76] A similar, although less severe, trend was also apparent in a subgroup analysis of the larger multicenter trial.[23]

Heterogeneity of findings is not unique to HFJV; two studies of HFOV published simultaneously in the *New England Journal of Medicine* used the same early intervention approach with optimal lung volume strategy in a virtually identical population and obtained very different results. The key differences between the "successful" Courtney study and the United Kingdom Oscillator Study (UKOS) that failed to show reduction in BPD were an early return to CMV and the use of a 1:1 I:E ratio in the UKOS trial.[50,51] Additionally, the UKOS trial did not specify the CMV strategy, whereas the North American study stipulated a lung protective approach with the goal of optimal lung volume recruitment in both arms and attention to exhaled tidal volume. Both these examples of contrasting findings in identical populations highlight the importance of ventilation strategy on outcome. Overall, grouped analysis of all randomized controlled studies to date would not support the selective use of early and elective HFV over CMV in premature babies with respiratory insufficiency unequivocally, although it remains a reasonable choice. The lack of clear benefit of HFOV is very likely due to the improved methods of CMV in use today, including volume-targeted ventilation (see Chapter 22).

Concerns about the safety of HFV were first raised by the HIFI study that compared early HFOV to CMV, as the HFOV-treated group demonstrated increased incidence of intraventricular hemorrhage (IVH) and/or PVL, as well as air leak.[44] More alarmingly, the neurodevelopmental outcomes at 16 to 24 months post–term age were significantly worse in the HFOV-treated group.[77] The study was done in the early days of HFV and once more may have failed to use an appropriate ventilatory strategy. Unfortunately, no $PaCO_2$ data were published, but alterations in $PaCO_2$ could theoretically explain these findings. The subsequent large RCTs by Courtney et al.[50] and Johnson et al.[51] demonstrated no difference in the rates of IVH or PVL, and nor did the individual patient meta-analysis by Cools et al.[70] Studies by Truffert et al.[78] and Marlow et al.[79] have provided reassuring long-term neurodevelopmental follow-up at 2 years of age from the UKOS trial. Interestingly, despite no apparent impact of HFOV on the outcome of BPD at 36 weeks' postmenstrual age, Zivanovic et al. found superior lung function at 11 to 14 years of age in the HFOV-treated infants from the UKOS trial.[80] Although valuable, more follow-up data are needed before definitive conclusion can be made regarding long-term outcomes. The Cochrane review also concluded that HFOV is associated with increased risk of air leak (combining PIE and gross air leak). That finding is driven by the HIFI trial, which did not use an appropriate ventilatory strategy, and the Thome trial,[62] which used the Infant Star HFFI device, which is not an oscillator but an HFFI device no longer in use. The Schreiber study,[81] which focused on iNO but also randomized infants to receive HFOV or CMV, also found increased incidence of air leak with HFOV when gross air leak and PIE were combined, but the published data reported PIE and pneumothorax separately as not being significantly different. The larger studies that used true HFOV devices and an optimal lung volume strategy did not suggest any evidence of increased air leak.

Because elective use of HFV has not demonstrated a clear advantage over CMV for RDS, what about the use of rescue HFV when CMV appears to be failing to provide adequate gas exchange? Four RCTs in premature and term infants have assessed HFV as a rescue technique after failing CMV.[24,31,82,83] The data are limited to older studies that include two studies using HFJV and two using HFOV. The HIFO trial demonstrated improved gas exchange and lower rate of new air leak with HFOV. There was no effect on existing air leak and no difference in overall pulmonary outcomes and a marginally increased rate of severe IVH.[82] Keszler et al. specifically enrolled infants with PIE and showed improvement of PIE in the HFJV group compared to those who remained on CMV.[31] In the two trials treating older preterm babies (more than 34 weeks), there was notable improvement in gas exchange and treatment success in the HFV groups; however, there was no significant difference in the incidence of BPD or death between those rescued with HFV and those who remained on CMV.[24,83] A meta-analysis of rescue HFV versus CMV in the Cochrane database demonstrates that

there is no clear long-term benefit of using rescue HFOV or HFJV over continued CMV.[84-86] However, lumping together results of studies using different modes of HFV in different populations may obscure important differences. The HFJV study did, in fact, demonstrate improved survival attributable to HFJV when the effect of crossover was taken into account.[31] These HFV rescue trials were performed when the administration of exogenous surfactant, maternal antenatal steroids, synchronized ventilation, and volume targeting were not routinely practiced, and therefore, the findings may not be applicable today. There have been no long-term neurodevelopmental or pulmonary outcome follow-up data published from these rescue trials. Nonetheless, early rescue use of both HFJV and HFOV remains the most common approach to HFV as of this writing.

Some conditions may respond to the use of HFV better than others. Persistent pulmonary hypertension secondary to meconium aspiration or other forms of lung disease often responds to iNO best when HFOV is used for support, likely because of improved lung aeration.[87] Over 90% of preterm infants treated with iNO for pulmonary hypertension were receiving HFV at the same time.[88] Anecdotally, HFJV appears to be equally effective for this purpose with less adverse effect on the circulation. Postsurgical support for infants with gastroschisis, omphalocele, necrotizing enterocolitis, and other conditions that restrict diaphragmatic excursion may benefit from HFOV or HFJV as well. Infants with pulmonary hypoplasia of various etiologies may benefit from the very small tidal volumes generated by various forms of HFV, potentially reducing the risk of air leak and volutrauma. Finally, HFV is experiencing a resurgence in first-intention use in the extremely low birth weight infant of 22 to 24 weeks' gestation. As more and more high-risk obstetric centers are offering resuscitation to these very tiny babies, interest in the possible protective effects of HFV has led to use of HFJV or HFOV as first-line respiratory support, often continued until extubation. It remains to be seen if this approach leads to less chronic lung disease and better outcomes.

LUNG PROTECTIVE STRATEGIES WITH HFV: LIMITING PRESSURE WHILE OPTIMIZING VOLUME

Much progress has been made in the treatment of neonatal respiratory failure over the past few decades, but BPD remains a persistent problem, in part because of increasing survival of the most immature infants.[89] HFV remains an attractive ventilation strategy with the potential to avoid large tidal volume (volutrauma), as well as uneven distribution of tidal volume and repetitive shear stress of the expansion and collapse with each CMV inflation (atelectrauma) that contributes to the development of BPD.

Animal models show that low V_T and increased PEEP during CMV lessen VILI.[90-93] Other preclinical studies show that recruiting lung volume to ensure open and stable alveoli attenuates VILI with both HFV and CMV.[94-98] The approach of recruiting and stabilizing the open alveoli is termed optimal lung volume or open lung strategy. The open lung strategy combined with mild permissive hypercapnia has been termed lung-protective ventilation. Most studies and reviews refer to an "open lung" strategy when there is a predefined FiO2 target of 0.25 to 0.30 being used as a surrogate for optimal lung recruitment.[99,100] It remains to be seen whether recruitment maneuvers and higher levels of PEEP could further optimize low V_T CMV and whether the use of HFV can decrease morbidity and mortality if the same lung-protective strategy is used in both groups.[101] However, it appears that lung volume recruitment may be easier to accomplish with HFV, at least psychologically, because there seems to be less resistance to using higher P_{aw} with HFOV than to increasing PEEP with CMV, an unfortunate mindset known as "PEEP-o-phobia." (For more in-depth discussion of lung-protective ventilation, please see Chapter 21).

CLINICAL APPLICATIONS OF HIGH-FREQUENCY VENTILATION IN SPECIFIC DISEASES

Respiratory Distress Syndrome

RDS continues to be the most common form of respiratory failure requiring treatment with mechanical ventilation in neonates. Because RDS is characterized by very short time constants, it is optimally suited to benefit from HFV. Treatment of acute RDS is based on principles of lung volume recruitment and avoidance of volutrauma, regardless of which device is used. Although not clearly shown to be superior to state-of-the-art CV, both HFJV and HFOV are nonetheless used as a first-line therapy in some neonatal intensive care units (NICUs), especially in the extremely low birth weight infant. Many other NICUs employ HFV in selected infants who are deemed at particularly high risk of complications, who require high inflation pressures, or who have already developed complications of mechanical ventilation, such as air leak.

High-Frequency Oscillatory Ventilation Strategy in Respiratory Distress Syndrome

Whether used as first-line therapy or in early rescue mode, the goal is to optimize lung volume, improve ventilation/perfusion matching, and reduce oxygen exposure. The open lung concept is key to preservation of lung architecture as well as preservation of endogenous and exogenous surfactant.[94,102-105] Because lung volumes are difficult to assess at the bedside, other surrogates must be employed. Electrical impedance tomography (EIT), which measures differences in electrical impedance from changes in lung tissue conductivity, may become a useful clinical adjunct for assessment of lung volume changes during mechanical ventilation but remains a research tool at this time.[106-108] Therefore, SpO2 (combined with FiO2) and chest radiographic findings are used most commonly as surrogates for assessment of lung volume.[100,109] Improved lung compliance can also be used to detect optimal lung recruitment and this is most easily recognized by a drop in high-frequency pressure amplitude when using HFOV + VG.

The airway pressures are measured within the oscillator circuit, not in the proximal airway. With a 33% inspiratory time (1:2 I:E ratio), an equal volume of gas must pass through the endotracheal tube in half as much time during inspiratory phase than during exhalation; thus, a higher pressure gradient is needed during inspiration than exhalation. This creates a pressure difference between the circuit pressure and tracheal pressure: the magnitude of the pressure difference increases nonlinearly with oscillatory amplitude but is about 2 to 3 cm H_2O at routine oscillatory pressures.[60] Thus, owing to the flow characteristics of the 1:2 I:E ratio, a set HFOV P_{aw} 2 to 3 cm H_2O above the conventional ventilator will provide a tracheal (P_{aw}) that is approximately equal to what was delivered on CV. This gradient does not exist when a 1:1 ratio is used, as is common with some devices. In theory, the longer expiratory time of the 1:2 I:E ratio means that the pressure during the active exhalation is less negative than when a 1:1 ratio is used, potentially making airway collapse less likely to occur. The sharper inspiratory flow profile may promote more efficient ventilation (because it is more penetrating), but this is achieved at risk of increased shear stress on the airways.

Optimizing lung volume is done by inflating the lung to near-maximum volume with stepwise increases in MAP. The lung is considered fully inflated when FiO_2 can be weaned to under 0.30. It is then deflated to the closing volume that is manifested by deterioration in S_PO_2. The lung is then reinflated to a point just above closing volume.[100] This technique allows ventilation to move from the inspiratory limb of the P-V curve to the expiratory limb, allowing effective ventilation and oxygenation at lower pressures (see also Chapter 21).[109] Surfactant distribution is improved when it is administered into an adequately aerated lung[110] and its benefits are further enhanced by subsequent lung volume recruitment.[111] In uncomplicated RDS, aggressive lung recruitment is seldom necessary with the currently available surfactant preparations, but persistent high oxygen requirement should trigger an attempt at optimizing lung inflation. However, some infants have coexisting neonatal pneumonia or other conditions that may preclude successful recruitment. As a general rule, if two consecutive increases in MAP fail to produce an improvement in oxygenation, the lung may not be recruitable. Furthermore, it is essential to verify that the cause of hypoxemia is diffuse microatelectasis, rather than pulmonary hypertension of the newborn (PPHN) or pneumothorax. Cautious attempts at weaning MAP should be made at least daily, as long as oxygen requirement remains low. If lowering MAP results in increased oxygen requirement, the MAP needs to briefly increase above the previous value to reinflate the lung and then be returned to the value that was adequate to maintain oxygenation previously. Tingay et al. demonstrated that many infants with RDS receiving HFOV could benefit from periodic reassessment of the optimal MAP, which changes over time (Fig. 24.15).[109] Routine suctioning should be avoided in the first week or two in infants with RDS, because secretions are seldom a problem and any disconnection/suctioning will result in derecruitment. Some experts advocate a sustained inflation (SI) maneuver (inflating the lungs with a high MAP for 15–20 seconds) to reinflate the lung after any disconnection, or when FiO2 increases, to reestablish adequate end-expiratory lung volume, but a more gradual lung volume recruitment maneuver as described earlier is likely a safer approach. If oxygenation does not improve or worsens, a chest radiograph may be

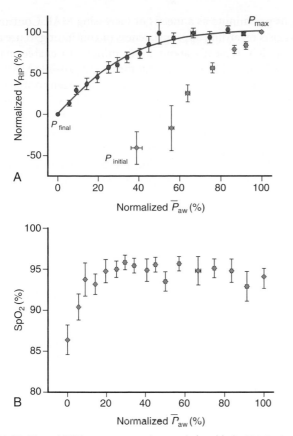

Fig. 24.15 (A and B) The pressure-volume relationship in 12 infants with respiratory failure during treatment with high-frequency oscillatory ventilation. *Diamonds* show the inflation limb; *circles*, the deflation limb of the curve. Inflation curves were established in individual patients by increasing $\overline{P}_{aw}$ from the baseline clinical value by 2 cm H_2O every 10 minutes until no further increase in SaO_2 was seen or SaO_2 decreased; deflation curves were established by decreasing $\overline{P}_{aw}$ from the maximum value by 2 cm $H2O$ until baseline pressures were reached, then decreases were continued by 1 cm H_2O until SaO_2 fell to 85% for more than 5 minutes or a $\overline{P}_{aw}$ of 5 cm H_2O was reached. Volume changes were estimated using respiratory impedance plethysmography. (From Tingay DG, Mills JF, Morley CJ, Pellicano A, Dargaville PA: The deflation limb of the pressure-volume relationship in infants during high-frequency ventilation. Am J Respir Crit Care Med 173:414, 2006.)

needed to evaluate possible other causes of increasing oxygen requirement. Avoiding the need to disconnect the infant when changing between conventional and HFOV ventilation is one of the advantages of the modern HFOV devices capable of both HFOV and CV that, as of this writing, are available only outside the United States.

Initial HFOV frequency for a premature infant with RDS is typically set between 10 and 15 Hz. There is seldom a need to change the frequency; however, if the frequency is altered, it is important to be mindful of the effect of frequency on delivered V_T as discussed earlier in this chapter. Some clinicians prefer to control V_T (and thereby $PaCO_2$) indirectly by manipulating frequency, rather than pressure amplitude. The relative merits of the two approaches have not been directly compared, but there is some evidence that lung injury may be minimized by using the highest frequency consistent with adequate CO_2 elimination,[112] which would suggest that increasing the

frequency to improve ventilation may not be the best approach early in the course of RDS.

The pressure amplitude, or ΔP, is the primary determinant of CO_2 removal. The initial amplitude setting is based on experience and estimation of lung compliance and subsequently adjusted based on adequacy of chest wall movement, transcutaneous CO_2, or measured V_T, when available. A commonly used, but not evidence-based, "rule of thumb" is to start with an amplitude that is twice the MAP value and adjust based on the subjective impression of adequate chest wall movement or "wiggle," which requires substantial experience. Increasing ΔP increases V_T and chest wall movement and decreases $PaCO_2$ values, sometimes dramatically. Use of a transcutaneous CO_2 monitor will provide important data on minute-to-minute gas exchange. Decreasing airway pressure amplitude decreases V_T and chest wall movement and increases $PaCO_2$ values. After assessment of the initial $PaCO_2$ value on HFOV, the amplitude is then adjusted up or down as necessary to produce the desired $PaCO_2$ levels. If a transcutaneous monitor is not available, frequent assessment of $PaCO_2$ values will be needed until the patient is stabilized within the goal range. In the absence of the ability to monitor V_T, continued vigilance is essential because changes in lung compliance may occur quite rapidly and result in large swings in $PaCO_2$ owing to the geometric relationship of V_T and CO_2 removal.

Several modern HFOV devices can monitor V_T and display a calculated value for CO_2 removal, termed DCO_2. Tracking DCO_2 allows the clinician to detect changes in ventilation and respond quickly, similar to what tracking transcutaneous CO_2 allows. Even more attractive is the ability of some of these devices to maintain a target V_T by means of a volume-targeted mode, analogous to volume-targeting with CMV. Once an appropriate V_T is identified, that V_T will be maintained by automatic adjustment of pressure amplitude, despite changes in lung mechanics, analogous to adjustment in PIP with CMV in volume-targeted mode.[113] When the volume-targeted mode is used with HFOV, changes in frequency will no longer produce the usual changes in minute ventilation, because the V_T will be unaffected by the frequency change. Consequently, with volume-targeted HFOV, changes in frequency will have the same effect as with CMV: increasing frequency decreases PCO_2.[114] Available data indicate that just as with CMV, ventilator frequency, patient size, age, as well as the nature and severity of the disease process influence the appropriate choice of V_T, which typically ranges between 0.8 mL/kg up to more than 2 mL/kg, with values around 1.6 to 1.8 mL/kg being a good starting point. As of this writing, there is limited information about the effectiveness of this important enhancement, but it appears to be effective and promises to greatly reduce the risk of hypocapnia during HFOV.[115-120]

Weaning from HFOV includes lowering of MAP as tolerated and manual or automated (i.e., with HFOV + VG) weaning of ΔP. If oxygen requirement remains low, cautious lowering of P_{aw} should be attempted daily or more often in the acute phase of the disease. As compliance improves, the $\overline{P}_{aw}$ may become excessive and compromise gas exchange as well as venous return/cardiac output. Excessive $\overline{P}_{aw}$ also increases pulmonary vascular resistance and can compromise pulmonary blood flow. Some authors recommend daily chest radiographs to monitor lung volume, with a target expansion indicated by the dome of the diaphragm projecting over 8½ to 9½ ribs. The appearance of the lung fields, heart size, and the shape of the diaphragm are perhaps even more important indicators of lung inflation. If volume-targeted HFOV is used, pressure amplitude is weaned automatically in response to improved lung compliance. $\bar{P}_{aw}$, however, needs to be weaned manually as needed. Available evidence suggests that the benefits of HFOV may be negated by early return to CV,[45] and therefore, it is recommended that HFOV is continued until extubation in most infants. Extubation directly to noninvasive support is usually possible, except in the most immature infants who never reach extubatable levels of support or fail extubation and go on to develop chronic lung disease of prematurity. There is no evidence that HFOV offers advantage over CV in infants with evolving BPD, and transitioning to CV is generally preferable after 2 to 3 weeks of mechanical ventilation if extubation is not feasible or fails.

High-Frequency Jet Ventilation Strategy in Respiratory Distress Syndrome

Although more widely understood to be an inherent aspect of HFOV, the same open lung approach can and should be used with HFJV when treating RDS or any other condition where atelectasis may occur. The MAP (we use this term here because that is what the Life Pulse ventilator labels this value) is increased by increasing PEEP (provided by the tandem conventional ventilator), using the same basic approach of stepwise increases in PEEP until an open lung is achieved, as evidenced by the ability to lower FiO$_2$ below 0.30. A study in preterm lambs showed decreased final pressure requirements, improved compliance, and reduced inflammatory markers using this technique.[121] When using HFJV in atelectasis-prone lung disease, the clinician needs to become comfortable with using PEEP levels that are substantially higher than those commonly used with CMV. The reason is the extremely short inspiratory time that results in I:E ratio of about 1:6 at the usual HFJV rate of 420 per minute. Thus, because the bulk of the ventilator cycle is spent at the level of PEEP, the MAP is only modestly above the set PEEP, which therefore has a disproportionately large impact on MAP. As with HFOV, once the lung is fully recruited, MAP (i.e., PEEP) must be lowered cautiously to avoid lung overexpansion. As with all ventilators, oxygenation is primarily determined by MAP. Unlike the traditional piston oscillator, the Bunnell jet ventilator provides the opportunity to deliver background "sigh" inflations using the tandem conventional ventilator. A rate of two to five inflations per minute may be used to facilitate lung recruitment if areas of atelectasis are present. If the PIP of the sighs is set slightly below the Jet PIP, the Jet ventilator will continue to cycle during the sigh. When the PIP of the sighs is close to or above the Jet PIP, the ventilator will pause and resume when the sigh is completed. There are no comparative data to inform the best choice here, but in the published RCTs, the former strategy was used. Sigh breaths should be given at a PIP that will not contribute to volutrauma or barotrauma and should not be used at a rate of more than 5 sighs per minute as a means of increasing MAP. Controversy also exists regarding appropriateness of continuing to use a low rate of sigh, typically about 2 per minute, to enable maintenance of optimal lung volume at the lowest possible MAP, or to discontinue sighs once lung recruitment has been completed, as the manufacturer recommends. One author (MK) favors continuing the sighs, as was done in the clinical trials for the following reasons: because there are gravity-dependent differences in closing pressure, it is impossible to keep the entire lung optimally inflated. A distending pressure that is sufficient to maintain full aeration of the dependent lung regions will inevitably overexpand the apical portion. Thus, an intermediate distending pressure with occasional sighs might allow more optimal lung aeration with a lower MAP and less hemodynamic impairment. Another author (SEC) uses sighs only if areas of atelectasis are present with areas of overdistension on chest radiographs, reasoning that with homogeneous lung disease, optimal MAP (with PEEP) should allow optimal lung aeration. However, no studies have been performed to resolve this controversy.

Historically, HFJV was primarily used to treat air leak, rather than atelectasis-prone lungs, and thus was typically used at a lower MAP than CMV. Predictably, this strategy resulted in greater ventilation/perfusion mismatch and higher oxygen requirement. Consequently, HFJV acquired a reputation for not being as good as HFOV for oxygenation. It is important to understand that this reputation was simply a function of the low pressure strategy that was used; oxygenation with HFJV is comparable to HFOV (and may be even better in some circumstances) when a similar MAP is used. The background sigh rate should not be increased further if oxygenation remains a problem; increasing PEEP is the appropriate way to achieve adequate lung recruitment.

PaCO$_2$ is controlled primarily by adjustments in pressure amplitude, which equals PIP minus PEEP. Tidal volume measurement with HFJV is currently not clinically available, so assessment of chest wall movement and transcutaneous CO$_2$ monitoring are used to monitor the adequacy of ventilation. Because of the unique nature of gas flow within the large airways, proper endotracheal tube position is critical. Optimal ventilation is achieved when the jet stream travels down the center of the airway unimpeded. This occurs when the head is in midline and slightly extended, with the endotracheal tube at least 1 cm above the carina. If the tube is too close to the carina, the jet stream either hits the carina and partially disperses or preferentially travels down one or the other mainstem bronchus, leading to uneven ventilation. Turning of the head sharply to one side results in the endotracheal tube entering the trachea at an angle, causing the jet stream to hit the wall of the trachea and disperse, causing deterioration of clinical status and possibly also contributing to mucosal injury. An acute change in PaCO$_2$ is almost always related to endotracheal tube malposition or secretions in the airway and must be promptly recognized and corrected. Because pressure amplitude is not set directly, it is important to remember to adjust PIP as needed to maintain the desired ΔP when changing PEEP. However, because changes in MAP may lead to changes in lung compliance, the need for PIP adjustment is not always predictable. The use of transcutaneous monitoring of $PaCO_2$ is therefore advised. HFJV is commonly used in the setting of hypercapnia and its use often results in dramatic drop in $PaCO_2$, prompting relatively rapid lowering of PIP, ideally based on visual assessment of chest wall movement and transcutaneous CO_2 monitoring. Such large drops in PIP, while appropriate, may lead to an inadvertent fall in MAP, if not compensated by an increase in PEEP. The danger is that after a period of relative alkalosis that necessitates rapid weaning of PIP, the loss of lung recruitment can lead to atelectasis, drop in lung compliance, and subsequent hypercapnia, increasing the risk of IVH. Failure to understand the interdependence of PIP changes on MAP and of PEEP changes on pressure amplitude is a common problem for clinicians more accustomed to HFOV, where amplitude and MAP are set independently.

Depending on clinician preference and availability of devices, patients can remain on HFJV until sufficiently low settings are achieved to allow for extubation directly to CPAP or another form of noninvasive ventilation or may be switched to CMV when lower pressures provide sufficient support. The benefits of HFOV appear to be negated by early return to CMV and the same likely applies to HFJV as well. However, after 2 to 4 weeks, if the infant cannot be extubated to noninvasive support, transition to CMV may be appropriate, as there is no clear evidence that HFJV is superior to CMV in chronic lung disease. If HFJV is continued beyond 7 to 10 days or if evidence of air leak or overdistension is present, the ventilator rate should be gradually lowered to provide sufficient expiratory time to avoid air-trapping that may develop as airway resistance begins to increase. A general schematic of the approach to lung volume optimization applicable to all modes of ventilation is shown in Fig. 24.16.

Air-Leak Syndromes

The presence of an air leak is perhaps the most common indication for HFV today and was the original clinical use of HFJV.[13,18,27] Although all forms of HFV are used in patients with air leak, the evidence is most definitive for HFJV. There are few RCTs evaluating the management of air-leak syndromes with HFV versus CMV, and those that have been done are now quite old. Keszler et al.[31] compared rapid CMV and HFJV in 144 infants with severe PIE. Some 61% of those treated with HFJV improved, compared to only 37% treated with rapid rate CMV. For ethical reasons, the study allowed for crossover when predefined failure criteria were reached. About half of the babies were successfully rescued after crossover from CMV to HFJV compared with only 9% going from HFJV to CMV. The multicenter HIFO study of infants with RDS also examined the effect of HFOV on air leak.[82] Although HFOV patients who entered the study with air leaks tended to do better than their counterparts treated with CMV, the differences were not significant.

HFJV with low ventilatory rates may be particularly good for air leaks because of the extremely short inspiratory time (0.02 seconds), with relatively long expiratory time. In the large airways, the jet stream moves rapidly past any disruption of the airway and exerts minimal pressure on the lateral wall of the airway, resulting in minimal loss of gas. At the small airway

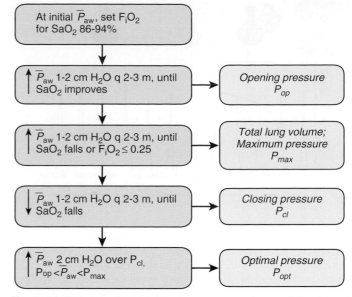

Fig. 24.16 Technique for defining the pressure-volume relationship of the lungs during treatment. Using systematic stepwise increases and decreases $\overline{P}_{aw}$ in, the clinician can find the opening pressure, maximum pressure (total lung volume), and closing pressure of each individual patient and target the optimal pressure for ventilation. (Modified from De Jaegere A, van Veenendaal MB, Michiels A, van Kaam AH: Lung recruitment using oxygenation during open lung high-frequency ventilation in preterm infants. Am J Respir Crit Care Med 174:639, 2006.)

level, an air leak will persist when gas is delivered at a pressure that opens the injured tissue, creating a low-resistance path for flow. The leak will continue during an inspiration for as long as the pressure exceeds that needed to stent the leak open. During CMV or HFOV, because of both the inspiratory time and the characteristics of gas flow, a leak may persist, whereas during HFJV, it may rapidly close (Fig. 24.17).

The low occurrence rates of bronchopleural and tracheoesophageal fistulas in neonates preclude the ability to perform adequately powered randomized clinical trials. However, a few studies have formally evaluated the amount of air leak through these types of fistulas using HFJV versus CMV. Gonzalez and colleagues[122] showed a decrease in chest tube air leak when using HFJV versus CMV in infants with bronchopleural fistula. Goldberg et al.[123] and Donn et al.[124] reported similar findings in managing infants with tracheoesophageal fistulas with HFJV. An animal study by Orlando et al. further supports the potential benefit to the use of HFJV in the ventilatory stabilization of patients with tracheoesophageal or bronchopleural fistula.[125] Although these studies were small and done many years ago, their findings do support use of HFJV for air leak especially in view of the pathophysiology of these conditions and the physics of HFJV.

High-Frequency Jet Ventilation Strategy in Air-Leak Syndromes

As discussed earlier, where available, HFJV is generally the treatment of choice for all forms of air leak. The general strategy includes minimal PIP necessary for acceptable CO_2 removal (recall that leak occurs during inflation) and somewhat lower ventilator rate (280–360 per minute in preterm infants; 240–320 per minute

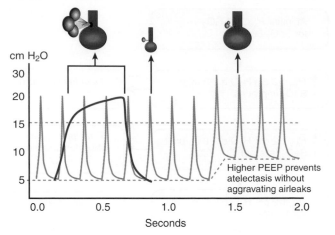

Fig. 24.17 Schematic representation of the impact of conventional inflations (red waveform) vs high-frequency jet ventilation "breaths" (blue waveform) on leakage through a tissue rent. Because airway pressure exceeds the threshold for leakage for a longer period with conventional ventilation, more air leaks and the rent is stented open. With jet ventilation, the threshold is exceeded only briefly, which limits the amount of leak and allows healing to occur. Traditional strategy employed very low end-expiratory pressure, but this resulted in generalized atelectasis (left side of the figure). Current approach utilizes higher end-expiratory pressure, which is still below threshold for leakage and thus does not worsen the leak while allowing better lung volume recruitment (right side of the figure). *PEEP*, Positive end-expiratory pressure.

in large infants) to further shorten the I:E ratio and ensure adequate expiratory time that may be needed because air trapped in the interstitium often impinges on the small airways and increases airway resistance. Background sigh should not be used and aggressive lung volume recruitment is contraindicated. However, the strategy has evolved to now include a higher PEEP level than was used in the early days of HFJV. The low PEEP approach was effective in resolving PIE, but it often resulted in progressive atelectasis

because PIE typically coexists with atelectasis-prone lung disease. Because loss of lung volume worsens lung compliance, a higher PIP would eventually be required. The current approach recognizes that air generally escapes from the airway only during peak inflation. A moderate level of PEEP sufficient to maintain adequate lung inflation will not cause air to escape during the expiratory phase, thus still allowing air leak to resolve. In practical terms, we typically use PEEP of 6 to 8 cm H_2O, but individual patients may need higher values to maintain adequate lung volume. In the presence of unilateral PIE (or other unilateral pathology), HFJV has a unique advantage because it is possible to selectively direct the jet stream into the unaffected lung, allowing the injured lung to recover, often dramatically (Fig. 24.18). This "virtual selective bronchus intubation" takes advantage of the unique flow characteristics of the jet ventilator and is accomplished by advancing the endotracheal tube to within 0.5 cm of the carina and turning the head to the opposite side, which angles the tube toward the lung we wish to preferentially ventilate (i.e., turn the head to the left to direct the jet stream toward the right mainstem bronchus). It is important to monitor for resolution of the problem and return to ventilating both lungs before the other lung becomes atelectatic.

High-Frequency Oscillatory Ventilation Strategy in Air Leak

NICUs that have access to HFJV usually switch to that modality when air leak develops. HFOV may offer some benefit when HFJV is not available.[126] The optimal strategy for the treatment of air leak with HFOV is less well established but generally follows the same principles as outlined earlier, namely, lower ventilator frequency, permissive hypercapnia, and acceptance of higher FiO_2 in exchange for a lower P_{aw}. With some of the newer HFOV devices, a 1:3 I:E ratio can be employed to mimic HFJV, but the benefit of that approach is unproven as the resulting shorter inspiratory times require higher oscillatory pressures to achieve adequate ventilation.

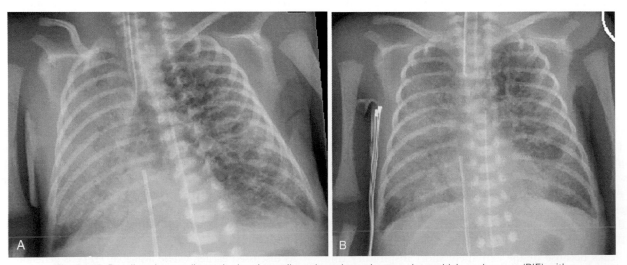

Fig. 24.18 Baseline chest radiograph showing unilateral tension pulmonary interstitial emphysema (PIE) with atelectasis of the right lung and partial herniation of the left lung across the midline **(A)**. Following 12 hours of selective right lung ventilation by aiming the jet ventilation stream into the right mainstem bronchus without actual mainstem bronchus intubation, there is improved aeration of the right lung with resolution of tension and substantial resolution of PIE on the left **(B)**.

Pulmonary Hypoplasia and Congenital Diaphragmatic Hernia

When the lungs are hypoplastic, the number of gas-exchanging units is decreased, and thus, it is reasonable to assume that ventilation at rapid rates using very low V_T would be less injurious, compared to ventilation with normal tidal volume that is likely to lead to volutrauma. Because of the variety of conditions associated with pulmonary hypoplasia and their relative rarity, controlled studies are difficult to design or perform, and clear evidence-based guidelines simply are not available. However, infants with various forms of pulmonary hypoplasia may derive at least short-term benefit from HFV.

Both HFOV and HFJV may be effective in congenital diaphragmatic hernia (CDH), but the evidence is equivocal. Early studies of HFV treatment before extracorporeal membrane oxygenation (ECMO) had varying results.[127-131] Despite ongoing widespread use of HFOV in this population and the sound rationale for its use, more recent studies do not clearly support the use of HFV in CDH. Migliazza and colleagues[132] retrospectively reviewed 111 babies with CDH treated with early HFOV for both preoperative stabilization and postoperative care. They saw a 69.4% survival overall, compared to a predicted 69% survival based on the CDH Study Group formula. A 2007 review summarizing "best-evidence practice strategies" for management of CDH discussed HFOV; they found no consistent approach and no clear evidence supporting HFOV over conventional approaches to respiratory support.[133]

The sole RCT evaluating the presumed benefits of HFOV in infants with CDH (the VICI trial) was challenged by slow recruitment and was abandoned when an interim analysis showed no hint of benefit of HFOV as applied in that trial.[134] A total of 41 patients (45%) randomized to CMV died or developed BPD compared with 43 patients (54%) in the high-frequency oscillation group. Patients initially ventilated by CMV were ventilated for fewer days ($P = .03$); less often needed ECMO support ($P = .007$), iNO ($P = .045$), or sildenafil ($P = .004$); had a shorter duration of vasoactive drug use ($P = .02$); and less often failed treatment ($P = .01$) as compared with infants initially ventilated by high-frequency oscillation.[134]

The poor response to HFOV in this study was likely related to the aggressive lung volume recruitment strategy used in the HFOV arm, in contrast to the appropriate gentle conventional strategy utilizing low PEEP. So, it is important to understand that although HFOV as used in that study was inferior to CMV, a more gentle HFOV approach appears to be more successful.[135] (See also Chapter 35.)

Preterm infants with a history of prolonged rupture of fetal membranes are another common condition that presents with pulmonary hypoplasia. Both HFOV and HFJV have been used in this scenario (often in conjunction with iNO) with anecdotal good response,[136,137] but randomized trials are lacking.

HFJV may be more effective when used with CDH.

High-Frequency Oscillatory Ventilation Strategy in Congenital Diaphragmatic Hernia and Other Lung Hypoplasia Conditions

Because of the concerning findings of the VICI trial, most clinicians initiate mechanical ventilation with conventional modes but have a low threshold to change to HFV if PIP greater than about 25 cm H_2O is needed. Because lung hypoplasia is often associated with pulmonary hypertension and because both overexpansion and underexpansion of the lungs increase pulmonary vascular resistance, it is critical to use the lowest $\bar{P}_{aw}$ that will achieve adequate lung inflation. Optimal lung volume is difficult to judge radiographically in the presence of pulmonary hypoplasia; the appearance of the lung fields, heart size, and diaphragms, not just the rib count, need to be taken into account. Trial-and-error adjustments of $\bar{P}_{aw}$ are sometimes necessary, but in any case, the goal is to avoid $\bar{P}_{aw}$ that worsens pulmonary hypertension. Other aspects of HFOV management are similar to infants with RDS, with the exception of more attention to hemodynamic consequences of ventilator adjustments and more permissive hypercapnia.

High-Frequency Jet Ventilation Strategy Congenital Diaphragmatic Hernia and Other Lung Hypoplasia Conditions

Despite the paucity of published data, HFJV may be better suited to treat pulmonary hypoplasia because of its ability to support effective gas exchange at low MAP, which should limit the risk of overexpansion and worsening pulmonary hypertension.[138] HFJV is used successfully during transport of unstable infants with CDH.[139] The ability of HFJV to ventilate effectively with lower MAP has less adverse effect on pulmonary blood flow in preclinical studies and after cardiac surgery in infants[140,141] and may aid in avoiding lung overexpansion and compromise of pulmonary blood flow in pulmonary hypoplasia. No direct comparisons between HFOV and HFJV are available, and the choice of modality is primarily based on personal preference and training.

Hypoxemic Respiratory Failure in Term Infants

Both HFOV and HFJV are commonly used, often in conjunction with iNO, as a treatment for severe respiratory failure secondary to meconium aspiration and other causes of hypoxemic respiratory failure. Kinsella et al. reported increased effectiveness of iNO when combined with HFOV when pulmonary hypertension was secondary to severe parenchymal lung disease, likely because of improved lung aeration.[87] The benefits of the combined use of iNO and HFV appear to also extend to HFJV. An observational study by Coates et al. found that fewer infants with PPHN required ECMO when treated with HFJV + iNO, compared with HFOV + iNO.[142] Evidence from randomized trials of HFOV and HFJV compared to CV is suggestive of benefit, but not conclusive,[24,45] Detailed discussion regarding management of PPHN in preterm and term neonates can be found in Chapter 34.

KNOWLEDGE GAPS AND RESEARCH DIRECTIONS

As mentioned on many occasions earlier in this chapter, the evidence base for clinical guidelines remains incomplete with many knowledge gaps that need answers. Although approved for general use, the role of HFV remains undefined in many respects.

Many different HFV devices are in use around the world. There are important differences in the capabilities of various ventilators and important differences in the dynamics of gas flow among HFOV, HFFI, and HFJV. There is a lack of adequate direct comparisons between various forms of HFV. Generalizations and recommendations developed for one ventilator may or may not apply to others. Some performance limitations are imposed by device design, although under normal clinical conditions and settings, these do not come into play.[143,144] Perhaps most importantly, the results of studies not only reflect the characteristics of the devices and the population under study but are greatly affected by the strategies and skill with which they are used, making interpretation of clinical trials complicated.

In the absence of a good technique for monitoring lung volumes at the bedside, there is concern that HFV could produce lung overdistention by quietly trapping gas. We know that under some circumstances, HFV may produce higher distal end-expiratory volumes and pressures at lower proximal airway pressures. Thome et al. showed that tracheal pressure was higher than circuit pressure with I:E ratio of 1:1, but lower when 1:2 I:E ratio was used.[145] Such silent distending pressure is commonly referred to as inadvertent PEEP (see Chapter 2). Because this pressure cannot be easily measured, the extent to which it produces problems is unknown but may have contributed to some of the disappointing results in HFOV studies that used the 1:1 I:E ratio.[44,51,54] In some circumstances, inadvertent PEEP may cause substantial difficulty with ventilation. Because HFJV depends on passive exhalation, the ventilator rate must be lowered to avoid this inadvertent PEEP in conditions of increasing airway resistance. For example, extremely small infants intubated with a 2.0mm endotracheal tube must be ventilated at rates of 240-280 to allow sufficient expiratory time necessitated by the high resistance of the tube. This possibility should always be considered when CO_2 retention develops in a baby beyond the first few days of life and/or overexpansion is noted on chest radiograph. HFOV may cause silent air trapping due to small airway collapse during the active exhalation phase if the pressure amplitude is relatively large, compared to the P_{aw}: large amplitudes relative to the P_{aw} produce negative pressure and choke points in small airways that are surrounded by terminal lung units that by definition must have a higher pressure in order to generate outward flow.

There is also a concern that HFV may lead to atelectasis. Under normal circumstances, small monotonous V_Ts delivered at relatively constant pressures result in progressive atelectasis. Early HFOV primate studies document that this atelectasis does occur, but the problem is almost always due to inadequate P_{aw} with resulting low end-expiratory lung volumes and lack of spontaneous breathing/sighs. Intermittent ventilator inflations (i.e., a background intermittent mandatory ventilation rate) or spontaneous sighs may overcome this concern but increasing P_{aw} may have the same effect. The knowledge base regarding appropriate V_T during HFV under different circumstances is still being accumulated. Newer machines provide volume targeting, which is not well studied in HFV but offers real promise.[120] It is not clear if SI is better

than gradual increase and then decrease in $\overline{P}_{aw}$. A 2009 study investigated four techniques for lung volume recruitment: stepwise increases in $\overline{P}_{aw}$, using a 20-second SI, using six 1-second repeated SIs, and setting a single higher $\overline{P}_{aw}$ without change.[146] The stepwise increases in $\overline{P}_{aw}$, followed by a reduction in pressure after the maneuver was completed, produced the greatest increase in thoracic gas volume, the best redistribution of aeration, and the greatest change in SaO2. A bedside technique for rapid accurate assessment of changes in lung volume is needed to assist the clinician no matter the technique.

High-frequency techniques have been associated with rare complications. A number of early reports linked tracheal inflammation and tracheal obstructions to various forms of HFV.[147] This unique tracheal injury, referred to as NTB, was to a large extent a function of inadequate humidification and has not been observed in contemporary neonatal care settings. Subsequent studies demonstrated that tracheal mucosal injury is also seen in other forms of mechanical ventilation, including HFOV, HFFI, and CV; excessive tracheal pressure and hypotension were identified as contributing factors.[32,148,149]

Previously, the most serious potential side effect of HFV was the concern that an increase in long-term neurologic injury may occur, resulting from an increase in early PVL or severe IVH. This concerning finding, originally reported in the HIFI trial,[44] was also seen in a study of HFJV reported by Wiswell et al.[75] These injuries seem to be linked to the strategy of ventilation used in these studies. Neither of these studies utilized a standardized technique for lung volume recruitment. Furthermore, hypocarbia during treatment was common, especially in the HFJV study. Meta-analyses of randomized trials of HFV have concluded that there is no evidence of increased neurologic injury in studies using an "optimal lung volume" strategy. Avoidance of inadvertent overventilation with the use of transcutaneous CO_2 monitoring or volume-targeted HFOV is likely to greatly reduce the risk of this serious complication.

SUMMARY

HFV is a unique and useful form of mechanical ventilation. Although not a panacea for all forms of neonatal respiratory failure, HFV is now a standard form of therapy for a wide variety of respiratory conditions. HFV can often produce excellent gas exchange at lower airway pressures than during CMV, and it allows safer application of high MAPs when necessary for lung volume recruitment and oxygenation. It is superior to CMV in air-leak syndromes and may be a useful rescue technique and/or bridge to ECMO. It has clear usefulness as a rescue or temporizing measure in pulmonary hypoplasia, persistent pulmonary hypertension, meconium aspiration and other forms of neonatal respiratory failure unresponsive to CMV. In neonatal RDS, early use of HFV, perhaps in association with surfactant therapy, may yet play a major role in improving long-term pulmonary outcomes. Volume-targeted HFV may provide even better therapy for neonatal respiratory diseases in the future.

KEY REFERENCES

10. Froese AB, Bryan AC: High frequency ventilation. Am Rev Respir Dis 135(6):1363–1374, 1987.
23. Keszler M, Modanlou HD, Brudno DS, et al: Multicenter controlled clinical trial of high-frequency jet ventilation in preterm infants with uncomplicated respiratory distress syndrome. Pediatrics 100(4):593–599, 1997.
31. Keszler M, Donn SM, Bucciarelli RL, et al: Multicenter controlled trial comparing high-frequency jet ventilation and conventional mechanical ventilation in newborn infants with pulmonary interstitial emphysema. J Pediatr 119(1 pt 1):85–93, 1991.
50. Courtney SE, Durand DJ, Asselin JM, et al: High-frequency oscillatory ventilation versus conventional mechanical ventilation for very-low-birth-weight infants. N Engl J Med 347(9):643–652, 2002.
51. Johnson AH, Peacock JL, Greenough A, et al: High-frequency oscillatory ventilation for the prevention of chronic lung disease of prematurity. N Engl J Med 47(9):633–642, 2002.
70. Cools F, Askie LM, Offringa M, et al: Elective high-frequency oscillatory versus conventional ventilation in preterm infants: a systematic review and meta-analysis of individual patients' data. Lancet 375(9731):2082–2091, 2010.
71. Cools F, Offringa M, Askie LM: Elective high frequency oscillatory ventilation versus conventional ventilation for acute pulmonary dysfunction in preterm infants. Cochrane Database Syst Rev (3):CD000104, 2015.
76. Wiswell TE, Graziani LJ, Kornhauser MS, et al: Effects of hypocarbia on the development of cystic periventricular leukomalacia in premature infants treated with high-frequency jet ventilation. Pediatrics 98(5):918–924, 1996.
103. Froese AB, McCulloch PR, Sugiura M, et al: Optimizing alveolar expansion prolongs the effectiveness of exogenous surfactant therapy in the adult rabbit. Am Rev Respir Dis 148(3):569–577, 1993.
121. Musk GC, Polglase GR, Bunnell JB, et al: High positive end-expiratory pressure during high-frequency jet ventilation improves oxygenation and ventilation in preterm lambs. Pediatric Res 69(4):319–324, 2011.

Mechanical Ventilation: Disease-Specific Strategies

Bradley A. Yoder and Peter H. Grubb

INTRODUCTION

When approaches to noninvasive respiratory support are insufficient to achieve adequate gas exchange, insertion of an endotracheal tube and mechanical ventilator support may be necessary. Once it is determined that mechanical ventilation is needed, a variety of factors should be considered. One factor is the type of mechanical ventilator to use, specifically either a more conventional approach or high-frequency ventilation. There are a number of conventional and high-frequency devices to choose from; most are covered in greater detail in other chapters and will not be specifically addressed here. A second factor to be considered is the mode of ventilator support to be applied. For conventional mechanical ventilation, several different support modes may be selected by device; again these are covered in more detail elsewhere in this book. A third factor to consider is the presumed benefits related to targeted gas exchange values and decreased work of breathing versus the relative risk of ventilator-induced lung injury (VILI). One also needs to incorporate the suspected underlying pathophysiologic features thought to be involved at the time of ventilator initiation, as well as the potential changes that may ensue over time. Finally, even from the time of initiating mechanical ventilator support, it is essential that the clinician has an active approach or plan for weaning and extubation (see also Chapter 26).

This chapter will discuss our approach to ventilator management in several of the most common neonatal respiratory disorders. It should be understood that there may be a variety of devices and approaches other than those described here that one could employ resulting in safe, effective respiratory support of the ill neonate. We firmly believe that the single most important factor associated with safe and successful ventilator management of the neonate is the person operating the device, not the device itself. A thorough understanding of the device, the mode applied, and the pathophysiology being managed, as well as a consistent, attentive approach to the specific infant being cared for, is essential to any success in managing respiratory problems in critically ill neonates.

RESPIRATORY DISTRESS SYNDROME

It is indeed ironic that over 40 years after the introduction of continuous positive airway pressure (CPAP) as the first effective therapy for neonatal respiratory distress syndrome (RDS), and despite the marked technological advances that have been made during that time span, there has been a renewed emphasis on the application of noninvasive approaches, such as nasal CPAP, for respiratory support of neonatal lung disease.[1] Despite the increasing success with noninvasive respiratory support, many neonates still require mechanical ventilator support for RDS, particularly those at the lowest gestational ages.

Key Pathophysiologic Features
Lung Surfactant

A comprehensive overview of surfactant and its role in neonatal RDS is beyond the scope of this presentation, and the reader is referred to Chapter 15 of this book and other publications for additional information.[2-5] Quantitative, qualitative, and metabolic disturbances in lung surfactant play key roles in the pathophysiology of neonatal RDS. The net effect is decreased compliance of distal airspaces that can lead to atelectasis, ventilation:perfusion mismatch, and intrapulmonary shunt.[2-5] Surfactant proteins play a critical role not only in the function of surfactant but also in the lung's response to infection. The indications for and approach to surfactant replacement therapy for neonatal RDS continues to be an area of very active investigation but will not be addressed in this chapter.[6-8]

Lung Liquid

Normal fetal lung growth is regulated, in part, via fluid secreted into the potential airspace across the alveolar epithelial cells. Fetal lung liquid secretion is generated via up-regulated Cl^- channels that actively transport Cl^- into the lung lumen, with Na^+ and H_2O following via an osmotic gradient.[9] During fetal life, the epithelial Na^+ channel that promotes Na^+ and fluid absorption from the airspace in postnatal life is down regulated. Delayed up-regulation of the all three subunits of the epithelial Na^+ channel has been found in preterm infants with RDS, persisting in some to at least 1 month of age.[10] Additional factors that may contribute to persistent fetal lung liquid formation and delayed reabsorption of airspace fluid following preterm delivery include variable expression and activity of aquaporin channel proteins and persistent function of the secretory Cl^- channels.[11]

Developmental Lung Biology

Development of the mammalian lung is a complex, highly orchestrated process that is subject to interruption from numerous insults, particularly premature birth. The progressive stages of lung development are well described and include embryonic, pseudoglandular, canalicular, saccular, and alveolar stages.[12] Vasculogenesis and angiogenesis, critical processes to lung growth and differentiation, are tightly coregulated throughout lung development. Postnatal viability first becomes possible for the human fetus during the latter phase of the canalicular stage, which occurs between 20 and 28 weeks' gestation, or approximately 50% to 70% gestation. During this stage, rudimentary air sacs begin to form off the terminal airways, simple interstitial capillaries begin to organize around these potential airspaces, and type I and type II epithelial cells begin to differentiate, with type II cells beginning to produce surfactant.[12] It must always be remembered that preterm birth, with subsequent exposure to increased ambient oxygen, unplanned gaseous inflation of the distal airspace, microbial colonization associated with prolonged tracheal intubation, and disturbances in nutrition, initiates a dramatic change in lung growth and development. The effect on lung growth and function, particularly at gestation under 30 weeks, may likely be lifelong, even for infants not diagnosed with bronchopulmonary dysplasia.[13,14] It is in the context of this immature stage of lung development, and the potential for adverse effects, that the following discussion on ventilatory support for neonatal RDS should be considered (Table 25.1).

Relevant Principles of Ventilation

In our neonatal intensive care unit (NICU) we most commonly use high-frequency oscillatory ventilation (HFOV) as the initial mode of support for those infants who require mechanical ventilation for neonatal RDS, at any gestational age. It is important to emphasize that there is no clear evidence that HFOV provides increased benefit (nor risk) compared with more conventional approaches to mechanical ventilation (i.e., volume-targeted, surfactant treated) in terms of short-term outcomes such as initial gas exchange and subsequent diagnosis of bronchopulmonary dysplasia (BPD) before initial discharge.[15] Our approach to conventional ventilation, which is primarily

TABLE 25.1 Pathophysiology of Respiratory Distress Syndrome of Prematurity

Factor	Effect	Possible Intervention
Surfactant	Reduced quantity	Antenatal steroid therapy
	Impaired metabolism	Surfactant replacement
	Reduced surfactant proteins	Surfactant specific proteins
	Disrupted function— proteins	Additional surfactant therapy
Lung liquid	Reduced clearance	Antenatal steroid therapy
	Sustained production	Postnatal steroid therapy
Mechanical	Reduced airspace compliance	Surfactant therapy
	High chest wall compliance	Positive end-expiratory pressure
	Increased airway compliance	Low inspiratory tidal volumes
Development	Canalicular-saccular stage	Antenatal steroid therapy
	Thickened mesenchyme	Maternal stress
	Immature capillary development	? Effect of subclinical chorioamnionitis
Inflammation	Altered surfactant metabolism	Antenatal steroid therapy
	Disrupted membrane integrity	Prevention/treatment of chorioamnionitis
	Interrupted lung development	Postnatal steroids and other antiinflammatories

TABLE 25.2 Indications for Trial of Noninvasive Respiratory Support

Indication	Comment
Consider noninvasive initially	• All infants >25 weeks' gestation
After 10 minutes of resuscitation if:	• Indication for intubation has resolved but requires FiO_2 0.3–0.5 to maintain targeted SpO_2
After surfactant administration if:	• $FiO_2 < 0.4$ & decreasing while maintaining targeted SpO_2
	• No marked retractions
	• No suspected airway obstruction
	• >5 minutes since surfactant delivered
While on mechanical ventilation if:	• On high-frequency oscillation (see Fig. 25.1)
	• On conventional ventilation (see Fig. 25.1)
Other	• Consider early/preextubation caffeine for infants <32 weeks' gestation
	• Wean/discontinue sedation/narcotics before extubation

FiO₂, Fraction of inspired oxygen; *SpO₂*, oxygen saturation.

volume targeted in nature, will also be discussed. Regardless of the mode of ventilation employed, the primary objective in the management of neonatal RDS is to minimize the initial use and/or duration of exposure to any form of invasive mechanical ventilation through aggressive application of early noninvasive modes of respiratory support (Tables 25.2 and 25.3), as well the application of written guidelines to promote weaning and extubation from mechanical ventilation when applied (Table 25.4). The key to management includes recognition of the predominant underlying pulmonary pathophysiology, which for RDS is

TABLE 25.3 Possible Indications for Intubation and Mechanical Ventilation in Neonates

Indication	Comment
Infant <25 weeks' gestation	Consider for prophylactic surfactant therapy
Apnea/bradycardia	Refractory; recurrent; unresponsive to BMV
Hypoxemia	FiO_2 >0.6 to maintain targeted PaO_2/SpO_2
Hypercapnia	$PaCO_2$ >65 mm Hg with pH <7.20
Severe distress	Marked retractions on noninvasive support
Suspected airway obstruction	Severe micrognathia, oropharyngeal mass, other
Cardiovascular collapse	Heart rate <60 or shock; CPR
Congenital malformations	Diaphragmatic hernia, choanal atresia, other

BMV, Bag mask ventilation; *CPR*, cardiopulmonary resuscitation; *FiO_2*, fraction of inspired oxygen; *PaO_2*, partial pressure arterial oxygen; *$PaCO_2$*, partial pressure arterial carbon dioxide; *SpO_2*, oxygen saturation.

TABLE 25.4 Guidelines for Recommending Extubation Based on Current Weight, Ventilator Mode, and Ventilator Settings (Assumes Stable Airway and Minimal Apnea)

	WEIGHT (g)			
	<1000	**1000–2000**	**2000–3000**	**>3000**
High-Frequency Ventilation				
P_{aw}	8	9–10	10–12	12
ΔP/amp	16	18	20	22
FiO_2	<0.40			
PC-SIMV and PSV				
PIP	<16	16–20	20	
PEEP	<6		<7	<8
PS	<6–8			
FiO_2	<0.40			
Rate	16–20 breaths per minute			
SIMV + VG and PSV				
PIP	<16	16–20	20	
PEEP	<6		<7	<8
V_T	4–5 mL/kg			
PS	<6–8			
FiO_2	<0.40			
Rate	16–20 breaths per minute			

FiO_2, Fraction of inspired oxygen; *ΔP/amp*, change in pressure amplitude; *P_{aw}*, mean airway pressure; *PC*, pressure control; *PEEP*, positive end expiratory pressure; *PIP*, peak inspiratory pressure; *PS*, pressure support; *PSV*, pressure support ventilation; *SIMV*, synchronized intermittent mandatory ventilation; *VG*, volume guarantee; *V_T*, tidal volume.

typically a diffuse "alveolar" disease, coupled with the underlying potential to disrupt immature lung development through pathways leading to or associated with VILI.[16-18] The management of the very preterm infant is additionally confounded by the underlying fetal inflammatory milieu that is often present in association with clinical/subclinical chorioamnionitis and impaired intrauterine growth.[19-21] The key to all lung-protective ventilation strategies in infants with diffuse alveolar disease (i.e., diffuse microatelectasis) is the recruitment and maintenance of optimal lung inflation and avoidance of excessive tissue stretch. In our NICU, we are comfortable achieving these goals with HFOV, but similar strategies can be achieved with conventional ventilation.

High-Frequency Ventilation

With HFOV, the key is to achieve initial airspace recruitment and then to maintain optimal lung inflation and gas exchange at the lowest acceptable mean airway pressure (P_{aw}) (Tables 25.5 and 25.6). The process for achieving this goal includes (1) an initial step-wise escalation in P_{aw} to recruit atelectatic airspaces indicated by the ability to significantly reduce fraction of inspired oxygen ([FiO_2] commonly referred to as the "opening pressure" for the lung); (2) a subsequent step-wise reduction in P_{aw} to a point at which FiO_2 needs to be again escalated to maintain targeted oxygen saturation ([SpO_2] commonly referred to as the "closing pressure" for the lung); and (3) increasing the P_{aw} back above the "closing pressure" (typically by 2–3 cm H_2O in surfactant treated infants) to maintain an end-expiratory lung volume (EELV) that allows effective gas exchange while minimizing pressure/volume effects on the cardiovascular system, thus "optimizing" oxygen delivery at the tissue/cellular level. A number of studies have described this approach using such measurements as SpO_2, respiratory inductance plethysmography, high-resolution computed tomography (CT) scan, and forced oscillatory exhalation.[22-25] Other than SpO_2, these tools are not currently available in most practice settings. Electrical impedance tomography (EIT) is a promising new technique that may facilitate this process in the future by enabling the clinician to visualize lung inflation and tidal ventilation in real time. However, as of this writing, EIT remains a research tool.[26,27] In clinical practice, we typically provide early surfactant replacement therapy to all preterm infants intubated for RDS, then begin the process of optimizing lung inflation. We do not usually reduce P_{aw} to "closing pressure" but more commonly will incrementally reduce P_{aw} by 1–2 cm H_2O once FiO_2 has been reduced to less than 0.25 (Table 25.7). Although radiographic lung volumes may not be ideal for assessing optimal lung inflation, when combined with clinical observations such as heart rate and blood pressure, as well as the temporal changes in FiO_2 and SpO_2, one can usually maintain adequate lung inflation and gas exchange while minimizing the risks of either overinflation or atelectasis.

Ventilation, or the removal of carbon dioxide (CO_2) during HFOV, is dependent on tidal volume (V_T) and rate. As described elsewhere in this book, during HFOV, V_T has a relatively greater effect on minute ventilation than rate. Factors affecting V_T during HFOV include lung compliance and resistance, inspiratory time, and the amplitude or power of the oscillatory breath. It is critical to remember that changes in frequency during HFOV can markedly affect V_T (increased as frequency decreases, and decreased as frequency increases). Dynamic changes in lung volume and compliance that accompany increased lung inflation can significantly impact not only oxygenation but also ventilation through effects on V_T.[24] As dramatic shifts can occur in partial

TABLE 25.5 Suggested Initial Approach to Mechanical Ventilation by Condition and Ventilatory Mode

Respiratory Disorder	Conventional Ventilation (Volume-Targeted, SIMV + PS, or AC)	High-Frequency Ventilation (HFOV, HFJV, Flow Interrupter)
RDS	Surfactant therapy Volume-target (V_T) @ 4–6 mL/kg; Rate 30–60 breaths per minute I-times 0.30–0.35 seconds PEEP @ 5–8 cm H_2O PS to achieve 2/3–3/4 set V_T	Surfactant therapy HFOV: Hz 8–12; P_{aw} 10–16; ΔP 2-x P_{aw} and adjust to vibrate chest/abd; I:E 1:2 HFJV: Rate 360–420; on-time 0.020 PEEP 7–10 cm H_2O (to optimize inflation) Minimal or no back-up rate
MAS	Surfactant therapy; ±iNO V_T 5–6 mL/kg Consider rate <30 I-time 0.35–0.50 seconds PEEP 4–7 cm H_2O; set/adjust based on lung inflation PS to achieve 2/3–3/4 set V_T	Surfactant therapy; ±iNO HFOV: Hz 6–8 w/ ΔP to vibrate chest/abd; P_{aw} as needed for 9 rib lung inflation HFJV: Rate 240–360; may need increased on-time; 0–5 back-up rate; PEEP 5–7 cm H_2O; PIP as needed Flow interrupter: Rate 240–360; convective rate 6–12; convective I-time >1 second; PEEP as needed
Lung hypoplasia	V_T 4–5 mL/kg; PIP < 26 cm H_2O Rate 40–60 breaths per minute I-time 0.25–0.40 seconds PEEP 3–5 cm H_2O Surfactant only for RDS features	HFOV: Hz 8–10; P_{aw} 10–13; ΔP 2-x P_{aw}; adjust to vibrate chest/abd; I:E 1:2 HFJV: Rate 360–420; PEEP @ 5–8 cm H_2O as needed to optimize lung inflation; minimal/no back-up rate
BPD Early/mild-moderate chronic-severe	Volume-targeted: V_T 6–8 mL/kg; Rate 20–40 breaths per minute I-time 0.35–0.45 seconds PEEP @ 5–8 cm H_2O PS to achieve 2/3–3/4 set V_T V_T: may need 7–12 mL/kg (or higher) Second increased dead space I-time: 0.50–1.00 seconds; longer to overcome airway resistance Rate: 15–30 breaths per minute; slower to allow adequate lung emptying PEEP: quite variable; may need 8–12 cm H_2O to "stent" airway open	HFOV: Similar to MAS HFJV: Similar to MAS; may need back-up rate to optimize lung recruitment HFV not commonly applied for managing "chronic-severe" BPD If used, consider MAS HFJV or "flow interrupter" approach
PPHN	iNO as indicated Minimize lung hyperinflation Adjunct therapies	iNO as indicated Minimize lung hyperinflation Adjunct therapies

abd, Abdomen; *AC*, assist-control; *HFJV*, high-frequency jet ventilation; *HFOV*, high-frequency oscillatory ventilation; *HFV*, high-frequency ventilation; *I:E*, inspiratory to expiratory ratio; *iNO*, inhaled nitric oxide; *I-time*, inspiratory time; *MAS*, meconium aspiration syndrome; ΔP, delta pressure (amplitude); P_{aw}, mean airway pressure; *PEEP*, positive end-expiratory pressure; *PIP*, peak inspiratory pressure; *PPHN*, persistent pulmonary hypertension of the newborn; *PS*, pressure support; *RDS*, respiratory distress syndrome; *SIMV*, synchronized intermittent mandatory ventilation; V_T, tidal volume.

TABLE 25.6 Initial Recommended Settings for Mechanical Ventilator Support of Infants With Respiratory Distress Syndrome by Current Weight and Ventilatory Mode

Mode	WEIGHT (g)		
	< 1000	1000–2500	>2500
HFOV Initial Settings			
Rate	10 Hz	10 Hz	8–10 Hz
P_{aw} (cm H_2O)	10–12	10–14	12–16
ΔP/amplitude	2 × P_{aw}	2 × P_{aw}	2 × P_{aw}
SIMV Initial Settings			
Rate	30–60	30–60	20–40
V_T (mL/kg)	5–6	~ 5	4–5
PEEP (cm H_2O)	5–8	5–8	6–9
I-time (sec)	Start at 0.3–0.4 seconds, adjust PRN based on graphics		
PS (cm H_2O)	Start at 8–12, adjust as needed to ~2/3 PIP for V_T		

HFOV, High-frequency oscillatory ventilation; *I-time*, inspiratory time; ΔP, change in pressure amplitude; P_{aw}, mean airway pressure; *PEEP*, positive end expiratory pressure; *PS*, pressure support; *SIMV*, synchronized intermittent mandatory ventilation; V_T, tidal volume.

TABLE 25.7 Recommended Adjustments for High-Frequency Oscillatory Ventilation by Ventilator Parameter Based on Oxygen Requirements and Ventilation

Parameter	Adjustment
Rate	Typically no change in frequency except: ↓↓ If ΔP > 2–3 × P_{aw} if ΔP < P_{aw}
P_{aw} (cm H_2O)	Increase/decrease as follows based on FiO_2 ↑ by 2–3 if FiO_2 > 50% ↓ by 1–2 if FiO_2 30%–50% No change or by 1 if FiO_2 <25% ↓ by 2–3 after surfactant therapy
ΔP	Increase/decrease based on PCO_2 or $TcPCO_2$[a] ↑ by 5–10 if PCO_2 >65 mm Hg ↑ by 2–5 if PCO_2 55–65 mm Hg ↓ by 2–5 if PCO_2 35–45 mm Hg ↓ by 5–10 if PCO_2 <35 mm Hg

[a]Must be assessed in the context of serum pH and base deficit/excess.

ΔP, Change in pressure amplitude; P_{aw}, mean airway pressure; $TcPCO_2$, transcutaneous partial pressure of carbon dioxide.

pressure of carbon dioxide (PCO_2) during HFOV, we recommend either frequent blood gas assessment or transcutaneous monitoring during the initial implementation of HFOV, particularly in the most immature infants. As shown in Table 25.7, adjustments in amplitude are more commonly made in response to measured PCO_2 than are changes in frequency. We practice a mild permissive hypercarbia approach at all gestational and postnatal ages.[28-30] More pronounced hypercarbia has not been shown to be of benefit in a randomized trial.[31]

Conventional Ventilation

Our approach to conventional ventilator support for neonatal RDS is almost always a volume-targeted synchronized intermittent mandatory ventilation (SIMV) mode, unless a large (>50%) air leak occurs around the endotracheal tube, in which case we will use a pressure-limited mode.[32] The same guiding principles should be used in initiating and adjusting support as noted previously. Typical initial ventilator settings for SIMV are shown in Tables 25.5 and 25.6. We prefer to initiate support with slightly higher positive end-expiratory pressure (PEEP) values, in the 6 to 8 cm H_2O range, in an effort to improve lung recruitment. Subsequent reductions in PEEP are based on FiO_2, SpO_2 and chest radiographs. V_T values are usually set at around 5 mL/kg; clinical assessment of chest movement as well as analysis of ventilator-derived lung mechanics are performed to ensure that V_T is adequate. If a pressure-limited mode is required, usually caused by excessive air leak around the endotracheal tube, we attempt to limit the peak pressure via clinical assessment as well as frequent monitoring of delivered V_T (again targeting volumes of 4–6 mL/kg). We employ early caffeine therapy in infants under 32 weeks' gestation and attempt to minimize sedation to encourage spontaneous respiratory efforts. Pressure support is commonly employed to minimize work of breathing, yet encourage diaphragmatic activity, while intubated (Tables 25.6 and 25.8).[33]

TABLE 25.8 Recommended Adjustments for Volume-Targeted Synchronized Intermittent Mandatory Ventilation by Ventilator Parameters

Parameter	Adjustment
Rate	Wean rate as tolerated for PCO_2 <50[a]
	Minimum SIMV rate 15–20
V_T (mL/kg)	Wean as indicated for PCO_2 <50[a]
	Do not wean V_T below 4 mL/kg
PEEP (cm H_2O)	Wean as indicated when FiO_2 <0.25
	Follow lung inflation by chest radiograph
	Typically we do not wean below 5 cm H_2O
I-time (s)	Typically we do not adjust for acute RDS
PS (cm H_2O)	Wean as indicated based on PIP for delivered V_T
	Change to tube compensation if <5 cm H_2O

[a]Must be assessed in the context of serum pH and base deficit/excess.
I-time, Inspiratory time; *PEEP*, positive end expiratory pressure; *PS*, pressure support; *RDS*, respiratory distress syndrome; *SIMV*, synchronized intermittent mandatory ventilation; *V_T*, tidal volume.

Extubation

An aggressive approach to weaning (Table 25.8) and extubation (Table 25.4) is encouraged. This includes (1) written guidelines for weaning from all modes of mechanical ventilation (Table 25.4); (2) encouragement of active weaning by respiratory therapists as well as physicians and nurse practitioners; (3) written extubation criteria for both conventional ventilation and HFOV; (4) a policy that mandates daily assessment during clinical rounds of whether the infant meets extubation criteria; and (5) promotion of all approaches to noninvasive respiratory support. With this approach, we have demonstrated a quality improvement process by which almost 90% of infants who meet criteria can be extubated within 24 hours of doing so, with an overall reduction in ventilator days by 40%, and a median duration of mechanical ventilation less than 1 day for infants over 27 weeks' gestation.

Evidenced-Based Recommendations

The best evidence base for management of RDS includes initial management with noninvasive modes of respiratory support and, for those infants requiring intubation, surfactant replacement therapy.[6,34] There is also evidence to support the use of a volume-targeted rather than pressure-limited approach to conventional mechanical ventilation.[30] Although there is evidence to support the use of a "lung protective" approach to mechanical ventilation in adults with RDS,[35] such trials do not exist (and likely may not be undertaken) for neonatal RDS.[17,18] Although we preferentially employ HFOV in the management of neonatal RDS, there is no convincing evidence from randomized controlled trials (RCTs) in the era of surfactant availability that HFOV using an "open lung" approach results in improved outcomes compared with "lung-protective," volume-targeted approach via conventional mechanical ventilators.[15]

Gaps in Knowledge

Despite over 50 years of experience with mechanical ventilation in the support of neonates with RDS, there remain important gaps in knowledge. One of the most important needs is the extension of pulmonary follow-up studies beyond the first few years of life. There is now compelling evidence, primarily from presurfactant survivors, that altered lung growth and function may persist into early adulthood, with the potential to result in significant functional issues as the lung undergoes normal age-related declines in physiologic function.[36] Some studies have suggested that the use of much later functional assessments, rather than the short-term definitions of BPD, support the early, sustained use of HFOV over more conventional modes of ventilation.[37-39] Nonetheless, at this time, there is not clear evidence to that effect and, when properly employed, one approach cannot be clearly advocated over the other. Additional studies are also needed to evaluate the potential benefits of newer approaches to mechanical ventilator support for neonatal RDS, such as neurally adjusted ventilator assist,[40] and the use of different approaches to early noninvasive support including high-amplitude bubble CPAP and high frequency nasal ventilation.[41,42]

MECONIUM ASPIRATION SYNDROME

Although meconium-stained amniotic fluid is a relatively common occurrence, particularly as gestation increases beyond 40 weeks, true meconium aspiration syndrome (MAS) is relatively infrequent and appears to be decreasing in frequency over the past couple of decades.[43-46] Despite a relatively low incidence, approximately 50% of infants diagnosed with MAS may require ventilator support.[47-49]

Key Pathophysiologic Features

MAS has a complex, multifactorial pathophysiology that is primarily inflammatory based.[43,43,50-52] Key features include altered surfactant metabolism/function, obstruction of the airways, and the pulmonary vascular response (Fig. 25.1). These components lead to disordered surfactant metabolism and function, epithelial and endothelial membrane injury, partial or complete obstruction of large and small airways, superimposed on an altered pulmonary vascular bed related to both inflammation, and prenatal/postnatal hypoxia-ischemia. Perhaps more than any other neonatal disorder, the clinical features of MAS may be quite variable from one infant to the next and can change fairly rapidly during the course of caring for a single infant. As such, the ventilatory approach must be individualized and frequently assessed based on the suspected pathophysiology at the time. Clinical examination, radiographic features, and echocardiography may all play a role in determining the variable dominant pathophysiologic processes. This section will focus on the ventilatory approach to MAS; other adjunctive therapies may also be indicated including surfactant replacement, antibiotics, pulmonary hypertension therapies, and antiinflammatory treatments, but will not be discussed in detail.

Surfactant Dysfunction

Disturbances in surfactant metabolism and function lead to decreased compliance of distal airspaces leading to atelectasis and intrapulmonary shunt.[51,53-55] From the perspective of ventilator management, the primary goal is attempting to establish an optimal functional residual volume through recruitment and maintenance of poorly inflated airspaces while attempting to minimize overinflation of unaffected regions of the lung and those areas where airway obstruction predisposes to air trapping. Beyond the use of surfactant replacement therapy in an effort to improve lung compliance, lung inflation is optimized through judicious application of PEEP and/or P_{aw}.

Airway Resistance

Severe MAS is often accompanied by elevated airway resistance because of obstruction from inhaled/aspirated meconium.[44,56] In animal models of MAS, there is an early acute phase of near complete obstruction of the large airways, followed by movement of the meconium into smaller more distal airways.[50,57] Given that the prenatal conditions that typically predispose to MAS are extant well before delivery, the vast majority of neonates with significant MAS have already moved the bulk of any inhaled meconium into the distal airways/airspaces.[43] Given the small diameter of more distal airways, the potential exists for partial or complete obstruction, or a "ball-valve" effect (Fig. 25.2). The former prevents gas getting into the distal gas-exchange space leading to atelectasis, while the latter allows some gas into the distal air space but impedes gas from escaping during the exhalation phase, leading to air trapping and overinflation. Lung overinflation not only directly impairs gas exchange but can also further aggravate oxygenation through compressive effects on the pulmonary microvasculature. It is this combination of disturbed airway mechanics coupled with

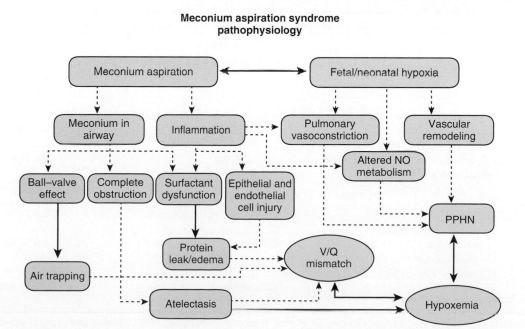

Fig. 25.1 Pathophysiology of meconium aspiration syndrome. *NO,* Nitric oxide; *PPHN,* persistent pulmonary hypertension of newborn; *V/Q,* ventilation-perfusion.

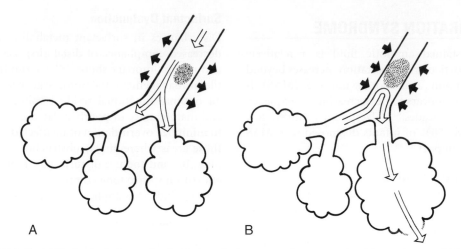

Fig. 25.2 Partial "ball-valve" air trapping behind particulate matter (i.e., meconium) in an airway, which leads to alveolar overexpansion and rupture. **(A)** Tidal gas passes beyond the meconium on inspiration when the airway dilates but **(B)** cannot exit on expiration when airways constrict. (From Goldsmith JP: Continuous positive airway pressure and conventional mechanical ventilation in the treatment of meconium aspiration syndrome. J Perinatol 28(suppl 3):S49–S55, 2008; used with permission.)

surfactant dysfunction, creating a nonhomogeneous lung disease, that makes severe MAS so difficult to manage.

Pulmonary Hypertension

Unlike most other neonatal lung disorders, pulmonary hypertension is a common and significant problem in infants with severe MAS.[58-60] Fetal hypoxemia and inflammation are thought to be primary contributors to underlying pulmonary hypertension.[50,51,60-62] Abnormalities in nitric oxide (NO) metabolism contribute to the underlying dysfunction in pulmonary vasomotor tone.[60,63,64] As noted previously, air trapping and compression of the pulmonary vascular bed can also contribute to pulmonary hypertension. Adjunct therapy with inhaled NO and other pulmonary vasodilators, as well as inotropic support of the systemic vascular system, may be required for management of the pulmonary hypertension.

Relevant Principles of Ventilation

Although we most commonly use HFOV, other approaches to high-frequency ventilation (HFV) and/or volume-targeted conventional ventilation are commonly used in the initial management of MAS (Tables 25.5 and 25.9). Key to management

---

TABLE 25.9 **Suggested Initial Approach to Ventilator Support of Meconium Aspiration Syndrome by Ventilatory Mode and Suspected Underlying Pathophysiology**

Ventilator Mode	Airway Obstruction w/ Gas Trapping	Alveolar Disease w/ Low Lung Volume	Pulmonary Hypertension
Pathophysiology	↑ Resistance ↑ Time constant Lung hyperexpansion	↓ Surfactant function ↓ Lung compliance ↑ V/Q mismatch	↓ NOS Hypoxemia Acidosis
Conventional (SIMV)			

Pressure-controlled	PIP to move chest; lower I-time
	—Adjust PIP to desired V_T
	PEEP 4–6 cm H_2O; PS ~¾ set PIP
		Surfactant therapy; monitor lung volume; higher
		  PEEP as needed
			iNO; SpO_2 92%–98%; consider
			  inodilators; optimize sedation

Volume-targeted	V_T 5–6 mL/kg; limit rate <30; PEEP 4–6 cm H_2O; PS ~¾ set PIP	Same as above	Same as above
High Frequency			
Oscillator	Hz 6–8 ΔP to vibrate chest/abdomen	P_{aw} as needed for ~9 rib expansion	Same as above
Jet	HF rate 240–360 May need longer on-time Minimal to no back-up rate	PEEP as needed for 9 rib expansion Consider back-up rate 3–5	Same as above
Flow interrupter	HF rate 240–360 Convective rate 6–10	PEEP as above Convective I-time ~1 second	Same as above

Hz, Hertz; *iNO,* inhaled nitric oxide; *I-time,* inspiratory time; *ΔP,* change in pressure/amplitude; *PEEP,* positive end expiratory pressure; *PIP,* peak inspiratory pressure; *PS,* pressure support; *NOS,* nitric oxide synthase; *SIMV,* synchronized intermittent mandatory ventilation; *V/Q,* ventilation/perfusion; *V_T,* tidal volume.

is recognition of the predominant underlying pulmonary pathophysiology. Although the majority of infants with MAS do not require ventilator support, those infants who do are usually quite ill and often have a mixed pattern of both over- and underinflated lung segments, as well as severe persistent pulmonary hypertension of the newborn (PPHN).

High-Frequency Ventilation

With HFOV, the key is to use a lower rate, typically 6 to 8 Hz, and to set the initial P_{aw} based on the overall pattern of lung inflation. For infants with significant air-trapping, we start at 6 Hz with a P_{aw} similar to that on conventional ventilation. Amplitude, or ΔP, is then adjusted to generate vibration of the chest to mid-abdomen. This approach provides a slightly greater oscillatory V_T and longer expiratory phase, both of which support improved ventilation. For those infants with MAS who have relatively poor lung inflation, the P_{aw} is typically started at 3 to 5 cm H_2O above that on conventional ventilation. Subsequent adjustments in P_{aw} are made based on FiO_2 response and radiographic assessment of lung inflation. In most babies with MAS, we typically adjust amplitude, not frequency, to further affect ventilation. If high-frequency jet ventilation (HFJV) is employed, it is important to use a lower rate (in the range of 240–360 cycles per minute) as exhalation is passive and air trapping is a significant risk at higher rates. On occasion, it may be helpful to increase the inspiratory time ("on-time," from 0.02 to as high as 0.03 seconds) to gain increased V_T with high-frequency pulses. When employing HFJV in the management of MAS, a back-up rate may also be helpful if additional lung recruitment is indicated, using V_T breaths rather than large increases in PEEP. However, back-up conventional breaths should be set at a relatively low frequency, typically 2 to 5 breaths per minute (Tables 25.5 and 5.9). On occasion, we also use the Bird VDR-4 high-frequency flow interruption ventilator. Although not as "user friendly" as other neonatal ventilators, this device can be quite effective to aid in the removal of airway secretions for infants with large amounts of airway meconium. It is important to again remember that exhalation is passive; thus, lower high-frequency rates (240–360 breaths per minute) should be used to minimize risk for air trapping. Typically, we use convective breaths between 5 and 10 breaths per minute and set the I-time for convective breaths close to 1 second (Table 25.5 and 25.9).

Conventional Ventilation

We almost always use a volume-targeted, SIMV-based approach to conventional ventilator support (Table 25.5 and 25.9). The same guiding principles should be used for initiating and adjusting support as described earlier. When air trapping is the predominant pathological problem, it is often caused by dynamic PEEP because of long expiratory time constant. Thus, set PEEP should be limited (typically <6 cm H_2O) and ventilator rate should be kept relatively low (typically <30 breaths per minute), with shorter I-times to ensure adequate expiratory time to minimize gas trapping. As inspiratory time constants can also be prolonged, attention must be paid to ensure that the I-time is long enough to complete V_T delivery. For infants in

whom the predominant pathology is alveolar disease with low lung volumes, PEEP should initially be set at higher levels (5–8 cm H_2O) and adjusted as needed to achieve an acceptable EELV. We also commonly use pressure support to assist spontaneous breaths with a goal of support between two-thirds and three-fourths the set V_T of the SIMV supported breaths. Because the pathophysiology of MAS includes increased alveolar dead space, these infants require slightly larger V_T/kg than similar infants with more homogeneous lung disease.[65]

Irrespective of the ventilatory approach used, frequent clinical, radiographic, and laboratory assessments are indicated to optimize gas exchange and minimize VILI. Close monitoring is even more important following surfactant therapy and during the initial 12 to 24 hours of support as the predominant pathophysiology can and does change quickly.

Evidenced-Based Recommendations

There is a very limited "evidence" base to support the multiple management schemes employed for MAS. Although numerous trials have been conducted comparing different modes of conventional ventilation, or conventional to high-frequency ventilation, in term and preterm neonates with respiratory failure, no randomized trials have specifically compared different approaches to mechanical ventilation in a population of babies limited to a diagnosis of MAS. Therefore, the use either oscillator or jet for HFV support, or different modes of conventional ventilation including volume- or pressure-targeted SIMV versus assist-control (AC) are a matter of practice preference, and not specifically evidence based. There is increasing evidence from RCTs involving mechanically ventilated infants diagnosed with MAS related to the potential benefit of surfactant therapy (including bolus and lavage approaches)[66-68] as well as early corticosteroid therapy (including systemic and inhaled approaches).[9,69,70] Evidence does suggest that optimizing lung inflation improves the effectiveness of inhaled NO therapy for pulmonary hypertension.[71]

Gaps in Knowledge

Although the evidence related to the benefits of surfactant therapy is compelling, additional studies are indicated to better define the optimal at-risk patient, timing, dose, and approach of this therapy. Corticosteroid-based trials are relatively few and small, additional trials are needed to further clarify the overall benefit-to-risk effect of this intervention. The lack of any RCTs comparing different approaches to mechanical ventilation in babies diagnosed with MAS (such as pressure controlled versus volume targeted, SIMV versus AC, conventional ventilation versus HFV, or HFOV versus HFJV) leaves a large gap in our knowledge about optimal ventilator management of this group of patients. Given the overall decreasing incidence of MAS and the relatively limited number of babies diagnosed with MAS who require mechanical ventilation, such studies may never be carried out but, at a minimum, will require a multicenter approach.

LUNG HYPOPLASIA DISORDERS

Pulmonary hypoplasia has remained one of the most challenging and frustrating neonatal lung disorders to manage. Lung hypoplasia is thought to arise from increased drainage of fetal lung liquid and/or extrinsic compression during key phases of fetal lung development (mostly late pseudoglandular to early saccular), or more rarely as an isolated, inherited defect.[72-74] Importantly, the arrest or impairment in normal development typically affects both airway and vascular structures. A wide variety of pathologies are associated with the development of fetal/neonatal lung hypoplasia[74-76] (Table 25.10). Working definitions of pulmonary hypoplasia rely on postmortem measures such as lung-to-body weight ratio and radial alveolar counts, or on fetal ultrasonographic or magnetic resonance comparisons of observed to expected lung cross-section or volume.[77-80] Physiological definitions for the ventilated neonate are sparse, but functionally can be thought of as inadequate pulmonary gas exchange surface to support minimal metabolic requirements for oxygen and carbon dioxide exchange.[17,81-83]

Since 1995, a number of treatment strategies for hypoplastic lungs have evolved, but even in the most common etiology, congenital diaphragmatic hernia (CDH), there are few RCTs systematically evaluating the management of pulmonary hypoplasia in the newborn. Nonetheless, a general "consensus" approach to management of CDH has emerged, with specific guidelines targeting early cardiopulmonary management, much of which is applicable to other etiologies of lung hypoplasia.[84-90] Adoption of a "gentle" approach to ventilator support has been associated with reported improvements in morbidity and mortality in both CDH and other etiologies of hypoplasia.[81-84,87-89] However, it remains unclear what the best ventilation mode is to provide "gentle" support. It was hoped that information from a large RCT comparing initial ventilator support with high-frequency oscillation to pressure-targeted conventional ventilation would help provide answers to this question in the CDH population.[90] Findings from this study included no significant difference in the combined outcome of mortality or BPD between the two ventilation groups for infants with prenatally diagnosed CDH. Of interest, there was a relative benefit with initial use of conventional ventilation, including shorter duration of ventilator support, less

inotrope use, and decreased need of extracorporeal membrane oxygenation (ECMO). Methodologically, however, the study was compromised by the use of much higher P_{aw} in the high-frequency group compared with the conventional mechanical ventilation group. Excessive mean pressure can result in lung overinflation and contribute to cardiopulmonary dysfunction in a variety of ways, including altered lung mechanics, direct compression of pulmonary vasculature, and limited ventricular preload owing to impaired venous return.[83,91-94]

Key Pathophysiologic Features
Lung Hypoplasia

The most obvious pathophysiologic problem is impaired lung growth. The severity of impact on airways, terminal respiratory units, and the pulmonary vascular bed depends on how early in gestation lung growth is affected. Compromised lung liquid formation and developmental defects in lung morphogenesis contribute to the severity of lung hypoplasia.[72-74] The specific mechanisms for impaired lung development in the context of processes promoting lung hypoplasia are beyond the scope of this chapter; the reader is referred to other reviews for more information.[95-99]

Pulmonary Vascular Bed

Given that angiogenesis and vasculogenesis of the pulmonary circulation and capillary network are closely linked, impaired vascular development accompanies the altered lung growth. A variety of pulmonary vascular abnormalities have been described in animal models and neonates with lung hypoplasia, most commonly associated with CDH. These include impaired growth and development of pulmonary arteries and arterioles, as well as increased arteriolar medial muscle thickness,[99,100] altered expression of angiogenic factors including vascular endothelial growth factor,[95-97,101-103] decreased endothelial NO synthase expression,[98,99] impaired response to NO metabolites,[101] increased expression and activity of phosphodiesterase 5,[102] and increased expression/levels of endothelin-1 and endothelin receptor A.[103,104] The effect of decreased vascular growth and impaired endothelial cell function is an impaired pulmonary vascular response at birth to inflation and oxygen. Additionally, the postnatal response to inhaled NO (iNO) also appears to be impaired.[105] PPHN continues to be a major contributor to the continuing relatively high mortality rate among infants with severe lung hypoplasia despite a variety of new therapeutic approaches.

Relevant Principles of Ventilation

Starting with the seminal publication by Wung et al. in 1985, there has been increasing acceptance of using a "lung-sparing" or "gentle" approach to mechanical ventilation of neonates with severe respiratory failure, including lung hypoplasia.[87,88] In our NICU, we use HFOV as the initial mode of support for all infants with lung hypoplasia disorders, an approach that continues to evolve (Table 25.11). Differences in our initial support parameters for HFOV compared with those established for the VICI Trial[90] include the following: (1) initiate HFOV with a lower P_{aw}, usually 11 cm H_2O, and rarely exceed maximum

TABLE 25.10 Possible Etiologies for Neonatal Lung Hypoplasia	
Major Mechanism	**Specific Diagnoses**
An/Oligohydramnios	Prolonged rupture of membranes
	Severe renal dysfunction (agenesis, cystic/multicystic/dysplastic lesions)
	Genitourinary obstruction
Thoracic compression	Intrathoracic: diaphragmatic hernia, cystic pulmonary abnormalities, teratoma, large pleural effusions
	Intra-abdominal: hepatomegaly, ascites, polycystic kidneys, genitourinary masses or obstruction
Thoracic wall abnormalities	Osteogenesis imperfecta, thanatophoric dysplasia, other skeletal dysplasias, rib and/or vertebral anomalies
Neuromuscular disorders	Myopathies, akinesia, arthrogryposis, syndromic
Abdominal wall	Omphalocele

TABLE 25.11 Recommended Initial Ventilator Settings for Neonates With Lung Hypoplasia Disorders, Including Diaphragmatic Hernia

	High-Frequency Oscillatory Ventilation	High-Frequency Jet Ventilation	Synchronized Intermittent Mandatory Ventilation
ΔP/PIP	24–28	20–25 cm H_2O	V_T 4–5 mL/kg
Max PIP			<25 cm H_2O
P_{aw}/PEEP	10–12 cm H_2O	10–12/6–8 cm H_2O	4–5 cm H_2O
Max P_{aw}	Rarely >16 cm H_2O	Rarely >16 cm H_2O	
Frequency	8–10 Hz	360–420 breaths per minute	40–60 breaths per minute
I:E/I-time	1:2	0.02 seconds	0.3 seconds
FiO_2	0.40	0.40	0.40
SpO_2			
preductal	>80%	>80%	>80%
First hour	92%–98%	92%–98%	92%–98%
Goal	>90%	>90%	>90%
"Tolerated"			
$PaCO_2$			
Goal	45–55 mm Hg	45–55 mm Hg	45–55 mm Hg
"Tolerated"	<65 mm Hg	<65 mm Hg	<65 mm Hg
Chest x-ray	9 rib inflation contralateral lung	9 rib inflation contralateral lung	9 rib inflation contralateral lung

FiO₂, Fraction of inspired oxygen; *I:E*, inspiratory to expiratory ratio; *ΔP*, delta pressure (amplitude); *PaCO₂*, partial pressure arterial carbon dioxide; *P_AW*, mean airway pressure; *PEEP*, positive end-expiratory pressure; *PIP*, peak inspiratory pressure; *SpO₂*, oxygen saturation; *V_T*, tidal volume.

P_{aw} under 16 cm H_2O; (2) we often start larger babies at a lower frequency, typically 8 Hz; (3) we use an inspiratory-to-expiratory ratio of 1:2 rather than 1:1; (4) we attempt to maintain lung inflation as close to 9 ribs as possible, trying to minimize both under- and over-inflation of the lungs. It is important to emphasize that there is no clear evidence that HFOV provides increased benefit (nor risk) compared with HFJV or conventional mechanical ventilation. We have recently published retrospective data contrasting the higher P_{aw} approach as used in the VICI Trial (start at 13–15 cm H_2O) to a lower P_{aw} approach (start at 10–12 cm H_2O).[106] Initiating HFOV support at a lower P_{aw}, in association with several other management changes, was associated with significantly lower use of iNO and inotropes, as well as significantly lower use of ECMO and improved survival. Although the use of HFJV has been reported by other investigators, most often, it has been used as a rescue therapy in lieu of HFOV, and the parameters employed have not been well described.[107-109] There is clinical evidence to suggest that HFJV may be the optimal approach for ventilation of babies with lung hypoplasia related to an ability to ventilate using small V_T and lower P_{aw} while minimizing adverse cardiovascular effects.[91-94,110]

Irrespective of the ventilatory approach used for managing lung hypoplasia, several key concepts must be kept in mind.

First, the lung is small, with a functional residual capacity that may be considerably less than normal.[111] Given the effects that both atelectasis and hyperinflation have on pulmonary microvasculature and vascular resistance, careful attention must be paid to optimizing lung inflation.[112-115] In that regard, the P_{aw} needed to achieve optimal lung inflation may be less than that required for a normal-sized lung, even with surfactant dysfunction as in preterm infants. It is also considerably more difficult to determine optimal P_{aw} and lung inflation under conditions of lung hypoplasia. Attempting to employ the stepwise increase in P_{aw} as suggested under the RDS section is not recommended in babies with lung hypoplasia as it may be easier to inadvertently provide a higher P_{aw} than is necessary without any identifiable improvement in oxygenation. This may be especially problematic with underlying pulmonary hypertension. An alternate, but unproven, approach is to start at a lower P_{aw} and gradually adjust upward based on radiographic lung inflation. Although the minute ventilation necessary to achieve normocarbia should be the same as for infants with normal lungs, use of a V_T on the higher end of "normal" (i.e., 6 mL/kg) may have greater risk for initiating lung injury secondary to inadvertent "volutrauma" in hypoplastic lungs.[116] The fact that studies by Landolfo and Sharma report relatively normal to high V_T to achieve effective ventilation should not be taken to indicate that V_T over 5 mL/kg ought to be employed in babies with CDH or lung hypoplasia attributed to other etiologies.[111,117] It is unclear whether higher rates (i.e., 60 breaths per minute) and lower V_T (4 mL/kg) or higher V_T (6 mL/kg) at lower rates have an effect on short- or long-term outcomes for lung hypoplasia disorders. However, given the implied decreased complement of alveoli in these disorders, physiologic V_T of 5 mL/kg could result in volutrauma, as this volume is directed into a fraction of the normal number of terminal airspace units; this reality provides a sound physiologic rationale for the use of HFV in such infants.[117] As of March 2020, there was an ongoing trial at King's College in London to compare the effectiveness and safety of conventional ventilation using 4, 5, and 6 mL/kg in babies with CDH (ClinicalTrials.gov Identifier: NCT0284905). In this context, it is also important to note that those infants with the greatest degree of lung hypoplasia have increased dead space-to-V_T ratios, suggesting that more of the applied V_T is "lost" as ineffective dead space ventilation.[118] Oxygenation is dependent as much on the impaired pulmonary vascular bed as it is on relative lung volumes. Adjustments in ventilator support must be made with the recognition that altered oxygenation could be attributed to increased pulmonary vascular resistance related to factors other than changes in ventilator support.

Pulmonary Hypertension

The management of pulmonary hypertension in lung hypoplasia disorders, including CDH, remains controversial.[119-125] There are no large RCTs demonstrating short- or long-term benefit for many of the approaches that have been used, including iNO[126-134] (Table 25.12). The reader is referred to Chapter 34 of this book and to review articles for a more thorough discussion of therapeutic approaches to PPHN.[60,126,135,136] As previously noted, a

TABLE 25.12　Potential Vasodilator Therapies Considered for Management of Pulmonary Hypertension in Lung Hypoplasia Syndromes

Therapy	Mechanism	Comments
Lung "Specific"		No proven benefit by RCTs
Inhaled NO	↑ cGMP production	Commonly used
Sildenafil	PDE5 inhibitor; ↓ cGMP breakdown	Often used later in course; EURO trial underway
Inhaled PGI2	↑ cAMP production	Highly alkaline
"Nonspecific"		No proven benefit by RCTs
Milrinone	PDE3 inhibitor; ↓cAMP breakdown	Inodilator, lusitrope; RCT underway
Intravenous PGI2	↑ cAMP production	Hypotension common
Bosentan	Blocks endothelin receptors	Low risk hepatotoxicity
Norepinephrine	α1,2 & β1 activation; ? NO	↑ SVR:PVR ratio
Vasopressin	Systemic vasoconstriction	↑ SVR:PVR ratio
Intravenous PGE1	Cyclooxygenase inhibitor	Open PDA "off-loads" RV
Cinaciguat	↑ cGMP; activates soluble guanylate cyclase	No neonatal studies

cAMP, Cyclic adenosine monophosphate; *cGMP,* cyclic guanosine monophosphate; *NO,* nitric oxide; *PDA,* patent ductus arteriosus; *PDE,* phosphodiesterase inhibitor; *PGI,* prostacyclin; *PVR,* pulmonary vascular resistance; *RCT,* randomized controlled trial; *SVR,* systemic vascular resistance.

critical component of PPHN management in all neonatal lung conditions includes optimization of lung inflation.[25,110,113,114,137,138] Currently, there is not a proven clinical approach to such lung optimization for infants with lung hypoplasia. The combination of clinical examination, monitoring indices of gas exchange and cardiac function, as well as serial chest radiographs is most commonly used.

Evidenced-Based Recommendations

There is almost no "evidence base" for the clinical management of lung hypoplasia disorders, including CDH.[81,83,85,87,88,106] There is universal agreement that "gentle ventilation," including tolerance to relative hypercarbia as well as avoidance of excessive V_T and relative lung inflation, should drive the ventilatory approach.

Gaps in Knowledge

Nearly all approaches to ventilatory and cardiovascular support of newborns with pulmonary hypoplasia require systematic investigation. There is a uniform consensus that "gentle ventilation" improves outcomes, although the optimal approach and device remain unclear. Identifying better clinical tools to determine "optimal" lung inflation, such as impedance tomography and forced oscillatory technique,[25] should be investigated in babies with lung hypoplasia. Another area of interest is the "optimal" preductal and/or postductal saturation to target. In an effort to prevent/manage pulmonary hypertension, many

centers target a higher SpO_2, whereas others suggest that a lower preductal SpO_2 may be reasonable. What the optimal SpO_2 targets should be across all etiologies of lung hypoplasia, and whether they should be adjusted over time, remain unknown. Finally, in addition to postnatal studies, investigations of maternal-fetal interventions to improve lung growth and/or vascular development continue to be studied. For example, a number of investigations related to fetal tracheal occlusion for CDH are ongoing.[139-141] Animal investigations suggest that pharmacologic approaches may also be an option to improve fetal lung and vascular development in CDH and possibly other forms of lung hypoplasia.[142-144]

BRONCHOPULMONARY DYSPLASIA

BPD is the most common morbidity affecting surviving preterm infants, described in various studies at rates of over 40% for infants of less than 29 weeks' gestation.[145-148] Efforts have been made to differentiate the "old" form of BPD, first described clinically by Northway and colleagues in 1967,[149] from a "new" form of BPD suggested from human and animal studies in the 1990s[150-152] (Fig. 25.3). The epidemiology of BPD has clearly changed over time, with the vast majority of infants diagnosed with BPD now at under 29 weeks and less than 1000 g birth weight, and most probably being of the new BPD variant with underlying impaired alveolarization.[146,147,150-152] Nonetheless, although much less common, preterm infants with an underlying pathophysiology consistent with old BPD continue to survive with severe chronic respiratory failure.[143,144,151,152] Any effort to discuss the ventilatory approach to BPD must take into consideration the wide range of clinical variability and diagnostic criteria used to make this diagnosis[146,153-155] (Box 25.1). Infants diagnosed with "mild" BPD may require supplemental oxygen for only the first few weeks of life, whereas infants with "severe-chronic" BPD continue to require positive pressure support beyond 36 to 40 weeks postmenstrual age. These represent distinctly different ends of the BPD spectrum. Additionally, in the context of BPD care, it is important to differentiate approaches aimed at BPD prevention versus management of established severe-chronic lung disease. This section will focus on the latter group of patients, requiring ongoing ventilator support beyond the initial weeks of life and extending into the first year or beyond. Approaches designed to prevent or ameliorate BPD are discussed elsewhere in this chapter as well as in other chapters throughout this book. Not specifically addressed in this chapter is the important concept that management of the infant with severe BPD is best served through a multidisciplinary approach to care including specialized nursing and respiratory therapy support, neonatal nutritionists, and occupational/physical therapists. Other pediatric subspecialty providers also need to be members of the severe BPD care team, including pulmonology, cardiology, radiology, and otolaryngology, as well as pediatric surgery.

Key Pathophysiologic Features

Infants with established chronic lung disease are very different from premature newborns with RDS and those with mild BPD,

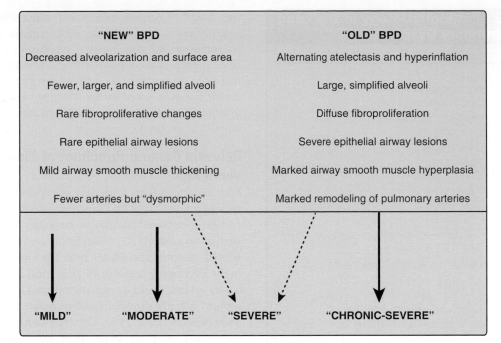

Fig. 25.3 Contrasting pathology for and relative association with definitions of bronchopulmonary dysplasia (*BPD*): "old" (presurfactant era) versus "new" (postsurfactant era).

BOX 25.1 Defining Bronchopulmonary Dysplasia—Contrasting 2001 National Institutes of Child Health Consensus Conference (NICHD) to Updated Criteria from 2018 NICHD and Neonatal Research Network Evidence-Based Definition

2001 NICHD Bronchopulmonary Dysplasia (BPD) Definition[151]

	Received supplemental O_2 for >28 days PLUS:
Mild BPD	Breathing room air at 36 weeks CGA or discharge
Moderate BPD	Need for <30% oxygen at 36 weeks CGA or discharge
Severe BPD	Need for >30% oxygen and/or positive pressure at 36 weeks CGA or discharge

2018 NICHD BPD Definition[153]

Persistent clinical/radiographic parenchymal lung disease and the following FiO_2/respiratory mode for >3 consecutive days:

	NC <1 L/min	NC 1–3 L/min	CPAP, NIPPV, NC >3 L/min	Invasive PPV
Mild BPD	22%–70%	22%–29%	21%	–
Moderate BPD	>70%	>30%	22%–29%	21
Severe BPD	–	–	>30%	>21%
Severe plus BPD	Early death (14 days PNA–36 weeks) attributed to persistent parenchymal lung disease and respiratory failure that is not attributable to other neonatal morbidities			

2019 NRN BPD Definition[144]

Mild BPD NC <2 L/min at 36 weeks CGA or discharge
Moderate BPD NC <2 L/min at 36 weeks CGA or discharge
Severe BPD invasive PPV

CGA, Corrected gestational age; *CPAP*, continuous positive airway pressure; *NC*, nasal cannula; *NIPPV*, nasal intermittent positive pressure ventilation; *PNA*, postnatal age; *PPV*, positive-pressure ventilation.

---

requiring an individualized ventilatory approach based on the underlying pathophysiology of the lung (Table 25.13). Other important factors to consider in their overall management include nutritional approaches,[156] assessment for pulmonary hypertension,[157] and the possible influence of gastroesophageal reflux and aspiration on injury to the airway and lung parenchyma.[158,159]

Lung Pathology

Abnormalities are well described for both the airways and the gas exchange areas of the lungs (Table 25.13). The most notable features include interrupted alveolarization with reduced number and increased size of the remaining saccular-alveolar structures, thickened mesenchymal/septal tissues, disrupted growth and development of the pulmonary microvasculature, and varying degrees of fibrosis.[150-152,160,161] More severe changes in airway pathology, similar to that reported in presurfactant era "old" BPD, are still a component of the severe-chronic type of BPD seen in infants requiring prolonged ventilatory support, although this appears to be relatively uncommon among infants with "new" BPD.[150-152,160] Additionally, infants with more severe forms of BPD may often have impaired cartilaginous development of the large and small airways, leading to tracheobronchomalacia.[162]

Lung Mechanics and Function

Decreased lung volumes and alveolar surface area resulting from the interrupted alveolarization and accompanying reduced lung microvasculature lead to impaired gas exchange[161,163 168] (Table 25.14). Most studies report decreased lung compliance in infants with BPD, although this may not be sustained into

TABLE 25.13   Pathophysiology of the Lung in Bronchopulmonary Dysplasia

Respiratory Site	Issues
Upper Airways	
Glottis	Arytenoid inflammation/edema
Trachea	Subglottic stenosis, malacia
	Infection
Bronchus	Granuloma, infection
	Stenosis
	Malacia
Lower Airways	
Bronchioles	Hyperplasia of epithelium and mucous glands
	• Bronchoconstriction; increased secretions
	• Smooth muscle hypertrophy
	• Increased vascular tone, reactivity
Distal air space	Interrupted alveolarization
	Reduced gas exchange surface area
	↓
	• Hypoxemia
	Altered capillary/vascular growth
	Pulmonary vascular resistance
	↑
	• Increased risk pulmonary hypertension
	Heterogeneous lung development/disease
	• Focal atelectasis, hyperinflation
	• Ventilation/Perfusion shunt

TABLE 25.14   Abnormalities of Lung Function among Infants With Bronchopulmonary Dysplasia[161–168]

Parameter	Abnormality
Lung Volume	
Overall lung volume	Decreased
Functional residual volume	Decreased
Compliance	Reduced
Gas exchange	Impaired diffusion
Airway Function	
Expiratory flow velocity	Decreased
Resistance	Increased

later life.[166-168] Among infants with more severe forms of BPD, heterogeneous lung disease with regions of atelectasis and air trapping can also impair oxygenation owing to increased ventilation/perfusion mismatch and intrapulmonary shunts.[165] Increased resistance related to airway injury can contribute to the air trapping noted earlier affecting ventilation.[166-170] Failure to adjust V_T owing to increased physiologic dead space also may impair gas exchange.[171]

Relevant General Principles of Mechanical Ventilation

Even among infants with less severe forms of BPD, there is increased anatomical and functional dead space. Thus, mild increases in delivered V_T may be necessary to achieve reasonable ventilation goals (PCO_2 values in the range of 45–55 mm Hg for arterial samples and 50–65 mm Hg for capillary samples).[171] In the developing stages of BPD, beyond 7 to 14 days of age but before several weeks of age, the optimal approach to ventilator support is fairly similar to that recommended for the management of RDS (Table 25.5). The exception may be the previously mentioned need for some slight increase in V_T. With more chronic, severe forms of BPD (typically these are preterms well beyond 34–36 weeks postmenstrual age), the severity of airway disease and more heterogeneous saccular-alveolar disease significantly changes the approach to ventilatory support (Table 25.15). With "chronic-severe" BPD, even higher V_T may be needed, sometimes as high as 10 to 12 mL/kg.[172] There are several potential reasons for this: (1) similar to infants with milder forms of BPD, there is interrupted/impaired alveolarization with reduced gas exchange surface area; (2) nonheterogeneous lung disease is accompanied by increasing nonfunctional lung volume because of increased areas of atelectasis coupled with areas of overinflation (increased alveolar dead space); (3) dilatation of large airways owing to exposure to cyclic stretch from positive-pressure ventilation (acquired tracheomegaly);[162,173] and (4) there may be loss of V_T-related to expansion of floppy large airways and/or to back-pressure leakage around the endotracheal tube related to high airway resistance. Increased airway resistance should be managed via longer inspiratory times to allow for more complete distribution of V_T. Additionally, modification of the "slope" of gas delivery from a square-wave form to a more

TABLE 25.15   Suggested Approaches to Mechanical Ventilation for Infants Diagnosed With Bronchopulmonary Dysplasia Based on Relative Severity of Disease

Mild/Moderate Bronchopulmonary Dysplasia	Severe-Chronic Bronchopulmonary Dysplasia
Tidal volume (V_T): 5–8 mL/kg	V_T: may need 6–12 mL/kg, 2nd dead space
PEEP: as needed to "optimize" lung inflation; often 6–8 cm H_2O	PEEP: quite variable; often 8–10 cm H_2O to "stent" open large airways
I-time: 0.35–0.45 seconds	I-time: 0.5–1.0 seconds; longer to overcome inspiratory airway resistance, enhance volume delivery to lung units with long time constants
Rate: 20–40 breaths per minute based on effort	Rate: 15–30 breaths per minute; need longer expiratory time to allow for adequate exhalation second long time constants
SpO₂ goals: 92–98	SpO₂ goals: 92–98
Target PaCO₂: 45–60 mm Hg	Target PaCO₂: 50–60 mm Hg

I-time, Inspiratory time; *PaCO₂*, partial pressure arterial carbon dioxide; *PEEP*, positive end-expiratory pressure; *SPO₂*, oxygen saturation; *V_T*, tidal volume.

bell-shaped form may also improve the flow of gas through these airways. Owing to the local and/or regional abnormalities in airway resistance and air space compliance, a longer expiratory time is also needed for the multicompartmental BPD lung to effectively empty during the exhalation phase. Thus, the combination of higher V_T, longer inspiratory times, and low rates (allowing for increased exhalation time) is indicated for infants who remain ventilator dependent with more chronic-severe forms of BPD.[172] Finally, both tracheal and bronchomalacia can develop in infants with chronic-severe BPD.[162,173] For infants with these lesions, increased PEEP levels are required to prevent closure of the larger airways before complete exhalation of the inspired V_T.[174,175] At times, we have used PEEP as high as 14 cm H_2O to prevent airway collapse, improve expiratory airway mechanics, and reduce trapped gas lung volumes. However, the application of high PEEP must be used cautiously because of the potential to further aggravate areas of localized/regional lung overinflation. Additional diagnostic studies may prove useful in helping to define both the severity of heterogeneous lung disease and the presence/location of significant airway lesions, including endoscopy[162,172] and dynamic high-resolution spiral CT scans.[172,173,176] Other evaluations that may be considered for infants with chronic-severe BPD include pulmonary function testing, echocardiography or cardiac catheterization to evaluate for pulmonary hypertension,[172,177] and testing for gastroesophageal reflux and aspiration.[158,159] In select cases, we have obtained a lung biopsy to evaluate for other processes that may contribute to severe chronic lung disease of infancy.[178]

The importance of airway dysfunction in the nonventilated as well as the mechanically ventilated infant with BPD is highlighted by studies evaluating the functional and mechanical effect of helium-oxygen mixtures. The low viscosity of the helium-oxygen allows for increased laminar flow and decreased turbulent flow through obstructed airways. In the study by Migliori and colleagues, helium-oxygen was associated with decreased peak inflation pressures, increased minute ventilation, and a 50% reduction in work of breathing; additionally, improved gas exchange PCO_2 and $TcPCO_2$ (partial pressure of transcutaneous carbon dioxide) was noted during both intubated and noninvasive support.[179] In a more recent study, relatively brief exposures (1 hour) to a helium-oxygen mixture again were accompanied by improvements in peak expiratory flow, dynamic compliance, exhaled V_T, and minute ventilation of 25% to 37%, with an associated 50% reduction in FiO_2 needs.[180] When the helium-oxygen mixture was discontinued, lung mechanics and FiO_2 needs returned to baseline values.

Tracheostomy

Some infants with chronic-severe BPD may require tracheostomy, with a reported rate of 3% to 5% in populations of very preterm infants at high risk for BPD.[153,181] The optimal time to move toward tracheostomy in terms of postnatal age and/or duration of mechanical ventilation is unclear at this time. Data from retrospective studies of large neonatal data sets suggest that most infants have been ventilator dependent for more than 2 to 3 months before tracheostomy is considered.[181,182] In our practice, we tend to delay tracheostomy unless we have evidence

for earlier development of trachea/bronchomalacia, but there appear to be developmental and other benefits to earlier tracheostomy. In one of these studies, tracheostomy after 120 days was associated with worse neurodevelopmental outcome,[181] but this was an observational study with many potential confounders. A prospective randomized trial would be required to determine the optimal time and conditions for this serious procedure. Nonetheless, clinical practice appears to already be shifting in favor of earlier tracheostomy placement.

Pulmonary Hypertension

Pulmonary hypertension is a relatively common problem among infants with more severe forms of BPD, with rates ranging from 20% to 50% depending on the population and approach to evaluation.[157,183-185] Mechanisms for pulmonary hypertension in this population include reduced vascular bed associated with impaired alveolarization, increased vascular smooth muscle proliferation and reactivity, and pulmonary vascular effects of localized areas of atelectasis or hyperinflation.[186,187] Diagnosis of pulmonary hypertension in babies with BPD requires a deliberate investigative approach. Echocardiography is the mainstay for diagnosis, but occasionally, cardiac catheterization is needed for both diagnosis and evaluation of response to various therapies.[172,177] Management of BPD-associated pulmonary hypertension includes adequate oxygenation (we recommend SpO_2 values >92%; but not hyperoxemia),[172,188,189] adjustment of support to prevent significant respiratory acidosis, avoidance of lung overinflation, and occasional use of adjunctive therapies. A number of potential pulmonary vasodilators are available and in use, including iNO,[185,189,190] sildenafil,[185,186,188-190] inhaled or intravenous prostacyclin, and bosentan.[185,187] It is important to note, however, that no RCTs have been performed as of this writing to establish the efficacy and safety of these therapies in the treatment of infants with BPD.[185] General management of infants with severe BPD is further discussed in Chapter 36.

Evidenced-Based Recommendations

There is almost no high-quality evidence base supporting a specific approach to mechanical ventilation for infants with significant BPD. Given the wide range of BPD phenotypes and relatively low incidence of severe disease, it is unlikely that adequately powered randomized trials are doable. The approaches described here are based on clinical experience linked to known/suspected underlying pathophysiology. The best approach for BPD is prevention,[191,192] but that has proved a difficult task to accomplish.[193-195]

Gaps in Knowledge

Given the fairly broad pathophysiologic spectrum and the relatively limited number of infants with chronic-severe BPD, even large specialized centers will have difficulty in performing randomized studies targeting specific ventilatory approaches to the care of this population of infants. Multicenter approaches, such as the Neonatal Research Network, the Children's Hospital Neonatal Database collaborative,[153] and the BPD Collaborative,[196] may be able to provide large enough patient populations to perform such studies.

Although comparative effectiveness studies of treatments for severe BPD are urgently needed, research also needs to focus on interventions aimed at the prevention of BPD. Although much effort and money have been expended in the pursuit of a single "magic bullet" for the prevention of BPD, given the multifactorial pathophysiology of BPD, studies designed around "systems" approaches to preventing BPD (i.e., "best demonstrated practices")[196-198] and/or combination therapy approaches[199,200] are more likely to prove useful.

Finally, trials must be sufficiently funded to evaluate not just relatively short-term outcomes such as BPD at 36 or 40 weeks' gestation, or even at 2 to 5 years of age, but well beyond those time points. Current long-term studies, primarily of infants born before the uniform availability of surfactant, suggest that even preterm infants not diagnosed with BPD have reduced lung growth and impaired lung function relative to infants born at term.[14,36,201,202] Given the fact that lung function normally begins to decline around the end of the third decade of life, minimizing the interruption of alveolarization associated with very preterm birth, and exacerbated through processes leading to "BPD," should be a top research priority.[38,203,204]

CONCLUSION

A variety of respiratory disorders may be encountered in the neonatal period, the most common of which have been discussed in this chapter. A firm understanding of the underlying pathophysiology, and how it may change over time, is necessary to optimally apply any approach to mechanical ventilation. A variety of ventilatory modes are available, and there is limited evidence to strongly support one mode or approach over another for most of these conditions. Given the limited evidence base for much of the care we provide, there is much to be gained through controlled interventional trials within collaborative networks. It is critical to recognize that the lungs of all newborns are not developmentally complete (not just the most premature) and may be more susceptible to VILI. Protocols for weaning and extubation are strongly recommended. The most important factor associated with safe and successful ventilator management of the sick neonate is the person operating the ventilator rather than the ventilator itself.

KEY REFERENCES

12. Nikolic MZ, Sun D, Rawlins EL: Human lung development: recent progress and new challenges. Development 145(16), 2018.
22. Tingay DG, Mills JF, Morley CJ, et al: The deflation limb of the pressure-volume relationship in infants during high-frequency ventilation. Am J Respir Crit Care Med 173(4):414–420, 2006.
32. Klingenberg C, Wheeler KI, McCallion N, et al: Volume-targeted versus pressure-limited ventilation in neonates. Cochrane Database Syst Rev 10:CD003666, 2017.
36. Vollsaeter M, Roksund OD, Eide GE, et al: Lung function after preterm birth: development from mid-childhood to adulthood. Thorax 68(8):767–776, 2013.
39. Greenough A, Peacock J, Zivanovic S, et al: United Kingdom Oscillation Study: long-term outcomes of a randomised trial of two modes of neonatal ventilation. Health Technol Assess 18(41):1–95, 2014.
52. van Ierland Y, de Beaufort AJ: Why does meconium cause meconium aspiration syndrome? Current concepts of MAS pathophysiology. Early Hum Dev 85(10):617–620, 2009.
73. Harding R, Hooper SB: Regulation of lung expansion and lung growth before birth. J Appl Physiol (1985) 81(1):209–224, 1996.
83. de Waal K, Kluckow M: Prolonged rupture of membranes and pulmonary hypoplasia in very preterm infants: pathophysiology and guided treatment. J Pediatr 166(5):1113–1120, 2015.
113. Shekerdemian L, Bohn D: Cardiovascular effects of mechanical ventilation. Arch Dis Child 80(5):475–480, 1999.
121. Chandrasekharan, Kozielski R, Kumar VH, et al: Early use of inhaled nitric oxide in preterm infants: is there a rationale for selective approach? Am J Perinatol 34(5):428–440, 2017.
146. Jensen EA, Dysart K, Gantz MG, et al: The diagnosis of bronchopulmonary dysplasia in very preterm infants. An evidence-based approach. Am J Respir Crit Care Med 200(6):751–759, 2019.
160. Coalson JJ: Pathology of new bronchopulmonary dysplasia. Semin Neonatol 8(1):73–81, 2003.
169. Thunqvist P, Tufvesson E, Bjermer L, et al: Lung function after extremely preterm birth—a population-based cohort study (EXPRESS). Pediatr Pulmonol 53(1):64–72, 2018.
185. Varghese N, Rios D: Pulmonary hypertension associated with bronchopulmonary dysplasia: a review. Pediatr Allergy Immunol Pulmonol 32(4):140–148, 2019.
204. Thébaud B, Goss KN, Laughon M, et al: Bronchopulmonary dysplasia. Nat Rev Dis Primers 5(1):78, 2019.

26

Weaning and Extubation From Mechanical Ventilation

Wissam Shalish, Guilherme Sant'Anna, and Martin Keszler

KEY POINTS

- Despite the general consensus that weaning of support and extubation at the earliest opportunity is desirable, there is little agreement regarding how to best wean from mechanical ventilation or the settings from which extubation is indicated.
- Both premature extubation leading to failure and the need for reintubation, as well as unnecessary prolongation of mechanical ventilation, may have adverse consequences.
- Despite many attempts, none of the proposed indicators of extubation readiness have stood the test of time; thus, wide practice style variation persists.
- The addition of analysis of the dynamics of cardiorespiratory signals to spontaneous breathing tests may enhance their predictive value for extubation readiness

BACKGROUND

Although a life-saving intervention, mechanical ventilation (MV) is associated with many complications (Box 26.1), making timely and safe weaning an important imperative. However, the process of discontinuing MV in newborn infants with significant pulmonary morbidity and those who are extremely premature remains a major challenge, made more complex by the variety of modes of respiratory support currently in use. There is no consensus about the most appropriate way to wean babies from MV, and their management remains largely subjective, depending on institutional practices and individuals' training or preferences. Unfortunately, many important gaps in knowledge remain in the science of weaning from MV and assessment of extubation readiness in neonates, resulting in significant variations in periextubation practices worldwide.[1] In this chapter, we provide a comprehensive review of this subject and some evidence-based recommendations to guide clinical practice for weaning from MV, assessment of extubation readiness, and postextubation management.

WEANING FROM VENTILATORY SUPPORT

Weaning from MV is the process of decreasing the amount of ventilatory support, with the patient gradually assuming a greater proportion of the overall work of ventilation. As mentioned in Chapter 19, weaning and extubation at the earliest possible time are among the a priori goals of mechanical respiratory support. In addition to the obvious goal of reducing ventilator-associated lung injury, early weaning will reduce the risk of nosocomial sepsis, reduce patient discomfort and need for sedation, minimize the development of oral aversion with subsequent feeding difficulties, and facilitate parental bonding and developmentally appropriate care. Therefore, as soon as the patient's condition stabilizes and the underlying respiratory disorder that led to the initiation of ventilation begins to improve, weaning should be initiated. This approach differs from that employed in the past (and persisting in some centers) when patients were heavily sedated or even paralyzed during the acute phase of the illness and weaning from MV did not begin until some arbitrary weaning criteria were met.[2,3] In the early days of MV of newborn infants, there was a widespread practice of keeping infants on MV until they reached the arbitrary weight of 1 kg. This practice, long ago abandoned, was based on the assumption that small preterm infants would expend too much energy to breathe and were unlikely to remain extubated. This concept was in large part related to the practice of extubating preterm infants to an oxygen hood rather than to continuous positive airway pressure (CPAP). Today, given the significant improvements in noninvasive respiratory support provision, some extremely preterm infants are successfully stabilized without MV after birth, and many of those requiring MV are able to be extubated within a few days and thrive. Those who remain ventilator dependent beyond the first week of life have a much higher risk of bronchopulmonary dysplasia (BPD).[4-6]

Many different modes of invasive respiratory support are used in neonates, and the specific mechanics of weaning from MV are to a large extent a function of the mode of support in use. The basic types of MV are (1) pressure-controlled ventilation, (2) volume-controlled or volume-targeted ventilation, and (3) high-frequency ventilation (HFV). The basic process of weaning for the various pressure-controlled synchronized modes is described in Chapter 20 and the basic steps for pressure-controlled ventilation and HFV are summarized in Table 26.1. A detailed discussion of weaning using volume-targeted ventilation is available in Chapter 22. Available data support the preferential use of (1) any mode of synchronized ventilation over unsynchronized intermittent mandatory ventilation (IMV),[7] (2) modes that support each spontaneous breath over synchronized IMV (SIMV),[2,8,9] and (3) volume-targeted over pressure-controlled ventilation.[10] Some important concepts that should be kept in mind to facilitate weaning include

---

BOX 26.1 Complications of Mechanical Ventilation in Newborns

Ventilator-induced lung injury (volutrauma)	Palatal deformities
Atelectasis	Nasal septal defects
Overdistention	Endotracheal tube complications
Bronchopulmonary dysplasia	Obstruction
Air-leak syndromes	Displacement
Pulmonary interstitial emphysema	Accidental extubation
Pneumothorax	Infection
Pneumomediastinum	Ventilator-associated pneumonia
Pneumopericardium	Late-onset sepsis
Airway trauma	Cardiovascular
Vocal cord injury	Decreased cardiac output
Subglottic stenosis	Neurologic
Subglottic cysts	Hypocarbia (cerebral vasoconstriction)
Granulomas	Neurodevelopmental impairment
Tracheobronchomalacia	

BOX 26.2 Ventilatory Settings at Which Extubation Should Be Considered in Infants 2 Weeks of Age and Under

Conventional Ventilation (AC, SIMV, PSV)
- SIMV: PIP $\leq$16 cm H_2O, PEEP $\leq$6 cm H_2O, rate $\leq$20, FiO_2 $\leq$0.30
- AC/PSV, BW <1000 g: MAP $\leq$7 cm H_2O and FiO_2 $\leq$0.30
- AC/PSV, BW >1000 g: MAP $\leq$8 cm H_2O and FiO_2 $\leq$0.30

Volume-Targeted Ventilation (Tidal Volume Measured at the Endotracheal Tube)
- Tidal volume $\leq$4.0–4.5 mL/kg (5–6 mL/kg if <700 g or >2 weeks of age) and FiO_2 $\leq$0.30

High-Frequency Oscillatory Ventilation
- BW <1000 g: MAP $\leq$7 cm H_2O and FiO_2 $\leq$0.30
- BW >1000 g: MAP $\leq$9 cm H_2O and FiO_2 $\leq$0.30

High-Frequency Jet Ventilation
- BW <1000 g: PIP $\leq$14 cm H_2O, MAP $\leq$7 cm H_2O, and FiO_2 $\leq$0.30
- BW >1000 g: PIP $\leq$16 cm H_2O, MAP $\leq$8 cm H_2O, and FiO_2 $\leq$0.30

Older infants may be able to be extubated from higher pressures or tidal volumes. Extubation should only be performed if the patient does not have significant tachypnea or increased work of breathing.
AC, Assist control; *BW*, birth weight; *MAP*, mean airway pressure; *FiO2*, fractional inspired oxygen concentration; *PEEP*, positive end-expiratory pressure; *PIP*, peak inflation pressure; *PSV*, pressure-support ventilation; *SIMV*, synchronized intermittent mandatory ventilation.

TABLE 26.1 Basic Weaning Strategies With Pressure-Controlled Modes and High-Frequency Ventilation

Desired Result	Action: SIMV	Action: AC or PSV	Action: HFV
Increase Pco₂	Reduce PIP, rate	Reduce PIP	Reduce Amplitude
Decrease Po₂	Reduce FiO₂, PEEP	Reduce FiO₂, PEEP	Reduce FiO₂, MAP

AC, Assist control; *FiO2*, fractional inspired oxygen concentration; *HFV*, high-frequency ventilation; *MAP*, mean airway pressure; *PEEP*, positive end-expiratory pressure; *PIP*, peak inflation pressure; *PSV*, pressure-support ventilation; *SIMV*, synchronized intermittent mandatory ventilation.

---

the following: (1) Weaning too slowly may be more dangerous than weaning too fast, as it may result in excessive lung injury and hypocarbia. (2) Weaning should be attempted throughout the day, not just during rounds. (3) When gas exchange is satisfactory and the work of breathing is not excessive, weaning should be attempted. (4) Volume-targeted ventilation effectively addresses concepts 1 to 3 by lowering inflation pressure in real time in response to improving lung mechanics and patient effort. Ventilatory settings at which to consider extubation readiness in infants 2 weeks of age or younger are provided in Box 26.2. These reflect general consensus and are based on values used as extubation criteria in many randomized controlled trials (RCTs), but not based on hard data. Older, more mature infants can usually be extubated from higher settings.

WEANING FROM PRESSURE-CONTROLLED VENTILATION

With SIMV, weaning is accomplished by reducing both peak inflation pressure (PIP) and the ventilator rate. The rate should not be reduced much until PIP has been reduced to relatively low values (<20 cm H_2O), which indicates improved lung compliance. PIP changes should be guided not only by blood gas values but also on monitoring of exhaled tidal volume (V_T), provided it is measured accurately at the airway opening. Lowering the SIMV rate while lung compliance is still low is likely to impose a high work of breathing and result in rapid shallow spontaneous breathing, which is inefficient, requiring high PIPs (and hence excessively large V_T) for the low-rate SIMV inflations to maintain adequate alveolar minute ventilation. In small preterm infants, it is advisable to add pressure support (PS) when SIMV rate is reduced below 30/minute. In one study, the combination of SIMV + PS resulted in more rapid weaning from mechanical respiratory support compared to SIMV alone in extremely low birth weight (ELBW) infants[9] and significantly lower work of breathing.[11] If SIMV is used without PS, the rate should not be reduced below 15 inflations per minute. There are no studies to inform the best method of weaning from SIMV + PS. It seems reasonable to reduce the SIMV rate gradually to 10 while also reducing the PIP as necessary to avoid excessive V_T and maintain PS at a level sufficient to achieve acceptable V_T for the spontaneous breaths, typically 4 to 5 mL/kg.

With assist control (AC) and PS ventilation as a stand-alone mode, each spontaneous breath is supported, but the infant controls the ventilator rate (as well as the inspiratory time in the case of PS). Therefore, lowering the set rate, which acts as a backup only in the case of apnea, has no real impact on reducing ventilator support. Weaning is accomplished by lowering the PIP or PS level and gradually transferring the work of breathing to the infant. For a brief period of several hours just before extubation, it may be reasonable to reduce the backup rate to 20 inflations per minute to better recognize any inconsistent respiratory effort that may have been masked by a normal backup rate. AC as a weaning mode has been more rigorously studied than PS, with evidence suggesting that it provides more homogeneous tidal volumes, reduces work of breathing, and shortens weaning duration compared to SIMV.[12,13] Recent data also suggest that AC may result in lower work of breathing compared to SIMV + PS, especially in the most immature patients.[14] Although PS ventilation may have the same benefits as AC, there is limited evidence to guide its use during the weaning phase. In fact, in the tiniest preterm infants with very short time constants, their inherently fast respiratory rates and short inspiratory times may theoretically lead to lower mean airway pressures (MAPs) and lung derecruitment.

WEANING FROM HIGH-FREQUENCY VENTILATION

Many clinicians are more comfortable changing from HFV to conventional modes before extubation under the premise that the infant's respiratory drive and breathing patterns can better be visualized. That being said, extubation directly from both jet and oscillatory ventilation has not only been shown to be feasible[15] but also may actually be desirable. Clark et al. reported that infants who remained on high-frequency oscillatory ventilation (HFOV) until extubation had a lower incidence of BPD than those ventilated conventionally, but infants who were changed to SIMV after 72 hours of HFOV did not seem to benefit equally.[16] Similarly, the large HFOV trial by Courtney et al., which required infants to remain on HFOV for 14 days or until extubation, reported a lower rate of BPD and shorter duration of ventilation compared with conventional ventilation,[17] whereas a comparable study published in the same issue of the *New England Journal of Medicine*, which allowed early crossover from HFOV to conventional ventilation, showed no such benefits.[18] The way HFOV support is reduced is based on empiric data and experience, with little experimental evidence to guide the clinician. With traditional HFOV modes, both pressure amplitude and MAP are reduced progressively as tolerated, the former to reduce minute ventilation, the latter to avoid overexpansion as lung compliance and oxygenation improve. However, when using the HFOV with volume guarantee, only weaning of the MAP is necessary, as pressure amplitude is reduced automatically (see Chapter 24 for details). There is no clear consensus regarding "extubatable" settings during HFOV, but in general, extubation is considered when MAP is 8 cm H_2O or under with FiO_2 0.30 or under. Frequency is not reduced as a means of reducing support during HFOV, because delivered V_T increases as frequency decreases during HFOV, so that reducing ventilator frequency has the opposite effect compared to that on conventional ventilation. Some clinicians increase the HFOV frequency as an indirect means of reducing V_T, but this approach of making ventilation more inefficient seems counterintuitive and not specifically supported by evidence. However, when HFOV + volume guarantee is used, frequency changes have the same effect as with conventional ventilation, because the V_T is held constant.

Weaning from high-frequency jet ventilation more closely parallels conventional ventilation, with stepwise reduction in peak and mean pressures. The primary means of decreasing support is via reduction of the pressure amplitude, which is the difference between PIP and positive end-expiratory pressure (PEEP). With both jet and oscillatory ventilation, when support is reduced enough to allow mild respiratory acidosis, spontaneous breathing will be observed as the infant begins to take over more of the respiratory effort. When there is good spontaneous effort and the settings are judged to be sufficiently low, extubation should be attempted.

GENERAL STRATEGIES TO FACILITATE WEANING

Permissive Hypercarbia

Permissive hypercarbia is a ventilatory strategy that accepts higher than normal $PaCO_2$ levels (between 45 and 65 mm Hg) as long as the pH is 7.20 or higher, while using lower rates and/or V_T. This strategy may reduce injury to the developing lung through a variety of mechanisms, which include more efficient CO_2 removal, better ventilation–perfusion matching, stabilization of (or increase in) respiratory drive, and improvement in cardiac output. Permissive hypercarbia appears to be an effective strategy to allow continued use of noninvasive support and avoidance of MV. This approach, although widely practiced, has not actually been directly evaluated as an isolated intervention in randomized trials. Nonetheless, it is generally accepted as appropriate and was an important part of several large trials comparing different delivery room management strategies.[19,20] It remains unclear if permissive hypercarbia is effective in facilitating weaning. Mariani et al. showed shorter duration of MV with a trend to less BPD in a single-center randomized pilot trial comparing target $PaCO_2$ of 35 to 45 mm Hg with 45 to 55 mm Hg during the first 96 hours of life.[21] A subsequent multicenter trial targeting an even higher level of hypercarbia failed to replicate these findings, possibly because unlike the pilot study, a clear separation between the two arms could not be achieved.[22]

The largest trial that incorporated permissive hypercarbia as part of a strategy to avoid MV and hasten extubation before and during the first 14 days of MV was the Surfactant, Positive Pressure, and Oxygenation Randomized Trial (SUPPORT).[19] The study compared a strategy of routine intubation and surfactant administration to primary use of noninvasive support in the delivery room along with permissive hypercarbia. The target PCO_2 was over 65 mm Hg with a pH over 7.20 in the group assigned to noninvasive support and under 50 mm Hg and a pH over 7.30 in the routine intubation group. Although no differences were found in the primary outcome of BPD/death, subgroup and secondary analyses showed decreased mortality among infants with gestational age (GA) between 24 and 25 weeks, lower rates of MV and surfactant supplementation, shorter duration of MV, and less use of postnatal corticosteroids for BPD in the noninvasive support group.[19] However, a secondary analysis of data from SUPPORT reported increased risk of adverse outcomes, including severe intraventricular hemorrhage

(IVH) and death, with both high $PaCO_2$ and fluctuating $PaCO_2$ levels.[23] A single-center trial focusing solely on permissive hypercarbia enrolled 65 infants of 23 to 28 weeks' gestation who received MV within 6 hours of birth.[24] Infants were randomized to a $PaCO_2$ target of either 55 to 65 or 35 to 45 mm Hg for the first week of life. The trial was stopped early after enrolling about one-third of the projected sample size, because of a concerning finding that permissive hypercarbia was associated with trends toward higher mortality and higher incidence of neurodevelopmental impairment, with a significantly increased combined outcome of mental impairment or death.[24]

As of this writing, the most recent randomized trial on the subject was the Permissive Hypercapnia in Extremely Low Birthweight Infants (PHELBI) trial, which compared permissive hypercarbia with more traditional PCO_2 targets.[25] The high-target group aimed for $PaCO_2$ values of 55 to 65 mm Hg on postnatal days 1 to 3, 60 to 70 mm Hg on days 4 to 6, and 65 to 75 mm Hg on days 7 to 14; the control group aimed for $PaCO_2$ values of 40 to 50 mm Hg on days 1 to 3, 45 to 55 mm Hg on days 4 to 6, and 50 to 60 mm Hg on days 7 to 14. The trial was stopped after it became evident from an interim analysis that the probability of showing a benefit from the intervention was vanishingly small. Ultimately, 359 infants with birth weights 400 to 1000 g were analyzed. The rate of the combined outcome of BPD or death in the permissive hypercarbia group versus control (36% vs. 30%; $P = .18$), death (14% vs. 11%; $P = .32$), and grade III to IV IVH (15% vs. 12%; $P = .30$) showed nonsignificant trends favoring the control group.[25] Moreover, there were no differences between groups with regards to weaning durations from MV. As with the previous randomized trials, the $PaCO_2$ in the hypercarbia group, although higher than in the control group, was generally below the target range despite the fact that infants were on significantly lower ventilator settings to achieve those targets. This highlights the practical limitation of targeting a significant respiratory acidosis in infants who are not heavily sedated or paralyzed; the baby's own respiratory drive will cause increased spontaneous respiratory effort, which may lower the $PaCO_2$ below the target range while also causing tachypnea, retractions, and possible agitation requiring sedation. Because very preterm infants have limited muscle strength and endurance, their effort to normalize their pH is often intermittent, leading to large fluctuations in PCO_2, which has been shown to be a strong predictor of severe IVH.[23] Thus, taking together results of the PHELBI trial with observational studies suggesting that $PaCO_2$ values over 60 to 65 mm Hg during the first few days of life are associated with increased risk of severe IVH (especially when rapid changes occur),[26-28] it appears that targeting marked permissive hypercarbia is not beneficial and may in fact be harmful. Instead, mild degrees of permissive hypercarbia similar to the control arm of the PHELBI trial[25] are based on sound physiologic principles and are generally accepted as safe and potentially effective in reducing the need for (and time on) MV.

Permissive Hypoxemia

Less aggressive oxygenation targets became incorporated into neonatal care without the benefit of large, randomized trials, in an effort to reduce oxidative stress and adverse effects on the lungs and other organs. Early observational studies suggested that lower oxygen saturation targets were associated with less retinopathy of prematurity, less chronic lung disease, and faster weaning from MV.[29-32] The safety of this permissive hypoxemia approach was called into question by a series of studies attempting to define the optimal target saturation as measured by pulse oximetry (SpO_2). Five trials with similar designs and a prespecified composite outcome of death/disability at 18 to 24 months' corrected GA were conducted to compare two different ranges of oxygen saturation (high, 91%–95%, and low, 85%–89%). A prospectively planned meta-analysis of individual patient data from 4965 infants below 28 weeks' gestation who participated in these five trials was recently completed and published.[33] Although infants randomized to the low oxygen saturation target group had a reduced relative risk (RR) of treated retinopathy of prematurity (RR, 0.74 [95% confidence interval (CI), 0.63–0.86]) and oxygen supplementation at 36 weeks' postmenstrual age (RR, 0.81 [95% CI, 0.74–0.90]), this came at the expense of an increased risk of mortality (RR, 1.17 [95% CI, 1.04–1.31]) and severe necrotizing enterocolitis (RR, 1.33 [95% CI, 1.10–1.61]) compared to the high oxygen saturation target group. As a result of this monumental endeavor, even though many questions still remain unanswered, it has been suggested that SpO_2 targets should be raised between 91% and 95% in infants with GA under 28 weeks until 36 weeks' postmenstrual age.[34] Therefore, permissive hypoxemia does not appear to be a suitable strategy to accelerate weaning from MV.

Weaning Protocols

The availability of a variety of ventilators and ventilatory modes, combined with the diversity in training backgrounds of neonatal practitioners, contribute to the highly variable intracenter and intercenter approaches to MV.[35] Such variability can be harmful, not only at the level of the patient (and her family), but also for health care providers, trainees, and the workplace at large. One solution to harmonizing practices and decreasing unnecessary variations is through the development and implementation of ventilation protocols driven by clinicians, nurses, and/or respiratory therapists.[36,37] In adults, the use of protocolized weaning has been demonstrated to accelerate weaning, reduce overall duration of MV, and decrease costs.[38,39] Similarly, several trials involving patients in the pediatric intensive care setting have indicated benefits from protocol-driven weaning.[40-42] In contrast, although no large RCTs have evaluated the usefulness of weaning protocols in neonates,[43] some evidence in favor of weaning protocols is available. In a retrospective study, Hermeto et al. demonstrated significant reductions in weaning time and MV duration in preterm infants (birth weights ≤1250 g) after a respiratory therapy-driven protocol was implemented.[44] Moreover, in a small RCT in 2002, experienced neonatal intensive care unit (NICU) nurses were found to be more effective at weaning infants from MV than physicians in training, thus suggesting another potential avenue for protocols to facilitate weaning.[45] Thus, despite the lack of solid evidence, weaning protocols appear to have a beneficial role in preterm infants. In fact, already 30% to 40% of NICUs around the world have adopted protocols for ventilator weaning in their respective units.[1,46]

Adjunctive Therapies

Adjunctive therapies are interventions designed to help preterm infants maintain adequate gas exchange and respiratory effort during the weaning and postextubation periods. Some of these therapies have been investigated by large RCTs, whereas for others, there is still a glaring lack of evidence to support or refute their use. A more complete discussion of pharmacologic therapies can be found in Chapter 32.

Caffeine

When given to infants receiving MV, caffeine has been associated with faster weaning, reduced MV duration, decreased BPD, and improved neurodevelopmental outcomes at 18 to 22 months of age.[47,48] The most appropriate dose is still not well defined and highly variable across centers, but the large Caffeine for Apnea of Prematurity (CAP) trial administered a loading dose of caffeine citrate of 20 mg/kg followed by a maintenance dose of 5 mg/kg/day once a day (with the possibility of increasing the dose to 10 mg/kg/day if apneas persisted).[47] Moreover, the most appropriate age at which caffeine should be initiated among mechanically ventilated infants is also not well established.[49] Although some centers prefer to initiate caffeine only around the time of extubation, an increasing number of clinicians prefer to initiate it soon after birth given the evidence from retrospective cohort studies that early caffeine may be associated with shorter duration of MV and improved long-term outcomes.[50-52] However, a recent trial addressed this question by evaluating the impact of early caffeine on weaning duration in preterm infants requiring MV.[53] Infants were randomized to receive either early caffeine or placebo in the first 5 days of life, and the placebo group later received a blinded dose of caffeine before extubation. Owing to an interim analysis at 75% enrollment showing a trend of increased mortality in the early caffeine group ($P = .22$), only 83 out of the intended 110 preterm infants were enrolled. Early initiation of caffeine did not reduce weaning or total MV duration, did not affect the rates of BPD, and was associated with a nonsignificant trend toward increased mortality before discharge, but no difference in the combined outcome of severe BPD or death.[53] Inadequate statistical power and some baseline imbalances in this study preclude definitive conclusions, but the study suggests that caution should be exercised in initiating caffeine early in mechanically ventilated infants.

Diuretics

High fluid intake and limited weight loss during the first 10 days of life are associated with an increased risk of death or BPD in preterm infants.[54] A meta-analysis on this subject concluded that restricted water intake reduces the risk of patent ductus arteriosus (PDA) and necrotizing enterocolitis with trends toward reduced risks of BPD, intracranial hemorrhage, and death.[55] These findings naturally led clinicians to consider therapies to address fluid overload as a means of improving lung function and reducing the need for respiratory support. However, diuretics have been shown to be ineffective in the

treatment of the acute phase of respiratory distress syndrome, even though the disease is clearly associated with fluid retention.[56] Furosemide is the most commonly used diuretic in the newborn period.[57] Furosemide decreases interstitial lung water and improves lung mechanics in the short term and thus is commonly used in infants who are difficult to wean from MV, especially when there is evidence of fluid overload. However, it is important to recognize the lack of objective evidence for its effectiveness in the acute and long term. In a secondary analysis from a multicenter prospective observational study (the Prematurity and Respiratory Outcomes Program [PROP]), extremely preterm infants started on any diuretic had a significantly greater probability of needing higher levels of respiratory support compared to nonexposed infants during the first 7 days after initiating the medication.[58] Given the nonrandomized nature of the intervention, it is possible that the perceived need to initiate diuretic therapy was a marker for more severe disease. In contrast, a recent retrospective cohort study of nearly 40,000 preterm infants suggested an association between greater furosemide exposure and decreased BPD risk.[59] Nevertheless, there are still no RCTs evaluating the impact of loop diuretics on weaning from MV. It is also important to note that furosemide stimulates the renal synthesis of prostaglandin E2,[60] a potent dilator of the ductus arteriosus, and therefore should be used with caution within the first days of life.[56]

Closure of Patent Ductus Arteriosus

Left-to-right shunting of blood through a wide PDA can cause pulmonary edema and decreased lung compliance. Moderate to large PDA has been associated with increased mortality and morbidities (including BPD) in preterm infants requiring prolonged MV,[61,62] and difficult weaning from the ventilator is commonly attributed to a "hemodynamically significant PDA." Although aggressive PDA treatment (pharmacologic and/or surgical) used to be routinely instituted as a means to facilitate weaning, such practice has been increasingly questioned after several analyses of individual RCTs and meta-analyses showed no impact of prophylactic or selective PDA treatment on preventing BPD.[63,64] The fact that both medical and surgical PDA closure have significant associated risks, that spontaneous PDA closure commonly occurs without intervention, and that meta-analyses have found no differences in mortality or morbidities in RCTs comparing active versus conservative PDA management all further support a more conservative approach.[64-66] It is possible that a select group of at-risk preterm infants may benefit from PDA treatment to facilitate weaning from MV; unfortunately, precise identification and targeting of these infants remain an unresolved issue.[67]

Avoidance of Routine Sedation

In preterm infants, there is currently insufficient evidence to recommend the routine use of opioids in neonates receiving MV.[68] In the largest multicenter randomized trial of its kind, the use of intermittent morphine boluses was independently associated with increased rates of IVH and air leaks as well as longer durations of MV, nasal CPAP, and oxygen therapy.[69,70] In another observational study, the use of morphine given preemptively or without ongoing patient-specific measures of pain was associated with prolonged MV and hospitalization.[71] In that study, the implementation of a nursing-driven comfort protocol significantly reduced this type of nonstandard morphine use. Moreover, morphine administration to ventilated preterm infants has been associated with subtle neurobehavioral changes during childhood.[72] Therefore, routine use of morphine analgesia/sedation cannot be recommended as it clearly impairs weaning from respiratory support and may confer long-term harm. In patients for whom nonpharmacologic therapy is not sufficient, an attractive alternative is dexmedetomidine, a highly selective alpha-2 adrenergic receptor agonist with both analgesic and sedative effects. Although dexmedetomidine does not appear to affect respiratory drive and does not prolong MV compared to opioids,[73,74] long-term safety data are still lacking. As such, routine use of dexmedetomidine should also be avoided.

Nutritional Support

Adequate nutritional support is critical to any patient receiving intensive care. Nutrition is interdependent with lung growth and development and plays a critical role in the prevention and management of BPD.[75,76] Most preterm infants with moderate or severe BPD experience growth failure predominantly because of suboptimal nutritional intake, which in turn can worsen BPD by further compromising lung repair and growth.[76] Indeed, high rates of extrauterine growth restriction have been described in critically ill preterm infants.[77,78] Therefore, adequate nutritional management of these infants should start immediately after birth to enhance ventilation weaning and lung repair and growth, thereby ultimately minimizing respiratory morbidities.

Chest Physiotherapy

Chest physiotherapy, such as percussion and vibration followed by suction, in infants receiving MV was assessed in a systematic review updated in 2008. A total of three trials involving 106 infants were included, and analysis identified insufficient evidence to adequately assess the efficacy and/or adverse effects of this therapy.[79]

Systemic Corticosteroids

The most recently updated Cochrane meta-analysis concluded that the use of early postnatal dexamethasone (before 8 days of age) facilitates weaning and decreases the risk of BPD in preterm infants but also increases the risk of short-term complications and long-term neurologic sequelae.[80] In contrast, early prophylaxis with low-dose hydrocortisone appears to improve BPD-free survival without affecting neurodevelopmental outcomes at 2 years,[81] but it also increases the risk of gastrointestinal perforation and late-onset sepsis.[82] Data about the role of prophylactic hydrocortisone on weaning from MV are not available. Evidence for later use of postnatal corticosteroids (beyond 7 days of age) summarized in the most recent Cochrane meta-analysis concluded that dexamethasone also facilitates earlier weaning, reduces BPD and reduces mortality at 28 days of life without significantly affecting long-term neurodevelopmental outcomes.[83] There was a trend toward a higher rate of cerebral palsy (CP), but this was offset by a trend toward lower mortality before follow-up.[83] In 2005, a

metaregression analysis of several RCTs demonstrated that the risk of death or CP conferred by postnatal dexamethasone decreased as the a priori risk of BPD increased.[84] An update of this analysis in 2014 showed that the results were unchanged by the addition of more studies, but a slightly narrower confidence interval was observed.[85] Based on this evidence, clinicians should use prediction equations or their own local data to identify the highest risk infants who are likely to have a net benefit from postnatal corticosteroid treatment with respect to survival free of CP. Unfortunately, the optimal timing and dosing regimen for dexamethasone when given after the first week of life remain unclear.[86] In a recent trial randomizing high-risk infants 27 weeks' gestation and under, requiring high settings on MV between days 10 and 21 of life to a 42-day course of dexamethasone (cumulative dose 8 mg/kg) versus 9-day courses repeated as necessary (cumulative dose 2.6 mg/kg/course), infants in the high-dose group were weaned faster, had shorter durations of MV, and had higher rates of intact survival at 7 years of age.[87] This study reinforces the notion that infants at the highest risk of long-term complications may selectively benefit from a larger total dose and duration of dexamethasone. Contrary to dexamethasone, data relating to the efficacy and safety of hydrocortisone administered after the first week of life are sparser and only beginning to emerge. In the recent Systematic Hydrocortisone to Prevent Bronchopulmonary Dysplasia in preterm infants (SToP-BPD) trial, hydrocortisone initiated between 7 and 14 days of life facilitated extubation and was associated with significantly reduced mortality at 36 weeks but did not affect the primary outcome of death/BPD at 36 weeks.[88] A follow-up on neurodevelopmental outcomes of the study cohort is underway. Furthermore, another large randomized trial conducted by the National Institute of Child Health and Human Development (NICHD) Neonatal Research Network evaluating the safety and effectiveness of hydrocortisone administered between 14 and 28 days of age in facilitating weaning and reducing BPD found that more babies in the hydrocortisone group were extubated during the treatment period, compared to the placebo group, but this did not translate into a significant reduction in the primary outcome of BPD at 36 weeks. There was no evidence of adverse effects on neurodevelopment.[89]

Inhaled and Intratracheal Corticosteroids

Inhaled steroids have long been used in the management of preterm infants on MV. Published reports indicate a relatively high and variable use of inhaled steroids in preterm infants with BPD,[90,91] despite the lack of evidence to support their routine use, whether given prophylactically[92] or after the first week of life.[93] In the largest multicenter trial from Europe (NEUROSIS), 863 extremely preterm infants were randomized to inhaled budesonide or placebo within the first 24 hours of life. Infants who received inhaled budesonide had significantly lower rates of reintubation and BPD, but their mortality rate was significantly higher at the 2-year follow-up.[94,95] Based on these concerning long-term results, the short-term pulmonary benefits conferred by inhaled steroids cannot justify their routine use for weaning from MV. The use of surfactant as a vehicle for administering steroids directly into the trachea has recently emerged as an alternative to inhaled and systemic corticosteroids. This practice, first reported in a pilot trial by Yeh and colleagues in 2008 and later reaffirmed in a larger yet still underpowered trial in 2016, showed promising results in terms of significantly reducing weaning duration, BPD, and the composite of death/BPD.[96,97] As of this writing, two large multicenter RCTs are underway to evaluate the safety and effectiveness of surfactant combined with budesonide, compared to surfactant alone, in preventing the risk of BPD in extremely preterm infants (the Budesonide in Babies [BIB] trial, ClinicalTrials.gov Identifier: NCT04545866, and the Preventing Lung Disease Using Surfactant + Steroid [PLUSS] trial, Australian New Zealand Clinical Trials Registry; ACTRN12617000322336).

ASSESSMENT OF EXTUBATION READINESS

With no clear evidence to guide extubation practices, the decision to extubate is most often based on the clinical judgment of the responsible physician, relying largely on personal training and experience while taking into account the infant's birth demographics (GA and birth weight), preextubation conditions (postnatal age, weight, and any other ongoing comorbidities), gas exchange (pH and pCO_2), and ventilatory parameters (MAP and FiO_2).[1] Although most clinicians attempt to extubate as soon as the infant has reached hemodynamic stability and "minimal ventilatory settings," many others rather rely on different philosophies about the optimal timing of extubation. For example, some clinicians have adopted the practice of immediate extubation following surfactant administration, while others still favor delaying extubation until the infant gains more maturity or reaches a higher weight threshold, irrespective of their clinical status. Even more recently, some clinicians have questioned the idea of extubation within the first 72 hours of life under the premise that a failed attempt may cause clinical instability and therefore increase the risk of IVH during this fragile postnatal transition period.[98,99]

Predictably, these subjective assessments of extubation readiness lead to substantial variations in practice and thus highly variable extubation outcomes across units. Reported rates of successful extubation range anywhere from 30% to 70% in ELBW infants,[4,100,101] and as high as 80% to 86% in some series that include larger preterm infants.[102,103] Infants who develop clinical instability postextubation (severe apneas, hypoxemia and/or hypercarbia) and require reintubation are exposed to significant risks and discomfort and may experience further deterioration of their respiratory status because of atelectasis. Reintubation in itself is technically challenging and can be associated with severe adverse events, including bradycardia, hypercarbia, alterations in cerebral blood flow and oxygenation, hypotension, and need for chest compressions.[104-106] It is, however, also worth noting that a relatively large number of infants experience inadvertent extubation and remain successfully extubated subsequently.[107] Those infants may have been exposed to MV and the associated ventilator-associated lung injury for longer than necessary. Protracted MV is clearly not benign; in preterm baboons, 5 days of elective MV resulted in a greater degree of brain injury compared to only 1 day of ventilation.[108] Based on data from the NICHD Neonatal Research Network, Walsh et al. showed that each week of additional MV was associated with a significant increase in the

likelihood of neurodevelopmental impairment.[109] Those findings have been reaffirmed in more contemporary cohorts, showing that prolonged MV exposure increases not only the odds of neurodevelopmental impairment at 18 to 24 months[110,111] but also mortality and several morbidities, including BPD, pulmonary hypertension, and severe retinopathy of prematurity.[5,6] Additionally, the endotracheal tube acts as a foreign body, quickly becoming colonized and acting as a portal of entry for pathogens, increasing the risk of ventilator-associated pneumonia and late-onset sepsis.[112] Clearly, both premature extubation and unnecessarily prolonged MV are undesirable. For those reasons, it is critical and highly desirable to determine extubation readiness in a timely and accurate manner to minimize MV duration while maximizing the chances of success.

Unfortunately, there is a striking paucity of high-quality data to guide the clinician regarding optimal ways to wean from respiratory support as well as judging an infant's readiness for extubation. Many attempts at developing tools to predict extubation readiness have been evaluated and are reviewed in this section.

Clinical Predictors

Over the years, many studies have attempted to identify clinical markers of extubation readiness in extremely preterm infants. Infants with successful extubation tended to have significantly higher GA and weight (at birth and at extubation), had less severe lung disease in the first 24 hours of life, and had lower oxygen requirements at the time of extubation compared with infants who failed extubation.[119-119] However, these results were not always consistent across studies, and even when they were statistically significant, there was considerable overlap between success and failure groups. As a result, it becomes very difficult to determine a cutoff for each clinical variable at which the extubation outcome can be accurately predicted. Nonetheless, a few studies have attempted to develop prediction models of extubation readiness using clinical variables, employing traditional methods such as multivariate logistic regression or more sophisticated machine-learning methodology (artificial neural networks, Bayesian classifiers, decision trees, and support vector machines).[116,120-122] Overall, these prediction models had low to modest accuracies in classifying extubation outcomes when compared to clinical judgment alone or were never validated and replicated in a second prospective cohort. Together, these results confirm that using a handful of clinical variables to determine extubation readiness is unlikely to mimic the complex decision-making process that goes into expert clinical judgment. At the same time, the findings imply that clinical variables alone are insufficient for capturing why infants succeed or fail extubation. Therefore, the use of additional physiological and/or clinical predictor tests, as adjuncts to clinical judgment, appear justifiable when assessing extubation readiness.

Extubation Readiness Tests

Extubation readiness tests are generally performed during a brief period on endotracheal CPAP (ET CPAP), or more rarely during temporary disconnection from the ventilator, while the patient is spontaneously breathing via the endotracheal tube without the assistance of mechanical inflations. During this imposed challenge, various physiological and/or clinical parameters are measured or monitored to assess whether the infant can successfully sustain breathing after extubation without the help of the ventilator. Physiological parameters include various measurements of lung mechanics, respiratory muscle strength, and breathing patterns, while clinical parameters involve assessments of the patient at the bedside for signs of clinical instability (e.g., apneas, desaturations, bradycardias, increased work of breathing, or increased oxygen needs). In a recent systematic review and meta-analysis, predictors of extubation readiness evaluated in preterm infants were described and their accuracies determined.[123] Included studies were small and single-center and had significant variations in their population characteristics and methodologies to assess extubation readiness. Assessments ranged anywhere from a few seconds to 24 hours, provided PEEP levels between 0 and 6 cm H_2O, and measured several different clinical and physiological parameters. A total of 31 extubation readiness tests were identified, showing overall good abilities to identify successful extubations (high sensitivities) but low abilities to detect failures (low specificity). Thus, none of the evaluated extubation readiness tests convincingly had sufficient accuracy, power, or external validity to justify recommending them in clinical practice. Box 26.3 lists the various extubation readiness tests evaluated in preterm infants, which are reviewed later.

Physiological Assessments

Measurements of respiratory rate, V_T, minute ventilation, and the rapid shallow breathing index have been the most extensively evaluated physiological parameters in preterm infants. Although certain measurements related to minute ventilation were significantly different between infants with extubation success and failure, the considerable overlap between groups limited their overall accuracy. Altogether, minute ventilation–related tests had a pooled sensitivity of 84% (95% CI, 77%–90%) and pooled specificity of 71% (95% CI, 57%–83%).[123] In the only RCT of its kind, infants extubated based on passing a minute ventilation test had faster extubation but also a higher reintubation rate compared to infants extubated based on clinical judgment alone.[124] Measurements of lung and respiratory system compliance and resistance, functional residual capacity, and lung volume have been investigated but not been shown to improve the ability to determine successful extubation.[102,125-128] Furthermore, most of these studies were performed long ago and may no longer apply to current clinical practice. Lastly, measurements of diaphragmatic and respiratory muscle function have shown some promise in differentiating infants with successful or failed extubation.[103,127] However, in the more recent studies, markers of respiratory muscle strength were found to have only modest accuracy in predicting successful extubation in preterm infants and performed no better than GA or birth weight alone.[130,131]

Clinical Assessments

Clinical assessments done during ET CPAP, also known as ET CPAP trials, have long been used to assess extubation readiness in a variety of populations, but the number of studies in

---

BOX 26.3 **Physiological and Clinical Parameters Evaluated During Extubation Readiness Tests in Preterm Infants**

Physiological Parameters
Pulmonary Function
Tidal volume
Minute ventilation
Compliance
Resistance
Functional residual capacity

Respiratory Muscle Strength
Maximum inspiratory pressure
Diaphragmatic pressure
Tension-time index of the diaphragm and respiratory muscles

Breathing Patterns
Respiratory rate
Inspiratory time
Expiratory time
Total respiratory cycle time

Cardiorespiratory Behavior
Heart rate variability
Respiratory variability

Clinical Parameters
Vital signs (heart rate, respiratory rate, oxygen saturation)
Oxygen requirements
Work of breathing
Apneas

---

newborn infants is small. Several early RCTs done more than 20 years ago used ET CPAP trials ranging from 6 to 24 hours; a meta-analysis of those studies concluded that preterm infants should be extubated directly from low ventilatory settings without a trial of ET CPAP, because the latter increased the risk of lung derecruitment without improving extubation outcomes.[132] Over time, ET CPAP trials continued to be investigated but became progressively shorter in duration to minimize the risk of adverse effects. Today, these short ET CPAP trials, commonly referred to as spontaneous breathing trials (SBTs), are usually done by having the patient to breathe through the endotracheal tube with PEEP (with or without PS) for 3 to 30 minutes while being monitored for various thresholds of clinical instability. In fact, of all predictors evaluated to date, SBTs have gained the most traction in clinical practice given that they are very easy to perform at the bedside and require no further equipment or sophisticated measurements. However, as highlighted in an international survey, SBTs are performed using widely variable test durations, PEEP levels, and SBT pass/fail definitions.[1] Based on results of the meta-analysis, SBTs were only evaluated in two small diagnostic studies, showing a pooled sensitivity of 95% (95% CI, 87%–99%) and pooled specificity of 62% (95% CI, 38%–82%) for predicting successful extubation in preterm infants.[123] The only study to evaluate the impact of daily SBTs as part of routine institutional practices showed that infants were extubated from higher ventilatory settings but had similar weaning durations and extubation failure rates compared to a historical control group.[133] More recently, in a secondary analysis from a large multicenter observation study, the safety and accuracy of a 5-minute SBT were evaluated in a cohort of 259 extremely preterm infants deemed ready for extubation.[134] Nearly 60% of infants developed signs of clinical instability during the 5-minute ET CPAP recording. In addition, after evaluating over 40,000 different combinations of clinical events to define SBT pass/fail, all definitions had low accuracies in predicting extubation success compared with clinical judgment alone. All in all, none of the evaluated SBTs so far have demonstrated convincing superiority over clinical judgment alone, either in terms of accelerating weaning or reducing extubation failure rates. Thus, SBTs cannot currently be recommended as part of routine use for the assessment of extubation readiness in preterm infants. Several aspects of SBTs, such as the optimal level of PEEP to be used, duration of the test, and definition of SBT pass or failure, remain uncertain and deserve further investigation.

Analysis of the Dynamics of Physiologic Signals Before Extubation

Several physiologic variables exhibit rhythms that are essential to life. These rhythms fluctuate irregularly over time and are characterized by a highly elaborate, apparently random output that arises from nonlinear biological mechanisms interacting with the fluctuating environment.[135] The application of physiologic variability measurements as markers of well-being has a long tradition in medicine. Unusually regular dynamics are often associated with disease, including periodic breathing, certain abnormal heart rhythms, cyclical blood diseases, and epilepsy. Analysis of biological signal variability has also been used in the prediction of clinical outcomes.[136] In adults, variations in cardiac and respiratory rhythms have been demonstrated to be good predictors of ventilation weaning and extubation readiness.[137-140] In preterm infants, investigations of the dynamics of physiologic signals, particularly using heart rate variability, have increasingly gained favor for the prediction or prognostication of later critical illness, such as sepsis, hypoxic ischemic encephalopathy, and death.[141-143] A few studies have also evaluated the usefulness of cardiorespiratory signal analysis for the prediction of extubation readiness in preterm infants. In a cohort of preterm infants with birth weight of 1250 g or less undergoing their first extubation attempt, measures of respiratory variability during a 3-minute ET CPAP period, used in combination with a successful SBT, led to a more accurate prediction of extubation failures compared to the SBT alone.[144] In another group of preterm infants, separate analyses of heart rate and respiratory variability calculated during a 3-minute SBT showed a good predictive ability to differentiate the outcome of extubation success and failure.[117,119] Using this same cohort and applying support vector machine methodology, a combined and more sophisticated analysis of cardiorespiratory variability was conducted. Results demonstrated an ability to identify 80% of the preterm infants who went on to fail their first extubation attempt.[145] Following these promising results, a large multicenter prospective collaborative study was initiated, aiming to develop an automated predictor of extubation readiness (APEX study) using machine-learning methods that combine clinical information with metrics of cardiorespiratory behavior derived from the analysis of cardiac and respiratory signals in extremely preterm infants (Clinicaltrials.gov—NCT01909947).[146] Infants classified as "success" by APEX had an improved probability of successful extubation compared to clinical judgment (positive prediction value of 94%), but this was at the cost of potentially prolonging ventilation in some infants classified as "failure" who were in fact successfully extubated following the APEX assessment (Shalish et al., Pediatric Academic Societies Meeting, 2019).

In summary, no single approach applied before disconnection from MV has been convincingly demonstrated to improve the assessment of extubation readiness or decrease the incidence of extubation failure in the extremely preterm population. Thus, the need to improve the clinician's ability to correctly predict extubation readiness in these infants continues to warrant further investigation.

POSTEXTUBATION MANAGEMENT

Some form of distending airway pressure should always be employed for at least 24 hours after extubation.[147] For the more immature infants, this period should be extended for much longer. The use of CPAP following extubation of preterm infants has been shown to reduce extubation failure compared to headbox or oxygen hood.[147] The rationale for using distending pressure relates to the excessively compliant rib cage of the ELBW infant, which is unable to maintain adequate functional residual capacity. The preterm infant normally uses grunting as a means to generate an internal distending pressure, but after being intubated for some time, the infant's vocal cords are edematous, preventing effective grunting.

The most commonly used noninvasive modalities for providing distending pressure are CPAP, nasal intermittent positive-pressure ventilation, and to a lesser extent the heated humidified high-flow nasal cannula therapy (Box 26.4). Details about these therapies are provided in Chapter 18 of this book. In addition, several adjunctive therapies may be useful during the postextubation period (see Box 26.4).

BOX 26.4 Key Elements of Postextubation Management

Respiratory Support
- Continuous positive airway pressure
- Nasal intermittent positive-pressure ventilation
- Heated humidified high-flow nasal cannula

Adjunctive Therapies
- Caffeine
- Racemic epinephrine
- Chronic diuretics
- Chest physiotherapy
- Inhaled and/or systemic steroids

Adjunctive Therapies

Caffeine

As previously discussed, caffeine became a common therapy in the management of preterm infants with respiratory problems following the positive results of RCTs.[47,148] With regard to the postextubation period, a Cochrane meta-analysis documented a significant reduction in the risk of failed extubations (RR, 0.48; 95% CI, 0.32–0.71) for infants exposed to methylxanthines.[149] Thus, in preterm infants at risk of apnea of prematurity, caffeine should virtually always be administered before extubation, if it has not been initiated previously. The optimal dose to achieve successful extubation may be higher than the standard dose used for apnea, but the overall evidence is not conclusive. Based on a recent meta-analysis comparing high (loading dose >20 mg/kg and maintenance dose >10/kg/day) with standard doses of caffeine citrate periextubation, a total of six RCTs were included.[150] Infants in the high dosing regimen had a significant reduction in extubation failures (18% vs. 36%; RR, 0.51; 95% CI, 0.36–0.71), fewer apneas, a shorter duration of MV, and less BPD compared to infants in the standard dosing regimen. Nevertheless, the limited number of studies, the wide variation in population characteristics and dosing regimens, and the absence of long-term safety data preclude from recommending routine use of high-dose caffeine for extubation.[151,152] Moreover, caffeine is not without side effects. Caffeine is associated with tachycardia, diuresis, increased metabolic rate, and gastroesophageal reflux (possibly via reduced intestinal blood flow velocity, reduced lower esophageal sphincter tone, and delayed gastric emptying).[47,153-155] In addition, early high-dose caffeine has been linked to increased seizure burden and increased risk of cerebellar injury with abnormalities on neurological examination at term equivalent age.[156,157] Therefore, high-dose caffeine should be reserved for those infants at the highest risk of a failed extubation after carefully weighing the risks and benefits and should be kept for the shortest necessary period.

Nebulized Racemic Epinephrine and Dexamethasone

Nebulized racemic epinephrine is commonly used to treat acute airway edema for postextubation stridor in newborn infants. Although anecdotal experience and short-term studies support its use,[158] a Cochrane meta-analysis failed to identify any randomized studies that evaluated important clinical outcomes.[159] There is a similar paucity of clear evidence in support of nebulized budesonide, but it is in common use for this indication based largely on anecdotal experience.

Postnatal Corticosteroids for the Prevention and Treatment of Postextubation Stridor

Two studies (published in 1989 and 1992) have examined the use of intravenous dexamethasone for the prevention of postextubation stridor in newborn infants. A meta-analysis revealed that the results were heterogeneous, with no overall statistically significant reduction in postextubation stridor (RR, 0.42; 95% CI, 0.07–2.32).[160,161] One of those studies, in which a selective high-risk group of neonates were treated with multiple doses of steroids around the time of extubation, showed a significant reduction in stridor.[162] Neither study had sufficient statistical

power to properly evaluate the need for reintubation, an outcome that deserves evaluation in further investigations. Despite the equivocal data, the use of a short burst of low-dose corticosteroids has become quite widespread, largely based on favorable anecdotal experience. Because corticosteroids have important side effects, it is prudent to reserve such therapy for infants who have been intubated for prolonged periods, who have a history of traumatic or multiple endotracheal intubations, or who previously failed extubation owing to subglottic edema.

Chest Physiotherapy

Four small RCTs have evaluated the effects of active respiratory physiotherapy, chest wall percussion, and vibration followed by oropharyngeal suctioning, during the periextubation period. A systematic review of these trials showed a lack of clear evidence to support the use of this therapy.[162] However, frequent chest physiotherapy performed every 1 to 2 hours was associated with a reduction in the need for reintubation within the first 24 hours post extubation. There was no decrease in the incidence of postextubation lobar collapse and insufficient information to adequately assess important short- and longer-term outcomes, including adverse effects. Caution is required when interpreting any possible positive effects of this therapy because the studies are old and enrolled a small number of larger, more mature infants and results were not consistent across the trials.

EXTUBATION FAILURE

When assessing whether an infant is ready for extubation, it is important to first establish what exactly is considered a clinically meaningful definition of extubation success or failure. Based on the literature, extubation failure has been defined either by using specific clinical criteria or by the perceived need for reintubation within a certain window of observation. Most studies report extubation failure rates within a single time frame after extubation, typically ranging from 24 to 72 hours but occasionally up to 1 week after extubation.[163] However, the increased use of aggressive noninvasive respiratory support during the postextubation period has further complicated the interpretation of the time frame for failure, because it may simply delay failure. The inconsistent reporting of extubation failure across studies makes it very challenging to compare the effectiveness of different extubation readiness tests or compare extubation outcomes between studies. Moreover, the lack of consensus on extubation failure definitions makes it difficult to determine acceptable failure rates for different GAs and better understand the risks associated with failure. The major risk factors for extubation failure in neonates are presented in Box 26.5.

In the extreme preterm population, an increasing body of literature over recent years has improved our understanding of the magnitude and clinical implications of extubation failure. To begin with, reintubations in this population are a dynamic phenomenon, occurring for various reasons throughout hospitalization and well beyond 72 hours from extubation. In a large cohort study of extremely preterm infants longitudinally followed from their first planned extubation until discharge from the NICU, reintubation rates increased considerably as a

BOX 26.5 Risk Factors for Extubation Failure in Neonates

General
- Sedation (narcotics or benzodiazepines)
- Multiple endotracheal intubations
- Difficult or traumatic intubation
- Neurologic or neuromuscular disorder
- Genetic disorders
- Airway abnormalities
- Positive fluid balance
- Acidosis before extubation (pH <7.20)
- Hemodynamic instability
- Sepsis and necrotizing enterocolitis

Preterm Infants
- Low gestational age (<26 weeks)
- Low postmenstrual age
- Extremely low birth weight (<1000 g)
- Low current weight
- Male gender
- Intraventricular hemorrhage (grade III and/or IV)
- Hemodynamically unstable patent ductus arteriosus
- Lack of caffeine administration preextubation
- Extubation from high ventilatory settings (FiO_2 and mean airway pressures)
- Inadequate provision of noninvasive respiratory support after extubation

function of time after extubation, going from 15% at 72 hours to 27% at 7 days and 47% by discharge.[101] The most commonly stated reasons for reintubation were apneas and bradycardias (in 65% of infants), followed by increased oxygen needs and increased work of breathing (in 35% and 29% of infants, respectively). Reintubations in the first 7 days post extubation were predominantly respiratory related, whereas reintubations caused by nonrespiratory-related diagnoses (such as sepsis or necrotizing enterocolitis) typically occurred after the first postextubation week. Thus, it is clear from this study that the commonly used time frames of 24 to 72 hours to define extubation failure underestimate the true occurrence of respiratory-related reintubations. Moreover, it is clear that no single observation window can accurately capture the true patterns of reintubation in any given cohort. For those reasons, it is preferable to report extubation failure rates in this population as a continuum, using a cumulative distribution graph, for at least the first 7 days postextubation.

Despite the earlier suggestions, a central question that remains is whether extubation failure independently contributes to increased morbidities and mortality or is simply a marker of the underlying disease severity. From the adult and pediatric literature, there is some evidence that extubation failure, reintubation, or prolongation of MV adversely affects survival independent of the underlying illness severity.[164-166] In extremely preterm infants, four studies have attempted to provide some insight into this problem, but with varying methodologies and results.[5,113,114,167] First, Jensen et al. retrospectively evaluated in a cohort of 3343 ELBW infants whether the number of reintubations, performed at any time interval after extubation, increased the risk of BPD, supplemental O_2 at discharge, tracheostomy,

and death.[5] After adjusting for confounders and including the total MV duration, only exposure to three or more reintubations was associated with an independently increased risk for BPD in survivors. Manley et al. and Chawla et al. performed secondary analyses of two RCTs in which they evaluated the outcomes associated with extubation failure, defined as the need for reintubation within 7 days and 5 days, respectively.[113,114] After adjusting for confounders but without including the total MV duration, extubation failure was associated with significantly increased risk of mortality, BPD, and longer duration of oxygen therapy, respiratory support, and hospitalization. In the most recent, secondary analysis from a prospective study, the relationship between reintubations at different time intervals after extubation and the composite outcome of death/BPD in extremely preterm infants was analyzed.[167] After adjusting for confounders, reintubation within any time frame between 24 hours and 3 weeks post extubation was associated with increased odds of death/BPD, independently of the cumulative duration of MV. Interestingly, reintubations occurring in the first 48 hours were associated with disproportionately higher odds of death/BPD compared with any other observation window. Also, the need for reintubation was associated with an additional 12 days of MV exposure, which in itself was independently associated with increased death/BPD. Thus, summarizing from the available four studies, although the need for reintubation appears to increase the risk of mortality and respiratory morbidities in extremely preterm infants, it may be mostly mediated by the extension of MV exposure that accompanies reintubation. However, results from the latest study indicate that reintubations occurring within 48 hours from extubation may carry the highest independent risk of complications and thus should be priority targets in future extubation studies. Moving forward, larger, well-designed multicenter trials are needed to better clarify this issue. In the meantime, we must continue to strive to extubate infants as early as possible, while attempting to optimize the chance of success. Despite those efforts, extremely preterm infants will frequently require reintubation. Therefore, both interventions need to be carefully planned and performed under well-controlled conditions by the most experienced personnel.

SUMMARY

Weaning from invasive ventilation and subsequent extubation continue to be challenging problems in urgent need of further study. Available evidence indicates that early extubation is desirable, but our ability to predict the level of support at which this can be accomplished safely remains limited, especially in very preterm infants. There is strong evidence that volume-targeted ventilation accelerates weaning from MV. There is also strong support for the use of caffeine and distending airway pressure following extubation. Evidence for other adjuncts to weaning and extubation is less well established. Improved tools for predicting successful extubation in this vulnerable population are currently being explored with the goal of reducing extubation failure and need for subsequent reintubation.

SUGGESTED READINGS

1. Al-Mandari H, Shalish W, Dempsey E, et al: International survey on periextubation practices in extremely preterm infants. Arch Dis Child Fetal Neonatal Ed 100(5):F428–F431, 2015.

6. Choi YB, Lee J, Park J, et al: Impact of prolonged mechanical ventilation in very low birth weight infants: results from a national cohort study. J Pediatr 194:34–39.e33, 2018.

25. Thome UH, Genzel-Boroviczeny O, Bohnhorst B, et al: Permissive Hypercapnia in Extremely Low Birthweight Infants (PHELBI): a randomised controlled multicentre trial. Lancet Respir Med 3(7):534–543, 2015.

46. Shalish W, Sant'Anna GM: The use of mechanical ventilation protocols in Canadian neonatal intensive care units. Paediatr Child Health 20(4):e13–e19, 2015.

99. Mukerji A, Razak A, Aggarwal A, et al: Early versus delayed extubation in extremely preterm neonates: a retrospective cohort study. J Perinatol 40(1):118–123, 2020.

101. Shalish W, Kanbar L, Keszler M, et al: Patterns of reintubation in extremely preterm infants: a longitudinal cohort study. Pediatr Research 83(5):969–975, 2018.

106. Venkatesh V, Ponnusamy V, Anandaraj J, et al: Endotracheal intubation in a neonatal population remains associated with a high risk of adverse events. Eur J Pediatr 170(2):223–227, 2011.

123. Shalish W, Latremouille S, Papenburg J, et al: Predictors of extubation readiness in preterm infants: a systematic review and meta-analysis. Arch Dis Child Fetal Neonatal Ed 104(1):F89–F97, 2019.

133. Kamlin CO, Davis PG, Argus B, et al: A trial of spontaneous breathing to determine the readiness for extubation in very low birth weight infants: a prospective evaluation. Arch Dis Child Fetal Neonatal Ed 93(4):F305–F306, 2008.

147. Ferguson KN, Roberts CT, Manley BJ, et al: Interventions to improve rates of successful extubation in preterm infants: a systematic review and meta-analysis. JAMA Pediatr 171(2):165–174, 2017.

27

Common Devices Used for Mechanical Ventilation

Robert L. Chatburn and Waldemar A. Carlo

KEY POINTS

- A wide variety of devices is available for invasive and noninvasive respiratory support of newborn infants. Some are primarily designed for adult and pediatric patients, while other devices are specifically designed for newborn infants.
- Contemporary ventilators used in neonatal intensive care units (ICUs) are complex microprocessor-controlled devices that offer many different modes, some of which have not been adequately evaluated in newborn infants. It is incumbent on the users to learn the advantages and limitations of the devices used in their neonatal ICU and to become familiar with the ventilation modes commonly used in newborn infants.
- The key to optimal outcomes is to understand that these complex tools need to be used with care, and there needs to be an understanding of the particular disease pathophysiology with a clear idea of the goals of mechanical ventilation.
- The ventilator descriptions in this chapter are meant to provide an overview of their functionality and available options. The reader is referred to the user's manual for each device for further details.

INTRODUCTION TO VENTILATORS

A ventilator is defined as an automatic machine designed to provide all or part of the work required to generate enough ventilation to satisfy the body's respiratory needs. Devices like resuscitation bags or a T-piece resuscitator are used to assist breathing but are not automatic and are not considered mechanical ventilators.

There was a time (the late 1970s) when textbooks[1,2] describing ventilators emphasized individual mechanical components and pneumatic schematics of mechanical ventilators. Today, ventilators are incredibly complex mechanical devices controlled by multiple microprocessors running sophisticated software. Fig. 27.1 shows a simplified pneumatic schematic diagram of a current-generation intensive care ventilator.

To keep this chapter practical, we restrict our description of ventilator design to a simplified discussion of general principles. From an engineering systems point of view, a ventilator can be viewed as having three main design characteristics: power inputs, power conversion and control, and power outputs. Beyond that, we need to understand some of the common design features of both the operator–ventilator interface (i.e., the control panels and displays) and the ventilator–patient interface (i.e., the tubing and adjunctive equipment that connects the ventilator to the patient).

Power Inputs

Work is force acting through a distance. For example, if you are asked to walk up a flight of steps, you do work in moving the mass of your body a certain distance above the earth. If you are asked to run up the steps, you may be disappointed to know that you are doing the same amount of work because it does not feel the same. What you are feeling is related to power, the rate of doing work. Similarly, it takes a certain amount of work as you inhale a breath. The larger the breaths and the faster you breathe, the more work you do per minute and the more power your body expends. Thus, power is a useful concept in understanding how ventilators are designed and operated and may be an important variable in the development of ventilator-induced lung injury.[3]

Modern ventilators are powered by either electricity or compressed gas (early iron lung ventilators could actually be manually powered). Power is defined as the rate of doing work and is usually expressed in units of watts. Electrical power is calculated as the product of voltage and current required to operate the ventilator (watts = volts × amperes).[4] Electricity, either from wall outlets (e.g., 110–220 V AC, at 50/60 Hz) or from batteries (e.g., 10–30 V DC), is used to run compressors or blowers of various types. Batteries are used for transport or emergency power.

Alternatively, the power to expand the lungs is supplied by compressed gas. Pneumatic power in watts is equivalent to a flow of 1 L/s moving in response to a pressure gradient of 1 kPa.[4] Compressed gas is usually supplied to ventilators from tanks or from wall outlets in the hospital (in the United States, hospitals supply about 50 psi from wall outlets). Some ventilators use compressed gas to power both lung inflation and the control circuitry, making them practical for transport and emergency use. Typically, ventilators are powered by separate sources of compressed air and compressed oxygen. This permits the control of oxygen concentrations between 21% (O_2 concentration in room air) and 100%. Although wall outlets supply air and oxygen at 50 psi, most ventilators have internal regulators to reduce this pressure to a lower level (e.g., 20 psi) to allow for safe operation in the case of fluctuating supply pressure. Compressed gas has all moisture removed. Otherwise, there could be condensed liquid in the tubing system, which could ruin ventilator pneumatic systems. Therefore, the ventilator gas output must be warmed and humidified before it reaches the patient to avoid drying out the airway and lung

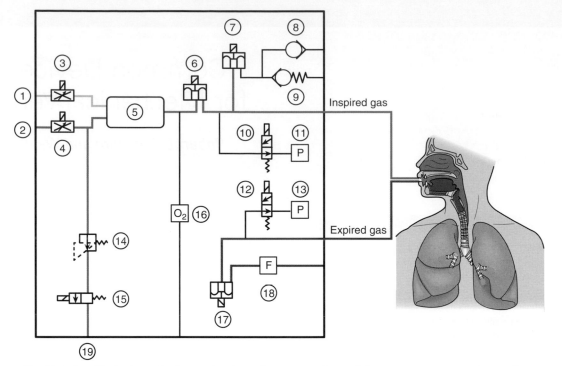

Fig. 27.1 Simplified schematic of a modern intensive care ventilator. High-pressure gas enters the ventilator through the gas inlet connections for oxygen and air (1, 2). Mixing takes place in a reservoir (5) and is controlled by two valves (3, 4). Inflation flow from the reservoir is controlled by a separate proportional valve (6). On the inspiratory circuit, there is a safety valve (7) and two nonreturn valves (8, 9). In normal operation, the safety valve is closed so that inflation flow is supplied to the patient's lungs. When the safety valve is open, spontaneous inspiration of atmospheric air is possible through the emergency breathing valve (8). The emergency expiratory valve (9) provides a second channel for expiration when the expiratory valve (17) is blocked. Also on the inspiratory circuit are an inflation pressure (*P*) sensor (11) and a pressure sensor calibration valve (10). The exhalation circuit consists of the expiratory valve (17), expiratory pressure sensor (13) with its calibration valve (12), and an expiratory flow (*F*) sensor (18). The expiratory valve is a proportional valve and is used to adjust the pressure in the patient circuit. It has an expiratory flow sensor. Conversion of mass flow to volume (barometric temperature and pressure saturated) requires knowledge of ambient pressure, measured by another pressure sensor (not shown). Pressure in the patient circuit is measured by two independent pressure sensors (11, 13). Oxygen flow to the nebulizer port (19) is controlled by a pressure regulator (14) and a solenoid valve (15). (Reproduced with permission from Mandu Press Ltd.)

tissues. A description of heating and humidification devices is beyond the scope of this chapter but is well described in current textbooks[5] and in Chapter 17.

Power Conversion and Control

Input power must be converted (e.g., from electrical to pneumatic) to get the desired outputs of pressure, volume, and flow. Electrical power is converted to pneumatic power with either a compressor or a blower. A compressor generates a relatively low flow of gas at ambient pressure to a storage container at a higher level of pressure (e.g., 20–50 psi). Compressors are used to create stores of compressed air in hospitals. Smaller versions are also built into intensive care ventilators (avoiding the need for connection to the hospital supply). In contrast, a blower (also called a turbine) is smaller, consumes less electrical power, and generates relatively larger flows of gas directly to the ventilator output with a relatively moderate increase of pressure (e.g., 2 psi). Blowers are typically built into home care and transport ventilators, and more powerful versions are starting to appear in intensive care unit (ICU) ventilators.

Flow Control Valves

Once pneumatic power is produced, it must be controlled to achieve the desired output of flow to the patient. Flow is manipulated in various ways to achieve predetermined patterns of patient–ventilator interaction called "modes of ventilation" (see Chapter 19). Inexpensive microprocessors became available in the 1980s and led to the development of digital flow control valves. Digital control allows a great deal of flexibility in shaping the ventilator's output pressure, volume, and flow.[6] Such valves are used in the current generation of intensive care ventilators used for neonates.

The output control valve works in coordination with another valve, called the expiratory valve or "exhalation manifold." When inflation is triggered, the output control valve opens, the expiratory valve closes, and the only path left for gas is into the patient. When inflation is cycled off, the output valve closes, flow from the ventilator ceases, and the exhalation valve opens, allowing the patient to exhale to the atmosphere. An additional function of the exhalation valve is to adjust the instantaneous expiratory flow path resistance to control the level of positive end-expiratory pressure (PEEP). There is a complex interaction between the output flow control valve and the exhalation valve enabling many different pressures, volume, and flow waveforms to be generated.

Control Subsystems

The output flow valve and the exhalation valve behavior are coordinated by the ventilator's control system.[7] Most ventilators use electronic control circuits with microprocessors and complex software algorithms to manage monitoring (e.g., from pressure and flow sensors) and control functions. The differences among modes of ventilation (and the ventilators themselves) are attributed to the control system software as much as to the hardware. Software determines how the ventilator interacts with the patient (i.e., the modes available).[8]

Power Outputs

As we have seen, the ventilator takes input power (e.g., electricity) and converts it to flow. Then it generates output as the power that supports the work of breathing for the patient. This output power is a function of the ventilator settings, such as frequency and preset inflation pressure, as are often used in the ventilation of infants.[9]

The clinically relevant outputs of a mechanical ventilator are the pressure, volume, and flow waveforms it generates in supporting the patient's work (or more accurately, power) of breathing along with the measured or calculated data it generates and displays to the operator. A "waveform" is simply a graphic representation of a variable as a function of time. Most modern ICU ventilators have graphic displays that plot the variables of interest (pressure, volume, or flow) on the vertical axis with time on the horizontal axis. The best way to understand this subject is to start with idealized waveforms, meaning the waveforms that would exist in an ideal world with perfect machines and no interferences from leaks or patient breathing efforts. These waveforms can be easily generated for educational purposes by using graphs of mathematical models using a spreadsheet program like Excel. Understanding idealized waveforms, one can more easily interpret real-world waveforms displayed on ventilators.

Idealized Pressure, Volume, and Flow Waveforms

Typical waveforms available on modern ventilators are illustrated in Fig. 27.2. These waveforms are defined by mathematical equations that characterize the ventilator's control system. They do not show the minor deviations, or "noise," caused by extraneous factors such as vibration, flow turbulence, or the patient's spontaneous breathing efforts. Remember that most ventilators have manual or automatic scaling of the horizontal and vertical axes, and this can dramatically affect the appearance of waveforms. Interpretation of ventilator waveforms requires an in-depth understanding of a number of underlying concepts (see Understanding Modes of Ventilation later).

Ventilator Alarm Systems

Ventilators used for neonates in the hospital environment have a wide range of alarms. The most important alarms cover events that are life-threatening, like loss of input power or microprocessor malfunction.[10] Other alarms cover events that can lead to life-threatening situations if not corrected quickly. These include things like high or low airway pressure, tidal volume, and minute ventilation or unusual ventilator settings such as an

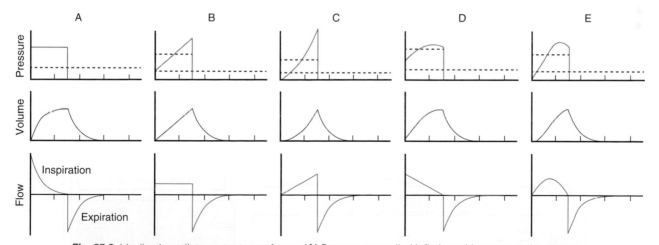

Fig. 27.2 Idealized ventilator output waveforms. **(A)** Pressure-controlled inflation with a rectangular pressure waveform. **(B)** Volume-controlled inflation with a rectangular flow waveform. **(C)** Volume-controlled inflation with an ascending-ramp flow waveform. **(D)** Volume-controlled inflation with a descending-ramp flow waveform. **(E)** Volume-controlled inflation with a sinusoidal flow waveform. The *short dashed lines* represent mean inflation pressure, and the *long dashed lines* represent mean pressure for the complete respiratory cycle (i.e., mean airway pressure). Note that mean inflation pressure is the same as the pressure limit in A. These waveforms were created as follows: (1) defining the control waveform using a mathematical equation (e.g., an ascending-ramp flow waveform is specified as flow = constant × time), (2) specifying the tidal volume for flow- and volume-control waveforms, (3) specifying the resistance and compliance, (4) substituting the preceding information into the equation of motion for the respiratory system, and (5) using a computer to solve the equation for the unknown variables and plotting the results against time. (Reproduced with permission from Mandu Press Ltd.)

I:E ratio greater than 1:1. The ventilator may also provide alarms for external monitors such as pulse oximeters and capnometers.

Operator–Ventilator Interface: Displays

The operator interface allows the operator to adjust settings and to monitor the status of the ventilator and patient. Interface designs vary widely, ranging from just a few hardware knobs and gauges to digital touch screen "virtual displays" and hybrids that have hardware knobs and buttons combined with digital displays. Obviously, the more complex the ventilator, the more complex the operator interface (e.g., a simple transport ventilator compared with an ICU ventilator). Yet among the complex ventilators, there is still a wide range of "user friendliness" of interface design, and there is a need for standardization.[11]

There are four basic ways to present monitored patient data: as numbers or text, as waveforms, as trend lines, and in the form of abstract graphic symbols.

Alphanumeric Values

Data represented in numeric form include both settings and measured values such as fraction of inspired oxygen (FiO_2), peak, plateau, mean and baseline airway pressures, inhaled/exhaled tidal volume, minute ventilation, and frequency. A wide range of calculated parameters may also be displayed, including resistance, compliance, time constant, percentage leak, I:E ratio, and peak inspiratory/expiratory flow, to name just a few.

Alarms and alerts are commonly displayed as text messages. Some ventilators also present brief instructions to the operator about settings and alarms, and there may even be excerpts from the operator's manual. See the later sections describing specific ventilators to see examples of the operator's interface.

Trends

Aside from the current values of ventilator settings and measured values, we are often interested in how parameters related to mechanical support change over time. Therefore, many ventilators provide trend graphs of just about any parameter they measure or calculate. These graphs show how the monitored parameters change over variable periods of time (Fig. 27.3). Significant events or gradual changes in patient condition can be easily identified. In addition, ventilators often provide an alarm log. This is usually a text-based list documenting such things as the date, time, alarm type, urgency level, and events associated with alarms including when activated and when canceled. Such a log could be invaluable in the event of a ventilator failure leading to a legal investigation.

Waveforms and Loops

Most ventilators display graphical depictions of pressure, volume, and flow waveforms (see Chapter 12). These waveforms are quite useful for adjusting ventilator settings or evaluating respiratory system mechanics.[12,13] They are essential for assessing sources of patient–ventilator asynchrony such as missed

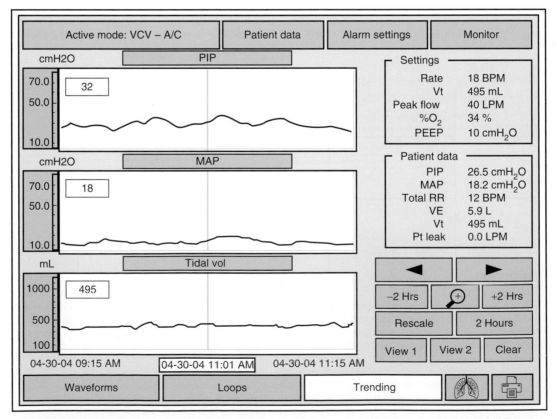

Fig. 27.3 Example of an operator interface showing trend data. *AC*, Assist-control; *LPM*, ***; *MAP*, ***; *PEEP*, positive end-expiratory pressure; *PIP*, peak inspiratory pressure; *RR*, ***; *VCV*, ***; *VE*, ***. (Reproduced with permission from Cleveland Clinic.)

triggers, flow asynchrony, and delayed/premature cycling and making appropriate corrections.[14] Sometimes, it is more useful to plot one variable against another as an *x–y* or "loop" display. Pressure–volume loop displays are useful for identifying optimum PEEP levels (to avoid atelectrauma) and optimum tidal volume (to avoid volutrauma).[15] Ideally, loop displays for such usage should be made with patients who are paralyzed or heavily sedated (to avoid errors caused by the effect of patient effort) and with very slow inflations (i.e., quasi-static curve), but that is rarely possible in newborn infants. Caution must be exercised because ventilators display loops under any ventilating circumstances, and hence, the display may be meaningless when the patient is actively breathing or when there is a large leak around the endotracheal tube. An example of a composite display showing numeric values, waveforms, and loops is shown in Fig. 27.4.

Patient–Ventilator Interface: Circuits

The ventilator output is connected to the patient input (i.e., the airway opening) by means of the *patient circuit*. There are four basic configurations (Fig. 27.5). Home care and transport ventilators often use only one tube, called a single limb circuit, with a pneumatically controlled exhalation valve (Fig. 27.5A) rather than having the exhalation valve built into the ventilator. The exhalation valve is controlled by a pressure signal from the ventilator, conveyed through small-bore tubing. This signal determines the timing of flow into and out of the patient for mandatory inflations and also may control the PEEP level.

Intensive care ventilators usually have the exhalation valve built into the ventilator and are connected to the patient with a double-limb circuit (Fig. 27.5B).

Noninvasive ventilation (NIV) may use a mask instead of an artificial airway. Ventilators designed specifically for mask ventilation often have single limb circuits that are used without an exhalation valve (Fig. 27.5C). In this case, the circuit or the mask has a carefully sized opening or port. The port provides a known leak. The relationship between circuit pressure and flow through the leak is programmed into the ventilator's microcontroller. Thus, the ventilator can estimate the flow and, hence, the volume delivered to the patient by measuring the pressure in the circuit, calculating the leak flow, and deducting that from the total flow delivered by the blower.

A single limb, coaxial circuit (sometimes called a Bain or F circuit) is often used on anesthesia machines as well as ICU ventilators (Fig. 27.5D).

Some intensive care ventilators measure flow at the airway opening using a small, usually disposable sensor. There are two basic types of flow sensors used with ventilators (Fig. 27.6). One is called a *pneumotachometer*. It has a flow-resistive element such as a screen or plastic flap in the flow path. The pressure on both sides of the resistor is conducted to pressure sensors in the ventilator through small-diameter stiff tubing. The difference between the two pressures is proportional to flow. The second type of flow sensor is called a *hot-wire anemometer*. Very thin wires are placed in the flow path and heated. Gas flow passing

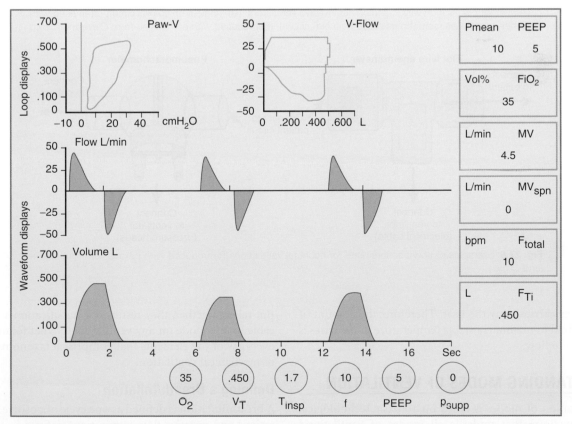

Fig. 27.4 Example of a composite ventilator display showing numeric data, waveforms, and loops. *PEEP*, Positive end-expiratory pressure. (Reproduced with permission from Cleveland Clinic.)

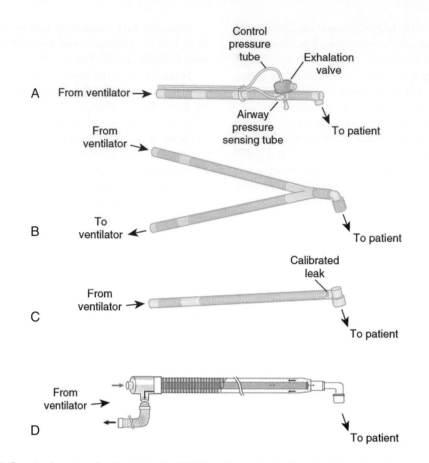

Fig. 27.5 Four basic types of patient circuits. **(A)** Single-limb circuit with exhalation valve often used on home care or transport ventilators. **(B)** Double-limb circuit usually used on intensive care ventilators. **(C)** Single-limb circuit without exhalation valve used on noninvasive ventilators. **(D)** Single-limb coaxial circuit often used with anesthesia machines (sometimes called Bain or F circuit). (Reproduced with permission from Cleveland Clinic.)

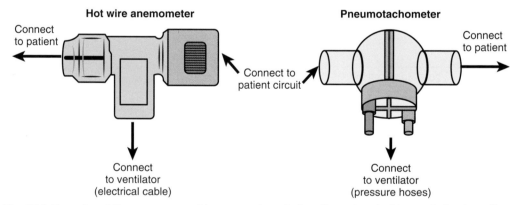

Fig. 27.6 Examples of flow sensors used for neonatal ventilation. (Reproduced with permission from Cleveland Clinic.)

over the wires carries away the heat. Therefore, the amount of energy required to maintain a stable temperature in the wires is proportional to flow.

UNDERSTANDING MODES OF VENTILATION

The classification of modes is based on 10 basic technological concepts (maxims) that underlie all modes of ventilation.[8] These concepts are each fairly simple and intuitively obvious.

But taken together, they result in a classification system applicable to any mode on any ventilator.[5,16] What follows is a brief overview of the elements that comprise a taxonomy for modes of mechanical ventilation.

Defining a Breath/Inflation

A breath/inflation is defined as one cycle of positive flow (inspiration) and negative flow (expiration) defined in terms of the flow–time curve (Fig. 27.7). A breath is a spontaneous breath.

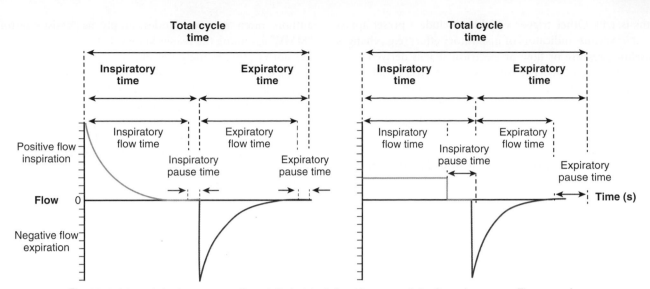

Fig. 27.7 A breath (or better, a ventilator inflation) is defined in terms of the flow–time curve. The curve for pressure control (with constant pressure) is shown on the left and for volume control (with constant flow) on the right. Important timing parameters related to ventilator settings are labeled. (Reproduced with permission from Mandu Press Ltd.)

An inflation (followed by exhalation) is a ventilator-generated "breath." For the purpose of the proposed classification, a "spontaneous breath" (inflation) is one for which inflation is started (triggered) and stopped (cycled) by the patient. A mandatory inflation is one for which inflation is either started or stopped (or both) by the ventilator independent of the patient.

Defining Assisted Breath

A breath is assisted if the ventilator provides some or all of the work of breathing. Graphically, this corresponds to airway pressure increasing above baseline during inspiration. In contrast, a "loaded" breath is one for which airway pressure decreases below baseline during inspiration and is interpreted as the patient doing work on the ventilator (e.g., to signal the ventilator to start inspiration).

Assistance With Volume or Pressure Control

A ventilator assists breathing using either pressure control (PC) or volume control (VC) based on the equation of motion for the respiratory system:

$$P(t) = EV(t) + R\dot{V}(t)$$

This equation relates pressure (P), volume (V), and flow ($\dot{V}$) as continuous functions of time (t) with the parameters of elastance (E) and resistance (R). If any one of the functions (P, V, or $\dot{V}$) is predetermined, the other two are derived. The term "control variable" refers to the function that is controlled (predetermined or preset) during a ventilator cycle. This form of the equation assumes that the patient makes no inspiratory effort and that expiration is complete (no auto-PEEP). VC means that *both* volume and flow (variables on the right-hand side of the equation) are preset. In the literature, the following terms are often used interchangeably to mean VC: volume targeted, volume limited, and volume preset. PC means that inflation pressure (the variable on the left-hand side of the equation) is preset.

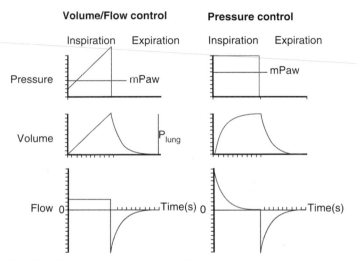

Fig. 27.8 Characteristic waveforms for volume control and pressure control. Note that mean airway pressure (*mPaw*) is less for volume control than for pressure control given the same tidal volume and inspiratory time. (Reproduced with permission from Mandu Press Ltd.)

In practice, this means one of two things: (1) the peak inflation pressure is preset (i.e., airway pressure rises to some target value and remains there until inflation time is complete) or (2) inflation pressure is controlled by the ventilator so that it is proportional to the patient's inspiratory effort. In the literature, PC is often referred to as *pressure controlled*, *pressure limited*, and *pressure preset*. Characteristic waveforms for VC and PC are shown in Fig. 27.8.

Trigger and Cycle Events

Ventilator inflations are classified according to the criteria that trigger (start) and cycle (stop) the inflation. The most common *trigger* variable during ventilation of the neonate is time, as in the case of a preset breath frequency (the period between breaths is 1/f). Other trigger variables include a preset apnea interval or various indicators of inspiratory effort (e.g., changes in baseline pressure or flow or electrical signals derived from diaphragm movement). The most common *cycle* variable is a preset inspiratory time. Other cycle variables include pressure (e.g., peak airway pressure), volume (e.g., tidal volume), flow (e.g., percent of peak inspiratory flow), and electrical signals derived from diaphragm movement.

Machine Versus Patient Trigger and Cycle Events

Trigger and cycle events can be either patient or ventilator initiated. Inflation can be patient triggered or patient cycled by a signal representing inspiratory effort (e.g., changes in baseline airway pressure, or changes in baseline bias flow, or the electrical signal derived from diaphragm activity as with neurally adjusted ventilatory assist [NAVA]).[7] *Patient triggering* means starting inflation based on a patient signal independent of a ventilator generated trigger signal. *Ventilator triggering* means starting inspiratory flow based on a signal (usually time) from the ventilator, independent of a patient trigger signal. *Patient cycling* means ending inspiratory time based on signals representing the patient determined components of the equation of motion (i.e., elastance, or resistance and including effects owing to inspiratory effort). Note that flow cycling (as used in the mode called Pressure Support) is a form of patient cycling because the rate of flow decay to the cycle threshold, and hence the inspiratory time, is determined by patient mechanics (i.e., the time constant and effort). *Ventilator cycling* means ending inspiratory time independent of signals representing the patient determined components of the equation of motion.

Spontaneous Versus Mandatory Breaths/Inflations

Inflations are classified as spontaneous or mandatory based on both the trigger and cycle events. A *spontaneous breath/inflation* is one for which inspiration is both triggered and cycled by the patient. Spontaneous breaths may or may not be assisted. A *mandatory inflation* is one for which inflation is either triggered or cycled by the ventilator (or both). A mandatory inflation is assisted by definition.

Breath Sequences

A breath sequence is a particular pattern of spontaneous and/or mandatory inflations. The three possible breath sequences are continuous mandatory ventilation (CMV), intermittent mandatory ventilation (IMV), and continuous spontaneous ventilation (CSV). CMV, commonly known as "assist-control" or "AC," is a breath sequence for which spontaneous breaths are not possible between mandatory inflations because every patient trigger signal produces a ventilator-cycled inflation (i.e., a mandatory inflation).

IMV is a breath sequence for which spontaneous breaths are possible between mandatory inflations. The term "SIMV" (synchronized intermittent mandatory ventilation) is commonly used to indicate that the machine triggering of mandatory inflations may be synchronized with the patient's inspiratory effort, but the "S" is irrelevant in the mode taxonomy. In the literature about neonatal and pediatric mechanical ventilation,

authors often refer to modes simply as "assist-control" or "SIMV," assuming the reader knows that they are talking about PC, not VC. Interestingly, the adult literature does the exact opposite. Over time, four different varieties of IMV have evolved in an effort to make modes more robust in serving, to some extent, all three of the goals of mechanical ventilation (i.e., safety, comfort, and liberation).[17] The legacy form of IMV, designated as IMV(1), allows the operator to set the frequency of mandatory inflations and they will be delivered regardless of inspiratory efforts of the patient.

Mandatory inflations (i.e., those which are either triggered or cycled by the ventilator independent of patient breathing efforts) increase the risk of patient–ventilator synchrony problems compared to spontaneous breaths (i.e., those for which inspiration is both triggered and cycled by the patient). This prompted engineers to invent a second variety of IMV, designated IMV(2). In this variety, mandatory inflations are suppressed if the frequency of spontaneous breaths is higher than the set rate.

Recognizing that safety may be compromised with IMV(2) if the patient takes rapid shallow breaths, yet another variety was created, IMV(3), where mandatory inflations are suppressed if minute ventilation because of spontaneous breaths exceeds the mandatory minute ventilation determined by the set rate and tidal volume.

Finally, in an effort to serve the goal of comfort in VC modes (i.e., with preset tidal volume and inspiratory flow), engineers invented the dual targeting scheme. With this, individual mandatory inflations are suppressed if the patient triggers inflation and if the inspiratory effort is large enough to switch the control variable from volume to pressure (with patient cycling at a predetermined flow threshold as in pressure support). This has important ramifications; modes that are designated by the manufacturer as volume control assist-control (i.e., VC-CMV) but use dual targeting are actually not CMV but rather the fourth type of IMV, IMV(4), because spontaneous breaths can appear between mandatory inflations (the definition of IMV). Note that dual targeting is also used for modes designed to be IMV (i.e., "SIMV + pressure support"). In this case, the classification is VC-IMV(1) d,s because it would be confusing to say IMV(1+4) and because the mode defaults to IMV(1) if no inflations switch from VC to PC (please see Full Mode Taxonomy later).

At this point, we should note that some ventilator designers consider the mode of ventilation to be simply the breath sequence. For example, the Medtronics Puritan Bennett (PB) 840 presents the operator with the option of first setting the "mode" as assist-control (AC), synchronized intermittent mandatory ventilation (SIMV), Bilevel, or Spont (being CMV, IMV, and CSV, respectively). Then the operator selects a combination of the control variable and targeting scheme for mandatory inflations and spontaneous breaths (Table 27.1). This is a logical paradigm for selecting settings on an individual ventilator; however, it is not a good paradigm for a general mode classification system. All manufacturers have (understandably) tended to see the problem of describing modes from the narrow vision of their particular product rather than from the larger issue of understanding, classifying, and comparing modes in general.

TABLE 27.1 Mode Setting Options for the Medtronic PB 980 Ventilator[a]

| Mode | BREATH CATEGORY | |
	Mandatory	Spontaneous
AC	VC PC VC+	NA
SIMV	VC	PS TC
	PC	PS VS PA TC
	VC+	PS TC
Bilevel	PC	PS TC
Spont	NA	PS VS PA TC

[a]The word "mode" in this case refers to the breath sequences (continuous mandatory ventilation, intermittent mandatory ventilation, and continuous spontaneous ventilation), which are given names (AC, SIMV, and spontaneous, respectively).

AC, Assist-control; NA, not applicable; PA, proportional assist; PC, power control; PS, pressure support; SIMV, synchronized intermittent mandatory ventilation; TC, tube compensation; VC, volume control; VC+, volume control plus; VS, volume support.

Although a standardized nomenclature and mode taxonomy will probably never be embraced by all manufacturers, we can still hope that they at least describe modes the same way in their operator manuals. And even if that never happens, end-users are now free to apply this knowledge on their own to understand and use the available technology.

Ventilatory Patterns

A ventilatory pattern is a sequence of inflations (CMV, IMV, or CSV) with a particular control variable (volume or pressure) for the mandatory inflations (or the spontaneous breaths for CSV or IMV). Thus, with two control variables and three breath sequences there are five possible ventilatory patterns: VC-CMV, VC-IMV, PC-CMV, PC-IMV, PC-CSV. The combination VC-CSV is not possible because VC implies that ventilator cycling and ventilator cycling make every inflation mandatory, not spontaneous (see Maxim 6).

Targeting Schemes

Within each ventilatory pattern, there are several types that can be distinguished by their targeting schemes. A targeting scheme is a model of the relationship between operator inputs and ventilator outputs to achieve a specific ventilatory pattern, usually in the form of a feedback control system.[4] Targets can be set for parameters during a breath (within-breath targets). These parameters relate to the pressure, volume, and flow waveforms. Examples of within-breath targets include peak inspiratory flow and tidal volume or inflation pressure and rise time (set-point targeting), pressure, volume, and flow (dual targeting) and constant of proportionality between inspiratory pressure and patient effort (servo targeting).

Targets can be set between breaths to modify the within-breath targets and/or the overall ventilatory pattern (between-breath targets). These are used with more advanced targeting schemes, where targets act over multiple breaths. In neonatal ventilation, the between-breath target is typically tidal volume (for PC, using adaptive targeting). For pediatric and adult ventilation, between-breath targets include work rate of breathing and minute ventilation (for optimal targeting) and combined end tidal PCO_2, volume, and frequency values describing a "zone of comfort" (for intelligent targeting, e.g., SmartCarePS or IntelliVent-ASV).

The targeting scheme (or combination of targeting schemes) is what distinguishes one ventilatory pattern from another. There are currently seven basic targeting schemes that account for the wide variety seen in different modes of ventilation:

Set-point: A targeting scheme for which the operator sets all the parameters of the pressure waveform (PC modes) or volume and flow waveforms (VC modes). The ventilator does not adjust any targets automatically.

Dual: A targeting scheme that allows the ventilator to switch between VC and PC *during a single inspiration* (not currently used for neonatal ventilation).

Bio-variable: A targeting scheme that allows the ventilator to automatically set the inflation pressure (or tidal volume) randomly to mimic the variability observed during normal breathing (not currently used for neonatal ventilation).

Servo: A targeting scheme for which the output of the ventilator (e.g., inflation pressure) automatically follows a varying input (e.g., inspiratory effort). Currently, the only example for neonatal ventilation is NAVA.[7]

Adaptive: A targeting scheme that allows the ventilator to automatically set one target (e.g., pressure within an inflation) to achieve another target (e.g., tidal volume). Modes that use PC with adaptive targeting are often referred to in the literature as "volume targeted" or "volume guarantee" modes.

Optimal: A targeting scheme that automatically adjusts the targets of the ventilatory pattern to either minimize or maximize some overall performance characteristic (e.g., work rate of breathing, not currently used for neonatal ventilation but applicable to pediatric patients).

Intelligent: A targeting scheme that automatically adjusts the targets of the ventilatory pattern using artificial intelligence programs such as fuzzy logic, rule-based expert systems. Artificial neural networks have been described in the literature but are not commercially available at this time.

Targeting schemes commonly used for neonatal ventilation are shown in Table 27.2.

Full Mode Taxonomy

A mode of ventilation is classified according to its control variable, breath sequence, and targeting scheme(s). Thus, the ventilator mode taxonomy has four hierarchical levels:

Control variable (pressure or volume, for the primary breath)

TABLE 27.2 Targeting Schemes Commonly Used for Neonatal Ventilation

Name	Abbreviation	Description	Advantage	Disadvantage	Example Mode Name	Ventilator	Manufacturer
Set-point	s	Operator sets all parameters of pressure waveform (pressure control modes) or volume and flow waveforms (volume control modes)	Simplicity	Changing patient conditions may make settings inappropriate	Pressure Control AC	Babylog VN500	Dräger
Servo	r	Output of the ventilator (pressure/volume/flow) automatically follows a varying input. Currently implemented as inspiratory pressure proportional to inspiratory effort	Proportion of total work of breathing supported by the ventilator is constant regardless of inspiratory effort	Requires estimates of artificial airways and/or respiratory system mechanical properties	Proportional Assist Ventilation Plus	PB 980	Medtronics
Adaptive	a	Ventilator automatically sets target(s) between breaths in response to varying patient conditions	Can maintain stable tidal volume delivery with pressure control for changing lung mechanics or patient inspiratory effort	Automatic adjustment may be inappropriate if algorithm assumptions are violated or they do not match physiology	Pressure-Regulated Volume Control	SERVO-U	Maquet

(Used with permission of Mandu Press Ltd.)

Breath sequence (CMV, IMV, or CSV)

Primary breath targeting scheme (for CMV or CSV)

Secondary breath targeting scheme (for IMV)

The "primary breath" is either the only breath there is (mandatory inflations for CMV and spontaneous breaths for CSV) or the mandatory inflation in IMV. We consider it primary because if the patient becomes apneic, it is the only thing keeping the patient alive. The targeting schemes can be represented by single, lower-case letters: set-point = s, dual = d, servo = r, bio-variable = b, adaptive = a, optimal = o, intelligent = i. More than one targeting scheme may be used for each type of breath.

How to Classify a Mode of Ventilation

Translating a name of a mode into a mode classification using the taxonomy is a simple three-step procedure:

Step 1: Identify the primary breath control variable. If the inspiratory pressure is preset, or if pressure is proportional to inspiratory effort, then the control variable is pressure. On the contrary, if the operator sets *both* tidal volume *and* inspiratory flow, then the control variable is volume.

Step 2: Identify the breath sequence.

Step 3: Identify the targeting schemes for the primary and (if applicable) secondary breaths.

For example, the mode that is commonly called "time-cycled pressure-limited" in the neonatal literature is classified as follows: (1) inflation pressure is preset, so the control variable is pressure;

(2) inspiratory time is preset, indicating machine cycling and thus the presence of mandatory inflations, plus the allowance for spontaneous breaths between mandatory inflations, indicating the breath sequence is IMV; and (3) all targets are operator preset so the targeting scheme is set-point. The "tag" (classification abbreviation) for this mode is hence PC-IMVs,s. In contrast, for a mode called "Volume Support," the operator sets a target tidal volume *but* flow is not preset; hence, the control variable is pressure. Every breath is both patient triggered (pressure or flow) and patient cycled (% of peak flow), and hence, the breath sequence is CSV. Finally, the ventilator automatically adjusts the inflation pressure between breaths to achieve (on average) the operator set target tidal volume.

To make this chapter practical for the user, we provide only a brief description of the unique features of the most common ventilators used for infants. We provide the list of available modes and their classification in the accompanying tables.

UNIVERSAL INTENSIVE CARE VENTILATORS USED FOR NEONATAL VENTILATION

Up until the 1980s, there was an unequivocal need to have separate adult and infant ventilators, mainly because of technological limitations related to delivering small volumes to children and newborns. Today, most of the high-end ICU ventilators used in the United States are able to ventilate the whole range of patients from premature infants (weighing a few hundred grams) up to obese adults (<400 kg). This is an amazing technological feat but by necessity involves certain compromises. Because the adult market is much larger than the neonatal and pediatric market, these devices are primarily adult ventilators that extend their reach into neonatal-size patients but do not address some of the unique aspects of neonatal physiology, allow for precise tidal volume measurement at the airway opening or ventilation in the presence of large leaks because of the use of uncuffed endotracheal tubes. Thus, some of these devices may not be optimal for the smallest preterm infants. The most common "universal" ventilators are described here.

Note that the tables showing the modes for each ventilator pair the arbitrary names created by the manufacturers with the standardized ventilator mode taxonomy.[8]

Modes commonly referred to as *volume-targeted* in the pediatric literature include both modes classified as VC and those that are classified as PC with adaptive targeting of tidal volume (either of which may have any of the three breath sequences).

AVEA CVS

The AVEA CVS (Vyaire Medical) is designed for intensive care ventilation of adult, pediatric, and neonatal patients (Fig. 27.9).

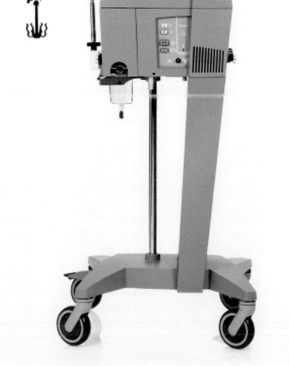

Fig. 27.9 Vyaire AVEA ventilator. (Reproduced with permission from Vyaire.)

Modes

Modes are selected by pressing the virtual button with the desired mode name. There are 10 basic mode names (Table 27.3). All modes can be flow or pressure triggered. In addition, there are "advanced settings" that can be used to modify the main modes (Table 27.4). Some of these advanced settings actually change the mode, resulting in many more modes by classification (Table 27.5).

The advanced settings increase both flexibility and confusion. For example, all VC breaths use dual targeting instead of set-point targeting. That means the mode labeled as Volume Control AC volume is not a form of CMV but is really VC-IMV(4), as explained earlier in the sections on dual targeting and IMV varieties. Furthermore, adding the "Vsync" and "Flow Cycle" advanced settings to this mode turns it into PC IMV with adaptive and set-point targeting (PC-IMVa,s), a completely different mode. Leak compensation is used to compensate for baseline leaks, which may occur at the patient–mask interface or around the patient's endotracheal tube. It provides only baseline leak compensation and is not active during breath delivery. Machine volume uses inspiratory tidal volume as its target and thus would overestimate actual tidal volume in the presence of a large leak around an uncuffed endotracheal tube.

When artificial airway compensation is turned on, the ventilator calculates the pressure at the airway opening required to deliver the set inflation pressure to the distal (carina) end of the endotracheal tube, as if the pressure drop across the artificial airway did not exist. This calculation takes into account flow, gas composition (e.g., heliox or nitrogen/oxygen), FiO_2, tube diameter, tube length, and pharyngeal curvature based on patient size (neonatal, pediatric, adult). This compensation occurs only during inflation. Artificial airway compensation is active in all pressure support (spontaneous) and flow-cycled PC inflations (spontaneous or mandatory depending on machine or patient triggering).

Airway pressure release ventilation/biphasic. Airway pressure is maintained at a relatively high level for most of the respiratory cycle with intermittent release to a lower value. This is in essence extreme inverse ratio ventilation with a very long inspiratory time and brief exhalation. Spontaneous breaths are permitted both between and during mandatory inflations and account for the bulk of minute ventilation; therefore, adequate respiratory effort is needed. (Please see Chapter 23 for a functional description of airway pressure release ventilation [APRV].)

Continuous positive airway pressure/pressure support. All spontaneous breaths are pressure supported if the pressure support level is set above zero.

Continuous positive airway pressure/pressure support with volume limit. All spontaneous breaths are pressure supported: When a patient-triggered inflation exceeds the set volume limit, inflation is terminated.

Infant nasal continuous positive airway pressure. This is available for the neonatal patient size setting only. This mode is designed to work with standard two-limbed neonatal patient circuits and nasal prongs.

Infant nasal intermittent mandatory ventilation. This mode is available for the neonatal patient size setting only. It is designed to work with standard two-limbed neonatal patient circuits and nasal prongs.

TABLE 27.3 The 10 Basic Mode Names for Vyaire AVEA

Setting	VOL/AC	VOL SIMV	PRES AC	PRES SIMV	PRVC AC	PRVC SIMV	CPAP/PSV	APRV/ BIPHASIC	TCPL AC	TCPL SIMV
Frequency	x	x	x	x	x	x			x	x
Volume	x	x			x	x				
Peak flow	x	x							x	x
Inspiratory pressure			x	x				x	x	x
Inspiratory time			x	x	x	x		x	x	x

TABLE 27.4 Advanced Modes for the Vyaire AVEA

Advanced Setting	Action
Volume limit	For pressure control modes, sets a volume cycle threshold. Note that volume cycling of a pressure support breath changes it from spontaneous to mandatory.
Machine volume	For pressure control modes, allows a volume target and flow and activates dual targeting. The operator sets the target volume and the ventilator calculates the target flow as the volume divided by the set inspiratory time. If flow decays to this flow target and the volume has not been delivered, then inspiration switches to volume control with constant flow until the volume has been delivered. Inspiratory time remains constant. Machine volume overrides flow cycle setting if activated.
Flow cycle	For pressure control modes, changes the cycle criterion from time to flow and sets the threshold for inspiratory flow termination as a percentage of peak flow.
Demand flow	For volume control modes, sets a ventilator-determined pressure target and activates dual targeting. If inspiratory pressure decreases 2 cm H_2O (because of patient inspiratory effort), volume control switches to pressure control. If the set volume is delivered and flow is equal to the set flow, inspiration is volume cycled. Otherwise, inspiration is flow cycled at 25% of peak flow.
Vsync	Switches the mode from volume control to pressure control with adaptive targeting. Inspiratory pressure is automatically adjusted to maintain an average tidal volume equal to the set volume.

TABLE 27.5 All Modes Available on the Vyaire AVEA

Mode Name	MODE CLASSIFICATION				
	Control Variable	Breath Sequence	Primary Breath Targeting Scheme	Secondary Breath Targeting Scheme	Tag
Volume AC	Volume	CMV	Set-point	N/A	VC-CMVs
Volume SIMV	Volume	IMV	Set-point	Set-point	VC-IMVs,s
Volume SIMV with artificial airway compensation	Volume	IMV	Set-point	Set-point/servo	VC-IMVs,sr
Volume AC with demand flow	Volume	IMV	Dual	Dual	VC-IMVd,d
Volume SIMV with demand flow	Volume	IMV	Dual	Set-point	VC-IMVd,s
Volume SIMV with demand flow and artificial airway compensation	Pressure	IMV	Dual	Set-point/servo	VC-IMVd,sr
Pressure AC	Pressure	CMV	Set-point	N/A	PC-CMVs
Time-cycled pressure-limited AC	Pressure	CMV	Set-point	N/A	PC-CMVs
Pressure AC with machine volume	Pressure	CMV	Dual	N/A	PC-CMVd
Pressure AC with volume guarantee	Pressure	CMV	Adaptive	N/A	PC-CMVa
Time-cycled pressure-limited AC with volume guarantee	Pressure	CMV	Adaptive	N/A	PC-CMVa
Volume AC with Vsync	Pressure	CMV	Adaptive	N/A	PC-CMVa
Regulated volume control AC	Pressure	CMV	Adaptive	N/A	PC-CMVa
Pressure AC with flow cycle	Pressure	IMV	Set-point	Set-point	PC-IMVs,s
Pressure AC with flow cycle and artificial airway compensation	Pressure	IMV	Set-point	Set-point/servo	PC-IMVs,sr
Pressure SIMV	Pressure	IMV	Set-point	Set-point	PC-IMVs,s
Pressure SIMV with artificial airway compensation	Pressure	IMV	Set-point	Set-point/servo	PC-IMVs,sr
CPAP/pressure support ventilation with volume limit	Pressure	IMV	Set-point	Set-point	PC-IMVs,s
CPAP/pressure support ventilation with volume limit and artificial airway compensation	Pressure	IMV	Set-point	Set-point/servo	PC-IMVs,sr
Infant nasal IMV	Pressure	IMV	Set-point	Set-point	PC-IMVs,s

TABLE 27.5 All Modes Available on the Vyaire AVEA—cont'd

Mode Name	MODE CLASSIFICATION				
	Control Variable	Breath Sequence	Primary Breath Targeting Scheme	Secondary Breath Targeting Scheme	Tag
Infant nasal IMV with artificial airway compensation	Pressure	IMV	Set-point	Set-point/servo	PC-IMVs,sr
Airway pressure release ventilation/biphasic	Pressure	IMV	Set-point	Set-point	PC-IMVs,s
Time-cycled pressure-limited AC with flow cycle	Pressure	IMV	Set-point	Set-point	PC-IMVs,s
Time-cycled pressure-limited SIMV with artificial airway compensation	Pressure	IMV	Set-point	Set-point/servo	PC-IMVs,sr
Time-cycled pressure-limited SIMV	Pressure	IMV	Dual	Set-point	PC-IMVs,s
Pressure SIMV with volume guarantee	Pressure	IMV	Adaptive	Set-point	PC-IMVa,s
Pressure SIMV with volume guarantee and artificial airway compensation	Pressure	IMV	Adaptive	Set-point/servo	PC-IMVa,sr
Time-cycled pressure-limited AC with flow cycle and volume guarantee	Pressure	IMV	Adaptive	Set-point	PC-IMVa,s
Time-cycled pressure-limited SIMV with volume guarantee	Pressure	IMV	Adaptive	Set-point	PC-IMVa,s
Time-cycled pressure-limited SIMV with volume guarantee and artificial airway compensation	Pressure	IMV	Adaptive	Set-point/servo	PC-IMVa,sr
Volume AC with Vsync and flow cycle	Pressure	IMV	Adaptive	Set-point	PC-IMVa,s
Volume SIMV with Vsync	Pressure	IMV	Adaptive	Set-point	PC-IMVa,s
Volume SIMV with Vsync and artificial airway compensation	Pressure	IMV	Adaptive	Set-point/servo	PC-IMVa,sr
Pressure-regulated volume control AC with flow cycle	Pressure	IMV	Adaptive	Adaptive	PC-IMVa,s
Pressure-regulated volume control SIMV with flow cycle	Pressure	IMV	Adaptive	Set-point	PC-IMVa,a
Pressure-regulated volume control SIMV	Pressure	IMV	Adaptive	Set-point	PC-IMVa,s
Pressure-regulated volume control SIMV with artificial airway compensation	Pressure	IMV	Adaptive	Set-point/servo	PC-IMVas,s
Time-cycled pressure-limited AC with flow cycle, volume guarantee, and artificial airway compensation	Pressure	IMV	Adaptive/servo	Set-point/servo	PC-IMVar,sr
Volume AC with Vsync, flow cycle, and artificial airway compensation	Pressure	IMV	Adaptive/servo	Set-point/servo	PC-IMVar,sr
Pressure-regulated volume control AC with flow cycle and artificial airway compensation	Pressure	IMV	Adaptive/servo	Set-point/servo	PC-IMVas,as
Pressure-regulated volume control SIMV with flow cycle and artificial airway compensation	Pressure	IMV	Adaptive/servo	Set-point/servo	PC-IMVar,sr
Time-cycled pressure-limited AC with flow cycle and artificial airway compensation	Pressure	IMV	Set-point/servo	Set-point/servo	PC-IMVsr,sr
CPAP/pressure support ventilation	Pressure	CSV	Set-point	N/A	PC-CSVs
CPAP/pressure support ventilation and artificial airway compensation	Pressure	CSV	Set-point/servo	N/A	PC-CSVsr

a, Adaptive; AC, assist-control; b, bio-variable; CMV, continuous mandatory ventilation; CPAP, continuous positive airway pressure; CSV, continuous spontaneous ventilation; d, dual; i, intelligent; IMV, intermittent mandatory ventilation; PC, pressure control; r, servo; s, set-point; SIMV, synchronized intermittent mandatory ventilation; VC, volume control.
(Used with permission of Mandu Press Ltd.)

Mandatory inflations are delivered at a set rate. Spontaneous breaths are allowed but receive no support.

Pressure assist-control. All inspiratory efforts trigger a pressure-controlled inflation (provided the ventilator detects the effort). A preset frequency of mandatory inflations provides a backup rate in case of apnea.

Pressure assist-control with flow cycle. Activation of flow cycle makes every inflation patient cycled. A backup rate will trigger the ventilator at the preset rate in case of apnea. Flow-cycled AC is equivalent to pressure support on many devices.

Pressure assist-control with machine volume. All inspiratory efforts trigger a pressure-controlled inflation. In this mode,

the ventilator switches from PC to VC if inflation flow decays to a machine-determined threshold before the preset tidal volume is reached. Inflation continues at a constant flow for preset inspiratory time until the set *inspiratory* tidal volume is delivered. Thus, this mode will not function well in the presence of a large endotracheal tube leak.

Pressure assist-control with volume guarantee. This mode is available for the neonatal patient size setting only.

All inspiratory efforts trigger a time-cycled, pressure-controlled inflation and are volume targeted, based on the *exhaled* tidal volume measured at the airway opening. An upper pressure limit and average tidal volume target are set by the user, and the device will adjust the delivered inflation pressure to maintain the set target tidal volume. A backup rate will trigger the ventilator at the preset rate in case of apnea.

Pressure-regulated volume control assist-control (not available for neonatal ventilation). Pressure-regulated VC (PRVC) delivers pressure-controlled inflations that support every breath for which the pressure level is automatically modulated to achieve a preset *inspiratory* volume. Initially, a decelerating-flow, volume-controlled test inflation to the set tidal volume is delivered to the patient. The ventilator then sets the target pressure based on the peak inflation pressure of the test inflation for the subsequent pressure-controlled inflations. The inflation pressure is then adjusted automatically by the ventilator to maintain the target volume. The maximum step change between two consecutive inflations is 3 cm H_2O. The maximum tidal volume delivered in a single inflation is determined by the volume limit setting.

Pressure-regulated volume control assist-control with flow cycle (not available for neonatal ventilation). This mode is as earlier, but flow cycled.

Pressure-regulated volume control synchronized intermittent mandatory ventilation with flow cycle (not available for neonatal ventilation). This mode is as earlier, but only a preset number of mandatory inflations is delivered in synchrony with inspiratory efforts (if present). Spontaneous breaths are possible between mandatory inflations. Machine-triggered inflations occur at the set rate if no respiratory effort is detected.

Pressure-regulated volume control synchronized intermittent mandatory ventilation (not available for neonatal ventilation). This mode is as earlier, but with time, not flow, cycling.

Pressure synchronized intermittent mandatory ventilation. This mode is pressure-controlled SIMV.

Pressure synchronized intermittent mandatory ventilation with volume guarantee (available for neonatal patient size setting only). The volume guarantee is the same as with AC. Mandatory inflations are delivered at a preset rate and synchronized with inspiratory effort (if present).

Time-cycled pressure-limited assist-control (available for neonatal patient size setting only). Every inspiratory effort triggers a time-cycled pressure-limited inflation. Pressure-limited modes are flow controlled with a pressure limit, as opposed to pressure-controlled modes that are directly pressure controlled. The practical implication of this distinction is that it is possible that the pressure limit may not be reached if inspiratory flow is low and the inspiratory time is long. On the other hand, peak inspiratory flow may be set higher than what may occur with a pressure-controlled inflation, perhaps improving patient–ventilator synchrony. A backup rate will cycle the ventilator at the preset rate in case of apnea.

Time-cycled pressure-limited assist-control with flow cycle. Every inspiratory effort triggers a flow-cycled pressure-limited inflation. This mode is equivalent to pressure support on other devices.

Time-cycled pressure-limited assist-control with flow cycle and volume guarantee. This mode is as earlier, but with volume guarantee.

Time-cycled pressure-limited assist-control with volume guarantee (available for neonatal patient size setting only). This mode is as earlier, but time, not flow, cycled.

Time-cycled pressure-limited synchronized intermittent mandatory ventilation (available for neonatal patient size setting only). Pressure-limited, time-cycled mandatory inflations are delivered at a preset rate and synchronized with inspiratory efforts (if present). Spontaneous breaths are possible between mandatory inflations.

Time-cycled pressure-limited synchronized intermittent mandatory ventilation with volume guarantee (available for neonatal patient size setting only). This mode is as earlier, but with volume guarantee.

Volume assist-control (with demand flow). Every inspiratory effort triggers a volume-controlled inflation. A set tidal volume is delivered using a constant flow over a specified amount of time during each mandatory inflation. The amount of pressure required to deliver the tidal volume will vary according to the compliance and resistance of the respiratory system. Tidal volume measurement is based on volume entering the ventilator circuit. Endotracheal tube leak will cause a problem. Note that all volume-controlled modes use dual targeting instead of set-point targeting by default. This feature is called "demand flow" and allows the patient to turn a mandatory volume-controlled inflation into spontaneous pressure-controlled inflation if the inspiratory effort is high enough. Thus, "volume AC" is not classified as VC-IMV(4), not VC-CMV (see earlier sections on IMV and dual targeting).

Volume assist-control with Vsync. Activation of Vsync makes this mode a form of PC, not VC, because inflation pressure is preset within each inflation. Vsync is a form of adaptive targeting that allows the ventilator to adjust inflation pressure between inflations to achieve an average preset tidal volume. Vsync is available only for adult and pediatric patients.

Volume assist-control with Vsync and flow cycle. Activation of Flow Cycle makes this mode a form of IMV, not AC. Flow cycling makes every inflation patient cycled. Hence, every patient-triggered inflation is spontaneous (i.e., patient triggered and cycled), whereas every machine-triggered inflation is mandatory (i.e., machine triggered and patient cycled) by definition.

Volume synchronized intermittent mandatory ventilation. Volume-controlled mandatory inflations are delivered at a preset rate and synchronized with inspiratory efforts (if present). Spontaneous breaths are possible between mandatory inflations. Machine-triggered inflations occur at the set rate if no respiratory effort is detected. A set amount of volume is delivered using a constant flow over a specified amount of time during each mandatory inflation. The amount of pressure required to deliver the tidal volume will vary according to the compliance and resistance of the respiratory system.

Volume synchronized intermittent mandatory ventilation with Vsync. Activation of Vsync makes this mode a form of PC, not VC, because inflation pressure is preset within each breath. Vsync is a form of adaptive targeting that allows the ventilator to adjust inflation pressure between inflations to achieve an average preset tidal volume. Vsync is available only for adult and pediatric patients.

PB 980

The PB 980 (Medtronic) is designed for invasive ventilation and NIV of adult, pediatric, and neonatal patients. It is electrically controlled and pneumatically powered (requires external compressor).

Modes

Modes on the PB 980 are set by selecting the breath sequence and the control variables separately. The operator interface uses the term "mode" to refer to what we have described previously as the breath sequence (i.e., CMV, IMV, CSV). Menu selections include AC (assist-control), SIMV (synchronized intermittent mandatory ventilation), Spont (spontaneous), CPAP (continuous positive airway pressure), and BILEVEL. Mandatory inflation types available are PC, VC, and VC+ (VC Plus). Spontaneous breath types available are PS (pressure support), TC (tube compensation), VS (volume support), PA (proportional assist), and NONE. An Apnea mode is available, with default settings based on the patient ideal body weight (entered during the setup routine), circuit type, and mandatory inflation type. These settings can be changed.

The modes available on the PB 980 are shown in Table 27.6.

Assist-control pressure control. Every inspiratory effort triggers a pressure-controlled, time-cycled inflation. A preset rate of backup apnea ventilation is available in case of apnea.

Assist-control volume ventilation plus. Every inspiratory effort triggers a pressure-controlled, time-cycled inflation with

adaptive pressure adjustment. Tidal volume measurement is at the ventilator end of the circuit using inspiratory tidal volume. The manufacturer's specifications indicate that with a set value of 5 mL, 95% of the time, the actual delivered tidal volume was between 2.3 and 3.9 mL on a test lung. Endotracheal tube leaks lead to further underestimation of tidal volume. An optional proximal sensor is available to monitor actual tidal volume. A preset rate of backup apnea ventilation is available in case of apnea.

Assist-control volume control. Every inspiratory effort triggers a volume-controlled inflation. A set amount of volume is delivered using a constant flow over a specified amount of time during each mandatory inflation. The amount of pressure required to deliver the tidal volume will vary according to the compliance and resistance of the respiratory system. A preset rate of backup apnea ventilation is available in case of apnea. Tidal volume measurement is at the ventilator end of the circuit using inspiratory tidal volume.

Bilevel + pressure support. This is a form of low-rate pressure-controlled IMV that allows spontaneous breathing throughout the ventilatory cycle. Inflation pressure and PEEP are called $PEEP_H$ and $PEEP_L$, respectively. The bulk of minute ventilation depends on the spontaneous respiratory effort.

Bilevel + tube compensation. This mode is as earlier. Spontaneous breaths occur throughout the entire cycle. Tube compensation reduces the work of breathing.

Synchronized intermittent mandatory ventilation pressure control + pressure support. A set number of spontaneous breaths trigger a pressure-controlled inflation. Machine-triggered inflations occur at the set rate if no respiratory effort is detected.

TABLE 27.6 Modes Available on the Medtronic PB 980

Mode Name	MODE CLASSIFICATION				
	Control Variable	Breath Sequence	Primary Breath Targeting Scheme	Secondary Breath Targeting Scheme	Tag
AC volume control	Volume	CMV	Set-point	N/A	VC-CMVs
SIMV volume control with pressure support	Volume	IMV	Set-point	Set-point	VC-IMVs,s
SIMV volume control with tube compensation	Volume	IMV	Set-point	Servo	VC-IMVs,r
AC pressure control	Pressure	CMV	Set-point	N/A	PC-CMVs
AC volume control plus	Pressure	CMV	Adaptive	N/A	PC-CMVa
SIMV pressure control with pressure support	Pressure	IMV	Set-point	Set-point	PC-IMVs,s
SIMV pressure control with tube compensation	Pressure	IMV	Set-point	Set-point	PC-IMVs,r
Bilevel with pressure support	Pressure	IMV	Set-point	Set-point	PC-IMVs,s
Bilevel with tube compensation	Pressure	IMV	Set-point	Servo	PC-IMVs,r
SIMV volume control plus with pressure support	Pressure	IMV	Adaptive	Set-point	PC-IMVa,s
SIMV volume control plus with tube compensation	Pressure	IMV	Adaptive	Servo	PC-IMVa,r
Spont pressure support	Pressure	CSV	Set-point	N/A	PC-CSVs
Spont tube compensation	Pressure	CSV	Servo	N/A	PC-CSVr
Spont proportional assist	Pressure	CSV	Servo	N/A	PC-CSVr
Spont volume support	Pressure	CSV	Adaptive	N/A	PC-CSVa

a, Adaptive; *AC,* assist-control; *CMV,* continuous mandatory ventilation; *CSV,* continuous spontaneous ventilation; *IMV,* intermittent mandatory ventilation; *N/A,* *******; *PC,* pressure control; *r,* servo; *s,* set-point; *SIMV,* synchronized intermittent mandatory ventilation; *VC,* volume control. (Reproduced with permission of Mandu Press Ltd.)

Spontaneous breaths in excess of the set rate are supported with a user set pressure above PEEP.

Synchronized intermittent mandatory ventilation pressure control + tube compensation. Pressure-controlled mandatory inflations are delivered at a preset rate and synchronized with inspiratory efforts (if present). Spontaneous breaths are possible between mandatory inflations and may be assisted with pressure support. Spontaneous breaths in excess of the set rate have reduced work of breathing with tube compensation that adjusts inflation pressure in proportion to inspiratory flow throughout inflation to overcome endotracheal tube resistance.

Synchronized intermittent mandatory ventilation volume control + pressure support. Volume-controlled mandatory inflations are delivered at a preset rate and synchronized with inspiratory efforts (if present). Spontaneous breaths are possible between mandatory inflations and may be assisted with pressure support. VC is based on tidal volume measurement at the ventilator end of the circuit using inspiratory tidal volume.

Synchronized intermittent mandatory ventilation volume ventilation plus + pressure support. Mandatory pressure-controlled inflations are delivered with adaptive targeting to automatically adjust inflation pressure to achieve the preset average tidal volume. Machine-triggered inflations occur at the set rate if no respiratory effort is detected. Tidal volume measurement is at the ventilator end of the circuit using inspiratory tidal volume, which leads to underestimation of delivered tidal volume. Endotracheal tube leaks lead to further underestimation of tidal volume. An optional proximal sensor is available to monitor actual tidal volume. Spontaneous breaths between mandatory breaths can be assisted with a user-set pressure above PEEP (i.e., Pressure Support).

Synchronized intermittent mandatory ventilation volume control plus + tube compensation. This mode is as earlier, but with tube compensation rather than pressure support.

Spont pressure support. This mode is spontaneous ventilation on CPAP with all spontaneous breaths supported by a set pressure above PEEP.

Spont volume support. This is the same as pressure support but with adaptive targeting such that inflation pressure is automatically adjusted to achieve the preset average tidal volume, based on inspiratory tidal volume measurement at the ventilator end of the patient circuit.

Neonatal ventilation. A NeoMode option determines values for allowable settings based on patient circuit type and ideal body weight (range for neonates is 0.3–7.0 kg or 0.66–15 lb).

Bellavista 1000

The Vyaire bellavista 1000 (Vyaire Medical, Fig. 27.10) is designed for invasive ventilation and NIV of adult, pediatric, and neonatal patients. It is electrically controlled and pneumatically powered (requires external compressor).

Modes

Modes are selected by pressing the virtual button with the desired mode name. The bellavista introduces some new concepts for setting modes. SingleVent corresponds to ventilation with a conventional ventilator with one ventilation mode, settings, and monitoring. Day/Night is used with patients who require ventilation support that is different at night from during the day. This feature allows the operator to set two ventilation modes, with sound intensity and screen brightness separately from one another. The bellavista switches to and from a timed basis (or manually on request) between Day (settings for the day) and Night (settings for the night). DualVent

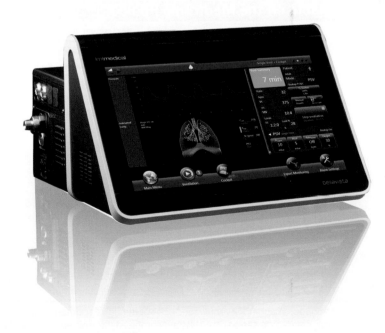

Fig. 27.10 Vyaire bellavista ventilator. (©2021 Vyaire Medical, Inc.; Used with permission.)

is a feature that makes it possible to switch between either of two set modes.

DualVent A means that the patient is breathing spontaneously. Modes that allow spontaneous breaths are available for selection. If no breath is triggered by the patient for an adjustable apnea time, bellavista automatically switches over to DualVent B (with no alarm).

DualVent B means that the patient does not have adequate spontaneous breathing and requires mandatory ventilation. If the patient triggers an adjustable number of inflations in succession, bellavista automatically switches over to DualVent A.

Note that DualVent produces a type 2 IMV breath sequence; that is, mandatory breaths may be suppressed by spontaneous breaths.

There are also some unique features applied to modes depending on the control variable. For all VC modes, the tidal volume is adapted to the currently measured tidal volume, which is calculated as the average of the inspired and expired volumes. Adaptation is breath based. The increment per breath is limited to 30% of the difference between set and actual tidal volumes. That creates the following advantages: accurate volume delivery based on proximal measurement, compensation for leakage and pneumatic nebulizer volume, and automatic compensation for patient circuit compliance.

Furthermore, a feature called Pressure Limited Ventilation (PLV) is always activated in VC modes. As soon as the inflation pressure rises to 5 cm H_2O below the set peak inflation pressure alarm, the inflation pressure is kept at that level until the set tidal volume has been reached, but until the end of the set inspiratory time at the latest. If the set tidal volume cannot be reached, an appropriate alarm message appears (Fig. 9.22). Note: this feature is what the taxonomy of modes refers to as dual targeting, meaning that the ventilator may switch from VC to PC during a single inflation.

For PC modes, there is an automatic pressure rise that minimizes the pressure rise rate, prevents pressure overshoots, and maximizes peak flow. For Pressure Support inflations, there is an automatic cycle algorithm that uses three separate criteria simultaneously for switching from inflation to expiration: (1) differential flow trigger: active expiratory effort on the part of the patient is recognized by a rapid drop in flow; (2) limit for expiration: the fuller the lungs, the lower the flow. As an expiratory trigger the ratio of increasing tidal volume to decreasing flow reduces the risk of hyperinflation; and (3) differential pressure trigger: substantial expiratory effort on the part of the patient (e.g., coughing) results in a sudden pressure rise that immediately initiates expiration.

Some PC modes offer adaptive targeting, called TargetVent. The ventilator determines the compliance for each inflation and sets the inflation pressure for the next inflation to achieve the selected target volume.

The bellavista offers automatic tube compensation (ATC) for both VC and PC modes. ATC compensates for tube resistance by increasing ventilation pressure in the breathing circuit during inflation on a flow-dependent basis or reducing it during expiration. Compensation can be set for 10% to 100% based on the input diameter of the artificial airway. ATC is active for both inspiration and expiration in PC modes but for expiration only in VC modes.

Finally, a sigh function can be enabled for most adult ventilation modes. The amplitude of a sigh is set as percent of the inflation pressure (for PC modes) or as percent of the tidal volume (for VC modes).

Table 27.7 shows the modes available on the Vyaire bellavista 1000 ventilator.

Adaptive ventilation mode. This mode is similar to adaptive support ventilation mode on the Hamilton ventilators. It is a

---

TABLE 27.7 Modes Available on the Vyaire bellavista 1000 Ventilator

| | | **MODE CLASSIFICATION** | | | | |
Mode Name	Abbreviation	Control Variable	Breath Sequence	Primary Targeting Scheme 1	Secondary Targeting Scheme 2	Tag
Pressure AC	P AC	Pressure	CMV	Set-point	N/A	PC-CMVs
Pressure AC + Automatic Tube Compensation	P AC + TC	Pressure	CMV	Set-point/servo	N/A	PC-CMVsr
Pressure AC + TargetVent	P AC + TV	Pressure	CMV	Adaptive	N/A	PC-CMVa
Pressure AC + TargetVent + Automatic Tube Compensation	P AC + TV + TC	Pressure	CMV	Adaptive/servo	N/A	PC-CMVar
Pressure Controlled Ventilation	PCV	Pressure	CMV	Set-point	N/A	PC-CMVs
Timed	Timed	Pressure	CMV	Set-point	N/A	PC-CMVs
Timed + TargetVent	Timed + TV	Pressure	CMV	Adaptive	N/A	PC-CMVa
Volume Controlled Ventilation	VC Ventilation	Volume	CMV	Dual	N/A	VC-CMVd
CPAP	CPAP	Pressure	CSV	Set-point	N/A	PC-CSVs
CPAP + Automatic Tube Compensation	CPAP + TC	Pressure	CSV	Servo	N/A	PC-CSVr
Nasal CPAP	Nasal CPAP	Pressure	CSV	Set-point	N/A	PC-CSVs
Pressure Support Ventilation (Backup Off)	PS (backup off)	Pressure	CSV	Set-point	N/A	PC-CSVs
Pressure Support Ventilation (Backup Off) + Automatic Tube Compensation	PS (backup off) + TC	Pressure	CSV	Set-point/servo	N/A	PC-CSVsr

Continued

TABLE 27.7 Modes Available on the Vyaire bellavista 1000 Ventilator—cont'd

Mode Name	Abbreviation	Control Variable	Breath Sequence	Primary Targeting Scheme 1	Secondary Targeting Scheme 2	Tag
Pressure Support Ventilation (Backup Off) + TargetVent	PS (backup off) + TV	Pressure	CSV	Adaptive	N/A	PC-CSVa
Pressure Support Ventilation (Backup Off) + TargetVent + Automatic Tube Compensation	PS (backup off) + TV + TC	Pressure	CSV	Adaptive/servo	N/A	PC-CSVar
Spontaneous	Spontaneous	Pressure	CSV	Set-point	N/A	PC-CSVs
Spontaneous + Automatic Tube Compensation	Spontaneous + TC	Pressure	CSV	Set-point/servo	N/A	PC-CSVsr
Spontaneous + TargetVent	Spontaneous + TV	Pressure	CSV	Adaptive	N/A	PC-CSVa
Spontaneous + TargetVent + Automatic Tube Compensation	Spontaneous + TV + TC	Pressure	CSV	Adaptive/servo	N/A	PC-CSVar
Spontaneous/Timed	S/T	Pressure	CSV	Set-point	N/A	PC-CSVs
Spontaneous/Timed (backup off) + TargetVent	S/T (backup off) + TV	Pressure	CSV	Adaptive	N/A	PC-CSVa
Spontaneous/Timed (backup off) + TargetVent + Automatic Tube Compensation	S/T (backup off) + TV + TC	Pressure	CSV	Adaptive/servo	N/A	PC-CSVar
Airway Pressure Release Ventilation	APRV	Pressure	IMV(1)	Set-point	Set-point	PC-IMV(1)s,s
Airway Pressure Release Ventilation + Automatic Tube Compensation	APRV + TC	Pressure	IMV(1)	Set-point/servo	Set-point/servo	PC-IMV(1)sr,sr
beLevel	beLevel	Pressure	IMV(1)	Set-point	Set-point	PC-IMV(1)s,s
beLevel + Automatic Tube Compensation	beLevel + TC	Pressure	IMV(1)	Set-point/servo	Set-point/servo	PC-IMV(1)sr,sr
Nasal Intermittent Positive Pressure Ventilation	Nasal IPPV	Pressure	IMV(1)	Set-point	Set-point	PC-IMV(1)s,s
PC-SIMV	PC SMV	Pressure	IMV(1)	Set-point	Set-point	PC-IMVs,s
PC-SIMV + Automatic Tube Compensation	PC SIMV + TC	Pressure	IMV(1)	Set-point/servo	Set-point/servo	PC-IMV(1)sr,sr
PC-SIMV + TargetVent	PC SIMV + TV	Pressure	IMV(1)	Adaptive	Adaptive	PC-IMV(1)a,a
PC-SIMV + TargetVent + Automatic Tube Compensation	PC SIMV + TV + TC	Pressure	IMV(1)	Adaptive/servo	Adaptive/servo	PC-IMV(1)ar,ar
Pressure Support Ventilation (Backup On)	PS (backup on)	Pressure	IMV(1)	Set-point	Set-point	PC-IMV(1)s,s
Pressure Support Ventilation (Backup On) + TargetVent	PS (backup on) + TV	Pressure	IMV(1)	Adaptive	Adaptive	PC-IMV(1)a,a
Spontaneous/Timed + TargetVent	S/T + TV	Pressure	IMV(1)	Adaptive	Adaptive	PC-IMV(1)a,a
Volume Controlled SIMV	VC SIMV	Volume	IMV(1)	Dual	Set-point	VC-IMV(1)d,s
Volume Controlled SIMV + Automatic Tube Compensation	VC SIMV + TC	Volume	IMV(1)	Dual/adaptive/servo	Set-point/servo	VC-IMV(1) dar,sr
Pressure Controlled DualVent	PC DualVent	Pressure	IMV(2)	Set-point	Set-point	PC-IMV(2)s,s
Pressure Controlled DualVent + Automatic Tube Compensation	PC DualVent + Tc	Pressure	IMV(2)	Set-point/servo	Set-point/servo	PC-IMV(2)sr,sr
Spontaneous/Timed + TargetVent + ATC	S/T + TV + TC	Pressure	IMV(2)	Adaptive/servo	Adaptive/servo	PC-IMV(2)ar,ar
Volume Controlled DualVent	VC DualVent	Volume	IMV(2)	Dual	Set-point	VC-IMV(2)d,s
Volume Controlled DualVent + Automatic Tube Compensation	VC DualVent + TC	Volume	IMV(2)	Dual/servo	Set-point/servo	VC-IMV(2)dr,sr
Adaptive Ventilation Mode	AVM	Pressure	IMV(3)	Optimal/intelligent	Optimal/intelligent	PC-IMV(3)oi,oi
Adaptive Ventilation Mode + Automatic Tube Compensation	AVM + TC	Pressure	IMV(3)	Optimal/intelligent/servo	Optimal/intelligent/servo	PC-IMV(3)oir,oir
Volume AC	Volume AC	Volume	IMV(4)	Dual	Dual	VC-IMVd,d

a, Adaptive; *AC*, assist-control; *ATC*, Automatic Tube Compensation; *CPAP*, continuous positive airway pressure; *CMV*, continuous mandatory ventilation; *CSV*, continuous spontaneous ventilation; *d*, dual; *i*, intelligent; *IMV*, intermittent mandatory ventilation; *N/A*, ***; *o*, optimal; *PC*, pressure control; *r*, servo; *s*, set-point; *SIMV*, synchronized intermittent mandatory ventilation; *VC*, volume control.
(Reproduced with permission of Mandu Press Ltd.)

form of PC type 3 IMV with a targeting scheme that minimizes power transmission from the ventilator to the patient.[18] The operator sets patient height and gender, % minute ventilation to support, PEEP, maximum inflation pressure, and pressure rise time. The ventilator automatically adjusts inflation pressure, and for mandatory inflations, inspiratory time, and frequency.

Airway pressure release ventilation. This is a form of pressure-controlled type 1 IMV that allows spontaneous breathing throughout the ventilatory cycle. Airway pressure is maintained at a relatively high level (P_{high}) for most of the respiratory cycle with intermittent release to a lower value (P_{low}). (Please see Chapter 23 for functional description of APRV.)

beLevel. The mode called beLevel is a highly flexible ventilation mode and can be set like CPAP, P-AC, PC-SIMV, PSV, or APRV, depending on the application.

Continuous positive airway pressure. All spontaneous breaths are pressure supported if the pressure support level is set above zero.

Nasal continuous positive airway pressure. The nCPAP mode is for spontaneously breathing neonates. It can be configured to be flow based or pressure based. For flow-based nCPAP, the operator sets a constant flow and pressure is generated by the nasal interface (i.e., CPAP pressure is proportional to flow). For pressure-based nCPAP, again, the airway pressure is generated by the nasal interface, but flow is regulated automatically by the ventilator to generate the operator-set CPAP level.

Nasal intermittent positive pressure ventilation. Like nCPAP, this mode is designed for neonates. It is a form of PC IMV with unrestricted spontaneous breathing.

Pressure control-synchronized intermittent mandatory ventilation. A set number of spontaneous breaths trigger a pressure-controlled inflation. Machine-triggered inflations occur at the set rate if no respiratory effort is detected. Spontaneous breaths in excess of the set rate are supported with a user set pressure above PEEP.

Pressure control-synchronized intermittent mandatory ventilation + TargetVent. Mandatory pressure-controlled inflations are delivered with adaptive targeting to automatically adjust inflation pressure to achieve the preset average tidal volume. Machine-triggered inflations occur at the set rate if no respiratory effort is detected. Spontaneous breaths between mandatory breaths may be assisted with a user-set pressure above PEEP (i.e., pressure support).

Pressure assist-control ventilation. Every inspiratory effort triggers a pressure-controlled, time-cycled inflation. Machine-triggered inflations occur at the set rate if no respiratory effort is detected.

Pressure assist-control + TargetVent. Mandatory pressure-controlled inflations with adaptive targeting to automatically adjust inflation pressure to achieve the preset average tidal volume. Machine-triggered inflations occur at the set rate if no respiratory effort is detected.

Pressure-controlled ventilation. This mode differs from pressure assist-control in that all inflations are machine triggered. Spontaneous efforts are ignored. The clinical utility of this mode is questionable, except perhaps for cardiopulmonary resuscitation where chest compressions might cause false triggering.

Pressure support ventilation. This mode differs from conventional pressure support because a backup rate can be set for mandatory inflations. It is like the Spontaneous/Timed mode in that spontaneous breaths will suppress mandatory inflations if the spontaneous breath frequency is higher than the set mandatory inflation rate.

Pressure support ventilation + TargetVent. This is like pressure support except that it uses adaptive targeting to achieve an average tidal volume according to the value set by the operator.

Spontaneous. This mode is spontaneous ventilation on CPAP with all spontaneous breaths supported by a set pressure above PEEP.

Spontaneous + TargetVent. This mode applies adaptive targeting to the spontaneous mode so that the inspiratory pressure is automatically adjusted to achieve an average tidal volume equivalent to the operator set value.

Spontaneous/Timed. This is the same as spontaneous except that it allows the user to set a mandatory inflation rate. Mandatory inflations are suppressed if the spontaneous breath rate is higher than the set rate.

Spontaneous/Timed + TargetVent. This mode applies adaptive targeting to the spontaneous/timed mode so that the inflation pressure is automatically adjusted to achieve an average tidal volume equivalent to the operator set value.

Timed. Although this mode is classified the same as pressure assist/control and pressure controlled ventilation (i.e., PC-CMVs) it is unlike them in that patient inspiratory efforts between mandatory inflations do not allow the patient to inspire, not even unsupported spontaneous breaths like PC-SIMV. The clinical utility of this mode is questionable, except perhaps for cardiopulmonary resuscitation where chest compressions might cause false triggering.

Volume assist-control. All VC modes on the bellavista use dual targeting (called pressure limited ventilation) rather than set-point targeting as used with conventional VC modes. Dual targeting allows the patient to turn a VC mandatory inflation into a PC spontaneous breath. Hence, this mode is not AC (or CMV) but actually type 4 IMV.

Evita Infinity V500, V600/800

The Evita Infinity V500 and the newer V600/800 (Dräger Medical, Fig. 27.11) series ventilators are designed for invasive

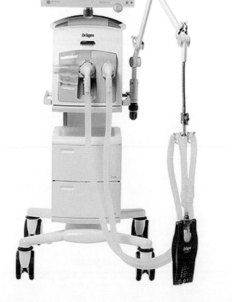

Fig. 27.11 Dräger Evita Infinity V800 ventilator. (Reproduced with permission from Dräger.)

ventilation and NIV of adult and pediatric patients. With additional software and optional flow measurement at the wye-piece, it can also ventilate neonatal patients, thus becoming one of the universal ventilators. It is electrically controlled and pneumatically powered (requires external compressor). A specialty neonatal version of these ventilators, the VN500 and VN600/800, is discussed in the next section.

Modes

Modes are selected by the mode name (e.g., VC-AC, VC-SIMV, etc.), using tabs on the touch screen. Relevant ventilator setting screens are displayed according to the mode tab. The settings are also grouped by tab, giving access to basic settings (e.g., tidal volume for VC modes and inflation pressure for PC modes) and additional settings. Some additional settings are simple, like trigger sensitivity or ATC. Others are more complex, such as AutoFlow. Activating AutoFlow changes the mode from VC with set-point targeting to PC with adaptive targeting, a completely different mode. All modes can be flow or pressure triggered. Table 27.8 shows the modes available on the Dräger Evita Infinity V500.

When ATC is active, the ventilator controls airway pressure such that the resistive load of breathing through the artificial airway is supported. Compensation may be independently

TABLE 27.8 Modes Available on the Dräger Evita Infinity V500 Ventilator

Mode Name	Control Variable	Breath Sequence	Primary Breath Targeting Scheme	Secondary Breath Targeting Scheme	Tag
Volume control continuous mandatory ventilation	Volume	CMV	Set-point	N/A	VC-CMVs
Volume control assist control	Volume	CMV	Set-point	N/A	VC-CMVs
Volume control assist control with pressure-limited ventilation	Volume	CMV	Dual	N/A	VC-CMVd
Volume control synchronized intermittent mandatory ventilation	Volume	IMV	Set-point	Set-point	VC-IMVs,s
Volume control synchronized intermittent mandatory ventilation with automatic tube compensation	Volume	IMV	Set-point	Set-point/servo	VC-IMVs,sr
Volume control synchronized intermittent mandatory ventilation with pressure-limited ventilation	Volume	IMV	Dual	Set-point	VC-IMVd,s
Volume control synchronized intermittent mandatory ventilation with pressure-limited ventilation and automatic tube compensation	Volume	IMV	Dual	Set-point/servo	VC-IMVd,sr
Volume control mandatory minute volume ventilation	Volume	IMV	Adaptive	Set-point	VC-IMVa,s
Volume control mandatory minute volume ventilation with automatic tube compensation	Volume	IMV	Adaptive	Set-point/servo	VC-IMVa,sr
Volume control mandatory minute volume with AutoFlow/volume guarantee	Volume	IMV	Adaptive	Set-point	VC-IMVda,s
Volume control mandatory minute volume with AutoFlow/volume guarantee and automatic tube compensation	Volume	IMV	Adaptive/servo	Set-point/servo	VC-IMVdar,sr
Volume control mandatory minute volume with pressure-limited ventilation	Volume	IMV	Dual/adaptive	Set-point	VC-IMVda,s
Volume control mandatory minute volume with pressure-limited ventilation and automatic tube compensation	Volume	IMV	Dual/adaptive	Set-point/servo	VC-IMVda,sr
Pressure control assist control	Pressure	CMV	Set-point	N/A	PC-CMVs
Pressure control assist control with automatic tube compensation	Pressure	CMV	Set-point/servo	N/A	PC-CMVsr
Volume control continuous mandatory ventilation with AutoFlow/volume guarantee	Pressure	CMV	Adaptive	N/A	PC-CMVa
Volume control continuous mandatory ventilation with AutoFlow/volume guarantee and automatic tube compensation	Pressure	CMV	Adaptive/servo	N/A	PC-CMVar
Volume control assist control with AutoFlow/volume guarantee	Pressure	CMV	Adaptive	N/A	PC-CMVa
Volume control assist control with AutoFlow/volume guarantee and automatic tube compensation	Pressure	CMV	Adaptive/servo	N/A	PC-CMVar
Pressure control continuous mandatory ventilation	Pressure	IMV	Set-point	N/A	PC-IMVs
Pressure control continuous mandatory ventilation with automatic tube compensation	Pressure	IMV	Set-point/servo	N/A	PC-IMVsr,sr
Pressure control synchronized intermittent mandatory ventilation	Pressure	IMV	Set-point	Set-point	PC-IMVs,s
Pressure control synchronized intermittent mandatory ventilation with automatic tube compensation	Pressure	IMV	Set-point/servo	Set-point/servo	PC-IMVsr,sr
Pressure control biphasic positive airway pressure	Pressure	IMV	Set-point	Set-point	PC-IMVs,s
Pressure control biphasic positive airway pressure with automatic tube compensation	Pressure	IMV	Set-point/servo	Set-point/servo	PC-IMVsr,sr
Pressure control airway pressure release ventilation	Pressure	IMV	Set-point	Set-point	PC-IMVs,s

TABLE 27.8 Modes Available on the Dräger Evita Infinity V500 Ventilator—cont'd

Mode Name	Control Variable	Breath Sequence	Primary Breath Targeting Scheme	Secondary Breath Targeting Scheme	Tag
Pressure control airway pressure release ventilation with automatic tube compensation	Pressure	IMV	Set-point/servo	Set-point/servo	PC-IMVsr,sr
Pressure control pressure support ventilation	Pressure	IMV	Set-point	Set-point	PC-IMVs,s
Pressure control pressure support ventilation with automatic tube compensation	Pressure	IMV	Set-point/servo	Set-point/servo	PC-IMVsr,sr
Volume control synchronized intermittent mandatory ventilation with AutoFlow	Pressure	IMV	Adaptive	Set-point	PC-IMVa,s
Volume control synchronized intermittent mandatory ventilation with AutoFlow and automatic tube compensation	Pressure	IMV	Adaptive/servo	Set-point/servo	PC-IMVar,sr
Spontaneous continuous positive airway pressure/pressure support	Pressure	CSV	Set-point	N/A	PC-CSVs
Spontaneous continuous positive airway pressure/pressure support with automatic tube compensation	Pressure	CSV	Set-point/servo	N/A	PC-CSVsr
Spontaneous continuous positive airway pressure/variable pressure support	Pressure	CSV	Bio-variable	N/A	PC-CSVb
Spontaneous continuous positive airway pressure/variable pressure support with automatic tube compensation	Pressure	CSV	Bio-variable/servo	N/A	PC-CSVbr
Spontaneous continuous positive airway pressure/volume support	Pressure	CSV	Adaptive	N/A	PC-CSVa
Spontaneous continuous positive airway pressure/volume support with automatic tube compensation	Pressure	CSV	Adaptive/servo	N/A	PC-CSVar
Spontaneous proportional pressure support	Pressure	CSV	Servo	N/A	PC-CSVr
SmartCare	Pressure	CSV	Intelligent	N/A	PC-CSVi

a, Adaptive; b, bio-variable; CMV, continuous mandatory ventilation; CSV, continuous spontaneous ventilation; d, dual; i, intelligent; IMV, intermittent mandatory ventilation; N/A, ***; o, optimal; PC, pressure control; r, servo; s, set-point; SIMV, synchronized intermittent mandatory ventilation; VC, volume control.

(Reproduced with permission of Mandu Press Ltd.)

deactivated for the expiratory breathing cycle. Depending on the direction of the patient flow, the airway pressure is increased during inspiration or decreased during expiration. Tube compensation may be applied to spontaneous breaths and mandatory inflations in PC modes.

There is a feature called Pressure Limitation that invokes dual targeting in VC. When inflation pressure reaches the operator set Pmax value, VC switches to PC with pressure limited to Pmax until inflation is time cycled by the set inspiratory time. An alert is issued if the preset tidal volume is not delivered by the end of inflation.

Pressure control assist-control. Every inspiratory effort triggers a time-cycled, pressure-controlled inflation. A backup rate of apnea ventilation ensures a minimum machine-triggered rate.

Pressure control airway pressure release ventilation. This is a form of pressure-controlled IMV that allows spontaneous breathing throughout the ventilatory cycle. Airway pressure is maintained at a relatively high level (P_{high}) for most of the respiratory cycle with intermittent release to a lower value (P_{low}). (Please see Chapter 23 for functional description of APRV.)

Patient triggering of mandatory inflations is possible using the AutoRelease feature. This triggers inflation once a preset expiratory flow threshold is reached. When AutoRelease is turned on, the switch from P_{high} to P_{low} is synchronized with the patient's breathing. Spontaneous breaths occur both between

and during mandatory inflations and provide the bulk of minute ventilation. Thus, a reliable respiratory effort is needed.

Pressure control continuous mandatory ventilation. The ventilator generates mandatory pressure-limited inflations at a set machine-triggered rate. Spontaneous breaths are permitted both during and between mandatory inflations, so this is a form of IMV, not CMV.

Pressure control pressure support. Every inspiratory effort triggers a pressure-controlled, flow-cycled inflation. A backup rate of apnea ventilation ensures a minimum machine-triggered rate.

Pressure control synchronized intermittent mandatory ventilation. Pressure-controlled mandatory inflations are delivered at a preset rate and synchronized with inspiratory efforts (if present). Spontaneous breaths are possible between mandatory inflations and may be assisted with pressure support if that option is selected.

SmartCare/pressure support. This mode is a specialized form of pressure support that is designed for true (i.e., ventilator-led) automatic weaning of patients. The targeting scheme uses artificial intelligence to determine acceptable ranges for spontaneous breathing frequency, tidal volume, and end-tidal carbon dioxide tension. These ranges are then used to automatically adjust the inflation pressure to maintain the patient in a respiratory zone of comfort.

The SmartCare/PS system divides the control process into three steps. The first step is to stabilize the patient within the zone of respiratory comfort, defined as combinations of tidal volume, respiratory frequency, and end-tidal CO_2 values considered acceptable by the targeting scheme. These values depend on the operator-set patient diagnosis (i.e., chronic obstructive pulmonary disease or neuromuscular disorder). The second step is to progressively decrease the inflation pressure while making sure the patient remains in the "zone." The third step tests readiness for extubation by maintaining the patient at the lowest level of inflation pressure. The lowest level depends on the type of artificial airway (endotracheal tube vs. tracheostomy tube), the type of humidifier (heat and moisture exchanger vs. a heated humidifier), and the use of ATC. Once the lowest level of inflation pressure is reached, a 1-hour observation period is started (i.e., a spontaneous breathing trial [SBT]), during which the patient's breathing frequency, tidal volume, and end-tidal CO_2 are monitored. Upon successful completion of this step, a message on the screen suggests that the clinician "consider separation" of the patient from the ventilator.

Spontaneous continuous positive airway pressure. This mode is continuous positive airway pressure but only available with NIV in the Neo. Patient setting on the ventilator.

Spontaneous continuous positive airway pressure/pressure support. This mode is spontaneous breathing on CPAP, with each breath receiving a set amount of pressure support above CPAP. Reliable respiratory drive is necessary.

Spontaneous continuous positive airway pressure/variable support. This is the same as pressure support but with biovariable targeting. The operator sets a percentage (0%–100%) of set pressure support level that acts as the range of values for individual breaths. The ventilator randomly varies the inspiratory pressure target within this range to achieve variable tidal volumes.

Spontaneous continuous positive airway pressure/volume support. This is the same as pressure support but with adaptive targeting such that inflation pressure is automatically adjusted to achieve the preset average tidal volume.

Spontaneous/proportional pressure support. This is a form of proportional assist ventilation for which the operator sets levels for flow assist (amount of resistance to be supported) and volume assist (amount of elastance to be supported).

Volume control assist-control. Every inspiratory effort triggers a VC inflation. A backup rate can be set in the case of apnea.

Volume control assist-control + AutoFlow/volume guarantee. Every inspiratory effort triggers a PC, time-cycled inflation with adaptive targeting to achieve an average volume delivery equal to the set target tidal volume (it is not volume control despite the name). A backup rate ensures a minimum machine-triggered rate.

Volume control assist-control + pressure limitation. This is volume AC with dual targeting instead of set-point targeting. The operator sets a maximum inflation pressure, Pmax, and when reached, VC switches to PC at that pressure. Inspiration is cycled off at the preset inspiratory time. A waning is activated if the preset tidal volume is not delivered.

Volume control continuous mandatory ventilation. Every inflation is machine triggered at a preset rate. Patient-triggered inflations are not allowed.

Volume control continuous mandatory ventilation + autoflow. Every inflation is machine triggered at a preset rate. Patient-triggered inflations are not allowed. Inflation is pressure controlled with adaptive targeting to achieve an average volume delivery equal to the set target tidal volume (it is not VC despite the name). A backup rate ensures a minimum machine-triggered rate.

Volume control continuous mandatory ventilation + pressure limitation. This is volume control continuous mandatory ventilation with dual targeting instead of set-point targeting. The operator sets a maximum inflation pressure, Pmax, and when reached VC switches to PC at that pressure. Inflation is cycled off at the preset inspiratory time. A waning is activated if the preset tidal volume is not delivered.

Volume control mandatory minute volume ventilation. Mandatory VC inflations are delivered at a preset tidal volume and rate. Spontaneous breaths are allowed, and if the minute ventilation exceeds the set value (i.e., volume and rate), then mandatory inflations are suppressed. This is type 3 IMV.

Volume control mandatory minute volume ventilation + autoflow/volume guarantee. Mandatory inflations delivered at a preset tidal volume and rate. Inflation is pressure controlled with adaptive targeting to achieve an average volume delivery equal to the set target tidal volume (it is not VC despite the name). A backup rate ensures a minimum machine-triggered rate. Spontaneous breaths are allowed, and if the minute ventilation exceeds the set value (i.e., volume and rate), then mandatory inflations are suppressed. This is type 3 IMV.

Volume control continuous positive airway pressure. Volume-controlled mandatory inflations are delivered at a preset rate and synchronized with inspiratory efforts (if present). Spontaneous breaths are possible between mandatory inflations and may be assisted with pressure support.

Volume control synchronized intermittent mandatory ventilation + autoflow/volume guarantee. Inflation is pressure controlled with adaptive targeting to achieve an average volume delivery equal to the set target tidal volume (it is not VC despite the name). Spontaneous breaths are permitted between mandatory inflations. A backup rate ensures a minimum machine-triggered rate.

Volume control synchronized intermittent mandatory ventilation + pressure limitation. This is Volume Control SIMV with dual targeting instead of set-point targeting. The operator sets a maximum inflation pressure, Pmax, and when reached VC switches to PC at that pressure. Inflation is cycled off at the preset inspiratory time. A waning is activated if the preset tidal volume is not delivered.

Neonatal Ventilation

The neonatal mode offers flow measurement at the wye-piece, which provides precise volume monitoring independent of compliance of the patient circuit in addition to accurate triggering. The measured values for minute ventilation and tidal volume are not corrected for leakage and are therefore lower than the actual minute and tidal volumes applied to the patient if a leakage occurs. When leakage compensation is activated, the measured volume and flow values as well as the curves for flow and volume are displayed with leakage correction. The Dräger Evita Infinity V500 compensates for leakages up to 100% of the set tidal volume. Exhaled tidal volume is used for volume targeting.

Evita Infinity V600/800

The latest generation of the Dräger Evita series features an enhanced user interface, improved alarm configuration, and more interactive features. The ventilation modes are similar to those described earlier with further refinements to the Smart-Care/PS function.

SERVO-I and SERVO-U

The Maquet SERVO ventilators (Getinge, Fig. 27.12) are intended for invasive ventilation and NIV of adults, children, and infants with respiratory failure or respiratory insufficiency in hospitals or health care facilities and for in-hospital transport.

Modes

Mode names are selected by pressing buttons on the touch screen. Once a mode name is chosen, the screen changes to show the available settings options. All modes can be flow or pressure triggered.

This ventilator offers three selections for inspiratory flow waveforms for VC inflations in CMV or IMV. One is constant flow and the other is a descending ramp flow. Both of these are achieved with set-point targeting. There is a third waveform associated with a feature called Flow Adaptation. This is achieved with dual targeting and has important clinical implications. The inflation starts out in VC with constant inspiratory flow. If the patient makes an inspiratory effort large enough cause inspiratory pressure to fall by 3 cm H_2O, the ventilator

automatically switches to PC. Depending on the size of the inspiratory effort, inflation may be volume cycled at the preset tidal volume or it may be flow cycled with whatever tidal volume the patient demands. If such an inflation was patient triggered, then it is classified as a spontaneous inflation (i.e., patient triggered and patient cycled). Hence, when Flow Adaptation is active (selectable as a flow waveform in the VC mode settings), the mode becomes IMV instead of CMV. This is an example of IMV(4). Note: if flow adaptation is activated in IMV(1), such as SIMV volume control, or IMV(2), automode volume control, then the mode is classified using the baseline IMV type because that is what will occur in the absences of patient-triggered breaths.

Automode is a term to describe the automatic transition between mandatory and spontaneous inflations, depending on the adequacy of respiratory effort. It is a form of IMV in which mandatory inflations are suppressed if the spontaneous breath rate is higher than the preset mandatory rate. This is classified as IMV(2).

The modes available on the SERVO-I and SERVO-U are shown in Table 27.9.

Automode (pressure control to pressure support). Mandatory pressure-controlled inflations are delivered at a preset rate. Spontaneous breaths are supported with pressure support. Mandatory inflations are suppressed if the spontaneous breath rate is greater than the set mandatory inflation rate.

Automode (pressure-regulated volume control to volume support). Mandatory inflations are delivered at a preset rate with adaptive targeting to achieve a preset average tidal volume. Spontaneous breaths are delivered with pressure support also using adaptive targeting. Mandatory inflations are suppressed if the spontaneous breath rate is greater than the set mandatory inflation rate.

Automode (volume control to volume support). Mandatory inflations are delivered at a preset rate with VC using either set-point or dual targeting, depending on the flow waveform setting. Spontaneous breaths are delivered with pressure support using adaptive targeting to achieve the preset average tidal volume. Mandatory inflations are suppressed if the spontaneous breath rate is greater than the set mandatory inflation rate.

BiVent. This is essentially PC-IMV(1) with unrestricted spontaneous breathing. Generally, it is expected that spontaneous breaths provide the bulk of minute ventilation; thus, the mode requires an intact respiratory drive.

Neurally adjusted ventilatory assist. NAVA uses the electrical activity of the diaphragm (EAdi) to trigger and cycle inflation and delivers pressure in proportion to patient inspiratory effort. A gain (the NAVA level) is applied to the electrical signal from the diaphragm to translate that signal to an inflation pressure. Triggering by EAdi ensures optimal synchronization, irrespective of circuit leaks; thus, it is ideal for noninvasive support. However, NAVA is a positive feedback mechanism that assumes mature respiratory control. Pressure and volume are variable and controlled by the patient's inspiratory effort.

Note: If the EAdi signal is lost, the ventilator switches to Pressure Support. It returns to NAVA if the signal is regained. If the patient becomes apneic, mandatory inflations at a preset inflation pressure, inspiratory time, and rate; these cease if the

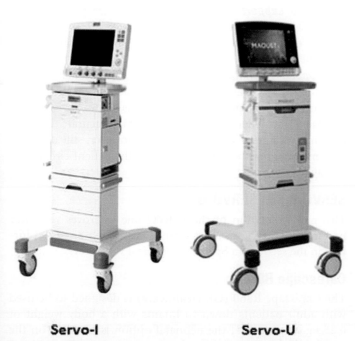

Servo-I   **Servo-U**

Fig. 27.12 Maquet SERVO ventilators. (Reproduced with permission from Getinge.)

TABLE 27.9 Modes Available on the Maquet SERVO Ventilators

Mode Name	MODE CLASSIFICATION				
	Control Variable	Breath Sequence	Primary Breath Targeting Scheme	Secondary Breath Targeting Scheme	Tag
Volume control	Volume	IMV	Dual	Dual	VC-IMVd,d
SIMV (volume control)	Volume	IMV	Dual	Dual	VC-IMVd,s
Automode (volume control to volume)	Volume	IMV	Dual	Adaptive	VC-IMVd,a
Pressure control	Pressure	CMV	Set-point	N/A	PC-CMVs
Pressure-regulated volume control	Pressure	CMV	Adaptive	N/A	PC-CMVa
SIMV (pressure control)	Pressure	IMV	Set-point	Set-point	PC-IMVs,s
BiVent	Pressure	IMV	Set-point	Set-point	PC-IMVs,s
Automode (pressure control to pressure support)	Pressure	IMV	Set-point	Set-point	PC-IMVs,s
SIMV pressure-regulated volume control	Pressure	IMV	Adaptive	Set-point	PC-IMVa,s
Automode (pressure-regulated volume control to volume support)	Pressure	IMV	Adaptive	Adaptive	PC-IMVa,a
Spontaneous/CPAP	Pressure	CSV	Set-point	N/A	PC-CSVs
Pressure support	Pressure	CSV	Set-point	N/A	PC-CSVs
Neurally adjusted ventilatory assist	Pressure	CSV	Servo	N/A	PC-CSVr
Volume support	Pressure	CSV	Adaptive	N/A	PC-CSVa

a, Adaptive; *CMV*, continuous mandatory ventilation; *CPAP*, continuous positive airway pressure; *CSV*, continuous spontaneous ventilation; *d*, dual; *IMV*, intermittent mandatory ventilation; *N/A*, ***; *PC*, pressure control; *r*, servo; *s*, set-point; *SIMV*, synchronized intermittent mandatory ventilation; *VC*, volume control.
(Reproduced with permission of Mandu Press Ltd.)

patient begins to trigger Pressure Support or NAVA breaths. NAVA itself is classified as PC-CSVr, but on this ventilator, because of the preset mandatory inflations (not a separate backup mode during an alarm event), NAVA is classified as IMV(2).

Pressure control. Mandatory pressure-controlled inflations are patient triggered or machine or triggered at a preset frequency, and machine cycled. Spontaneous breaths are not allowed.

Pressure-regulated volume control. PRVC delivers pressure-controlled inflations with adaptive targeting. The inflation pressure is adjusted automatically based on the exhaled tidal volume of the previous inflation to maintain the average preset target volume. The maximum step change between two consecutive inflations is 3 cm H_2O.

Pressure support. Every inspiratory effort triggers a pressure-controlled, flow-cycled inflation.

Synchronized intermittent mandatory ventilation (volume control). Mandatory VC inflations are delivered at a preset rate. Spontaneous breaths are permitted between mandatory inflations but receive no support. This mode uses either set-point or dual targeting, depending on the flow waveform setting.

Synchronized intermittent mandatory ventilation (pressure-regulated volume control). Mandatory inflations are pressure controlled with adaptive targeting, such that the inflation pressure is automatically adjusted to achieve the average tidal volume setting. Spontaneous breaths are allowed between mandatory inflations and may be assisted with Pressure Support.

Synchronized intermittent mandatory ventilation (pressure control). Mandatory inflations are pressure controlled with set-point targeting. Spontaneous breaths are allowed between mandatory inflations and may be assisted with Pressure Support.

Spontaneous/continuous positive airway pressure. This is spontaneous breathing on a set level of CPAP. Minute ventilation is fully dependent upon patient effort.

Volume control. Every inspiratory effort triggers a volume-controlled inflation. This mode uses either set-point or dual targeting, depending on the flow waveform setting. Spontaneous breaths are not permitted between mandatory inflations if constant flow or descending ramp flow waveforms are selected. However, if the flow adaptation waveform is selected (i.e., dual targeting) then mandatory VC inflations may be converted to spontaneous pressure support breaths if the inspiratory effort is high enough. Hence, activation of flow adaptation turns volume control from CMV to IMV(4).

Volume support. Spontaneous breaths are pressure controlled with adaptive targeting to achieve an average tidal volume equal to the set value. Mandatory inflations are not available.

Neonatal ventilation with SERVO-I. An optional neonatal flow sensor is available with an airway adapter dead space of less than 0.75 mL and weight of 4 g. This allows flow readings as close to the patient as possible to provide accurate tidal volume measurement. Volume targeting, however, still uses volume measured at the ventilator end of the patient circuit, not airway opening.

SERVO-n and SERVO-U

This new generation of the SERVO line improves ventilator performance in the smallest infants and thus is discussed further in the section on Specialty Neonatal ventilators.

Carescape R860

The Carescape R860 (GE Healthcare) is designed to be used with adult patients down to infants with a body weight of 0.25 kg or greater. If the neonatal option is installed on the ventilator, patients weighing down to 0.5 kg may be ventilated with the device.

Modes

Modes on the CARESCAPE R860 are selected by mode name (e.g., VCV, PCV, SIMV-VC, etc.) using a menu. Ventilation mode settings are separated into four categories: main parameters, breath timing, patient synchrony, and safety. Available modes are shown in Table 27.10.

By default, all VC inflations use dual targeting. This means that with sufficient inspiratory effort, the patient can turn a mandatory VC inflation into a spontaneous pressure support breath. Hence, the mode called "assist-control volume control" is actually IMV(4), not CMV.

There is also an additional way to implement dual targeting involving the pressure limit setting (Plimit). During VC, if the airway pressure reaches the Plimit setting, the ventilator switches to PC for the remainder of the preset inspiratory time.

TABLE 27.10 Modes Available on the GE Healthcare Carescape R860

Mode Name	Abbreviation	Control Variable	Breath Sequence	Primary Targeting Scheme 1	Secondary Targeting Scheme 2	Tag
AC Pressure Control	AC PC	Pressure	CMV	Set-point	N/A	PC-CMVs
AC Pressure Control + Tube Compensation	AC PC + TC	Pressure	CMV	Set-point/servo	N/A	PC-CMVsr
AC Pressure Regulated Volume Control	AC PRVC	Pressure	CMV	Adaptive	N/A	PC-CMVa
AC Pressure Regulated Volume Control + Pressure Minimum	AC PRVC + P Min	Pressure	CMV	Adaptive/set-point	N/A	PC-CMVas
AC Pressure Regulated Volume Control + Tube Compensation	AC PRVC + TC	Pressure	CMV	Adaptive/servo	N/A	PC-CMVar
AC Volume Control	AC VC	Volume	CMV	Dual	N/A	VC-CMVd
AC Volume Control + Pressure Limit	AC VC + PL	Volume	IMV(4)	Dual	Dual	VC-IMV(4)d,d
Airway Pressure Release Ventilation	APRV	Pressure	IMV(1)	Set-point	Set-point	PC-IMV(1)s,s
BiLevel	BiLevel	Pressure	IMV(1)	Set-point	Set-point	PC-IMV(1)s,s
BiLevel + Tube Compensation	BiLevelt + VG + TC	Pressure	IMV(1)	Set-point/servo	Set-point/servo	PC-IMV(1)sr,sr
BiLevel + Volume Guarantee	BiLevel + VG	Pressure	IMV(1)	Adaptive	Set-point	PC-IMV(1)a,s
BiLevel + Volume Guarantee + Tube Compensation	Bilevel + VG + TC	Pressure	IMV(1)	Adaptive/servo	Set-point/servo	PC-IMV(1)ar,sr
CPAP/Pressure Support	CPAP + PS	Pressure	CSV	Set-point	N/A	PC-CSVs
CPAP/Pressure Support + Tube Compensation	CPAP + PS + TC	Pressure	CSV	Set-point/servo	N/A	PC-CSVsr
Noninvasive Ventilation	NIV	Pressure	CSV	Set-point	N/A	PC-CSVs
Noninvasive Ventilation + backup rate	NIV + backup rate	Pressure	IMV(2)	Set-point	Set-point	PC-IMV(2)s,s
Pressure Support + backup rate	PS + backup rate	Pressure	IMV(2)	Set-point	Set-point	PC-IMV(2)s,s
SIMV Pressure Control	SIMV PC	Pressure	IMV(1)	Set-point	Set-point	PC-IMV(1)s,s
SIMV Pressure Control + Tube Compensation	SIMV PC + TC	Pressure	IMV(1)	Set-point/servo	Set-point/servo	PC-IMV(1)sr,sr
SIMV Pressure Control + Tube Compensation	SIMV PC + TC	Pressure	IMV(1)	Set-point	Set-point/servo	PC-IMV(1)sr,sr
SIMV Pressure Regulated Volume Control	SIMV PRVC	Pressure	IMV(1)	Adaptive	Set-point	PC-IMV(1)a,s
SIMV Pressure Regulated Volume Control + Pressure Minimum	SIMV PRVC + P Min	Pressure	IMV(1)	Adaptive/set-point	Set-point	PC-IMV(1)as,s
SIMV Pressure Regulated Volume Control + Tube Compensation	SIMV PRVC + TC	Pressure	IMV(1)	Adaptive/servo	Set-point/servo	PC-IMV(1)ar,sr
SIMV Volume Control	SIMV VC	Volume	IMV(1)	Dual	Set-point/dual	VC-IMV(1)d,sd
SIMV Volume Control + Pressure Limit	SIMV VC + PL	Volume	IMV(1)	Dual	set-point/dual	VC-IMV(1)d,sd
SIMV Volume Control + Pressure Limit + Tube Compensation	SIMV VC + PL + TC	Volume	IMV(1)	Dual	set-point/dual/servo	VC-IMV(1)d,sdr
SIMV Volume Control + Tube Compensation	SIMV VC + TC	Volume	IMV(1)	Dual	set-point/dual/servo	VC-IMV(1)d,sdr
Spontaneous Breathing Trial	SBT	Pressure	CSV	Set-point	N/A	PC-CSVs
Spontaneous Breathing Trial + Tube Compensation	SBTI + TC	Pressure	CSV	Set-point/servo	N/A	PC-CSVsr
Volume Support	VS	Pressure	CSV	Adaptive	N/A	PC-CSVa
Volume Support + backup rate	VC + backup rate	Pressure	IMV(2)	Set-point	adaptive	PC-IMV(2)s,a
Volume Support + Tube Compensation	VS + TC	Pressure	CSV	Adaptive/servo	N/A	PC-CSVar

a, Adaptive; *AC*, assist-control; *CMV*, continuous mandatory ventilation; *CPAP*, continuous positive airway pressure; *CSV*, continuous spontaneous ventilation; *d*, dual; *IMV*, intermittent mandatory ventilation; *N/A*, ***; *PC*, pressure control; *r*, servo; *s*, set-point; *SIMV*, synchronized intermittent mandatory ventilation; *VC*, volume control.

(Reproduced with permission of Mandu Press Ltd.)

Tube compensation adjusts the target delivery pressure to compensate for the resistance caused by the endotracheal tube or tracheostomy tube used. The compensation is applied to the inspiratory phase of all pressure-controlled, CPAP, and pressure-supported breaths.

When the modes use adaptive targeting (e.g., pressure regulated volume control), a pressure minimum setting can be used to place a lower limit on the automatic adjustment of inflation pressure (i.e., it turns adaptive targeting back into set-point targeting).

Assist-control pressure control. Every inspiratory effort triggers a pressure-controlled, time-cycled inflation. A preset rate of backup apnea ventilation is available in case of apnea.

Assist-control pressure regulated volume control. Every inspiratory effort triggers a pressure-controlled, time-cycled inflation with adaptive targeting to automatically adjust inflation pressure to meet the average tidal volume setting. Spontaneous breaths are not allowed.

Assist-control volume control. Every inspiratory effort triggers a VC mandatory inflation. A backup rate may be set, but spontaneous breaths are not allowed. Note that by default, all VC inflations use dual targeting, which means a large inspiratory effort can turn a mandatory VC inflation into a spontaneous Pressure Support breath. Hence, this mode is not really AC but rather IMV(4).

Assist-control volume control + pressure limit. Every inspiratory effort triggers a VC mandatory inflation. A backup rate may be set, but spontaneous breaths are not allowed. Note that by default, all VC breaths use dual targeting, which means a large inspiratory effort can turn a mandatory VC inflation into a spontaneous Pressure Support breath. Hence, this mode is not really AC but rather IMV(4). Furthermore, in this mode, if the airway pressure reaches the Plimit setting, the ventilator switches to PC for the remainder of the preset inspiratory time.

Airway pressure release ventilation. This is a form of pressure-controlled IMV(1) that allows spontaneous breathing throughout the ventilatory cycle. Inflation pressure and PEEP are called $PEEP_{high}$ and $PEEP_{low}$, respectively. The bulk of minute ventilation depends on the spontaneous respiratory effort.

Bilevel airway pressure ventilation. Pressure-controlled mandatory inflations are delivered at a preset rate. Inflation pressure and PEEP are called P_{high} and P_{low}, respectively; this mode is commonly referred to as bilevel CPAP. The patient can breathe spontaneously while at either of the pressure levels. Spontaneous breaths provide most of the minute ventilation.

Bilevel airway pressure ventilation + volume guaranteed. This mode is as earlier but uses adaptive targeting so that the P_{high} level is automatically adjusted to achieve an average value equal to the set inspired tidal volume.

Continuous positive airway pressure/pressure support. This mode requires reliable respiratory drive, allowing the patient to breathe on CPAP. The ventilator provides a set pressure level above the CPAP level to support each spontaneous breath. Inspiratory effort determines the rate, tidal volume, and inspiratory timing.

Noninvasive ventilation. The ventilator provides Pressure Support on top of CPAP. Because flow triggers are affected by patient circuit leaks, flow and pressure triggers are applied simultaneously in NIV mode to improve trigger detection. If the patient does not meet the set minimum rate for spontaneous breaths, the ventilator delivers a backup inflation based on the backup inflation pressure and inspiratory time settings.

Synchronized intermittent mandatory ventilation pressure controlled. Mandatory pressure-controlled inflations are delivered at a preset rate and synchronized with inspiratory efforts (if present). Spontaneous breaths are allowed between mandatory inflations.

Synchronized intermittent mandatory ventilation pressure regulated volume control. Mandatory pressure-controlled inflations are delivered with adaptive targeting to automatically adjust inflation pressure to achieve the preset average tidal volume. Machine-triggered inflations occur at the set rate if no respiratory effort is detected. Spontaneous breaths between mandatory inflations may be assisted with Pressure Support.

Synchronized intermittent mandatory ventilation volume control. Mandatory volume-controlled inflations are machine triggered at a preset frequency or patient triggered and machine cycled. VC uses dual targeting so that a large inspiratory effort will change a mandatory VC inflation into a spontaneous pressure support breath.

Synchronized intermittent mandatory ventilation volume control + pressure limit. Mandatory volume-controlled inflations are machine triggered at a preset frequency or patient triggered and machine cycled. VC uses dual targeting so that a large inspiratory effort will change a mandatory VC inflation into a spontaneous pressure support breath. Furthermore, in this mode, if the airway pressure reaches the Plimit setting, the ventilator switches to PC for the remainder of the preset inspiratory time.

Spontaneous breathing trial. The SBT mode is intended to be used to evaluate the patient's ability to breathe spontaneously during a specified duration of time. The SBT feature will place the ventilator in CPAP/PSV mode at the settings defined in the SBT menu. Before the SBT evaluation, the following setting limits must be entered: SBT Duration, Apnea Time, High and low minute ventilation alarm, and High and low respiratory rate alarm. If the minute volume, respiratory rate, or apnea alarm limits are exceeded during the SBT, the trial will immediately end and the ventilator will return to the previous mode and settings. The SBT Split Screen displays the minute ventilation, respiratory rate, and end-tidal CO_2 for the trial. A message appears while the SBT is running indicating the amount of time remaining. The trial will automatically end at the time set and the ventilator will return to the previous mode and settings.

Volume support. Spontaneous breaths are pressure controlled with adaptive targeting to achieve an average tidal volume equal to the set value. Mandatory inflations are not available.

Neonatal ventilation. The neonatal option on the Carescape R860 provides ventilation for intubated neonatal patients weighing down to 250 g. This is accomplished by using a proximal flow sensor at the patient wye-piece, which connects to the ventilator with a cable.

Hamilton G5

The G5 (Hamilton Medical, Fig. 27.13) is designed for intensive care ventilation of adult and pediatric patients, and optionally infant and neonatal patients. The device is intended for use in the hospital and institutional environment where health care professionals provide patient care. This ventilator has an electronically controlled pneumatic ventilation system with electrical power from an AC source with internal battery backup. The device's pneumatic system delivers gas, and its electrical systems control the pneumatics, monitor alarms, and distribute power. The Hamilton G5 receives inputs from a disposable, proximal flow sensor (required) and other sensors within the ventilator. Based on these monitored data, the device adjusts gas delivery to the patient. This sensor lets the ventilator sense even weak patient breathing efforts. The flow sensor is highly accurate even in the presence of secretions, moisture, and nebulized medications.

Modes

Modes on the G5 are selected by mode name (e.g., SIMV, SPONT, ASV, DuoPAP, etc.) using a menu. Specific mode settings are selected using other menus. Available modes are shown in Table 27.11.

Tube resistance compensation adjusts the target delivery pressure to compensate for the resistance caused by the endotracheal tube or tracheostomy tube used. The compensation is applied to the inspiratory phase of all pressure-controlled, CPAP, and pressure-supported inflations/breaths.

IntelliSync is an optional feature. The ventilator monitors incoming sensor signals from the patient and reacts dynamically to initiate inspiration and expiration in real time to improve patient–ventilator synchrony.

Adaptive support ventilation. This mode is similar to adaptive ventilation mode on the bellavista ventilator. It is a form of PC type 3 IMV with a targeting scheme that minimizes power transmission from the ventilator to the patient.[18] The operator sets patient height and gender, % minute ventilation to support, PEEP, maximum inflation pressure, and pressure rise time. The ventilator automatically adjusts inflation pressure and, for mandatory inflations, inspiratory time, and frequency.

Airway pressure release ventilation. This is a form of pressure-controlled IMV(1) that allows spontaneous breathing throughout the ventilatory cycle. Inflation pressure and PEEP are called $PEEP_{high}$ and $PEEP_{low}$ respectively. The bulk of minute ventilation depends on the spontaneous respiratory effort.

Adaptive pressure ventilation continuous mandatory ventilation (APVCMV). Every inspiratory effort triggers a pressure-controlled, time-cycled inflation with adaptive targeting to automatically adjust inflation pressure to meet the average tidal volume setting. Spontaneous breaths are not allowed.

Adaptive pressure ventilation intermittent mandatory ventilation (APVIMV). Mandatory pressure-controlled inflations are delivered with adaptive targeting to automatically adjust inflation pressure to achieve the preset average tidal volume. Machine-triggered inflations occur at the set rate if no respiratory effort is detected. Spontaneous breaths between mandatory inflations may be assisted with Pressure Support.

DuoPositive airway pressure. This is a form of pressure-controlled IMV(1) that allows spontaneous breathing throughout the ventilatory cycle. Inflation pressure and PEEP are called $PEEP_{high}$ and $PEEP_{low}$, respectively. The bulk of minute ventilation depends on the spontaneous respiratory effort.

INTELLiVENT adaptive support ventilation. An optional mode, IntelliVent-ASV is a complete fully closed-loop ventilation algorithm for oxygenation and ventilation as a form of PC-IMV(3). It relies on adaptive support ventilation to select an optimal tidal volume and mandatory inflation frequency targets based on lung mechanics. It uses a rule-based expert system in conjunction with volumetric CO_2 and SpO_2 measurements to select targets for minute ventilation, PEEP, and F_1O_2. It covers all applications from intubation until extubation with simplicity for an early weaning.

Nasal continuous positive airway pressure/pressure support. This mode is designed to apply CPAP and intermittent positive pressure support with a nasal interface (mask or prongs).

Noninvasive ventilation. NIV is an adaptation of the SPONT mode. The primary difference is that NIV is designed to compensate for leaks when using a mask or other noninvasive patient interface.

Noninvasive ventilation-spontaneous/timed. NIV is an adaptation of the SPONT mode, whereas NIV-ST is an adaptation of the PSIMV+ mode. The primary difference is that NIV modes are designed to compensate for leaks when using a mask or other noninvasive patient interface. This mode is PC IMV(2),

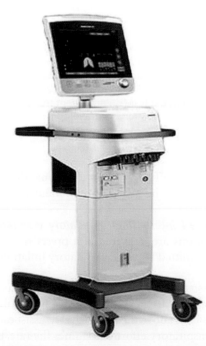

Fig. 27.13 Hamilton G5 ventilator. (© Hamilton Medical.)

TABLE 27.11 Modes Available on the Hamilton G5 Ventilator

Mode Name	Abbreviation	Control Variable	Breath Sequence	Primary Targeting Scheme 1	Secondary Targeting Scheme 2	Tag
(S)CMV	AC	Volume	CMV	Set-point	N/A	VC-CMVs
Adaptive Support Ventilation	ASV	Pressure	IMV(3)	Optimal/intelligent	Optimal/intelligent	PC-IMV(3)oi,oi
Adaptive Support Ventilation + Tube Resistance Compensation	ASV + TC	Pressure	IMV(3)	Optimal/intelligent/ servo	Optimal/intelligent/ servo	PC-IMV(3) oir,oir
Airway Pressure Release Ventilation	APRV	Pressure	IMV(1)	Set-point	Set-point	PC-IMV(1)s,s
Airway Pressure Release Ventilation + Tube Resistance Compensation	APRV + TC	Pressure	IMV(1)	Set-point/servo	Set-point/servo	PC-IMV(1)sr,sr
APVcmv (also called (S)CMVplus) + Tube Resistance Compensation	APVcmv	Pressure	CMV	Adaptive/servo	N/A	PC-CMVar
APVcmv (also called (S)CMVplus)	APVcmv	Pressure	CMV	Adaptive	N/A	PC CMVa
APVsimv (also called SIMVplus)	APVimv	Pressure	IMV(1)	Adaptive	Set-point	PC-IMV(1)a,s
APVsimv (also called SIMVplus) + Tube Resistance Compensation	APVimv	Pressure	IMV(1)	Adaptive/servo	Set-point/servo	PC-IMV(1)ar,sr
Duo Positive Airway Pressure	Duo PAP	Pressure	IMV(1)	Set-point	Set-point	PC-IMV(1)s,s
Duo Positive Airway Pressure + Tube Resistance Compensation	Duo PAP + TC	Pressure	IMV(1)	Set-point/servo	Set-point/servo	PC-IMV(1)sr,sr
INTELLiVENT ASV	INTELLiVENT ASV	Pressure	IMV(3)	Optimal/intelligent	Optimal/intelligent	PC-IMV(3)oi,oi
Nasal CPAP/Pressure Support	Nasal CPAP + PS	Pressure	IMV(2)	Set-point	Set-point	PC-IMV(2)s,s
Noninvasive Ventilation	NIV	Pressure	CSV	Set-point	N/A	PC-CSVs
Noninvasive Ventilation Spontaneous/ Timed	NIV S/T	Pressure	IMV(2)	Set-point	Set-point	PC-IMV(2)s,s
P-CMV	PC AC	Pressure	CMV	Set-point	N/A	PC-CMVs
P-CMV + IntelliSync	PC AC + IntelliSync	Pressure	IMV(2)	Set-point	Set-point	PC-IMV(2)s,s
P-CMV + Tube Resistance Compensation	PC SIMV + TC	Pressure	CMV	Set-point/servo	N/A	PC-CMVsr
P-SIMV	PC SIMV + IntelliSync	Pressure	IMV(1)	Set-point	Set-point	PC-IMV(1)s,s
P-SIMV + IntelliSync + Tube Resistance Compensation	PC SIMV + IntelliSync + TC	Pressure	IMV(2)	Set-point/servo	Set-point/servo	PC-IMV(2)sr,sr
P-SIMV + Tube Resistance Compensation	PC SIMV + TC	Pressure	IMV(1)	Set-point/servo	Set-point/dual/ servo	PC-IMV(1)sr,sr
SIMV	SIMV	Volume	IMV(1)	Set-point	Set-point	VC-IMV(1)s,s
Spontaneous	Spontaneous	Pressure	CSV	Set-point	N/A	PC-CSVs
Spontaneous + Tube Resistance Compensation	Spontaneous + TC	Pressure	CSV	Set-point/servo	N/A	PC-CSVsr
Volume Support	VS	Pressure	CSV	Adaptive	N/A	PC-CSVa

a, Adaptive; *APV*, adaptive pressure ventilation; *(S)CMV*, synchronized controlled mandatory ventilation; *CPAP*, continuous positive airway pressure; *CMV*, continuous mandatory ventilation; *CSV*, continuous spontaneous ventilation; *d*, dual; *i*, intelligent; *IMV*, intermittent mandatory ventilation; *N/A*, ***; *o*, optimal; *PC*, pressure control; *r*, servo; *s*, set-point; *SIMV*, synchronized intermittent mandatory ventilation; *VC*, volume control.

where mandatory breaths are suppressed if the spontaneous breath rate exceeds the set rate.

Positive-continuous mandatory ventilation. This is pressure controlled ventilation where every inspiratory effort triggers a pressure-controlled, time-cycled inflation. A preset rate of backup apnea ventilation is available in case of apnea.

Positive-synchronized intermittent mandatory ventilation. This is pressure controlled synchronized intermittent mandatory ventilation. Mandatory pressure-controlled inflations are delivered at a preset rate and synchronized with inspiratory efforts (if present). Spontaneous breaths are allowed between mandatory inflations.

Synchronized continuous mandatory ventilation. This is synchronized controlled mandatory ventilation, (S)CMV.

Every inspiratory effort triggers a VC mandatory inflation. A backup rate may be set but spontaneous breaths are not allowed.

Synchronized intermittent mandatory ventilation. Mandatory VC inflations are delivered at a preset rate. Spontaneous breaths are permitted between mandatory inflations but receive no support.

Spontaneous. This mode requires reliable respiratory drive, allowing the patient to breathe on CPAP. The ventilator provides a set pressure level above the CPAP level to assist each spontaneous breath. Inspiratory effort determines the rate, tidal volume, and inspiratory timing. Mandatory inflations are not available.

Volume support. Spontaneous breaths are pressure controlled with adaptive targeting to achieve an average tidal volume equal to the set value. Mandatory breaths are not available.

SPECIALIZED NEONATAL VENTILATORS

Specialized neonatal ventilators are more common outside the United States, and there are many brands to choose from. Within the United States, until recently, there has been only one specialized ICU infant ventilator available, the Dräger VN500 Babylog, and one specialized noninvasive ventilator, the Vyaire Infant Flow SiPAP device. The SERVO-n has now joined the ranks of ventilators specifically designed to be suitable for small preterm infants, although as of this writing, there is limited published evidence about performance in the clinical setting.

Babylog VN500 and 600/800

The Babylog VN500 (Dräger Medical; Fig. 27.14A and B) is the most extensively used and studied specialty neonatal ventilator available in the United States. It differs from the universal ventilators in a number of features specifically designed to address the unique needs of the neonatal patient described in Chapter 19. The VN500 shares the basic layout, controls, and hardware components with its adult counterpart, the V500, but its software provides excellent leak compensation to allow for ventilation with uncuffed endotracheal tubes with precise flow sensing and triggering as well as leak-adapted breath termination in the face of endotracheal tube leaks as large as 80%. The Babylog is intended for the ventilation of neonatal patients from 0.4 kg up to 10 kg and pediatric patients from 5 kg up to 20 kg body weight. It is electrically controlled and pneumatically powered (requires an external compressor).

Modes

Modes are selected by mode name (e.g., pressure control AC, pressure control pressure support, etc.), using tabs on the touch screen. The settings screens are also tabbed, giving access to basic settings and additional settings. The additional settings include trigger sensitivity, ATC, and volume guarantee. There are no VC modes available on this ventilator. Table 27.12 shows the modes that are available on the Babylog VN500.

Pressure control-assist-control. Every inspiratory effort triggers a pressure-controlled inflation. A set rate provides mandatory inflations in case of apnea.

Pressure control-assist-control + volume guarantee. This mode is as earlier, but with adaptive targeting to automatically adjust inflation pressure to achieve the target tidal volume. Effective dynamic leak compensation allows accurate tidal volume calculation even with moderately large endotracheal tube leak.

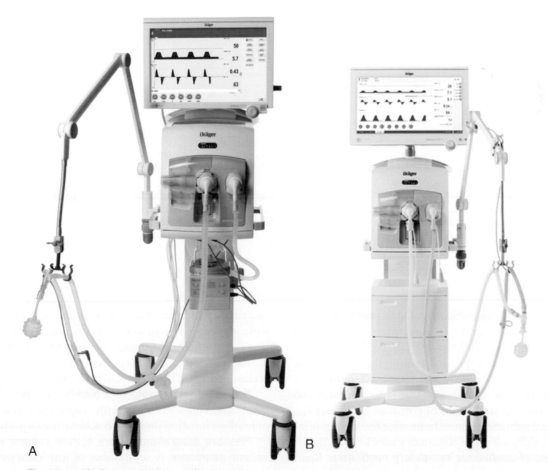

Fig. 27.14 (A) Dräger VN500 and **(B)** VN800Babylog ventilator. (Reproduced with permission from Dräger.)

TABLE 27.12   Modes Available on the Dräger Babylog VN500

Mode Name	Control Variable	Breath Sequence	Primary Breath Targeting Scheme	Secondary Breath Targeting Scheme	Tag
Pressure control AC	Pressure	CMV	Set-point	N/A	PC-CMVs
Pressure control AC with automatic tube compensation	Pressure	CMV	Set-point/servo	N/A	PC-CMVsr
Pressure control AC with volume guarantee	Pressure	CMV	Adaptive	N/A	PC-CMVa
Pressure control AC with volume guarantee and automatic tube compensation	Pressure	CMV	Adaptive/servo	N/A	PC-CMVar
Pressure control continuous mandatory ventilation	Pressure	IMV	Set-point	Set-point	PC-IMVs,s
Pressure control continuous mandatory ventilation with automatic tube compensation	Pressure	IMV	Set-point/servo	Set-point/servo	PC-IMVsr,sr
Pressure control SIMV	Pressure	IMV	Set-point	Set-point	PC-IMVs,s
Pressure control SIMV with automatic tube compensation	Pressure	IMV	Set-point/servo	Set-point/servo	PC-IMVsr,sr
Pressure control pressure support ventilation	Pressure	IMV	Set-point	Set-point	PC-IMVs,s
Pressure control pressure support ventilation with automatic tube compensation	Pressure	IMV	Set-point/servo	Set-point/servo	PC-IMVsr,sr
Pressure control airway pressure release ventilation	Pressure	IMV	Set-point	Set-point	PC-IMVs,s
Pressure control airway pressure release ventilation with automatic tube compensation	Pressure	IMV	Set-point/servo	Set-point/servo	PC-IMVsr,sr
Pressure control mandatory minute volume ventilation with volume guarantee	Pressure	IMV	Adaptive	Set-point	PC-IMVa,s
Pressure control continuous mandatory ventilation with volume guarantee	Pressure	IMV	Adaptive	Set-point	PC-IMVa,s
Pressure control continuous mandatory ventilation with volume guarantee and automatic tube compensation	Pressure	IMV	Adaptive/servo	Set-point/servo	PC-IMVar,sr
Pressure control SIMV with volume guarantee	Pressure	IMV	Adaptive	Set-point	PC-IMVa,s
Pressure control SIMV with volume guarantee and automatic tube compensation	Pressure	IMV	Adaptive/servo	Set-point/servo	PC-IMVas,sr
Pressure control pressure support ventilation with volume guarantee	Pressure	IMV	Adaptive	Set-point	PC-IMVa,s
Pressure control pressure support ventilation with volume guarantee and automatic tube compensation	Pressure	IMV	Adaptive/servo	Set-point/servo	PC-IMVar,sr
Spontaneous CPAP/pressure support	Pressure	CSV	Set-point	N/A	PC-CSVs
Spontaneous CPAP/pressure support with automatic tube compensation	Pressure	CSV	Set-point/servo	N/A	PC-CSVsr
Spontaneous proportional pressure support	Pressure	CSV	Servo	N/A	PC-CSVr
Spontaneous proportional pressure support with automatic tube compensation	Pressure	CSV	Servo	N/A	PC-CSVr
Spontaneous CPAP/volume support	Pressure	CSV	Adaptive	N/A	PC-CSVa
Spontaneous CPAP/volume support with automatic tube compensation	Pressure	CSV	Adaptive/servo	N/A	PC-CSVar

a, Adaptive; *AC*: assist-control; *CMV*, continuous mandatory ventilation; *CPAP*, continuous positive airway pressure; *CSV*, continuous spontaneous ventilation; *IMV*, intermittent mandatory ventilation; *N/A*, ***; *PC*, pressure control; *r*, servo; *s*, set-point; *SIMV*, synchronized intermittent mandatory ventilation. (Used with permission of Mandu Press Ltd.)

Pressure control-airway pressure release ventilation. This is basically PC-IMV(1) but with unrestricted spontaneous breathing throughout the ventilatory period. Patient triggering of mandatory inflations is possible using the AutoRelease feature. This triggers inflation once a preset expiratory flow threshold is reached. The purpose of this is to maintain end expiratory lung volume using autoPEEP instead of a preset P_{low} value above zero. Spontaneous breaths provide the bulk of minute ventilation—thus, adequate respiratory effort is required.

Pressure control-continuous mandatory ventilation. Mandatory inflations occur at a set rate and are machine triggered and time-cycled. Synchronization of mandatory inflations with patient effort is not available; that is, patient trigger efforts are ignored. Spontaneous breaths are permitted both between and during mandatory inflations. Because of this feature, the mode is classified as IMV(1), not CMV, despite the name.

Pressure control-continuous mandatory ventilation + volume guarantee. This is PC-CMV with adaptive targeting to automatically adjust inflation pressure to achieve the target tidal volume.

Pressure control-mandatory minute volume ventilation + volume guarantee. A set number of inspiratory efforts trigger pressure-controlled, time-cycled inflations with adaptive targeting to automatically adjust inflation pressure to achieve the target tidal volume. Mandatory inflations are suppressed if minute ventilation from spontaneous breaths is above the preset minute ventilation target (i.e., product of tidal volume and frequency). This is IMV(3). Spontaneous breaths in excess of the set rate are not volume guaranteed.

Pressure control-pressure support ventilation. Every inspiratory effort triggers a pressure-controlled, patient-triggered, flow-cycled inflation.

Pressure control-pressure support ventilation + volume guarantee. This mode is as earlier, but with volume guarantee.

Pressure control-synchronized intermittent mandatory ventilation. Pressure-controlled mandatory inflations are delivered at a preset rate and synchronized with patient effort, if any. Machine-triggered inflations occur at the set rate if no respiratory effort is detected. Spontaneous breaths are allowed between mandatory inflations, IMV(1).

Pressure control-synchronized intermittent mandatory ventilation + volume guarantee. This PC-SIMV with adaptive targeting to automatically adjust inflation pressure to achieve the target tidal volume.

Spontaneous continuous positive airway pressure/pressure support. This mode provides for spontaneous breathing with pressure support of every spontaneous breath to a fixed level above CPAP. Pressure support is pressure-controlled inflation with patient triggering and patient (flow) cycling.

Spontaneous continuous positive airway pressure/volume support. This is the same mode as earlier, but with adaptive targeting (instead of set-point targeting) to achieve a target tidal volume. This is not really a neonatal mode, but it may be used in pediatric patients.

Spontaneous proportional pressure support. Every inspiratory effort triggers a pressure-controlled inflation with servo targeting (instead of set-point targeting) that makes inflation pressure proportional to inspiratory effort. This mode assumes mature respiratory control and thus is probably not ideal for preterm infants.

Automatic tube compensation (ATC). This is an available option providing dynamic compensation for endotracheal tube resistance.

High-frequency oscillatory ventilation (with volume guarantee). Outside the United States, the VN500 ventilator has a high-frequency oscillatory ventilation (HFOV) option that has the ability to measure tidal volume and maintain a set tidal volume by means of a volume guarantee option, which maintains a stable tidal volume by means of automatic adjustment of pressure amplitude. As of this writing, the HFOV option is not available in the United States, but a clinical trial designed to obtain US Food and Drug Administration approval has been completed (https://clinicaltrials.gov/; NCT02445040). See also Chapter 24 for further details.

Babylog VN600/800

This latest generation of the Babylog series features an enhanced user interface, improved configuration of alarms, and more interactive features. The ventilation modes are similar to those described earlier, including the proprietary leak compensation and leak adaptation technologies, and HFOV with volume guarantee. As of this writing, this latest generation of the VN series is pending US Food and Drug Administration approval in the United States.

SERVO-n and SERVO-U

The Maquet SERVO-U and SERVO-n (Getinge, see Fig. 27.12) improve the functionality of the SERVO line for use in newborn infants and feature a modern touch-screen operator interface and more interactive decision-support features. The SERVO-U is intended for the full range of adult, pediatric, and neonatal patients, while the SERVO-n is intended for use in pediatric and neonatal patients. The range and functionality of ventilation modes are similar to the SERVO-I, as described in detail earlier, except that VC and SIMV (VC) + PS and Automode VC ↔ VS are not available in the neonatal patient category. The main difference is the availability of the optional "Y-sensor module," which makes it possible to accurately measure and regulate tidal volume at the airway opening, rather than at the ventilator end of the circuit, eliminating the major drawback of the SERVO-I ventilator when used in small newborn infants. This Y-sensor should not be considered optional when ventilating newborn infants. Better leak compensation is also implemented.

fabian High-Frequency Oscillatory

The Vyaire fabian HFO (Vyaire Medical, Fig. 27.15) is intended for premature infants, newborns, as well as children weighing up to 30 kg. This device offers HFOV but is not currently available in the United States. The device works with a neonatal flow sensor as well as oximeter and CO_2 sensors.

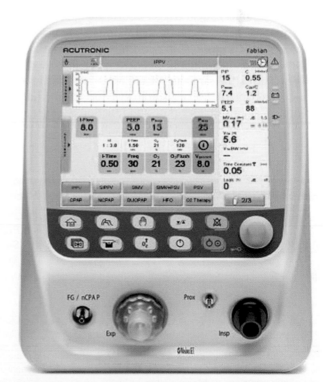

Fig. 27.15 Vyaire fabian HFO ventilator. (©2021 Vyaire Medical, Inc.; Used with permission.)

Modes

Modes are selected by mode name using a touch screen. There are no VC modes available on this ventilator. However, PC is implemented as a form of dual targeting. This means that if the inspiratory pressure target is set high enough, the ventilator will deliver a constant inspiratory flow until the pressure target is reached, when flow enters an exponential decay. Thus, if the pressure target is high enough and inspiratory time is low enough, it is possible to deliver VC because inspiratory flow is preset and tidal volume become the product of the set inspiratory time and inspiratory flow. Volume guarantee (i.e., adaptive targeting) is achieved with a proximal air flow sensor with the target being the exhaled tidal volume to avoid errors because of airway leaks. The ventilator also has a feature called Volume Limit. This is a setting that signals the ventilator to cycle off inspiration when the default tidal volume has been reached.

This ventilator offers an O_2 Therapy option, which allows the use of a continuous flow of blended gas, from 1 to 15 L/min. Nasal cannulas of various can be used. There are no alarm functions active in this mode, except for the set FiO_2

The modes available on the fabian are shown in Table 27.13.

Intermittent positive-pressure ventilation (continuous mandatory ventilation). This is intermittent positive-pressure ventilation (CMV). It delivers mandatory inflations that are machine triggered by a preset frequency and machine cycled by a preset inspiratory time. Patient trigger efforts are ignored. The operator's manual recommends that this mode should be used only if no spontaneous breathing from patient is expected.

Intermittent positive-pressure ventilation (continuous mandatory ventilation) + volume guarantee. This is IPPV(CMV) with adaptive targeting (instead of set-point targeting) that automatically adjusts inflation pressure to achieve the average preset tidal volume. Patient trigger efforts are ignored. The operator's manual recommends that this mode should only be used if no spontaneous breathing from patient is expected.

Synchronized intermittent positive pressure ventilation (ASSIST). This is the same as IPPV(CMV) but patient trigger efforts are recognized. Every inspiratory effort triggers an inflation with a fixed inspiratory time and inflation pressure.

Synchronized intermittent positive pressure ventilation (ASSIST) + volume guarantee. This is SIPPV(ASSIST) with adaptive targeting (instead of set-point targeting) that automatically adjusts inflation pressure to achieve the average preset tidal volume.

Synchronized intermittent mandatory ventilation. Pressure-controlled mandatory inflations are delivered at a preset rate and synchronized with patient effort, IMV(1). Machine-triggered inflations occur at the set rate if no respiratory effort is detected. Spontaneous breaths are allowed between mandatory inflations but are not assisted with Pressure Support.

Synchronized intermittent mandatory ventilation + pressure support ventilation. Pressure-controlled mandatory inflations are delivered at a preset rate and synchronized with patient effort, IMV(1). Machine triggered inflations occur at the set rate if no respiratory effort is detected. Spontaneous breaths are allowed between mandatory inflations and may be assisted with Pressure Support.

Pressure support ventilation. Every inspiratory effort triggers a pressure-controlled, patient-triggered, flow-cycled inflation. The apnea backup ventilation will start after the preset apnea delay set in the alarm menu. If apnea is set to OFF, the ventilator starts backup after E-Time.

Pressure support ventilation + volume guarantee. This is PSG with adaptive targeting for pressure. Inflation pressure is automatically adjusted to achieve the average preset target tidal volume.

High-frequency oscillatory ventilation. In this mode, HFOV, the operator may preset the bias flow, mean airway pressure, oscillatory pressure amplitude, oscillatory frequency, and I:E ratio.

Continuous positive airway pressure. This mode is unlike conventional continuous positive airway pressure because in the event of apnea, the ventilator performs a default number of mandatory inflations to stimulate spontaneous breathing. After breathing commences, stimulation stops and only commences with the next apnea event.

Nasal continuous positive airway pressure/duo positive airway pressure. The nCPAP mode supplies CPAP with automatic leak compensation. It is intended for use with a mask or

TABLE 27.13	**Modes Available on the Vyaire fabian High-Frequency Oscillation**					
			MODE CLASSIFICATION			
Mode Name	**Abbreviation**	**Control Variable**	**Breath Sequence**	**Primary Targeting Scheme 1**	**Secondary Targeting Scheme 2**	**Tag**
SIMV	SIMV	Pressure	IMV(1)	Dual	Set-point	PC-IMV(1)d,s
SIMV + PSV	SIMV + PSV	Pressure	IMV(1)	Dual	Dual	PC-IMV(1)d,d
SIMV + PSV +VG	SIMV + PSV +VG	Pressure	IMV(1)	Dual/adaptive	Set-point	PC-IMV(1)da,s
SIMV +VG	SIMV +VG	Pressure	IMV(1)	Dual/adaptive	Set-point	PC-IMV(1)da,s
SIPPV (ASSIST)	SIPPV	Pressure	CMV	Dual	N/A	PC-CMVd
SIPPV(ASSIST) + VG	SIPPV + VG	Pressure	CMV	Dual/adaptive	N/A	PC-CMVda

a, Adaptive; *d*, dual; *CMV*, continuous mandatory ventilation; *IMV*, intermittent mandatory ventilation; *IPPV*, intermittent positive pressure ventilation; *N/A*, ***; *PC*, pressure control; *PSV*, ***; *s*, set-point; *SIMV*, synchronized intermittent mandatory ventilation; *VG*, ***.
(Used with permission of Mandu Press Ltd.)

nasal prongs. DUPAP is the same as nCPAP but with the option of positive pressure ventilation with adjustable frequency and inspiratory time.

Leoni plus

The Leoni plus (Löwenstein Medical, Fig. 27.16) is among a family of neonatal ventilators that includes the Leoni plus CLAC and the Leoni plus transport. This ventilator is intended for invasive ventilation and NIV of premature babies, neonates, and infants up to 30 kg body weight for stationary use. As of this writing, this ventilator is not available in the United States.

Modes

Modes are selected with the integrated touchscreen, the rotary pulse encoder, the hard keys, or a combination of these elements. The ventilator has a feature called Volume Limit. This is a setting that signals the ventilator to cycle off inspiration when the default tidal volume has been reached. Modes available on the Leoni plus are shown in Table 27.14.

Continuous positive airway pressure. This mode is unlike conventional continuous positive airway pressure because in the event of apnea, the ventilator delivers mandatory inflations if the Backup option has been enabled.

High-frequency oscillation. In this mode, HFOV, the operator may preset the oscillatory pressure amplitude, mean airway pressure and oscillatory frequency, and I:E ratio. A volume guarantee option is available.

Intermittent positive-pressure ventilation/intermittent mandatory ventilation. The IPPV or IMV mode will be active depending on the mode settings. If an expiratory time of more than 1.5 seconds results from the set inspiratory time and the frequency, the device will be in IMV mode; otherwise, it will be in IPPV mode. Inflation is pressure controlled. The manual says, "ventilation follows a pattern set in the device without

reference to any spontaneous breathing by the patient." Thus, it is not clear if the patient can inspire during the preset expiratory time (some ventilators impose an occlusion in this situation). Therefore, it is unclear if this mode CMV or IMV. Given that the manual also describes IMV as "the patient is allowed the option of spontaneous breathing between the ventilation strokes," we will assume IPPV is classified as CMV.

When IMV is in effect, mandatory inflations are pressure controlled and delivered with preset inspiratory time and frequency. Spontaneous breaths are permitted. Spontaneous breaths cannot be assisted with Pressure Support.

Intermittent positive-pressure ventilation/intermittent mandatory ventilation + volume guarantee. The same as IPPV or IMV but delivered with adaptive targeting. Inflation pressure is automatically adjusted to deliver the average preset target tidal volume.

Nasal continuous positive airway pressure. In nCPAP mode, the flow sensor is automatically switched off because with the expected high leakage rate, VC would produce incorrect information. The flow does not change in response to leaks. However, the device is able to maintain the pressure even with high leakage rates by controlling the expiratory valve.

Nasal intermittent positive pressure ventilation. nIPPV is designed for use of the Neojet generator, which allows the patient to breathe spontaneously at both pressure levels. In nIPPV mode, the flow sensor is automatically switched off as with CPAP. The flow does not change in response to leaks. However, the device is able to maintain the pressure even with high leakage rates by controlling the expiratory valve.

Pressure support-intermittent mandatory ventilation. Like with S-IMV, only certain spontaneous breaths are supported within the time interval derived from the set frequency.

Pressure support-intermittent mandatory ventilation + volume guarantee. Like with PS-IMV but delivered with adaptive targeting.

Fig. 27.16 Löwenstein Leoni plus ventilator. (Reproduced with permission from Löwenstein.)

TABLE 27.14 **Modes Available on the Heinen and Löwenstein Leoni plus**

		MODE CLASSIFICATION				
Mode Name	Abbreviation	Control Variable	Breath Sequence	Primary Targeting Scheme 1	Secondary Targeting Scheme 2	Tag
CPAP	CPAP	Pressure	CSV	Set-point	N/A	PC-CSVs
CPAP (backup off)	CPAP (backup off)	Pressure	CSV	Set-point	N/A	PC-CSVs
CPAP (backup on)	CPAP (backup on)	Pressure	IMV(1)	Set-point	Set-point	PC-IMV(1)s,s
High-Frequency Oscillation	HFO	Pressure	IMV(1)	Set-point	Set-point	PC-IMV(1)s,s
IMV	IMV	Pressure	IMV(1)	Set-point	Set-point	PC-IMV(1)s,s
IMV + VG	IMV + VG	Pressure	IMV(1)	Adaptive	Set-point	PC-IMV(1)a,s
IPPV	IPPV	Pressure	CMV	Set-point	N/A	PC-CMVs
IPPV + VG	IPPV +VG	Pressure	CMV	Set-point	N/A	PC-CMVa
nCPAP	nCPAP	Pressure	CSV	Set-point	N/A	PC-CSVs
nIPPV	nIPPV	Pressure	IMV(1)	Set-point	Set-point	PC-IMV(1)s,s
Pressure Support Ventilation-SIMV	PS-SIMV	Pressure	IMV(1)	Set-point	Set-point	PC-IMV(1)s,s
Pressure Support Ventilation-SIMV + VG	PS-SIMV + VG	Pressure	IMV(1)	Set-point	Set-point	PC-IMV(1)a,s
Pressure Support Ventilation-S-IPPV	PS-SIPPV	Pressure	IMV(1)	Set-point	Set-point	PC-IMV(1)s,s
Pressure Support Ventilation-SIPPV + VG	PS-SIPPV + VG	Pressure	IMV(1)	Adaptive	Set-point	PC-IMV(1)a,s
S-IMV	S-IMV	Pressure	IMV(1)	Set-point	Set-point	PC-IMV(1)s,s
S-IMV + VG	S-IMV + VG	Pressure	IMV(1)	Adaptive	Set-point	PC-IMV(1)a,s
S-IPPV	S-IPPV	Pressure	CMV	Set-point	N/A	PC-CMVs
S-IPPV + VG	S-IPPV + VG	Pressure	CMV	Adaptive	N/A	PC-CMVa

a, Adaptive; *CMV*, continuous mandatory ventilation; *CPAP*, continuous positive airway pressure; *CSV*, continuous spontaneous ventilation; *d*, dual; *I*, intelligent; *IMV*, intermittent mandatory ventilation; *IPPV*, intermittent positive pressure ventilation; *N/A*, ***; *nCPAP*, nasal continuous positive airway pressure; *nIPPV*, nasal intermittent positive pressure ventilation; *o*, optimal; *PC*, pressure control; *r*, servo; *s*, set-point; *SIMV*, synchronized intermittent mandatory ventilation.
(Used with permission of Mandu Press Ltd.)

Inflation pressure is automatically adjusted to deliver the average preset target tidal volume.

Pressure support-S intermittent positive pressure ventilation. Pressure-controlled inflations are patient triggered and patient cycled (by flow). If a patient trigger is not detected during the expiratory time interval set by the set frequency, a mandatory inflation will be triggered by the ventilator, similar to other neonatal ventilators.

Pressure support-intermittent positive pressure ventilation + volume guarantee. The same as PS-IPPV but delivered with adaptive targeting. Inflation pressure is automatically adjusted to deliver the average preset target tidal volume.

S-intermittent mandatory ventilation. This is the same as IMV except that mandatory inflations are synchronized with inspiratory efforts. Spontaneous breaths may be assisted with Pressure Support.

S-intermittent mandatory ventilation + volume guarantee. The same as S-IMV but delivered with adaptive targeting. Inflation pressure is automatically adjusted to deliver the average preset target tidal volume.

S-intermittent positive pressure ventilation. This is the same as IPPV but patient trigger efforts are recognized. Every inspiratory effort triggers an inflation with a fixed inspiratory time and inspiratory pressure.

S-I intermittent positive pressure ventilation + volume guarantee. The same as S-IPPV but delivered with adaptive targeting. Inflation pressure is automatically adjusted to deliver the average preset target tidal volume.

Vyaire Infant Flow SiPAP

The Vyaire Infant Flow SiPAP (Fig. 27.17) is designed for NIV of infants using either nasal prongs (Fig. 27.18) or a nasal mask (Fig. 27.19). The Infant Flow SiPAP is available in a Plus or a Comprehensive configuration. The Plus configuration provides nCPAP (nasal CPAP) and time-triggered BiPhasic modes with and without breath rate monitoring. Vyaire defines "BiPhasic" as time-triggered, time-cycled pressure assists at two separate pressure levels (i.e., bilevel CPAP). Using the ventilator mode taxonomy described in this book, the name Bi-Phasic is classified as PC IMV, although for the purpose of the US Food and Drug Administration, SiPAP is not a ventilator. The Comprehensive configuration offers these features plus a patient-triggered BiPhasic mode with apnea backup inflations.

Modes

Modes on the Infant Flow SiPAP are selected by name—that is, CPAP, BiPhasic, and BiPhasic *tr* (triggered). The available modes are shown in Table 27.15.

BiPhasic. The device cycles between two levels of CPAP (e.g., 6 and 9 cm H_2O) at an operator-selected rate, with spontaneous breathing occurring throughout and accounting for the bulk of minute ventilation.

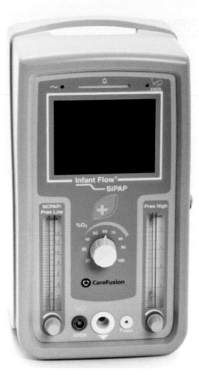

Fig. 27.17 Vyaire Infant Flow SiPAP noninvasive ventilator. (Reproduced with permission from Vyaire.)

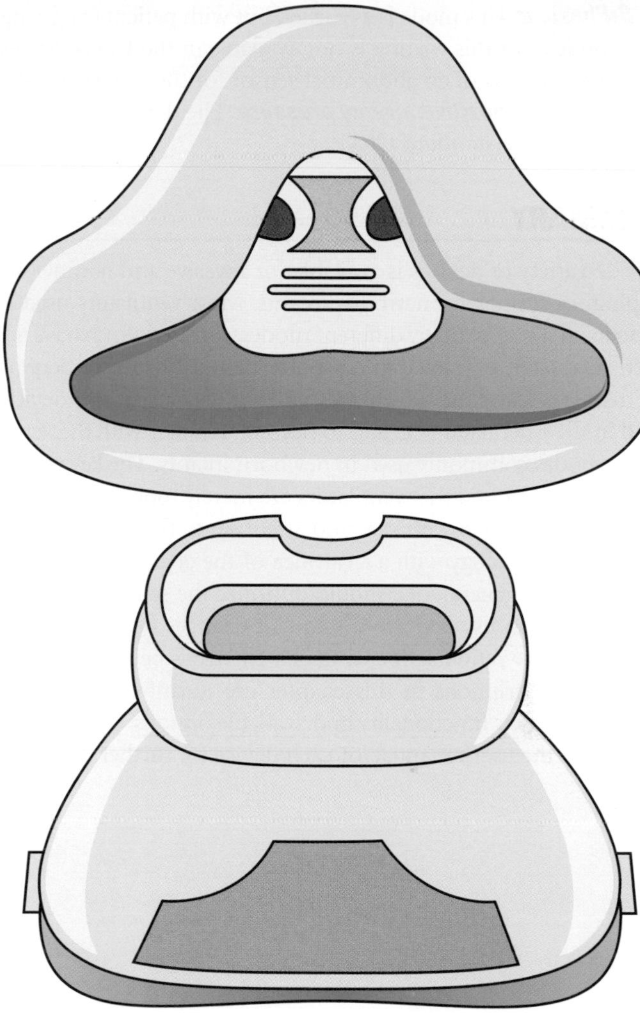

Fig. 27.19 Nasal mask for noninvasive ventilation. (Reproduced with permission from Cleveland Clinic.)

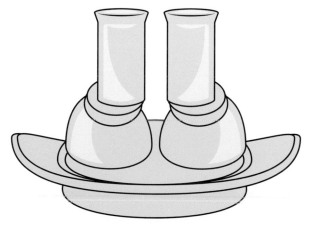

Fig. 27.18 Nasal prongs for noninvasive ventilation. (Reproduced with permission from Cleveland Clinic.)

TABLE 27.15	Modes on the Vyaire Infant Flow SiPAP				
			MODE CLASSIFICATION		
Mode Name	**Control Variable**	**Breath Sequence**	**Primary Breath Targeting Scheme**	**Secondary Breath Targeting Scheme**	**Tag**
BiPhasic	Pressure	IMV	Set-point	Set-point	PC-IMVs,s
Nasal CPAP	Pressure	IMV	Set-point	N/A	PC-CSVs

CPAP, Continuous positive airway pressure; *CSV*, continuous spontaneous ventilation; *IMV*, intermittent mandatory ventilation; *N/A*, ***; *PC*, pressure control; *s*, set-point.
(Used with permission of Mandu Press Ltd.)

BiPhasic tr. This mode is as earlier, but with patient triggering. This mode as of this writing is not available in the United States. It requires the use of an abdominal sensor for the trigger signal.

Continuous positive airway pressure. The device can also be used to provide standard CPAP.

SUMMARY

A wide variety of devices is available for invasive and noninvasive respiratory support of newborn infants. Most ventilators used in neonatal ICUs offer many different modes, some of which have not been adequately evaluated in newborn infants. It is incumbent on the users to learn the advantages and limitations of the devices used in their neonatal ICU and to become familiar with the ventilation modes commonly used in newborn infants. The key to success is to understand that ventilators are merely tools in our hands that need to be used with care and attention to the particular disease pathophysiology with a clear idea of the goals of mechanical ventilation. In general, one should optimize the settings on whatever mode is in use and avoid frequent changes between modes, without a clear rationale for why such change is being made. The ventilator descriptions in this chapter are meant to provide an overview of their functionality and available options. The reader is referred to the user's manual for each device for further details.

KEY REFERENCES

3. Tonna JE, Peltan I, Brown SM, et al, University of Utah Mechanical Power Study Group: Mechanical power and driving pressure as predictors of mortality among patients with ARDS. Intensive Care Med. Published online 2020.

5. Volsko TA, Chatburn RL, El-Khatib MF: Equipment for Respiratory Care. 1st ed. Jones & Bartlett Learning, 2016.

6. Sanborn WG: Microprocessor-based mechanical ventilation. Respir Care 38(1):72–109, 1993.

7. Chatburn RL, Mireles-Cabodevila E: Closed-loop control of mechanical ventilation: description and classification of targeting schemes. Respir Care 56(1):85–102, 2011.

8. Chatburn RL, Carlo WA: A taxonomy for mechanical ventilation. In: Berhardt LV (ed): Advances in Medicine and Biology. Vol 78. Nova Biomedical, 2014, pp. 2–70.

12. de Wit M: Monitoring of patient-ventilator interaction at the bedside. Respir Care 56(1):61–72, 2011.

16. Tobin MJ: Principles and Practice of Mechanical Ventilation. McGraw Hill Medical, 2013.

17. Mireles-Cabodevila E, Hatipoglu U, Chatburn RL: A rational framework for selecting modes of ventilation. Respir Care 58(2): 348–366, 2013.

18. van der Staay M, Chatburn RL: Advanced modes of mechanical ventilation and optimal targeting schemes. Intensive Care Med Exp 6(1):30, 2018.

28

Extracorporeal Membrane Oxygenation

Robert M. Arensman, Billie Lou Short, Nathaniel Koo, and Andrew Mudreac

KEY POINTS

- Extracorporeal membrane oxygenation (ECMO) is a method of cardiopulmonary bypass that provides oxygen support as well as carbon dioxide extraction and cardiovascular support without toxic ventilatory settings.
- Conditions in which ECMO may be beneficial include meconium aspiration syndrome, pneumonia, neonatal sepsis, primary and secondary persistent pulmonary hypertension of the newborn, congenital diaphragmatic hernia (CDH), perinatal asphyxia, respiratory distress syndrome, barotrauma with air-leak syndrome, and preoperative support of newborns with congenital cardiac lesions. Reversibility of the disease process is the major criterion for ECMO selection. In addition to neonates, older children and adults have also benefited from the application of ECMO.
- Contraindications to ECMO are those clinical situations that preclude either a quality outcome or a successful ECMO run.
- Technically, one accomplishes ECMO through arterial/venous or venous/venous connections, generally in a neonate's neck, which allows the blood flow to accomplish cardiopulmonary bypass.
- As of 2019, the Extracorporeal Life Support Organization Registry has recorded 27,728 neonates with respiratory failure having been treated with ECMO; 84% were successfully decannulated and 74% survived to discharge. The cumulative survival statistics are highest for meconium aspiration syndrome at 94% and lowest for CDH at 51%.

INTRODUCTION

The field of assisted ventilation continues to evolve, with new computer-assisted ventilators that are equipped with numerous modalities and feedback mechanisms, pulmonary function measurements and graphics, as well as drugs to modulate the pulmonary vascular bed and to manage the complications of ventilation. However, even with these advances, some neonates continue to deteriorate and are at risk of death from hypoxic respiratory failure without alternative treatment. Certain conditions, such as persistent pulmonary hypertension of the newborn (PPHN) and congenital diaphragmatic hernia (CDH), may not improve with assisted ventilation and require alternative therapy.

In children who receive aggressive ventilatory support, there are unacceptably high rates of nonsurvival and ventilator-induced pulmonary complications: baro/volu-trauma including pulmonary air leak, bronchopulmonary dysplasia, and chronic lung disease. Because of the short- and long-term morbidity and mortality associated with ventilator-induced pulmonary complications, extracorporeal membrane oxygenation (ECMO)

should be considered in selected term or near-term newborns requiring respiratory support (Figs. 28.1 and 28.2).

ECMO is a method of cardiopulmonary bypass that provides oxygen support as well as carbon dioxide extraction and cardiovascular support without injurious ventilator settings. These processes may also be referred to as extracorporeal life support (ECLS). ECLS expands the definition of extracorporeal

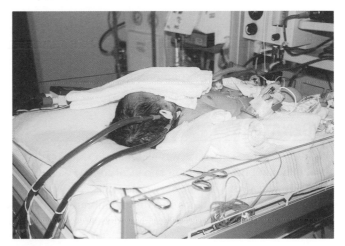

Fig. 28.1 Photograph of a neonate on extracorporeal membrane oxygenation.

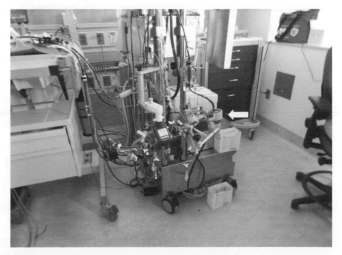

Fig. 28.2 Photograph of the bed space for an infant on extracorporeal membrane oxygenation (ECMO) showing a centrifugal ECMO pump in the foreground.

support to include many newer cardiac support systems such as ventricular assist devices and pumpless extracorporeal support with hollow fiber oxygenators only. When discussing neonatal support systems, both terms are frequently used.

HISTORY OF CARDIOPULMONARY BYPASS

In 1934, John and Mary Gibbon pioneered artificial maintenance of circulation.[1] Their technique was first reported in 1937, but it was not until the 1950s that it became widely used by cardiac surgeons. Shortly thereafter, they discovered that use of the device for more than 1 to 2 hours led to lethal protein denaturation, thought to be caused by the gas exchange device.[2] Consequently, the biologic lung was used as the oxygenator for extracorporeal circulation, as described by Lillehei and colleagues.[3] Because the oxygenator was the primary issue with artificial circulation until this point, many new devices such as the membrane oxygenator[4] and the bulb oxygenator (also known as a bubble oxygenator)[5] were developed, which became the standard for cardiac surgery.

When these oxygenators were used for prolonged bypass, it was found that cells and proteins became damaged because of direct oxygen exposure to blood, which manifested as coagulopathy and anemia a few hours after initiating bypass. Moreover, the large reservoir used for oxygenation had complicated volume management and necessitated complete suppression of coagulation in the low-flow component.

DEVELOPMENT OF MEMBRANE OXYGENATORS

The direct blood-gas interface was eliminated using streamlined units that did not have a reservoir and incorporated a membrane oxygenator instead of a bubble oxygenator (Fig. 28.3). Polyethylene and Teflon were used for the first membranes, but these materials required large surface areas for adequate oxygenation.[6]

Silicone, a polymer of dimethylsiloxane, was reported to have excellent gas transfer properties by Kammermeyer in 1957.[7] Subsequently, many new oxygenators were developed and the first trials in infants soon followed.[8] Newer modifications have eliminated the membrane oxygenator for the more commonly used hollow-fiber oxygenators to further reduce surface area, priming volume, and eliminate stagnant flow areas.

Once blood runs through the circuit and membrane lungs, they become coated with a protein monolayer. This provides a barrier between the blood and the thrombogenic foreign surface, thereby minimizing cellular trauma, prolonging gas exchange, eliminating the need of the reservoir, and allowing for the use of low-dose anticoagulation. For most patients, bleeding events are reduced and manageable.

Development of a Pump

Most neonatal ECMO devices were adapted from existing devices used by cardiac surgery teams.[9,10] Initially, multiactivated Sigma motor pumps were used. Soon thereafter, roller pumps became popular because of easier use and greater reliability. These devices compress blood-conducting tubing and force fluid forward. The disadvantages of roller pumps were increased hemolysis and pressurization of the circuit if leak or rupture occurred. Partially occluding systems reduce hemolysis but often increase clotting and the need for membrane changes. Currently, most ECMO centers use the centrifugal pump, as these devices allow for a wider range of flows and generally carry a lower risk of hemolysis and air embolus.

None of the currently available pumps provide pulsatile blood flow to the patient, which may have detrimental physiologic effects on end organs (e.g., impairment of cerebral autoregulation).[11] Consequently, the use of venovenous bypass whenever possible with preservation of endogenous pulsatile flow possible may be advantageous to the sick neonate (see further discussion of venovenous cannulation later in this chapter).

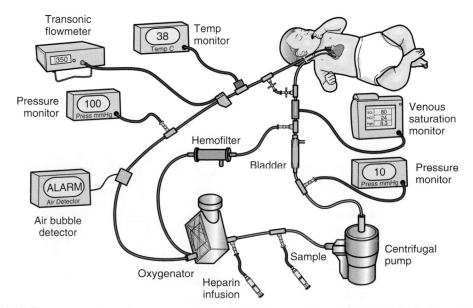

Fig. 28.3 Extracorporeal membrane oxygenation circuit diagram. (From *CNMC ECMO Training Manual.* Washington, DC, 2014.)

Vascular Access

After the resolution of issues related to the oxygenator and pump, the final major problem hindering the development of successful bypass techniques in the neonate was vascular access. The umbilical vessels were used by early investigators, but these vessels did not provide sufficient flow for adequate respiratory and cardiac support. Later, investigators cannulated the internal jugular vein and the common carotid artery, which allowed sufficient flow to permit near-total cardiopulmonary bypass if necessary. With these multiple problems successfully solved, Bartlett and his colleagues[9] were able to complete the first successful application of ECMO for respiratory failure in a neonate in 1975.

PHYSIOLOGY OF EXTRACORPOREAL CIRCULATION

Membrane Lung

As of this writing, the membrane lungs currently in use are the diffusion, hollow-fiber membrane oxygenators composed of poly-4-methyl-1-pentene. Unlike other hollow-fiber oxygenators, these membranes are nonporous and therefore a "true" membrane lung—they do not develop a plasma leak like the microporous hollow fiber oxygenators. Oxygen (O_2) and carbon dioxide (CO_2) diffuse across the membrane at the molecular level (Fig. 28.4), shown for a silicone membrane; hollow-fiber membrane is essentially the same process. The difference between the O_2 content in the ventilating gas and that in the venous blood of the patient provides a gradient for O_2 diffusion across the membrane.

Oxygen and Carbon Dioxide Transfer

Red blood cells closest to the membrane fibers are saturated with oxygen first, thereby increasing the local partial pressure of O_2 (PO_2). The bundled fibers provide adequate surface area for gas exchange. The blood film must remain in contact with the membrane long enough for O_2 to diffuse to the center of the film in order for complete saturation to occur. For any given membrane lung, the amount of venous blood that can be completely saturated is a function of the O_2 content of the venous blood returning to the membrane and the amount of time spent in the membrane. As flow increases, blood spends less time in the membrane. Oxygen transfer increases in proportion to the flow rate until O_2 transfer becomes limited by the thickness of the blood film. Once venous blood entering the membrane is 75% saturated, the flow rate at which blood leaving the membrane is 95% saturated is termed the "rated flow" of that device, a number that allows for standardization of various membrane lungs (Fig. 28.5). If the membrane is assumed to be large enough, O_2 delivery is predominately dependent on available blood flow, not on the membrane capacity to transfer O_2.

Compared with O_2, CO_2 is much more diffusible through plasma, and CO_2 transfer is limited by its diffusion rate across the membrane. Because newer hollow-fiber membranes have excellent gas transfer at low gas flow rates (0.25–0.5 L/min), addition of CO_2 gas to the membrane gas mixture going across the membrane is not usually needed, as was the case with the older silicone membrane lung. Carbon dioxide transfer is dependent on surface area of the membrane and independent of blood flow; thus, an

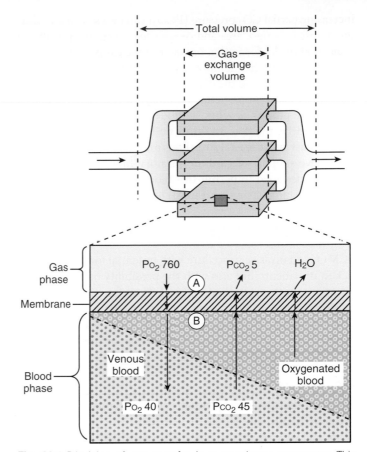

Fig. 28.4 Principles of gas transfer in a membrane oxygenator. This expanded view shows interactions across the gas-exchange membrane. Venous blood enters from the left and becomes arterialized as O_2 diffuses through the membrane and blood film and as CO_2 diffuses from the blood film into the gas phase. (From Bartlett RH, Gassaniga AB: Extracorporeal circulation for cardiopulmonary failure. Curr Prob Surg 15:9, 1978.)

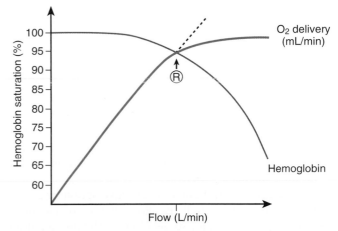

Fig. 28.5 Rated flow. As flow through the membrane increases, actual oxygen (O_2 transfer increases proportionally until the residence time of the venous return prevents complete hemoglobin saturation. At this point, the absolute O_2 transfer becomes fixed, but as the flow continues to increase, a smaller percentage of the venous return to the membrane becomes saturated. ® represents the rated flow, which is the flow at which the blood leaving the membrane is 95% saturated. (Modified from Galletti PM, Richardson PD, Snider MT: A standardised method for defining the overall gas transfer performance of artificial lungs. Trans Am Soc Artif Intern Organs 18:359, 1972.)

increasing partial CO_2 pressure (PCO_2) can be a sensitive indicator of loss of surface area and oxygenator function (typically an indication of clot formation or water in the gas phase).

Blood flow to the membrane is limited by the total circulating blood volume and the diameter of the venous catheter. With the older roller pumps, venous drainage was driven by gravity; centrifugal pumps develop a modest negative pressure that serves to drive the flow and thus no longer depend on gravity. There must be at least 120 mL/kg/min of flow in the system to achieve support of cardiorespiratory function. The ECMO circuit is designed to permit this blood flow volume, with the membrane lung having a greater rated flow.

PATIENT SELECTION

ECMO is an invasive procedure with potential for benefit in the sickest of patients, but also with the possibility of serious complications, both medical and ethical. Therefore, it is of utmost importance to consider the appropriate criteria in patient selection. This can be approached in two ways: Which patients would receive significant benefit from this therapy? and When should this therapy be instituted?

Disease States

Reversibility of the disease process is the major criterion for ECMO selection. Ideally, this should be achievable within 2 to 4 weeks, although ECLS beyond this time has been successful in many cases. Disease processes that may fall within this spectrum include meconium aspiration syndrome, pneumonia, neonatal sepsis, primary and secondary PPHN,[11-14] CDH, perinatal asphyxia, respiratory distress syndrome, barotrauma with air-leak syndrome, and preoperative support of newborns with congenital cardiac lesions. In addition to neonates, older children and adults have also benefited from the application of ECMO (Fig. 28.6).

Although congenital cardiac defects can generally be managed and corrected without the need for ECMO, one example that may mimic some of the other conditions listed earlier by causing clinical signs of PPHN is total anomalous pulmonary venous return. Two-dimensional echocardiogram can be misleading in this case, as the heart itself may appear normal unless there is an associated intracardiac defect. Noninvasive techniques may be necessary to determine the absence of pulmonary veins entering the left atrium and the common pulmonary venous channel. Pulmonary hypertension would then arise from obstruction of the anomalous pulmonary venous drainage, most commonly in the infradiaphragmatic variety.[11]

In severe cases, ECMO can be an effective option for perioperative stabilization, as well as allowing for completion of workup and preparation for surgery in more hemodynamically stable patients. ECMO can also be used as a ventricular assist device in the management of infants with perioperative ventricular failure, allowing many babies to survive who would otherwise be unable to come off operative bypass.

Selection Criteria

Optimal use of selection criteria for ECMO would recognize the patients on traditional therapy at risk of life-threatening

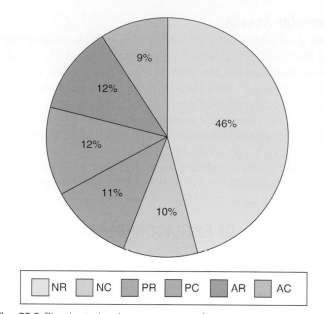

Fig. 28.6 Pie chart showing percentage of extracorporeal membrane oxygenation patients by category. *AC*, Adult cardiac; *AR*, adult respiratory; *NC*, neonatal cardiac; *NR*, neonatal respiratory; *PC*, pediatric cardiac; *PR*, pediatric respiratory. (Data from the ECMO Registry of the Extracorporeal Life Support Organization. Ann Arbor, Michigan; 1980–2014. Data from 2014 are incomplete.)

complications or irreversible lung injury before those occurring and identify the point when the risk-benefit balance tips to ECMO. In practice, this is often a gray area without a universally clear set point. Box 28.1 describes criteria used for scoring systems at a number of centers. These systems can be useful for guidance when making the decision for ECMO use.[14-16] In certain specific situations, there appears to be broad consensus among practitioners. For example, for neonates with CDH, a commonly used threshold is preductal O_2 saturation <80% that is refractory to ventilator support and medical therapy.[16]

Alveolar-Arterial Oxygen Gradient

One of the original, and therefore oldest, predictors of mortality in the neonate with respiratory failure is the alveolar-arterial O_2 gradient:

$$A\text{-}aDO_2 = P_AO_2 - PaO_2 \qquad \textbf{(Eq. 28.1)}$$

where P_AO_2 is the alveolar O_2 tension and PaO_2 is the arterial O_2 tension.

The PaO_2 is measured directly from a postductal arterial blood sample, and the P_AO_2 can be calculated from the alveolar gas equation:

$$Pao_2 - PIO_2 - P_ACO_2/R \\ + PaCO_2 \times FiO_2 \, (1\text{-}R)/R \qquad \textbf{(Eq. 28.2)}$$

where PIO_2 is the partial pressure of inspired O_2 and is calculated by the following equation:

$$PIO_2 = FiO_2 \times (P_{ATM} - PH_2O) \qquad \textbf{(Eq. 28.3)}$$

BOX 28.1 Extracorporeal Membrane Oxygenation Selection Criteria

Indications
- A-aDo$_2$ > 610 × 8 hours or > 605 × 4 hours, if PIP is >38 cm H$_2$O
- Oxygen index >40
- Acute deterioration with partial pressure of oxygen (PaO$_2$) < 40 × 2 hours and/or pH < 7.15 × 2 hours
- Unresponsive to treatment: PaO$_2$ < 55 and pH < 7.4 × 3 hours
- Barotrauma (any four concurrently)
  Pulmonary interstitial emphysema
  Pneumothorax or pneumomediastinum
  Pneumoperitoneum
  Pneumopericardium
  Subcutaneous emphysema
  Persistent air leak for >24 hours
  MAP >15 cm H$_2$O and subcutaneous emphysema
- Postoperative cardiac dysfunction
- Bridge to cardiac transplantation

Relative Contraindications
- Prolonged severe hypoxia >7 days
- Structural cardiac disease

- History or evidence of ischemic neurologic damage
- Lack of parental consent

Absolute Contraindications
- Lack of parental consent
- Inadequate conventional therapy
- Weight <2000 g
- Gestational age <35 weeks
- Contraindications to anticoagulation
  Severe pulmonary hemorrhage
  IVH ≥grade II
  Gastrointestinal hemorrhage
  Head trauma
- Prolonged mechanical ventilation >7–14 days
- History of severe asphyxia or severe global cerebral ischemia
- Lethal genetic condition or unrelated fatal diagnosis (trisomy 13, trisomy 18, untreatable malignancy)
- Untreatable nonpulmonary disease, significant untreatable congenital cardiac malformation or disease

IVH, Intraventricular hemorrhage; *MAP*, mean airway pressure; *PIP*, peak inspiratory pressure.

---

where P$_{ATM}$ is the atmospheric pressure, PH$_2$O is the partial pressure of water vapor, P$_A$CO$_2$ is the alveolar CO$_2$ tension, and R is the respiratory exchange ratio (respiratory quotient).

Assuming that fraction of inspired oxygen (FiO$_2$) is 1.0 during maximum ventilation therapy, that the P$_A$CO$_2$ is equal to PaCO$_2$, and that R is 1.0, substitution of Eq. 28.2 and 28.3 into Eq. 28.1 yields a simplified equation for calculation of the gradient:[13]

$$P_AO_2 - PaO_2 = (P_{ATM} - PH_2O) - (PaO_2 + P_aCO_2) \quad \textbf{(Eq. 28.4)}$$

Krummel et al.[14] and Ormazabal et al.[15] showed that a gradient greater than 620 mm Hg for 12 consecutive hours predicted a 100% mortality rate, even in the presence of maximum conventional therapy, including alkalinization (no longer practiced) and tolazoline (Priscoline®; no longer available). However, by the time one-third of patients met this criterion, they were so moribund that ECMO salvage was no longer possible. Similarly, a gradient of 600 mm Hg for 12 consecutive hours predicted a mortality rate of 94%. Again, in a retrospective study of 30 infants with PPHN by Beck et al.,[16] a gradient of 610 mm Hg for eight consecutive hours predicted a 79% mortality rate (see Box 28.1). Other studies for this criterion have shown some variations for the value, but it is clear that elevated gradient pressures over prolonged periods indicate high probability of a poor outcome.

Oxygenation Index

The sensitivity of the alveolar-arterial O$_2$ gradient as a predictor of outcome was somewhat blunted by the ventilator management improvements in the 1980s. Dworetz et al.[17] showed that the previous gradient criterion predicted only 10% mortality for their cohort of patients. Thus, new indices were developed with the goal of providing greater precision, including one of the most commonly used in ECMO centers today, the oxygenation index (OI). This criterion assesses a neonate's oxygenation status but also accounts for the amount of ventilator support needed to achieve it by measuring the mean airway pressure (MAP) on conventional ventilation.

The OI is calculated by dividing the product of the FiO$_2$ (×100) and the MAP by the postductal PaO$_2$:

$$OI = FiO_2 \times MAP \times 100/PaO_2 \quad \textbf{(Eq. 28.5)}$$

If it is assumed that the FiO$_2$ is 1.0, as it is in most patients who are candidates for ECMO, the equation can be simplified to read as follows:

$$OI = \frac{MAP \times 100}{PaO_2} \quad \textbf{(Eq. 28.6)}$$

In a patient population of candidates for ECMO where the alveolar-arterial O$_2$ gradient did not accurately predict mortality, Ortega et al.[18] showed that an OI greater than 40 for 2 hours predicted a mortality rate of 82%. This was supported by Ortiz et al.,[19] who found the mortality rate to be 80% to 90% for patients with an OI of 40 or higher for more than 2 hours. It should be stressed that strict reliance on historical criteria is not without risk, and constant reassessment of criteria for ECMO therapy at each ECMO center is strongly recommended.

Acute Deterioration

The standard ECMO criteria are based on gas exchange deficits, but increasingly, it has become evident that cardiovascular decompensation may be an important pathway to requirement for ECMO support. It is not an uncommon situation to have a previously stable neonate have a sudden and drastic deterioration of their clinical status, often as a result of acute right ventricular decompensation, which manifests by hypotension, clinical signs of poor perfusion, and development of lactic acidosis. Such a precipitous decline may not allow the 3 to 12 hours needed to calculate an accurate alveolar-arterial O_2 gradient or OI. Because of this, many ECMO centers have adopted criteria that address this issue. A pH less than 7.15 and a PaO_2 less than 40 mm Hg for two consecutive hours are common simplified criteria that would suggest ECMO candidacy for an infant.[20] In addition, if the baby is in severe distress or cardiac arrest, clinical judgment supervenes, and a decision must be made as to whether ECMO may be used to attempt life salvage.

Ventilator-Associated Lung Injury

Although important, gas exchange is not the only consideration when evaluating an infant's suitability for ECMO therapy. Mechanical ventilation can lead to pulmonary injury caused by the high pressure or volume created by the ventilator, known as baro/volu-trauma. To account for this problem, specific indicators are identified:

1. Pulmonary interstitial emphysema or pseudocyst
2. Pneumothorax or pneumomediastinum
3. Pneumoperitoneum
4. Pneumopericardium
5. Subcutaneous emphysema
6. Persistent air leak for 24 hours
7. MAP of 15 cm H_2O or greater

Significant baro/volu-trauma, which significantly increases the morbidity and mortality of the patient, is determined if four or more of these criteria are met. To reduce the risk of pulmonary damage and chronic lung disease in a neonate demonstrating these problems, ECMO therapy should be seriously considered.

Contraindications

The contraindications to ECMO are those clinical situations that preclude either a quality outcome or a successful ECMO run (see Box 28.1). Infants who weigh less than 2000 g are at increased risk of intraventricular hemorrhage. These patients are generally premature and have an immature germinal matrix that is susceptible to vascular rupture.[21] In their pilot study, Bartlett and Andrews[22] treated 15 infants weighing less than 2000 g and had only three (20%) survivors. Patients with an estimated gestational age of less than 35 weeks have been found to have an almost 100% incidence of intracranial hemorrhage (ICH).[23] Further evaluations of this population have shown survival rates between 40% and 70% and an ICH risk between 40% and 50%.[24,25] Many centers consider these high-risk patients and use a cut-off of 2000 g and/or 34 weeks' gestation. However, there is some support more recently to push the bounds to 1500 g and/or 30 weeks. Of course, the physical limitations of cannula size remain for those potential candidates.

Other exclusion criteria include neonates with chromosomal abnormalities or syndromes known to be associated with profound neurodevelopmental impairment or a fatal outcome in infancy. Severe ICH is another contraindication, but grade I or II hemorrhage may be acceptable with close monitoring (low activated clotting times and high platelet counts), because it

may be possible to avoid extension of the bleed. Determination of the severity of pulmonary hypoplasia may be difficult, but important because ECMO may not change the outcome. Some centers have used the inability to reduce $PaCO_2$ to less than 70 to 80 pre-ECMO as a measure of hypoplastic lungs. These patients may still receive ECMO therapy, but parents are made aware of the potential irreversibility of the lung disease and how that may affect decisions about further treatment. To date, there are no specific criteria for the use of $PaCO_2$, just institutional experience.

Evaluation before Extracorporeal Membrane Oxygenation

It is important to carefully evaluate an infant who may be a candidate for ECMO, paying special attention to the cardiovascular and neurologic systems. A thorough physical examination is mandatory to exclude congenital defects. Laboratory abnormalities are to be expected, but baseline values, such as those of the platelet count and coagulation studies, will play an important role in management decisions.

A cardiovascular evaluation is performed to rule out congenital heart disease (CHD). Obtaining a two-dimensional echocardiography study can indicate the presence of pulmonary hypertension: elevated right heart pressure, septal bulging, tricuspid valve regurgitation, and right-to-left shunting at the ductal or foramen ovale sites. It can also note the degree of ventricular dysfunction and any structural abnormalities. Poor ventricular function secondary to hypoxia in the setting of pulmonary hypertension is often seen and is not a contraindication to ECMO. ECMO will actually improve the hypokinesia by increasing myocardial oxygenation, as well as decreasing preload to lower the ventricular workload. If CHD is strongly suspected in an unstable patient, the patient should be placed on ECMO in most circumstances with plans for a reevaluation on ECMO for CHD including a potential cardiac catheterization. The stress of cardiac catheterization would not be tolerated by most of these patients before being placed on ECMO. If a congenital lesion is found, then discussion should be undertaken with the cardiac surgery team to determine the optimal timing of the operation and potential risks and benefits of ECMO in the perioperative period.

An accurate neurologic evaluation that can determine the severity of damage before ECMO can be difficult. Apgar scores are a commonly used shorthand for neurologic status; however, there are three points to consider. First, Apgar scores often do not correlate with intrauterine hypoxia/ischemia.[26] Second, neonatal hypoxia/ischemia is not the only cause of depressed Apgar scores.[27] Third, because an infant can have good Apgar scores and then experience a prolonged period of hypoxia/ischemia, Apgar scores cannot predict neurologic outcome and are of limited value in the determination of candidates for ECMO.[28]

Because many infants under consideration for ECMO are paralyzed, sedated, or both, as part of their ventilator management, seizure activity and focal neurologic deficits can be difficult to assess. Head ultrasounds are regularly done to rule of ICH but may not detect ischemic lesions. A finding of ICH is concerning, as the systemic anticoagulation required during ECMO may cause a rapid extension of the hemorrhage. Von

Allmen et al.[29] found that grade I ICH is not associated with a significant risk for major intracranial complications after ECMO, but that severe edema and periventricular leukomalacia are associated with a 63% incidence of major intracranial complications. Grade II necessitates close management of anticoagulation and daily head ultrasound studies. Any patient with an ICH grade III and above should not be considered a candidate for ECMO secondary to risk for rapid increase in the hemorrhage and associated major morbidity and/or mortality.

An electroencephalogram (EEG) is a reliable indicator of severe hypoxic-ischemic encephalopathy in the paralyzed term infant. The presence of low-voltage or burst-suppression on the EEG indicates a poor neurologic outcome[30] and is therefore a relative contraindication to ECMO. True isoelectric pattern is uncommon in neonates but would constitute an absolute contraindication. In the absence of those findings, however, seizure activity alone on the EEG is not an absolute contraindication to ECMO. Okochi et al.[31] did find that nearly a quarter of the neonatal and pediatric ECMO patients at their institution had seizure activity on continuous EEG, and there was a correlation with survival to hospital discharge, so it is still a significant factor to consider in the decision to initiate ECMO. In questionable cases, it is helpful to consult with a pediatric neurologist.

TECHNIQUE FOR BEGINNING EXTRACORPOREAL MEMBRANE OXYGENATION

Before Cannulation

When a neonatal unit believes a baby is approaching the need for ECMO, a communication chain should be activated to notify the surgical service, the operating room, the perfusion service, the blood bank and any service that may assist in the ECMO process. Blood samples should go urgently to the blood bank for preparation of the blood elements that will be needed.

ECMO is an invasive surgical procedure, so surgical consent is required. Care should be used to see that parents are well informed of the seriousness of their child's illness. The myriad complications of ECMO should be fully revealed and explained: hemorrhage, infarctions of various tissues, chronic neurological deficits, chronic lung disease, and possible death.

There is no "off-the-shelf" ECMO device, rather, each institution assembles their own equipment according to local needs and preferences from equipment that is for the most part designed primarily for short-term cardiopulmonary bypass. Circuits can be assembled in advance and kept sterile until needed. The system consists of polyvinyl chloride tubing, a hollow fiber membrane lung, a small venous bladder or compliance chamber, multiple ports for sampling and infusions, a heat exchanger, and computer aided perfusion system (several models are available). The tubing runs through a centrifugal or roller pump (ECMO center choice), which is servo regulated to decrease or stop flow when volume in the compliance reservoir is inadequate. This reduces the chance of negative pressure causing gas to come out of solution (foaming) and red cell damage if the vortex pump is in use. In addition, many pressure

monitoring systems are available to monitor pressure throughout the system adjusting the flow minutely to match the volumes available for perfusion.

The ECMO circuit is primed with packed cells, fresh frozen plasma, and platelets. The pH and electrolytes in the priming solution are corrected if time allows so that an adverse reaction associated with sever electrolyte/pH shifts can be prevented because priming volumes may be two to three times the neonatal blood volume.

Venoarterial Versus Venovenous Cannulation

ECMO can be done via a double lumen cannula (venoarterial [VA]) (Fig. 28.7) or a single lumen cannula (venovenous [VV]) (Fig. 28.8). In certain cases, a combination is used, generally commencing with VV and then converting to VA if needed. VV generally requires good cardiac action in the child whereas VA is used when cardiac function is severely compromised.

In VA bypass, venous outflow is established from the right atrium via the internal jugular vein, usually with a 10- to 16-French cannula. Blood is returned to the aortic arch through an 8- to 12-French cannula within the right common carotid artery. Both cardiac support and oxygenation occur; therefore, if a neonate has an asphyxiated myocardium or requires maximum pressor support, this is generally the procedure of choice.

VV ECMO provides gas exchange but relies on the neonatal patient's cardiac output. VV ECMO does not decompress the pulmonary circulation to the same extent as does VA ECMO. Managing an ECMO run with a VV cannula may be more difficult and require conversion to VA ECMO. Thus, this modality is often best used in those infants who come early

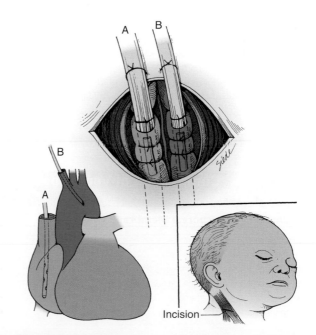

Fig. 28.7 Vessel cannulation for venoarterial extracorporeal membrane oxygenation. Both the internal jugular vein (*A*) and the carotid artery (*B*) are ligated. The cannulae are then secured in the vessels with two ligatures over a small piece of vessel loop. When these ligatures are removed, they are cut over the vessel loop without risking damage to the vessels or the cannulae. Both cannulae are also secured to the skin of the neck.

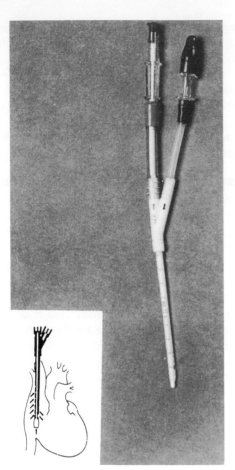

Fig. 28.8 Double-lumen venovenous catheter for single-site access. The indwelling obturator is seen in the venous drainage lumen. The two lumens, separated by an eccentrically located septum, allow both venous blood drainage and reinfusion of warmed oxygenated blood. The catheter is inserted through a venotomy in the internal jugular vein such that the tip of the catheter, and thus the reinfusion port, is located in the right atrium (*inset*). (From Anderson HL, Snedecor SM, Otsu T, et al: Multicenter comparison of conventional venoarterial access versus venovenous double-lumen catheter access in newborn infants undergoing extracorporeal membrane oxygenation. J Pediatr Surg 28:530, 1993.)

to ECMO, are in the more stable category, and require help primarily with gas exchange.

Venous drainage still occurs via the internal jugular vein with a 12- to 16-French cannula, but venous return is via the second lumen of the double lumen cannula. Alternatively, in rare cases, venous return can be directed through a femoral vein. Clearly, VV is less invasive than VA, so this approach should be chosen unless there is a clear advantage for VA bypass.

Operative Procedure

Operative cannulation is usually done in the neonatal intensive care unit. Full surgical preparation, drapes, gown, and gloves are used with the addition of some form of good anesthesia technique. Obviously, these children are intubated and ventilated, so paralysis is added if not already required to prevent spontaneous ventilation and possibility of air embolus. Surgical teams today have all the lighting, cautery, and supplies required to do this procedure in the nursery, usually under a radiant warmer.

The incision is made over the lower third of the sternocleido-mastoid muscle. The carotid sheath is exposed. The artery and vein are identified and isolated, taking care to preserve the vagus nerve that also runs within the sheath. At this point, the neonate is given an intravenous bolus of heparin, 100 to 200 units/kg.

For VA bypass, the common carotid artery is ligated distally and controlled proximally. Through a transverse arteriotomy, the arterial cannula is passed a premeasured distance into the common carotid artery almost to the aortic arch. The venous cannula is inserted in a similar manner into the right atrium through the right internal jugular vein. The cannulae are secured by a variety of methods—an important step in the surgery because accidental decannulation is probably a fatal event. Care must be taken to avoid air embolization or air within the circuit.

VV bypass is much the same procedure; however, the carotid artery although usually visualized and exposed for possible future use is left intact. The jugular vein is opened, and the single, double lumen catheter is advance into the atrium, taking care to direct the venous return orifices toward the tricuspid valve (Table 28.1).

TABLE 28.1 **Comparison of Venovenous and Venoarterial Extracorporeal Membrane Oxygenation**	
Venovenous Extracorporeal Membrane Oxygenation	**Venoarterial Extracorporeal Membrane Oxygenation**
Advantages	
• Requires venous access only	• Good oxygenation and CO_2 removal
• Pulsatile flow to organs preserved via native cardiac function in series with extracorporeal membrane oxygenation (ECMO) circuit	• ECMO circuit both in parallel and in series with native cardiopulmonary circuit. The fraction of blood flowing in parallel is dependent upon the ECMO pump velocity.
• Good carbon dioxide (CO_2) removal	• Can provide partial cardiac bypass and cardiac rest
• Easy to wean off ECMO support	• Rapid wean off ventilator, inotropes, and pressors
Disadvantages	
• Dependence on native cardiac function for cardiac output	• Nonpulsatile pump flow
• Flow through circuit may be limited by smaller cannula compared with single-lumen VA venous cannula	• Cannulation of right carotid artery support
• Decreased oxygen delivery to periphery compared with VA ECMO	• Somewhat more difficult to wean off ECMO
• Decreased flow if mediastinum is displaced	

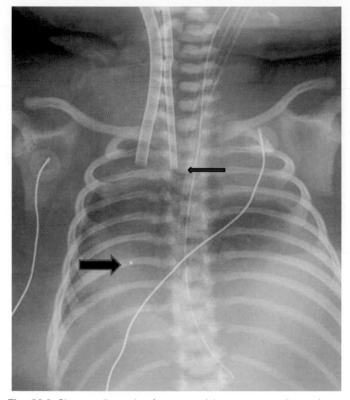

Fig. 28.9 Chest radiograph of venoarterial extracorporeal membrane oxygenation patient showing the venous cannula tip (*large arrow*) in the right atrium, with the tip at the right atrium– inferior vena cava junction, and the arterial cannula (*small arrow*) in the aortic arch. Note that the venous catheter has a small metal dot at the end.

A chest x-ray is required to confirm correct placement. An echocardiogram may also be helpful to establish correct placement of the cannulae and to exclude placement too close or across the aortic valve (Fig. 28.9).

DAILY MANAGEMENT

Once a child is on ECMO, gas manipulation occurs via the ECMO circuit. Consequently, ventilatory settings are set low to avoid lung damage: FiO_2 of 0.21 to 0.40, rate of 10 to 20 breaths per minute, peak inflation pressure of 15 to 20 cm H_2O, and a positive end-expiratory pressure (PEEP) of 5 to 6 cm H_2O. Typically, an ECMO patient's lungs worsen on the first few days of the ECMO run. The lungs "white out" on chest x-ray. In a multicenter randomized trial, Keszler et al.[32] demonstrated that increased PEEP during bypass shortened the ECMO run and improved lung compliance during the first 72 hours of bypass. This high-PEEP group also had fewer complications, so many centers manipulate this parameter toward values of 10 to 15 mm H_2O pressure.

Activated clotting time is measured hourly and maintained between 160 and 200 seconds with continuous infusion of heparin (30–70 units/kg/hour). Many centers are also using UFH (unfractionated heparin level: Anti-Xa), a measure of the bound UFH-AT complex which inhibits coagulation immediately. The goal level is 0.4 to 0.6 U/mL and should be measured

every 4 to 8 hours. Activated clotting time and blood heparin levels correlated well in infants undergoing ECMO.[33] Hematocrit is maintained between 35% and 45% and supported with saline-washed red blood cells as needed. Likewise, the platelet count is maintained above 75,000/mm³ unless there is unusual bleeding or a surgical procedure is anticipated (adjust upward to 100,000–150,000/mm³). Fibrinogen levels can be supported with cryoprecipitate and other clotting factors with fresh frozen plasma as needed. A full discussion of anticoagulation methods is beyond the scope of this chapter.

Complete intravenous nutritional support is established with standard calculations for protein, lipids, carbohydrate, trace elements, and vitamins. Some centers start enteral feeds, but the abdominal examination needs to be followed closely, and if distension occurs, the feeding should be held.

Echocardiography is extremely useful during ECMO therapy. It may be needed initially for corroboration of cannula placement, but its major contribution is determination of pulmonary vascular resistance as evidenced by shunts and flow across the ductus arteriosus. Resolution of this problem heralds the ability to wean from ECMO. This is less evident in children with CDH who have greater persistence of high pulmonary pressures after ECMO runs, but an improving echocardiogram assists with the decision to wean from ECMO.[34]

Serial cranial ultrasound examinations to screen for ICH are generally done during the first 5 to 7 days of an ECMO run. Experience suggests that bleeds occur within this time frame if they are going to occur. However, some centers continue twice-weekly cranial ultrasound until cessation of ECMO. In addition, an immediate study is indicated whenever a clinical change suggests a bleed (seizure, bulging fontanelle, sudden unexplained fall in hematocrit). Severe bleeds are indication for cessation of ECMO. Smaller bleeds (grade I and II) require a tighter control of coagulation and platelet support but may not extend, allowing the ECMO run to continue to successful wean and decannulation.

Fig. 28.10 demonstrates that many of the complications seen on ECMO are related to either bleeding or clotting complications.

Chest X-rays are generally a daily event to monitor position of lines, endotracheal tube, cannulae, and any other invasive lines. Airleak events may occur, including pneumothoraxes, which may require chest tube placement or simple observation. Any surgical procedure while on the ECMO circuit requires meticulous attention to hemostasis and to levels of anticoagulation and platelets.

WEANING

During ECMO bypass, a neonate's mixed PaO_2 is a combination of contributions from the pump and the infant's heart and lungs. Arterial O_2 content, measured in the distal aorta represents a mixture of pump blood and blood that traverses the pulmonary circuit. Because the pump blood is greater than 99% saturated, any increase in distal aorta PaO_2 represents an increase in the contribution of the patient's cardiovascular system, provided the pump flow remains constant.

At the initiation of ECMO, pump flow is generally between 100 and 120 mL/kg/min. This is enough to achieve good gas exchange via the oxygenator. As the infant's lungs improve, the

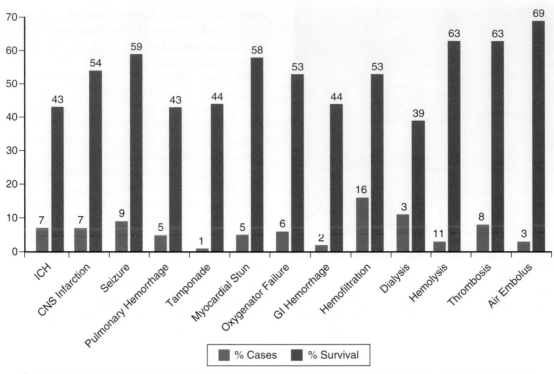

Fig. 28.10 Incidences of the most commonly seen complications in neonatal respiratory extracorporeal membrane oxygenation. *CNS*, Central nervous system; *GI*, gastrointestinal; *ICH*, intracranial hemorrhage. (Data from the ECMO Registry of the Extracorporeal Life Support Organization. Ann Arbor, Michigan; 1980–2014. Data from 2014 are incomplete.)

additional oxygenation taking place via the lungs increases the systemic PaO₂, allowing the flow through the ECMO circuit to be reduced. This process continues stepwise, gradually reducing flow to 50 to 80 mL/kg/min. This flow rate, often called idling, is maintained for 4 to 6 hours. If gas exchange and hemodynamic status remain stable during this period, the infant is ready for removal from the ECMO circuit. Alternatively, the child can be excluded from the circuit by clamping the cannulae and observing the child for stability and good gases. If the child's condition deteriorates, he or she can be quickly returned to bypass support.

Volume status during bypass and weaning is a critical parameter. It can be easily monitored by blood pressure, heart rate, capillary refill, skin turgor and color, urine output, and venous blood gas levels. Venous pH and O₂ content are sensitive indicators of adequate perfusion (aerobic cellular respiration), and changes in these parameters may be seen before any changes in arterial blood gas values. Blood volume increase or decrease can be easily controlled through addition or removal of volume from the circuit. But increases in volume are generally in extracellular fluid and manifest as increase in weight and edema.[35] When natural diuresis occurs, pulmonary status generally improves, and weaning begins.

DECANNULATION

Removal of cannulae is a surgical procedure at the neonate's bedside, similar to the cannulation process. Stabilizing sutures

are cut and cannulae are removed. Once again, care to prevent air embolus is critical. Most centers simply ligate the vessels used for the cannulation. Retrograde flow has been demonstrated[36] in the ligated vessels, but ultimate long-term neurological and vascular outcomes are unknown.

When the ECMO run is short, it is possible to reconstruct the transverse arteriotomy.[37] However, two pseudoaneurysms have been reported (verbal communication from Adolph), and Moulton and colleagues[38] have reported greater than 50% transmural necrosis in the areas of ligatures. Consequently, resection and anastomosis or simple ligation may be safer alternatives. Many centers convert the site to a central line as needed to support the neonate in the post ECMO period.

OUTCOME

As of 2019, the Extracorporeal Life Support Organization Registry has recorded 27,728 neonates with respiratory failure having been treated with ECMO; 84% were successfully decannulated and 74% survived to discharge.[39] The cumulative survival statistics are highest for meconium aspiration syndrome at 94% and lowest for CDH at 51% (Fig. 28.11). This relationship continues when looking at late death and comorbidities.[40] Changes in intensive care and the introduction of new therapies such as surfactant, selective antibiotic prophylaxis for mothers and babies, high-frequency ventilation, and inhaled nitric oxide have reduced the numbers of infants who require ECMO annually, but those who do may be sicker and at higher risk for poor outcome. As of this writing,

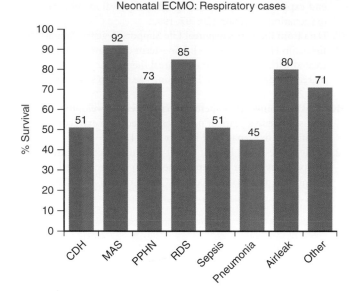

Neonatal ECMO: Respiratory cases

Fig. 28.11 Distribution of extracorporeal membrane oxygenation between neonatal respiratory diagnoses and survival rates to hospital discharge with each diagnosis. *CDH*, Congenital diaphragmatic hernia; *MAS*, meconium aspiration syndrome; *PPHN*, persistent pulmonary hypertension of the newborn; *RDS*, respiratory distress syndrome. (Data from the ECMO Registry of the Extracorporeal Life Support Organization. Ann Arbor, Michigan; 1980–2014. Data from 2014 are incomplete.)

approximately 800 infants per year are placed on ECMO for respiratory failure. Newer therapies and the greater use of a gentle ventilation approach have reduced the number infants requiring ECMO.[41]

Medical and neurodevelopmental outcomes of the ECMO patient are encouraging considering the severity of illness in the newborn period.[42,43] Analysis of outcome studies performed in PPHN survivors treated with conventional medical therapy, inhaled nitric oxide, and ECMO yield grossly equivalent morbidities and longer-term outcomes.[41,43] These findings suggest that neurodevelopmental outcome is more related to the underlying illness than to the therapeutic interventions used.[44]

Chronic lung disease (defined as oxygen use at 28 days) is seen in 15% of ECMO survivors, but long-term oxygen use is uncommon except in infants with CDH. Hospitalization for respiratory problems in the first year of life is needed in approximately 25% of survivors.[45] Normal somatic growth is seen in ECMO-treated children, except those with CDH.

Progressive high-frequency sensorineural hearing loss is seen in 3% to 21% of ECMO-treated infants.[46] An important aspect of this morbidity is the delayed onset, making diagnosis problematic. The position statement by the Joint Committee on Infant Hearing in 2000 added PPHN and ECMO as risk indicators for hearing loss and stated that babies with these risk factors should receive audiologic evaluation every 6 months until 3 years of age.[47]

Numerous investigators have studied the neurodevelopmental outcomes of ECMO patients and consistently report Bayley scores in the normal range in the first 2 years of life.[48-51] The UK trial has the most organized follow-up and showed that severe disability was found in only 4% at 1 year of age but later at 4 years of age was found in 17%.[52] They also found that 33% experienced hyperactivity or behavioral difficulties at age 7. Fewer studies of ECMO survivors at older ages have been performed. By 5 years of age, mean IQ scores remain in the normal range but are lower than normal controls (96 vs. 115, $P < .001$).[50] Glass et al. reported that approximately 15% of ECMO survivors at age 5 years had a major handicap, most commonly mental retardation, whereas less than 5% had severe or profound impairment.[51] Nevertheless, 50% of ECMO survivors have an increased risk of learning and behavioral problems compared with normal controls.[44] As a result of these deficits, ECMO survivors are vulnerable to academic and psychosocial difficulties. All ECMO patients and the near-miss ECMO population should be followed closely into school age so that interventions can be started early if needed. But, in general, the ECMO population is doing quite well, and if patients are selected appropriately, the risk of short-term and long-term morbidities and mortality should not deter the initiation of this procedure.

The only study that has examined outcomes in the young adult population treated with ECMO as infants is the one by Engle et al.[52] This multicenter study evaluated, using a questionnaire modified from the Behavioral Risk Factor Surveillance System and the 2011 National Health Interview Survey with additional unique questions added, a cohort of 146 young adults, average age 23.7 years, with an age matched cohort from the National Behavioral Risk Factor Surveillance System and National Health Interview Survey. The ECMO cohort differed statistically from the national cohort by being more satisfied with life (93% vs. 84%), more educated (80% vs 58% with some college), and less frequent users of the healthcare system (47% vs. 58%) despite being more limited because of physical, mental, and developmental problems (20% vs. 11%). Some 29% of the ECMO cohort had learning problems. Of note, asthma was noted in 34% of the ECMO population and only 16% of the study cohort non-ECMO population. Hearing was also noted to be an issue in 13% of the ECMO population, requiring hearing aids in 2.7%. Gastroesophageal reflux, scoliosis, and slow growth were more common in the CDH study cohort compared with other diagnostic groups. Although the study was limited, as surveys are, and with only 146 patients, it did show that most young adult survivors treated with ECMO were satisfied with their lives, working and/or in college, in good health, and having families.

KEY REFERENCES

9. Bartlett RH, Gazzaniga AB, Jefferies MR, et al: Extracorporeal membrane oxygenation (ECMO) cardiopulmonary support in infancy. Trans Am Soc Artif Intern Organs 22:80, 1976.
12. Krummel TM, Greenfield LJ, Kirkpatrick BV, et al: Alveolar-arterial oxygen gradients versus the neonatal pulmonary insufficiency index for prediction of mortality in ECMO candidates. J Pediatr Surg 19:380, 1984.
14. Krummel TM, Greenfield LJ, Kirkpatrick BV, et al: Clinical use of an extracorporeal membrane oxygenator in neonatal pulmonary failure. J Pediatr Surg 17:525, 1982.

16. Beck R, Anderson KD, Pearson GD, et al: Criteria for extracorporeal membrane oxygenation in a population of infants with persistent pulmonary hypertension of the newborn. J Pediatr Surg 21:297, 1986.

17. Dworetz AR, Moya FR, Sabo B, et al: Survival of infants with persistent pulmonary hypertension without extracorporeal membrane oxygenation. Pediatrics 84:1, 1989.

18. Ortega M, Ramos AD, Platzker AC, et al: Early prediction of ultimate outcome in newborn infants with severe respiratory failure. Pediatr Res 113:744, 1988.

22. Bartlett RH, Andrews AF, Toomasian JM, et al: Extracorporeal membrane oxygenation for newborn respiratory failure: forty-five cases. Surgery 92:425, 1982.

32. Keszler M, Ryckman FC, McDonald JV, et al: A prospective, multicenter, randomized study of high versus low positive end-expiratory pressure during extracorporeal membrane oxygenation. J Pediatr 120:107, 1992.

39. Data from the Extracorporeal Life Support Registry. January 2020.

44. Ijsselstijn H, van Heijst ARJ: Long-term outcome of children treated with neonatal extracorporeal membrane oxygenation: increasing problems with increasing age. Semin Perinatol 38: 114, 2014.

51. Glass P, Wagner AE, Papero PH, et al: Neurodevelopmental status at age five years of neonates treated with extracorporeal membrane oxygenation. J Pediatr 127:447–457, 1995.

52. Engle B, West KW, Hocutt GA, et al: Adult outcomes after newborn respiratory failure treated with extracorporeal membrane oxygenation. Pediatr Crit Care Med 18(1):73, 2017.

Respiratory Care of the Newborn

Robert DiBlasi

KEY POINTS

- Optimal respiratory care of a neonate provides the infant with the level of respiratory support required, avoids discomfort and complications, and is weaned off as the infant improves.
- A wide variety of equipment is used to provide respiratory support to neonates, including different types of face masks, devices to provide positive-pressure ventilation by hand, devices to provide continuous positive airway pressure and inhaled gas flow, endotracheal tubes, and humidification devices. Health professionals caring for neonates should be familiar with the design and use of devices used in their unit.
- Infants receiving respiratory support should be monitored and periodically assessed. Infants requiring greater support require more frequent and closer monitoring.
- Secure fixation of the endotracheal tube is important to prevent accidental extubation and to minimize tube movement during patient care. It can be performed by several different methods, including the use of specially designed devices.
- Endotracheally intubated infants should undergo periodic endotracheal suction, preferably without instillation of normal saline, with appropriate precautions to avoid complications from such suction.
- Chest physiotherapy is a common but controversial procedure for airway clearance in the neonatal intensive care unit.
- Several medications are administered into the respiratory tract by instillation, aerosolization, or nebulization, including surfactant, bronchodilators, and inhaled steroids.
- The use of ventilator-weaning protocols driven by bedside clinicians, including respiratory therapists, has the potential to improve compliance with clinical guidelines, decrease variation in care, and improve respiratory outcomes.

INTRODUCTION

Respiratory care encompasses a set of clinical practices, usually implemented by a multidisciplinary team (physician, respiratory therapist, nurse), to ensure the optimal delivery of respiratory support to newborn infants with respiratory distress or other problems. These practices include resuscitation, artificial airway management, invasive and noninvasive monitoring of

gas exchange, airway clearance, and aerosolized drug administration. A thorough understanding of these techniques will help clinicians provide optimal invasive and noninvasive respiratory support to sick neonates and simultaneously avoid iatrogenic injury such as skin breakdown, airway injury and inflammation, infection, ventilator-induced lung injury, and other complications. Unfortunately, many of these interventions have not been rigorously studied, and the recommendations and suggestions in this chapter are often based on low-quality evidence and experience.

TECHNIQUES TO PROVIDE POSITIVE-PRESSURE VENTILATION

Manual Ventilation

Positive-pressure ventilation can be provided through a face mask or through an endotracheal tube (ETT), either with a mechanical ventilator or with one of the three commonly used manual resuscitators: the self-inflating bag, the flow-inflating ("anesthesia") bag,[1] and the T-piece resuscitator.[2] Each possesses inherent features that distinguish one from the other. The clearest differences are found in their ability to control ventilating pressures, their reliance upon a gas source, and their potential to deliver free-flow oxygen, continuous positive airway pressure (CPAP), positive end-expiratory pressure (PEEP), and sustained inflations.

Both flow-inflating and self-inflating bags come in a wide variety of configurations, but all configurations share some basic attributes, including an oxygen inlet, patient outlet, flow-control valve, and pressure manometer attachment site. The self-inflating bag, as the name implies, reinflates after squeezing and does not require the flow of oxygen to reinflate. However, this bag with an oxygen source can deliver only about 40% oxygen because as the bag reinflates, room air is drawn into the bag and mixes with 100% oxygen from the oxygen source. A reservoir will not allow room air to come into the bag; therefore, the self-inflating bag attached to an oxygen source with a reservoir is able to deliver 90% to 100% oxygen to the baby.

TABLE 29.1 **Neonatal Manual Resuscitators**		
	Self-Inflating Bag	**Non-Self-Inflating Bag**
Types	Laerdal, Hope II, PMR 2, and a host of disposable equivalents	"Anesthesia bag" with spring-loaded or variable-orifice bleed port
Operator	Requires education on bag characteristics	Requires both experience and knowledge of bag characteristics for adjustment of flow and bleed
Oxygen-air source positive fraction of inspired oxygen (FiO$_2$) delivery	Operates with room air	Requires compressed gas
	Efficacy of oxygen (O$_2$) delivery dependent on correct use of closed reservoir system and closure of pop-off valve (use of open reservoir or pop-off valve reduces FiO$_2$)	Delivers FiO$_2$ of gas source unambiguously
	Many brands deliver room air on spontaneous breaths (in-house verification of brand performance is recommended)	O$_2$ delivery same on spontaneous breaths as it is on mandatory breaths
Pressure delivery	Having excessive trust in pop-off feature is unwise; occlusion of pop-off valve and use of manometer allow performance equal to that of non-self-inflating bags	With manometer attached, any pressure can be easily given
Comments	Relatively complex mechanism with possibility of failure, particularly when reusable units are reassembled	Simple, reliable mechanism dependent on gas supply
	If pop-off pressure is adequate, allows removal of bulky manometer for transport	Manometer is bulky

Two other important characteristics of most self-inflating bags are a pressure-relief ("pop-off") valve, which is set at 30 to 40 cm H$_2$O, and a nonrebreathing valve, which is built into the bag and prevents the reliable delivery of free-flow oxygen.[3] To deliver free-flow oxygen, the operator needs to disconnect the oxygen tubing from the bag and hold the oxygen tubing close to the nose of the baby. In contrast, the flow-inflating bag is an excellent source of free-flow oxygen, especially with the use of the appropriate-sized mask attached to the bag. Finally, both of these bags require a pressure manometer to provide safe and effective ventilation to the newborn.[3] Table 29.1 compares the two ventilation bags (or manual resuscitators).

The self-inflating bag is the only resuscitator that can operate with or without a gas source, making it ideal for transport. Because of its design, however, it cannot deliver free-flow oxygen or "blow-by oxygen." Some devices incorporate a reservoir hose coming from the back that can be used for this purpose. Improvements in sensitive valve mechanisms now allow spontaneous breathing and CPAP without having to squeeze the bag and at a relatively low work of breathing. Sustained inflations are not reliably given across all available models of self-inflating bags.[4] PEEP can be delivered with a self-inflating bag, but only with an adjunctive PEEP valve affixed to the exhalation port on the resuscitator. The self-inflating bag does not reliably control ventilating pressures and volumes even when the device is equipped with a manometer and pressure-relief valve.[5]

A flow-inflating bag, as the name suggests, requires flow from a pressurized gas source to operate. Its design allows for free-flow oxygen delivery as well as CPAP during spontaneous breathing and PEEP during positive-pressure ventilation. Inspiratory pressure, PEEP, and/or CPAP are very difficult to maintain with these systems because the clinician must coordinate a mask seal and regulate egress of flow using the thumb valve while observing chest rise and pressure readings on a manometer. One study showed more excessive PEEP (defined as >10 cm H$_2$O for >10 seconds) with the flow-inflating bag than with the self-inflating bag.[6] Flow-inflating bags have traditionally been believed to be superior to self-inflating bags because they allow the clinician to feel changes in lung compliance better than with a self-inflating bag.[7-9] Repeated laboratory scenarios have found that the flow-inflating bag produced more variable tidal volume and PEEP than the self-inflating bag.[10] Studies have also shown that this sense of "feeling compliance changes" with a flow-inflating bag is less reliable than with a self-inflating bag.[11] In fact, experienced physicians were unable to detect when an ETT was occluded in a lung model 75% of the time. Additionally, experienced respiratory therapists specializing in neonatology were shown not to distinguish changes in compliance better with a flow-inflating bag than with a self-inflating bag.[10]

Most manual ventilation devices used during resuscitation have been shown to result in variability in delivered volumes and pressures. Displayed tidal volume permits better detection of compliance changes than monitored or preset pressures.[12] Future devices are needed to display or limit volume to avoid hypo/hyperventilation and lung injury in neonates.

The T-piece resuscitator is the newest and most sophisticated of the manual resuscitator designs. Similar to the flow-inflating bag, it requires a pressurized gas source to operate and can be used to administer free-flow oxygen and CPAP to a spontaneously breathing patient. Its greatest advantage lies in its ability to regulate ventilating pressures.[13]

Face Masks for Ventilation

In cases in which the baby requires manual ventilation before endotracheal intubation, a ventilation bag with a manometer and the appropriate-sized mask should be used. The mask should be clear and have a soft, form-fitting cushion that extends around the circumference. The alternative is the rigid but anatomically shaped Rendell-Baker/Soucek mask, which may have less dead space but has been demonstrated to be more difficult to use, often resulting in ineffective ventilation.[14]

Endotracheal Intubation

Endotracheal intubation is commonly required during neonatal resuscitation at birth or postnatally in an infant with apnea or severe respiratory failure. Certain anatomic lesions may cause obstruction at the level of the nasopharynx, larynx, and upper trachea and may necessitate endotracheal intubation of affected neonates during initial resuscitation.[15] Beginning at the nasal level, these lesions include bilateral or severe unilateral choanal atresia or stenosis, pharyngeal hypotonia, and micrognathia, such as may be seen in the Robin sequence (which may include cleft palate and glossoptosis). At the level of the larynx, obstructive problems may include laryngomalacia (or laryngotracheomalacia), laryngeal web, bilateral vocal cord paralysis, and congenital subglottic obstruction. In addition, critical airway obstruction may be secondary to other lesions that may compress the airway and impair normal respiration. These may include cystic hygroma, goiter, or hemangioma. Many of these lesions, particularly those causing significant fixed obstruction at the level of the larynx or below, may render endotracheal intubation extremely difficult and may require emergency tracheostomy.

Infants in the neonatal intensive care unit (NICU) may require endotracheal intubation and positive-pressure ventilation because of respiratory failure related to a variety of causes. Two common scenarios that merit particular consideration include preterm infants with worsening respiratory distress syndrome and infants with postextubation respiratory failure.

A variety of competing factors will influence the decision to intubate an infant who has worsening respiratory distress syndrome (RDS). The symptoms of untreated RDS will tend to worsen during the first 48 to 72 hours of life, until the infant begins to make significant amounts of endogenous surfactant. Therefore, an infant with moderately severe respiratory insufficiency and distress during the first 24 hours of life may merit intubation and ventilation in anticipation of worsening disease, whereas an infant with comparable disease severity at 3 or 4 days of life may avoid intubation in anticipation of spontaneous improvement.

Although the optimal timing of surfactant administration for treatment of RDS is controversial, the available data suggest that early treatment and multiple doses are more effective, and this observation may thus lead to earlier intubation. On the other hand, positive-pressure ventilation delivered through an ETT is well known to cause lung injury, particularly if large tidal volumes are used. Some centers that make extensive use of nasal CPAP to avoid intubation and mechanical ventilation have reported fewer apneic events, less need for (re)intubation, and low rates of chronic lung disease.[16] However, these finding were not duplicated in randomized controlled trials.[17,18] Different practitioners will weigh these competing factors differently, and the indications for intubation of an infant with RDS will vary depending on the clinical circumstances and local practices.

Postextubation respiratory failure is a common occurrence in preterm infants, occurring in as many as one-third of infants. Causes of respiratory failure in these infants include central or obstructive apnea, respiratory insufficiency leading to progressive atelectasis, and early chronic lung disease. Although premature infants represent a large percentage of the patient population treated in NICU, term or postterm babies can become critically ill and develop life-threatening respiratory failure. This can result from congenital diaphragmatic hernia, primary pulmonary hypertension, meconium aspiration, sepsis, and pneumonia. Early application of nasal CPAP directly following extubation has been shown to result in lower incidence of respiratory failure, need for mechanical ventilation, and risk of developing bronchopulmonary dysplasia (BPD) in preterm neonates than extubation to no respiratory support, but CPAP may fail in 25% to 40% of infants.[19-21] Some evidence suggests that intermediary forms of noninvasive ventilation (NIV) or noninvasive intermittent mandatory ventilation may be more effective in preventing postextubation respiratory failure.[22] Other techniques to avoid reintubation include the use of methylxanthines. Indications for reintubation include progressive respiratory acidosis, increased work of breathing, grunting, stridor, significant oxygen requirement, or severe apnea.

It is not uncommon to have significant respiratory failure following extubation because of upper airway edema or subglottic stenosis, especially if the patient received prolonged ventilator support or multiple intubations or had traumatic intubation. Patients who develop respiratory failure following extubation often present with stridor, grunting, nasal flaring, and prolonged exhalation. These infants are at significant risk for severe clinical deterioration and cardiopulmonary arrest. Often, infants with a known risk of failed extubation attempts will be given intravenous steroids to reduce inflammation before extubation. Many clinicians will monitor the ETT leak displayed on the ventilator to determine the degree of airway edema present. However, this practice may not accurately reflect whether the neonatal patient will develop distress following extubation. Also, cuffed ETTs have been introduced into the NICU arena. Attempts should be made to reduce the cuff volume and prevent excessive pressure on the tracheal mucosae, but only if the patient is able to be ventilated appropriately. In the event that there is airway compromise from edema following extubation, inhaled aerosolized racemic epinephrine can be delivered to reduce swelling, but there are no data to support or refute this practice.[23] Nonetheless, many NICUs will have supplies ready at the bedside of high-risk neonates in the event that they develop stridor and respiratory distress. Additionally, clinicians should also have reintubation supplies ready at the bedside in case the patient develops severe respiratory failure. If the baby is unable to maintain adequate ventilation despite interventions, then reintubation and suctioning should be accomplished. There are multiple reasons for extubation failure; Box 29.1 provides a comprehensive list. Extubation failure should prompt a search for a cause that can be corrected before the next extubation attempt.

Routes of Intubation

Intubation can be performed orally or nasally. The choice of route depends on the circumstances and the preference of the clinician. Both oral and nasal endotracheal intubations have their unique complications and share a few as well.[24-26] Oral intubation is easier, faster, and less traumatic to perform, and it may be preferable in an emergency. Available data have failed to demonstrate statistically significant differences between oral and nasal intubation with respect to tracheal injury, frequency of tube retaping, or tube replacement.[27] However, a higher incidence of postextubation atelectasis has been noted in nasally intubated patients,

BOX 29.1 Major Causes of Extubation Failure

I. Pulmonary
   A. Primary disease not resolved
   B. Postextubation atelectasis
   C. Pulmonary insufficiency of prematurity
   D. Bronchopulmonary dysplasia
   E. Eventration or paralysis of diaphragm
II. Upper airway
   A. Edema and/or excess tracheal secretions
   B. Subglottic stenosis
   C. Laryngotracheomalacia
   D. Congenital vascular ring
   E. Necrotizing tracheobronchitis
III. Cardiovascular
   A. Patent ductus arteriosus
   B. Fluid overload
   C. Congenital heart disease with increased pulmonary flow
IV. Central nervous system
   A. Apnea (extreme immaturity)
   B. Intraventricular hemorrhage
   C. Hypoxic ischemic brain damage/seizures
   D. Drugs (phenobarbital)
V. Miscellaneous
   A. Unrecognized diagnosis (e.g., nerve palsy, myasthenia gravis)
   B. Sepsis
   C. Metabolic abnormality

especially in preterm infants with birth weight less than 1500 g; atelectasis was associated with a marked reduction in nasal airflow through the previously intubated nares and stenosis of the nasal vestibule.[28,29] Midface hypoplasia has been reported to be associated with long-term intubation for BPD.[30]

On the other hand, proponents of nasal intubation believe that fixation of the tube to the infant's face is easier and more stable because it minimizes the chance for accidental dislodgment and decreases tube movement, which can result in subglottic stenosis. Prolonged oral intubation can result in palatal grooving[31] and defective dentition.[32] Furthermore, there is evidence that acquired subglottic stenosis is increased in patients who were orally intubated and whose birth weight was less than 1500 g. The same study and one other offer evidence that the nasotracheal tube is easier to stabilize than an oral tube and that extubation occurs less frequently than in oral intubation.[26,33] Acquired subglottic stenosis secondary to oral intubation may be a sequela of tracheal mucosal damage from the ETT itself or from repeated intubations. Most significantly, severe damage can occur from the up-and-down movement of the ETT.[27] Even with perfect fixation of the tube, up-and-down movement of 7 to 14 mm has been reported owing to the varying degrees of flexion of the neck. The caretaker team can minimize palatal grooving and defective dentition by rotating the fixation site from side to side during periodic retaping. Devices are available commercially that serve as palate protectors for prolonged intubation of very low birth-weight infants (Gesco Pla-nate, MedChem Products, Woburn, MA, USA). Continuing attention to the quality of fixation, together with stabilization of the

infant's head position, minimizes tube shifting and accidental extubation with the oral approach. However, both the oral and the nasal techniques will continue to have a place in the care of the ventilated neonate. Problems associated with oral and nasal ETT use are summarized in Box 29.2.

Equipment

The equipment needed for intubation is listed in Box 29.3, and the guidelines for choosing the correct tube size and suction catheters are listed in Tables 29.2 and 29.3.[1]

BOX 29.2 Problems in Newborn Infants With Oral and Nasal Endotracheal Tubes

Common Problems
- Postextubation atelectasis—more common with nasal endotracheal tubes
- Pneumonia/sepsis
- Accidental extubation
- Intubation of main stem bronchus
- Occlusion of tube from thickened secretions
- Tracheal erosion
- Pharyngeal, esophageal, tracheal perforation
- Subglottic stenosis

Problems Unique to Nasal Endotracheal Tubes
- Nasal septal erosion
- Stricture of the nasal vestibule

Problems Unique to Oral Endotracheal Tubes
- Palatal grooving
- Interference with subsequent primary dentition

(Data from Spitzer AR, Fox WW: The use of oral versus nasal endotracheal tubes in newborn infants. J Calif Perinatol Assoc 4:32, 1984.)

BOX 29.3 Equipment Needed for Intubation

- Laryngoscope with premature (Miller No. 0) and infant (Miller No. 1) blades; Miller No. 00 optional for extremely premature infant
- Batteries and extra bulbs
- Endotracheal tubes, sizes 2.5, 3.0, 3.5, and 4.0 mm internal diameter
- Stylet
- Suction apparatus (wall)
- Suction catheters: 5.0, 6.0, 8.0, and 10.0 F
- Meconium aspirator
- Oral airway
- Stethoscope
- Non-self-inflating bag (0.5 L), manometer, and tubing; self-inflating bag with reservoir, manometer optional for self-inflating bag
- Newborn and premature mask
- Source of compressed air/oxygen (O_2) with capability for blending
- Humidification and warming apparatus for air/O_2
- Tape: ½-inch pink (Hy-Tape)
- Scissors
- Magill neonatal forceps
- Elastoplast (elastic bandages)
- Cardiorespiratory monitor
- Carbon dioxide monitor or detector
- Pulse oximeter (oxygen saturation [SpO_2])

TABLE 29.2 Selecting the Appropriate-Sized Endotracheal Tube

Tube Size (Inside Diameter in mm)	Weight (g)	Gestational Age (week)
2.5	<1000	<28
3.0	1000–2000	28–34
3.5	2000–3000	34–38
3.5–4.0	>3000	>38

(From Kattwinkel J, ed: Neonatal Resuscitation Textbook. 5th ed. Elk Grove Village, IL, American Academy of Pediatrics and the American Heart Association, 2006. Used with permission of the American Academy of Pediatrics.)

TABLE 29.3 Selecting the Appropriate-Sized Suction Catheter

Endotracheal Tube Size (Inside Diameter in mm)	Catheter Size (French)
2.5	5 or 6
3.0	6 or 8
3.5	8
4.0	8 or 10

(From Kattwinkel J, ed: Neonatal Resuscitation Textbook. 5th ed. Elk Grove Village, IL, American Academy of Pediatrics and the American Heart Association, 2006. Used with permission of the American Academy of Pediatrics.)

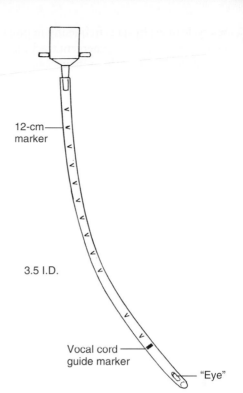

Fig. 29.1 Murphy-type endotracheal tube. The Murphy type is straight and relatively soft, with markings to show depth of insertion in the airway and in the trachea. An "eye" is present at the tip.

The use of tubes of appropriate size minimizes trauma, airway resistance, and excessive leak around the tube. A standard kit containing all of the equipment, as listed in Box 29.3, can be prepared and stocked, but it must be checked regularly to ensure that all of the necessities are present. The infant should be placed under a radiant warmer for endotracheal intubation. A laryngoscope with a Miller No. 0 or No. 1 blade should be used to visualize the vallecula, epiglottis, and glottis. The No. 0 blade is used for almost all newborns. The No. 1 blade is used for infants who are several months of age or newborns whose birth weight is greater than 4 to 5 kg.[1,34] A Miller No. 00 blade has been touted for use in extremely low birth-weight infants because its smaller blade is more easily accommodated in the mouths of micropreemies. However, because the light source is set back farther from the blade tip, some clinicians believe that the visualization is not as good as with the No. 0 blade.

Types of Tubes

The ETT should be made of a nontoxic, thermolabile, nonkinking material that molds to the airway. The tube should meet the standards of the American Society for Testing and Materials F1242-89 and be radiopaque or have a radiopaque line. Cuffed ETTs are not routinely used in neonates because the bulk of the cuff may prevent the practitioner from inserting a tube with as large a diameter as would otherwise be possible. There is always a serious concern that the inflated cuff may damage the very sensitive airway mucosa of the small baby. If sealing the space around the tube becomes a priority, cuffed tubes are now available (Sheridan, Teleflex, Morrisville, NC, USA).

The type of ETT used most commonly is the Murphy ETT (Fig. 29.1). The Murphy tube is preferred for long-term ventilation. Most often, Murphy tubes have centimeter markers to show the overall depth of the tube, as well as vocal cord guide markers near the tip. These markers, under laryngoscopic visualization, show the clinician the depth within the trachea. Standard default markers should be used with caution because of the range of anatomic variation. In one review of the length of the black area at the tip of ETTs produced by four major manufacturers, the marker length varied by 10 mm in 2.5-mm internal-diameter tubes.[35]

A Murphy tube has a tip bevel that allows smooth passage through the nares and a side hole whose purpose is to allow ventilation even if the tip is partially obstructed or is placed in the right main stem bronchus. Some clinicians avoid using side-hole ("Murphy eye") tubes for prolonged ventilation because of anecdotal evidence that these tubes can abrade the trachea and cause scarring. Exclusive use of these ETTs in one institution was associated with an increased incidence of subglottic stenosis that ended when use of the tubes was discontinued. It can be adequately maintained in the correct position if the lip marker is placed on the tube at the lip level and it is fixed to the face. After proper placement is determined, the marker can be used as a reference to ensure that the tube's position remains constant. The Murphy tube is pliable (and becomes even less firm when it is allowed to remain under a radiant warmer while preparations are made for resuscitation). Many clinicians prefer to use an obturator or stylet to facilitate insertion. The stylet should not extend beyond the distal tip of the tube to avoid tracheal damage from the insertion process.

The vicious cycle of asphyxia is frequently in progress in the critically ill neonate who requires emergent tracheal intubation. The process of intubation in such an infant can exacerbate the difficulties that he or she is already experiencing. Intubation is associated with severe bradycardia, hypoxia, and elevation of arterial blood pressure and intracranial pressure.[36]

Depth of Tube Insertion

In addition to direct visualization of the tube as it passes through the glottis, there are a number of suggested "rules of thumb" for initial estimation of proper depth of tracheal tube placement. These rules use the centimeter markings on the side of an ETT to gauge the depth of placement. The most common rule uses birth weight and a simple formula, the rule of 7-8-9. An ETT is advanced 7 cm to the lip for a 1-kg infant, 8 cm for a 2-kg infant, and 9 cm for a 3-kg infant. Nasotracheal tube insertion is generally governed by adding 1 cm to the 7-8-9 rule. The rule of 7-8-9 is not appropriate for infants with hypoplastic mandibles (e.g., those with Pierre Robin syndrome) or short necks (e.g., those with Turner syndrome).[37] Although the 7-8-9 rule appears to be an accurate clinical method for oral ETT placement in neonates with more than 750 g birth weight, especially between 1500 and 2500 g, in infants weighing less than 750 g, it may lead to an overestimated depth of insertion and potentially result in clinically significant consequences.[38] New guidelines from the Neonatal Resuscitation Program (NRP)[1] suggest determining the optimal depth of the ETT placement by measuring the newborn's nasal tragus length (NTL) and adding 1 cm or by using a table with predetermined numbers for depth of placement. The NTL is described as the distance from the base of the nasal septum to the tragus of the ear. The use of marks on the ETT such as the vocal cord guide to determine initial depth of placement of the ETT below the vocal cords is no longer recommended by the NRP.

Determination of Placement

Placement of the ETT after intubation is determined first clinically and then by chest radiograph. Clinical determination includes the following:
- Improvement or maintenance of heart rate in the normal range
- Good color, pulses, and perfusion after the intubation
- Good bilateral chest wall movement with each breath
- Equal breath sounds heard over both lung fields
- Breath sounds heard much louder over the lung fields than are heard over the stomach
- Presence of inspiratory and expiratory tidal volume measurements
- No gastric distention with ventilation
- Presence of vapor in the tube during exhalation
- Direct visualization by laryngoscope of the tube passing between the vocal cords
- Presence of exhaled carbon dioxide (CO_2) as determined by a CO_2 detector and/or an end-tidal CO_2 monitor or capnography[39]
- Measurement: Add 6 to the newborn's weight in kilograms (rule of 7-8-9), or use the NTL, or a predetermined depth from a printed guide, as described earlier

The chest radiograph should be performed to demonstrate that the tube is in the mid-trachea. Tube position can change during the x-ray procedure if the infant's neck is in a flexed or extended position. ETT position can be confirmed on x-ray by following both of the main stem bronchi back to the carina and cephalad to the tip of the tube.[1] Occasionally a lateral radiograph is necessary to confirm placement in the trachea. Only one study has been conducted to compare differences in outcomes related to radiographic placement of the ETT.[40] They concluded that the ETT tip should be kept at the level of the first or second thoracic vertebrae in extremely premature babies to reduce the incidence of nonuniform lung aeration and adverse pulmonary outcomes.

Tube Fixation

Secure fixation of the ETT is important, not only to prevent accidental extubation but also to minimize tube movement during ventilation and other interventions such as suctioning, chest physiotherapy (CPT), surfactant administration, and positioning the patient. An insecure fixation of the tube is one of the most common reasons accidental extubation can occur. Accidental extubation and repeated intubations have been demonstrated to be associated with the development of subglottic stenosis, as well as increased mortality.[24,25] The likelihood of accidental extubation also has been associated with younger gestational age, higher level of consciousness, higher volume of secretions, and slippage of the tube.[25] It also is clear that there is no consensus as to which tube fixation method is most effective. The technique shown in Fig. 29.2 represents a modification of the method originally described by Gregory.[41] Another approach that was initially described by Cussel et al.[42] is to secure an umbilical clamp with a drilled hole in the center with tape to the face. Several modifications have been described using this technique. Compared with standard taping to the upper lip, methods using a modified umbilical clamp have been shown to substantially reduce unplanned or accidental extubation in neonatal patients (Fig. 29.3 and Box 29.4).[43]

Other studies have compared standard taping to approved commercially available fixation devices, and the ETT location was shown to be directly attributable to the type of fixation being used.[44] Another important development is that tincture of benzoin is no longer used, especially in extremely low birth-weight infants (micropreemies). Also, some of these techniques can be used to secure nasotracheal tubes (Fig. 29.4) without the use of tincture of benzoin. Several devices for fixation of neonatal ETTs and adhesive materials are available from various manufacturers.

Acquisition and Maintenance of Intubation Skills

Intubation of the trachea is a complex psychomotor skill taught to a variety of health care professionals. Although ventilation can be accomplished successfully using a bag and mask, there are many instances in which neonatal tracheal intubation is required. The challenge is maintaining a high skill level for a procedure that may be performed only sporadically by individual providers.

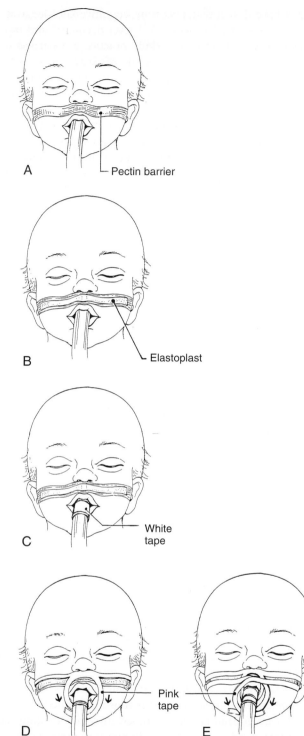

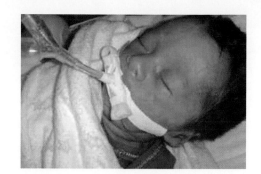

Fig. 29.3 A 32-week-old infant (birth weight 1840 g) with cord clamp in place. (From Loughead JL, Brennan RA, DeJuilio P, et al: Reducing accidental extubation in neonates. *Jt Comm J Qual Patient Saf.* 34(3): 164–170, 125, 2008.)

BOX 29.4 Using a Modified Umbilical Clamp

1. Umbilical cord clamps are converted into ETT stabilizers by drilling holes through their center such that when closed, they will snugly accommodate ETTs of 2.5-, 3.0-, 3.5-, 4.0-, and 4.5-mm inside diameters.
2. The clamps are opened, cleaned, individually packaged, and marked with size.
3. With the infant orally intubated, the clamp is secured around the ETT just above the lip with the ETT fitting within the predrilled hole. The clamp fits snugly but does not narrow the internal diameter of the ETT.
4. Skin barrier is applied to the infant's clean buccal surfaces bilaterally.
5. Adhesive tape is applied over the skin barrier and the tube is secured using the Y-tape method. The base portion of the Y tape is secured to the face, and the top arms are wrapped one around the ETT and one around the clamp. The second Y tape is applied in a mirror fashion to the other cheek.
6. Appropriate placement of the clamp allows the child to fully close lips and mouth.
7. NICU RNs and RCPs are accountable for assessing ETT placement and stability with every vitals check, position change, and suction and as needed. Repositioning and/or retaping of the ETT occur as needed and are performed with two caregivers to minimize accidental dislodgment during the procedure. During retaping, the clamp and ETT remain in place and only the tape and skin barrier are replaced. Tape reinforcement is discouraged.

ETT, Endotracheal tube; *NICU,* neonatal intensive care unit; *RNs,* registered nurses; *RCPs,* respiratory care practitioners.
(Data from Loughead JL, Brennan RA, DeJuilio P, et al: Reducing accidental extubation in neonates. Jt Comm J Qual Patient Saf 34(3): 164–170, 125, 2008.)

Fig. 29.2 Technique for securing an endotracheal tube. **(A)** Pectin barrier is applied to the infant's face from ear to ear and over the upper lip. **(B)** A ¼-inch-wide elastic bandage (Elastoplast) is applied over the pectin barrier. **(C)** A short strip of cloth tape or elastic bandage is wrapped around the tracheal tube to mark its point of passage at the mouth. The centimeter marking under the tape should be charted. **(D)** Pink tape cut in the shape of an H is applied over the elastic bandage, with its ends extending beyond the bandage. The lower arms of the H are then wrapped around the tube. **(E)** Single, ¼-inch strips of pink tape are secured over the lower part of the elastic bandage and wrapped around the tube. As an alternative to using an H-shaped piece of tape, the entire taping procedure can be done with a series of single strips of tape.

Depending on the clinical setting, intubation skill may be required of attending physicians, residents, nurses, respiratory therapists, and paramedics. Institutional or departmental policies may require or expect that certain individuals be proficient at intubation yet may be unable to provide opportunities to maintain proficiency. The challenge is that, without regular practice, individual intubation skill level decreases over time,[45] and the complications from an unskilled intubation may be severe.[46,47]

Initial training in intubation often occurs in a clinical skills lab using plastic manikins made specifically for the purpose of intubation. This is typically the first exposure to the skill of intubation for medical students as well as for other disciplines. Courses such as the NRP and the Pediatric Advanced

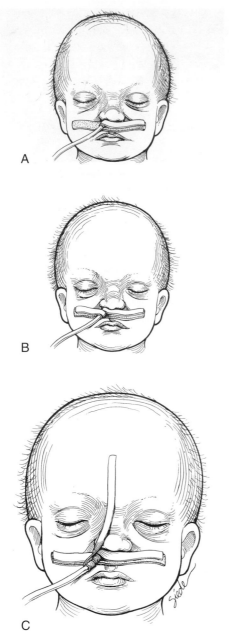

Fig. 29.4 Technique for securing a nasotracheal tube. **(A)** A ¼-inch strip of elastic bandage is applied over the upper lip, and a ¼-inch strip of Hy-Tape (*pink*) is applied from the right side of the face and around the tube. **(B)** A second piece of tape is applied from the left side of the face and around the tube. **(C)** A third piece of tape is applied down the bridge of the nose and around the tube.

Life Support course include intubation education, practice, and testing on a manikin. The fact that students are "tested" on their ability to intubate a plastic manikin airway model may lead some to think that they are now "proficient." It is important to emphasize that such courses provide only limited exposure to the intubation skill and that the ability to intubate a plastic manikin does not immediately translate to the bedside. However, improvements in the manikin, especially the anatomy and "feel" of the airway, have made this simulation experience more readily transferable to actual clinical situations.

Studies have shown that, over time, cognitive knowledge remains but the actual hands-on skill level declines[48] and that ongoing review and proctored skills practice are needed to maintain a level of proficiency.[49] A 10-year study of neonatal intubations performed by pediatric residents at one institution showed that median success rates varied from 33% for PL 1 residents to 40% for PL 2 and PL 3 residents. Success rates for residents with greater than 20 intubation attempts was 49%, whereas those residents with fewer than 20 attempts had a 37% success rate.[50] These same pediatric residents may go on to take positions in which they are expected to and need to have intubation proficiency, yet the study showed that they did not have the opportunity during their training to achieve a high level of success at the procedure. Another study found that, although pediatric residents stated that they felt confident with neonatal intubation skills, objective findings showed that they did not meet the study-specified definition of technical competence.[51]

Neonatal and pediatric transport teams typically use a combination of registered nurses, respiratory therapists, paramedics, and physicians, and there are some teams that run primarily as nurse-therapist or nurse-paramedic. Because team members are expected to perform advanced-level skills, team training generally includes skills such as intubation, umbilical line, and needle aspiration/chest tube insertion. In addition to a didactic and skills practice orientation, transport team members should attend regular update and competency sessions. Experts recommend that team members perform a minimum number of transports to maintain skills, and if the number of transports is low, there be other mechanisms to simulate transport team function.[52]

Since 1990, there have been many changes related to the indications for intubation of the neonate. Historically, all newly born infants with meconium staining of the amniotic fluid were subjected to intubation and suctioning. The latest NRP recommendations call for intubating only those infants with meconium staining who are not vigorous.[1] Newer oxygen delivery methods, such as high-flow nasal cannula (HFNC) and nasal CPAP, allow more infants to be cared for without the need for intubation. Ready availability of high-risk perinatal units and NICUs ensures that more critically ill neonates are born at a center with high-level skills. All of these advances are good for the neonate, but they have unfortunately resulted in a decreased number of intubations available for pediatric residents and other practitioners, necessitating alternate methods to ensure that competence in airway management is maintained.

Health care educators need to be creative in providing the initial intubation education and also in monitoring and facilitating the continuing education of those individuals expected to respond to a neonatal emergency. A blended learning approach can integrate online learning with supervised manikin practice. Although expensive, animal intubations (usually cats) can provide an excellent practice model but must be done adhering to the National Institutes of Health Office of Animal Care and Use guidelines. The airline industry has long been using simulators for initial training and for continuing education and competency evaluation. The simulator manikin setup is expensive but provides an excellent learning model that functions in real time. Patient simulations are generally enjoyed by students (generic and professional) and are perceived by the students to be of benefit.[53,54] The newest neonatal simulator manikins, although expensive, provide an excellent resource for this training.

Looking to the future, educators should consider the use of virtual reality simulation. Virtual reality simulators are available to teach trauma assessment and skills and also diagnostic bronchoscopy. In one study, the virtual reality bronchoscopy simulator was used to train new students in doing a diagnostic bronchoscopy. With minimal time practicing on the simulator, the new students were able to attain a level of proficiency similar to that of more experienced bronchoscopists.[55] Virtual reality simulation can be used for initial education and practice and at regular intervals to reinforce skills.

Laryngeal Mask Airway

The laryngeal mask airway (LMA) has been available for a number of years as an alternative to endotracheal intubation in babies, infants, children, and adults.[1] It is mentioned but not recommended for routine use in the new NRP textbook,[1] and a variety of papers discuss its use in various clinical scenarios, including the following:

- In neonatal resuscitation of term and larger preterm infants (size 1 LMA)
- In the difficult airway, such as in the Robin sequence, and other situations when micrognathia is profound
- As an aid to endotracheal intubation
- As an aid in flexible endoscopy
- In surgical cases in place of endotracheal intubation[56-59]

The success rate of insertion of the LMA has been reported to be greater than 90% in a number of descriptive studies of small series of infants and children.[60]

NONINVASIVE VENTILATION AND CONTINUOUS POSITIVE AIRWAY PRESSURE

Avoiding ventilator-induced lung injury is a common goal of neonatal intensive care and has led to considerable interest in less invasive means of providing effective respiratory support. Neonates who might require respiratory support short of intubation and mechanical ventilation include those with apnea of prematurity, mild to moderate RDS, and atelectasis caused by respiratory insufficiency, as well as recently extubated infants at risk for postextubation respiratory failure. Nasal CPAP has traditionally been a widely used support modality in these infants. It has the advantage of being well studied and is known to improve pulmonary mechanics and to stabilize the upper airway.[61] The use of CPAP and NIV is discussed in more detail in Chapter 18.

HEATED HUMIDIFIED HIGH-FLOW NASAL CANNULA

Humidified high-flow nasal cannula (HHFNC) devices have come into widespread use in NICUs. These devices differ from traditional nasal cannula therapy in that the gas flow to the patient is warmed and humidified up to the point of patient contact, allowing the use of higher gas flows without causing nasal drying, mucosal trauma, and patient cooling. Gas flow

rates used in neonatal HHFNC therapy may range between 2 and 8 L/min. The higher gas flows that can be attained with HHFNC have led many to view this therapy as a viable alternative to nasal CPAP that is less bulky and easier to maintain.

The level and consistency of CPAP that can be attained with HHFNC have been examined in several small case series reports, with variable results.[62-65] There is general agreement that HHFNC can produce a clinically significant level of CPAP, particularly at higher flow rates. However, several variables appear to play an important role in determining the level of CPAP attained, including patient size,[62] cannula diameter,[66] and whether the mouth is open or closed.[62] In some instances, particularly when the nasal cannula completely occludes the nares, dangerously high levels of CPAP may be produced.[66] It should be noted that, unlike nasal CPAP devices, most HHFNC devices at this time do not incorporate a safety pop-off valve in their design, raising the possibility that very high pressures could be transmitted to the lungs. Many HFNC strategies have been derived from study protocols or are based on expert opinion or both.[66a] In the NICU, many centers have commonly used HFNC at 2 to 8 L because these settings have been shown to result in around 2 to 8 cm H_2O CPAP in the lungs of infants.[66b-66d] A growing body of evidence supports that HFNC can be used safely and effectively as an alternative to CPAP in NICU for term and preterm infants following extubation. A meta-analysis from six randomized control trials ($n = 934$ subjects) comparing outcomes between HFNC and CPAP postextubation in term and preterm newborns showed no differences in death or chronic lung disease or rate of treatment failure or reintubation.[66e] Also, infants randomized to HFNC had lower nasal trauma and pneumothorax and trend toward lower necrotizing enterocolitis than other forms of noninvasive therapy.

MONITORING DURING RESPIRATORY SUPPORT

Monitoring During Noninvasive Respiratory Support

Infants are supported with noninvasive respiratory support using nasal HFNC, CPAP (NCPAP), or NIV to prevent intubation or following weaning and extubation from invasive support. Such patients may require more attention at the bedside than a patient who is being ventilated invasively. Patients receiving this form of support do not have accurate or reliable mechanics or tidal volume measurements. Also, many of these devices are limited by a lack of alarms. As such, ongoing assessment, gas exchange, and evaluation of work of breathing are vital to the management and success of this form of support. Patients receiving noninvasive approaches can be instrumented with physiologic monitoring to include oxygen saturation (SpO_2), transcutaneous CO_2, heart rate, and blood pressure. Routine blood gases are not frequently obtained and are reserved for situations in which the patient has developed clinical deterioration and for correlating values with noninvasive monitoring. Chest x-rays are a poor surrogate for determining lung volumes during noninvasive support. Unfortunately, there are no approved devices for monitoring inspiratory and end-expiratory lung volumes. Novel technology using electrical impedance tomography may prove to be useful once it has been developed for newborns. Because of the lack of physiologic monitoring, many institutions have embraced respiratory scoring tools (i.e., Silverman-Anderson Respiratory Severity Score) to guide clinical management. These scores have been shown to have good interrater reliability among clinicians and can be useful for determining when the patient requires support or ongoing settings adjustments and for weaning.

Airway management is a time-consuming endeavor but perhaps the single most important aspect for improving outcomes and reducing complications in infants receiving noninvasive support. This detailed approach is more art than science, and the increased use of noninvasive support since 2005 has provided new experience that is summarized in some excellent resources.[67,68] Many neonates are being supported for weeks and sometimes months with this support. Briefly, clinicians caring for infants receiving CPAP should select prongs of the optimal size and ensure that the prongs are not displaced. Prongs that are too small increase the resistance to gas flow and work of breathing and are associated with excessive leaks. An optimally sized prong fills the entire opening without blanching the external nostril. The infant's nostrils should be suctioned periodically, and the nasal airway evaluated for skin breakdown. There are many approaches that are used to prevent nasal breakdown, including (1) alternating between nasal prongs and mask, (2) nasal barrier devices, and (3) nasal airway interfaces/fixation that are less likely to cause sustained pressure on the nasal airway.

As mentioned previously, many noninvasive devices do not provide clinical monitoring of pressure or alarms. Disconnection of the patient from the device (e.g., dislodged prongs) may not result in an alarm to indicate low pressure. Two such devices, bubble NCPAP and HHFNC, do not have integrated alarms as a standard system component. Thus, it is important to provide continuous physiologic monitoring. In a bench model, condensation forming in the expiratory limb of a commercially available bubble NCPAP system resulted in substantially higher CPAP levels than desired.[69] Whenever possible, stand-alone pressure manometers, alarms, and pressure-relief devices should be used. Also, bedside clinicians must provide measures to frequently empty the exhalation limb of condensate, provide water traps, or use circuits that incorporate heated wires or are constructed from material that wicks moisture to the environment.

Monitoring During Conventional and High-Frequency Ventilation

Electrocardiography, blood pressure, and serial arterial and/or capillary blood gases have been the traditional mainstays of bedside monitoring of the newborn, and they still have an important role. In general, the emphasis on noninvasive monitoring has resulted in the development and availability of new technologies that allow close monitoring without invasive procedures. The following is a list of those instruments:

- Transcutaneous monitoring of partial pressure of oxygen (PO_2) and partial pressure of carbon dioxide (PCO_2)
- Pulse oximetry to provide continuous measurement of hemoglobin saturation with oxygen (O_2)
- End-tidal CO_2 monitoring

See Chapter 11 for a more in-depth discussion of these noninvasive monitoring techniques.

Nearly all of the neonatal mechanical ventilators that are currently available provide airway graphics monitoring. A complete understanding of airway graphics can be vital for determining response to different therapies (i.e., surfactant and bronchodilators), clinical improvement and deterioration, equipment malfunction, and appropriate setting changes. In the NICU, there is also the additional difficulty of dealing with ETTs that are uncuffed, leading to large positional leaks around the ETT, which can lead to autocycling and missed trigger attempts by the patient. Assessing airway graphics can be useful, in cases such as these, for providing improved patient comfort. Airway graphics and tidal volume monitoring are best accomplished using a proximal flow sensor in neonates. Tidal volume monitoring and targeting have steadily become a widely accepted practice in most NICUs. Seminal animal studies have shown that ventilation for 15 minutes with a volume of 15 mL/kg has been shown to cause lung injury and as few as three overdistending breaths at birth have been shown to compromise the therapeutic effect of subsequent surfactant replacement.[70-72] Conversely, small or inadequate volumes can also cause lung injury.[73,74] Tidal volume is also an important measurement in volume-targeted ventilation. Compared with pressure ventilation, volume-targeted ventilation has been shown to reduce pneumothorax, days of ventilation, hypocarbia, periventricular leukomalacia or grade 3 to 4 intraventricular hemorrhage, and combined outcome of death/BPD. Monitoring expiratory volumes at the level of the ventilator valves may overestimate tidal volume delivery and reduce the accuracy of airway graphics, despite attempts to adjust for circuit tubing compliance with the ventilator.[75] Proximal flow sensors are prone to accumulating secretions, malfunctioning, creating torque on the ETT, and adding mechanical dead space. The benefit of a flow sensor outweighs all of these risks. Flow sensors may not accurately predict the delivered volumes when tube leaks are present but measured expiratory volume is usually more accurate than inspiratory tidal volumes for predicting the delivered volume in these cases. Appropriate bedside maintenance of flow sensors, calibration, and standardized cleaning procedures are important clinical quality measures.

For infants on high-frequency ventilation (HFV), pulmonary care involves new technology and keen observation.[76,77] These critically ill babies require a definite team approach, including an experienced respiratory therapist and nurse, and the traditional tools, including cardiorespiratory monitoring, intermittent arterial blood gases (from an arterial line), and "wiggle" assessment. A sample of a protocol used in the infant special care unit at one institution includes the following:

Assessments every hour:
- Vital signs from monitors, including heart rate, arterial blood pressure, body temperature
- Vibration (or wiggle) assessment (scale +1 to +3)
- Capillary refill
- Comfort level
  Assessments every 4 hours—"hands-on assessment":
- Auscultation of breath sounds on oscillator
- Palpation of pulses

- Nasogastric tube placement can be assessed without having to take the baby off of the ventilator

Assessments every 8 hours—ventilator is turned off, but the patient remains on the circuit or backup rate (high-frequency jet ventilation):

- Heart rate, position of point of maximum intensity of heart, presence or absence of a heart murmur
- Bowel sounds
  Other assessments:
- Arterial blood gases after initiation of HFV: hourly for 6 hours, every 2 hours for 6 hours, and every 4 hours and as needed thereafter
- Tidal volumes (when available)
- Chest radiograph schedule: just before being placed on HFV, within 1 hour of initiation of HFV, every 12 hours twice, and then daily and as needed
  - Continuous monitoring of oxygen saturation using the pulse oximeter

HUMIDIFICATION AND WARMING DURING RESPIRATORY SUPPORT

The ETT bypasses the normal humidifying, filtering, and warming systems of the upper airway; therefore, heat and humidity must be provided to prevent hypothermia, inspissation of airway secretions, and necrosis of airway mucosa. Filtration of dry gases before humidification also is needed because of the contamination sometimes found in medical gas lines.

Assuming all other forms of infant warming are provided, ventilation with nonhumidified gases is a major reason for the development of hypothermia[78] in neonates. Inadequate humidification of the respiratory tract may reduce mucociliary clearance and predispose infants to airway obstruction by secretions, thereby increasing the risk of gas trapping and air leak.[79] Also, dry gases have been associated with severe lung injury in animal models.[80] Higher inspired gas temperatures are associated with a lower incidence of pneumothorax and a decreased severity of chronic lung disease in ventilated very low birth-weight infants compared with lower temperatures.[79]

The use of heat-moisture exchangers, or artificial noses, in neonates should be discouraged because they have been shown to increase ventilation requirements, increase CO_2 levels, lower body temperature, and increase artificial airway blockage. They are particularly ineffective in the presence of large ETT leaks. In most cases, heat-moisture exchangers are reserved for short-term use, such as neonatal transport. A heated water humidifier is necessary to ensure that inspired gases are delivered at or near body temperature (37° C) and that they achieve near-total saturation with water vapor. In the past, nebulizers were used in some applications, particularly with oxygen administration with a hood after extubation. Use of this system has been discarded because of impairment in oxygenation and the possibility of water intoxication caused by excess delivery of particulate water droplets and because of the presence of excessive noise.

A modern servo-controlled heated humidifier, with high- and low-temperature alarms and heated wires that prevent accumulation of condensation, should provide adequate humidification with proper operation. O'Hagan et al.[81,82] observed wide variation in the delivery of relative humidity, even when the temperature was maintained above 34.7° C; this variation resulted in failure to meet the American National Standards Institute guidelines for humidifier performance.[83] This may account for the findings of O'Hagan et al.,[82] who observed a significant increase in morbidity when temperatures below 36.5° C were maintained at the airway. These studies have led to the recommendation that relative humidity, as well as temperature, be monitored continuously. Miyao et al.[84] suggest that even maintenance of the Institute's standards (70% humidity at 37° C) may be inadequate, particularly if heated wire circuits are used. Use of circuits with heated wires was adopted primarily because of the frequency with which condensation needed to be drained and because of infection control considerations. The heated wire circuits were intended to enable the clinician to heat the gas inside the circuit to a temperature above that at which it left the humidifier, ensuring adequate absolute humidity without condensation in the circuit. This feature, which results in delivery of a hot gas with a lower relative humidity, may have caused the problems noted earlier.[84]

The increased temperature of a gas shifts the isothermal boundary (the point at which the gas completes equilibrium to body temperature and humidity levels) to a point closer to the airway opening. At first glance, this seems beneficial because less mucosa is exposed to the humidity deficit of the gas. However, because the effect of a given humidity deficit is concentrated on a smaller area of the mucosa, there is the potential for a greater degree of damage. Moreover, use of higher airway temperatures means that, even with lower humidity, there is relatively less opportunity for humidified air from within the lung to recondense some of its humidity upon exhalation. The result is an increase in the humidity deficit (the difference in total water content of inspired gas and the water content it achieves within the lung). The potential for adverse effects with use of the heated wire circuit is exacerbated by inadequate monitoring of humidity levels. If the wire is so hot that the circuit is dry, it is not known whether the relative humidity is 70% (the nominally acceptable American National Standards Institute value) or less.[82]

Traditionally, probes for monitoring inspired gas have been placed as close as possible to the patient connection so that the effect of the trip down the inspiratory line on the inspired gas can be monitored. Unfortunately, in some neonatal circumstances, the probe is continuously in the presence of a heated field and may register the effect of this heat by radiation and/or convection, totally apart from the effect of the inspired gas. If this temperature is sensed by a servo controller, the humidifier and the heated wires may automatically heat less because the temperature is actually being controlled by another heat source (Fig. 29.5). An extension adapter, which is provided by most manufacturers, allows the probe to be placed outside of the heating field, thus remedying this problem. This extension does not need to incorporate heated wires because the gas temperature is maintained by the heated field on entry.

The use of inline water traps is recommended for decreasing the resistance to flow caused by condensate and for ensuring

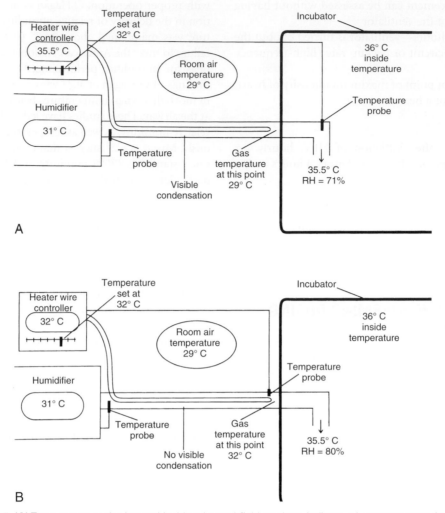

Fig. 29.5 (A) Temperature probe located inside a heated field tends to indicate a heat representative of the heated field rather than of the inspiratory gas before entry into the field. The humidifier does not provide the heat that is being detected by the wire controller. The heat source is particularly difficult to assess because most heated wire circuits operate with humidifiers that do not provide a display of the temperature of the gas immediately after it leaves the humidifier. **(B)** Proper placement of the probe. If the probe is only slightly outside a radiant warmer field, it may need to be shielded, particularly if phototherapy is in use. *RH*, Relative humidity. (From Chatburn RL: Principles and practice of neonatal and pediatric mechanical ventilation. *Respir Care* 36:560, 1991.)

stability of oxygen concentrations. Novel materials have been used in the latest generation of infant ventilator circuits to minimize mobile condensate in the expiratory limb by allowing water vapor to diffuse through the tubing wall. In theory, these circuits may minimize alarms, excessive pressure and volume delivery to the infant, and work of breathing.

Ventilator-acquired pneumonia (VAP) and other respiratory infections can arise and are prevalent in neonates because of prolonged mechanical ventilation, frequent reintubation, low gestational age, and low birth weight.[85] VAP has been associated with higher mortality rates than in those unaffected by this disease. There is concern that the frequency at which ventilator circuits and humidifiers are changed may affect the rate of VAP.[86] However, one study showed that there were no differences in VAP between a 7-day circuit change and a 14-day change.[85] Some sources suggest changing the patient circuit only when visibly soiled to avoid opening the circuit. Other attempts at reducing VAP include changing manual resuscitators once per week, changing equipment on stand-by every 12 hours, elevating the head of the bed, and draining circuit fluid frequently.

AIRWAY CLEARANCE TECHNIQUES

Patients who have an ETT are predisposed to damage to the airway lining, weak or ineffective cough, and improper humidification of the airways. This can result in accumulated secretions in the airways and consequent gas trapping, air leak, and poor gas exchange. Based on two extensive literature reviews, "successful suctioning of an intubated patient improves air exchange and breath sounds, decreases the peak inspiratory pressure, decreases airway resistance, increases compliance, increases tidal volume delivery, improves arterial blood gas values, improves oxygen saturation, and removes secretions."[87,88]

There are significant risks to endotracheal suctioning, including atelectasis and loss of lung volume because of high negative suction pressures,[89-92] hypoxemia,[93-95] cardiovascular instability,[96,97] and changes in cerebrovascular volume.

One study showed that ETT suctioning significantly increases intracranial pressure in preterm infants on assisted ventilation in the first month of life. These changes appear to be independent of changes observed in oxygenation and ventilation.[98,99] ETT suctioning has been found to be a risk factor for VAP in ventilated infants.[100]

Use of a closed "inline" suctioning system has been promoted to decrease respiratory contamination and pulmonary infections. Inline suction systems use a suction catheter integrated into the patient circuit using a specialized adapter, and the catheter is protected with a transparent sleeve. Closed suction is perceived by nursing staff to be easier, less time consuming, and better tolerated by patients. The suction depth is determined by the length of the tube, the adapter, and the preferred suction depth using colored markings that can be visualized in a small window. Deep suctioning should be avoided, and attempts should be made to remove secretions from within the tube and slightly beyond (~0.5 cm). Visual bedside charts, like the one used at the authors' center (Fig. 29.6), can be useful for guiding proper suction depths using inline or closed suction devices.

Disadvantages of these systems include increased expense and potential increase in system air leaks. Also, the catheter or portion of the catheter can be left in the airway accidentally, causing airway obstruction.

Closed suction obviates the physiological disadvantage of ventilator disconnection. In one study, a total of 39% of infants in the supported with closed suction devices group and 44% of infants in the disconnected from the ventilator to use and open airway suction technique group had significant differences in airways colonized with gram-negative bacilli. Also, closed suction is perceived by nursing staff to be easier, less time consuming, and better tolerated by small premature infants requiring mechanical ventilation for a week or longer.

Depending on the severity of lung disease, ETT suction may cause transient loss of lung volumes throughout the lung. It has been suggested that the lowest possible suction pressure that adequately removes secretions from the tube should be used. Suction pressures of 50 to 100 cm H_2O have been shown to be safe and effective in neonates, and suction time should not exceed 10 to 15 seconds.[88] The number of catheter passes should be minimized to less than three to avoid irritation to the airway mucosa.[101] The patient should also be allowed to recover between each catheter pass.

One study investigated whether closed endotracheal suctioning reduces the frequency of hypoxemia and bradycardia in extremely low birth-weight neonates compared with open suctioning. There were no differences in heart rate between the two treatment strategies. The magnitude and frequency of hypoxemic events were lower with the closed suction than with the open suction technique.[102] Despite significant derecruitment with ETT suction, there was rapid recovery resulting in an increase in end-expiratory lung volume immediately after suction. The lung volume remained increased for the next 2 hours, suggesting that the benefit of suction persists much longer than many of the previous studies have described.[103]

ETT suction causes transient loss of lung volume. Catheter size exerts a greater influence than suction method, with closed suction protecting against derecruitment only when a small catheter is used, especially in the nondependent lung.[104]

Routine endotracheal suctioning with an open system has increasingly become less desirable not only for infection control purposes but also because intermittent manual ventilation is needed. As mentioned previously, this practice is typically associated with variable tidal volume ventilation. Removing a patient from the ventilator and initiating hyperinflation and hyperoxygenation with 100% fraction of inspired oxygen (FiO_2) may produce oxygen free radicals and may be associated with the development of retinopathy of prematurity and lung injury. Preoxygenation has been shown to result in less hypoxemia and faster return to baseline oxygenation before suction than no preoxygenation.[105] The latest guidelines suggest that the FiO_2 is adjusted to 10% to 20% above the current FiO_2 on the ventilator. Many ventilators have a suction key that can be configured to deliver a preset FiO_2 for oxygenation before suctioning. Manual ventilation with excessive tidal volumes can also initiate lung injury in the developing lung. Also, removing the patient from the ventilator can cause clinical destabilization and introduce bacteria into the circuit, placing infants at greater risk for developing ventilator-acquired infections. The use of manual resuscitation and sigh breaths should be avoided whenever necessary in neonates.

Suctioning should be performed by experienced personnel because complications from the trauma of this procedure may

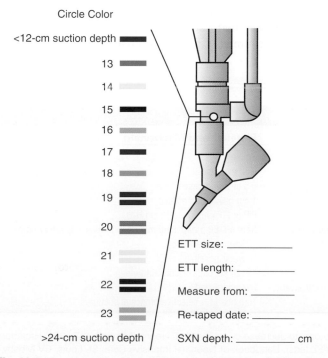

Circle Color

<12-cm suction depth
13
14
15
16
17
18
19
20
21
22
23
>24-cm suction depth

ETT size: _____

ETT length: _____

Measure from: _____

Re-taped date: _____

SXN depth: _____ cm

Fig. 29.6 Visual bedside chart. *ETT,* Endotracheal tube; *SXN,* suction.

lead to hypoxemia,[106-108] cardiovascular compromise, barotrauma, and intraventricular hemorrhage. The frequency of ETT suctioning of infants ventilated in the NICU has been widely debated. One study showed that a low-frequency suctioning regimen (every 8 hours plus as needed) and a higher frequency suctioning regimen (every 4 hours plus as needed) were associated with similar frequencies of nosocomial bloodstream infections, VAP, bacterial airway colonization, frequency of reintubation, need for postural drainage, severity of BPD, neonatal mortality, duration of mechanical ventilation, and duration of hospitalization.[109]

The interval should be individualized and documented at the bedside; an example of a suctioning regimen is illustrated in Fig. 29.7. Following are a few suggestions on how to optimize benefits and prevent complications (Table 29.4).

Many clinicians will use bulb suction during deliveries or to suction the upper airway before endotracheal suctioning. There is evidence that suggests that most bulb suction devices will not provide pressures under 100 mm Hg. Excessive pressure may be damaging to the sensitive oral mucosa of the infant's upper airway.

The once routine practice of instilling normal saline before endotracheal suctioning is now discouraged. With the present focus on VAP, studies that have shown a marked increase in the number of bacteria present in the lower airway after normal saline administration versus no normal saline have forced nurses and respiratory therapists to reevaluate suction procedures.[110]

An American Association of Respiratory Care guideline has provided excellent information for suctioning and may be useful to optimize benefits and prevent complications during suctioning of a ventilated patient:[87]

1. Endotracheal suctioning should be performed only when secretions are present and not routinely.
2. Preoxygenation should be considered if the patient has a clinically important reduction in oxygen saturation with suctioning.
3. Performing suctioning without disconnecting the patient from the ventilator is suggested.

4. Use of shallow suction is suggested instead of deep suction, based on evidence from infant and pediatric studies.
5. Routine use of normal saline instillation before endotracheal suction should not be performed.
6. Endotracheal suctioning without disconnection (closed system) is suggested for neonates.
7. It is suggested that a suction catheter that occludes less than 70% of the lumen of the ETT is used.

FRONT

ET TUBE PLACEMENT AND SUCTIONING RECORD
Baby's Name _____   Weight (g) _____
Date Tube Inserted _____
Tube Position _____ cm Above Carina
ET Tube Size _____   Catheter Depth _____ cm

BACK

INTERTECH / OHIO		
TUBE SIZE	CUT (cm)	CATHETER DEPTH (cm)
2.5	11	14.5
3.0	13	17.0
3.5	13	17.0
4.0	14	18.0

Fig. 29.7 Bedside "suction card" with values to be reverified after every chest radiograph has been obtained. Values are based on tube position relative to the carina. Suction depth must be reduced if the tip is not 2 cm above the carina. The table on the back of the card allows compensation for the extra length of the endotracheal tube's 15-mm adapter.

TABLE 29.4	**Endotracheal Suctioning in Newborn Infants**		
	Hodge	**Hagedorn et al.**	**Fletcher and MacDonald**
Irrigation solution	Saline, but not routinely	Saline	Saline
Amount for irrigation	0.1–0.2 mL/kg	0.25–0.5 mL	Not specified
Catheter size	0.5–0.66 of tube diameter	Not specified	0.5 of tube diameter
Depth of insertion	Length of tube only	Length of tube only	1 cm beyond tip of tube
Hyperinflation	PIP 10%–20% above baseline	Match PIP	PIP or PIP plus up to 10 cm H_2O
Hyperventilation	Equal to total respiratory rate	Equal to ventilatory rate	Rate 40–60 breaths per minute with long inspiratory time
Oxygen enhancement	10%–20% above baseline	If clinically indicated	10% above baseline
Suction pressure	50–80 cm H_2O	80–100 mm Hg	"Lowest possible"
Duration	Not specified	5–10 seconds	15–20 seconds disconnect time
Intermittent vs continuous	Not addressed	Continuous on withdrawal	Not addressed
Head turn	No	No	Turn head for selective bronchial suction

PIP, Peak inspiratory pressure.
(Data from Hodge D: Endotracheal suctioning and the infant: a nursing care protocol to decrease complications. Neonat Network 9:7, 1991; Hagedorn MI, Gardner SL, Abman SH: Respiratory diseases. In: Merenstein GB, Gardner SL (eds): Handbook of Neonatal Intensive Care. St. Louis, CV Mosby, 1989, 381; Fletcher MA, MacDonald MG: Atlas of Procedures in Neonatology. 2nd ed. Philadelphia, JB Lippincott, 1993, p. 292.)

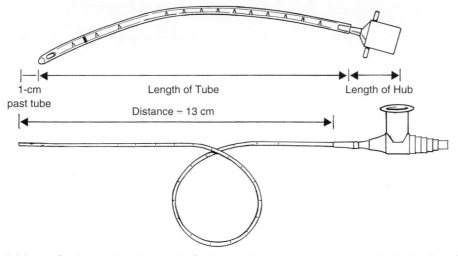

Fig. 29.8 Method for determining the length of catheter advancement in an endotracheal tube. Knowledge of the placement of the tube and of the length of the tube can be applied to the use of a calibrated suction catheter for providing consistent catheter advancement to a level 1 cm above the carina.

8. The duration of the suctioning event is limited to less than 15 seconds.

Other guidelines that may be useful include (1) providing the proper equipment; (2) awareness of FiO_2 settings and ventilator parameters; (3) performing noninvasive monitoring of oxygenation before, during, and after suctioning; (4) having the proper suction catheter size; and (5) using normal saline for irrigation, 0.1 to 0.5 mL/kg only if secretions are deemed to be thick and tenacious upon assessment (see Tables 29.1 and 29.2 and Figs. 29.7 and 29.8).

Many hospitals have embraced practices to prevent VAP (called "bundles") such as (1) strict hand hygiene, (2) limited circuit breaks, (3) inline suction, (4) palate protectors, (5) circuit changes for new equipment, (6) weaning protocols, (7) taping and confirmation of tube placement, and (8) scheduled oral care. These strategies have been shown to reduce VAP rates, need for reintubations, and length of hospital stay,[111] as well as having substantial cost savings.[112]

Chest Physiotherapy

CPT is a common but controversial airway clearance technique for infants in the NICU. Generally, appropriate indications for CPT include (1) evidence of retained pulmonary secretions, (2) weak or ineffective cough, (3) focal lung opacity on chest x-ray consistent with mucous plugging and/or atelectasis, and (4) intrapulmonary shunt requiring oxygen. CPT involving postural drainage in concert with percussion or vibration has been shown to be beneficial in removing secretions and preventing atelectasis in recently extubated neonates.[113] It also has been shown to result in removal of more secretions from intubated neonates.[114] Furthermore, oxygenation has been shown to be enhanced after completion of CPT.[113] The benefit of this procedure may lie in the periodic redistribution of the gravity-dependent regions of the lung from positioning, rather than in the physical removal of secretions.

Two systematic reviews found no evidence from randomized controlled trials to support the use of CPT to improve oxygenation, reduce length of time on the ventilator, reduce stay in the intensive care unit, resolve atelectasis/consolidation, and/or improve respiratory mechanics versus usual care.[115,116]

CPT was traditionally thought to assist in clearance of secretions in infants with bronchiolitis, but according to a Cochrane meta-analysis, CPT did not improve the severity of the disease or the respiratory parameters or reduce the length of hospital stay or oxygen requirements in hospitalized infants with acute bronchiolitis not on mechanical ventilation.[117] It is unclear at this time whether there is a benefit in infants with other respiratory infections receiving mechanical ventilation.[118] Another review found that routine use of CPT in ventilated neonates does not improve outcomes and may induce hypoxemia and increase oxygen requirements.[119] Two separate studies compared short-term outcomes between neonates supported with CPT and those without CPT after extubation and found no differences in radiologic evidence of atelectasis.[120] While the benefit of such techniques remains in question, CPT does not go entirely without some risk to the patient. CPT has also been found to be poorly tolerated, with side effects such as esophageal reflux, tachypnea, tachycardia, hypoxemia, rib fracture, and severe central nervous system complications, especially in newborns.[121,122]

CPT use should be individualized in each baby because, as noted earlier, the use of these techniques has been associated with a variety of negative effects, especially in infants born weighing less than 1000 g. This group of extremely low birth-weight infants frequently is on a minimal stimulation plan of care for the first 3 to 5 days of extrauterine life, thus minimizing any pulmonary care interventions.[123] The paucity of airway secretions in this group of infants during this time has led some clinicians to suction only on an "as needed" basis or not at all.

Positioning of the Patient

Postural drainage involves the use of different positions in which the different main stem bronchi are positioned vertically so that drainage from the smaller bronchi moves into the larger bronchi (Figs. 29.9 to 29.16). The approach has been combined

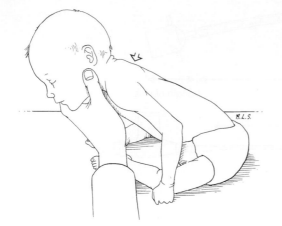

Fig. 29.9 Drainage of the posterior segments of the upper lobe. The infant is leaned over at a 30-degree angle from the sitting position. The clinician claps and vibrates over the upper back on both sides.

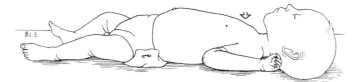

Fig. 29.10 Drainage of the anterior segments of the upper lobe. While the infant is lying flat on their back, the clinician claps and vibrates between the nipples and the clavicle on both sides.

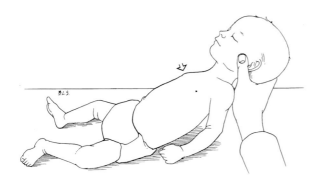

Fig. 29.11 Drainage of the apical segment of the upper lobe. The infant is leaned backward about 30 degrees from the sitting position, and the clinician claps or vibrates above the clavicle on both sides.

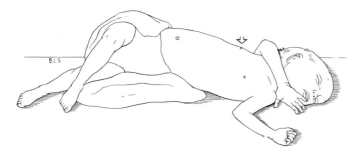

Fig. 29.12 For drainage of the right middle lobe, the caregiver elevates the hips to about 5 inches above the head. He or she rolls the infant backward one-quarter turn and then claps and vibrates over the right nipple. For drainage of the lingular segments of the left upper lobe, the caregiver places the infant in the same position but with the left side lifted upward; he or she then claps and vibrates over the left nipple.

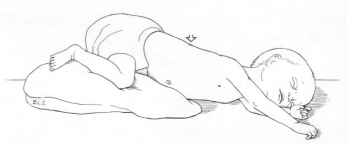

Fig. 29.13 Drainage of the lateral basal segments of the lower lobes. The caregiver places the infant on the left side with the hips elevated to a level about 8 inches above that of the head. The caregiver rolls the infant forward one-quarter turn and then claps or vibrates over the lower ribs. Note that the position shown is for draining the right side. For draining the left side, the same procedure is followed, except that the infant is placed on his or her right side.

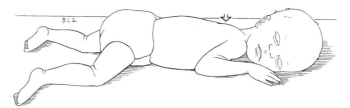

Fig. 29.14 Drainage of the superior segments of the lower lobe. The clinician places the infant flat on the stomach and then claps or vibrates at top of the scapula on the back side of the spine.

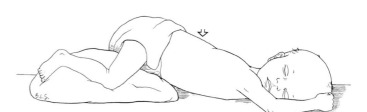

Fig. 29.15 Drainage of the posterior basal segments of the lower lobe. The clinician places the infant on the stomach with the hips at a level 8 inches above that of the head. He or she then claps and vibrates over the lower ribs close to the spine on both sides.

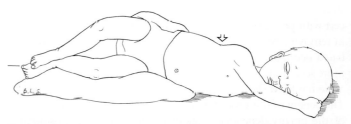

Fig. 29.16 Drainage of the anterior basal segment of the lower lobes. The caregiver places the infant on the left side with the hips at a level about 8 inches above that of the head. He or she then claps and vibrates just beneath the axilla. Note that for drainage of the opposite anterior basal segment, the infant is turned on the right side.

with CPT in the past. The two forces at work during this procedure are gravity and airflow. Any area of the bronchial tree that is to be drained (with the exception of the medial basal segment) must be uppermost.[124] These positions may not be practical for implementation in critically ill babies who have chest tubes or ETTs, who have undergone surgery, or who are at great risk for intraventricular hemorrhage. Optimally, the infant should be monitored during CPT; potential monitors include transcutaneous O_2 or CO_2 or pulse oximeter. Significant oxygen desaturation during the procedure should cause the caretaker to pause and initiate measures necessary to correct hypoxemia.

Percussion and Vibration

Two types of hand pressure can be applied to the neonatal chest to expedite adequate drainage: percussion and vibration. Percussion (chest physiotherapy) in the neonate can be performed with small plastic cups with padded rims or with soft circular masks with their adapters plugged so that the air pockets are maintained. The chest is percussed over the area to be drained for 1 to 2 minutes. Percussion may be reserved for infants who weigh more than 1500 g and are older than 2 weeks of age because of the potential risk for intraventricular hemorrhage.

The traditional view of vibration is that it is effective only during exhalation because it causes secretions to move from the periphery of the lungs with the outflow of air. This technique requires careful observation of chest movements. For vibration, the wrist is extended and the arm muscles are contracted in a manner similar to that used for isometric exercises. The result can be described as a controlled quiver. The placement of fingers flat against chest walls of infants suffices. A light touch with rapidly vibrating fingers has been considered effective in mobilizing secretions in neonates.[123] Because few practitioners feel comfortable with this manual technique, vibrations can be done with a small hand vibrator or a commercially available pulmonary vibrator. It is unclear whether gentle vibrations produced by these devices are transmitted to the lungs. Nonetheless, clinicians prefer them simply because they "soothe" the patient.

Vibration is tolerated by a greater number of patients than is percussion. The duration of vibration therapy is subject to the infant's tolerance and can be monitored on the basis of the parameters discussed previously.[123]

ADMINISTRATION OF MEDICATIONS INTO THE RESPIRATORY TRACT

Surfactant Treatment

Surfactant treatment of established RDS has been shown to decrease the incidence of air-leak complications and death.[124]

Intratracheal surfactant replacement therapy, administered via the ETT, has been an essential component of the prevention and treatment of RDS in premature infants since the early 1990s (also see Chapter 15). Multiple trials have compared prophylactic surfactant administration, usually given within the first 10 minutes of life in the delivery room, with later rescue treatment of established RDS in infants at substantial risk for the development of RDS. A meta-analysis of these trials demonstrated that prophylactic surfactant administration leads to

significant reductions in the risk of air-leak complications and death.[125] More recent trials have further demonstrated that prophylactic surfactant administration reduces the incidence of RDS and length of time on mechanical ventilation compared with rescue treatment.[126] These benefits are most pronounced in those infants born at less than 30 weeks of gestation who have not been exposed to antenatal steroids.[127,128] Current recommendations from the American Academy of Pediatrics (AAP) Committee on the Fetus and Newborn suggest that prophylactic surfactant be considered for those premature infants at highest risk for RDS.[129] However, the use of prophylactic surfactant is quite variable in neonatal units across the country.[130] One reason for this variation in practice is the widespread interest in early application of NCPAP, rather than prophylactic intubation and surfactant treatment, for the prevention and early treatment of RDS. Early NCPAP may have the potential to reduce the incidence of BPD without an increase in other morbidities.[16] However, a 2008 randomized controlled trial demonstrated that early NCPAP, compared with early intubation, did not significantly reduce the rate of death or BPD.[17]

Surfactant Administration

This section addresses the technical aspects of surfactant administration, including dosage forms, amounts, and administration techniques. Other aspects of surfactant treatment are discussed in Chapter 15.

The surfactant pool size in the lungs of healthy, full-term neonates is about 100 mg/kg.[131] Infants with RDS have a surfactant pool size that is approximately 10% of that seen in the healthy, full-term lung.[132] Surfactant doses for prevention or treatment of RDS are aimed at achieving a surfactant pool size comparable to that in the full term lung while also allowing for some uneven distribution of exogenous surfactant and surfactant inactivation by protein exudates. Thus, surfactant doses in the range of 50 to 200 mg/kg have been used in various clinical studies.[133] Currently available commercial surfactant preparations contain varying amounts of phospholipids, but the recommended dosage amounts give 100 to 200 mg/kg phospholipids per dose (Table 29.5). All currently available surfactant preparations are obtained by extraction from animal lungs and are available in a liquid form for intratracheal instillation, although a new, completely synthetic surfactant (lucinactant) has been tested in humans. Compared in clinical trials, lucinactant was found to have rates of mortality and morbidity similar to those of beractant and poractant alfa.[134] Differences in recommended

TABLE 29.5 Surfactant Preparations Data From Package Inserts

Surfactant	Source	Phospholipid Content, mg/mL	RECOMMENDED DOSE (mL/kg)	
			Initial	Repeat
Calfactant	Calf lung	35	3	3
Beractant	Cow lung	25	4	4
Poractant	Pork lung	80	2.5	1.25

dosage volume may lead the clinician to favor a particular surfactant preparation in certain clinical situations.

Surfactant replacement therapy should be performed only by clinicians who are proficient at administering surfactant and capable of handling adverse events. Recommended modes of surfactant administration are based on those used in research protocols, but there are limited human data comparing techniques of surfactant administration. Surfactant is generally administered through a small-bore catheter inserted into the ETT, although the Infasurf package insert suggests instillation through a side-port adapter.[135] Animal data suggest that administering surfactant by bolus or rapid intratracheal infusion results in a more even distribution of surfactant than giving the surfactant by very slow continuous intratracheal infusion.[136] Surfactant doses are typically divided into two or four aliquots. In animal studies, the distribution of intratracheally instilled surfactant has been largely determined by gravity and unaffected by the position of the chest.[137] As such, leaving the chest in a horizontal position may result in even distribution of surfactant to the lungs. Placing the infant in a reverse Trendelenburg position should be avoided to avoid increased intracranial pressures.

Tracheal suctioning should be avoided immediately following surfactant administration and as long as 6 hours if ventilation can be adequately maintained. Safe and effective administration and monitoring by the respiratory therapist or nurse at the bedside are critical to the success of surfactant administration in infants. Careful patient assessment and continuous monitoring of work of breathing, FiO_2, compliance, pulmonary airway graphics and tidal volumes with a proximal flow sensor, chest radiograph, and SpO_2 are useful for clinicians when responding to deterioration or improvement in the patient's condition.[138] These tools may provide important information for stopping therapy, weaning, and/or escalation of mechanical respiratory support and assessing the need for subsequent dosing.

Very limited data suggest that delivery of surfactant by nebulization might result in improved distribution of surfactant,[139] and recent clinical investigations suggest safety and feasibility for delivery with nasal CPAP,[139a-139c] but this approach requires further study in humans. It was discovered that surfactant delivery could be accomplished sooner by nebulization in an LMA group, with efficacy equal to that of direct instillation with an ETT. Although far from conclusive, this method holds hope for areas in which ETT intubation skills are lacking.[140] Also, new research focused on minimizing invasive ventilation by injection of surfactant through the nasopharynx during delivery[141] or by using a thin catheter[142] may show promise in the future.

Optimization of Aerosol Drug Delivery

The common practice of administering aerosolized medications before bronchopulmonary hygiene and suctioning is based on custom more than scientifically verified practice.

Although delivery of aerosolized medication has a number of advantages over systemic dosing, recent information has helped in the design of a few reliable aerosol delivery systems (Boxes 29.5 and 29.6 and Table 29.6).[143] The basic fundamental characteristics of factors that influence neonatal aerosol delivery and deposition are listed in Box 29.5. These factors can be

---

BOX 29.5 Overview of Factors That Influence Neonatal Aerosol Delivery and Deposition

Host-Related Factors
- Anatomic (nasal breathing, size of oropharynx, airways, lung development)
- Physiologic (breathing pattern, inspiratory flow rate, tidal volume, pulmonary mechanics)
- Pathophysiologic (inflammation, mucus, atelectasis, fibrosis)

Aerosol System–Related Factors
- Characteristics of the medication (particle size, shape, density, output)
- Generator (pressurized metered-dose inhaler [pMDI] or nebulizer)
- Delivery device–patient interfaces (face mask or endotracheal tube)
- Conditions (ventilatory, environmental)
- Provider technique (optimum use of pMDI with spacer)

(Data from Cole C: The use of aerosolized medicines in neonates. Neonat Respir Dis 10:4, 2000.)

BOX 29.6 The Ideal Aerosol Delivery System

- High efficiency in aerosol delivery
- Predictable and reproducible (in same patient and different patients)
- Easy to use and maintain
- Efficient to administer
- Convenient
- Cost effective
- Environmentally safe

(Data from Cole C: The use of aerosolized medicines in neonates. Neonat Respir Dis 10:4, 2000.)

---

divided into two groups: host-related factors and aerosol system–related factors.[143] Box 29.6 lists the characteristics of "the ideal aerosol delivery system." Table 29.6 compares the advantages and disadvantages of the three most frequently used aerosol delivery systems: the pressurized metered-dose inhaler (pMDI) and the jet and ultrasonic nebulizers.[143] However, even with the progress being made in the design of aerosolized medication delivery systems, the clinician may need to test a variety of delivery devices and decide which system is most efficacious for each individual patient. The same may have to be done with the type and dose of aerosol medication[144,145] to establish a bronchodilator dose, that is, measuring a patient's response to a specific drug and dose using bedside pulmonary function methods, detailed in Chapter 12, rather than using predetermined dose tables. Apart from bronchodilators, novel inhaled drugs are being delivered via the aerosolization pathway, including hypertonic saline, surfactant, pulmonary vasodilators, and antibiotics. It is important to understand the variables unique to the aerosol route that can affect the drug delivery device. The small internal diameter and high resistance of the neonatal ETT and humidity impair aerosol delivery in the intubated patient compared with the nonintubated patient. In studies with animals, humans, and bench models, from 0.19% to 2.14% of the total drug amount in the nebulizer cup was administered to the lung or lung model when conventional

TABLE 29.6 Advantages and Disadvantages of Aerosol Generators in Neonates

Aerosol Generator	Advantages	Disadvantages
Pressurized metered-dose inhaler (pMDI)	• More consistent aerosol particle size and output • Less time consuming • Less preparation time • Less contamination • Less expensive than single-use nebulizers • Some hydrofluoroalkane formulations have more optimal aerosol particle size	• Technique problems • Lack of pure medications • Not all medications available in pMDI • New hydrofluoroalkane formulations need clinical studies
Jet nebulizer	• Tidal breathing • Passive cooperation • Can be used for long periods to deliver high doses • Wide range of medications	• Expensive and inconvenient • Inefficient and highly variable aerosol output • Numerous environmental factors affect aerosol particle size and output • Poor aerosolization of suspensions and viscous solutions • Preparation time • Time consuming to administer • Contamination potential • Requires compressed gas
Ultrasonic nebulizer	• Potentially more efficient than jet nebulizer and pMDI • Tidal breathing • Passive cooperation • Can be used for long periods to deliver high doses	• Expensive and inconvenient • Requires power source • Contamination potential • Limited medications available for use • Preparation time • Time consuming to administer

(Data from Cole C: The use of aerosolized medicines in neonates. Neonat Respir Dis 10:4, 2000.)

jet nebulizers were used[144,145] compared with 10% of the total dose that was shown to be deposited in the lungs of nonintubated patients.[146] There are several different approaches for delivering inhaled drugs to patients. A review of aerosol practices in infants reviews the safety and efficacy of these disparate practices.[147] Briefly, spontaneously breathing patients who receive blow-by, face mask, and infant hood treatments should receive the treatments using a nebulizer that uses a gas source to direct the aerosol to the infant's airway opening or a pMDI with a valved holding chamber. Vibrating mesh nebulizers should be used for drug delivery during HHFNC, CPAP, NIV, and invasive mechanical ventilation.

The greatest challenge with drug delivery in infants is getting the patient to tolerate a mask treatment. The mask should have low dead space and should be tightly fitted to the face. A crying infant receives substantially lower drug deposited in the lungs (<1%) and more on the face than one who is resting or sleeping (~5%).[148-150] Blow-by aerosol[151] therapy is accomplished using a gas-powered jet nebulizer placed within a reasonable distance from the patient, and the aerosol plume is directed toward the oral or nasal airway opening with an aerosol mask or T-piece. Although this practice may result in less crying or distress, it has been shown to result in negligible drug delivery in patients and anatomically accurate lung/airway models (~0.3%).[150,152] Drug delivery using a jet nebulizer attached to a hood may be as effective as a face mask treatment and better tolerated by the patient.[153,154]

With currently available methods, the placement and operation of a nebulizer are important for maximizing drug delivery to the lung. The nebulizer should be placed in the inspiratory limb and proximal to the patient wye-piece (not directly between the ventilator Y and the ETT) during invasive infant ventilation. If using a gas-powered jet nebulizer with a time-cycled pressure-limited ventilator with a fixed flow, the operational flow used with the nebulizer should be adjusted from a blended gas source, and the ventilator flow should be reduced transiently to maintain pressure and volume delivery to the patient.[155] On the other hand, for more sophisticated microprocessor-controlled ventilators, a gas-powered jet nebulizer may cause the ventilator to alarm and/or affect the patient's ability to flow trigger-assisted ventilator inflations. A vibrating mesh nebulizer does not add flow to the ventilator system. This may improve triggering and reduce excessive pressure and volume delivery to the patient. Bench and animal studies have shown that the vibrating mesh nebulizer is capable of providing between 10.74% and 12.6% of the drug placed in the nebulizer during neonatal ventilation.[156] Although it appears that vibrating mesh nebulizers represent a potentially safer and more efficient drug delivery system than jet nebulizers during ventilation, the cost of this drug delivery system may not be feasible for many institutions. Reports have also shown that drug delivery is more efficient with a vibrating mesh nebulizer during neonatal high-frequency compared with conventional ventilation.[156]

Most infant ventilators now require proximal flow sensors to be placed at the airway under normal operation. Medication condensate from a nebulizer treatment can accumulate within these sensitive flow sensors, affecting patient triggering, quality of airway graphics, tidal volume accuracy, ventilator operation, and drug delivery. As such, the proximal flow sensor is typically removed for a short-term nebulizer treatment. Although humidity has been shown to reduce aerosol delivery, a humidifier should not be disabled during a nebulizer treatment.

There is renewed interest in providing aerosolized drugs to patients supported by noninvasive support. Several studies have evaluated aerosol drug delivery during HFNC in neonatal lung models, but this practice cannot be suggested at this time.[157-160] A 2014 study compared bronchodilator drug delivery using a vibrating mesh nebulizer between HFNC, sigh intermittent mandatory ventilation (synchronized inspiratory positive airway pressure [SiPAP]), and bubble CPAP.[161] Drug delivery to a lung model was quite low (<1.5%) with all testing conditions. Overall, SiPAP provided lower drug mass than HFNC and bubble CPAP, probably because of drug loss in the nasal pressure generator. There were also no differences between different nebulizer circuit positions for HFNC and SiPAP, but during bubble CPAP, nebulizer placement at the humidifier provided greater drug delivery than when placed proximal to the patient nasal airway interface.

Improvements in nebulizer efficiency and safety as well as a better understanding of how nebulizers can be integrated in the array of delivery options for infants will be useful for future drug preparations and research. Owing to the improved efficiency of nebulizers and the small particle size, many investigators are intensely focused on ways to deliver aerosolized surfactant. Preclinical studies in mechanically ventilated preterm animals have shown improved outcomes and are likely to be used more frequently in the NICU in the future.[162]

CLINICIAN-BASED VENTILATOR AND WEANING PROTOCOLS

High variability in medical practice may have contributed, in part, to higher health care costs and poor adherence to evidence-based interventions. Evidence-based protocol strategies have been developed to reduce the lack of concordance in an attempt to improve clinical outcomes. Where evidence is lacking, expert opinion has been used to guide the development of management guidelines or protocols and reduce unnecessary variations in practice. In the respiratory care setting, non-physician-driven protocols have been shown to result in improvement in cost and allocation of appropriate resources to patients when respiratory therapy protocol–based care was used in adults.[163-168] The message is less clear in neonates receiving mechanical ventilation, and this is probably because of the array of lung diseases treated in the NICU.

Only one study has evaluated the impact of the implementation of a ventilation protocol driven by registered respiratory therapists on respiratory outcomes of premature infants. This included strict guidelines for outcomes, which were assessed at 1 and 2 years following implementation of the protocol and compared with historic controls. Following implementation of the protocol, there were significant and sustained reductions in time of first extubation attempt, duration of mechanical ventilation, and rate of extubation failure.

A protocol that used early extubation to NCPAP after 24 hours of ventilation has been shown in animals to result in less apnea and need for more intubations compared with those supported with invasive ventilation for 5 days.[169] However, outside of animal studies, mechanical ventilator weaning protocols are scant in the medical literature. The one study that has compared outcomes in infants between a weaning protocol and no intervention failed to show any differences.[170] As such, weaning practices vary widely from one institution to the next.

According to a survey among NICUs in the United States, weaning decisions are frequently physician dependent and not evidence based, with only 36% of respondents having a guideline (31%) or written protocol (5%) for ventilator weaning.[171] Reasons for this lack of definitive data may include the fact that there is no single reliable physiologic parameter or pulmonary function test in neonates that determines readiness for extubation. Further, many neonates have leaky ETTs, making tidal volume and minute ventilation difficult to measure. The optimal time for extubation is determined by a variety of parameters, including mean airway pressure, oxygen requirement, ventilatory requirements, estimation of negative inspiratory force, static compliance, and, most importantly, the appearance of the baby. Gillespie et al.[172] have suggested placing the infant on endotracheal CPAP for 10 minutes while monitoring the spontaneous minute ventilation. The ability of the infant to spontaneously generate at least 50% of the minute ventilation that was seen during assisted ventilation predicted readiness for extubation and shortened the time to successful extubation. The baby's primary problem and the clinical course and duration of assisted ventilation can provide helpful information regarding the appropriate timing for extubation. Some experts believe that a transition period from assist mode, pressure support, and/or extubation to CPAP is an excellent way to facilitate extubation. Sometimes, methylxanthine is used during the weaning process because its effects include "reminding the newborn to breathe" and increasing the efficiency of the diaphragm, especially in very low birth-weight infants.[173,174] If the infant has been on assisted ventilation for several days and there is concern about edema and inflammation in the upper airway, one or two doses of dexamethasone, given 24 to 48 hours before extubation, may be helpful.

All caretakers involved in the management of these babies need to be aware of the safety issues with regard to the transmission of pathogenic organisms by bodily fluids and closely follow the Occupational Safety and Health Administration standards outlined in Appendix 30.

RESUSCITATION AND STABILIZATION AT DELIVERY

The NRP is a training program for providers of newborn resuscitation created by the AAP and the American Heart Association to provide a comprehensive stepwise algorithm for the assessment and resuscitation of the newborn infant at delivery.[1] A core feature of this algorithm is the provision of adequate respiratory support and establishing effective ventilation using a variety of resuscitation devices, while repeatedly assessing the patient's response to the support provided and adjusting the technique of respiratory support.

Furthermore, endotracheal intubation may be considered at several points during a resuscitation; however, the timing of intubation may be influenced by the skill and experience of the provider as well as the clinical circumstances. Potential indications for endotracheal intubation during delivery room resuscitation include (1) tracheal suctioning of meconium (this is no longer recommended by the NRP), (2) need for prolonged positive-pressure ventilation, (3) administration of prophylactic surfactant, (4) presence of obstructive upper airway lesions requiring an artificial airway, and (5) cases in which air distention of the gastrointestinal (GI) tract is undesirable, such as with congenital diaphragmatic hernia.

Positive-pressure ventilation should be initiated during neonatal resuscitation when the infant is bradycardic (heart rate >100 beats per minute) or apneic despite stimulation or when there is persistent hypoxemia despite supplemental oxygen administration.[1] Under these circumstances, positive-pressure ventilation should be initially provided with a resuscitation bag and mask or T-piece resuscitator. Ultimately, intubation for positive-pressure ventilation should be considered if bag and mask ventilation is ineffective or if the need for prolonged positive-pressure ventilation is anticipated.

A recent approach to manual ventilation of the newborn has been the introduction of the sustained lung inflation.[175] The process involves using one of the resuscitation devices previously discussed to administer a single high pressure to the infant's lungs in an effort to better establish the functional residual capacity. The pressure is sustained for a designated amount of time and then reduced to a standard CPAP level to assist spontaneous breathing. Although there was initial evidence suggesting that such a maneuver may decrease the need for mechanical ventilation in the first few days of life,[176,177] randomized trials (summarized in a systematic review with a meta-analysis)[177] showed a lack of benefit with this maneuver and an increased risk of death. Therefore, sustained inflation should not be routinely used in preterm infants at birth.

Infants born with congenital diaphragmatic hernia frequently require positive-pressure ventilation at delivery because of respiratory distress with cyanosis. Provision of positive-pressure ventilation with bag and mask will drive large amounts of air into the upper GI tract, causing distention of a bowel that has herniated into the chest. Such bowel distention will cause further lung compression and compromise respiratory function. For this reason, infants with diaphragmatic hernia should be promptly intubated in the delivery room if resuscitation is required.[1] Some clinicians also advise that these infants should be paralyzed with a muscle relaxant to prevent spontaneous breathing from causing bowel distention. An orogastric tube should also be placed to evacuate any air that does enter the stomach. The diagnosis of diaphragmatic hernia is often confirmed by antenatal ultrasound studies and should be suspected in any infant with a scaphoid abdomen, unilaterally diminished breath sounds, and persistent respiratory distress.

A complete reference list is available at https://expertconsult. inkling.com/.

KEY READINGS

10. Salyer JW: Manual resuscitators: some inconvenient truths. Respir Care 54(12):1638–1643, 2009.
12. Kattwinkel J, Stewart C, Walsh B: Responding to compliance changes in a lung model during manual ventilation: perhaps volume, rather than pressure, should be displayed. Pediatrics 123(3):e465–e470, March 2009.
40. Thayyil S, Nagakumar P, Gowers H: Optimal endotracheal tube tip position in extremely premature infants. Am J Perinatol 25(1):13–16, January 2008.
76. Avila K, Mazza L, Morgan-Trukillo L: High-frequency oscillatory ventilation: a nursing approach to bedside care. Neonatal Network 13:23–29, 1994.
78. Meyer MP, Hou D, Ishrar NN, et al.: Initial respiratory support with cold, dry gas versus heated humidified gas and admission temperature of preterm infants. J Pediatr 166(2):245–250, February 2015.
88. Gardner DL, Shirland L: Evidence-based guideline for suctioning the intubated neonate and infant. Neonatal Network 28(5):281–302, September–October 2009.
101. Glass CA, Grap MJ: Ten tips for safer suctioning. Am J Nurs 95(5):51–53, May 1995.
119. Hough JL, Flenady V, Johnston L: Chest physiotherapy for reducing respiratory morbidity in infants requiring ventilatory support. Cochrane Database Syst Rev(3)CD006445, July 16, 2008.
147. DiBlasi RM: Clinical controversies in aerosol therapy for infants and children. Respir Care 60(6):894–914, 2015.
168. Kollef MH, Shapiro SD, Clinkscale D, et al.: The effect of respiratory therapist-initiated treatment protocols on patient outcomes and resource utilization. Chest 117(2):467–475, 2000.

Nursing Care

Debbie Fraser

INTRODUCTION

Neonates needing respiratory support require close monitoring to detect subtle changes that can signal either the need for weaning or a deterioration requiring additional intervention. Managing small and sick infants requires the expertise of a skilled interdisciplinary team. It is important that all care providers, including nurses, have a good understanding of developmental physiology, pathophysiology, pharmacotherapeutics, and the needs of the newborn and family.

As we learn more about the morbidities experienced by very low birth weight (VLBW) infants and other newborns requiring respiratory assistance, it has become clear that technology alone will not result in further improvements in outcome unless accompanied by exquisite attention to the neonate's environment and the small details that result in an optimal outcome. Because nurses spend the most concentrated period of time at the bedside, they are likely to be the most familiar with the neonate and most likely to detect changes in the patient's condition.

ASSESSMENT OF THE NEONATE

Newborns should be assessed at the time of admission to the neonatal intensive care unit (NICU) and also at regular intervals each day. A complete assessment of all body systems should be done, and the findings documented in the medical record at least once per shift and according to unit policy. Before assessing the infant, it is important to review the history, including that of the family, mother, labor and delivery, and problems and interventions since birth (Box 30.1). Expected findings will vary according to the infant's gestational and chronologic age.

Assessment begins with a period of observation before disturbing the infant and is followed by auscultation and palpation. General observation encompasses the infant's color, tone, and activity levels. Note the presence of cyanosis of the lips or mucous membranes. All infants should be centrally pink; acrocyanosis is common especially in the first hours and days after birth. Term infants are normally flexed and cycle through periods of sleep and activity. Premature infants are more likely to have decreased tone and activity levels; therefore, it is important to observe each infant for subtle changes over time.

In appropriately grown term infants, the chest circumference is approximately 2 cm less than the occipital-frontal head circumference, or approximately 33 cm in diameter.[1] A small or bell-shaped chest may be seen in infants with pulmonary hypoplasia or neuromuscular abnormalities, whereas a barrel chest with an increase in the anteroposterior diameter is seen in conditions associated with air trapping such as meconium aspiration, advanced chronic lung disease, or transient tachypnea of the newborn.

BOX 30.1 Elements of a Neonatal History

Family history
  Genetic conditions
  Maternal and paternal occupations
  Siblings—ages, health status
  Socioeconomic status, living conditions
  Environmental risks/exposures
Maternal history
  Age, previous pregnancies including complications in those pregnancies
  Blood type, Rh status, Group B *Streptococcus* status, serology results, human immunodeficiency virus, and hepatitis B status
  Results of prenatal screening tests including glucose tolerance testing
  Preexisting medical conditions
  Complications of pregnancy
  Exposure to teratogens, tobacco, alcohol, and drugs
  Prenatal steroids
Labor and delivery
  Onset of labor (premature, spontaneous or induced)
  Complications during labor—maternal fever, bleeding, fetal heart tracing
  Time of membrane rupture, amniotic fluid quantity and quality
  Medications during labor (pain medications, magnesium sulfate, other)
  Type of delivery (spontaneous vaginal, operative)
  Apgar scores and resuscitation required

TABLE 30.1 Examination of Newborn Chest

	Normal Findings	Abnormal Findings
Inspect	Oval chest shape, narrow at top and flares at bottom with narrow anteroposterior diameter	Bulging of chest
	Prominent xiphoid process	Concavity of chest
	Flexible chest wall, mild retractions with crying	Increased anteroposterior diameter (barrel chest)
	Symmetric chest movement in synchrony with abdomen during respirations	Depressed sternum (pectus excavatum/funnel chest)
	Breath rates 30–40/min in term infants and 40–60/min in preterm infants	Protuberant sternum (pectus carinatum/pigeon breast)
	Nipples well formed and prominent, symmetrically positioned; may have milk secretion	Asymmetric chest wall movement, flail chest
		Asynchronous respirations/paradoxical breathing ("seesaw")
	Pink color; harlequin color change	Retractions
Palpate	Clavicles and ribs intact	Tachypnea
	Breast nodule 3–10 mm	Supernumerary nipples
	PMI left of lower sternum	Erythema and tenderness of breasts
Auscultate	Equal bronchovesicular breath sounds	Widely spaced nipples
	Lusty cry	Central cyanosis, jaundice, pallor, mottling
	No murmur or soft murmur	Precordial impulse visible beyond first hours of life in term infant
		Lump over clavicle
		Crepitus
		Lack of breast tissue
		Shifts in point of maximal intensity
		Fremitus
		Crackles, rhonchi, wheeze, stridor, rubs, bowel sounds in chest
		Grunting
		Cough
		Weak, whining, or high-pitched cry
		Hoarseness, stridor
		Harsh murmur (grade 2–3) in the first hours of life

(Data from Koszarek K, Ricouard D: Nursing assessment and care of the neonate in acute respiratory distress. In Fraser D (ed): Acute Respiratory Care of the Neonate. 3rd ed. Petaluma, CA, NICU INK Books, 2012, pp. 65–108.)

Examine the chest for symmetry, shape, and movement. Pay attention to work of breathing, use of accessory muscles, and chest wall movement. Normal respiratory rate is 30 to 60 breaths per minute with relaxed diaphragmatic movements. Tachypnea is one of the most common manifestations of respiratory disease, especially diseases with decreased compliance such as respiratory distress syndrome (RDS). Infants are preferential nose breathers but will breathe through their mouth in the presence of nasal obstruction. In infants receiving mechanical ventilation, excessive chest wall excursion may be seen when ventilator pressure exceeds what is required for adequate gas exchange.[2] Diminished chest wall movement may signal a loss of lung volume related to atelectasis or obstruction of the airway. Asymmetrical chest movement may indicate the presence of a pneumothorax.

Auscultate breath sounds over both the anterior and the posterior surfaces of the chest, comparing one side to the other. Breath sounds are diminished in the presence of air leaks, atelectasis, or fluid in the pleural space. Infants with RDS may have faint breath sounds with a sandpaper-like quality in the latter part of inspiration. Sounds may be accentuated in the presence of consolidation such as occurs with pneumonia. Fine crackles are a normal finding in the first few hours after birth as fetal lung fluid is cleared. Beyond that period, crackles may be heard in infants with RDS or bronchopulmonary dysplasia (BPD). More prominent crackles reflect fluid in the alveoli and airways. Wheezes are not common in neonates but may be heard in infants with BPD. Stridor occurs in the presence of upper airway obstruction and is most common after extubation. Both wheezes and rubs are more common in ventilated infants because of narrowing of the airway in the presence of an endotracheal tube (ETT). Infants receiving high-frequency ventilation (HFV) will have altered breath sounds that range from jackhammer in nature (jet ventilation) to more high pitched and vibratory. Higher-pitched or musical sounds are heard when secretions are present. Auscultation of the chest includes an assessment of heart sounds listening for any irregularities, extra beats, or murmurs.

Palpate the chest to assess for the presence of masses, edema, or subcutaneous emphysema. It is also a useful technique to assess air entry in infants receiving HFV. Using the palm of the hand, compare one side of the chest to the other. Differences in the strength of the vibrations between one side of the chest and the other may indicate an air leak, secretions, or a displaced ETT. Chest examination findings are summarized in Table 30.1.

PAIN ASSESSMENT

Pain is considered by many to be the "fifth vital sign"; the importance of pain assessment cannot be overemphasized. It is well recognized that neonates in the NICU experience numerous painful treatments and procedures on a daily basis.[3,4] There are a number of pain assessment tools that have been validated for use in the neonatal population.[5,6] However, there are gaps and shortcomings in current practice in regard to the selection of, use of, and response to pain assessment tools.[6,7] Each NICU should use a validated assessment tool that is appropriate for its patient population. Staff should be educated on the use of the tool, and protocols should be in place to provide guidance regarding the appropriate response to elevated pain scores. Regular audits should be undertaken to ensure compliance with pain assessment and management protocols.

RESPIRATORY CARE

Providing care to an infant in the NICU is best accomplished through the efforts of a multidisciplinary team. When the infant is receiving respiratory support, additional monitoring of both the patient and the equipment is essential. Special concerns while caring for infants requiring assisted ventilation include maintaining targeted oxygen saturation parameters, positioning and containment, providing nasal continuous positive airway pressure (NCPAP) or noninvasive ventilation, maintaining a secure and patent airway, addressing challenges related to high-frequency ventilators and inhaled nitric oxide (iNO), preventing ventilator-acquired pneumonia, and detecting and intervening in cases of sudden respiratory deterioration.

Oxygen Saturation Monitoring

Neonates receiving respiratory support should have their oxygen status monitored on a continuous basis. The optimal oxygen saturation targets, especially in extremely preterm infants, have not been definitively determined and are usually set by unit protocol. Earlier studies, including one in 2014 by Bizzarro and colleagues, found that reducing the targeted oxygen saturation ranges in premature infants to between 85% and 93% substantially decreased rates of grades III and IV retinopathy of prematurity.[8] More recently, two systematic reviews examining optimal targets for oxygen saturation in extremely preterm infants have found higher rates of death and necrotizing enterocolitis in infants born at less than 28 weeks gestation whose SpO_2 target range was 85% to 89% compared with those with a range of 91% to 95%.[9,10] The meta-analysis by Manja and associates[9] did not demonstrate a difference in BPD or retinopathy of prematurity (ROP) between the groups; however, the review by Askie and colleagues[10] found that infants in the higher oxygen saturation (SpO_2) target range group had a significantly increased risk of requiring oxygen therapy at the 36 weeks postmenstrual age and of ROP requiring treatment. The results of these reviews led to a recommendation from the American Academy of Pediatrics (AAP) and others that, until more research is available, an oxygen saturation target range of 90% to 95% may be safer than lower ranges in very premature infants.[11,12]

Target saturation levels are also dependent on the infant's underlying condition and the goals of care. In infants with persistent pulmonary hypertension (PPHN), it may be desirable to maintain a higher oxygen saturation level, whereas in those infants with cyanotic congenital heart disease, a target saturation as low as 75% may be acceptable.[13]

Maintaining tight control of oxygen levels presents a significant challenge for clinicians. Among the challenges is the lability displayed by ventilated premature infants related to their disease conditions, responses to environmental stimuli, and need for ongoing interventions such as suctioning and other invasive procedures. For this reason, it is recommended that the oxygen saturation alarm limits be set at a slightly wider range than the target saturation levels. The AAP Clinical Report recommends setting the upper limit at 95 with a lower limit set just below the lower saturation target. This report also raises the issue of excessive alarms, which can result if alarm limits are set too narrowly.[12] In 2013, The Joint Commission issued a sentinel alert statement related to medical device alarm safety that highlighted the potential danger of alarm fatigue, a problem familiar to those responding to repeated oxygen saturation alarms.[14]

Several successful quality improvement projects designed to address oxygen targeting and alarm fatigue have been reported. One of the early reports came from Chow and colleagues,[15] who developed an oxygen targeting policy followed by an extensive staff education and audit process. The authors describe an initial resistance to change among staff, difficulties in consistency in implementation on different shifts, and the need for initial training, followed by retraining. Since Chow and colleagues reported on the results of their initiative, many NICUs have undertaken similar quality improvement projects to remind staff of the need to carefully monitor oxygen saturation and maintain much tighter control of parameters, avoiding hyperoxia in infants at high risk of retinopathy of prematurity (Fig. 30.1). Carefully evaluating the number and types of

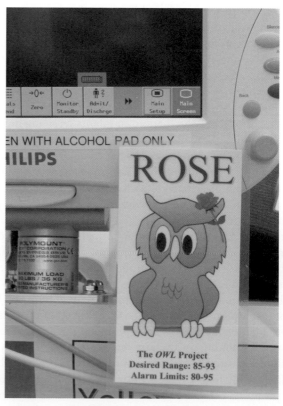

Fig. 30.1 Pulse oximetry sign.

procedures that a ventilated neonate receives is also necessary to reduce episodes of hypoxia and resulting hyperoxia when increased fraction of inspired oxygen (FiO$_2$) is administered.

Positioning and Containment

Premature and seriously ill neonates undergo a large number of hands-on assessments or procedures in a 24-hour period. A 2014 study found that infants in NICU experienced a median of 75 painful procedures during their NICU stay, with an average of 10 procedures per day.[16]

Procedures such as heel sticks, intravenous (IV) starts, and intubation often result in significant and prolonged reductions in oxygenation.[17-19] The extent of hypoxemia and overall distress can be dramatically reduced when personnel modify their caregiving according to the infant's responses. Careful observations of oxygenation and behavioral reactions in infants receiving NCPAP or mechanical ventilation with appropriate, individualized interventions can reduce the amount of stress the infant experiences. Many NICUs have moved to cue-based care, providing routine care only during times when the infant is awake.

Supporting the infant's body position can also reduce the stressful effects of procedures and other interventions. Swaddling, rolls, and the use of other containment techniques have been shown to improve physiologic and behavioral organization during weighing, suctioning, and heel sticks and provide pain relief.[18,20]

A study examining the effects of positioning on physiologic variables and comfort scores in neonates receiving NCPAP found that there was no difference between lateral, prone, and supine positioning on heart rate, respiratory rate, and oxygen saturation but that infants positioned prone scored highest on assessment of comfort.[21]

Positioning has also been found to affect oxygenation in neonates requiring both invasive and noninvasive respiratory support. Miller-Barmak and colleagues studied the histograms of 23 VLBW infants receiving noninvasive respiratory support. Each infant was positioned prone and supine in alternating 3-hour blocks with 11 starting supine and 12 starting in the prone position. These authors found that the infant's histograms were more stable with improved oxygenation while in a prone position compared with the time spent in supine position.[22] Similarly for ventilated infants, a Cochrane review of 19 trials (516 infants) comparing various positions for ventilated infants found that prone positioning slightly improved oxygenation, but the trials included in the review did not demonstrate evidence of sustained improvement for infants who were positioned prone. This review also found that there may be a further benefit in facilitating expansion of the lungs when the head of the bed is elevated.[23]

Infant positioning may also impact the risk of intraventricular hemorrhage (IVH) in VLBW infants. It has been postulated that positioning a neonate with the head turned to the side may decrease jugular venous drainage, hence increasing the risk of IVH in the first 72 hours of life.[24] A Cochrane review on the topic identified three trials that met the inclusion criteria (290 infants) and found no effect on the rates of moderate to severe IVH but did find a lower rate of neonatal mortality in infants positioned with their head midline.[25] Neutral or midline head positioning has been bundled with other interventions to reduce IVH, including elevating the head of the bed, minimal handling, and avoiding raising the infant's legs above midline in the first 72 hours of life. There has been limited research evaluating these bundles. One recent Dutch study of 280 VLBW infants matched with 281 historical controls found that implementation of an IVH bundle in the first 72 hours of life resulted in a lowered risk of mortality and of developing a new/progressive (severe) IVH or cystic periventricular leukomalacia.[26]

Noninvasive Ventilation

One of the key strategies in preventing barotrauma and chronic lung disease is avoiding ETT-mediated mechanical ventilation. As a result of the shift away from intubation, the use of noninvasive ventilation strategies including NCPAP and high-flow nasal cannula has increased dramatically. Caring for an infant receiving noninvasive ventilation is challenging. A major factor contributing to success or failure of noninvasive therapies, especially NCPAP, is the comfort level and knowledge of the team providing the care.[27,28] For example, one study reported significant decrease in the risk of nasal injury in infants receiving NCPAP when cared for by nurses and physicians who received comprehensive training as part of a continuous positive airway pressure (CPAP) bundle.[29]

Assessment of infants receiving noninvasive ventilation includes overall evaluation of respiratory status including retractions and respiratory effort, breath sounds, oxygenation, and partial pressure of carbon dioxide (PCO$_2$) levels. Although there may be retractions and PCO$_2$ levels in the range of 45 to 65 torr, if the infant generally appears comfortable, he or she can be maintained on NCPAP. Signs of impending treatment failure include a pH of less than 7.2, PCO$_2$ greater than 65, hypoxia despite an FiO$_2$ of greater than 60%, and increased retractions, tachypnea, and apnea.[30] These signs may be indications that the infant is failing noninvasive support and that surfactant or intubation and mechanical ventilation are needed.

Additional assessment includes monitoring the cheeks, philtrum, and nasal structures for any evidence of redness, erythema, or injury.[31] Additionally, the abdomen should be evaluated for distension and signs of feeding intolerance.

Complications from noninvasive ventilation include blocking of the airway or prongs by secretions, injury to the skin and nasal septum, abdominal distension, feeding intolerance, and pneumothorax.[30,32] Careful auscultation of breath sounds is needed, as well as attention to the pressure limits on the CPAP delivery device. Excessive abdominal distension is addressed by gastric decompression with an orogastric tube,[30] although this complication may hinder the advancement of enteral feedings and lead to numerous abdominal x-rays. Of note, one study documented that gastric emptying occurred earlier in infants receiving NCPAP.[33]

Maintenance of continuous-flow and appropriate CPAP pressures is affected by the infant's position and overall comfort. To maintain appropriate CPAP levels, the prongs or mask interface needs to be properly positioned, and the infant's mouth closed. To reduce the risk of the infant developing atelectasis, avoid removing the mask or prongs for routine care in the first

24 to 48 hours and minimize the disruption of CPAP as much as possible until the infant is ready for weaning.

One of the biggest challenges encountered while caring for the infant on NCPAP is protecting the nasal septum and surrounding structures from injury. Nasal injury is more common in more premature infants and in those infants requiring CPAP for long periods of time. Types of nasal injury include nasal snubbing, flaring or widening of the nares, and necrosis of the columella nasi.[34] The nasal septum is fragile, and the interfaces between the infant's nose and the CPAP system, either prongs or mask, may cause pressure on facial structures. There are limited data examining the use of a mask to deliver NCPAP in premature infants. One study of 175 infants born at less than 30 weeks' gestation found that the use of a mask significantly reduced the risk of nasal injury when compared with either nasal prongs or the rotation of prongs and a mask.[35] A systematic review of seven trials of mask versus prongs for the delivery of CPAP in infants born at less than 37 weeks found a decrease in the rate of CPAP failure and nasal injury when CPAP was delivered by mask rather than prongs.[36]

Be diligent in ensuring the appropriate positioning of prongs relative to the nose and reposition the infant and CPAP interface frequently. The CPAP hat should fit snugly and should rest just above the infant's eyebrows. Prongs should be the correct size to fit snugly in the nares without excessive pressure on the septum and should be positioned to avoid blanching of the skin around the nose. Straps should be snug but not to the point of creating indentations on the cheeks.

Despite meticulous care practices, tissue injury may occur on the philtrum of the lip or the nasal septum (Fig. 30.2).[28]

Hydrocolloid "shields" have been shown to offer some protection against injury[37,38] but do not prevent all injuries because pressure is often the problem, rather than friction. Application of an antimicrobial ointment such as mupirocin may be beneficial to reduce the risk of infection through this portal of entry.[39]

Administration of oxygen under pressure through nasal prongs can be excessively irritating to the nasal mucosa, resulting in increased production of secretions, especially in the first few hours after initiation.[37] The use of warmed, humidified gas is imperative. Although there is currently no empirical evidence for exactly how best to care for the airway of infants on NCPAP,[40] suctioning of the nares to maintain patency is usually required. Suctioning should be based on assessment of the patient and not routinely scheduled. Frequent suctioning causes trauma to the nares and nasopharynx and may increase the risk of edema, bleeding, and infection through skin breakdown.[40] Other hazards of suctioning include bradycardia or cardiac dysrhythmias. Using specialized equipment such as a round-tipped plastic suction device can minimize trauma, mucosal bleeding, and swelling. Saline or sterile water drops instilled before suctioning may be helpful in loosening secretions and lubricating the catheter.

Repositioning is essential for a number of reasons, including to improve neurodevelopmental outcomes, and is recommended every 3 to 4 hours.[30] Care should be taken in positioning both the infant and the prongs or mask as well as any tubing to avoid undue pressure on the nasal septum. Prone positioning may also be beneficial in infants receiving NCPAP because lying prone aids in keeping the infant's mouth in a closed position, decreases abdominal distension, and keeps the infant calmer. Offering a pacifier and providing containment using swaddling or nesting

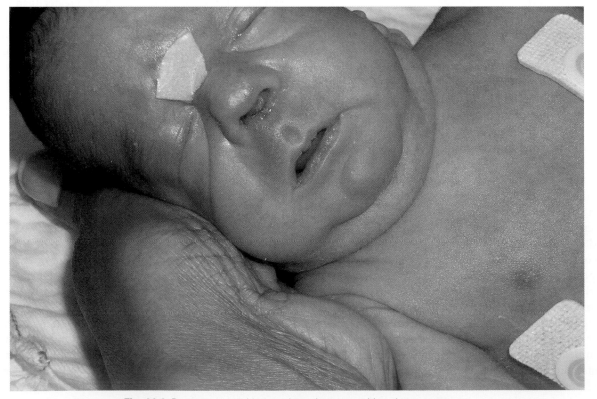

Fig. 30.2 Damage caused by nasal continuous positive airway pressure.

techniques can be beneficial in both promoting comfort and improving respiratory support. The use of a chin strap may prevent air leaks and loss of CPAP pressure.[30]

Mechanical Ventilation

There are a wide variety of neonatal ventilators on the market, each with unique properties and settings. Everyone providing care to the infant on mechanical ventilation should understand the machine and the interface between the machine and the baby. Carefully assess the infant's breathing pattern, chest movement, respiratory rate, and oxygenation each shift and whenever ventilator parameters are adjusted. Document the assessment findings in the patient record along with any diagnostic tests (x-rays or blood gases) that are performed. There are some issues unique to mechanical ventilation that should be considered in the care of the infant. These include airway security, ETT movement and position, suctioning of the ETT, and prevention of ventilator-acquired pneumonia.

Airway Security

Accidental dislodgment of the ETT can result in serious complications, including acute hypoxia, bradycardia, and potential damage to the trachea or larynx. Factors increasing the risk of accidental extubation include agitation, ETT suctioning, weighing, turning the patient's head, loose tape, and retaping the ETT.[41] The incidence of accidental extubations reported in the literature is variable, with a range of 0.14 to 5.3 per 100 ventilator days,[42] although quality improvement projects have reduced this rate to below the benchmark rate of 1 per 100 ventilator days.[43]

Strategies used to reduce unplanned extubations in neonatal patients include ensuring that the tip of the ET tube is below the first thoracic vertebrae (T1), using standardized anatomic reference points and securement methods, having multiple providers present for tube retaping, ensuring adequate comfort and sedation, and debriefing after unplanned extubation events.[43,44]

Many different techniques have been described to secure ETTs, ranging from adhesives with bonding agents or pectin barriers to using metal or plastic bows to prevent slipping of the ETT. A systematic review of taping methods identified five trials, but methodologic issues and small study sizes prevented the authors from drawing conclusions regarding the superiority of any particular strategies for tube securement.[45] Some commercially available products for securing neonatal ETTs have incorporated similar ideas in their products. Because the common link in all these methods is the use of adhesives, an in-depth review of adhesive application and removal in the neonate is in the section on skin care later.

Endotracheal Tube Movement and Malposition

The position of the ETT may be altered with inadequate fixation of the tube, changes in patient position, and flexion and extension of the head. Because the trachea of a term newborn is quite short and even shorter in premature infants, small movements of the ETT can result in displacement, causing the tube to move into the right main stem bronchus or into the esophagus with (Fig. 30.3).[46] In addition to potentially altering ventilation and blood gas parameters and causing tracheal damage, ETT movement can result in misinterpretation of the ETT position

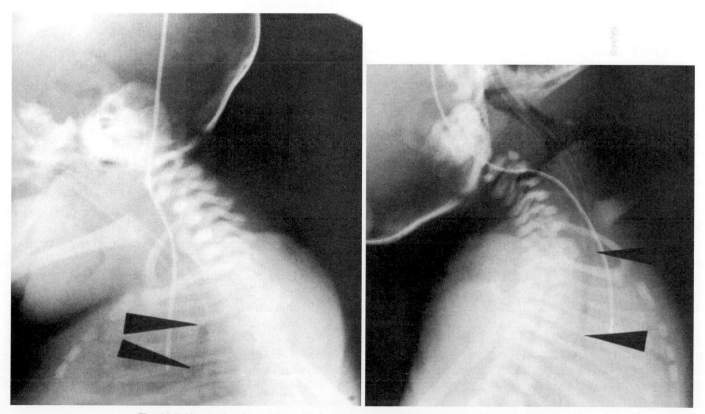

Fig. 30.3 X-rays showing endotracheal tube position changes with head position changes.

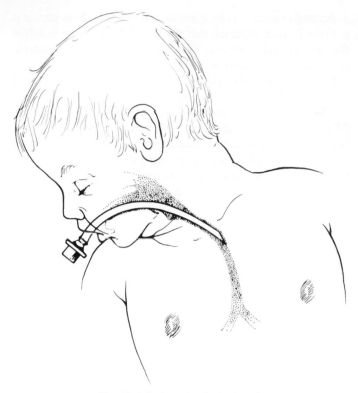

Fig. 30.4 Endotracheal tube bevel.

on x-rays. The infant's head should be carefully positioned when obtaining x-rays and placed in a "neutral" position to avoid extension or flexion. The ETT should be positioned with the bevel opening to the same side the head is facing to avoid having the bevel abut against the tracheal wall with head movement or position changes (Fig. 30.4).[47]

Each NICU should develop a standard practice that is consistently used to avoid confusion during intubations and ETT retaping. Using consistent anatomical reference points, post a card specifying the depth at which the ETT is inserted at each bedside, with the centimeter marking that is at the agreed upon reference point (i.e., lip, gum). Inspect the ETT tapes often to ensure adequate adhesion and retape the ETT whenever necessary to prevent accidental dislodgment. Two care providers should be present for tube retaping. Regular monitoring of unplanned extubations should be incorporated into quality improvement audits.[43]

Suctioning

The presence of an ETT is irritating to tissue and increases secretions. It is necessary to clear this artificial airway periodically to maintain ventilation for the infant. ETT suctioning has been associated with a number of complications in infants including hypoxemia, bradycardia, atelectasis, airway trauma, and pneumothorax.[48] Systemic effects are also of concern, including increased blood pressure, changes in intracranial pressure, and an increased risk of infection.[48] Neonates should be suctioned only when needed, that is, when breath sounds are moist or congested, when secretions are visible, when there is a change in the infant's respiratory rate and pattern, or when the infant is bradycardic, hypoxic, or agitated with no known

cause.[48,49] During high-frequency oscillatory or jet ventilation, it is not always obvious when suctioning is needed, and some nurseries implement routine suctioning every 4 to 8 hours for patients on HFV.

To reduce trauma to the tracheal mucosa, the suction catheter should not extend beyond the tip of the ETT.[2] Normal saline has been used for many years to lubricate the ETT; however, there is limited quality research examining the effects of normal saline instillation in the neonatal population.[50] A systematic review of normal saline instillation for endotracheal suctioning found only three studies that met the inclusion criteria; in those studies, a transient drop in oxygen saturation following saline instillation was noted.[50] Similarly, a meta-analysis of five studies examining saline instillation in adult ICU patients found that oxygen saturation was significantly lower in the 5 minutes following saline instillation.[51] In addition, there is concern that saline instillation does not lead to increased secretion recovery and may be a risk factor in ventilator-associated pneumonia (VAP) by releasing the biofilm that occurs in the ETT, moving it further into the distal airway.[52]

Suctioning techniques have also been examined to determine the least harmful method of suctioning. Closed suctioning (CS) systems that are placed in-line with the ETT and ventilator circuit are widely used in the NICU (Fig. 30.5). In addition to requiring less nursing time, proposed benefits of CS include reducing the physiologic disturbances associated with suctioning and the potential for introduction of microorganisms into the trachea and decreasing the potential loss of positive end expiratory pressure (PEEP).[53] The research comparing open suctioning and CS practices has not been definitive in determining which system is more advantageous.[54,55] A Cochrane review evaluated four studies using a crossover design that included 252 infants and found a reduction in the number and severity of hypoxic events and a decrease in the number and severity of bradycardic episodes with CS. The authors concluded, however, that the evidence was not strong enough to recommend CS as the only acceptable method for suctioning ventilated neonates.[55]

Ventilator-Associated Pneumonia

Preventing nosocomial infection, including VAP and catheter-related bloodstream infections, in hospitalized patients is now mandated by The Joint Commission (formerly the Joint Commission on Accreditation of Healthcare Organizations). The assumption is that these complications can be prevented by measures undertaken by care providers in the NICU.

Little evidence exists about how to best prevent VAP in the NICU. One of the most pressing challenges is diagnosing VAP. Barriers to diagnosis include a lack of objective criteria specific to VAP in neonates, the coexistence of other respiratory conditions, and the impracticality of obtaining a lung specimen in a neonate, where a lower airway culture is the gold standard for diagnosing VAP in adults.[56] Longer duration of mechanical ventilation, low birth weight (LBW), low gestational age, and numbers of reintubation increase the likelihood of a patient developing a VAP.

Risk factors specific to neonatal VAP include prematurity, LBW, days of mechanical ventilation, and the need for reintubation, with days of mechanical ventilation being the most significant risk.[57]

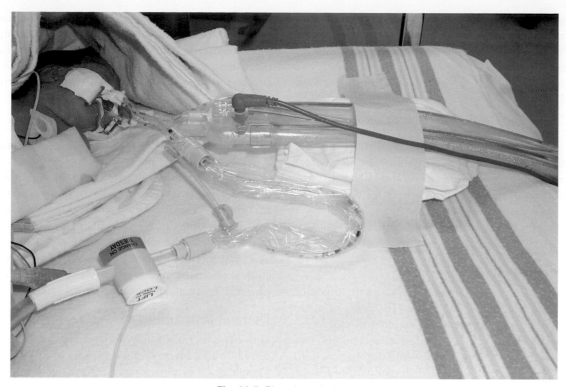

Fig. 30.5 Closed suctioning.

Although the presence of a bloodstream infection has been identified as a risk for VAP, it appears that most infections are attributed to exogenous sources such as the hands of health care workers, biofilm on the ETT, and contamination from the ventilator circuit.[58]

A number of VAP-prevention guidelines have been developed for neonates and, in many cases, have been extrapolated from the adult or pediatric populations.[59,60] VAP prevention strategies for neonates on assisted ventilation include the following: (1) avoiding the use of mechanical ventilation and daily assessment of readiness to extubate, (2) avoiding repeated intubations, (3) changing the ventilator circuit only when visibly contaminated, (4) draining condensation from the ventilator circuit every 2–4 hours, (5) daily interruption of sedation, (6) keeping the head of the bed elevated 30 degrees, (7) performing mouth care routinely, and (8) performing appropriate hand hygiene.[59,60] A systematic review examining VAP-prevention bundles in the neonatal and pediatric ICUs identified eight studies and found that, overall, these bundles reduced the incidence of VAP. These authors noted that there was considerable variation in the bundle components, making it difficult to draw strong conclusions.[59] VAP is discussed in more detail in Chapter 30.

High-Frequency Ventilation

Nursing care for the infant on HFV, either via oscillator or via jet ventilators, requires a unique set of knowledge and skills.[61] The condition of the infant receiving HFV can change very rapidly because of both the infant's underlying pulmonary pathology and the device in use. Assessment of the infant receiving HFV should be done frequently and differs from routine nursery assessment because of the nature of the equipment and its effects on the infant's breathing. Auscultation is aimed at detecting changes in the pitch of breath sounds, with high-pitched sounds suggestive of secretions. It is not possible to auscultate the apical pulse or to detect the presence of a heart murmur while the infant is on HFV. In addition to auscultation, observe the infant's chest movement and palpate the chest, looking for equal vibrations. In some cases, it may be necessary to interrupt or pause the ventilator briefly during the assessment process to auscultate spontaneous breath sounds and listen for heart murmurs; however, this can also destabilize the infant. Coordination among multidisciplinary team members is recommended for these assessment periods, so that the infant's time without HFV is kept to a minimum.

CS should be used to prevent disconnecting the infant from ventilation during suctioning. Many NICUs use in-bed scales, weigh infants infrequently, or simply do not weigh patients receiving HFV to prevent destabilizing the respiratory system or accidental extubation. Depending on which high-frequency ventilator is used, positioning and turning infants on HFV may require two people, one to rotate the infant and another to briefly disconnect the ventilator circuit while the ventilator itself remains in a fixed location. The infant should be positioned to maintain the head in alignment with the body rather than turned to the side. This prevents obstruction of the flow of gases and disruption in ventilation.

Inhaled Nitric Oxide

The use of iNO is now commonplace for newborns receiving assisted ventilation. Originally approved for the treatment of pulmonary hypertension, iNO is now also used to treat premature infants with PPHN[62] and BPD.[63] The Cochrane review examining iNO for respiratory failure in preterm infants included 17 studies on the subject and concluded that iNO was not effective as a rescue therapy but may offer some benefit in preventing BPD. The authors recommended further study.[63]

Care of the newborn receiving iNO includes careful monitoring of the gas administration and preventing any interruption of iNO administration during hand ventilation, turning, moving, or suctioning; CS systems are recommended. Gradual weaning from iNO is necessary even in patients who are "nonresponders" because of the downregulation of the patient's endogenous nitric oxide production during treatment with iNO and the potential for destabilizing patients with marginal oxygenation and reserves.

Sudden Deterioration

A sudden deterioration can occur as a result of a multitude of factors in the ventilated neonatal patient. The cause of acute deterioration is not always apparent and requires prompt investigation. Sudden changes in a ventilated infant's condition can result from mechanical issues including ventilator malfunction, displacement, or obstruction of the ETT or complications such as an air leak or pericardial effusion.

Begin by auscultating the infant's breath sounds; if equal bilaterally, the tube is likely to be in proper position and free from obstruction. If the breath sounds are distant, or if air entry is detected in the gastric areas accompanied by distension, or an audible cry is heard, the ETT may have slipped into the esophagus. An end-tidal CO_2 monitor or detection device will show an absence of CO_2 during expiration. The ETT should be immediately removed and bag and mask ventilation provided until it is determined whether reintubation is necessary. If replaced, the ETT should be securely taped at the same level as the previous tube, and an x-ray obtained to confirm appropriate ETT position.

If the breath sounds are louder on the right side, the ETT may have slipped into the right mainstem bronchus. A chest x-ray can confirm this diagnosis or perhaps identify an air leak in the left lung. If the ETT extends into the right bronchus, the left lung or the upper lobe of the right lung may appear to have atelectasis on x-ray. The appropriate adjustment to the ETT position is determined by measuring the tube position from the x-ray and then repositioning and taping the ETT securely.

If the ETT is plugged with secretions, breath sounds may be diminished bilaterally, with decreased rise of the chest wall during hand ventilation. Suction the ETT to remove the secretions. If this measure is unsuccessful, remove the ETT and initiate bag and mask ventilation until the ETT is replaced.

A large pneumothorax typically presents with cyanosis, bradycardia, decreased blood pressure, narrowing pulse pressure, and diminution of the QRS complex on electrocardiography. The point of maximal impulse of the heart may be shifted away from the side with the air leak, and breath sounds may be diminished or absent on the affected side. The diagnosis of a pneumothorax can be confirmed with transillumination of the chest with a high-density fiber-optic light source or with a chest

x-ray. When the infant is significantly compromised, it may be necessary to decompress the chest with needle aspiration before the diagnosis is confirmed radiographically. Once the air is evacuated and the patient stabilized, a chest tube is inserted and attached to a drainage system to assist in air removal.

GENERAL CARE OF THE NEONATE

Infants requiring care in the NICU, especially those ill enough to need respiratory support, require expert assessment and ongoing care. Respiratory diseases, with the potential for episodes of hypoxemia, predispose infants to complications such as retinopathy of prematurity, necrotizing enterocolitis, infection, and chronic lung disease. Optimizing the infant's environment to reduce the likelihood of complications is an important part of caring for these infants. Issues requiring special consideration include temperature management, nutrition, skin care, pain management, and developmental care.

Thermal Instability

Both hyperthermia and hypothermia place neonates at risk of complications. Hyperthermia is more likely to be iatrogenic as a result of exogenous sources of heat such as too many layers of clothing or blankets, an elevated incubator temperature, or excessive radiant heat. Hyperthermia increases the neonate's metabolic rate, leading to tachycardia, tachypnea, increased oxygen consumption, increased insensible water loss, and poor weight gain.[64]

Because of the large surface area-to-body weight ratio and an inability to generate heat through shivering, all newborn infants are more susceptible to hypothermia. The risk of hypothermia is accentuated in premature infants who have limited subcutaneous tissue, reduced brown fat stores, and decreased tone and muscle activity. Evaporative heat losses are higher in VLBW infants as a result of the thin epidermal skin layer.

Hypothermia increases the risk of morbidity and mortality especially in VLBW infants. In a study of 1764 infants born between 22 and 33 weeks' gestation, hypothermia on admission increased the likelihood of early neonatal death 1.64-fold.[65] These findings are similar to a more recent prospective study of 4356 VLBW infants that confirmed a higher risk of early neonatal death in infants who were hypothermic on admission to the NICU.[66] Cold stress results in increased oxygen consumption and an increased risk of worsening respiratory distress, hypoxemia, hypoglycemia, and metabolic acidosis.[64] Longer term hypothermia slows postnatal growth because calories are used for heat production rather than weight gain.

Monitor the temperature of all neonates frequently, especially those at increased risk of hypothermia. Providing a neutral thermal environment is critical in minimizing oxygen consumption and caloric expenditure. Use double-walled incubators or servo-controlled radiant warmers to provide additional thermal support. Increased humidity is recommended for VLBW infants as a means of reducing transepidermal evaporative heat loss. Polyethylene bags or wraps should be used for VLBW infants immediately after birth in the delivery room to reduce both evaporative and convective heat losses.[67]

Nutrition

The contribution of nutrition and growth to long-term neuro-developmental outcomes in premature infants has been clearly recognized.[68-70] In addition, altered growth patterns have been implicated in the development of adult-onset conditions such as diabetes and cardiovascular disease.[68,71] The increased work of breathing common to infants with respiratory disease results in increased caloric consumption and may prevent adequate oral intake of nutrients. Adequate growth has been identified as an important strategy in mitigating the risk of BPD in VLBW infants.[72,73]

Attaining adequate growth rates in premature infants is challenging. Most fat and energy stores are accrued in the third trimester, leaving preterm infants with limited caloric reserves at birth. These infants often experience a delay in achieving adequate intake of nutrients and may have periods of relative undernutrition related to feeding intolerance or fluid restrictions. Prematerm and sick infants require increased calories for tissue repair, generation of heat, and work of breathing. Early optimal nutrition for VLBW infants is a key pillar in preventing postnatal growth restriction and the related complications. Strategies to optimize nutrition include early parenteral nutrition with adequate protein and lipid intake, initiating parenteral nutrition immediately after birth and continuing until oral feeding reaches adequate levels, minimal enteral feedings introduced on day 1 of life, advancement of feeds at a rate of 30 mL/kg/day, use of maternal or donor breast milk, and the appropriate fortification of calories and nutrients beginning when oral feeds are progressing well.[70,74] Growth rates should be monitored carefully and individual adjustments made when anticipated growth rates are not achieved.

Skin Care

In premature infants, the uppermost layer of the epidermis, the stratum corneum, is histologically thinner, and there are fewer and more widely spaced fibrils that connect the epidermis and the dermis compared with term infants.[75] Thus, premature infants are more vulnerable to skin injury and stripping of the epidermis. Risk factors for skin injury include gestational age less than 32 weeks, edema, and adhesives applied to the skin to secure tubes, lines, and monitoring equipment. Although pressure sores are very rare in neonates, they may occasionally be seen on the ears or occiput of critically ill neonates on HFV or extracorporeal membrane oxygenation unless appropriate preventative measures are employed.

Assessment of preterm infants should include frequent inspection of the skin for color, perfusion, turgor, edema, pressure points, and evidence of injury. A breech in skin integrity is a risk factor for sepsis, and attention should be given to preventing damage to the skin. Acutely ill infants should have their skin cleansed when it is soiled, with full baths reserved for more stable infants. To avoid drying out the skin, pH-neutral soaps should be used sparingly. Any product applied to the skin should be evaluated to determine if it contains dyes, perfumes, or drying agents and should be assessed for potential absorption of any chemically active ingredients. Emollients are not routinely used in some NICUs because of concern for infection[76] but may be needed when the infant's skin is dry and cracking.[77] Again, care should be taken to select agents that have been tested in the neonatal population.

The use of products for skin antisepsis before invasive procedures such as intravenous starts, line placement, or heel sticks is an important part of preventing infection. Most products capable of killing bacteria are potentially harmful to the fragile skin of premature infants. Alcohol products are drying; products containing iodine may be absorbed systemically. Topical antiseptic products should be approved for use in neonates and should be removed from the skin after the procedure using sterile water.[78]

Adhesive Application and Removal

The traumatic effects of adhesive removal on premature infant skin include reduced barrier function, increased transepidermal water loss, erythema, and skin stripping.[78,79] Moistened gauze or saline wipes are recommended for gentle removal of adhesives. Silicone-based adhesive removers have been shown to be safe and effective in removing adhesives in premature infants. Alcohol-, organic-, or oil-based solvents are not recommended for adhesive removal in newborns because these products have potential toxicity when absorbed.[78] Hydrocolloid or pectin barriers are sometimes used between the skin and the adhesive to protect the skin. A study using direct measurements of skin barrier function found that pectin barriers caused a degree of trauma similar to that of plastic tape.[80] Despite this finding, pectin barriers and similar hydrocolloid adhesive products continue to be used in the NICU because they mold well to curved surfaces and adhere even with moisture.[78,80] Silicone-based liquid barrier films do not leave a residual on the skin and can also be used as a barrier between the skin and adhesives.[78]

Hydrogel- and silicone-based adhesive products have been shown to reduce skin trauma, with hydrogel having an analgesic effect on wounds.[81] Silicone-based adhesives do not adhere well to plastics such as cannulas, thereby limiting their use in those applications.[78] The use of bonding agents, such as tincture of benzoin or Mastisol, increases the adherence of adhesives and may result in skin stripping and damage because they cause the adhesive to adhere more tenaciously to the epidermis than the fragile bond between epidermis and dermis, especially in the premature infant.[82]

Prevent trauma from adhesives by minimizing use of tape when possible, dabbing cotton on tape to reduce adherence, and using hydrogel adhesives for devices such as electrodes. Delaying tape removal may be helpful, because many adhesives attach less well to skin when in place for over 24 hours. Remove adhesives slowly and carefully, using water-soaked cotton balls and pulling the adhesive parallel to the skin surface, folding the adhesive onto itself.[79]

Pressure Ulcers and Skin Injury

Although the incidence of ischemic injury related to pressure ulcers is low in NICU patients compared with adults, infants at risk for this complication include those on HFV, therapeutic cooling and extracorporeal membrane oxygenation because they are more difficult to turn or move. In addition, they are generally critically ill and may be hypotensive, which can lead to peripheral tissue hypoperfusion. They may also be edematous because of leaking capillaries and may need excessive fluid or blood products to maintain blood pressure. Paralyzing medications such as pancuronium and vecuronium, or high levels of sedation, create poor tone and decreased movement,[83] which also increases the risk of skin breakdown.

Sites for pressure ulcers in newborns on assisted ventilation include the nares and gums secondary to pressure from delivery devices (prongs, masks, ETT), and the occiput of the head and the ears, because of the heavy weight of the infant's head compared with the body. In addition, the circuit connected to the ETT is often secured to avoid displacing the tube, and thus, the infant cannot turn or move the head without assistance.[84] Although less common, pressure injuries can also occur with the use of monitoring devices such as oxygen saturation probes, blood pressure cuffs, arm boards, and vascular catheter hubs.[78]

Prevention of skin injury begins with assessing the skin at least once per shift using a validated skin assessment tool.[85] Skin rounds has been suggested as a method of bringing further awareness to the issue of skin injury in the NICU.[86] To prevent skin injury, the infants should be repositioned on a regular basis, with gentle massage on pressure points. Even when turning side to side is not feasible, lifting the head, shoulders, and hips and supporting these areas with pressure-reducing surfaces are helpful. Positioning aids such as water mattresses or pillows, air and gel mattresses, pillows, and wedges that equalize the pressure around the head and ears can be useful in infants at high risk of pressure injuries.[78] If a pressure ulcer occurs, wound care should be based on the type of injury, stage of healing, and the presence of eschar or infection, as well as the amount of moisture present.[78,85]

Managing Pain

There are a variety of interventions that have been shown to reduce pain and agitation in NICU patients; strategies should be put in place to both reduce and manage infant pain and agitation. Exposure to painful procedures in infants has been shown to result in short-term hyperanalgesia.[87] Repeated exposure to stress and pain in the neonatal period has long-term detrimental effects, including postnatal growth impairment, early neurodevelopmental delay, and altered brain development and long-term responses to pain.[6,88] Early pain exposures in premature infants has also been found to result in changes in childhood, including delayed visual-perceptual development, lower neurocognitive scores, internalizing behaviors, and reduced cortical thickness.[89,90]

The first and most important strategy should be to decrease the number of stressful procedures (Box 30.2). Skin-to-skin care,[91] facilitated tucking,[92,93] and swaddling[92] have been found to reduce agitation and pain responses to acute painful procedures and may be useful as adjunctive strategies for the management of ongoing pain.[92,94]

Oral sucrose has been shown to reduce crying when offered to newborns during painful procedures such as heel-stick blood sampling.[87,94,95] However, there is controversy regarding the efficacy and long-term effects of repeated doses of sucrose.[95]

BOX 30.2 **Strategies to Minimize Stress and Overstimulation**

- Swaddle or provide boundaries to promote flex position.
- Place prone with arms and knees flexed or side-lying with hands in midline.
- Move the infant slowly during position changes and contain limbs to avoid startle response.
- Avoid hyperextending neck or arms.
- Coordinate care activities to reduce handling and sleep disruptions.
- Provide care during times when the infant is awake rather than according to a fixed schedule.
- Before handling, bring the infant to a quiet alert stage by talking in a soft voice and touching the infant gently.
- Reduce environmental noise in the unit.
- Implement periods of "quiet time" on each shift with lights dim and noise minimized.
- Cover the incubator to reduce exposure to bright lights.
- If medically stable, dress and bundle the infant.

(Data from Koszarek K, Ricouard D: Nursing assessment and care of the neonate in acute respiratory distress. In Fraser D (ed): Acute Respiratory Care of the Neonate. 3rd ed. Petaluma, CA, NICU INK Books, 2012, pp. 65–108.)

Routine administration of opiates and sedatives for ventilated infants remains controversial.[87,96] Use of opiates for ventilated infants during routine caregiving procedures has been reported to be effective in the treatment of moderate to severe pain.[97] However, opioids may increase the risk of hypotension, interfere with the infant's own respiratory effort, and prolong weaning from assisted ventilation as well as the time to reach full enteral feeds.[96,98,99] Earlier studies examining the use of opioids in preterm infants failed to show a decrease in pain scores or a reduction of adverse effects (death, IVH, and periventricular leukomalacia).[100,101]

In addition, the safety profile for morphine in preterm infants has not been established. A secondary analysis of infants in the NEOPAIN (Neurologic Outcomes and Pre-emptive Analgesia in Neonates) trial found that head circumference and body weight at 5 to 7 years of age were smaller/lower in premature infants treated with morphine compared with infants receiving a placebo.[102]

Narcotic withdrawal is a risk when higher doses of opioids are administered over a prolonged period. Signs of withdrawal including irritability, tachypnea, jitteriness, increased tone, vomiting, diarrhea, sneezing, hiccoughs, and skin abrasions may be seen when narcotics are weaned rapidly.[103] Avoid abrupt discontinuation of opioids and wean these infants in a slow and planned manner. Monitoring for signs of abstinence should also be part of the weaning plan.

Medications are best used judiciously, considering the stage of illness, therapeutic goals, and individual infant characteristics. Other causes of agitation should be considered, including inadequate ventilation. In many cases, patient comfort is often the best indicator of the appropriateness of selected ventilator support modes, perhaps more useful than blood gases. The infant's response to all interventions should be assessed and documented. Clear communication among health care team members is critical to ensure that pain is appropriately managed and the potential side effects of pain medication limited.

Developmental Care

The NICU environment is bright, noisy, and overstimulating to premature or sick infants who may not have the capacity to cope. The seminal work of Heidelise Als[104] provided the basis for our understanding of newborn adaptation as an integration of physiologic and behavioral systems. An inability to cope with environmental stimuli causes dysfunctional autonomic, state, and motor responses. The ability to cope with stimuli such as light, noise, touch, and pain is inversely proportional to gestation age, with very preterm infants lacking the self-regulatory mechanisms to promote stability. Studies have examined various interventions aimed at modifying the NICU environment to support optimal preterm infant development.[105] Attempts at systematically reviewing developmental care interventions have been hampered by a lack of consistency among interventions. Two systematic reviews of the Newborn Individualized Developmental Care and Assessment Program (NIDCAP) failed to demonstrate a clear benefit;[106,107] however, there is evidence to support a number of individual interventions to support neurodevelopment in VLBW infants.[105,108]

A comprehensive plan of care for VLBW infants should include strategies to promote uninterrupted sleep, reduce stressful procedures, and promote self-regulation through supportive positioning, nonnutritive sucking, and hand-to-mouth behaviors. Parents should be taught to recognize both approach and avoidance signals displayed by their infant and should be encouraged to modify their interactions according to the infant's developmental stage.

Skin-to-Skin Holding

Skin-to-skin or kangaroo care confers significant benefits for both newborns and their parents. Short-term benefits include stabilizing heart rate, oxygen saturation, and breathing patterns;[109] decreased risk of sepsis and hypothermia;[109] improved sleep-wake cycles;[110] increased growth rate;[109,111] decreased response to pain;[110] improved breast-feeding duration;[111] and greater maternal attachment.[110] Longer-term benefits of kangaroo care include decreased mortality and rates of hospital readmission.[109,111] Kangaroo care in the NICU has been identified as an important factor in reducing parental stress, promoting maternal milk production, and facilitating parent-infant bonding.[110]

Kangaroo care can be done with ventilated infants[110] (Fig. 30.6) and is an integral part of family-centered care (FCC). A feasibility study of 20 LBW infants with a mean birth weight of 1390 ± 484 g who required respiratory support found that during kangaroo care, no significant changes in respiratory rate, temperature, or oxygen saturation were noted. No unplanned extubations were reported.[112] Practical issues during skin-to-skin holding include transfer techniques from bed/incubator to parent, selecting chairs that support the parent and infant comfortably, and monitoring during holding. Transfer techniques include carefully moving the baby to the seated parent or having the parent stand while the infant is placed on his or her chest, then the parent carefully lowers himself or herself with

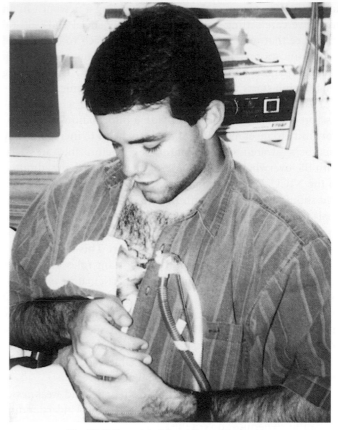

Fig. 30.6 Parent holding infant skin-to-skin.

the infant onto the chair. Some NICUs have invested in special lounge or reclining chairs that can be raised to the level of the infant's incubator, which then provide a comfortable way for the parent to relax during holding for prolonged periods. Carefully monitor all physiologic parameters during skin-to-skin holding to assess each infant's response to this valuable experience and to determine when nursing intervention is needed.

The knowledge level and comfort with skin-to-skin care among nurses and other health care providers have been identified as a barrier to the implementation of skin-to-skin holding.[113,114] Education programs to enhance knowledge and comfort should be undertaken to increase the utilization of skin-to-skin holding for infants receiving respiratory support.

CARE OF THE FAMILY

Providing support for the family is the responsibility of all members of the health care team, and that family should be viewed as an integral part of the team. Most NICUs have adopted an FCC approach to neonatal care that recognizes the importance of integrating family members in care decisions. FCC is based on principles of participation and partnership that come from empowering family members to be involved in their infant's care.[115] Providing open access to the unit for parents, having parents participate in infant caregiving, and maintaining open communication are basic principles of FCC.[116,117]

Having an infant who requires NICU care is an extremely stressful event for parents and extended family members. It is important to recognize the impact of having a newborn in an intensive care setting and to recognize the social and cultural influence that may shape the parents' approach to coping and communication. True FCC is built on a trusting relationship between parents and health care team members. That trusting relationship starts with open and honest communication.

Fostering parental partnership should begin when a high-risk pregnancy is identified. Providing information and an opportunity to meet members of the team helps to increase family members' awareness and comfort level before they are faced with the overwhelming situation of having their baby admitted to the NICU. Parents should receive an orientation to the unit and should be provided with written (and sometimes audiovisual) material that they can refer to. Material should include an overview of visiting policies, an introduction to members of the health care team, and contact information. This written material is the ideal place to reinforce important roles the parents can play, such as providing breast milk, participating in skin-to-skin holding, and helping to provide care for their infant. In many NICUs, parents are given the opportunity to participate in rounds at their infant's bedside and/or to meet with the team on a regular basis to discuss their infant's care. Where available, parent or peer-support groups are valuable, especially for families who do not have extended family nearby.[116,117]

Each family presents with unique strengths and weaknesses and has a varying capacity for coping in a crisis. Understanding the family dynamics and coping strategies will assist care providers in meeting the family "where it is at" and working together to build capacity for providing care for the family's infant.

CONCLUSION

In conclusion, the daily care of newborns who are receiving respiratory support involves knowledge that extends beyond pulmonary anatomy, physiology, and technology. Care of these infants requires advanced knowledge of multiple organ systems, precision in caregiving, and creative problem solving. Also critical to successful outcomes is attention to developmental care and FCC during this vulnerable period for infants and their families.

A complete reference list is available at https://expertconsult. inkling.com/.

KEY REFERENCES

6. Eriksson M, Campbell-Yeo M: Assessment of pain in newborn infants. Semin Fetal Neonatal Med 24(4), 2019.

12. Cummings JJ, Polin RA, Committee on Fetus and Newborn: Oxygen targeting in extremely low birth weight infants. Pediatrics 138(2):e20161576, 2016.

17. Maheshwari R, Tracy M, Badawi N, et al: Neonatal endotracheal intubation: how to make it more baby friendly. J Paediatr Child Health 52(5):480–486, 2016.

22. Miller-Barmak A, Riskin A, Hochwald O, et al: Oxygenation instability assessed by SpO_2 histograms during supine vs. prone position in very low birthweight infants receiving non-invasive respiratory support. J Pediatr. Epub June 29, 2020. S0022-3476 (20)30819–2.

26. de Bijl-Marcus K, Brouwer AJ, De Vries LS, et al: Neonatal care bundles are associated with a reduction in the incidence of intraventricular haemorrhage in preterm infants: a multicentre cohort study. Arch Dis Child Fetal Neonatal Ed 105(4):419–424, 2020.

28. Nasef N, Rashed HM, Aly H: Practical aspects on the use of non-invasive respiratory support in preterm infants. Int J Pediatr Adolesc Med 7(1):19–25, 2020.

30. Sahni R, Schiaratura M, Polin RA: Strategies for the prevention of continuous positive airway pressure failure. Semin Fetal Neonatal Med 21(3):196–203, 2016.

43. Klugman D, Melton K, Maynord PO, et al: Assessment of an unplanned extubation bundle to reduce unplanned extubations in critically ill neonates, infants, and children. JAMA Pediatr 174(6):e200268, 2020.

78. AWHONN: Neonatal Skin Care Evidence-based Clinical Practice guideline. 4th ed. Washington, DC, AWHONN, 2018.

87. Committee on Fetus and Newborn and Section of Anesthesiology and Pain Medicine: Prevention and management of procedural pain in the neonate: an update. Pediatrics 137(2):e20154271, 2016.

96. McPherson C, Inder T: Perinatal and neonatal use of sedation and analgesia. Semin Fetal Neonatal Med 22(5):314–320, 2017.

105. Griffiths N, Spence K, Loughran-Fowlds A, et al: Individualised developmental care for babies and parents in the NICU: evidence-based best practice guideline recommendations. Early Hum Dev 139:104840, 2019.

117. Davidson JE, Aslakson RA, Long AC, et al: Guidelines for family-centered care in the neonatal, pediatric, and adult ICU. Crit Care Med 45(1):103–128, 2017.

31

Nutritional Support

Laura D. Brown, Camilia R. Martin, and Sarah N. Taylor

KEY POINTS

- Nutrition and lung growth during the saccular and alveolar stage of development are closely interrelated. Poor nutritional delivery and growth disturbances in utero result in increased susceptibility to developing bronchopulmonary dysplasia (BPD), and preterm infants with BPD demonstrated poorer growth velocities, including reduced accretion of both lean mass and fat mass. Meticulous attention must be given to optimizing nutritional delivery, with balanced protein and energy, in these vulnerable patients.
- Energy intakes from enteral nutrition of 110 to 130 kcal/kg/day and from parenteral nutrition of 90 to 120 kcal/kg/day are required to support normal growth and metabolism in preterm infants, provided protein intake is adequate. Those infants with respiratory disease and those on mechanical ventilation have a higher energy expenditure and thus may require energy delivery on the higher end of the recommended ranges.
- Enteral feedings should begin as soon after birth as is safely possible in preterm and critically ill infants, including those who require assisted ventilation. Maternal or donor human milk, fortified with macronutrient supplements for preterm infants, is the preferred enteral feeding of choice.
- Few medical interventions offer as much advantage to preterm and critically ill infants as human milk feeding. Human milk stimulates the establishment of the commensal gastrointestinal (GI) microbiome, modulates the critical inflammatory balance of the immature GI tract, and provides hormones and growth factors to stimulate organ growth and health, including lung growth.

THE IMPORTANCE OF NUTRITION DURING CRITICAL STAGES OF LUNG DEVELOPMENT

Optimal nutritional support is required for the survival, good health, growth, and development of newborn infants who require intensive care, particularly those who require assisted ventilation. Most of these infants suffer disorders that place them at risk for poor nutrition as a result of increased metabolic rate, limited gastrointestinal function, and limited capacity for metabolic processing of nutrients. Hypoxia, circulatory insufficiency, fluid and electrolyte imbalance, acid-base disorders, and deficiencies in anabolic hormones also complicate the ability to sustain optimal growth. Furthermore, physiologically unstable preterm or term infants often face limitations in the tolerance and processing of enterally and parenterally delivered nutrients. As a result of poor nutrition, impaired somatic growth is common in these infants and exacerbates poor pulmonary and neurodevelopmental outcomes.[1]

Nutrition and lung growth during the saccular and alveolar stage of development are clearly interrelated.[2] During the prenatal period, conditions such as placental insufficiency that restrict nutrient delivery to the fetus result in intrauterine growth restriction (IUGR). Several studies have shown that the preterm infant with a history of IUGR is at higher risk for development of bronchopulmonary dysplasia (BPD) compared with the appropriately grown preterm infant.[3-9] IUGR also is an independent risk factor for higher airway resistance in infants[10] and lower forced expiratory volume and diffusion capacity in school aged children,[11] indicating that the effects of IUGR on lung function extend beyond the neonatal period. Animal studies in pregnant sheep have shown that lower nutrient delivery rates from placental insufficiency decrease alveolarization and vascular growth,[12] decrease total gas-exchange surface area,[12] and lead to a thicker pulmonary blood-air barrier due to a thickened basement membrane[13] in late gestation fetal lambs. Decreased alveoli per respiratory unit and thickened basement membranes were persistent in IUGR lambs at 8 weeks and 2 years after birth, which correlated with decreased pulmonary functional outcomes.[14,15]

In preterm infants, even those who are appropriately grown at the time of delivery, the saccular and alveolar stages of lung development occur after birth such that nutritional deficiencies during the postnatal period can impact lung growth and function. Extremely low birth weight (ELBW) preterm infants under 1000 g who demonstrated lower growth velocities relative to higher growth velocities had a higher rate of BPD.[1] Although there have been no randomized controlled trials on the effects of early nutrition on the risk of developing BPD,[16] there is evidence that improved nutritional status can provide beneficial effects for lung growth. Infants who received more nutritional support during the first 3 weeks of life (and who were less critically ill, defined as having required mechanical ventilation for <7 days) were less likely to develop moderate to severe BPD.[17] Severity of illness and early nutritional practices were both independently associated with morbidity, including BPD.[18] When energy and protein intakes over the first 7 to 27 days of life were measured in ELBW infants, higher energy and protein intakes were associated with a lower risk of BPD.[19] Poor intrauterine growth is an additive burden to poor pulmonary outcomes as a result of preterm birth.[10]

The most widely accepted standard for developing nutritional goals for preterm infants is the intrauterine growth rate of a fetus of corresponding postmenstrual age.[20] Intrauterine growth rates, body composition, and energy expenditure are all used to define the nutritional requirements of the healthy, growing preterm infant. For term infants, the growth rate and nutrient intakes of healthy breast-fed infants are used as the standard. Much less attention has been paid to how the physiology of illness, such as evolving BPD, affects growth, metabolism, and nutrient requirements.[21] For example, the goals of nutritional support for infants who require assisted ventilation are to prevent catabolism and exhaustion of endogenous energy resources, to achieve growth in lean body mass, and to promote healing, growth, and maturation of the lungs, brain, and other vital organs. These nutritional goals must be met without impairing respiratory gas exchange or tissue oxygen delivery. Thus, nutritional support for infants with respiratory distress syndrome (RDS) and BPD requires special consideration.

NUTRITIONAL REQUIREMENTS

Water Requirement

Water is a key element in nutritional management because energy, protein, and other nutrients cannot be delivered without water, and optimal water intake is important for all infants who require assisted ventilation.[22] Water is required for growth and is produced in small amounts as a by-product of cellular metabolism. Water comprises a large fraction of body weight in preterm and term infants,[23] declining after birth with improvement in renal function[24] triggered, at least in part, by atrial natriuretic peptide.[25] Body water balance and, thus, weight may not decrease, however, and in fact often increase with aggressive fluid intake from intravenous (IV) solutions. Normal infants with good kidney and lung function generally can tolerate high rates of IV fluid. In contrast, physiologically unstable infants with limited renal function who receive excessive water can accumulate fluid in the lung and develop compromised pulmonary function, which, in turn, increases the need for potentially injurious oxygen and ventilator support. Pulmonary edema caused by fluid overload can contribute to decreased pulmonary compliance and increased airway resistance.[26] A Cochrane review showed that restricted water intake reduced the risk of patent ductus arteriosus but did not reduce the risk of BPD in preterm infants.[27] The clinical trials included in this review, however, are over 20 years old and may not reflect current ventilatory practices. If fluid restriction is applied, the delivery of goal daily nutrients should not be compromised.

Insensible Water Loss

Preterm infants lose more water by evaporation because of greater surface area–to–body weight ratios, thinner and more permeable skin, dry ambient air, higher respiratory rates, and increased humidity gradient between the upper respiratory airway and the gas mixture they breathe. Antenatal corticosteroids given to promote fetal maturation reduce the insensible water loss (IWL) of preterm infants during the first few days of life, presumably by enhancing epidermal barrier function.[28] Several practices also have been shown to decrease IWL. Polyethylene occlusive skin wrapping reduces the IWL of infants under radiant warmers during resuscitation in the delivery room.[29] IWL has been reduced with improved humidification of incubators,[30] ventilators, and respiratory gas circuits used for

noninvasive ventilation, such as continuous positive airway pressure (CPAP), heated high-flow nasal cannula, or noninvasive positive pressure ventilation (NIPPV).[31] In addition to minimizing IWL, the use of heated, humidified gas during delivery room resuscitations and during transport to the neonatal intensive care unit (NICU) has been shown to improve admission temperature.[32]

Renal Function and Water Excretion

Fluid balance and renal function in the critically ill infant who requires assisted ventilation are important issues. Most preterm infants have an increase in urine volume on the second or third day of life,[33,34] which is accompanied by a rise in plasma atrial natriuretic peptide[35] and contraction of the extracellular water compartment.[25] Hypoxia or hypotension during the first week of life may compromise kidney function by causing tubular or cortical injury. During the anuric or oliguric phase of acute kidney injury (AKI), renal water excretion is reduced, and its allowance in the maintenance water calculation should be reduced accordingly. In the diuretic phase of AKI, water excretion through the kidney is increased. Data from the Assessment of Worldwide Acute Kidney Injury Epidemiology in Neonates (AWAKEN) study group show that the incidence of AKI (defined as an increase in serum creatinine of 0.3 mg/dL or >50% of the previous lowest value, or a urinary output of <1 mL/kg per hour on postnatal days 2–7) in preterm neonates under 36 weeks' gestational age was 30% and that AKI was associated with increased mortality and length of hospital stay.[36] RDS itself has been shown to be an independent predictor of AKI.[37] Furthermore, in both preterm[38] and term[39] neonates, those neonates with AKI were less likely to have negative fluid balance, and higher fluid balance on postnatal day 7 was independently associated with need for mechanical ventilation. Higher fluid intake and less weight loss in ELBW neonates during the first 10 days of life also were associated with an increased risk of BPD.[40] These findings indicate that careful attention to fluid balance might be an important means to reduce the incidence of BPD. However, fluid restriction must be balanced with providing adequate delivery of nutrition for growth and lung development.

There is no evidence, however, that renal function is affected by specific methods of assisted ventilation, such as conventional ventilation or high-frequency oscillation.[41] Furthermore, there is no evidence to support routine administration of diuretic therapy to promote diuresis in preterm infants with RDS.[42]

Energy Requirement

Energy from the diet that is not lost in the stool or urine (~10% of intake) is either expended for metabolism or stored in the body for growth. Energy is expended during rest (~50 kcal/kg/day for preterm infants) and also for activity, thermoregulation, postprandial or synthetic energy expenditure, and growth.[43] The energy expended during growth in human infants has been estimated to be 5.5 kcal/g of new tissue deposited for protein and 1.6 kcal/g for fat.[44] Estimates of the overall energy cost of growth range from about 2.9 to 6.0 kcal/g.[45] The energy cost of physical activity in healthy, preterm infants accounts for only about 3% of the total daily energy expenditure.[46]

TABLE 31.1 Energy, Protein, and Nutrient Requirements for Enterally Fed Preterm Infants

Nutrient	ADVISABLE INTAKE (PER KG/DAY)	
	<1000-g Infant	1000- to 1500-g Infant
Energy (kcal)	110–130	110–120
Protein (g)	3.3–4.3	3.0–4.0
Sodium (mg)	82	69
Potassium (mg)	98	86
Chloride (mg)	113	92
Calcium (mg)	150–220	120–200
Phosphorus (mg)	60–140	60–140
Magnesium (mg)	8–15	8–15
Iron (mg)	2.0–3.0	2.0–3.0
Zinc (mg)	1.0–3.0	1.0–3.0
Copper (mg)	0.2	0.2

Healthy preterm infants gain weight at rates similar to the fetus of corresponding postmenstrual age (15–20 g/kg/day). An average intake of 110 to 130 kcal/kg/day from preterm infant formula or fortified human milk and 90 to 120 kcal/kg/day for parenterally fed preterm infants because of better efficiency are generally sufficient to support normal growth and metabolism of very low birth weight (VLBW) preterm infants, provided protein intake is adequate (see Table 31.1).[43] This broad range of energy intake is designed to accommodate the needs of rapidly growing, ELBW infants, who may need higher energy delivery for growth, as well as larger, more mature preterm infants who may require less. Low energy intake (<100 kcal/kg/day) has been shown to increase the risk of severe retinopathy of prematurity (ROP) and BPD in extremely preterm infants.[19,47]

Energy expenditure is 15% to 25% higher in infants with respiratory disease such as apnea, RDS, and BPD and those on mechanical ventilation,[48,49] an important factor to consider when providing nutrition to this vulnerable population. Energy expenditure is increased during therapy with caffeine for apnea of prematurity.[50] Energy expenditure is increased with more severe RDS requiring higher levels of ventilatory support and oxygen administration, which together are associated with higher risk of BPD.[51-54] Spontaneously breathing infants with BPD also have increased rates of energy expenditure,[55-58] in conjunction with lower energy intake and poor weight gain.[59] Increased energy expenditure is not entirely attributed to increased work of breathing, however, as strategies implemented to improve pulmonary function do not necessarily decrease oxygen consumption.[60]

Targeting total energy delivery is a balance between sufficient but not excessive. If sufficient amounts of glucose and lipid are not able to be delivered when preterm infants are acutely ill, this can lead to a cumulative energy deficiency and require higher energy delivery to avoid postnatal growth failure during the convalescent phase of growth.[61] In the converse, infants receiving high energy intakes develop excess body fat without accelerating their gain in fat-free mass.[62-64]

Protein Requirement

The provision of parenteral or enteral protein soon after birth is essential to prevent negative nitrogen balance and promote protein accretion. Preterm infants have lower lean mass and higher body fat by postmenstrual age 40 weeks compared with normally growing fetuses at term.[65] Specifically, infants with BPD have decreased lean body mass, indicating that current levels of protein intake might be inadequate.[66,67] Providing an optimal balance of protein and energy is critically important to maximize lean tissue and organ growth.[62] The protein requirement of the healthy term infant in the first month of life is approximately 2.0 g/kg/day. Estimates of the protein requirement of preterm infants are higher than for term infants and range between 3 and 4 g/kg/day depending on gestational age (see Table 31.1).[49,68,69] These estimates are supported by experimental studies of protein turnover, nitrogen balance, tissue accretion, and growth.

Preterm infants, including those who require assisted ventilation, benefit from IV amino acids starting as soon after birth as possible.[70-72] In a retrospective analysis of a large multicenter database, early initiation of IV amino acids was associated with better growth, as assessed by gain in weight, length, and head circumference from birth to 36 weeks' postmenstrual age.[73] Although this study did not evaluate lung growth specifically, linear and head growth measurements are better indicators of lean tissue growth (including the lung) than weight measurements alone. Furthermore, the severity of BPD was reduced among infants who received more nutrition during the first 3 weeks after birth.[17] In adults, branched-chain amino acids such as leucine in IV nutrient solutions can modulate respiratory distress, decrease PCO_2 and stimulate the ventilatory response to hypercarbia, corresponding to an enhanced ventilatory sensitivity.[74] In preterm infants of about 30 weeks' gestation, providing higher concentrations of branched-chain amino acids in parenteral nutrition results in increased dynamic lung compliance, decreased pulmonary resistance, and fewer episodes of apnea,[75] findings also observed in neonatal piglet studies.[76] Finally, infants given a nutrient-enriched formula through 3 months of age demonstrate greater linear growth and lean and bone mass growth when fed higher intakes of protein, calcium, phosphorus, and zinc than are provided in standard formulas.[66]

Lipid Requirement

Lipids are important as a source of energy for metabolism and growth. Only two fatty acids are known to be essential (cannot be synthesized in the body) for humans: α-linolenic acid (ALA), an ω3 fatty acid (18:3ω3), and linoleic acid (LA), an ω6 fatty acid (18:2ω6). These two essential fatty acids are metabolized downstream into two biologically important very long chain polyunsaturated fatty acids (LC-PUFAs) of docosahexaenoic acid (DHA, 22:6ω3) and arachidonic acid (ARA, 20:4ω6). DHA and ARA play particularly important biological roles in development as immune modulators and components of membrane phospholipids and are essential for normal development of the central nervous system.[77,78] In preterm infants, however, there is a reduced ability and/or lower efficiency to adequately metabolize the essential fatty acids to DHA and ARA.[79] Given the biological importance of these fatty acids and the fact that preterm infants have insufficient capacity for de novo synthesis of downstream very long chain fatty acids, even despite the provision of the essential fatty acids, DHA and ARA are often referred to as conditionally essential for the preterm infant. Like all humans, it is required that preterm infants receive the essential fatty acids in their diet. Recommendations also have been proposed to supplement the conditionally essential fatty acids of DHA and ARA in the diet to minimize the postnatal deficiency of these fatty acids;[78] however, the ideal preparation, dosing, and health benefit of a supplemental strategy has not been determined.

During the parenteral phase of nutrition, the dietary requirement for the essential fatty acids can be met by providing 1.0 g/kg/day intake in the form of an 100% soybean oil IV lipid emulsion.[80] If a mixed oil lipid emulsion (i.e., a lipid emulsion with multiple oil sources including one or more of olive oil, medium-chain triglycerides, and/or fish oil in addition to soybean oil) is used, it is recommended that 2.5 g/kg/day intake is provided given the lower content of soybean oil.[81,82] The type of IV lipid emulsion to use as part of early provision of maintenance parenteral emulsion has emerged as a controversial decision. The use of either a 100% soybean oil or a mixed oil solution each possess pros and cons. Soybean oil emulsions have been implicated in detrimental effects on pulmonary gas exchange and hemodynamics,[83,84] although a metaanalysis of this practice did not show beneficial or adverse effects on growth, death, or chronic lung disease (CLD).[85] In small studies using mixed oil emulsions, a decreased incidence of BPD was found in the infants receiving fish oil–containing lipid emulsions compared with infants receiving 100% soybean oil,[86-88] but this conclusion failed to be a robust, significant finding in a meta-analysis of the data.[89] Potentially concerning is the reduction in ARA levels with fish oil–based emulsions[90,91] as low systemic levels of ARA have been linked to nosocomial sepsis and ROP.[92,93] Most importantly, providing a parenteral lipid emulsion is a key component of parenteral feeding regimens for infants who require assisted ventilation and provides an important source of energy during the early postnatal period that may help reduce the vulnerability to chronic lung injury.[17,64]

For preterm infants, a reasonable range of fat intake during the enteral phase of nutrition is 4.8 to 6.6 g of fat per 100 kcal (40% to 55% of energy intake).[49] Mother's own milk and formulas contain the essential fatty acids and DHA and ARA. Mother's milk though, unlike formula, has lipase, which aids the preterm infant in the hydrolysis and absorption of these lipids. In the absence of lipase, preterm infants demonstrate an impaired absorption of fat and fatty acids, specifically for the fatty acids greater than 14 carbons in length.[94] This includes the conditionally essential fatty acids of DHA and ARA. Pasteurization of human milk destroys the lipase, and thus, the incomplete absorption of fats and fatty acids can be seen with donor milk as well.[95]

Despite the known biological importance of DHA and ARA in fetal development, especially of the neural tissues of the brain and eye, there is no evidence from clinical trials that adding LC-PUFAs to commercial term infant formulas confers benefits.[96] Based on theoretical benefits that they could improve visual acuity,[97] neurodevelopmental outcomes,[98] and lung development[99]

and on evidence from studies that show no harm,[77] they are commonly added to commercial infant formulas. It might be that LC-PUFA requirements for ELBW infants are much higher than what is seen in term breast milk; thus, higher supplemental doses of DHA might be of greater benefit and require further investigation.[78] However, despite a clinical association with decreased DHA and ARA levels in preterm infants and an increased risk of BPD,[92] a recent clinical trial of DHA supplementation found that the risk of BPD and/or death was actually increased compared with the control group.[100] Thus, it is currently not recommended to add additional DHA or ARA beyond what is already present in human milk and formula diets.

There are several physiologically relevant reasons as to why DHA- and ARA-supplemented diets have not shown health benefits in the preterm infant, including (1) the presence of developmental exocrine pancreatic insufficiency and decreased primary bile acid pools, limiting lipid hydrolysis and absorption; (2) an incomplete understanding of the necessary target dose to achieve adequate tissue levels of these fatty acids; and (3) an incomplete understanding of the desirable fatty acid composition or blend to achieve optimal balance. The biological potential of long chain fatty acids is mediated by the relative presence of both DHA and ARA, and the lack of benefit in some studies may be attributed to supplementing one fatty acid, typically DHA, without the other, ARA.

Carbohydrate Requirement

Approximately half of an infant's energy needs are normally provided by carbohydrate metabolism. Moreover, glucose is the primary energy source for brain metabolism. In the preterm infant, glucose is largely derived from exogenous carbohydrate sources once glycogenolysis has exhausted stored hepatic glucose. The normal glucose utilization rate in the term newborn is 3 to 5 mg/kg/min, but slightly higher, 5 to 7 mg/kg/min, in preterm infants.[101,102] Maintenance of normal plasma glucose concentrations is important, as the vital organs (brain and heart) take up glucose according to plasma concentration and not IV infusion rates or rates of hepatic glucose production. When plasma glucose concentrations decline, the newborn brain may use ketone bodies as additional energy sources, but these are usually limited in very preterm and IUGR infants who have low body stores of fat.[103]

Preterm and stressed infants are at risk for developing hyperglycemia, especially those with respiratory distress, mechanical ventilation, and restricted cardiac output and circulation. Such infants often are intermittently hypoxic, which adds to increased glucagon, adrenaline, and glucocorticoid secretion. These stress-reactive hormones reduce insulin secretion and insulin action and promote glucose production from both glycogenolysis (acutely) and gluconeogenesis (over a sustained period). They also contribute to protein breakdown. Hyperglycemia leads to increased cellular allostatic load, in which excess carbon cannot be fully oxidized, producing increased amounts of reactive oxygen species that cause cellular breakdown (Box 31.1).[104]

Other complications of hyperglycemia frequently develop in neonates when maximal glucose oxidative capacity (>12 mg/kg/min) is exceeded, including increased energy expenditure

BOX 31.1 Toxicity From Hyperglycemia and Excess Allostatic Load

Excess glucose, cortisol, and mitochondrial allostatic load (acute as well as chronic)
Increased cortisol and catecholamine levels
Hyperglycemia
Increased insulin[a]
Increased cell glucose uptake
Increased mitochondrial allostatic load
Mitochondrial fragmentation
Increased reactive oxygen species production
Accumulation of mitochondrial DNA damage
Decreased energy-producing capacity
Increased susceptibility to cell death
Cellular dysfunction
Oxidative stress
Molecular damage
Telomere shortening
Cell loss, apoptosis
Energy deficiency
Systemic Inflammation
Increased circulating proinflammatory cytokines

[a]Also antiinflammatory, by suppressing proinflammatory transcription factors (nuclear factor B, activator protein-1, and early growth response-1).

(glucose-to-fat synthesis is energy expensive), increased oxygen consumption (and hypoxia), increased carbon dioxide production,[58,105] increased fat deposition in excess of lean mass, and increased fatty infiltration of heart and liver.[106,107] Such problems may underlie the increased morbidity and mortality in infants with severe and/or persistent hyperglycemia.[108]

Mechanisms for enteral carbohydrate digestion and absorption mature in a defined sequence in the human fetus. Sucrase, maltase, and isomaltase are usually fully active by 24 to 28 weeks' gestation, but lactase lags behind the others and is not fully active until term.[109] For this reason, most preterm formulas contain lower lactose content than that in human milk. However, there is evidence that intestinal lactase activity increases to adequate functional levels within a few days after the initiation of enteral feedings, even in infants born as early as 28 weeks' gestation.[110,111] Furthermore, despite the late gestational rise in lactase activity, both term and preterm infants seem to tolerate the carbohydrates in human milk and commercial formulas quite well. Activity of pancreatic amylase remains low until after term.[109] Salivary amylase activity is present even in VLBW preterm infants.[112]

Other carbohydrates such as mannose and inositol, as well as oligosaccharides (prebiotics), play an important role in nutrition and organ development for the preterm infant. Mannose is an essential carbohydrate for protein glycosylation and normal neural development.[113] Mannose is a component of oligosaccharides, which contribute to the establishment of nonpathogenic intestinal flora and play a major role in intestinal health for both term and preterm infants.[114] Inositol is particularly important for lung development, as it is integral in the formation of surfactant phospholipid production. Inositol is present in high concentrations in human milk and can be synthesized by newborn infants of gestational age 33 weeks or more.[115] Early studies showed that lower inositol concentrations were associated with more severe RDS[116] and that inositol supplementation may reduce the incidence of RDS.[117] However, a large, randomized controlled trial of inositol supplementation in preterm infants under 27 weeks' gestational age was terminated because of an increased mortality rate in the myo-inositol supplemented group compared with placebo and no difference in the incidence of BPD between groups.[118]

Mineral Requirements

Recommended sodium, potassium, and chloride requirements are shown in Table 31.1, with the caveat that sodium requirements vary based on gestational age at birth and postnatal age.[119] The requirement of sodium is higher for preterm infants, as the immature kidney lacks fully functional regulatory systems, including the inability to retain salt.[120] Urinary excretion of electrolytes depends on intake. Typical urinary concentrations of sodium are 20 to 40 mmol/L and of potassium are 10 to 30 mmol/L.[22] When an infant is receiving diuretic therapy, urinary sodium concentrations can reach 70 mmol/L or higher, and these large losses must be considered when electrolyte needs are assessed.[121] This is particularly important as insufficient sodium intake impairs longitudinal growth and weight gain; thus, sufficient sodium intake should be provided to maintain serum sodium values between 135 and 140 mEq/L to promote adequate growth early in life.[119] A recent randomized controlled trial of sodium supplementation in the first month of life in preterm infants born less than 32 weeks' gestational age showed improvement in weight gain, but not length or head circumference gain.[122] The outcomes of sodium supplementation as they relate to effects on lung function in preterm infants are lacking.

The recommended intakes of calcium and phosphorus depend on the route of administration. If given enterally, absorption rates might be limiting. The fraction of calcium absorbed depends on the type of milk or formula and the infant's gestational and postnatal age. If given parenterally, the limits of mineral solubility become a significant factor. Adequate enteral intake of calcium for term infants in the first 6 months of life is about 70 mg/kg/day. The calcium requirement for ELBW preterm infants is much higher, 150 to 220 mg/kg/day, because of more active bone formation and remodeling (see Table 31.1).[123,124] Adequate enteral intake of phosphorus for term infants is about 30 mg/kg/day but is higher for preterm infants (60–140 mg/kg/day) to ensure adequate bone mineralization. Fortification of human milk is necessary to ensure adequate intakes of calcium and phosphorus to preterm infants, particularly with mature mother's milk and donor milk.[125,126] Recommended IV intakes of calcium and phosphorus are lower than enteral requirements, ranging from 65 to 100 mg/kg/day for calcium and 50 to 80 mg/kg/day for phosphorus.[123] The risk factors in preterm infants for calcium and phosphorus deficiency and subsequent rickets are gestational age less than 27 weeks or birth weight less than 1000 g, long-term parenteral nutrition (>4–5 weeks), severe BPD requiring diuretics and fluid restriction, long-term steroid treatment, a history of necrotizing enterocolitis (NEC), and intolerance to enteral formula or fortified human milk.[124]

Adequate intake of magnesium for enterally fed term and preterm infants is about 10 mg/kg/day (see Table 31.1). IV intake of 7 to 10 mg/kg/day is recommended for infants receiving total parenteral nutrition (TPN) for prolonged periods.[123]

Iron intake should be 2 to 3 mg/kg/day beginning at 2 weeks of age in growing preterm infants who are enterally fed[127] but increased to 5 mg/kg/day for some preterm infants with anemia of prematurity who are receiving recombinant erythropoietin.[80] Iron supplementation is required to counter anemia of prematurity and to ensure adequate iron supply to the growing brain, as iron is preferentially taken up by red blood cells.[127] Meta-analyses have shown that supplementation with iron for more than 8 weeks resulted in increased hemoglobin and ferritin concentrations and a reduction in iron deficiency and anemia but highlighted the need for long-term effects of supplementation on functional health outcomes.[128,129] One study found improved neurocognitive outcomes when iron supplements were started at 2 weeks versus 8 weeks after birth.[130] Risk of iron overload and toxicity from unnecessary iron supplementation following red blood cell transfusions also must be considered;[131] commonly, iron supplementation is delayed for 2 weeks after a transfusion. Each red blood cell transfusion in preterm infants typically adds 8 mg/kg iron, and hepatic iron stores as well as serum ferritin concentrations are highly correlated to the number of blood transfusions received.[132,133] Because individual infants vary considerably in their hematocrit at birth, delayed cord blood clamping, transfusions, blood sampling, and erythropoietin treatment, it is helpful to monitor their iron status and need for iron supplementation by following serum ferritin concentrations.[132]

The advisable enteral intakes of zinc are 1 to 3 mg/kg/day (Table 31.1). Zinc has been shown to improve growth, specifically in ELBW preterm infants with CLD receiving human milk.[134] The recommended enteral intake of copper is 0.2 mg/kg/day. Other minerals such as selenium, manganese, iodine, chromium, and molybdenum are also required in trace amounts.[135]

Vitamin Requirements

Vitamin A is essential for growth and differentiation of epithelial tissues, including those in the lung. Preterm infants have low stores of vitamin A at birth, and preterm infants with lung disease have lower plasma vitamin A levels than those without lung disease.[136] Thus, vitamin A deficiency may contribute to the development of BPD. A large randomized clinical trial showed a reduction in the risk of death or BPD with vitamin A supplementation, 5000 IU given intramuscularly three times a week for 4 weeks.[137] A systematic review of eight clinical trials of vitamin A supplementation to preterm infants confirmed the beneficial effect of vitamin A in reducing the risk of death or oxygen requirement at 1 month of age by 7% (relative risk, 0.93; 95% confidence interval, 0.88–0.99).[138] Neurodevelopmental assessment of surviving infants showed no differences between groups at 18 to 22 months' corrected age.[139] The number needed to treat was 20 to allow survival of one more infant without BPD. In the review, other morbidities and mortality

TABLE 31.2 Vitamin and Mineral Requirements for Preterm Infants	
	Advisable Intake (per day)
Vitamin A	400–3330 IU/kg
Vitamin D	400–1000 IU
Vitamin E	3.3–16.4 IU/kg
Vitamin K	4.4–28 μg/kg
Vitamin C	20–55 mg/kg
Thiamin (B_1)	140–300 μg/kg
Riboflavin (B_2)	200–400 μg/kg
Niacin (B_3)	1.0–5.5 mg/kg
Pyridoxine (B_6)	50–300 μg/kg
Biotin	1.7–16.5 μg/kg
Pantothenic acid	0.5–2.1 mg
Folic acid	35–100 μg
Cobalamin (B_{12})	0.1–0.8 μg/kg

were not significantly reduced by vitamin A supplementation. Despite its efficacy, vitamin A supplementation has not become standard practice,[140] in part because of the need for repeated intramuscular injections and cost.

Vitamin D is essential for bone health. As with other fat-soluble vitamins, the body stores of vitamin D are low at birth, especially in preterm infants.[141] Infants who require assisted ventilation have no exposure to ultraviolet light in the hospital and limited exposure after discharge and thus have minimal cutaneous synthesis of vitamin D. The recommended enteral intake of vitamin D is 400 to 1000 IU per day (Table 31.2).[123,124,142] A dose of 400 IU per day has been shown to maintain adequate (>50 nmol/L) serum concentrations of vitamin D in the majority of preterm infants.[143] However, higher doses (800–1000 IU per day) have been recommended for vitamin D–deficient newborns.[49,142] The major circulating metabolite of vitamin D after its 25-hydroxylation in the liver is 25-hydroxyvitamin D. Levels may be monitored in infants at risk for developing rickets, including those infants with extreme prematurity, short bowel syndrome, cholestasis, and long-term exposure to diuretics and/or steroids. The potential role of vitamin D in the protection against the development of BPD is currently being investigated.[144-146]

Vitamin E is a natural antioxidant in the body. It protects lipid-containing cell membranes against oxidative injury and is thought to play a role in preventing neonatal oxygen toxicity. The recommended enteral vitamin E intake, 3.3 to 16.4 IU/kg/day, is sufficient to compensate for variation in vitamin E absorption and distribution and in the intake of other nutrients known to influence vitamin E requirement, such as iron and LC-PUFAs.[135] The amount of vitamin E required to prevent lipid peroxidation in vulnerable tissues depends on the PUFA content of the tissues and diet.[147] Thus, it also is advisable to keep the dietary ratio of vitamin E to PUFAs at or above the level of 0.6 mg of d-α-tocopherol (0.9 IU) per gram of PUFAs.[147] Recommended IV doses of vitamin E are 2.8 IU/kg/day as α-tocopheryl acetate.[148] Although studies have shown efficacy of vitamin E supplementation in reducing the risk of ROP and intraventricular hemorrhage, excessive intake of vitamin E has the potential for severe toxicity including risk of sepsis.[149] Consequently, routine administration of high-dose vitamin E supplements is not recommended, even though a single enteral dose of vitamin E at birth may help correct the relative vitamin E deficiency that has been found in some VLBW preterm infants in the first days of life.[150]

Vitamin K is essential to prevent hemorrhagic disease of the newborn in the first weeks of life.[151,152] A single dose of intramuscular vitamin K (1.0 mg) is effective in the prevention of classic hemorrhagic disease of the newborn.[153] Vitamin K prophylaxis also is recommended for the preterm newborn, although further research on appropriate dose is warranted.[154] Subsequent supplementation with vitamin K is necessary to prevent deficiency, especially for critically ill infants, who often receive broad-spectrum antibiotics (reducing vitamin K synthesis by gut bacteria) and may have other abnormalities of hemostasis or hepatic function.

Infants with fat malabsorption because of cholestatic liver disease or short bowel syndrome are at risk for developing fat-soluble vitamin deficiency. Thus, additional fat soluble vitamin supplementation may be necessary in these patients. Additional nutrients, such as water-soluble vitamins and other trace substances, are required for recovery and healthy growth of preterm infants (see Table 31.2).

PARENTERAL NUTRITION

Parenteral nutritional support is essential for providing a continuous supply of both macro- and micronutrients to the preterm infant starting immediately after birth and as enteral feedings are being advanced, particularly in those infants who cannot tolerate enteral feedings. However, parenteral nutrition requires IV access. Indwelling short polyvinyl chloride catheters provide safe and convenient access to the peripheral venous circulation. The most common significant complication of peripheral IV infusions is tissue necrosis at the site of extravasation.[155] The infusion site must be carefully observed to detect extravasation as soon as possible. Infusions with glucose concentrations greater than 12.5 g/dL should be avoided in peripheral veins.

Central vein catheters, including umbilical vein and percutaneously inserted central catheters, are used for longer-term IV delivery of nutrients to newborn infants. Prevention strategies, including central catheter line care bundles and removing lines as soon as possible, are essential to reduce rates of line sepsis and other complications such as thrombosis or extravasation of infused fluid into the pleural or pericardial space.[156,157] The surgically placed central vein catheter is typically used for infants who have short bowel syndrome from gastrointestinal malformations or NEC and for whom extensively prolonged parenteral nutrition is anticipated.

Composition of Total Parenteral Nutrition

Preterm infants who are ill enough to require assisted ventilation should receive IV nutrition as soon as possible after birth. The initial infusion should consist of adequate energy and amino acids to improve protein balance.[158,159] Most NICUs now use a "starter" TPN solution that provides 2–3 g/kg/day of amino acids in addition to 10% dextrose. A relative restriction

of water intake during the first day or two of life allows for a physiologic state of negative water and sodium balance that accompanies the mobilization of extracellular water.[22] A standard starting rate for IV fluids is 80 mL/kg/day, with titration of the infusion rate based on environmental humidity, use of humidified air-oxygen mixtures in ventilator or CPAP circuits, and when the onset of diuresis and natriuresis develops.[34]

Full IV amino acid nutrition, including carbohydrate, protein, minerals, and vitamins, should be started as soon as possible after birth using standard guidelines.[145] To approximate intrauterine lean mass protein accretion and growth, total energy delivery should be 90 to 120 kcal/kg/day, which is slightly less than enteral requirements as no energy has to be added for enteral absorption.[160] Dextrose concentration should be titrated to deliver a glucose infusion rate of 6 to 8 mg/kg/min, with rates not to exceed 12 mg/kg/min and/or 50% of total caloric delivery. Protein in the form of amino acid solutions should range from 3 to 3.5 g/kg/day, depending on the gestational age of the neonate.[161] Lipid emulsions should be delivered in the range of 2 to 3 g/kg/day, with rates not to exceed 40% of total caloric delivery.[162] The standard IV lipid product is derived from soybean oil; although it does contain the essential fatty acids, LA and ALA, it lacks their downstream products, AA, eicosapentaenoic acid (EPA), and DHA. This product also contains relatively large amounts of phytosterols, which induce hepatic inflammation and lead to cholestasis and parenteral nutrition–associated liver disease (PNALD).[163] Lipid emulsions must be started within the first few days of life at a minimum dose of 1.0 g/kg/day to avoid essential fatty acid deficiency in infants who cannot be fed enterally. The maximum infusion rate should not exceed 3 g/kg/day, and the infusion is usually administered over 20 or more hours each day. Hypertriglyceridemia and/or hyperglycemia can result from parenteral lipid administration.[164] Plasma triglyceride levels should be monitored periodically, especially in ELBW infants, to assess lipid tolerance. Additionally, IV lipid intake may be associated with decreased binding affinity of bilirubin for plasma protein and increased free bilirubin concentration in VLBW preterm infants.[165]

Newer generation lipid emulsions that contain fish oil as one component of their oil blend contain ω3 LC-PUFAs such as EPA and DHA and ω6 LC-PUFAs such as ARA. However, despite the presence of these downstream LC-PUFAs, the use of mixed oil lipid emulsions has not shown to correct the postnatal fatty acid deficits in DHA and ARA seen in the early postnatal period and no clear health benefits have been documented in a meta-analysis of the clinical trial data published to date.[165] The use of mixed oil emulsions in certain circumstances such as ameliorating the risk of development and progression of PNALD also has not shown a clear benefit,[166] but a large, prospective, clinical trial is still under investigation (ClinicalTrials.gov Identifier: NCT02412566).[167-171]

Electrolytes, calcium, magnesium, and phosphorus are individually tailored in daily TPN. Sodium is usually given as sodium chloride or sodium acetate, depending on the degree of metabolic acidosis, and usually started on day 2 or 3, depending on degree of diuresis, natriuresis, fluid balance, and serum sodium concentrations.[172] Potassium chloride or acetate also is added to the infusate, provided the serum potassium concentration is normal and adequate urine flow is established. IV calcium and phosphorus supplementation should be started in high-risk infants as soon as possible after birth, given high rates of calcium and phosphorus accretion that occur normally in the third trimester.[173] The Ca/P ratio should be kept at 1:1 on a molar basis and 1.3:1 on a mg/mg basis to maximize accretion of both minerals during the first week of life. After the first week, the Ca/P ratio should be 1.3:1 on a molar basis and 1.6:1 on a mg/mg basis to provide the best supply of calcium and phosphorus for bone mineralization. Caution should be used if calcium is infused into a peripheral IV catheter, as tissue necrosis and sloughing can occur. Some intensive care units avoid peripheral calcium administration entirely except in emergencies.

ENTERAL NUTRITION

Most preterm infants, even those who require assisted ventilation, can and should be fed enterally by gavage tube, starting as soon as possible after birth, using the mother's own colostrum and subsequent maternal or donor human milk. Most early feeding protocols start with minimal enteral feedings, or small amounts (<24 mL/kg/day) of trophic feedings for intestinal priming and advancing as tolerated over several days toward full enteral feeding.

Advantages of Enteral Nutrition

Enteral feeding provides nutrients to support growth and metabolism but also, even in very small amounts, promotes intestinal development and function.[174] Feeding stimulates secretion of gut hormones and regulatory peptides,[175] motility,[176] and intestinal growth.[177] These effects are most prominent with feeding of maternal milk,[177] which also contributes to gut health by facilitating and augmenting the innate gut immune system[178] and establishing a more normal gut microbiome, which is increasingly being recognized as essential for both short- and long-term health.[179-181] Enteral feeding, even in small amounts, helps to prevent the cholestasis that often develops with TPN.[182]

Enteral feedings are contraindicated in those infants with active NEC or hemodynamic instability (marked hypotension). Caution must be exercised when considering enteral feeding of infants with poor intestinal motility or ileus, such as those who are postoperative, on extracorporeal membrane oxygenation, or if there is concern for compromised intestinal perfusion such as with congenital heart disease. Use of paralytics, per se, is not an absolute contraindication to enteral feeding because nondepolarizing neuromuscular blocking agents block transmission at the neuromuscular junction in skeletal muscle[183] but not in smooth muscle.

Methods of Gavage Feeding

Gavage feedings are indicated in infants who are unable to be fed by nipple or in infants requiring tracheal intubation, noninvasive ventilation, or higher levels of CPAP. Either oral or nasal feeding tubes can be used. Nasal tubes are easier to secure. Nasal feeding tubes partially obstruct the infant's airway and may not be feasible for those infants requiring CPAP, but they offer no disadvantage for infants who are intubated. Those infants who require noninvasive ventilation, such as single-level support with CPAP and heated high-flow nasal cannula or bilevel support with NIPPV, may have associated gaseous abdominal distension, commonly termed as "CPAP belly."[184] Investigation into how noninvasive ventilation might impact mesenteric flow, gastric emptying, and feeding tolerance has been relatively limited and somewhat conflicting.[185]

Intermittent ("bolus") gavage feeding at 2- or 3-hour intervals is the most commonly used method for enteral feeding. An alternative method of intragastric feeding is to infuse the milk or formula continuously through an indwelling nasogastric or orogastric tube at a constant rate controlled by an infusion pump. This method may offer the advantage of allowing greater volumes to be absorbed without compromising tidal volume and minute ventilation in preterm infants.[186] Unpredictable nutrient and energy delivery, however, is a significant problem with continuous feeding, because human milk fat separates from the nonfat milk and is left in the tubing or syringe, along with fat-soluble vitamins and calcium.[187,188] This problem can be minimized by positioning the infusion pump so that the opening of the syringe is pointed upward, ensuring that the fat is still delivered even if it separates, and by shortening the length of the extension tubing. Analysis of clinical trials did not find consistent differences in the effectiveness of continuous versus intermittent bolus intragastric feeding in terms of feeding intolerance, duration of hospitalization, growth outcomes, and risk of NEC.[189]

For most infants, intragastric feedings are preferred to transpyloric feedings, or a feeding tube positioned in the duodenum or jejunum. Transpyloric feeding is technically more difficult and requires x-ray or ultrasound confirmation of tube placement, and some evidence of harm exists, including gastrointestinal (GI) disturbances and mortality.[190] There also is risk of fat malabsorption when bypassing the stomach and upper portion of the duodenum. This technique, therefore, is not recommended as a primary feeding method for ventilated infants and should be restricted to short-term use in those infants who cannot tolerate gastric feedings because of excessive gastroesophageal reflux with aspiration, pneumonia, and apnea.

Nonnutritive sucking of a pacifier during gavage feedings has been tested as a way of compensating for the lack of oral stimulation in tube-fed infants. A systematic review based on published studies showed improvements with the transition from gavage to full oral feeding, transition from start of oral feeding to full oral feeding, and length of hospital stay with nonnutritive sucking.[191] When an infant no longer requires mechanical ventilation or CPAP, has achieved stable cardiorespiratory status, and has demonstrated adequate sucking and swallowing of secretions, nipple feedings may be introduced. The transition to oral feedings typically requires more time for infants who required assisted ventilation and those who were most preterm at birth.[192]

Minimal Enteral Feedings and Enteral Feeding Advancement

Low-volume enteral feedings (<24 mL/kg/day; "minimal enteral feeding," "gastrointestinal priming," or "trophic feeds") should be started as soon as possible after birth, preferably with maternal colostrum. Minimal enteral feedings over a short but defined period of time promote GI development, motility, and function in the preterm infant and can improve growth and time to reach full enteral feedings.[193-196] Minimal enteral feeding has not been shown to increase the risk of NEC.[197] Nearly all studies support the use of minimal enteral feedings compared with enteral fasting, although an evaluation of the current literature could not define specific benefits or exclude harmful effects of trophic enteral feedings for VLBW infants.[198] Studies that compare a period of trophic enteral feedings to immediate but slow advancement of enteral feedings are more limited.[199] The duration that minimal enteral feeds are provided depends on several factors, including degree of prematurity, presence of intestinal underperfusion in utero (such as in the IUGR infant), degree of perinatal hypoxic-ischemic injury, or need for medications after birth that might reduce intestinal perfusion (inotropic support, indomethacin).

Enteral feeding advancement is usually by 15 to 40 mL/kg/day. No advantage has been demonstrated in terms of protection from NEC by slower (15–20 mL/kg/day) versus faster (30–40 mL/kg/day) feeding advancement in VLBW preterm infants, ELBW infants, or IUGR infants with antenatal absent or reversed end-diastolic flow, particularly when fed with mother's milk or donor milk.[200] Furthermore, a recent trial of over 2000 VLBW infants randomized to receive either a slower (18 mL/kg/day) or faster (30 ml/kg/day) increment of enteral feedings showed no difference in survival without moderate or severe neurodevelopmental disability at 24 months.[201] If the enteral feeding advancement at an unnecessarily slow rate spans several days, this method must be combined with parenteral nutrition, results in several days of delay in establishing full enteral feeds, and may increase the risk of invasive infection.

Screening gastric residual volumes before every feeding has historically been used as a sign of worsening feeding intolerance, but avoidance of this routine practice was associated with earlier attainment of full enteral feedings without increasing risk for NEC.[202] Full enteral feedings (approximately 140–160 mL/kg/day, depending on caloric density) usually can be achieved over 5 to 7 days.

Human Milk

Few medical interventions offer as much advantage to preterm and critically ill infants as human milk feeding. Human milk stimulates the establishment of the commensal GI microbiome, modulates the critical inflammatory balance of the immature GI tract, and provides hormones and growth factors to stimulate organ growth and health.[203-210] The American Academy of Pediatrics states that human milk is the recommended basis of nutrition for the preterm infant.[211] The most compelling early benefit of human milk is its dose-related protective effect against NEC in preterm infants.[212-215] The most important long-term benefit is the favorable impact of human milk feeding on neurodevelopmental outcome.[216-224] Specific to respiratory outcomes, studies have demonstrated a decrease in BPD associated with mother's milk intake,[225] but this has not been observed in a systematic review of the literature.[226]

With improved prenatal education regarding the benefits of mother's milk, more women and women of diverse backgrounds are choosing to breastfeed.[227] NICU care should be designed to sustain maternal lactation goals. Thus, good lactation support services are required. These services should include parent education and information, electric breast pumps, convenient pumping and storage facilities, and the services of trained lactation specialists. The factors most associated with sustaining a maternal milk supply are milk expression by 6 hours postbirth, pumping both breasts simultaneously, expressing milk at least 5 times per day, producing 500 mL per day by postnatal day 10, and maintaining a NICU environment with adequate lactation support especially through education of nursing staff.[228-231]

Mothers of infants who require intensive care including assisted ventilation should be strongly encouraged to provide their milk for their infants. The importance of mother's milk can be emphasized early, even for ventilated infants through gavage feeding but also through oral immune therapy.[232] Oral immune therapy is the placement of mother's milk on the infant's buccal mucosa and is best performed with a syringe.[233] The practice is associated with a shorter duration to full enteral feeds and increased urinary immune markers, potentially demonstrating a systemic immune benefit.[234]

Donor Human Milk

Donor human milk is a pasteurized product from accredited milk banks. It is used when maternal milk is insufficient or unavailable, because of the multitude of benefits associated with the use of human milk in preterm infants as described earlier.[235] Donor milk is pasteurized to prevent the transmission of infection in the milk, but pasteurization also affects beneficial components of human milk. For example, enzymes such as lysozyme are inactivated and immune-functioning proteins such as immunoglobulins and lactoferrin are decreased.[236] Furthermore, donor human milk used for preterm infants commonly is donated by women who delivered full-term infants and from a later stage of lactation, which means this milk is lower in immune-functioning components even before pasteurization. Despite these differences in immune activity, when compared with preterm infant formula feeding, donor human milk is associated with significantly lower risk for NEC.[237] Therefore, infants should preferentially be fed mother's milk. When mother's milk is not available, VLBW preterm infants should be fed donor human milk instead of formula during the time that the infant is most at risk for NEC, which is commonly until 34 weeks' gestational age. When using donor human milk, attention should be given to nutrient fortification because infant growth can falter on donor human milk compared with formula. This likely is owing to less fat content, because (1) milk from mothers who delivered term infants contains less energy, specifically fat; (2) fat is lost during milk processing as it adheres to plastic containers; and (3) bile salt-stimulated lipase is inactivated during pasteurization.[236,238-240] Thus, close attention must be paid to appropriate fortification of donor human milk to meet the nutritional requirements for optimal growth of preterm infants.

Human Milk Fortification

Carefully controlled randomized trials demonstrate that the preterm infant will not grow at the normal rate of fetal growth if fed human milk alone. Multicomponent fortification of human milk is required for preterm infants to meet their increased daily requirements of energy, protein, vitamins, and minerals.[241] However, commercially available multicomponent fortifiers may provide inadequate and/or excess doses of specific vitamins and minerals, and clinicians should be aware of the concentrations of components when providing multicomponent fortification.[242] With new methods to analyze human milk macronutrients in the clinical setting, additional fortification may be added depending on the macronutrient concentrations in mother's milk or donor human milk to achieve specific intake, otherwise known as targeted fortification.[243] Further investigation is required to identify how targeted fortification can be performed to optimize benefit and efficiency.

Available multicomponent fortifiers differ in form (liquid vs. powder), protein concentration, protein state (hydrolyzed vs. intact), protein source (human vs. bovine), and other nutrients, most notably iron. No specific multicomponent fortifier has been identified as superior. In a meta-analysis, when receiving fortified human milk, preterm infants exhibit improved growth, no difference in neurodevelopment, and no difference in NEC when compared with infants receiving no fortification.[241] Research regarding the optimal enteral protein delivery to promote VLBW preterm infant growth points to 3.3 to 4.3 g/kg/day when assuming an approximately 1 g/dL concentration in human milk.[244-250]

The human milk–based human milk fortifier provides an opportunity to deliver an exclusive human milk diet. Currently available evidence demonstrates equivocal outcomes, with studies favoring benefit of exclusive human milk diet especially when compared with formula, but with no randomized trials demonstrating definitive benefit when compared with bovine-based fortifier.[251-253]

Formulas

Cow's milk–derived formulas have been modeled after the composition of human milk to provide biologically available protein mixtures with appropriate protein/energy ratios for normal growth. In general, formulas designed for term infants contain 19 to 20 kcal/oz and are adequate to meet the needs of term infants with an intact GI tract. Protein-hydrolyzed formulas are now available and are designed to treat GI disorders. They are generally well tolerated but do not lessen feeding intolerance or the rate of NEC in preterm infants and may result in slower weight gain.[254,255] Preterm formulas are designed to meet the additional protein, energy, and micronutrient requirements of the preterm infant. They have higher protein contents than those of term formulas, contain less lactose as a carbohydrate source and substitute corn syrup (largely sucrose), and provide some of the fat in the form of medium-chain triglycerides. Calcium and phosphorus content is increased, which allows for improved bone mineralization. Other minerals and vitamins also are present in higher concentrations to reflect the special nutritional needs of the VLBW infant. Preterm formulas are available in 20, 24, and 30 kcal/oz preparations, with similar osmolalities and renal solute loads.

SPECIAL NUTRITIONAL CONSIDERATIONS FOR INFANTS WITH ESTABLISHED BRONCHOPULMONARY DYSPLASIA

BPD is the most common pulmonary morbidity seen in VLBW preterm infants, with an incidence approaching 50% among infants born before 29 weeks' gestation.[256] Preterm infants who develop BPD are at risk of poor growth. In a cohort of ELBW infants with BPD, postnatal growth failure rates, defined as weight under the 10th percentile, were 53%, 67%, 66%, and 79% for postmenstrual ages of 36, 40, 44, and 48 weeks, respectively, despite a mean in-hospital weight gain of 30 g/kg/day.[257] Preterm infants with BPD demonstrated poorer growth velocities,[258-260] including reduced accretion of both lean mass and fat mass, that extend through the first year of life.[261] There are several plausible mechanisms of growth failure in infants with BPD: failure to meet nutritional requirements because of intolerance or fluid restriction, increased caloric expenditure with increased work of breathing, intermittent hypoxia, diuretic and postnatal steroid therapy, and comorbidities such as sepsis and pneumonia.[258] Meticulous attention must be given to optimizing nutritional delivery in these vulnerable patients. Exclusive use of mother's own milk may reduce the incidence of BPD.[262] In a prospective, nonrandomized study, preterm infants with BPD fed individually tailored fortified breast milk and/or preterm formula (with 130 kcal/kg/day energy intake and 3.2 g/kg/day protein intake) versus standard fortification showed greater weight gain velocity and less postnatal growth restriction.[263] Dietary supplements such as Ω-3 LC-PUFA supplementation was not associated with a decreased risk of BPD.[264] Box 31.2 summarizes the nutritional factors that are important to consider for infants who are developing and/or who have developed BPD.

BOX 31.2 Considerations for the Preterm Infant With Respiratory Insufficiency

Poor nutrition is associated with abnormal lung development

Careful fluid management during the first postnatal days may reduce the risk of BPD

Excessive fluid volumes increase pulmonary edema and contribute to lung injury

RDS and BPD increase the infant's metabolic needs for energy and protein

Steroid therapy and chronic disease have negative effects on protein balance

Diuretic therapy can waste electrolytes (Na, K) and calcium

Early nutritional support and feeding guidelines are associated with the prevention of BPD

Excessive carbohydrates (>12.5 mg/kg/min) will increase carbon dioxide production disproportionate to oxygen consumption

Lipids (ω3 LC-PUFAs) are a good alternative source of concentrated energy

Adequate provision of amino acids prevents catabolism of respiratory and diaphragmatic muscle protein

BPD, Bronchopulmonary dysplasia; *LC-PUFAs*, long-chain polyunsaturated fatty acids; *RDS*, respiratory distress syndrome.

Certainly, it is difficult to tease apart the cause-and-effect relationships between the provision and utilization of nutrients and the impact of lung disease on an infant's growth capacity. However, it is critically important to provide adequate nutrition to all infants requiring assisted ventilation, thereby allowing each infant the best possible chance for recovery of lung function and normal growth and development.

A complete reference list is available at https://expertconsult. inkling.com/.

KEY REFERENCES

1. Ehrenkranz RA, Dusick AM, Vohr BR, et al: Growth in the neonatal intensive care unit influences neurodevelopmental and growth outcomes of extremely low birth weight infants, Pediatrics 117:1253–1261, 2006.

5. Bose C, Van Marter LJ, Laughon M, et al: Fetal growth restriction and chronic lung disease among infants born before the 28th week of gestation. Pediatrics 124(3):e450–e458, 2009.

17. Ehrenkranz RA, Das A, Wrage LA, et al: Early nutrition mediates the influence of severity of illness on extremely LBW infants. Pediatr Res 69(6):522–529, 2011.

19. Klevebro S, Westin V, Sjöström ES, et al: Early energy and protein intakes and associations with growth, BPD, and ROP in extremely preterm infants. Clin Nutr 38(3):1289–1295, 2019.

49. Agostoni C, Buonocore G, Carnielli VP, et al: Enteral nutrient supply for preterm infants: commentary from the European Society of Paediatric Gastroenterology, Hepatology and Nutrition Committee on Nutrition. J Pediatr Gastroenterol Nutr 50(1): 85–91, 2010.

65. Johnson MJ, Wootton SA, Leaf AA, et al: Preterm birth and body composition at term equivalent age: a systematic review and meta-analysis. Pediatrics 130:E640–E649, 2012.

67. deRegnier RA, Guilbert TW, Mills MM, et al: Growth failure and altered body composition are established by one month of age in infants with bronchopulmonary dysplasia. J Nutr 126(1):168–175, 1996.

73. Poindexter BB, Langer JC, Dusick AM, et al: Early provision of parenteral amino acids in extremely low birth weight infants: relation to growth and neurodevelopmental outcome. J Pediatr 148:300–305, 2006.

78. Lapillonne A, Groh-Wargo S, Gonzalez CH, et al: Lipid needs of preterm infants: updated recommendations. J Pediatr 162: S37–S47, 2013.

89. Kapoor V, Malviya MN, Soll R: Lipid emulsions for parenterally fed preterm infants. Cochrane Database Syst Rev 6(6):CD013163, 2019.

129. McCarthy EK, Dempsey EM, Kiely ME: Iron supplementation in preterm and low-birth-weight infants: a systematic review of intervention studies. Nutr Rev 77(12):865–877, 2019.

201. Dorling J, Abbott J, Berrington J, et al: Controlled trial of two incremental milk-feeding rates in preterm infants. N Engl J Med 381(15):1434–1443, 2019.

219. Vohr BR, Poindexter BB, Dusick AM, et al: Persistent beneficial effects of breast milk ingested in the neonatal intensive care unit on outcomes of extremely low birth weight infants at 30 months of age. Pediatrics 120:e953–e959, 2007.

235. Bertino E, Giuliani F, Baricco M, et al: Benefits of donor milk in the feeding of preterm infants. Early Hum Dev 89(suppl 2): S3–S6, 2013.

253. O'Connor DL, Kiss A, Tomlinson C, et al: Nutrient enrichment of human milk with human and bovine milk-based fortifiers for infants born weighing <1250 g: a randomized clinical trial. Am J Clin Nutr 108(1):108–116, 2018.

257. Natarajan G, Johnson YR, Brozanski B, et al: Postnatal weight gain in preterm infants with severe bronchopulmonary dysplasia. Am J Perinatol 31:223–230, 2014.

32

Pharmacologic Therapies

Jegen Kandasamy and Waldemar A. Carlo

KEY POINTS

- Routine use of corticosteroids—either systemic or inhaled—postnatally to prevent or reduce severity of bronchopulmonary dysplasia (BPD) cannot be recommended at this time, and further evidence is awaited from recently concluded large trials.
- Use of dexamethasone or hydrocortisone to prevent BPD should be reserved for extremely preterm infants who continue to require considerable assisted ventilation support beyond 2 weeks of life and be preceded with a thorough discussion of the risks of possible neurodevelopmental sequelae and other risks with the parents.
- Prolonged use of sedatives and analgesics in extremely preterm infants is associated with significant risks of injury to the developing brain and requires careful consideration as well as the institution of weaning protocols designed to limit their use as much as possible.
- Although diuretics, bronchodilators, mucolytics, and other agents have been occasionally shown to produce transient or short-term physiological improvements in pulmonary function, none of these agents have demonstrated utility in preventing or reducing long-term pulmonary morbidity in extremely preterm infants.
- Caffeine (and theophylline) is effective in reducing apnea of prematurity as well as BPD incidence in preterm infants.

INTRODUCTION

Pharmacologic agents are often used during mechanical ventilation of newborn infants to achieve various therapeutic goals, including sedation and analgesia, neuromuscular paralysis, maintenance of fluid balance, and treatment of ventilator-associated inflammatory injury. Dosing, frequency, duration of use, and adverse effect profiles have not been studied well for most drugs used in neonates. Neonatal pharmacokinetics and pharmacodynamics exhibit considerable interindividual variability among neonates and also differ considerably from those of adults, so extrapolation of animal and adult studies to this age group is often fraught with errors.[1] Because of the limited data from studies, many of these drugs are used off-label as they have not undergone the rigorous testing in this age group required by the US Food and Drug Administration (FDA).[2] This chapter deals with several pharmacologic adjuncts to neonatal mechanical ventilation that are not covered in more detail elsewhere in the book.

STEROIDS

Maternal antenatal steroid administration for pregnancies at risk for preterm delivery to improve fetal lung maturity has become a well-established practice and has led to interest in using steroids postnatally for mechanically ventilated preterm infants at risk for bronchopulmonary dysplasia (BPD). Prolonged mechanical ventilation and its associated complications of volutrauma and biotrauma are some of the most important etiologic factors in the initiation and augmentation of the inflammatory processes that contribute to BPD.[3] As potent antiinflammatory agents, corticosteroids can potentially play a role in reducing its incidence and severity; indirect evidence for such a role is seen in infants with adrenal insufficiency, who have been shown to be at higher risk for developing BPD.[4] They increase the synthesis of annexin-1, a protein that inhibits phospholipase A2–induced release of arachidonic acid, the source of eicosanoid inflammatory mediators such as prostaglandins and leukotrienes.[5] Steroids also inhibit other enzymes such as cyclooxygenases 1 and 2, which are also involved in eicosanoid synthesis[6] and the influx of innate immune cells such as eosinophils into the pulmonary epithelium, thereby reducing inflammation and the concentration of inflammatory cytokines such as interleukin-1 in bronchoalveolar lavage.[7] Steroids accelerate lung maturation by promoting alveolar wall thinning and microvascular maturation and promote surfactant production, especially when given during the first week after birth.[8,9] They decrease elastase activity and collagen formation in the developing lung and increase antioxidant status and activity.[10,11] A small study ($n = 21$ per group) that compared early versus later administration of dexamethasone to mechanically ventilated preterm infants found decreased neutrophil numbers, activity and reduced concentrations of interleukin-1, leukotriene-B4, and albumin in the tracheobronchial aspirates collected from the former group.[12] Such evidence indicates that modulation of a broad range of inflammatory pathways is likely the major mechanism through which postnatal corticosteroid administration could reduce risk for subsequent BPD in prematurely born infants.

Postnatal steroid regimens have been categorized as early (less than 8 days, postnatal age) or late (≥ 8 days of life) depending on the timing of their initiation.

Early Postnatal (<8 Days) Steroid Therapy for Prevention of Bronchopulmonary Dysplasia

Although adopted enthusiastically by many clinicians in the late 1980s, early steroid therapy has become more controversial today, with the results of several studies raising concern for neurodevelopmental sequelae. The vast majority of these studies evaluated dexamethasone, which is a more potent steroid compared with hydrocortisone. In a large trial, 384 infants of less than 30 weeks' gestation were randomized to receive an early short course (two doses beginning at 12 hours of age) of dexamethasone or placebo.[13] This trial showed that a short course of early dexamethasone reduced later prolonged dexamethasone treatment and ventilator and/or oxygen use but did not reduce death or BPD at 36 weeks of gestation. The largest trial that evaluated early dexamethasone was conducted in 2001 by the Vermont Oxford Network. In this multicenter trial, 542 extremely low birth weight (ELBW) infants on mechanical ventilation soon after birth were randomized to receive either dexamethasone or placebo for 12 days, with the first dose administered at 12 hours of age.[14] The trial had to be stopped early before the completion of the predetermined sample size because of an increased incidence of complications, including gastrointestinal perforation, hyperglycemia, poor weight gain, and hypertension, in the early dexamethasone group. Furthermore, this trial also showed that early dexamethasone therapy increased periventricular leukomalacia (PVL) and did not decrease the risk for BPD or death. Studies of early hydrocortisone therapy to prevent BPD were also carried out around this time. A multicenter trial randomized 360 mechanically ventilated ELBW infants at 12 to 48 hours of life to receive either hydrocortisone or placebo for 15 days.[15] This trial, which was also stopped early as the authors discovered increased incidence of gastrointestinal perforation in the hydrocortisone group, found that survival without BPD and mortality were similar between the two groups. Another multicenter trial published in 2016 (the PREMILOC study) that enrolled 523 infants found that prophylactic hydrocortisone given for the first 10 days of life administration reduced the risk for BPD or death (number needed to treat = 12; odds ratio [OR], 1.48; 95% confidence interval [CI], 1.02–2.16) without any significant increase in risk for neurodevelopmental impairment at 2 years of age or other short-term adverse effects, with the exception of increased sepsis in infants born between 24 and 25 weeks' gestation when compared with placebo.[16,17]

The most recent Cochrane Collaboration systematic review that evaluated early postnatal steroid use for preterm infants at risk for developing BPD and included a total of 4395 participants from 32 trials concluded that early (<8 days) steroid treatment (either hydrocortisone or dexamethasone) decreases BPD risk at 28 days and 36 weeks' postmenstrual age (PMA) and facilitates extubation but also increases the risk for complications including intestinal perforation, hypertension, gastrointestinal bleeding, hyperglycemia, cardiomyopathy, and growth failure.[18] The meta-analysis also reported that several studies described adverse neurologic effects including cerebral palsy, especially with dexamethasone, but that there was no overall increase in major neurosensory disability for infants who received corticosteroids early. Despite these findings, the authors of the review have concluded that routine use of early steroids cannot be recommended for preterm infants at this time because of the heterogeneity of available studies regarding the evaluation of neurologic outcomes and recommend more extensive follow-up data regarding long-term neurodevelopmental outcomes from these studies.

Late (≥8 Days) Postnatal Steroid Therapy for Prevention or Therapy of Bronchopulmonary Dysplasia in Preterm Infants

The Cochrane Collaboration systematic review[19] that included 21 trials with a total of 1424 infants who were randomized to receive steroids or placebo when older than a week concluded that steroid regimens initiated on or after 8 days of life reduced neonatal mortality rate at 28 days' and at 36 weeks' PMA and decreased BPD at 36 weeks' PMA in addition to facilitating earlier extubation. Although there was a trend toward an increase in cerebral palsy rates, there was also an opposing and larger trend for decreased mortality in the steroid group at the latest follow-up. The review concluded that corticosteroid therapy should be restricted to infants who are unable to be weaned off mechanical ventilation and that such exposure be limited to minimal dosing and duration of treatment. The Canadian Pediatric Society has also taken a similar stand on the use of postnatal corticosteroids, by recommending against the use of routine dexamethasone or hydrocortisone therapy for ventilated infants.[20] These authors suggest short-term low-dose dexamethasone therapy as an alternative for infants with BPD who are on maximal ventilator and oxygen therapy and, further, that such therapy be initiated only after providing parents of such infants with information about the known short-term and long-term risks of such therapy. Another study from the National Institute of Child Health and Human Development Neonatal Research Network (NRN) that examined the association between age at first postnatal steroid exposure and risk for BPD in a cohort of 951 infants born at less than 27 weeks' gestation concluded that administering such therapy before 50 days after birth was associated with the lowest odds for risk of severe BPD. The study also concluded that the age at which steroids were given did not significantly impact the risk for subsequent neurodevelopmental impairment.[21] A more recent NICHD-NRN study assessed the utility of a 10 day tapering course of hydrocortisone in 800 very preterm infants who remained intubated between 14-28 days of life. This study showed that hydrocortisone use at this age in these infants was associated with neither growth nor neurodevelopmental impairment at 2 years of age (indicating it is safe to use at this time point) and improved extubation rates. However, the study also showed that hydrocortisone did not improve rates of survival without BPD compared to placebo.

In summary, very early prophylactic use of systemic steroids to prevent BPD in all prematurely born very low birth weight (VLBW) infants is considered a practice to be discouraged, as is the use of high doses and prolonged treatment courses. Additionally, despite evidence from the PREMILOC study indicating that early hydrocortisone therapy may decrease BPD and mortality at 36 weeks without increasing risk for cerebral palsy, its use also cannot be recommended until its impact on long-term survival and neurodevelopmental outcomes can be fully examined through further studies[259]. Additional questions such as whether certain subpopulations of infants could benefit more from systemic steroids compared with others, as well as the most appropriate dose regimen, also remain unanswered and corticosteroid administration for BPD risk reduction continues to be highly variable across centers around the country and globally. In the authors' practice, dexamethasone is considered for infants who continue to require mechanical ventilation at or beyond 28 days of life and is given according to the DART (Dexamethasone: A Randomized Trial) protocol, whereas hydrocortisone is preferred for infants between 14 and 28 days of life if the use of steroids is considered necessary by the clinician.[22]

In addition to management of BPD, steroids have also been used in attempts to facilitate and improve success rates of extubation for mechanically ventilated preterm infants. Studies have used up to three doses of 0.25 to 0.5 mg/kg dexamethasone given intravenously for this purpose. Infants included in these studies weighed at least 1 kg, had a mean GA greater than 30 weeks, and had been intubated for at least 7 days.[23-25] A Cochrane Collaboration systematic review that analyzed these studies concluded that because dexamethasone use for facilitating extubation has not been adequately evaluated in ELBW infants and is associated with adverse effects such as hyperglycemia, its use can be approved only for infants at high risk for airway edema and obstruction such as those with repeated or prolonged intubations.[26]

As an alternative to systemic steroid therapy, inhaled corticosteroids (ICSs) offer the advantage of minimal or limited adverse systemic effects. A survey found that ICS therapy has been used for infants with BPD in 25% of US children's hospitals.[27] However, variable and inefficient drug delivery and deposition in the lower airways of premature infants, secondary to factors such as small endotracheal tube diameters, short inspiratory times, and device limitations (type and placement of nebulizer

TABLE 32.1 Published Randomized, Placebo-Controlled Trials of Inhaled Steroids

Reference	Sample Size	Dosage	Recruitment Criteria	Delivery Method	Placebo	Positive Results in Steroid-Treated Infants
Laforce et al.[260]	13	Beclomethasone 3 × 50 mg for 28 days	>14 days, CXR BPD, VLBW	Nebulization through ventilator circuit or face mask	No blinded placebo	CRS; R(aw); no difference in infection
Giep et al.[261]	19	Beclomethasone 1000 mg daily for 7 days or until extubated	>14 days, VLBW CXR BPD	MDI + spacer	Double blind	Extubation
Arnon et al.[262]	20	Budesonide 600 mg twice daily for 7 days	14 days, BW <2000 g, IPPV	MDI + spacer	Double blind	Significant PIP; no difference in serum cortisol levels
Ng et al.[263]	25	Fluticasone propionate 1000 mg per day for 14 days	First 24 hours, <32 weeks' GA, VLBW	MDI + spacer	Double blind	Basal and poststimulation plasma ACTH and serum plasma cortisol concentrations significantly suppressed
Fok[264]	53	Fluticasone 500 mg bid for 14 days	<24 hours, VLBW MDI + spacer IPPV		Double blind	17/27 vs. 8/26 extubated at 14 days; CRS
Cole et al.[265]	253	Beclomethasone 40 mg/kg/day, decreasing to 5 mg/kg over 4 weeks	3–14 days, <33 weeks' GA, ≤1250 g, IPPV	MDI + spacer neonatal anesthesia bag + ET tube (even when extubated)	Double blind	Rescue dexamethasone, RR, 0.6 (0.4–1.0); IPPV at 28 days, RR, 0.8 (0.6–1.0) at 28 days
Jangaard et al.[31]	60	Beclomethasone (250 μg/puff), one to two puffs every 6–8 hours depending on birth weight	28 days	Inline in respiratory limb of ventilator circuit with Medilife spacer via aerochamber with mask	Double blind	Similar incidence of growth failure, IVH, infection as well as long-term outcomes including NDI compared with placebo
Bassler et al.[257] (NEuroSIS trial).	863	Budesonide (200 μg/puff), two puffs every 12 hours for the first 14 days, followed by one puff every 12 hours from day 15 until the enrolled infant no longer required PPV or reached 32 weeks' PMA	<12 hours, ELBW requiring PPV	MDI + spacer, inserted into the ventilator circuit or face mask	Double blind	Reduced BPD incidence in the inhaled steroid group, RR, 0.74 (0.6–0.91), P < .05, accompanied by increased mortality, RR, 1.24 (0.91–1.69), P > .1

ACTH, Adrenocorticotropic hormone; *bid,* twice a day; *BW,* birth weight; *CRS,* compliance; *CXR BPD,* chest radiograph appearance consistent with bronchopulmonary dysplasia; *ELBW,* extremely low birth weight; *ET,* endotracheal; *GA,* gestational age; *IPPV,* ventilator dependent (intermittent positive-pressure ventilation); *IVH,* intraventricular hemorrhage; *MDI,* metered-dose inhaler; *NDI,* neurodevelopmental impairment; *PIP,* peak inspiratory pressure; *PMA,* postmenstrual age; *PPV,* positive-pressure ventilation; *R(aw),* airway resistance; *RR,* relative risk; *VLBW,* very low birth weight.
(Data from Greenough A. Neonat Respir Dis 10:1–7, 2000.)

used, particle size, aerosol flow, and other factors), have been serious limitations to the use of ICS for preterm infants.[28] Although previously available data (Table 32.1) suggested that the use of ICS does not prevent BPD, either compared with placebo or with systemic steroid use, a large multinational clinical trial in which infants were randomized to receive either inhaled budesonide or placebo has found that ICS therapy does reduce BPD incidence in ELBW infants. However, this study also found an increased rate of mortality, albeit statistically nonsignificant, in the inhaled steroid group compared with the placebo group.[29,30,257] A Cochrane systematic review of 10 qualifying trials that included 1644 neonates found that early (within 2 weeks of birth) initiation of ICSs reduced the risk for the combined outcome of death or BPD at 36 weeks' PMA but did not reduce risk for BPD alone for VLBW infants.[29] More evidence regarding the effectiveness and safety of such early and prolonged use of ICS is required before their routine use can be recommended for the ELBW infant population.

SEDATION AND ANALGESIA

About 20% of all infants and 50% of all ELBW infants admitted to tertiary neonatal intensive care units (NICUs) receive endotracheal intubation and/or mechanical ventilation.[32-34] Sedation and analgesia may be important for the management of pain in neonates receiving respiratory support. In a 1997 survey, neonatologists and nurses rated their assessment of pain for intubation and endotracheal suctioning in neonates at 2 on a scale of 4 (not painful to very painful).[35] Consequences of episodic pain related to procedures like intubation include physiologic responses such as hypoxemia; pulmonary and systemic hypertension; release of stress hormones like cortisol, catecholamines, and glucagon; and increased markers of oxidative stress such as malondialdehyde.[36-42] In addition, agitation during endotracheal intubation can cause increased intracranial pressures that can lead to intraventricular hemorrhage (IVH); trauma to gingival, orolabial, and glottic structures; and increased number of attempts required for any provider irrespective of their level of training and experience.[41,43-48]

Despite the potential for adverse effects of pain during respiratory support, the management of procedural pain and sedation during endotracheal intubation remains an area of controversy and debate. For example, in a survey, only 44% of US neonatal units reported routine use of premedication for elective intubations.[49] First, pain assessment in the neonate is imperfect, and there is a poor correlation between individual tools that are used to attempt to objectively estimate pain.[50,51] Facial expressions of pain, high activity levels, poor response to routine care, and poor ventilator synchrony were associated with inadequate analgesia in one study of preterm ventilated infants.[52] Second, there are limited safety data regarding most drugs used for sedation and analgesia, especially regarding long-term neurodevelopmental outcomes when such medications are used for extremely premature infants.[53,54] An American Academy of Pediatrics guidance statement published in 2010 recommends routine administration of premedication, including sedatives and analgesics, for infants that undergo nonemergent intubations but also recognizes these and other knowledge gaps and stresses the importance of continued

research before such practice can become routine in all facilities that take care of such critically ill neonates.[55]

Invasive mechanical ventilation in infants appears to be associated with chronic pain and/or stress, as supported by the increased serum levels of β-endorphins.[39] Stress can lead to long-term consequences such as impaired motor and cognitive development at 8 and 18 months of corrected GA, lower IQ at 7 years, as well as internalizing behaviors at 18 months of age and decreased pain thresholds in adult life.[56-59] These outcomes are thought to be secondary to frontoparietal cortical thinning, reduced development of white matter and subcortical gray matter, and increased activation of the somatosensory cortex associated with repeated or prolonged exposure to painful stimuli, especially in the early neonatal period.[60,61] On the other hand, prolonged or repeated analgesic exposure can lead to excessive and prolonged need for ventilation, hypotension, and enhanced neuronal cell death.[62-66] Current evidence indicates that the use of sedatives and analgesic agents for premature neonates should be a carefully considered decision that takes into account the safety and effectiveness of such agents. Nonpharmacologic interventions such as administration of oral sucrose, swaddling, containment, kangaroo care, facilitated tucking, and reduction of environmental stressors such as light and noise along with intermittent music therapy are variously effective for reducing stress associated with acutely painful procedures such as endotracheal suctioning and can be attempted as adjuncts or as first-line measures before the use of pharmacologic agents.[67-71] However, there are limited data regarding the utility of these nonpharmacologic interventions for infants on mechanical ventilation. Typical dosages for sedatives and analgesics used in neonates are listed in Table 32.2. Individual drugs are discussed in the following.

Opioids

From the time it was first isolated from *Papaver somniferum* in 1803, the alkaloid opioid morphine and its related drugs have been the standard against which all other agents with analgesic effects have been measured. The analgesic effect of opioids is attributed to their activation of the endorphin μ, κ, and/or δ receptors in the central nervous system (CNS), which initiates signal transduction and activation of inhibitory G proteins and reduction of cyclic adenosine monophosphate (cAMP) levels, leading to reduced neuronal excitability and decreased neurotransmitter release.[72] Spinal and supraspinal activation of

TABLE 32.2 Sedation and Analgesia for Neonates

Agent	Bolus Dose	Dose Frequency	Infusion Dose
Sedation			
Lorazepam	0.05–0.1 mg/kg	4–12 hours	Not recommended
Midazolam	0.05–0.15 mg/kg	2–4 hours	10–60 mg/kg/hour
Analgesia			
Morphine	0.05–0.2 mg/kg	2–4 hours	10–15 μg/kg/hour
Fentanyl	1–4 mg/kg[a]	2–4 hours	1–2 mg/kg/hour

[a]Slowly, over approximately 5 minutes.

these pathways inhibits ascending nociceptive pathways, reduces pain thresholds, and alters the individual's perception of pain.[72,73]

Morphine

Morphine is one of the first-line agents for analgesia in adults and is also one of the most frequently used agents for this purpose in neonates. Morphine is a strong agonist of the μ opioid receptor (MOR) through which it mediates effects such as analgesia and respiratory depression.[72] Tolerance of and dependence on morphine are also mediated through this receptor.[74] Morphine acts as a weak agonist of the κ and the δ opioid receptors, unlike naturally occurring endorphins, which mediate most of their effects through these receptors rather than the MOR. The major effects of morphine are on the CNS and organs containing smooth muscle such as the gastrointestinal and urinary tracts.[72,73,75]

Although morphine can be administered through oral, subcutaneous, and rectal routes, intravenous administration is the most common route of use for premature infants. Morphine has a quick onset of action and peaks at about 1 hour after injection.[73] Its duration of action in neonates may be 2 to 4 hours.[76] After an initial loading infusion of 100 mcg/kg over the first hour, standard doses used for continuous infusion range between 5 and 15 mcg/kg/h. Analgesia, the primary therapeutic indication for morphine, is achieved with morphine plasma concentrations of 15 to 20 ng/mL; some studies, however, suggest that the effective plasma morphine concentration to produce analgesia may be variable in preterm neonates.[77] However, respiratory depression is often noted at levels not much more than this range in young infants ages 2 to 570 days.[76,78,79] Respiratory depression, which is attributed to effects on respiratory centers in the brain stem, may be marked but is not usually of clinical significance in ventilated infants unless weaning from the ventilator is anticipated. Sedation, another therapeutic effect of morphine, occurs at much higher plasma levels (125 ng/mL), so morphine does not provide sedation at doses that are used to provide analgesia.[80]

Rapid morphine bolus infusions can induce histamine release from mast cells, a common effect seen with other opioids as well, leading to vasodilation, hypotension, and bradycardia.[73] Morphine infusions can be used safely for most preterm infants, but caution is required for infants 23 to 26 weeks' gestation, especially those with preexisting hypotension.[63,81] There are both interindividual and intraindividual variations in the effects of morphine. The metabolism of morphine matures with increasing GA; therefore, morphine infusion should be carefully titrated to the effect in preterm infants.[77,82] Other effects of morphine include bronchoconstriction, decreased gastric motility, and increased anal sphincter tone and urinary tract smooth muscle tone. With prolonged morphine administration, some degree of tolerance develops, necessitating an increase in dosage.[74,83] Following extended use, a weaning regimen that reduces the dose by 10% to 20% per day is recommended to prevent withdrawal symptoms. Morphine effects can be reversed by a naloxone dose of 0.1 mg/kg.[72] Hepatic UDP-glucuronosyl transferase 2B7 converts morphine into morphine 6-glucuronide (responsible for both the analgesic and the respiratory depressant effects of morphine) and morphine 3-glucuronide (M3G), which acts as an antagonist to morphine and contributes to morphine tolerance.[78,84] Both metabolites are eliminated through urinary and biliary excretion. Data suggest that preterm neonates metabolize morphine to form the M3G derivative predominantly, because of which accelerated development of tachyphylaxis to continuous morphine infusion may be noted.[85] Morphine clearance reaches adult rates only at 6 to 12 months corrected postconceptual age.[86] Morphine is not highly protein bound even in adults, so its metabolism is relatively unaffected by plasma protein levels, but whether this is also true in preterm infants, who often have decreased albumin levels, remains unclear.[87,88]

The effectiveness and safety of morphine as a continuous infusion in ventilated infants remain to be established. The Neurologic Outcomes and Preemptive Analgesia in Neonates (NEOPAIN) trial was a large multicenter study that randomized 212 infants undergoing mechanical ventilation to receive placebo or morphine infusions (ranging from 10 to 30 mcg/kg/h), along with open-label intermittent morphine used for additional analgesia based on physician discretion. Reduction of pain score and smaller increases in heart rate and respiratory rate were noted in the morphine group. However, these infants took longer to tolerate full enteral feeds, had significant hypotension more often, and required mechanical ventilation for longer duration than infants in the placebo group. Mortality rates, the primary outcome of the NEOPAIN study, and morbidities related to prematurity such as IVH and PVL were similar between the two groups.[62] Neurologic outcomes also did not differ between the infants given morphine (up to 10 mcg/kg/h) or placebo in another study of 150 ventilated term and preterm infants.[89] A systematic meta-analysis of 13 studies (1505 infants) found that the reduction in pain scores achieved with continuous morphine infusion was clinically insignificant. This analysis also found that very preterm infants who received morphine took longer to achieve full enteral feeds and had more hypotensive episodes that required treatment. Other outcomes such as mortality, duration of mechanical ventilation, BPD, IVH, and PVL did not differ between infants who received morphine and those who received placebo. Overall, the systematic review concluded that there was insufficient evidence to recommend routine use of continuous morphine infusions for infants undergoing mechanical ventilation.[90]

Preclinical animal studies have provided evidence that morphine can alter hippocampal development in the developing brain.[91] Data regarding the impact of routine morphine use for preterm infants with regard to their long-term neurodevelopmental outcomes have shown that while overall intelligence may not be affected, effects on other neurodevelopmental outcomes may be of concern. A follow-up study of 19 infants who were part of the NEOPAIN trial showed that while there were no differences in IQ or school performance between the groups, head circumference was smaller for infants who received morphine compared with those who received placebo. Infants from the morphine group also required longer time to complete tasks compared with those from the placebo group.[92] A 5-year follow-up of mechanically ventilated preterm infants who were randomized to receive continuous morphine infusion or placebo also found that overall IQ scores, executive function, visual-motor integration, and intelligence did not differ between the morphine and the control groups, but the visual analysis subtest component score was noted to be lower for infants from the morphine group.[89,93] Other studies have also highlighted subtle adverse effects on long-term motor development and neurobehavior when morphine was routinely used for analgesia for preterm infants.[59,94]

Thus, based on the currently available data, morphine administration, especially as a continuous infusion, should not be considered routine for mechanically ventilated infants. Instead, opioids such as morphine should be used judiciously, either as intermittent doses or as continuous infusions, appropriately titrated for each infant to measurements of pain based on well-validated scales.

Fentanyl

Fentanyl is a synthetic opioid with higher lipophilicity compared with morphine. This higher lipid solubility allows fentanyl to cross the blood-cerebrospinal fluid barrier more rapidly and produce analgesic effects more quickly than morphine. In addition, the analgesic effects of fentanyl are 80 to 100 times more potent than the morphine effects. Fentanyl is oxidized by hepatic microsomal cytochrome P450 into norfentanyl, an inactive metabolite that is then renally excreted.[72,73] Fentanyl clearance matures quickly after birth, reaching 70% of adult levels by 2 weeks' postnatal age in term infants.[95,96] Clearance of fentanyl can be reduced secondary to decreased hepatic blood flow.[97] Owing to faster redistribution and an elimination half-life of 3 to 5 hours, fentanyl also has a shorter duration of action (30–40 minutes) than morphine, making it ideal for scenarios like intubation that require rapid induction and recovery from sedation and analgesia.[98,99] Fentanyl also has reduced propensity to cause histamine release from mast cells, as well as decreased activity on the vasomotor center. These advantages of fentanyl make it theoretically less likely to cause significant hypotension compared with morphine.[100,101] In addition, when used before endotracheal suctioning, fentanyl blunts increases in pulmonary arterial pressure, as shown in a study of infants recovering from cardiac surgery, who are often prone to such crises.[102] In contrast to morphine, studies of fentanyl pharmacodynamics also show that its therapeutic effects may be more predictable using serum levels.[96] Because of these advantages, fentanyl has emerged as the most commonly used synthetic opioid for procedural analgesia in neonates.[55]

Continuous fentanyl infusion is also often used to achieve more prolonged analgesia for mechanically ventilated infants. Currently available data suggest that fentanyl offers analgesia equivalent to that produced by morphine, as shown in a trial of 163 mechanically ventilated newborn infants between 29 and 37 weeks' gestation at birth randomized to receive continuous infusions of either fentanyl or morphine in the first 2 days of life. Adverse effects such as decreased gastrointestinal motility were also less commonly observed in the fentanyl group.[103] However, similar needs for vasopressors to treat hypotension were observed in both groups. Another important, although

rare, disadvantage that appears to be more common with fentanyl use than with morphine is chest wall rigidity, especially when it is administered as a rapid bolus infusion.[104] In addition, when used as a continuous infusion, the serum half-life of fentanyl is prolonged in preterm infants.[105] This may be secondary to the high lipid solubility of fentanyl that allows it to accumulate in adipose and other lipid-rich tissue. When discontinued after prolonged use, redistribution of fentanyl from such stores can prolong respiratory depression and delay the recovery from sedation.[98] Severe gastrointestinal adverse effects can also be seen with fentanyl, showing that the choice of fentanyl over morphine for analgesia may not be as advantageous as is sometimes believed.[106]

Prolonged opioid use can lead to the development of tolerance, tachyphylaxis, and withdrawal symptoms when such use is discontinued. In one study of infants on extracorporeal membrane oxygenation, fentanyl infusion was associated with more rapid development of tolerance and requirement for higher doses over time, along with increased incidence and severity of withdrawal effects, leading to significantly longer hospital stay compared with continuous morphine infusion.[83] Fentanyl use is also associated with more severe tachyphylaxis compared with morphine.[107] In another study, a fentanyl total dose greater than 415 mcg/kg predicted withdrawal with 70% sensitivity and 78% specificity, whereas a fentanyl infusion duration greater than 8 days predicted withdrawal with 90% sensitivity and 67% specificity.[108] Both fentanyl and morphine require weaning from the total daily dose by 10% to 20% per day to prevent such withdrawal.

As an analgesic agent, fentanyl is associated with disadvantages, as shown in several trials that compared it to placebo. Fentanyl was noted to be associated with a need for higher, rather than lower, ventilator support in a randomized trial of 20 infants with respiratory distress syndrome (RDS), possibly secondary to decreased chest wall compliance because of fentanyl-induced chest wall rigidity.[109] In a multicenter trial of 131 mechanically ventilated infants between 22 and 32 weeks' GA at birth randomized to receive either fentanyl or placebo, short-term pain scores were lower for infants who received fentanyl, but there were no long-term differences in either the pain scores or the need for open-label fentanyl use, which was also similar between the two groups. Fentanyl use also prolonged the duration of mechanical ventilation and the time to first meconium passage in this study.[110] Data available from a randomized placebo-controlled trial of 27 preterm ventilated infants regarding the impact of fentanyl infusion on mortality or the incidence of short-term adverse neurologic effects such as IVH indicate that it has no advantages over placebo; as of this writing, there are no data regarding its effects on long-term neurodevelopmental outcomes.[111]

Dexmedetomidine

As an analgesic agent with additional anxiolytic and sedative properties and the additional advantage of very minimal potential to cause respiratory depression, dexmedetomidine has been extensively used in adults, often beyond the 24 hours of use that it has been approved for by the FDA.[112] Dexmedetomidine is an imidazole derivative and the active isomer of medetomidine. It is a selective central α_2-adrenergic receptor agonist. α_2-Adrenergic receptors are found in a number of supraspinal and spinal neuronal sites in the central and peripheral nervous systems, where they modulate both presynaptic and postsynaptic sympathetic output. One of the areas of the CNS with a high density of this receptor is the locus coeruleus, the primary site of norepinephrine synthesis in the brain, with functions that include maintenance of sleep-wake cycle, attention, memory, and arousal. Blocking sympathetic outflow from the locus coeruleus is the primary mechanism behind the sedative and analgesic effects of dexmedetomidine. This area is also the origin of several descending spinal nociceptive pathways that converge on the substantia gelatinosa in the dorsal horn of the spinal cord. At this level, dexmedetomidine stimulates α_2 receptors to inhibit release of substance P, a nociceptive mediator.[113] Whereas other drugs that act on α_2-adrenergic receptors such as clonidine exist, dexmedetomidine is unique in its high specificity for the α_{2A} subtype of this receptor, which is primarily responsible for its very effective sedative and analgesic effects.[114,115]

Dexmedetomidine is increasingly being used in the pediatric population, especially in the postoperative cardiac intensive care environment.[116] In the first-ever study of its use in preterm infants, a study with historic controls (for whom fentanyl had been used as analgesic) assessed the use of dexmedetomidine in 24 preterm infants with a mean GA of 25 weeks.[117] This study showed that dexmedetomidine use was associated with less need for adjunctive sedation, shorter duration of mechanical ventilation, and lower incidence of culture-positive sepsis episodes compared with fentanyl use. The lower incidence of sepsis noted with dexmedetomidine is believed to be secondary to its promotion of macrophage activity and reduction of inflammatory mediators such as tumor necrosis factor-α and interleukin-6 that has been noted in animal studies.[118,119] This antiinflammatory effect of dexmedetomidine, if confirmed in large randomized trials, may be a significant advantage for mechanically ventilated preterm infants who are at high risk for BPD. Another difference was the lack of signs of withdrawal for infants in the dexmedetomidine group, whereas infants in the fentanyl group often required slower weaning.

Other potential advantages of dexmedetomidine use in preterm mechanically ventilated infants may include its minimal potential to cause respiratory depression and gastrointestinal dysmotility.[120] Adverse effects associated with dexmedetomidine also are a result of its α_2-adrenergic agonist activity. Like clonidine, which has a similar receptor activity albeit with lesser specificity, dexmedetomidine can cause hypotension, bradycardia, decreased secretion, bowel motility, and excessive diuresis.[121] In the study of dexmedetomidine use in preterm infants, the incidence of significant hypotension or bradycardia was similar between the dexmedetomidine group and the control group (fentanyl), indicating that dexmedetomidine may not be inferior to other currently used sedatives and analgesics with respect to this adverse effect. Although no differences were noted between the two groups with respect to short-term neurologic outcomes such as IVH, large randomized trials that include long-term neurodevelopmental outcomes of its use

need to be conducted before dexmedetomidine can be recommended for use in premature infants without reservation.[117]

Benzodiazepines

As sedative-hypnotics, the benzodiazepines cause CNS depression to reduce anxiety, produce drowsiness, and maintain a state of reduced awareness. Benzodiazepines are widely used for such purposes in the NICU. However, benzodiazepines do not possess analgesic effects. By increasing the affinity of γ-amino butyric acid (GABA) binding to the GABA-A receptors, benzodiazepines increase neuronal inhibition at various levels of the nervous system including the cerebral cortex, hypothalamus, hippocampus, and substantia nigra. Side effects of benzodiazepine use include respiratory depression and, especially in infants with hypovolemia or impaired cardiac function, hypotension.[122] The most commonly used benzodiazepines in the NICU are discussed here.

Midazolam

Because of its pH-dependent water and lipid solubility, midazolam combines decreased incidence of thrombophlebitis or discomfort during intravenous administration with rapid onset of action (<3 minutes) and time to peak sedative effects (<20 minutes) compared with other benzodiazepines, making it a preferred drug for use in emergent situations in which rapid onset and termination of sedative effects may be required.[123,124] It is also frequently used as a continuous infusion for sedation of mechanically ventilated neonates. Midazolam is converted by hepatic cytochrome P450 3A4 hydroxylation to form active and inactive metabolites. Owing to relatively lower levels of this enzyme at birth, midazolam has a longer elimination half-life (6.3 hours) and lower clearance rate (1.8 mL/kg/min) in healthy neonates.[125,126] In a study of 187 neonates between 26 and 42 weeks' GA who underwent mechanical ventilation, the midazolam elimination half-life was 1.6-fold greater than normal.[127] Preterm infants have a longer elimination half-life compared with term infants, indicating that midazolam clearance increases with postnatal age and is decreased by critical illness as well as mechanical ventilation.[128] Oral midazolam use in neonates is rare and associated with reduced clearance; bioavailability via the oral route was estimated to be around 50% in one study.[129] Midazolam is highly protein bound; low serum albumin concentrations may lead to increased fractions of unbound midazolam available to enter the CNS and potentiate its therapeutic as well as adverse effects.[130]

The adverse effects of midazolam in neonates include respiratory depression, hypotension, hypotonia, hypertonia, dyskinetic movements, myoclonus, and paradoxic agitation.[131] The decreased number of GABA-A receptors seen in the neonate is believed to be the cause of the hyperexcitability instead of sedation that is often seen with midazolam use. Young age, female gender, and reduced serum albumin levels have been reported to be risk factors for the development of such adverse short-term neurologic effects.[132] Withdrawal associated with discontinuation of midazolam use has been noted in rodent studies and may be the cause of the neurologic adverse effects seen in older infants, children, and adults.[133] Finally, the usual parenteral preparation contains 1% benzyl alcohol as a preservative; this may need to be taken into consideration when dosing this drug. Use of the more concentrated 5 mg/mL preparation will reduce exposure to benzyl alcohol per milligram of midazolam used. Newer preparations of midazolam are preservative-free.[123]

A randomized trial of the use of continuous midazolam infusion as sedation for mechanical ventilation in 46 preterm infants found that whereas midazolam was an effective sedative compared with placebo, it did not reduce duration of ventilation, supplemental oxygen use, or incidence of severe lung disease or mortality compared with placebo. In addition, midazolam use prolonged NICU stay and tended to increase the incidence of hypotension and bradycardia in preterm infants when its use was continued beyond 48 hours.[134] Another multicenter study of sedation in the NICU randomized 67 mechanically ventilated infants between 24 and 32 weeks' GA to receive morphine, midazolam, or dextrose placebo infusions for up to 14 days (the Neonatal Outcome and Prolonged Analgesia in Neonates trial). In addition to finding results similar to those of the previous study, this trial also found that midazolam use led to increased incidence of neurologic adverse effects such as IVH and PVL compared with morphine or placebo use.[64] A meta-analysis of three such studies by Ng et al.[135] concluded that in light of the currently available evidence, the increased risks of adverse neurologic effects seen with midazolam use outweigh any benefits and therefore preclude its recommendation for use as a continuous infusion for sedation in the preterm infant.

Lorazepam

Lorazepam is a longer acting, highly lipophilic benzodiazepine compared with midazolam with a serum half-life of 24 to 56 hours and a duration of action of 8 to 12 hours in critically ill neonates.[136] Lorazepam is metabolized by hepatic glucuronidation into inactive metabolites, which are then eliminated through biliary excretion.[122] Apnea, somnolence, and stereotypic movements are complications associated with lorazepam use in neonates.[137,138] In adults and older children, prolonged administration or continuous infusion of lorazepam causes metabolic acidosis secondary to accumulation of toxic alcohols such as propylene glycol, an agent that is used to increase the solubility of lorazepam in currently available lorazepam formulations.[139] Therefore, lorazepam cannot be recommended for administration as a continuous infusion in neonates. As lorazepam is a longer-acting agent, prolonged sedation can be achieved with intermittent dosing to achieve sedation in mechanically ventilated infants. However, like other benzodiazepines, routine use of lorazepam for sedation in preterm infants has not been adequately characterized with respect to its long-term neurodevelopmental effects and cannot be recommended at this time.

Diazepam

Diazepam has anxiolytic, hypnotic, anticonvulsant, muscle relaxant, and amnesic effects that are characteristic of benzodiazepines and, like other benzodiazepines, has no analgesic properties. Diazepam is absorbed rapidly after oral administration but irregularly after intramuscular administration. The elimination half-life approximates 75 hours in preterm infants and 30 hours in term infants.[140] Diazepam is metabolized in the liver and, along with its metabolites, is slowly excreted in the urine. Simple correlations do not exist between plasma level and clinical response. Diazepam can cause respiratory depression, which may actually help infants to "settle" on the ventilator. Diazepam can be useful as a long-acting sedative when given in doses ranging from 0.10 to 0.25 mg/kg every 6 hours.

Other Sedative Agents

Propofol is an intravenous alkylphenol sedative-hypnotic without analgesic effects. It is a rapid-acting agent with short half-life and low propensity to cause respiratory depression.[141] Pharmacokinetic studies have determined that 0.7 to 1.4 mg/kg of propofol is appropriate for its use as part of the INSURE (intubation, surfactant, extubation) protocol for premature infants.[142] A study of 63 neonates that compared a combination of succinylcholine, atropine, and morphine to the use of only propofol for sedation before intubation found that propofol use led to shorter time required for successful intubation and less associated oral/nasal trauma as well as shorter recovery times. Infants in the propofol group also experienced less hypoxemic events during the endotracheal intubation attempts.[143] Despite these advantages, the use of propofol in neonates as an induction agent for endotracheal intubation has been associated with a high incidence of hypotension.[144] In addition, continuous infusion of propofol has been associated with fatal complications secondary to metabolic acidosis, bradycardia, rhabdomyolysis, and renal failure (the propofol infusion syndrome) when used in children and adults.[145] Thus, continuous infusion of propofol for sedation is strongly discouraged.

Chloral hydrate, a commonly used sedative agent, has the major advantages of excellent oral bioavailability and minimal respiratory depression.[66,146] Although it is well suited to procedural sedation, particularly for radiologic procedures, electroencephalography, and echocardiography, with prolonged use, accumulation of trichloroethanol leads to life-threatening arrhythmias, hypotension, and paradoxic CNS stimulation.[147] This disadvantage of chloral hydrate, along with its tendency to displace various drugs and bilirubin from their protein-bound sites, as well as its propensity to cause direct hyperbilirubinemia,[148] preclude its use for sedation in neonates.

MUSCLE RELAXANTS

Neuromuscular blockade is sometimes required for the care of critically ill infants, especially during procedures that often require their immobilization. Such blockade can be achieved either through excessive depolarization at the neuromuscular junction (depolarizing agents) or through a blockade of transmission at the neuromuscular junction achieved by acetylcholine antagonists (nondepolarizing agents). The use of muscle relaxants is not routinely indicated during mechanical ventilation of neonates, but muscle relaxants are sometimes used as part of premedication regimens and in certain patient populations such as infants with persistent pulmonary hypertension of the newborn (PPHN).[149] Although paralysis may improve oxygenation and ventilation of severely hypoxemic term infants with PPHN, it may have adverse effects on preterm infants with RDS.[150] The use of synchronized ventilation using ventilator rates above the spontaneous rate of the patient frequently will accomplish the goals of paralysis (see Chapter 18).[151] Muscle relaxants may be useful in selected preterm infants whose own respiratory efforts interfere with ventilation and may reduce the incidence of pneumothorax in these infants.[152]

Perlman et al. demonstrated that the elimination of fluctuating cerebral blood flow velocity by muscle paralysis reduced the incidence of IVH in selected preterm infants with RDS, but this has not been tested in a large trial and is not practiced commonly. Because muscle paralysis may reduce oxygen consumption, paralysis may be advantageous to infants with compromised oxygenation.[153,154] Prolonged paralysis of greater than 2 weeks' duration has been associated with disuse atrophy and subsequent skeletal muscle growth failure. Importantly, in terms of pulmonary mechanics, Bhutani et al.[155] have shown a decrease in dynamic lung compliance and an increase in total pulmonary resistance only after more than 48 hours of continuous paralysis with pancuronium. Both parameters improved by 41% to 43% at 6 to 18 hours after discontinuation of paralysis.

Spontaneous respiratory efforts appear to contribute little to minute ventilation in the severely ill preterm infant with very low lung compliance.[154] These infants are at risk of decreased functional residual capacity after paralysis, possibly through loss of upper airway braking mechanisms.[150] In infants with lung compliance that is less compromised and in larger infants, spontaneous respiratory efforts contribute markedly to total ventilation. Thus, ventilator adjustments (usually increases in rate) are necessary to prevent significant hypoventilation when paralysis is instituted. Monitoring gas exchange is recommended. Although loss of intercostal muscle tone may lead to an increase in intrathoracic pressure, this does not appear to cause an increase in respiratory resistance.[156]

The primary hazard during paralysis appears to be accidental inconspicuous extubation. The paralyzed neonate is entirely dependent on mechanical ventilation, and careful observation is required. Also, paralysis obscures a variety of clinical signs whose expression depends on muscle tone and movement, such as seizures. Finally, paralysis does not alter the sensation of pain; thus, analgesics should be administered under circumstances in which their use would be indicated in a nonparalyzed infant.

In practice, the decision to administer a muscle relaxant is most often based on clinical observation of an infant in combination with arterial blood gas measurements. Muscle relaxants are used frequently to facilitate hyperventilation therapy (see Chapter 18 and the section entitled Persistent Pulmonary Hypertension of the Newborn in Chapter 23). Analysis of ventilator or esophageal pressure waveforms is a more objective method of assessing whether an infant is in phase with the ventilator and whether mean intrathoracic pressure is increased.[152] However, there is no reliable way of predicting which infants in this circumstance will benefit from paralysis. Thus, muscle relaxants should be administered as a therapeutic trial and their use continued if blood gas values improve during the trial, if nursing care is greatly simplified, or if there is obvious improvement in patient synchrony with the ventilator and comfort. If

TABLE 32.3 Neuromuscular Blocking Agents for Neonates

Agent	Initial Dose (mg/kg)	Dose Frequency	Infusion Dose (mg/kg/hour)
Pancuronium	0.04–0.15	1–4 hours	Not recommended
Vecuronium	0.03–0.15	1–2 hours	0.05–0.10
Rocuronium	0.3–0.6	0.5–1 hours	0.4–0.6

the complications of prolonged paralysis are to be prevented, periodic assessment of the infant in the nonparalyzed state is essential. The short-acting depolarizing muscle relaxant succinylcholine is infrequently used in the care of neonates, except when paralysis for intubation is necessary; therefore, only the commonly used nondepolarizing agents are discussed in this section. Recommended dosages are listed in Table 32.3.

Pancuronium

Pancuronium bromide, a long-acting, competitive neuromuscular blocking agent, is the muscle relaxant most frequently used in neonates. Gallamine and d-tubocurarine are seldom used because of significant cardiovascular effects, sympathetic ganglionic blockade, and, in the case of the former, obligatory renal excretion. All of these agents block transmission at the neuromuscular junction by competing with acetylcholine for receptor sites on the postjunctional membrane.[157] Pancuronium has vagolytic effects, and an increase in heart rate is commonly observed during its use. Administered intravenously, pancuronium produces maximum paralysis within 2 to 4 minutes. The duration of apnea after a single dose is variable and prolonged in neonates and can last from one to several hours. Incremental doses increase the duration of respiratory paralysis. In addition, the duration of paralysis is prolonged by acidosis, hypokalemia, use of aminoglycoside antibiotics, and decreased renal function. Alkalosis can be expected to antagonize blockade. Although renal excretion is the major route of elimination of pancuronium, hepatobiliary excretion and metabolism may account for the elimination of a significant portion of an administered dose.

The recommended dosage of pancuronium in neonates varies from 0.06 to 0.10 mg/kg.[157] Although it is customary to administer repeat doses that are of the same magnitude as the initial dose, subsequent doses of half the initial dose may be effective in prolonging paralysis when muscular activity or spontaneous respiration returns. Continuous infusion of pancuronium in neonates is associated with the potential for accumulation because of these patients' slow rate of excretion; thus, this method of administration is best avoided unless electrophysiologic monitoring is available.

The long-term benefits of respiratory paralysis need to be balanced with potential complications. Prolonged use of pancuronium bromide has been implicated in sensorineural hearing loss in childhood survivors of congenital diaphragmatic hernia.[158,159] In a cohort study of head trauma patients in a pediatric intensive care unit setting, patients treated with and without pancuronium were compared.[160] In the 15 patients with isolated intracranial pathology who received continuous paralysis, compliance progressively dropped by 50% over 4 days. Compliance normalized after discontinuation of paralysis. Compliance did not change in the patients who were ventilated but not paralyzed. The paralyzed patients required mechanical ventilation longer than the nonparalyzed patients, and 26% of these patients developed nosocomial pneumonia, a complication that was not seen in the nonparalyzed patients. Prolonged use of pancuronium has also been associated with weight gain and third-space accumulation from lack of movement and urinary retention.

Despite the reported complications, pancuronium is still frequently used in the NICU population.[161] A systematic review[162] summarized the literature by stating that in ventilated preterm infants with evidence of asynchronous respiratory efforts, neuromuscular paralysis with pancuronium seems to be associated with less IVH and possibly less pulmonary air leak. The authors went on to stress that long-term pulmonary and neurologic effects are uncertain.

The effects of pancuronium can be rapidly reversed with the use of the anticholinesterase agent neostigmine at 0.08 mg/kg intravenously, preceded by the administration of glycopyrrolate at 2.5 to 5 mcg/kg, which blocks the muscarinic side effects. Although rapid reversal is seldom needed for medical reasons in neonates receiving assisted ventilation, reversal may occasionally be useful diagnostically in infants considered to have suffered a CNS insult during paralysis.

Vecuronium

Vecuronium is a short-acting nondepolarizing muscle relaxant that is structurally related to pancuronium, with time to onset of action of 1.5 to 2.0 minutes after intravenous bolus infusion, with a duration of effect that lasts only 30 to 40 minutes.[157] It has few cardiovascular side effects and is cleared rapidly by biliary excretion. Thus, it is safer than pancuronium in the presence of renal failure. Interference with excretion or potentiation of effect has been suggested when vecuronium is used in combination with metronidazole, aminoglycosides, and hydantoins. However, no problems have been observed in infants receiving these agents and vecuronium in its usual dosage.[157] Acidosis can be expected to enhance the neuromuscular blockade provided by vecuronium and alkalosis to antagonize it.

Vecuronium usually is given by continuous intravenous infusion at a rate of 0.1 mg/kg/hr after an initial paralyzing bolus dose of 0.1 mg/kg. Intermittent bolus dosing would need to be so frequent (i.e., every 30-60 minutes) that this type of regimen usually is impractical. Continuous infusion is preferred for certain postoperative cardiac patients whose respiratory or other muscular movement may jeopardize the success of the repair. The effects of vecuronium can be reversed by neostigmine administration, as described earlier for pancuronium.

Rocuronium

Rocuronium is a rapid-acting but less potent desacetoxy analogue of vecuronium. Like other steroidal drugs, it is mostly (70%–90%) metabolized in the liver and excreted through the biliary tract, which accounts for its shorter duration of action,

reported to be 20 to 35 minutes, compared with agents that are mostly excreted through the renal system.[163] A trial of 44 intubations in preterm infants who were randomized to receive either atropine or fentanyl alone or rocuronium added to these agents found that infants in the latter group were more likely to be successfully intubated on the first attempt. Onset of paralysis was 22 to 106 seconds after administration of a 0.5-mg/kg dose of rocuronium. Complete paralysis was noted to last for 3 to 29 minutes after administration of the above dose. Adverse effects noted in this study included transient tachycardia (7%) and bronchospasm in one infant.[164] Recommended dosages for rocuronium can be found in Table 32.3.

Cisatracurium

Atracurium is an isoquinoline nondepolarizing neuromuscular blocker that is metabolized mostly by Hofmann elimination, a nonenzymatic spontaneous degradation process that occurs at physiologic pH and temperature. Cisatracurium is an enantiomer of atracurium that is four times more potent, slower in its onset of action, but similar to atracurium in its duration of action. Like atracurium, it undergoes Hofmann elimination but is not hydrolyzed by plasma cholinesterase. Unlike atracurium, cisatracurium does not provoke histamine release, thereby minimizing adverse effects such as hypotension and bradycardia. Its metabolism also produces less laudanosine, a CNS stimulant that can provoke seizures.[163] A study of continuous cisatracurium infusion for neuromuscular blockade compared with vecuronium in 19 infants recovering from cardiac surgery found that infants in the cisatracurium group recovered their neuromuscular function faster compared with infants in the vecuronium group. This study used doses of cisatracurium ranging between 0.75 and 4.5 mcg/kg/min. In these dosage ranges, cisatracurium had an elimination half-life between 15 and 468 minutes for the nine infants in this study.[165] Routine use of cisatracurium in newborn infants, especially for ELBW premature infants, requires more evidence regarding its pharmacokinetic and pharmacodynamic profiles in this patient group.

BRONCHODILATORS AND MUCOLYTIC AGENTS

Bronchospasm was long believed to play a minimal if any role in contributing to airway resistance in the newborn, especially in preterm infants. Anatomic studies that demonstrated lack of smooth muscle in the distal airways of premature infants strengthened this opinion.[166] However, studies that confirmed the presence of airway smooth muscle even in the lungs of 23-week gestation infants have disproved such misconceptions. The airways of 25-week-old infants have smooth muscle relative to airway circumference that is similar to that of term infants, indicating that bronchospasm is possible in preterm infants within the first few days after birth.[167] It is now known that mechanically ventilated infants with BPD have airway smooth muscle hypertrophy that often plays a significant role in increasing airway resistance.[168] In addition to contributing to resistance to airflow, the tracheobronchial tree of preterm infants compared with term infants and adults also possesses a relatively higher number of goblet cells that express mucus and

TABLE 32.4 Aerosolized Medications for Neonates

Agent	Dose	Dose Frequency	Comments
Salbutamol	0.20 mg/kg	Every 3–6 hours	With 0.5% solution, dilute 0.04 mL/kg in 1.5 mL NS 18-mg/puff, one or two puffs/dose with metered-dose inhaler[a]
Ipratropium bromide	0.025 mg/kg	Every 8 hours	
N-acetylcysteine	10–20 mg	Every 6–8 hours	Add bronchodilator if bronchospasm occurs; restricted use advised in view of undesirable effects
Cromoglycic acid (cromolyn sodium)	10 mg	Every 6 hours	Dilute 1 mL of 10-mg/mL solution up to 1.5 mL NS

[a]Only available metered-dose inhaler in the United States.
NS, Normal saline.

fewer ciliated airway cells to assist in the mobilization of airway secretions and mucus.[169] In addition to effecting bronchodilation, some agents such as aminophylline improve diaphragmatic and inspiratory muscle contractility, which may result in both improved ventilation and a greater likelihood of successful and earlier extubation, the goals for which the clinician should be striving.[170] Thus, bronchodilators to decrease airway resistance and mucolytic agents that promote mucin breakdown are often used as aids to mechanical ventilation of the neonate. Typical dosages for commonly used aerosolized medications are listed in Table 32.4.

Albuterol (Salbutamol)

Albuterol is a selective β_2-adrenergic agonist. By enhancing cAMP production, which then decreases intracellular calcium in smooth muscle cells, albuterol causes bronchodilation. Although other formulations exist, albuterol is primarily used as an aerosol, further enhancing its selectivity.[171,172] At high doses, inhaled albuterol loses such bronchial β_2 selectivity and leads to adverse effects such as vasodilation, hypotension, reflex tachycardia, hyperglycemia, and hypokalemia, secondary to its effects on other β_2-adrenergic receptor systems.[173]

Infants with established or developing BPD often have increased airflow resistance, decreased forced expiratory flow, and increased functional reserve capacity compared with normal cohorts.[174,175] Albuterol improves static lung compliance in VLBW infants as early as the second postnatal week.[176] Some 35% of infants with BPD, especially those with clinically noted symptoms such as wheezing, exhibited responsiveness to albuterol inhalation.[175]

Most of the previously mentioned studies, however, did not assess longer-term clinical outcomes of albuterol therapy for premature infants with BPD. In the only study as of this writing that assessed longer term outcomes in 173 infants of less than 28 weeks' GA, albuterol treatment started on day 11 and continued for 28 days did not reduce supplemental oxygen or mechanical ventilation, mortality, or the severity of BPD.[177] An important caveat to note is that all of these studies predate the use of surfactant and antenatal steroids and may not be applicable to infants with "new BPD." Controversy also exists regarding long-term β-agonist stimulation of nonpulmonary tissues, possible adverse effects of long-term bronchodilation on healing lung tissue, and theoretical concerns over the development of tolerance.[178] A large nonrandomized comparison of bronchodilators versus placebo in infants who were enrolled for the Neonatal European Study of Inhaled Steroids (NEuroSIS) study found no differences in rates of BPD or death between the two groups. A 2016 Cochrane collaboration systematic review identified only two trials of albuterol that met criteria for inclusion concluded that available data are insufficient to reliably assess the effectiveness of albuterol in improving clinical outcomes for infants with BPD.[179]

Cromoglycic Acid

Cromoglycic acid (cromolyn sodium) is an antiinflammatory agent that prevents mast cell activation and degranulation by inhibiting chloride transport and protein kinase C. Cromoglycic acid can also inhibit neutrophil chemotaxis and free radical–induced neutrophil nicotinamide adenine dinucleotide phosphate oxidase.[180] As cromoglycic acid is a highly ionized water-soluble compound, it does not cross cell membranes and can be effectively administered only by inhalation.[181] Interest in using cromolyn as a therapy for mechanically ventilated infants was created by a small cohort study that found that cromolyn sodium therapy administered to infants with BPD was associated with decreased need for invasive ventilation and an increase in dynamic lung compliance.[182] The antiinflammatory effects of cromolyn sodium that were postulated in this study led to two small trials that attempted to use cromolyn early in life for preterm infants to mitigate their risk for lung inflammation. In the first of these small studies, a trial of 38 infants with mean GA of 26 weeks who required mechanical ventilation at birth, nebulized cromolyn sodium given every 6 hours for the duration that the infants remained intubated did not reduce risk for BPD or mortality compared with placebo.[183] Another small trial of 26 infants randomized to receive either cromolyn or placebo for 28 days after birth also showed no difference in BPD or death.[184] Neither study found beneficial effects for the antiinflammatory effects of cromolyn for outcomes such as IVH, sepsis, necrotizing enterocolitis, or patent ductus arteriosus (PDA). A Cochrane review that included both of these studies ($n = 64$) found no evidence to recommend routine use of cromolyn sodium for prevention of BPD in preterm infants.[185] Because there is some evidence for a decrease in inflammatory markers associated with BPD when sodium cromolyn is used in conjunction with surfactant, diuretics, and steroids, cromolyn sodium may be an important adjunct therapy when used with other agents such as steroids and warrants further clinical trials.[186]

Ipratropium Bromide

Atropine, a potent inhibitor of acetylcholine at postganglionic muscarinic receptors, is known to produce bronchodilation and reduce the production of airway mucin. Ipratropium bromide is a quaternary ammonium derivative of atropine that when administered by inhalation into the airways is poorly absorbed into the circulation and can be used as a selective bronchodilator.[173] Because functional muscarinic airway receptors have been demonstrated in the airways of premature infants, ipratropium bromide has been used as a bronchodilator for infants with BPD.[187] A study that used inhaled ipratropium bromide for infants with BPD found that muscarinic receptors contributed to the increased bronchomotor tone seen in these infants and that a combination of ipratropium and albuterol produced effective and long-lasting bronchodilation.[188] However, similar to inhaled β agonists, there is no evidence as of this writing for long-term benefits of ipratropium bromide use for the natural course of BPD in preterm infants.

Racemic Epinephrine

The subglottis is the narrowest portion of the airway in neonates. The presence of a foreign body, as occurs with prolonged intubation, produces edema in the subglottic region, which can produce further narrowing of the airway when the neonate is extubated. Racemic epinephrine stimulates both α- and β-adrenergic receptors. It acts on vascular smooth muscle to produce vasoconstriction, which markedly decreases blood flow at the capillary level. This shrinks upper respiratory mucosa and reduces edema. Racemic epinephrine is a useful agent in patients with established postextubation stridor; however, its efficacy for the prevention of postextubation stridor has not been proven.[189] Racemic epinephrine may also be considered as an adjunct to therapy for pulmonary hemorrhage.[190] When using racemic epinephrine, one should be aware of the side effects, which include tachycardia, arrhythmias, hypertension, peripheral vasoconstriction, hyperglycemia, hyperkalemia, metabolic acidosis, and leukocytosis.[189]

N-Acetylcysteine

N-acetylcysteine (NAC) is a well-known thiol compound that possesses a free sulfhydryl group through which it reduces disulfide bonds present in mucoproteins, thereby reducing the elasticity and viscosity of mucus.[191] NAC also interacts directly with oxidants such as hydrogen peroxide and the hydroxyl radical through its role as a modulator of cellular redox status.[192] This role may also contribute to the efficacy of NAC in improving lung function in adults with chronic obstructive pulmonary disease.[193] However, experience with the use of NAC in neonates is fairly limited. A small study of NAC found that hourly doses of up to 0.2 mL of endotracheally administered NAC did not alter postmortem histology of trachea or bronchi in preterm infants.[194] Another study evaluated the effects of intratracheal NAC administration on lung function in mechanically ventilated infants with a mean GA of 27 weeks and mean postnatal age of 22 weeks. This study found that NAC administration was associated with an increase in airway resistance by the third day of treatment. The authors concluded that NAC administration was not associated with any improvement in lung function for infants with BPD and also that its administration may indeed be associated with adverse effects such as increased airway resistance and cyanotic spells.[195] Thus, the use of NAC in preterm infants should be undertaken cautiously, and when used, NAC should be administered along with bronchodilators to offset these reported adverse effects.

Although NAC held promise as an effective antiinflammatory agent secondary to its antioxidant properties, this too has not been borne out in studies. A study of 33 preterm infants between 24 and 28 weeks' gestation randomized them to receive either NAC or placebo during the first week of life. Measurements of lung function conducted when these infants were close to discharge from the NICU did not show any differences between the groups. The authors concluded that prophylactic NAC treatment for preterm infants at risk for BPD does not improve their lung function at term.[196]

Combination Therapies

In addition to the use of bronchodilators and ICS in isolation, their use in combination, using delivery devices like metered-dose inhalers (MDIs) and jet nebulizers, as therapy for BPD has also been evaluated. In a study of 173 infants of less than 31 weeks' GA randomized to receive albuterol, beclomethasone, their combination, or placebo delivered through an MDI or a jet nebulizer, no differences in the duration of oxygen therapy or ventilator support, or the incidence and severity of BPD, were noted among the various groups.[183] In addition, the combined use of such medication may not provide any additional effects than when administered individually, as was shown by a small study of 15 infants in which combined administration of β agonists and anticholinergics failed to demonstrate any synergy between these two agents in improving airway function.[197]

In summary, as concluded by a review that reported on 22 trials involving the use of inhaled β agonists, anticholinergics, and corticosteroids for infants with BPD, no clear long-term benefits have been demonstrated as of this writing.[198] Newer modalities of drug-delivery devices and combinations of such medications need to be evaluated, and as suggested by the authors of the review, stratification of infants who respond to such medications could help identify specific infant subgroups that could benefit from such therapy.

DIURETICS

Neonates have increased alveolar and interstitial fluid in the lungs. "Classic" BPD has also been associated with the exudative-inflammatory process in its earliest stages. Such excessive pulmonary interstitial fluid reduces lung compliance, increases airway resistance, and is followed by subacute and chronic fibroproliferative changes that further exacerbate its pathogenesis.[199] Factors responsible for this excessive pulmonary fluid accumulation include increased pulmonary epithelial, capillary permeability, and overcirculation secondary to a persistent PDA.[200,201] Diuretics decrease work of breathing and aid mechanical ventilation by decreasing pulmonary interstitial fluid and improving lung compliance.[202,203] In a 2013 survey, wide between-hospital variations for overall diuretic usage as well as specific agents used for infants under 29 weeks' GA were reported.[204] Although several classes of diuretics exist, the most commonly used agents in premature infants include the loop diuretic furosemide and the thiazides.

Furosemide

Furosemide is a sulfonamide derivative and is the most commonly used diuretic in the neonate. By blocking the NaCl reabsorption by the Na/K/2Cl symporter in the thick ascending loop of Henle (TAL), furosemide and other similar "loop" diuretics can produce highly efficacious diuresis. In addition, furosemide induces increased prostaglandin E2 (PGE2) synthesis by renal cyclo-oxygenase 2.[205] PGE2 is also a direct inhibitor of salt transport across the TAL and also acts as a vasodilator to increase renal blood flow and glomerular filtration, thereby enhancing the diuretic actions of furosemide.[206] Through such diuresis, furosemide decreases intravascular volume, increases systemic venous capacitance, and decreases lung lymph flow to decrease pulmonary interstitial fluid accumulation.[207] In addition to its diuretic effect, furosemide-induced PGE2 synthesis also causes pulmonary vasodilation and decreases pulmonary interstitial fluid accumulation.[208] Additionally, furosemide decreases inflammatory mediators such as leukotrienes and histamine in lung tissue.[209] Furosemide can be administered through enteral, intravenous, or intramuscular routes; oral bioavailability has been reported to be about 84% in term newborn infants.[210] The usual dosage is 1 to 2 mg/kg intravenously, but it may also be given intramuscularly or orally. A study of 10 preterm infants whose mean GA at birth was 27 weeks showed that plasma $T_{1/2}$ was greater than 24 hours in infants under 32 weeks and declined to approximately 4 hours by term corrected age, implying that furosemide clearance increases with maturity.[211]

Major adverse effects include hypokalemia, hypocalcemia, hypercalciuria, nephrocalcinosis (risk is especially higher with exposure to more than 10 mg/kg cumulative dose of furosemide in preterm infants), hypomagnesemia, hypochloremic alkalosis, and hyponatremia.[212] Coadministration of a thiazide diuretic along with furosemide can decrease the incidence of nephrocalcinosis.[213] Ototoxicity has been reported with furosemide exposure especially in preterm infants for whom a 12-hour interval dosing of furosemide often produced furosemide accumulation to potentially ototoxic levels (>25 mcg/mL).[210] Although such hearing loss is often transient and reversible, additive damage secondary to concomitant use of other ototoxic agents such as gentamicin should be taken into consideration during furosemide pharmacotherapy.[214] In addition, infants with BPD are often fluid restricted in an attempt to reduce pulmonary edema, and brisk diuresis with furosemide administration has the potential to cause hypotension in these infants. Elevated PGE2 levels secondary to furosemide use can also decrease closure of the ductus arteriosus and increase risk for hemodynamically significant PDA.[215,216] In addition, chronic use of loop diuretics may have the paradoxic effect of raising PCO$_2$ because they work by retaining bicarbonate at the expense of the excretion of chloride.

Furosemide-induced diuresis for preterm infants with RDS who required mechanical ventilation has been shown to improve lung compliance, improve functional residual capacity, and reduce peak inspiratory pressure required for ventilation.[217] Daily furosemide use for 3 days at 1 mg/kg/day improved diuresis and facilitated quicker extubation in a trial of 57 low birth weight infants who required mechanical ventilation for RDS.[218] In another randomized trial of 99 infants of less than 30 weeks, furosemide use led to decreased duration of mechanical ventilation and increased survival compared with thiazide-use or no-diuretic-use groups.[219] However, these investigators found in a subsequent study that routine use of prophylactic furosemide for infants with RDS did not improve pulmonary outcomes and, furthermore, led to volume depletion and increased requirement for vasopressors.[220] The most recent Cochrane review of diuretic use for preterm infants with RDS concluded that the risk of clinically significant hypotension and PDA associated with furosemide use outweighed the benefits of improved short-term pulmonary outcomes and recommends against the routine use of furosemide for infants with RDS.[221]

Similar to its effects on pulmonary function in younger infants with RDS, furosemide may also improve pulmonary compliance, airway conductance, and resistance in older infants with established BPD. A small randomized study in which pulmonary function of 17 infants with BPD was measured before and after administration of daily doses of 1 mg/kg of furosemide or placebo for 7 days found decreased ventilator requirements, increased pulmonary compliance, and improved alveolar ventilation for infants in the furosemide group but not for those in the placebo group.[222] A more recent retrospective analysis of a large cohort of VLBW preterm infants ($n = 37,693$) found that a 10% increase in number of days of furosemide exposure was associated with a 3.7% reduction in risk for BPD or death, but these results should be interpreted with caution.[223] A Cochrane review of loop diuretic use for infants with BPD concluded that all six studies eligible to be included in the review focused only on pathophysiologic parameters and not long-term clinical outcomes. Despite finding that long-term administration of furosemide did improve oxygenation and lung compliance, the authors do not recommend routine use of long-term furosemide to prevent or treat BPD.[224]

Furosemide has also been administered as an aerosol to preterm infants with BPD. When administered directly to the lung as an aerosol furosemide has been shown to decrease bronchospasm by decreasing smooth muscle contractility through several possible mechanisms that include modification of mast cell and sensory epithelial activation in the airways, decreased release of inflammatory mediators such as leukotrienes and histamine, increased vascular endothelial release of prostaglandins, and inhibition of cholinergic bronchoconstriction.[209,225-227] This mode of delivery offers the advantage of possibly decreasing systemic side effects while maintaining desired pulmonary effects. However, in view of the lack of data from randomized trials on the effects of aerosolized loop diuretics on important clinical outcomes, routine or sustained use of this mode of delivery cannot be justified based on the current evidence.[228]

Bumetanide

Bumetanide is also a loop diuretic, about 40 times more potent than furosemide. Owing to its high lipid solubility, bumetanide is able to diffuse passively to its site of action, unlike furosemide, which requires active tubular secretion. Bumetanide is highly effective in producing rapid diuresis and relieving pulmonary edema. Bumetanide also causes less renal potassium loss and is less ototoxic compared with furosemide. In a study of bumetanide metabolism in 14 neonates between 26 and 40 weeks' GA, its half-life was noted to be about 1.74 to 7 hours and the volume of distribution was 0.22 L/kg (range, 0.11–0.32 L/kg).[229] The authors suggest that bumetanide dosing may need to be higher and the dosing interval prolonged for neonates compared with adults. At plasma concentrations above those achieved during routine therapeutic use, the binding of bumetanide to neonatal plasma proteins is approximately 97%. Hence, saturation of albumin-binding sites is unlikely at therapeutic doses.[230] Nonrenal clearance is responsible for 58% to 97% of bumetanide metabolism. In a random crossover trial of 17 premature infants, bumetanide was found to produce lower sodium loss per urine volume, but higher urinary calcium loss, compared with furosemide.[231] There are currently no randomized trials that have compared bumetanide to furosemide use with respect to their safety profiles or their efficacy in preventing or reducing the severity of BPD in ventilated preterm neonates.

Thiazides and Potassium-Sparing Diuretics

Derived from sulfonamides, the thiazides are less potent diuretics compared with furosemide. They act at the distal tubule to inhibit reabsorption of NaCl through the apical luminal transporter. Because 90% of sodium reabsorption occurs proximal to their site of action in the distal nephron, thiazides are only moderately effective diuretics compared with the more potent loop diuretics. Spironolactone, a potassium-sparing diuretic, competes with aldosterone in the distal convoluted tubule. Because of the nature of aldosterone's mode of action, which is dependent on protein synthesis, the onset of action of spironolactone is delayed. In addition to increasing renal sodium excretion, thiazides can also cause hypokalemia, hypomagnesemia, and hypophosphatemia by increasing urinary loss of these electrolytes. However, in contrast to the loop diuretics, thiazides and spironolactone do not cause increased urinary calcium loss. Serum electrolyte monitoring should be considered when long-term use of thiazide diuretics is required. The usual dosages of chlorothiazide and spironolactone are 10 to 20 and 1 to 2 mg/kg, respectively.

Thiazide diuretic use for infants with BPD has become widespread. In one survey of diuretic use in children's hospitals in the United States, chlorothiazide was found to be the diuretic with the longest median duration of use, approximately 21 days.[204] A study that assessed the effect of combined chlorothiazide and spironolactone in 10 nonventilated infants with BPD found that the use of these diuretics was associated with decreased airway resistance and improved lung compliance compared with placebo.[232] Several other small studies have also concluded that thiazide diuretics improve lung function. A Cochrane collaboration

systematic review included six such studies to assess the impact of distal renal tubular diuretic use in improving outcomes for infants with BPD. As most of these studies focused on pathophysiologic parameters and did not sufficiently assess clinical outcomes or potential complications related to diuretic therapy, the reviewers concluded that there is no strong evidence for benefit from the routine use of thiazide diuretic therapy in preterm infants with BPD.[233]

RESPIRATORY STIMULANTS

Whereas apnea of prematurity continues to remain the primary indication for the use of respiratory stimulants such as caffeine in the NICU, these agents have shown benefits for other outcomes such as duration of mechanical ventilation, need for PDA ligation, and incidence of BPD at 36 weeks.[234] This has expanded their indications for use to include assistance with weaning mechanical ventilation and facilitating earlier extubation in neonatal units around the United States.[235] Methylxanthines, including caffeine and theophylline, are the most commonly used respiratory stimulants for treatment of apnea. By inhibiting phosphodiesterase (PDE) enzyme isoforms (especially PDE4) and through cell surface adenosine receptor antagonism, methylxanthines stimulate the medullary respiratory center and therefore increase minute ventilation. They also cause bronchodilation and enhanced diaphragmatic contractility. Research also suggests that methylxanthines enhance histone deacetylation, an epigenetic process that decreases genetic transcription.[173] Because some of the antiinflammatory effects of corticosteroids are mediated by histone deacetylation of several inflammatory genes, methylxanthines could enhance the effects of corticosteroids when these two therapies are used together, as is often the case in premature infants with BPD.[236,237] The pharmacology of theophylline and caffeine, the major methylxanthines in therapeutic use, and doxapram, which is a nonmethylxanthine respiratory stimulant, are discussed in detail in the following, and the usual dosages for methylxanthines are listed in Table 32.5.

Theophylline

Theophylline is a methylated xanthine alkaloid (1,3-dimethylxanthine) that is found naturally in tea. Its half-life is approximately 30 hours in the neonate, compared with 7 hours in adults.[238] Theophylline has more potent inotropic, vasodilator, bronchodilator, and diuretic actions compared with caffeine because of its more efficacious PDE inhibition and adenosine antagonism. Theophylline may cause less respiratory center stimulation than caffeine but enhances diaphragmatic contractility to a greater extent by facilitating increased neuromuscular transmission with increased tidal volumes.[170] It is also an inhibitor of lymphocyte function as well as mast cell histamine release; by these mechanisms, it can reduce airway inflammation.[239] In the adult, theophylline is eliminated by hepatic biotransformation and urinary excretion. In the newborn, however, the hepatic biotransformation with N-demethylation is absent; instead, the occurrence of N-7-methylation produces caffeine.[240] The therapeutic plasma concentration is about 7 to 20 mg/L. In one study, levels greater than 6.6 mg/L controlled apneic spells,

TABLE 32.5 Methylxanthines for Neonatal Apnea

Drug	Loading Dose (IV, mg/kg)	Maintenance Dosage (IV)[a]	Plasma Concentration (mg/L)	Toxicity
Theophylline	5.5–6.0	1 mg/kg every 8 hours or 2 mg/kg every 12 hours	7–20[b] (~10 ideal)	Cardiovascular: tachycardia CNS stimulation: seizures, jitteriness Gastrointestinal: vomiting, distention
Caffeine	10	2.5–5 mg/kg every 24 hours	7–20[b]	Unlikely with plasma levels <50 mg/L
Caffeine citrate	20	5–10 mg/kg every 24 hours		As for caffeine

[a]Oral dosage = intravenous (IV) dosage × 1.25.
[b]Monitor levels and screen for signs of toxicity.

whereas cardiovascular toxicity with tachycardia was noted only at levels greater than 13.0 mg/L.[241] Some newborns manifested toxicity at levels of 9.0 mg/L of transplacentally acquired theophylline. Because of the problems at these lower levels and because of the potential additive effects of the caffeine produced from theophylline, 10 mg/L may be a desirable level. Signs of toxicity may include irritability, diaphoresis, diarrhea, seizures, gastroesophageal reflux, and tachycardia.[242] The usual intravenous loading dose of theophylline is 4.0 to 6.0 mg/kg, with a maintenance dose of 1 mg/kg every 8 hours or 2 mg/kg every 12 hours. Its low cost makes its use especially advantageous in low-resource settings.

Caffeine

The addition of another methyl group to theophylline produces caffeine (1,3,7-trimethylxanthine), an agent with a plasma half-life of approximately 100 hours. This modification allows for caffeine to be administered once daily compared with theophylline, which needs to be administered two or three times daily.[239] Preterm infants have limited capacity to metabolize caffeine through the hepatic cytochrome P450 pathway; therefore, most of the drug is excreted unchanged in the urine. Caffeine has similar efficacy compared with theophylline for most therapeutic effects but may have less propensity for adverse effects such as tachycardia. Plasma levels of 5 to 20 mg/L are considered therapeutic, and studies suggest that higher levels (up to 50 mg/L) may not be associated with adverse effects.[240] Toxic manifestations of caffeine include excessive jitteriness and rarely seizures. The usual loading dose of caffeine is 10 mg/kg, with a daily maintenance dose of 2.5 to 5 mg/kg. The usual form of caffeine, the citrate in a 20-mg/mL solution, is equivalent to a 10-mg/mL solution of the base and may be administered intravenously or orally.[240]

A 2010 meta-analysis that reviewed five trials comparing theophylline and caffeine for apnea of prematurity found reduced risk of tachycardia and feeding intolerance for caffeine (relative risk, 0.17; CI, 0.04–0.72).[243] Because of these advantages, caffeine has become the most commonly used methylxanthine in the NICU.[161] In a study of 234 infants randomized to receive low-dose (2.5 mg/kg/day) versus high-dose (10 mg/kg/day) caffeine, significantly lower risk for extubation failure and disability at 12 months as well as documented apneic events was noted for infants who received the higher dose. However, risk for BPD remained similar between the two

groups.[244] The largest study of the effects of caffeine use in preterm neonates was the Caffeine for Apnea of Prematurity (CAP) trial, which enrolled 2006 infants to receive either caffeine or placebo when caffeine was indicated.[245] This study found that caffeine use led to reduced requirements for various forms of respiratory support, including intubation, positive-pressure support, and need for supplemental oxygen. Decreased duration of mechanical ventilation was another significant advantage noted with early initiation of caffeine therapy (up to 3 days of life), a benefit that was lost when caffeine was started beyond this age. In addition, caffeine use also reduced the incidence of BPD as well as the need for surgical ligation of PDA compared with placebo in infants with indications to give caffeine. One of the initial follow-up studies of the CAP trial showed that caffeine offered a significant benefit in reducing risk for death or disability at 18 months' corrected GA as well as reducing the risk for cerebral palsy compared with placebo.[246] Infants receiving respiratory support appeared to derive more neurodevelopmental benefits from caffeine than infants not receiving support.[247] However, a follow-up study of these infants at 5 years of age somewhat dampened the initial enthusiasm by showing no significant differences in neurodevelopmental indices between the two groups of infants at this age.[248] The timing of caffeine initiation remains a controversial issue. Whereas post hoc analyses of the CAP trial and other independent nonrandomized studies with large number of participants have shown a lower incidence of death or BPD when caffeine is started early (1–3 days of life) versus late (>3 days), a recent single-center randomized controlled trial (RCT) of early versus late caffeine was stopped early when an interim safety analysis found a trend toward higher mortality in the early caffeine group. However, further analyses indicated that this increased trend was not statistically significant. Although larger multicenter RCTs may be required to definitively answer this question, there are at least two small single-center trials currently in progress.[30,249]

Doxapram

Doxapram is a pyrrolidinone derivative with CNS-stimulant (analeptic) effects. Its mechanism of action, although still unclear, is believed to involve stimulation of both central and peripheral chemoreceptors, which then leads to stimulation of ventral brainstem nuclei and subsequent increased depth and rate of respiration.[250] In a study of 83 full-term infants, doxapram given at doses of 2 to 3 mg/kg immediately after birth hastened the recovery from respiratory depression secondary to maternal narcotic or anesthetic exposure.[251] Another study of 31 infants with apnea of prematurity with a mean GA of 30 weeks that randomized them to receive placebo, theophylline, or doxapram showed fewer treatment failures with theophylline or doxapram compared with placebo.[252] A smaller study of 15 infants showed that although both doxapram and aminophylline were equally efficacious for the treatment of apnea of prematurity, of 10 infants who failed treatment with aminophylline, eight responded to the addition of doxapram with complete cessation of apnea.[253] There are, however, no large trials of doxapram versus aminophylline or caffeine use for premature infants with apnea. A Cochrane Collaboration systematic review concluded that there are insufficient data to recommend doxapram for use as treatment to reduce apneic episodes in premature infants.[254]

Doxapram has been used primarily as a second-line agent in addition to methylxanthines for refractory apnea of prematurity. It is most often administered as a continuous intravenous infusion, although an intermittent intravenous bolus regimen has been proposed. Loading doses of 2.5 to 3 mg/kg are used, followed by maintenance infusion of 0.5 to 2.5 mg/kg/hr. Because many doxapram preparations contain benzyl alcohol or butorphanol, the use of doxapram should be exercised with caution. Ideal plasma therapeutic levels have been suggested to be between 2 and 5 mg/L, with adverse effects seen beyond this level. Potential side effects include hypertension, gastrointestinal disturbances that can lead to emesis and feeding intolerance, hypokalemia, jitteriness, hyperglycemia, and glycosuria.[255,256]

SUMMARY

The goal of mechanical ventilation for neonates, especially ELBW infants, should be to provide the least support required for adequate support of their cardiorespiratory status. Such a strategy will reduce the lung injury that accrues from volutrauma and barotrauma associated with mechanical ventilation. Pharmacologic adjuncts that are used to support mechanical ventilation such as sedative and analgesic agents should be used sparingly and with judiciousness to prevent prolonged mechanical ventilation. With the exception of caffeine and, to a limited extent, late administration of corticosteroids and thiazide diuretics, none of the other drug classes has proven effective in reducing ventilator-associated lung injury or BPD to date. More important, several of these agents have not yet been adequately evaluated for their efficacy as aids to mechanical ventilation and in reducing the severity or incidence of BPD in large randomized trials. Well-designed trials for these drugs that are adequately powered to test for differences in long-term outcomes such as BPD or neurodevelopmental impairment are required to make further recommendations regarding these medications. Until then, all of the drugs discussed should be dispensed by personnel who are competent in their administration, know their effects, and are aware of the attention required for patient monitoring. Techniques for the monitoring of many serum drug levels now are available in many centers. The information that such monitoring provides may allow the clinician to use these agents with greater accuracy and safety.

A complete reference list is available at https://expertconsult.inkling.com/.

KEY READINGS

18. Doyle LW, Cheong JL, Ehrenkranz RA, et al: Late (> 7 days) systemic postnatal corticosteroids for prevention of bronchopulmonary dysplasia in preterm infants. Cochrane Database Syst Rev 10:CD001145, 2017.
19. Doyle LW, Ehrenkranz RA, Halliday HL: Late (>7 days) postnatal corticosteroids for chronic lung disease in preterm infants. Cochrane Database Syst Rev 5:CD001145, 2014.
29. Shah VS, Ohlsson A, Halliday HL, et al: Early administration of inhaled corticosteroids for preventing chronic lung disease in very low birth weight preterm neonates. Cochrane Database Syst Rev 1:CD001969, 2017.
64. Anand KJ, Barton BA, McIntosh N, et al: Analgesia and sedation in preterm neonates who require ventilatory support: results from the NOPAIN trial. Neonatal outcome and prolonged analgesia in neonates. Arch Pediatr Adolesc Med 153:331–338, 1999.
179. Ng G, da Silva O, Ohlsson A: Bronchodilators for the prevention and treatment of chronic lung disease in preterm infants. Cochrane Database Syst Rev 12:CD003214, 2016.
249. Moschino L, Zivanovic S, Hartley C, et al: Caffeine in preterm infants: where are we in 2020? ERJ Open Res 6(1):00330-2019, 2020.

33

Common Hemodynamic Problems in the Neonate Requiring Respiratory Support

Keith J. Barrington and Eugene M. Dempsey

KEY POINTS

- The neonatal myocardium is metabolically, structurally, and functionally very different from that of older age groups. Responses to all cardiovascular medications are affected by this immaturity, which may lead to significant pharmacodynamic and pharmacokinetic differences.
- Echocardiography provides an insight into the underlying pathophysiology and allows one to assess the potential response to various interventions.
- There is very limited evidence on the short- and long-term efficacy of the majority of cardiovascular agents used in neonatal care, in particular in the setting of persistent pulmonary hypertension of the newborn, sepsis, and low blood pressure in the extreme preterm infant in the first days of life.
- Conducting clinical trials in hemodynamic support in the neonatal intensive care unit has proved exceptionally difficult and, as such, we remain limited in our evidence base.
- Defining low blood pressure in the preterm population needs to move beyond blood pressure values alone and include an overall global assessment of hemodynamic status of the newborn.
- Further evidence on noninvasive continuous monitoring techniques such as near infrared spectroscopy and noninvasive cardiac output monitoring may provide reliable objective assessment tools to both direct and assess the effect of interventions at the bedside.

INTRODUCTION

Hemodynamic problems are frequent in infants undergoing neonatal intensive care. The evaluation and treatment of such problems must take into account the developmental physiology of the neonatal cardiovascular system; cardiac structure, microstructure and function differ in many important and fundamental ways from mature humans. For example, the myocardium of the newborn has a greater concentration of noncontractile elements, such as mitochondria, and an irregular orientation of the myofibrils.[1] Neonatal myocardium uses glucose and lactate[2] rather than the preferential metabolism of fatty acids of the mature myocardium. Calcium-induced calcium release, which marks the function of sarcoplasmic reticulum, is absent in immature myofibrils.[1]

As a result of its structural and metabolic immaturity, the neonatal heart is functionally limited; basal contractility is already close to maximal levels and therefore there is little "contractile reserve," and the neonatal myocardium is largely incapable of responding to further demands on its function.[3]

One important implication of this is the afterload sensitivity of the circulation. An increase in afterload commonly leads to a reduction in cardiac output.[4] Many inotropic/vasopressor agents directly increase afterload and may therefore result in a decrease, rather than an increase, in systemic perfusion. Responses to all cardiovascular medications are affected by metabolic immaturity, functional immaturity, and pharmacokinetic differences. Some drugs that are positive inotropes in the mature myocardium have negative inotropic effects on the immature. Milrinone and other phosphodiesterase-3 inhibitors act by blocking the third fraction of phosphodiesterase; however, phosphodiesterase-3 and -4 are unbalanced in immature myocardium,[5] and therefore, blocking phosphodiesterase-3 may have relatively unpredictable effects in the immature newborn.[6] Extrapolation from studies in older subjects is of little or no value; only studies investigating specifically neonatal populations are relevant.[7]

Similarly, immature responses are also seen in the neonatal vasculature; we have little information about the development of the adrenergic vascular receptors that determine the responses to catecholamines. Vasoconstrictors, like dopamine, have been shown to increase systemic vascular resistance (SVR) in the preterm newborn;[8] however, the stage of maturation at which such responses appear and the gestational age at which vasodilator responses may appear in response to other agents are unknown.

Another important factor that limits extrapolation of data from older patients is the presence of shunts. Both ductal and intracardiac shunts are frequent; there is therefore no single value for "cardiac output" in the sick neonate; left ventricular output, right ventricular output, systemic perfusion, and pulmonary blood flow are all potentially different numbers. In addition, interventions that differentially affect systemic and pulmonary vascular resistance (PVR) may significantly affect systemic perfusion. Total systemic perfusion is equal to systemic venous return, that is, the sum of superior vena cava (SVC) and inferior vena cava (IVC) flow; pulmonary blood flow is equal to the sum of all of the pulmonary venous return to the left atrium. So in the absence of an intracardiac shunt, we have what seems initially to be paradoxical: systemic perfusion is equal to right ventricular output, whereas pulmonary blood flow is equal to left ventricular output; when there are significant shunts across the foramen ovale, these statements have to be modified. Finally, left ventricular output is equivalent to systemic perfusion only when the ductus arteriosus has closed.[9]

NORMAL TRANSITION

PVR is very high before birth, and less than 15% of the combined ventricular output perfuses the lungs during most of gestation; in human fetuses, this proportion may increase before delivery at term. Right ventricular output mostly crosses the ductus arteriosus (from right to left) and perfuses the lower body and the low-resistance placental circulation. Right ventricular afterload is therefore low in utero; afterload increases at birth with clamping of the umbilical cord and then falls again as the PVR decreases with respiration and lung inflation.

Recent physiologic investigations have shown that clamping of the umbilical cord before initiation of breathing in a neonatal lamb model, when the PVR is still high, causes a reduction in left ventricular preload, in addition to the increase in right ventricular afterload. Delayed clamping until after breathing has commenced may avoid these changes, thus avoiding cardiovascular compromise around the time of birth. A recent meta-analysis confirmed the benefits of delayed cord clamping in reducing mortality in preterm infants less than 32 weeks' gestational age. Umbilical cord milking in preterm infants less than 28 weeks has been associated with an increase in severe intraventricular hemorrhage.[10-12]

HEMODYNAMIC PROBLEMS IN THE NEONATE

Persistent Pulmonary Hypertension of the Newborn

When the PVR is persistently increased, or when it increases after an initial fall, there may be clinical consequences, known as persistent pulmonary hypertension of the newborn (PPHN). The most common underlying pulmonary disorders causing PPHN are meconium aspiration, septicemia, pneumonia, and pulmonary hypoplasia. In addition, it can be seen occasionally in newborns with clear chest x-rays, as so-called "primary" or "idiopathic" PPHN.

Clinical Evaluation

The clinical presentation is of hypoxic respiratory failure with the clinical signs of one of the underlying pulmonary conditions detailed earlier. In some patients, this may be accompanied by a gradient in the saturations from pre- to postductal sites, indicating bidirectional or right to left ductal shunting, usually in the most severely affected patients.

On echocardiography, many infants will be shown to have intracardiac shunting across a patent foramen ovale or they may have hypoxia from intrapulmonary shunting, that is, ventilation-perfusion mismatch.[12] Intra-atrial shunting will occur when right atrial pressure is above left atrial pressure; right atrial pressures increase when right ventricular failure occurs, usually as a result of high right ventricular afterload. Studies have shown that right ventricular function is an important predictor of outcome in infants with this condition.[12] Novel echocardiography techniques provide an insight into the underlying pathophysiology and potential response to various interventions.[13,14]

Intervention

Initial interventions should be supportive, including oxygen, fluid administration, warmth, and assisted ventilation. Infants who are agitated may benefit from sedation. Oxygen should be given to achieve normal saturations, but hyperoxia should be avoided. Oxygen is toxic when given in higher concentrations, may increase pulmonary vascular reactivity,[15] and may even decrease the response of the pulmonary circulation to nitric oxide.[16] It does not appear that increasing FiO_2 beyond that required to achieve normal saturations has any effect on decreasing PVR. As for sedation, it is not clear which sedative agent is preferable. A hemodynamic study of infants with pulmonary artery catheters undergoing surgery showed that fentanyl reduces pulmonary vascular responses to endotracheal suctioning,[17] which suggests that fentanyl may reduce pulmonary vasoreactivity and have a benefit in some infants with PPHN.

Hyperventilation should be avoided as it risks increasing pulmonary damage and causes cerebral vasoconstriction. Persistent respiratory alkalosis seems to cause progressive systemic hypotension, at least in some animal models.[18] Bicarbonate should be avoided, as its use has been associated with an increase in mortality and an increased need for extracorporeal membrane oxygenation (ECMO).[19] Optimizing lung inflation and ventilation to achieve a "normal" pH is reasonable, but going beyond this to alkalinize the patient, even if this might lead to a short-term improvement in PO_2, is not supported by any evidence.

Specific therapy. The only specific evidence-based therapy for PPHN is inhaled nitric oxide (iNO).[20] Nitric oxide can be commenced at between 2 and 20 parts per million;[21] there is little evidence that increasing beyond the initial concentration improves any clinical responses. More than 50% of children with PPHN will have a definite increase in the oxygen saturation after starting nitric oxide. Nitric oxide decreases the number of infants who will deteriorate to the point of needing ECMO; the number needed to treat to prevent one case of ECMO, among term newborns and the late preterm with hypoxic respiratory failure who have reached an oxygenation index of 25, is five.[20]

Cardiovascular support. Cardiovascular support including the use of inotropes may be required for infants with PPHN, but there is little evidence to support a choice of agent over another. The most appropriate agent would have no pulmonary vasoconstrictor effects, or be a pulmonary vasodilator, one which would increase contractility and cardiac output without increasing vascular resistance. No agent is known to have all these effects.

In animal models, dopamine increases both SVR and PVR equally, unless enormous doses are used,[22] suggesting that it may not be the best choice. In some animal models, epinephrine has a greater systemic than pulmonary pressor effect, and norepinephrine also may be reasonable choice; a small observational study in full-term infants showed a good response to norepinephrine.[23] Other agents such as milrinone[24] and levosimendan[25] have been suggested, and some animal models do show possible pulmonary vasodilatation with milrinone,[26] but there is limited clinical research data to support their use. The use of milrinone in the setting of PPHN is limited to case series demonstrating an improvement in oxygenation when used in infants failing to respond to iNO. Its inotropic, lusitropic, and pulmonary vasodilator properties make it a potential candidate in this setting. A pilot randomised trial of milrinone versus placebo is currently enrolling.[27]

Research Needs

Comparative studies of different agents among those who require hemodynamic support are needed. It will be important to determine which agents increase systemic pressures more than pulmonary pressures, which increase systemic perfusion, and most importantly if any choice of agent affects clinical outcomes. However, clinical trials in this area remain challenging.[28]

Septic Shock

The hemodynamic features of septic shock in the newborn have not been well described. Adults with gram-negative septic shock often present with so-called warm shock; this is a combination of excessive vasodilatation with incomplete cardiac response; cardiac output may be increased or within the normal range, and the patient often presents with hypotension. Many of the changes are attributed to the endotoxins (in particular lipopolysaccharides) produced by the causative organisms. Newborn infants with their different cardiovascular physiology and different bacteriology may present with a more variable profile. Newborn animals (such as piglets) with group B streptococcus more commonly have cold shock, with marked reductions in cardiac function (as a result of exotoxins produced by the organisms) and blood pressure is maintained initially with profound vasoconstriction, hypotension being a preterminal event.[29] Some infants with *Escherichia coli* or other gram-negative sepsis seem to present with typical warm shock, but there are very few descriptions of the hemodynamics of sepsis in the literature. One study from the group of Nick Evans in Sydney, Australia, described hemodynamic features in several septic infants,[30] but only a minority had signs of circulatory compromise or shock, as evidenced by the fact that several received neither fluid boluses nor inotropes. The organisms involved were variable; the infants tended to have low SVR and relatively high left and right ventricular outputs. A more recent study of preterm infants with septic shock with mostly gram-negative organisms suggested that they had mostly warm, vasodilatory shock, but this study had a number of limitations.[31]

Clinical Evaluation

If the previous considerations are appropriate, we can divide the clinical presentations into warm and cold shock: Infants with sepsis and cold shock are vasoconstricted with prolonged capillary filling, adequate blood pressure, and oliguria. They are often lethargic and may have biochemical signs of poor oxygen delivery. Infants with warm shock, on the other hand, have bounding pulses, hypotension, and normal capillary filling but may also be oliguric with lactic acidosis.

Evaluation of the circulatory status with echocardiography may well be important in such patients and may aid with targeted management strategies. Echo evaluation should include an analysis of cardiac filling, contractility, and systemic blood flow. Such an evaluation aids in providing more rational treatment, but it must be said that there is no clear evidence that this improves outcomes, largely because there are very little reliable data on which to base different interventions.

A reasonable therapeutic approach is to use physiology-based medicine; this implies examining the abnormalities found on clinical evaluation combined with echocardiography. Therefore, an infant with echocardiographic signs of reduced cardiac filling should receive a fluid bolus; an infant with reduced perfusion but adequate blood pressure may benefit from dobutamine or low-dose epinephrine (which increases systemic perfusion with little effect on blood pressure). Infants with shock and hypotension may receive moderate-dose epinephrine, which appears to increase both blood pressure and systemic perfusion. Norepinephrine has been little studied in the newborn, but one published study[32] and our own experience[33] suggest that it may have a very favorable hemodynamic profile.

Pharmacokinetics of the drugs is extremely variable; in addition, the concentration, affinity, and activity of the adrenoceptors are extremely variable. There is no consistent relationship between plasma catecholamine concentration and target organ effect. Thus, in general, for individual catecholamine infusions, the hemodynamic response to therapy is not related to plasma concentrations in a simple linear fashion. The response to a particular plasma catecholamine concentration varies with the functional state and density of adrenergic receptors. This means that dose responses are unpredictable and doses need to be carefully individualized.

Norepinephrine is now the first-line inotropic agent advocated in adult sepsis. However, a systematic review of data from adults with septic shock does not conclude that there is any difference in survival or other clinically important outcomes from trials comparing different inotropic agents, despite differences in short-term hemodynamic responses. There is one small trial comparing dopamine versus epinephrine in newborns with septic shock.[34] In this study, both agents appeared as efficacious at reversing signs of shock; however, the 28-day mortality overall was 75%, with a small difference between the two agents.

Even in the absence of signs of inadequate preload, septic patients are often considered to have "functional hypovolemia"; they therefore receive fluid boluses, often multiple. However, a recent trial in older infants showed an increase in mortality in the group of children with early septic shock who were randomized to a fluid bolus, compared with controls who did not. If we decide to give a fluid bolus, what fluid should we use? Acute responses to crystalloids and to colloids are different; the increase in systemic perfusion with colloids appears to be greater and more prolonged compared to that with saline. There is, however, no evidence that clinical outcomes are different. In the adult, in whom also colloids have a preferable short-term hemodynamic profile, the evidence suggests that crystalloids are preferable for improving clinical outcomes; therefore, the choice of fluid in the newborn remains uncertain.

Research Needs

Further studies are clearly needed. Interventions for septic shock will probably need to be individualized according to the hemodynamic profile of the patient. Mortality of septic shock in the newborn is very high,[35] so research in this area is clearly warranted. These studies should determine whether gram-negative and gram-positive shocks have similar or differing profiles in the newborn. The role of bedside targeted neonatal echocardiography in the setting of neonatal sepsis needs to be investigated.[36] The place of fluid bolus therapy in the newborn needs to be evaluated, and the hemodynamic effects and clinical responses to various agents need to be evaluated. Finally, the role and place of steroids, which are often given in treatment of septic shock, should be determined.

Hypoxic Ischemic Encephalopathy

Infants with hypoxic ischemic encephalopathy (HIE) may have a number of serious cardiovascular challenges, with myocardial insufficiency, leading to cardiogenic shock, as well as bradycardia, hypotension, and pulmonary hypertension. Infants with HIE often receive therapy with hypothermia, which leads to a further reduction in heart rate and blood pressure and may be associated with a worsening of pulmonary hypertension. Infants undergoing hypothermia therefore are more likely to receive inotrope/vasopressor therapy, but it is not clear what the effects of hypothermia are on the pharmacokinetics and pharmacodynamics of the commonly used agents. Thresholds for (and goals of) intervention during hypothermia treatment are also not certain. Cardiovascular instability with its potential impairment of brain blood flow may contribute to adverse outcome, including mortality and adverse neurodevelopmental outcome. Therefore, treatment aimed at preventing hypotension, poor myocardial contractility, and reduced cardiac output may have long-term benefits. However, we have no data to determine the most appropriate agent to use in the setting of cardiovascular instability associated with HIE.

Cardiogenic Shock

Cardiogenic shock is encountered most commonly after perinatal asphyxia. Other causes include following cardiac surgery or in infants with hypoplastic left heart syndrome who may have profound shock, usually following closure of the ductus arteriosus. Aberrant coronary artery origins, although rare, should be considered in the absence of other clear etiologies. Other causes such as cardiomyopathy and myocarditis are also possible but uncommon.

Usually, such infants have poor perfusion and often tachycardia (not always in the asphyxiated infant) seen in primary cardiac dysfunction; increasing serum lactate, often leading to a frank acidosis, and oligo-anuria may occur. This is one situation when echocardiography is essential. As well as an analysis of cardiac function, the cardiac structure, including a verification of normal coronary artery distribution, should be examined.

As mentioned, even the healthy neonatal myocardium is intolerant of increases in afterload. When the primary problem is cardiac dysfunction, it is essential to avoid increasing afterload. Agents that support cardiac function and decrease afterload, such as dobutamine and low-dose epinephrine, are reasonable first choices. Newer agents such as levosimendan, and perhaps milrinone, warrant further investigation. Excessive fluid administration should be avoided; even single fluid boluses should be carefully considered and given only if there is a good reason to suppose that there is hypovolemia.

Hypotension in the Extremely Low Gestational Age Newborn

In the first few days of life, preterm infants of less than 28 weeks' gestation are often treated with fluid boluses and inotropes after a diagnosis of hypotension. One large prospective cohort study[37] showed that, among infants born at 23 weeks' gestation, 93% received a fluid bolus and over half were treated with an inotrope (usually dopamine). Even at 27 weeks, 73% received a fluid bolus and 25% were treated with dopamine.[37] There was a huge variation between hospital centers, but the variation was not related to differences in patient characteristics, rather to variations in practice patterns.[37] The most consistent finding is that in the majority of circumstances, intervention commenced on the first day of life (90%, 89%, 91%, and 89% of infants born at 23 to 24 weeks, 25 weeks, 26 weeks, and 27 weeks of gestation, respectively). This is a time period where notable cardiorespiratory changes occur. Long-term outcome data from the same cohort show no evidence of benefit from more aggressive treatment of hypotension.[38,39]

Many extremely immature babies are being treated with fluid boluses and inotropic agents despite there being no clinical or other objective evidence that they are underperfused. A number of studies have shown a poor correlation between indicators of systemic blood flow or oxygen delivery and mean arterial blood pressure in the preterm infant.[40] Most hypotensive preterm infants have flows in the superior vena cava and/or right ventricular output which are within the normal range.[41] The converse of this is that infants with low systemic flow may well have normal blood pressure, and thus, patients who may benefit most from appropriate intervention are often underrecognized.

The combination of low numerical blood pressure with adequate systemic flow means that the SVR is low. On the first day of life, this low SVR is unlikely to be attributed to an open ductus arteriosus; PVR is high and shunting across the ductus is relatively limited for the most part. A low SVR with adequate oxygen delivery appears therefore to be part of the normal postnatal adaptation of the (very abnormal) extremely low gestational age neonate (ELGAN). Low numerical blood pressure without signs of poor perfusion may well not require any treatment; a small retrospective cohort study showed that good results can be seen with a permissive approach, avoiding active intervention for well-perfused infants who have low blood pressure.[42] Treating normal transition may not be the best course of action.

Therefore, a global assessment of hemodynamic status is critical before deciding if intervention is required or not. Bedside evaluation incorporating clinical assessment (skin color, capillary refill time and urinary output), physiological data (heart rate and blood pressure parameters) and point of care lactate values provide an overall picture of the cardiovascular status. Historically, the focus has been on the presence of a low mean blood pressure, and although this remains a very important element of the decision-making process, we would advocate a shift away from treating mean blood pressure values alone. Kluckow and colleagues have shown that a capillary refill time of more than 4 seconds improved the specificity and positive predictive value of identifying low flow states compared with a shorter duration of 3 seconds.[43] A prolonged capillary refill time of more than 4 seconds in addition to an elevated lactate values provide a better reflection of systemic blood flow.[44] Sequential lactate values provide more information about the overall status than isolated single lactate values.[45,46] Critically, the important element of each of these assessments is that they involve very little "handling" of the infant.

Echocardiography provides detailed estimates of cardiac output and cardiac function. Japanese data suggest that echo plays a very important management role in the care of extremely preterm infants.[47] Toyoshima et al. describe an individualized approach to echocardiography assessment, tailoring management plans based on specific echo findings and reporting enhanced outcome in a time series study adopting this approach.[48] McNamara highlights the role of echo in this population of infants.[49]

Cerebral near-infrared spectroscopy may prove to be an important monitoring tool for the preterm infant.[50] However, its role in the setting of low blood pressure requires further evaluation. The SafeBoosC III trial is currently enrolling. Likewise, there has been a growing interest in the role of noninvasive cardiac output monitoring in neonatal care.[51] However, there remain many unanswered questions with this technology and further research is required before it could be considered in the clinical care setting.

Research Needs

Intervention algorithms and surveys of practice are characterized by a very similar approach, volume administration followed by dopamine. However, we need evidence whether treating low blood pressure as such in the preterm infant is beneficial, and safe. Prospective randomized trials of intervention based on current commonly used thresholds for intervention are limited. The HIP trial set out to determine whether a restricted approach to the management of hypotension compared to a standard approach with volume and dopamine would result in an improved outcome in infants less than 28 weeks. However, this trial ended early owing to challenges with enrollment. Only 58 patients were enrolled, with no difference in outcome between the two approaches.[52] The Neocirc group performed a pilot trial of dobutamine therapy compared to placebo in low SVC flow states. They enrolled 28 patients as part of this feasibility trial.[53] The larger study has yet to commence and has encountered regulatory and formulation challenges. These studies highlight the significant challenges in conducting trials of cardiovascular support in preterm infants.

Until further evidence becomes available, we are left with the conundrum of whether to treat or not. We would suggest a holistic approach to management, including an assessment of the factors outlined previously. The decision to treat should rarely be based on absolute blood pressure values alone, being mindful of the fact that low flow states can be associated with normal blood pressure values. It is not unreasonable to administer one bolus of normal saline, but further volume administration needs to be carefully considered. The HIP trial confirmed that dopamine will increase blood pressure more readily compared to placebo. Infants in receipt of dopamine are less likely to require the administration of a further inotrope. The corollary is that almost half of the infants in receipt of placebo

did not receive an inotrope. This highlights the importance of a global approach to assessment. However, the overall number of included infants in this study was low and precludes one from making any definitive recommendations.

Therefore, we would advocate a global approach to assessment. Considering the available human and animal data,[54-56] if one is to commence an inotrope in the setting of low blood pressure in the first day of life, low-dose epinephrine may be a suitable agent to consider,[57] but it must be acknowledged that there is very little evidence to support any particular inotrope in this population of infants.

CONCLUSION

Hemodynamic problems are frequent in the neonate who requires respiratory support. Unfortunately, evidence-based recommendations for therapy remain limited for all the clinical scenarios outlined earlier. Although the patients involved are often unstable, research networks must be created to perform the trials that will form the basis of future evidence-based practice.

KEY REFERENCES

7. Paradisis M, Evans N, Kluckow M, et al: Randomized trial of milrinone versus placebo for prevention of low systemic blood flow in very preterm infants. J Pediatr 154(2):189–195, 2009.

10. Fogarty M, Osborn DA, Askie L, et al: Delayed vs early umbilical cord clamping for preterm infants: a systematic review and meta-analysis. Am J Obstet Gynecol 218(1):1–18, 2018.

11. Katheria A, Reister F, Essers J, et al: Association of umbilical cord milking vs delayed umbilical cord clamping with death or severe intraventricular hemorrhage among preterm infants. JAMA 22(19):1877–1886, 2019.

13. de Boode WP, Singh Y, Molnar Z, et al: Application of neonatologist performed echocardiography in the assessment and management of persistent pulmonary hypertension of the newborn. Pediatr Res 84(suppl 1):68–77, 2018.

32. Tourneux P, Rakza T, Abazine A, et al: Noradrenaline for management of septic shock refractory to fluid loading and dopamine or dobutamine in full-term newborn infants. Acta Paediatr 97(2):177–180, 2008.

37. Laughon M, Bose C, Allred E, et al: Factors associated with treatment for hypotension in extremely low gestational age newborns during the first postnatal week. Pediatrics 119(2):273–280, 2007.

42. Dempsey EM, Al Hazzani F, Barrington KJ: Permissive hypotension in the extremely low birthweight infant with signs of good perfusion. Arch Dis Child Fetal Neonatal Ed 94(4):F241–F244, 2009.

48. Toyoshima K, Kawataki M, Ohyama M, et al: Tailor-made circulatory management based on the stress-velocity relationship in preterm infants. J Formos Med Assoc 112(9):510–517, 2013.

50. da Costa CS, Greisen G, Austin T: Is near-infrared spectroscopy clinically useful in the preterm infant? Arch Dis Child Fetal Neonatal Ed 100(6):F558–F561, 2015.

52. Dempsey EM, Barrington KJ, Marlow N, et al: Hypotension in Preterm Infants (HIP) randomised trial. Arch Dis Child Fetal Neonatal Ed 106(4):398–403, 2021.

Diagnosis and Management of Persistent Pulmonary Hypertension of the Newborn

Satyan Lakshminrusimha and Martin Keszler

KEY POINTS

- Persistent pulmonary hypertension of the newborn (PPHN) can be idiopathic (without lung disease) or secondary to parenchymal (such as meconium aspiration syndrome) or hypoplastic (such as congenital diaphragmatic hernia) lung conditions.
- A gentle ventilation strategy (tolerating PaO_2 of 50–70 mm Hg or preductal SpO_2 of 90%–97% and $PaCO_2$ of 45–60 mm Hg) accompanied by lung recruitment with adequate airway pressure and/or surfactants for parenchymal lung disease and lung protection to minimize volutrauma for hypoplastic lung disease is recommended in PPHN.
- Inhaled nitric oxide (iNO) is the only US Food and Drug Administration–approved selective pulmonary vasodilator in term and late preterm infants with PPHN and is associated with reduced need for extracorporeal membrane oxygenation.
- Adjuvant pulmonary vasodilators such as sildenafil, milrinone, and bosentan can be used as second-line agents if there is a suboptimal or ill-sustained response to iNO or if there is no access to iNO.

INTRODUCTION

The fetus is in a state of relative hypoxemia and high pulmonary vascular resistance. It is dependent on the placenta for gas exchange. A successful transition at birth is dependent on establishing the lungs as the organ of gas exchange.[1] This process involves ventilation of the lungs and pulmonary vasodilation, resulting in a precipitous drop in pulmonary vascular resistance (PVR). In some neonates, this circulatory transition is impaired, resulting in persistence of fetal pulmonary hypertension into the neonatal period, which leads to "persistent" pulmonary hypertension of the newborn (PPHN).[2] The incidence of PPHN has not changed much over the years, ranging from 1.9 per thousand live births in the late 1990s[3] to 1.8 per thousand live births between 2007 and 2011.[4] This chapter outlines "cardiocentric" management of PPHN, focusing on gentle ventilation, optimization of lung inflation, pulmonary vasodilation limiting right ventricular afterload, maintaining systemic blood pressure (BP), and minimizing cardiac stress.

ETIOLOGY

Hypoxemic respiratory failure (HRF) is often associated with PPHN.[5] PPHN and HRF can be primary (no lung disease, also called black-lung PPHN) or secondary to lung disease (such as meconium aspiration syndrome [MAS]). From a pathophysiological perspective, causes of PPHN can be secondary to lung disease with loss of alveolar space (e.g., MAS, respiratory distress syndrome [RDS], transient tachypnea of the newborn,[6] pneumonia etc., and hence amenable to therapeutic lung recruitment) or hypoplasia (such as oligohydramnios, congenital diaphragmatic hernia [CDH]), where lung protection and gentle ventilation are important and lung volume recruitment may be counterproductive. Cardiac dysfunction contributes to pulmonary venous hypertension and exacerbates PPHN. The primary therapeutic strategy will depend on the etiology of PPHN (Fig. 34.1). Recent data from California suggest that infection (30%), MAS (24%), idiopathic (20%), RDS (7%), and CDH (6%) were the five leading causes of PPHN.[4]

CLINICAL FEATURES

The typical presentation of PPHN is based on primary pathology but is often associated with labile hypoxemia and, in some cases, differential cyanosis.[7] Cyanosis is secondary to extrapulmonary right-to-left shunting at the patent foramen ovale (PFO) and patent ductus arteriosus (PDA). Unlike cyanotic congenital heart disease with fixed shunts and hypoxemia, the shunts in PPHN are variable and dependent on the relative difference in right- and left-sided pressures. In patients with bidirectional or a right-to-left shunt at the PDA, preductal oxygenation (using SpO_2 from the right upper limb) is higher than the postductal oxygenation (SpO_2 from any lower limb). Systemic hypotension is common in PPHN because of multiple factors and can cause reduced afterload, reduced preload, or pump failure (Fig. 34.2).

Extremely preterm infants are at risk of developing HRF with physiological and clinical features similar to PPHN in term and late preterm infants.[8-10] Prolonged rupture of membranes

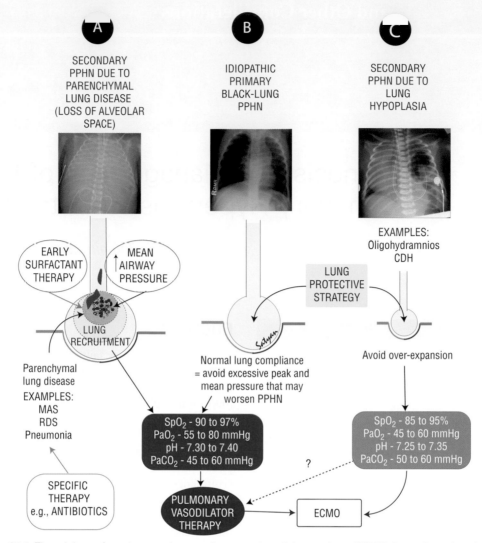

Fig. 34.1 The etiology of persistent pulmonary hypertension of the newborn (*PPHN*) determines the primary therapeutic strategy: Primary, idiopathic, or "black-lung" PPHN is mainly secondary to vascular remodeling and constriction. Optimal oxygenation, gentle ventilation targeting normocapnia, and vasodilator therapy with inhaled nitric oxide and sildenafil are the primary strategies for managing primary PPHN (B). Increasing mean airway pressure may be counterproductive. PPHN secondary to parenchymal lung disease (A) is mainly managed with lung recruitment with adequate airway pressures and surfactant replacement therapy. Pulmonary vasodilator therapy is used if lung recruitment fails to improve oxygenation in parenchymal lung disease such as meconium aspiration syndrome (*MAS*), respiratory distress syndrome (*RDS*), and pneumonia. In patients with lung hypoplasia (e.g., congenital diaphragmatic hernia [*CDH*], C), minimizing volutrauma with lung protective ventilation and avoidance of lung overdistension is the primary strategy of management. All these categories can be complicated by right and left ventricular dysfunction and pulmonary venous hypertension. Inotropes, vasodilators, and maintaining ductal patency are strategies to address cardiac dysfunction in PPHN. *ECMO,* Extracorporeal membrane oxygenation. (Copyright 2020 Satyan Lakshminrusimha.)

(PROM), oligohydramnios, delivery by C-section, and extreme prematurity increase the risk of PPHN in preterm infants. Preterm infants are also at risk for late pulmonary hypertension associated with bronchopulmonary dysplasia (BPD).[11,12]

HYPOXEMIA IN PERSISTENT PULMONARY HYPERTENSION OF THE NEWBORN

HRF is common in PPHN and creates a vicious cycle (Fig. 34.3). Lung disease (parenchymal or hypoplastic) and/or factors such as asphyxia trigger hypoxemia and hypercarbia

with acidosis. The pre–capillary pulmonary arteriole is the sensing site for hypoxic pulmonary vasoconstriction (HPV).[13] The primary determinant of HPV is the oxygen tension surrounding the pre–capillary pulmonary arteriole and is influenced by alveolar P_AO_2 and pulmonary arterial PO_2 (usually same as mixed venous PvO_2). Intrapulmonary shunts (secondary to ventilation-perfusion mismatch or intrapulmonary anastomotic vessels[14]) and extrapulmonary right-to-left shunts at the PFO or PDA exacerbate hypoxemia. Increased PVR causes right ventricular hypertrophy, dilation, and eventually failure. Hypoxemia contributes to lactic acidosis and

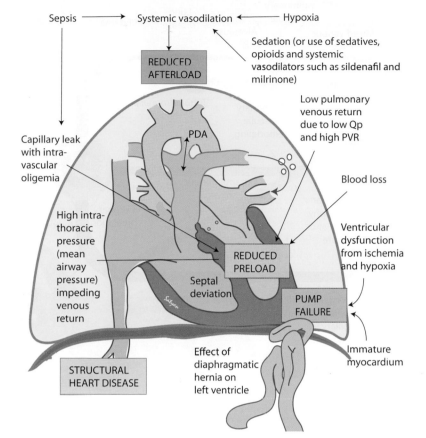

Fig. 34.2 Etiology of systemic hypotension in persistent pulmonary hypertension of the newborn (PPHN). Systemic hypotension exacerbates right-to-left shunting worsening hypoxemia in PPHN and can be secondary to reduced afterload, reduced preload, associated structural heart disease, and pump failure. *PDA,* Patent ductus arteriosus; *PVR,* pulmonary vascular resistance; *Qp,* pulmonary blood flow. (Copyright 2020 Satyan Lakshminrusimha.)

myocardial dysfunction. Left ventricular dysfunction leads to systemic hypotension (Fig. 34.2) and pulmonary venous congestion and edema aggravating hypoxia and hypercarbia. This vicious cycle can be interrupted with correction of hypoxemia and acidosis, therapy with selective pulmonary vasodilators and systemic vasoconstrictors, and reducing cardiac stress. Supplemental oxygen to increase alveolar and mixed venous oxygen levels minimizes pulmonary vasoconstriction.

Diagnosis

Any infant presenting with respiratory distress or HRF should be investigated with pre- and postductal pulse oximetry, arterial blood gas, and a chest x-ray. Cyanotic congenital heart disease is characterized by "fixed" hypoxemia and normal or low PCO_2. "Labile" hypoxemia with normal or high PCO_2 is seen in PPHN secondary to lung disease. Arterial PaO_2 is used to calculate oxygenation index (OI) (Fig. 34.4). OI = (fraction of inspired oxygen [FiO_2] * P_{aw} * 100) ÷ PaO_2 (mm Hg), where P_{aw} is mean airway pressure in cm H_2O. As arterial blood gases cannot be obtained on a continuous basis, oxygen saturation index (OSI) can be used. OSI = (FiO_2 * P_{aw} * 100) ÷ SpO_2.[15-17] Excluding high SpO_2 values enhances the correlation between OSI and OI. Approximately, OI is 1.8 to 2 times higher than OSI.

The results of a hyperoxia test can be equivocal in PPHN and depend on both the degree of right-to-left extrapulmonary shunt and the severity of lung disease. A hyperoxia-hyperventilation test may show an increase in PaO_2 because of the combined vasodilator effect of alkalosis and hyperoxia on pulmonary circulation.[18] However, with easy access to bedside echocardiography, these tests are no longer done in tertiary centers. In community hospitals, hyperoxia test or hyperoxia-hyperventilation test may be useful in determining empiric therapy before transfer in an infant with HRF. The response to these tests, if any, will occur in less than 30 minutes. Thus, prolonged exposure to excessive FiO_2 should be avoided.

Chest x-ray may be suggestive of a specific lung disease based on distribution (focal/diffuse), degree of lung expansion, and characteristic pattern (Table 34.1).[19]

ECHOCARDIOGRAPHY AND HEMODYNAMIC ASSESSMENT IN PERSISTENT PULMONARY HYPERTENSION OF THE NEWBORN[20]

The primary purpose of obtaining an echocardiogram is to rule out cyanotic congenital heart disease. Left-sided obstructive

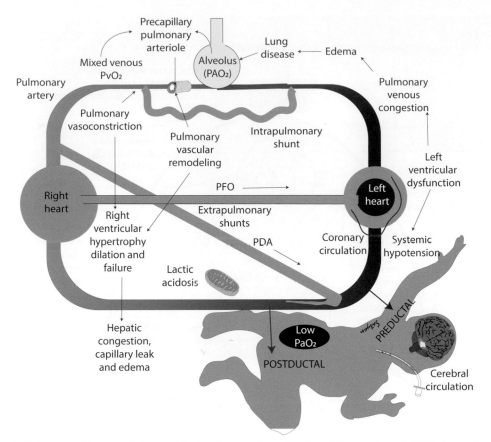

Fig. 34.3 Causes of hypoxemia in persistent pulmonary hypertension of the newborn (*PPHN*). Parenchymal lung disease, pulmonary vascular constriction, and remodeling with intrapulmonary shunts (ventilation-perfusion mismatch and intrapulmonary pulmonary artery-to-vein anastomoses) cause hypoxemia and hypercarbia. Increased pulmonary arterial pressure leads to right-to-left extrapulmonary shunts at the patent foramen ovale (*PFO*) and patent ductus arteriosus (*PDA*) levels. The precapillary pulmonary arteriole is the site of hypoxic pulmonary vasoconstriction and is influenced by a combination of alveolar (PAO$_2$) and mixed venous oxygen tension (PvO$_2$). (Copyright 2020 Satyan Lakshminrusimha.)

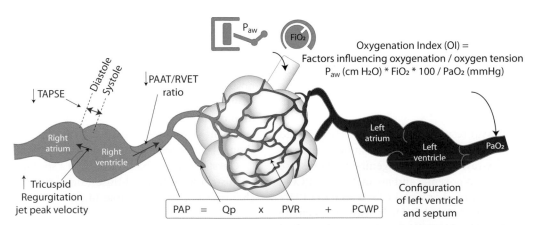

Fig. 34.4 Assessment of severity of hypoxemic respiratory failure (HRF) and persistent pulmonary hypertension of the newborn (PPHN). Oxygenation index (OI) is derived by dividing factors that facilitate oxygenation (mean airway pressure [P$_{aw}$]) and FiO$_2$ by PaO$_2$. OI under 15 is considered mild HRF, 15 to 25 as moderate HRF, over 25 as severe HRF, and more than 40 as critical. The severity of PPHN is assessed by estimating pulmonary arterial pressure (*PAP*) by echocardiography. Tricuspid regurgitation jet velocity, pulmonary arterial acceleration time (*PAAT*)/right ventricular ejection time (*RVET*) ratio, and configuration of the left ventricle and interventricular septum are commonly used to assess PAP. *PCWP*, Pulmonary capillary wedge pressure; *TAPSE*, tricuspid annular plane systolic excursion. (Copyright 2020 Satyan Lakshminrusimha.)

TABLE 34.1   Chest X-Ray Patterns in Lung Disease Associated With Persistent Pulmonary Hypertension of the Newborn

Low Inflation (<8 ribs)	Normal Inflation (8–9 ribs)	Hyperinflation (>9 ribs)
Diffuse, hazy, grainy, ground-glass with air bronchograms—RDS	Black lungs—primary PPHN (or pulmonary oligemia because of pulmonary stenosis/tetralogy of Fallot	Streaky—TTN
Patchy, hazy—pneumonia[a]	Hazy—pulmonary edema or hemorrhage	Fluffy—MAS
White—atelectasis		White—effusion (including chylothorax)
Clear/relatively clear—pulmonary hypoplasia		Black or bubbly appearance—pneumothorax or PIE

Expansion is evaluated using the level of the anterior diaphragm. The level of expansion may be altered by positive pressure ventilation.
[a]Pneumonia may mimic all patterns of lung disease shown in this table.
MAS, Meconium aspiration syndrome; *PIE*, pulmonary interstitial emphysema; *PPHN*, persistent pulmonary hypertension of the newborn; *RDS*, respiratory distress syndrome; *TTN*, transient tachypnea of the newborn.

lesions (coarctation of aorta, interrupted aortic arch, and hypoplastic left heart syndrome) can present with a preductal-to-postductal SpO_2 gradient. Cyanotic lesions such as obstructed total anomalous pulmonary venous return (TAPVR), transposition of great arteries, tricuspid atresia, and severe Ebstein anomaly can mimic PPHN. An echocardiogram can also assist in evaluating the severity of PPHN; assessing ventricular function, shunt direction, and end-diastolic volumes; and differentiating precapillary PPHN from postcapillary or pulmonary venous hypertension.

Severity of Persistent Pulmonary Hypertension of the Newborn

The essential feature of PPHN is elevated pulmonary arterial pressure (PAP). PAP is calculated by:

PAP = (Qp × PVR) + PCWP (where Qp is pulmonary blood flow and PCWP is pulmonary capillary wedge pressure). Based on this equation (Fig. 34.4), elevated PAP can be the result of three causes.

1. Elevated Qp: large left-to-right shunt (PDA, atrial septal defect, ventricular septal defect, etc., often in combination with a lung condition such as BPD).
2. Elevated PVR: owing to constriction, hypoplasia, or remodeling of pulmonary vasculature.
3. Elevated PCWP: pulmonary venous hypertension because of left heart failure or dysfunction and pulmonary vein stenosis.

Elevated PAP can be estimated in the presence of tricuspid regurgitation (by modified Bernoulli's equation) using the following formula: pressure gradient = $4v^2$ in m/s, where v is the tricuspid regurgitation jet velocity in meters per second. This gradient measures the systolic pressure difference between the right ventricle and the right atrium in mm Hg. It is customary to add 5 mm Hg as the arbitrary right atrial pressure to this number to estimate systolic PAP. Other echocardiographic findings such as pulmonary regurgitation peak velocity, transductal right-to-left peak blood flow velocity, or subjective estimation of the position of interventricular septum are commonly used to assess PAP. If the left ventricular configuration is O shaped, the estimated right ventricular pressure is less than 50% of systemic; D shaped, 50% to 100% of systemic and crescent shaped-systemic (Fig. 34.5).

PVR can be estimated by the ratio of pulmonary artery acceleration time (PAAT) to right ventricular ejection time (RVET). The normal value is 0.31 or more, and values under 0.23 are suggestive of elevated PVR.[20]

Ventricular Function

Biventricular dysfunction is seen in 70% of patients with PPHN and is related to increased right ventricular afterload, decreased left ventricular preload, and myocardial ischemia. Ventricular dysfunction leads to reduced cardiac output, further decreasing Qp and myocardial perfusion, setting up a vicious cycle (Fig. 34.6). Left ventricular failure with low stroke volume is associated with a need for advanced therapies such as high-frequency ventilation (HFV) and extracorporeal membrane oxygenation (ECMO).[21] Right ventricular function is assessed by tricuspid annular plane systolic excursion (TAPSE) and fractional area change. TAPSE is a measure of right ventricular longitudinal function and is obtained from the four-chamber view using M-mode. It refers to the distance traveled by the tricuspid annulus from diastole to systole in millimeters. TAPSE <4 mm is associated with increased need for ECMO or death in PPHN.

Shunt Direction

Right-to-left or bidirectional shunt at the PFO and PDA is commonly observed in 73% to 100% and 73% to 91% of patients with PPHN, respectively.[20] A left-to-right shunt is possible at the PFO with PPHN secondary to left ventricular dysfunction (see later). A pure left-to-right shunt at the PFO in the absence of tricuspid regurgitation is suspicious for TAPVR.[22] At the PDA level, right-to-left shunt ≥30% of total heart cycle is likely to represent PPHN. In the presence of significant right and left ventricular dysfunction, pop-off right-to-left shunting at the PFO and PDA offsets right ventricular afterload, improves left ventricular preload, and supports systemic blood flow. Maintaining ductal patency with intravenous prostaglandin E1 (PGE1) can potentially improve outcomes in severe PPHN with right ventricular dysfunction with high afterload by providing this pop-off.[23]

Precapillary Versus Pulmonary Venous Hypertension

Classic PPHN secondary to pulmonary parenchymal disease such as MAS is characterized by increased PAP and PVR, low PCWP, and right ventricular dilation with a normal or small left

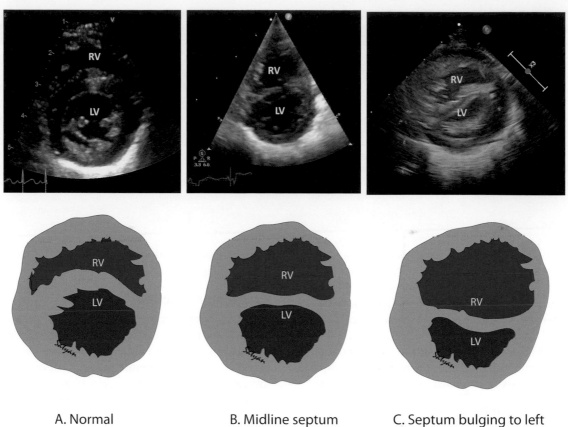

A. Normal   B. Midline septum   C. Septum bulging to left

Fig. 34.5 Interventricular septal position and severity of pulmonary hypertension. (A) Normal position of the septum (bulging to the right) with an O-shaped left ventricle (*LV*) and a crescentic right ventricle (*RV*). (B) Midline septum with D-shaped LV. (C) Septum bulging to the left with a crescentic LV. (Echo images courtesy of Jay Yeh, MD. Copyright Satyan Lakshminrusimha.)

ventricle. The shunt at PDA and PFO is right-to-left or bidirectional. This condition is essentially a precapillary disorder and responds well to pulmonary vasodilator therapy such as inhaled nitric oxide (iNO).[20] Pulmonary venous hypertension is a postcapillary disorder and often secondary to left ventricular dysfunction with elevated PCWP. It does not respond well to pulmonary vasodilator therapy. In this condition, a dilated left ventricle and elevated left atrial end-diastolic pressure can lead to a left-to-right shunt at PFO, although PAP is high with a right-to-left shunt at PDA.[24]

Serial echocardiography provides important ongoing information to assess the severity of PPHN, guide therapy, and evaluate the response to therapy. It is an important component of the "cardiocentric" management of PPHN.

Supportive Management

To optimize cardiac function and pulmonary vasodilation, maintaining euglycemia, normothermia, and acid-base balance is important. Infants with PPHN can be on trophic feeds in the absence of significant acidosis, hypotension, or hypoperfusion. Total parenteral nutrition (TPN) to maintain optimal caloric intake and blood glucose is important. There is some evidence to suggest that intravenous lipids (1.5–3 g/kg/d) can increase PVR in neonates.[25] Early initiation of TPN (<24 hours of intensive

care unit [ICU] admission) compared with late initiation (>7 days of ICU admission) was associated with lower incidence of hypoglycemia but an increased mortality and a trend toward increased infections among critically ill late-preterm and term infants in one study.[26,27] We recommend early initiation of TPN with moderate quantities of amino acids, lipids, and glucose to prevent essential fatty acid (EFA) deficiency and hypoglycemia with close attention to infection-prevention measures with central lines pending further studies. Minimal stimulation (quiet room with earmuffs and eye cover) and sedation are important, but excessive narcotic analgesia can be associated with systemic hypotension and aggravation of right-to-left shunt and should be avoided. Paralysis is not routinely recommended as it may exacerbate edema and has been associated with increased mortality.[3]

Optimal oxygen delivery to the tissues is dependent on maintaining adequate hemoglobin concentration and blood oxygen–carrying capacity. Delayed cord clamping and placental transfusion at birth increase fetal hemoglobin (HbF) levels and pulmonary blood flow in animal models of PPHN secondary to CDH.[28]

Severe anemia is associated with PPHN.[29,30] Low hemoglobin levels at birth are observed in babies with PPHN, suggesting a role of lack of placental transfusion in the etiology of PPHN.[31] However, there is no evidence that delayed cord clamping alters the incidence of respiratory distress from randomized clinical

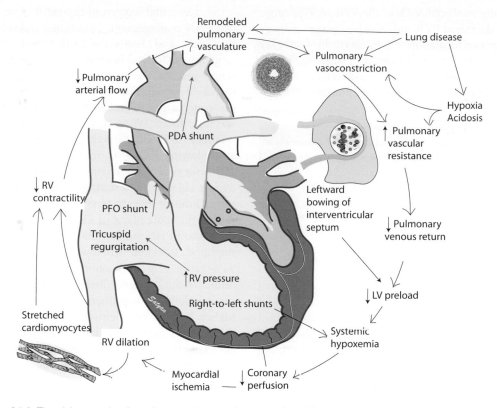

Fig. 34.6 The vicious cycle of persistent pulmonary hypertension of the newborn (PPHN). Pulmonary disease and/or vascular remodeling leads to elevated pulmonary vascular resistance. Increased right ventricular afterload initially leads to right ventricular hypertrophy but subsequently causes dilation and poor contractility of the right ventricle (*RV*). Bowing of the interventricular septum and reduced pulmonary venous return lead to reduced left ventricular (*LV*) preload. Diminished systemic perfusion and right-to-left shunts at the patent foramen ovale (*PFO*) and/or patent ductus arteriosus (*PDA*) contribute to systemic hypoxemia. Systemic hypoxemia and hypoperfusion reduce coronary perfusion pressure and exacerbate myocardial ischemia and ventricular dysfunction. (Modified from Care of the critically ill neonate with hypoxemic respiratory failure and acute pulmonary hypertension: framework for practice based on consensus opinion of Neonatal Hemodynamics Working Group. J Perinatol, 2021 (under review))

trials or metanalysis.[32] Minimizing iatrogenic blood losses and keeping hemoglobin levels of 10 g/dL or more (and preferably in the 13–17 g/dL range) may be prudent in HRF.

ASPHYXIA, HYPOTHERMIA, AND PERSISTENT PULMONARY HYPERTENSION OF THE NEWBORN

Perinatal asphyxia interferes with the fall in PVR and increases the risk for PPHN.[33] Fetal hypoxemia, ischemia, meconium aspiration, ventricular dysfunction, and acidosis contribute to pulmonary vasoconstriction. Therapeutic hypothermia at 33.5° C in asphyxiated infants with moderate to severe hypoxic-ischemic encephalopathy (HIE) does not alter the incidence of PPHN. However deeper cooling to 32° C increases the prevalence of PPHN and need for ECMO.[34] Among infants with moderate to severe HIE, the presence of PPHN is associated with higher mortality (~27% vs. 16% in a study from the Neonatal Research Network).[35] The four factors that increase the prevalence of PPHN following asphyxia include severe asphyxial insult, need for chest compressions or epinephrine,

preexisting lung disease such as MAS/pneumonia, and finally, need for high FiO_2 before onset of therapeutic hypothermia.[35] Most centers use blood gases corrected for core temperature (pH stat method) during hypothermia.[36]

Oxygen

Oxygen is a specific and potent pulmonary vasodilator, and increased alveolar oxygenation is a central mediator of the reduction in PVR at birth (Box 34.1). Alveolar hypoxia and hypoxemia increase PVR, resulting in HPV, and contribute to the pathophysiology of PPHN. Furthermore, animal studies demonstrate exaggerated HPV with PaO_2 under 45 to 50 mm Hg.[37] Although normoxemia (PaO_2 in the 50–80 mm Hg range) results in pulmonary vasodilation, hyperoxia with PaO_2 greater than 100 mm Hg does not result in additional vasodilation.[7,38,39] HPV is aggravated by pH below 7.25, suggesting that acidosis should be avoided during the acute phase of PPHN.[37] Exposure to extreme hyperoxia promotes the formation of reactive oxygen species and may lead to lung injury. Brief exposure to 100% oxygen in newborn lambs increases the contractility responses of pulmonary arteries[40] and the formation of superoxide anions[41] and reduces response to iNO.[42] Recent data from lambs with MAS and PPHN suggest that achieving preductal SpO_2 in the 93% to 97% range was associated with decreased PVR and increased oxygen delivery to the brain but increased formation of 3-nitrotyrosine (a marker of oxidative and nitrosative stress). In contrast, targeting 90% to 94% SpO_2 was associated with lower FiO_2 requirement and the best PaO_2/FiO_2 ratio and low brain 3-nitrotyrosine levels.[43]

BOX 34.1	**Supplemental Oxygen**
Indication	Hypoxemia with preductal oxygen saturation (SpO_2) <90% or PaO_2 <45 mm Hg
Dose/concentration	22%–100% (preferably <60%); titrate to achieve PaO_2 50–70 mm Hg or SpO_2 90%–97%[38]
Monitoring	Pulse oximetry, blood gases; avoid desaturations (<85%) and hyperoxia (≥98% SpO_2); lactate (maintain <3–5 mM/L)
Precautions	Achieve adequate lung recruitment with surfactants or mean airway pressure/positive end-expiratory pressure in the presence of parenchymal lung disease; avoid hyperinflation or atelectasis
	During whole-body hypothermia (core temperature 33°C–34°C), a leftward shift in hemoglobin oxygen dissociation curve may necessitate higher SpO_2 targets (95%–99%) to achieve desired corrected PaO_2 of 50–70 mm Hg
Class of recommendation	I[44]—evidence and/or general agreement that a given treatment or procedure is beneficial, useful or effective
Level of evidence	B[44]

Supplemental oxygen to correct hypoxemia is the mainstay of PPHN management. Traditional management of PPHN in the 1980s and 1990s included hyperoxic hyperventilation[45] targeting postductal PaO_2 in the more than 100 to 120 mm Hg range and $PaCO_2$ as low as 16 mm Hg (Fig. 34.6).[18] With increased recognition of the deleterious effects of hyperoxia, the concept of "tolerable" hypoxemia with gentle ventilation was introduced. Wung et al. reported successful management of infants with PPHN targeting PaO_2 between 50 and 70 mm Hg and allowing $PaCO_2$ to increase as high as 60 mm Hg with 100% survival.[46] We recommend preductal PaO_2 in the 50 to 80 mm Hg range and setting a lower alarm limit of 89% and an upper limit of 98% to target a preductal PaO_2 of 90% to 97% during the acute phase of PPHN. Recent data from lambs with MAS and PPHN suggest that targets in the 93% to 97% range might be associated with lower PVR compared with the 90% to 94% range (Fig. 34.7), but clinical corroboration is needed. Similarly, SpO_2 targets during the management of PPHN during whole-body hypothermia may also need to be slightly higher. Because of a leftward shift in the hemoglobin oxygen dissociation curve with hypothermia and HbF, to achieve a corrected PaO_2 of 50 to 70 mm Hg, SpO_2 targets are in the mid to high 90s.[36]

Carbon Dioxide and pH Targets

Similar to oxygen, there has been a significant shift in $PaCO_2$ targets in the management of PPHN in the last two decades (Fig. 34.8). The traditional approach before the availability of

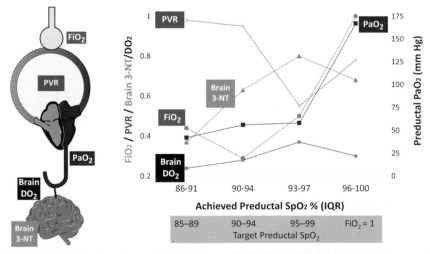

Fig. 34.7 Preductal oxygen saturation and pulmonary vascular resistance (*PVR*) in lambs with meconium aspiration and pulmonary hypertension based on Rawat et al.[43] Term lambs with asphyxia, meconium aspiration, and pulmonary hypertension were randomized to preductal SpO_2 target of 85% to 89%, 90% to 94%, 95% to 99%, and fixed inspired oxygen at 100%. The achieved SpO_2, PVR in the left pulmonary circuit (in mm Hg/mL/kg/min), oxygen delivery to the brain (DO_2 in mL/g of brain tissue), brain 3-nitrotyrosine (3-NT ng/mcg protein as a measure of oxidative and nitrosative stress), preductal PaO_2 (mm Hg), and FiO_2 are shown. The achieved SpO_2 interquartile ranges (*IQRs*) are shown on the horizontal axis. Achieving preductal 93% to 97% SpO_2 resulted in the lowest PVR and highest brain DO_2. However, 90% to 94% SpO_2 was associated with the lowest FiO_2 requirement and lower brain 3-NT levels. Targeting 85% to 89% SpO_2 was associated with high PVR and low brain DO_2. A fixed inspired FiO_2 of 1.0 resulted in a median SpO_2 of 100% (IQR, 96%–100%) with supraphysiological PaO_2 (mean, 167 mm Hg). However, in spite of high FiO_2 and PaO_2, no further reduction in PVR was observed compared with 93% to 97% achieved SpO_2. Optimal oxygenation in PPHN is a delicate balance between pulmonary vasodilation and oxidative stress. (Modified from Rawat M, Chandrasekharan P, Gugino SF, et al: Optimal oxygen targets in term lambs with meconium aspiration syndrome and pulmonary hypertension. Am J Respir Cell Mol Biol 63:510–518, 2020. Copyright 2020 Satyan Lakshminrusimha.)

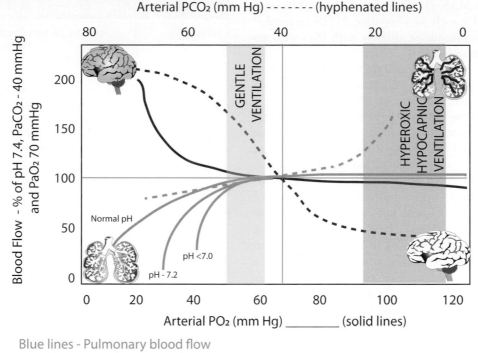

Fig. 34.8 Patterns of ventilation in persistent pulmonary hypertension of the newborn (PPHN) and effect on pulmonary and cerebral circulation (hypothetical, not drawn to scale). Arterial PaO_2 (*solid lines*) data are graphed along the primary horizontal axis. Arterial $PaCO_2$ (*dashed or hyphenated lines*) data are graphed along the secondary horizontal axis (*top*). Cerebral circulation is shown in *red* and pulmonary circulation is shown in *blue*. The intersection of the two *green lines* demarcates pH 7.40, $PaCO_2$ of 40 mm Hg, and PaO_2 of 70 mm Hg ("normal" parameters for a healthy term neonate). Percentage changes in response to changes in PaO_2 and $PaCO_2$ are depicted on the vertical axis. *Pink bar* represents hyperoxic, hypocapnic ventilation ("classic" approach in the 1980s and 1990s). The *blue bar* represents "gentle" ventilation with tolerable hypoxemia and permissive hypercapnia. (Copyright 2020 Satyan Lakshminrusimha.)

iNO was to focus on alkalosis (both metabolic and respiratory) to achieve pulmonary vasodilation with $PaCO_2$ target.[18] Metabolic alkalosis induced with sodium bicarbonate or tromethamine infusion was associated with increased use of ECMO and a higher incidence of chronic lung disease with oxygen need at 28 days of postnatal age.[3] Infants managed with hyperventilation and alkalosis were observed to have a higher risk of sensorineural deafness.[47] Among infants with moderate to severe HIE, management with $PaCO_2$ under 35 mm Hg was associated with lower survival without neurodevelopmental impairment (NDI). Hypocarbia is a cerebral vasoconstrictor, and cerebral ischemia may play a role in the pathogenesis of NDI observed a follow-up in these infants.[48] Although permissive hypercapnia with tolerance of $PaCO_2$ of 60 mm Hg is currently common practice and is accepted by current guidelines,[44] it is important to avoid acidosis with pH under 7.25. Acidosis increases the PaO_2 threshold at which vasoconstriction is observed in the pulmonary circulation and exacerbates HPV (Fig. 34.8).[37]

Noninvasive Ventilation

Patients with primary or idiopathic PPHN can be managed with noninvasive ventilation through nasal cannula, high-flow nasal cannula, continuous positive airway pressure, or nasal intermittent positive pressure ventilation. If hypoxemia without respiratory acidosis is observed, increased oxygen concentration and, if necessary, iNO can be administered through noninvasive ventilation.[49,50] However, the presence of severe respiratory distress, apnea or respiratory acidosis, intubation, and mechanical ventilation may be needed.

Invasive Ventilation

The goal of respiratory support in PPHN is to optimize lung inflation.[51] The optimal ventilation mode depends on the nature of lung disease (Fig. 34.1). Idiopathic and PPHN secondary to lung hypoplasia are managed with gentle ventilation with an initial positive end-expiratory pressure (PEEP) of 4 to 5 cm H_2O (lower values for hypoplastic lungs).[52] Open lung recruitment with adequate PEEP or P_{aw} is essential in PPHN secondary to parenchymal lung disease. Maintaining lung volume at normal functional residual capacity (FRC) lowers PVR whereas both atelectasis with low lung volumes and hyperinflation of the lung increase PVR (Fig. 34.8A). In infants with parenchymal lung disease such as MAS and RDS, recruitment of the lung with high-frequency oscillator improved oxygenation.[53] The combination of iNO and HFV had a synergistic effect among infants with PPHN secondary to parenchymal lung disease such as MAS. On the other hand, infants with other causes of PPHN such as idiopathic PPHN responded better to pulmonary vasodilator therapy with iNO with no incremental benefit from HFV.

There is minimal evidence regarding the initial choice of ventilation in infants with PPHN. Most centers start with conventional ventilation using appropriate PEEP (initial setting, 5–7 cm H_2O) to achieve lung recruitment to FRC. Volume-targeted or volume-guarantee ventilation with a targeted exhaled tidal volume of 5 to 6 mL/kg is the preferred mode of initial ventilation to minimize volutrauma. Recruitment and maintenance of underinflated air spaces (to prevent atelectotrauma during expiration) while minimizing overinflation of more compliant lung sections with air-trapping are important in PPHN secondary to parenchymal lung disease. If respiratory acidosis cannot be resolved in spite of PIP exceeding 25 to 28 cm H_2O or if lungs cannot be recruited to maintain oxygenation, a switch to high-frequency oscillator or jet ventilator is recommended. A trial of exogenous surfactant (see next section) is beneficial to recruit the lungs in secondary PPHN because of MAS, RDS, or pneumonia.

SURFACTANTS IN PERSISTENT PULMONARY HYPERTENSION OF THE NEWBORN

Lotze et al. demonstrated that early use of surfactants when OI was in the 15 to 22 range was associated with reduced need for ECMO in PPHN in a multicenter trial.[54] Konduri et al. have shown a similar association with the early use of surfactants in a post hoc analysis of a multicenter randomized trial of early versus standard use of iNO in PPHN.[55,56] More recently, Gonzalez et al. performed a randomized trial of iNO versus surfactant + iNO in PPHN. Surfactant + iNO slowed progression of HRF and reduced ECMO/death.[57]

How do surfactants and lung recruitment improve outcomes in PPHN (Box 34.2)? In parenchymal lung disease, asymmetric inflation leads to areas of collapse interspersed with areas of overdistension because of LaPlace's law. Overdistension compresses the alveolar vessels, increasing PVR (Fig. 34.9A). Similarly, collapse kinks extra-alveolar vessels and increases PVR.[58] In addition, V/Q mismatch contributes to hypoxemia and HPV. The administration of iNO to a poorly recruited lung will lead to asymmetric distribution of iNO to ventilated and distended alveoli (Fig. 34.9B). Homogenous lung recruitment enhances the ability of oxygen and inhaled vasodilators such as iNO to reach their target,[59] the pulmonary vasculature, thereby promoting pulmonary vasodilation (Figs. 34.9C and 34.10). The European Pediatric Pulmonary Vascular Disease Network recommends ventilatory support and/or surfactants if needed to achieve optimal oxygenation in PPHN through avoiding lung hyperinflation or atelectasis, or lung collapse (class of recommendation [COR] I and level of evidence [LOE] B).[44] Intratracheal surfactant is also recommended in PPHN with pulmonary diffusion impairment in all causes except CDH (COR IIa, LOE B; Fig. 34.11).

BOX 34.2	**Intratracheal Surfactant**
Indication	Intubated patient with parenchymal lung disease with OI >5 to 7 or requiring >40% oxygen to maintain SpO_2 ≥90%
Dose	Standard dose as per manufacturer (similar dose as preterm infants/kg); repeat as needed
Monitoring	Chest x-ray, FiO_2, pulse oximetry, blood gases; wean ventilator if compliance improves after administration (if on pressure control settings) or use volume-targeted ventilation, closely watch $PaCO_2$ as hypocapnia can occur
Precautions	Hypocapnia; avoid hyperinflation
Contraindications	CDH, idiopathic PPHN
Class of recommendation	IIa—Weight of evidence/opinion is in favor of usefulness/efficacy[44]
Level of evidence	B—data derived from single/few randomized trials[54] or large nonrandomized/post hoc analysis[44,55]

CDH, Congenital diaphragmatic hernia; *FiO₂*, fraction of inspired oxygen; *OI*, oxygenation index; *PPHN*, persistent pulmonary hypertension of the newborn.

INHALED NITRIC OXIDE

iNO is the only US Food and Drug Administration–approved selective pulmonary vasodilator and is indicated for term and near-term infants with HRF with clinical or echocardiographic evidence of PPHN (Box 34.3). It reduces the incidence of ECMO/death in PPHN attributed to all etiologies except CDH.[61] NO acts by stimulating soluble guanylyl cyclase (sGC) in vascular smooth muscle to produce cyclic guanosine monophosphate (cGMP), which in turn reduces cytosolic concentration of ionic calcium leading to vasodilation (Fig. 34.10). cGMP is broken down by phosphodiesterase 5 enzyme (PDE5), limiting its relaxation. Oxidative stress can limit the effectiveness of iNO through several mechanisms: (1) superoxide anions combine with NO to form peroxynitrite, a vasoconstrictor agent;[62] (2) oxygen free radicals can oxidize sGC;[63] (3) superoxide anions stimulate PDE 5 activity and catabolize cGMP;[64] and finally, (4) uncoupling of NO synthase can result in superoxide anion formation instead of NO.[65] It is imperative that prolonged exposure to hyperoxia and high FiO_2 be limited before initiation of iNO to maximize its effectiveness.[38]

The vasodilatory effect of iNO is selective to the pulmonary circulation partly because of its inactivation by combining with hemoglobin to form methemoglobin (MHb) once it diffuses into the circulation. In addition, iNO is microselective to ventilated portions of the alveoli as it only dilated blood vessels adjacent to ventilated alveoli, thereby improving V/Q matching. Hence, iNO is effective in improving oxygenation in HRF even in the absence of clinical or echocardiographic evidence of PPHN.[61]

Initiation of Inhaled Nitric Oxide

If optimization of lung volume, pH, hemodynamics, and sedation do not alleviate PPHN, iNO therapy is indicated. In all

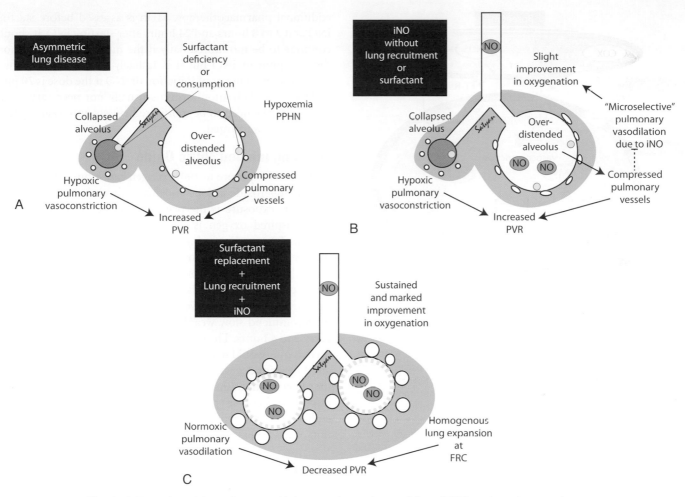

Fig. 34.9 Parenchymal lung disease with hypoxemic respiratory failure (HRF) and persistent pulmonary hypertension of the newborn (*PPHN*) in term neonates. **(A)** In surfactant deficiency without lung recruitment, because of the LaPlace effect, alveoli with a smaller diameter have high pressure and empty into alveoli with larger diameter. Asymmetric lung expansion results in collapsed and overdistended alveoli, resulting in stretching of extra-alveolar vessels and compression of alveolar vessels respectively increasing high pulmonary vascular resistance (*PVR*). **(B)** When treated with inhaled nitric oxide (*iNO*) without surfactant or alveolar recruitment. Alveolar collapse leads to extra-alveolar pulmonary vasoconstriction. In addition, hypoxia and decreased distribution of iNO (microselective effect) lead to constriction of alveolar vessels, further contributing to (PVR). Overdistension of the alveolus compresses alveolar pulmonary vessels, increasing PVR. In addition, overdistension results in volutrauma and air leaks, both of which contribute to high PVR and exacerbation of PPHN with poor response to iNO. Overdistention also compromises systemic venous return and left ventricular output, potentially exacerbating right to left shunting at the ductal level. **(C)** Treated with early surfactant and iNO: early surfactant and lung recruitment results in homogenous lung distension at or near functional residual capacity with effective distribution of iNO, improved tidal volumes because of increased compliance, and pulmonary vasodilation. The net result is low PVR and improved oxygenation. *FRC*, Functional residual capacity; *NO*, nitric oxide. (Modified from Konduri GG, Lakshminrusimha S: Surf early to higher tides: surfactant therapy to optimize tidal volume, lung recruitment, and iNO response. J Perinatol 41.1–3, 2021. Copyright Satyan Lakshminrusimha 2020.)

cases of PPHN, except CDH and pulmonary venous hypertension, we recommend initiation of iNO at 20 parts per million (ppm) for HRF with OI of 15 to 20.[55,56] In approximately two-thirds of cases, a sustained improvement in oxygenation with an increase in PaO_2/FiO_2 ratio by 20 mm Hg is seen within 20 minutes or less (the 20-20-20-20 rule).[70] A dose of 5 ppm shows improvement in oxygenation in some infants, in part because of improvement in V/Q matching.[71] However, the use of 20 ppm leads to peak reduction in pulmonary artery-to-systemic

artery pressure ratio.[71] Among patients with no or partial response to 20 ppm iNO, increasing dose from 20 ppm to 80 ppm improves oxygenation in only 6% of patients.[72] However, use of 80 ppm iNO increases the risk of methemoglobinemia and elevated nitrogen dioxide.[66] Thus, because of very limited benefit and increased risk, use of doses >20 ppm is generally not recommended.

Inadequate or poorly sustained oxygenation response to iNO is usually because of inadequate lung recruitment or poor

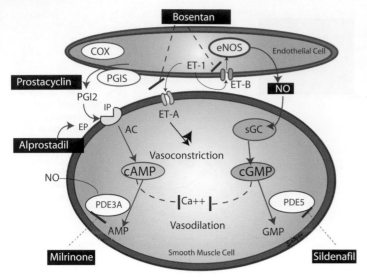

Fig. 34.10 Pathways of vasoactive agents in the pulmonary circulation and agents used for therapy of persistent pulmonary hypertension of the newborn (PPHN), including endothelium derived vasodilators—prostacyclin (*PGI₂*) and nitric oxide (*NO*) and blockers of vasoconstrictors (endothelin, ET-1). The enzymes cyclooxygenase (*COX*) and prostacyclin synthase (*PGIS*) are involved in the production of prostacyclin. Prostacyclin acts on its receptor (*IP*) in the smooth muscle cell and stimulates adenylate cyclase (*AC*) to produce cyclic adenosine monophosphate (cAMP). Similarly, alprostadil acts on prostaglandin E (*EP*) receptors to stimulate cAMP production. cAMP is broken down by phosphodiesterase 3A (*PDE 3A*) in the smooth muscle cell. Milrinone inhibits PDE 3A and increases cAMP levels in pulmonary arterial smooth muscle cells and cardiac myocytes, resulting in pulmonary (and systemic) vasodilation and inotropy. Endothelin is a powerful vasoconstrictor and acts on ET-A receptors in the smooth muscle cell and increases ionic calcium concentration. A second endothelin receptor (*ET-B*) on the endothelial cell stimulates nitric oxide release and vasodilation. Endothelin receptor blockers such as bosentan are beneficial in intractable PPHN. Endothelial nitric oxide synthase (*eNOS*) produces NO, which diffuses from the endothelium to the smooth muscle cell and stimulates soluble guanylate cyclase (*sGC*) enzyme to produce cyclic guanosine monophosphate (*cGMP*). cGMP is broken down by PDE 5 enzyme in the smooth muscle cell. Sildenafil inhibits PDE5 and increases cGMP levels in pulmonary arterial smooth muscle cells. Cyclic AMP and cGMP reduce cytosolic ionic calcium concentrations and induce smooth muscle cell relaxation and pulmonary vasodilation. (Copyright 2020 Satyan Lakshminrusimha.)

hemodynamics (e.g., hypovolemia). Optimal lung recruitment with adequate PEEP or P_{aw} and/or surfactants is a prerequisite before initiation of iNO. Hemodynamic management to avoid severe systemic hypotension and optimize left ventricular preload and right ventricular afterload is also important in PPHN (Fig. 34.1). If response to iNO does not improve despite optimizing lung recruitment and hemodynamics, iNO should be stopped, because infants who did not improve with the use of iNO can nonetheless deteriorate when it is stopped after prolonged use, likely because of suppression of endogenous NO synthase.

Monitoring response to iNO is usually done with SpO_2, PaO_2, FiO_2, and OI. Repeat echocardiograms to assess right ventricular afterload, ductal patency, sepal position, and direction of PFO and PDA shunts can assist in assessing the need for

additional pharmacotherapy. MHb is assessed before starting iNO and 2 to 8 hours and 24 hours after starting iNO. It should continue to be monitored daily if the infant is receiving more than 20 ppm of iNO but it is unlikely that MHb levels will increase after 24 hours of initiation of iNO if the dose is 20 ppm or less; thus, daily monitoring is usually not necessary. MHb levels over 2% need to be monitored closely and weaning iNO dose may be warranted.

Weaning Inhaled Nitric Oxide

Even a brief exposure to 100% oxygen can stimulate the formation of superoxide anions and free radicals.[40] Hence, limiting hyperoxic exposure is the primary goal before weaning iNO. Once inspired oxygen is weaned to 60% or less, and PaO_2 remains 50 mm Hg or higher or preductal SpO_2 consistently is 90% or higher, iNO can be weaned in steps of 5 ppm every 2 to 4 hours (from 20 ppm to 15 ppm, subsequently 10 ppm and 5 ppm). There is a risk of rebound pulmonary hypertension with rapid weaning especially during the last steps. Hence, we recommend slow weaning from 5 ppm at a rate of 1 ppm every 2 to 4 hours. The effect of reducing iNO concentration, if there is one, would manifest within 10 to 20 minutes. If oxygenation deteriorates well past that time period, other reasons for the deterioration should be sought. Expeditious weaning is important because prolonged exposure to iNO suppresses endogenous NO synthase[73] and may hinder final discontinuation of iNO therapy.

SILDENAFIL

Sildenafil is the most commonly used PDE 5 inhibitor in the pediatric age group (Box 34.4). Inhibition of PDE5 by sildenafil enhances cGMP levels generated in response to both endogenous and exogenous NO (Fig. 34.9). Sildenafil is a nonselective vasodilator and thus can lead to systemic hypotension. A small randomized trial suggested that oral sildenafil reduces mortality when patients with PPHN have no access to iNO or ECMO.[74] Sildenafil is commonly used in many areas as the first-line medication for PPHN in the absence of access to iNO. Oral absorption of sildenafil is approximately 40% in adults. In neonates, a nasogastric dose of 4.2 mg/kg/day results in an area under the curve pharmacokinetic profile similar to that of 20 mg TID in adults with pulmonary hypertension.[75] However, significant interpatient variability exists among neonates because of coexisting morbidities (such as cardiac failure) and medications (such as fluconazole that can interfere with the CYP pathway). Enteral sildenafil is reasonably well tolerated in term infants with a low incidence of systemic hypotension.[76]

Intravenous sildenafil improves oxygenation in patients with PPHN both as an adjunct to iNO and also without iNO.[77] Patients with an inadequate response to iNO in spite of optimal lung recruitment require an assessment of hemodynamics. If BP is within normal range and there is no evidence of ventricular dysfunction, IV sildenafil is the first adjunct to enhance response to iNO. In the presence of ventricular dysfunction and PPHN, milrinone might be a more appropriate adjunct to iNO (see next section).

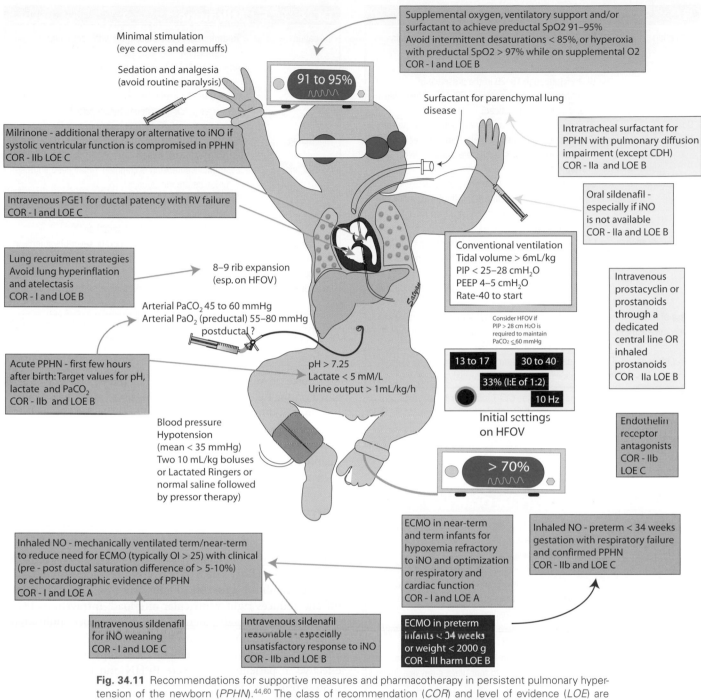

Minimal stimulation
(eye covers and earmuffs)

Sedation and analgesia
(avoid routine paralysis)

91 to 95%

Supplemental oxygen, ventilatory support and/or
surfactant to achieve preductal SpO2 91–95%
Avoid intermittent desaturations < 85%, or hyperoxia
with preductal SpO2 > 97% while on supplemental O2
COR - I and LOE B

Surfactant for parenchymal lung
disease

Milrinone - additional therapy or alternative to iNO if
systolic ventricular function is compromised in PPHN
COR - IIb LOE C

Intratracheal surfactant for
PPHN with pulmonary diffusion
impairment (except CDH)
COR - IIa and LOE B

Intravenous PGE1 for ductal patency with RV failure
COR - I and LOE C

Oral sildenafil -
especially if iNO
is not available
COR - IIa and LOE B

Lung recruitment strategies
Avoid lung hyperinflation
and atelectasis
COR - I and LOE B

8–9 rib expansion
(esp. on HFOV)

Conventional ventilation
Tidal volume > 6mL/kg
PIP < 25–28 cmH$_2$O
PEEP 4–5 cmH$_2$O
Rate-40 to start

Intravenous
prostacylin or
prostanoids
through a
dedicated
central line OR
inhaled
prostanoids
COR IIa LOE B

Arterial PaCO$_2$ 45 to 60 mmHg
Arterial PaO$_2$ (preductal) 55–80 mmHg
postductal ?

Consider HFOV if
PIP > 28 cm H2O is
required to maintain
PaCO2 ≤60 mmHg

Acute PPHN - first few hours
after birth: Target values for pH,
lactate and PaCO$_2$
COR - IIb and LOE B

pH > 7.25
Lactate < 5 mM/L
Urine output > 1mL/kg/h

13 to 17   30 to 40
33% (I:E of 1:2)
10 Hz

Initial settings
on HFOV

Endothelin
receptor
antagonists
COR - IIb
LOE C

Blood pressure
Hypotension
(mean < 35 mmHg)
Two 10 mL/kg boluses
or Lactated Ringers or
normal saline followed
by pressor therapy)

> 70%

Inhaled NO - mechanically ventilated term/near-term
to reduce need for ECMO (typically OI > 25) with clinical
(pre - post ductal saturation difference of > 5-10%)
or echocardiographic evidence of PPHN
COR - I and LOE A

ECMO in near-term
and term infants for
hypoxemia refractory
to iNO and optimization
or respiratory and
cardiac function
COR - I and LOE A

Inhaled NO - preterm < 34 weeks
gestation with respiratory failure
and confirmed PPHN
COR - IIb and LOE C

Intravenous sildenafil
for iNO weaning
COR - I and LOE C

Intravenous sildenafil
reasonable - especially
unsatisfactory response to iNO
COR - IIb and LOE B

ECMO in preterm
infants < 34 weeks
or weight < 2000 g
COR - III harm LOE B

Fig. 34.11 Recommendations for supportive measures and pharmacotherapy in persistent pulmonary hypertension of the newborn (*PPHN*).[44,60] The class of recommendation (*COR*) and level of evidence (*LOE*) are based on American Heart Association definitions. Recommendations with class I (benefits >>> risk, *green box*), class IIa (benefit >> risk, *yellow box*), class IIb (benefit ≥ risk, *orange box*), and Class III (no benefit or harm, *red box*) are shown. *CDH*, Congenital diaphragmatic hernia; *ECMO*, extracorporeal membrane oxygenation; *HFOV*, high frequency oscillatory ventilation; *iNO*, inhaled nitric oxide; *NO*, nitric oxide; *PEEP*, positive end-expiratory pressure; *PIP*, peak inflation pressure. (Modified from Polin and Fox, Fetal and Neonatal Physiology 6th edition, Elsevier, Chapter 154. Copyright 2020, Lakshminrusimha.)

MILRINONE

Milrinone is a PDE 3 inhibitor that increases cyclic adenosine monophosphate levels in the myocardium and vascular smooth muscle cells, resulting in inotropy and vasorelaxation and hence is called an inodilator (Box 34.5).[79] It is effective in improving left ventricular and right ventricular dysfunction often associated with PPHN. However, it is not selective to pulmonary circulation and a loading dose can be associated with a mean 9 mm Hg drop in systemic BP in neonates.[80] Hence, caution must be exercised when milrinone is used in patients with systemic hypotension on vasopressors. Prolonged iNO therapy increases PDE 3 activity in animal models,[81,82] potentially increasing the efficacy of milrinone. In patients with inadequate oxygenation response to iNO,

BOX 34.3	Inhaled Nitric Oxide
Indication	Mechanically ventilated term or near-term infants with HRF with clinical or echocardiographic evidence of PPHN
	OI $\geq$25 (although 15–20 in the presence of echocardiography confirmed PPHN is reasonable and commonly practiced)
Dose	20 ppm—wean if there is an oxygenation response
Monitoring	Chest x-ray, FiO_2, pulse oximetry, blood gases wean FiO_2 first to <0.6 before weaning iNO, Methemoglobin
Precautions	Optimize lung inflation with adequate positive end-expiratory pressure or P_{aw} (high-frequency ventilator) or surfactants in the presence of parenchymal lung disease
Contraindications	CDH, left ventricular dysfunction, presence of ductal dependent systemic circulation (e.g., hypoplastic left heart syndrome)
	Note: Use in infants <34 weeks' gestation is COR IIb with level of evidence-C
Class of recommendation	I[44]—evidence and/or general agreement that a given treatment or procedure is beneficial, useful or effective
Level of evidence	A[44]—data derived from multiple randomized clinical trials[53,56,58,66,67-69] and meta-analysis[61]

CDH, Congenital diaphragmatic hernia; *COR*, class or recommendation; *HRF*, hypoxemic respiratory failure; *iNO*, inhaled nitric oxide; *LOE*, level of evidence; *OI*, oxygenation index; *PEEP*, positive end-expiratory pressure; *PPHN*, persistent pulmonary hypertension of the newborn; *ppm*, parts per million.

BOX 34.4	Sildenafil (IV or Oral)
Indication	Treatment of PPHN or BPD associated pulmonary hypertension especially if
	1. iNO is not available[74]
	2. Suboptimal response to iNO—especially if associated with normal blood pressure and good ventricular function
	3. Difficulties in weaning iNO
Dose	IV—0.14 mg/kg/hr for 3 hours followed by 0.07 mg/kg/hr maintenance[77]
	PO/OG—Start at 0.5 to 1 mg/kg/dose and increase to 2 mg/kg/dose, three to four times a day (maximum dose: 8 mg/kg/day)
Monitoring	Systemic blood pressure, perfusion, lactate, FiO_2, pulse oximetry, blood gases
Precautions	Systemic hypotension is common—may need fluid bolus before initiation
	Black-box warning from FDA—caution regarding use in older children[78]
Contraindications	Severe liver dysfunction, Shock or severe hypotension
Class of recommendation	II a for oral and II b for IV[44]
Level of evidence	B—data derived from single/few randomized trials or large nonrandomized /post-hoc analysis

BPD, Bronchopulmonary dysplasia; *FDA*, US Food and Drug Administration; *FiO₂*, fraction of inspired oxygen; *iNO*, inhaled nitric oxide; *IV*, intravenous; *OG*, orogastric; *PO*, per oral; *PPHN*, persistent pulmonary hypertension of the newborn.

BOX 34.5	Milrinone
Indication	Treatment of PPHN associated with ventricular dysfunction
	Adjunct to iNO if there is an inadequate oxygenation response to iNO
Dose	IV—50 to 75 mcg/kg load over 1–3 hours[84] (optional, carries a risk of systemic hypotension)
	Maintenance—0.33 to 1 mcg/kg/min
Monitoring	Systemic blood pressure, perfusion, lactate, FiO_2, pulse oximetry, blood gases
Precautions	Systemic hypotension is common—may need fluid bolus before initiation
	One case series of increased risk of intracranial hemorrhage[85]
	Clearance improves with postnatal age[86]
Contraindications	Severe renal dysfunction, shock, or severe hypotension
Class of recommendation	II b[44]—Usefulness/efficacy is less well established by evidence or opinion
Level of evidence	C—consensus of opinion of the experts and/or small studies, or retrospective studies[87]

FiO₂, Fraction of inspired oxygen; *iNO*, inhaled nitric oxide; *IV*, intravenous; *PPHN*, persistent pulmonary hypertension of the newborn.

the choice of milrinone or sildenafil as the second-line drug is based on the following factors. The presence of cardiac dysfunction, liver dysfunction (milrinone is not metabolized in the liver), and prolonged prior exposure to iNO[83] favor the use of milrinone. Normal cardiac function, renal dysfunction (sildenafil is mainly metabolized in the liver), and prolonged prior exposure to hyperoxia[64] favor the use of sildenafil.

PROSTAGLANDIN E1

In PPHN, persistently elevated right ventricular afterload initially leads to enhanced contractility and increased function (Fig. 34.12A) (Box 34.6). When PVR is suprasystemic, the right-to-left shunt across the ductus arteriosus serves as a pop-off and reduces right ventricular afterload. Intravenous PGE1 can maintain ductal patency and also induce pulmonary vasodilation. A combination of iNO and IV PGE1 to reduce afterload and milrinone to enhance inotropy and lusitropy is effective in patients with severe PPHN and right ventricular dysfunction (Fig. 34.12B).[88]

ENDOTHELIN RECEPTOR ANTAGONISTS

Endothelin is a powerful vasoconstrictor acting through endothelin-A (ET-A) receptors in vascular smooth muscle cells (Fig. 34.10). Acting via endothelin-B receptors, endothelin can exert a pulmonary vasodilation. Nonselective endothelin receptor antagonists such as enteral bosentan (Box 34.7) are commonly used as third-line therapy in the management of both acute and chronic PPHN. A small randomized trial in late-preterm and term infants with PPHN did not show any significant benefit with the use of bosentan in acute PPHN.[92] Selective ET-A receptor antagonists are used in adults with pulmonary arterial hypertension, but the safety and efficacy of their use in PPHN are not known.

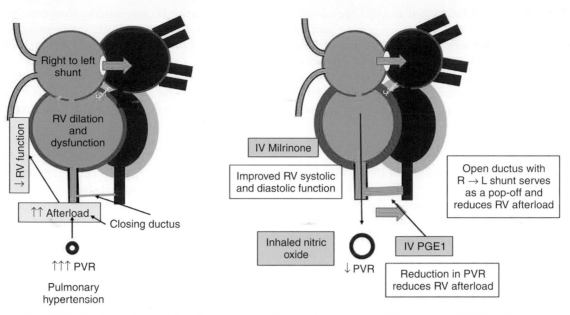

Fig. 34.12 Cardiac pathophysiology in persistent pulmonary hypertension of the newborn (PPHN). (A) In severe PPHN, the patent foramen ovale (PFO) and patent ductus arteriosus (PDA) shunt right to left with intraventricular septum bulging to the left, decreasing left ventricular (LV) preload. Extremely high right ventricular (RV) afterload leads to uncoupling of RV function, leading to RV dilation. An open PDA might benefit the RV by providing a pop-off mechanism to reduce RV afterload. (B) Inhaled nitric oxide reduces pulmonary vascular resistance (PVR) and reduces RV afterload, and milrinone can improve RV function, leading to synergy with ductal patency maintained by IV prostaglandin E1 (PGE1). (Copyright Satyan Lakshminrusimha.)

BOX 34.6	**Prostaglandin E1**
Indication	PPHN with right ventricular failure because of afterload to maintain ductal patency, reduce RV afterload[89] and promote pulmonary vasodilation[90]
Dose	IV—usual dose: 0.01 to 0.05 mcg/kg/min (range: 0.005 to 0.1 mcg/kg/min)[90]
Monitoring	Systemic blood pressure, perfusion, lactate, FiO$_2$, pulse oximetry, blood gases
Precautions	Apnea, temperature elevation, rash from cutaneous vasodilation
Contraindications	Shock or severe hypotension
Class of recommendation	I[44]—evidence and/or general agreement that a given treatment or procedure is beneficial, useful or effective
Level of evidence	C—consensus of opinion of the experts and/or small studies, or retrospective studies[90,91]

FiO$_2$, Fraction of inspired oxygen; *IV*, intravenous; *PPHN*, persistent pulmonary hypertension of the newborn; *RV*, right ventricular.

BOX 34.7	**Bosentan**
Indication	PPHN not responding to oxygen, iNO and sildenafil Chronic management of pulmonary hypertension especially associated with CDH or BPD as a second-line drug after sildenafil
Dose	PO 2 mg/kg/dose BID[92]
Monitoring	Liver function tests—check bilirubin, ALT, and AST before starting therapy and frequently (at least monthly) thereafter
Precautions	Hepatotoxicity
Contraindications	Elevated liver enzymes
Class of recommendation	II b—usefulness/efficacy is less well established by evidence or opinion
Level of evidence	C—consensus of opinion of the experts and/or small studies, or retrospective studies[92]

ALT, ***; *AST*, ***; *BID*, ***; *BPD*, bronchopulmonary dysplasia; *CDH*, congenital diaphragmatic hernia; *iNO*, inhaled nitric oxide; *IV*, intravenous; *PO*, ***; *PPHN*, persistent pulmonary hypertension of the newborn.

MANAGEMENT OF SYSTEMIC HYPOTENSION IN PERSISTENT PULMONARY HYPERTENSION OF THE NEWBORN

High PVR combined with low SVR and systemic hypotension requiring treatment is common in infants with PPHN, with nearly two-thirds of ventilated infants with PPHN and 87% infants requiring ECMO on three or more inotropes.[93] For practical purposes, systemic BP values 2 standard deviations below the mean are considered low. For practical purposes, most term babies with BP values below 55/25 with a mean of 35 mm Hg may need therapy if associated with signs of hypoperfusion. Low systemic BP will increase right-to-left shunting across the PDA and potentially decrease pulmonary blood flow. In the past, clinicians often strove to achieve higher-than-normal systemic BP to alleviate ductal shunting, but that practice is not evidence based and may contribute to RV decompensation. Efforts need to be directed toward reducing PVR, not increasing SVR. Hypotension may be attributed to poor cardiac output and/or hypovolemia, especially in infants with perinatal asphyxia or sepsis. Capillary leak is common and, coupled with high ventilator pressure that elevates venous pressure and increases the hydrostatic filtration pressure, often leads to intravascular volume depletion even as the patient is becoming edematous and gaining weight. Therefore, adequate volume replacement is essential when capillary leak is present (Fig. 34.3).

Fluid Management

Many infants with systemic hypotension and PPHN with poor perfusion and/or low central venous pressure receive fluid boluses before initiation of vasoactive agents.[93] The optimal fluid type is not known. Common choices include normal saline (NS), lactated Ringer's solution (LR), 5% albumin, and blood products such as fresh frozen plasma (FFP) or packed red blood cells. There appears to be no advantage of 5% albumin over NS.[94] NS has a low pH (~5.0) and can cause hyperchloremic acidosis. LR has less chloride compared with NS (109 vs. 154 mEq/L) and has lactate (28 mM/L) that corrects acidosis. There is no evidence that FFP is beneficial in the absence of coagulopathy and should be avoided owing to the risk and expense associated with blood products.

Sodium Bicarbonate

The use of small doses of sodium bicarbonate (1–2 mEq/kg) over 20 to 30 minutes in neonates with PPHN and metabolic acidosis with normal $PaCO_2$ has been common practice in the past but is not supported by current evidence.[95,96] Additionally, administration of sodium bicarbonate may raise $PaCO_2$ requiring further increase in ventilator settings and paradoxically decrease intracellular pH. Metabolic acidosis most commonly reflects poor tissue perfusion and will self-correct once circulatory status has improved.

Vasoactive Infusions

Several vasopressors and/or inotropic medications may be useful in treating hypotension associated with PPHN in neonates. All vary in mechanisms of action, and a good understanding of the physiology behind the neonate's hypotension and the medication's mechanism of action is necessary to choose the best treatment. Please see Chapter 33 for a review on vasopressor medications.

Dopamine has conventionally been the first-line therapy for hypotension in neonates including management of septic shock.[18] However, its nonspecific mechanism of action can cause pulmonary vasoconstriction, especially at high doses. For example, in a neonatal lamb model, dopamine selectively increased systemic arterial pressure at lower doses without significantly increasing PAP, thus increasing pulmonary blood flow in lambs without PPHN.[97] However, in lambs with PPHN, the pulmonary vasculature is remodeled and PAP is more sensitive to vasoconstrictor effects of dopamine, and therefore, dopamine did not increase pulmonary blood flow.[97] Thus, in a newborn with PPHN requiring dopamine infusion, especially when the dose exceeds 15 mcg/kg/min, monitoring of the directionality of PDA flow and PAP with serial echocardiograms is necessary.

Norepinephrine is more selective than dopamine, acting primarily on α_1 receptors resulting in vasoconstriction and minimal inotropic effect on β_1 receptors. In newborns with PPHN, norepinephrine increases PAP; however, unlike dopamine, the ratio of pulmonary/systemic arterial pressure decreased following norepinephrine infusion (0.98–0.87, $P < .001$).[98] This study also noted decreased oxygen requirement and increased postductal oxygen saturation, supporting the notion of increased pulmonary blood flow following norepinephrine infusion.[24]

Epinephrine is less selective than norepinephrine, and its stimulation on α and β receptors varies by dose. At lower doses, epinephrine has predominant β effect causing chronotropy and inotropy. Thus, for an infant with depressed myocardial function, epinephrine may be useful. However, epinephrine was associated with more metabolic disturbances such as hyperglycemia and lactic acidosis.[99,100]

Vasopressin is being increasingly used to treat systemic hypotension in PPHN.[101] There are three subtypes of vasopressin receptors, V_1, V_2, and V_3 (Fig. 34.13). V_1 receptors are located in the vasculature beds and are commonly known for their potent vasoconstrictive properties on systemic vasculature with minimal increase or even a potential decrease in PVR, leading to a decrease in the pulmonary/systemic arterial pressure ratio. The mechanism of vasodilation in the pulmonary vasculature is thought to be from stimulation of oxytocin endothelial receptors and subsequent NO pathway activation. Specifically in newborns, Mohamed et al. reported improved oxygenation and reduction in iNO in a case series of newborns with PPHN in which vasopressin was used as a "rescue" therapy for refractory pulmonary hypertension and systemic hypotension despite iNO and vasoactive infusions.[102] Acker et al. reported a case of 13 newborns with CDH that received vasopressin for refractory hypotension.[101] All 13 newborns in this series met ECMO criteria before vasopressin initiation. Eleven patients received vasopressin before initiation of ECMO (the other two received vasopressin concurrently with ECMO initiation). In 6 of those 11, ECMO was no longer indicated owing to overall improved hemodynamics.[49] In both the Acker and Mohamed series, vasopressin was used essentially as a rescue therapy after other interventions failed. Thus, earlier initiation of vasopressin in newborns with pulmonary hypertension warrants additional research. The effect vasopressin has on sodium and water balance has to be considered before initiation. Vasopressin can alter sodium and water balance via two mechanisms—V_1 receptors result in peripheral vasoconstriction and, thus, improved renal blood flow, and V_2 receptors have antidiuretic effects resulting in reabsorption of free water. This last mechanism has the potential to cause hyponatremia.

Hydrocortisone

Cases demonstrating response to exogenous glucocorticoids in catecholamine-resistance hypotension are reported.[103] In addition to increasing BP, glucocorticoids might have an effect on the lung in PPHN (Box 34.8). Glucocorticoids may have beneficial effects in MAS,[104] but there is a concern of exacerbation of infection and lack of multicenter randomized trials. Animal studies have shown that high-dose hydrocortisone inhibits

BOX 34.8	**Hydrocortisone**
Indication	Catecholamine-resistant systemic hypotension
	Refractory pulmonary hypertension not responsive to inhaled nitric oxide
Dose	Acute crisis: 1 mg/kg/dose q 6 h
	Maintenance: 1 mg/kg/day in divided doses
	Severe PPHN not caused by infection—4 mg/kg/dose × 1 followed by 1 mg/kg q 6h × 4 doses followed by maintenance (limited data)
Monitoring	Blood glucose, blood pressure, sodium, watch for infection
Precautions	Occult infection—fungal, viral (herpes simplex, CMV etc.), bacterial can be exacerbated with steroid therapy
Contraindications	Known or suspected infection
Class of recommendation	Class IIb—Usefulness/efficacy is less well established by evidence/opinion. May be considered
Level of evidence	C—consensus of opinion of the experts and/or small studies, retrospective studies, registries

CMV, Cytomegalovirus; *PPHN*, persistent pulmonary hypertension of the newborn.

PDE 5 and enhances oxygenation response in PPHN.[105] A single-center case series using 4 mg/kg loading dose followed by 1 mg/kg/dose q 6h in PPHN resistant to conventional therapy showed significant improvement in oxygenation and BP with a reduction in the need for vasopressors.[106]

PRETERM INFANTS WITH EARLY PULMONARY HYPERTENSION (PRETERM PERSISTENT PULMONARY HYPERTENSION OF THE NEWBORN)

Following extremely preterm birth (<26 weeks' gestation), PVR decreases at a slower rate compared with term neonates.[107] PROM and chorioamnionitis are associated with preterm PPHN (pPPHN).[9,108] The use of iNO in ELBW infants with HRF has resulted in contradictory responses[109,110] but overall has not improved mortality or neurologic outcomes.[111] Based on these results and systematic reviews[112] and meta-analyses,[113,114] the American Academy of Pediatrics has stated that the current evidence does not support treating preterm infants with respiratory failure with iNO for rescue or routine use to improve survival.[115,116]

There appears to be a subset of preterm infants with pPPHN that respond well to iNO.[117] These infants have preterm PROM with oligohydramnios and some degree of pulmonary hypoplasia.[118] Preterm infants with PROM presenting with HRF were noted to have low nitrate/nitrite levels in the tracheal aspirate, suggesting a specific deficiency of NO; these infants responded well to iNO.[108] However, an evaluation of extremely preterm infants with early HRF (without a diagnosis of pPPHN) did not associate long-term neurological benefit with use of iNO or PROM.[119]

CONCLUSION

Although significant progress has been made in the acute management of PPHN, there are some cases that fail medical management requiring ECMO (see Chapter 28). The overall mortality among infants with PPHN in California was 7.3%. After discharge from the hospital, 0.8% of PPHN infants died and 29% needed at least one readmission during infancy.[120] Close respiratory and neurological follow-up including hearing assessment is important for all infants with PPHN.

KEY REFERENCES

3. Walsh-Sukys MC, Tyson JE, Wright LL, et al: Persistent pulmonary hypertension of the newborn in the era before nitric oxide: practice variation and outcomes. Pediatrics 105(1 Pt 1):14–20, 2000.
34. Shankaran S, Laptook AR, Pappas A, et al: Effect of depth and duration of cooling on deaths in the NICU among neonates with hypoxic ischemic encephalopathy: a randomized clinical trial. JAMA 312(24):2629–2639, 2014.
35. Lakshminrusimha S, Shankaran S, Laptook A, et al: Pulmonary hypertension associated with hypoxic-ischemic encephalopathy—antecedent characteristics and comorbidities. J Pediatr 196: 45–51 e3, 2018.
37. Rudolph AM, Yuan S: Response of the pulmonary vasculature to hypoxia and H+ ion concentration changes. J Clin Investig 45(3):399–411, 1966.
44. Hansmann G, Koestenberger M, Alastalo TP, et al: 2019 updated consensus statement on the diagnosis and treatment of pediatric pulmonary hypertension: the European Pediatric Pulmonary Vascular Disease Network (EPPVDN), endorsed by AEPC, ESPR and ISHLT. J Heart Lung Transplant 38(9):879–901, 2019.
46. Wung JT, James LS, Kilchevsky E, et al: Management of infants with severe respiratory failure and persistence of the fetal circulation, without hyperventilation. Pediatrics 76(4):488–494, 1985.
56. Konduri GG, Solimano A, Sokol GM, et al: A randomized trial of early versus standard inhaled nitric oxide therapy in term and near-term newborn infants with hypoxic respiratory failure. Pediatrics 113(3 Pt 1):559–564, 2004.
57. Gonzalez A, Bancalari A, Osorio W, et al: Early use of combined exogenous surfactant and inhaled nitric oxide reduces treatment failure in persistent pulmonary hypertension of the newborn: a randomized controlled trial. J Perinatol 41:32–38, 2021.
67. Neonatal Inhaled Nitric Oxide Study G: Inhaled nitric oxide in full-term and nearly full-term infants with hypoxic respiratory failure. N Engl J Med 336(9):597–604, 1997.
77. Steinhorn RH, Kinsella JP, Pierce C, et al: Intravenous sildenafil in the treatment of neonates with persistent pulmonary hypertension. J Pediatr 155(6):841–847 e1, 2009.

35

Care of the Infant with Congenital Diaphragmatic Hernia

Satyan Lakshminrusimha, Martin Keszler, and Bradley A Yoder

KEY POINTS

- Herniation of abdominal contents into the thoracic cavity is associated with severe hypoplasia of the ipsilateral lung, variable degrees of hypoplasia on the contralateral side, making the lungs uniquely susceptible to injury.
- Decreased pulmonary vascular bed, pulmonary vascular remodeling, and various degrees of hypoplasia of the left ventricle (when the hernia is on the left side) lead to pulmonary hypertension and cardiac dysfunction.
- The overall goal of ventilation in congenital diaphragmatic hernia (CDH) is to protect the lung while maintaining acceptable gas exchange and avoiding worsening of persistent pulmonary hypertension of the newborn. Gentle ventilation, mild permissive hypercapnia, acceptance of lower PaO_2, and avoidance of overexpansion of the lungs are key elements of the ventilation strategy in CDH.
- Treatment of pulmonary hypertension includes optimizing gas exchange and lung inflation, adequate sedation, and the use of inhaled nitric oxide. Milrinone, sildenafil, and PGE1 are useful adjuncts in specific circumstances, and extracorporeal membrane oxygenation remains the ultimate rescue strategy.

INTRODUCTION

Congenital diaphragmatic hernia (CDH) is characterized by a defect in the diaphragm, leading to herniation of abdominal contents into the thoracic cavity (Fig. 35.1). The incidence of CDH is approximately 1 in 3000 live births and continues to be associated with high mortality (approximately 22%–27%).[1] The precipitous decrease in pulmonary vascular resistance (PVR) seen in normal term infants at birth does not occur in infants with CDH because of decreased vascular bed associated with pulmonary hypoplasia.[2] Hence, the pathophysiology of CDH is characterized by pulmonary hypoplasia (ipsilateral and contralateral), persistent pulmonary hypertension of the newborn (PPHN), and cardiac dysfunction (Fig. 35.1). The management of PPHN because of causes other than CDH is outlined in Chapter 34. This chapter focuses on ventilatory management of pulmonary hypoplasia and modifications to pulmonary vasodilator therapy in CDH. The following guidelines for "gentle" ventilation and pulmonary vasodilation are based on recent reviews,[3-5] guidelines from the American Heart Association,[6] and expert opinion from publications and personal management preferences of the authors. The overall quality of evidence for these recommendations, in general, is relatively low and provided by the clinical practice guideline from the Canadian CDH collaborative.[5]

ANTENATAL ASSESSMENT OF SEVERITY AND FETAL MANAGEMENT

Fetal lung volume assessment by ultrasound is typically performed by measuring and calculating the observed-to-expected lung-to-head ratio (O/E LHR) (please refer to Fig. 35.2 legend for details). Fetal magnetic resonance imaging can also assess total fetal lung volume (TFLV). The presence of liver herniation, side of the hernia, and O/E LHR and O/E TFLV are some of the antenatal predictors that determine outcome in CDH.[5] Poor outcome is predicted if O/E LHR is less than 25% with left-sided CDH and under 45% with right-sided CDH.[5] An O/E TFLV of less than 25% and the presence of liver in the thorax also carry poor prognosis.[5] Two large multicenter, randomized trials comparing fetal endoscopic tracheal occlusion ([FETO]; temporary occlusion of the fetal trachea allowing lung liquid expansion of both lungs with some reduction of intrathoracic bowel content back into the abdomen) to standard care were recently completed (www.TOTALtrial.eu). Published results were not available at the time of this writing to determine efficacy and safety for fetuses with moderate or severe risk based on the previously noted fetal measures.[5,10]

INITIAL TREATMENT AND PROCEDURES IN THE DELIVERY ROOM

Delivery as close to the due date as possible (39–40 weeks' gestation) is preferred in CDH to achieve optimal lung maturation (Fig. 35.3).[11,12] Delivery at a tertiary center with pediatric surgical and extracorporeal membrane oxygenation (ECMO) capabilities is preferred. A discussion with the obstetrician and perinatologists regarding assessment of fetal lung volume (see earlier and Fig. 35.2) will help in managing resources in the delivery room. Resuscitation in the delivery room is mainly based on modifications to the Neonatal Resuscitation Program and American Academy of Pediatrics/American Heart Association guidelines.[13-15]

1. Before delivery, appropriate plans for cord management should be made with the obstetrician. Delayed cord clamping appears to be feasible in human pilot studies and beneficial by increasing pulmonary blood flow soon after birth in ovine studies.[16-18] Further clinical trials are being conducted, and these results might identify optimal cord management strategies in CDH (NCT04373902 and NCT03314233).

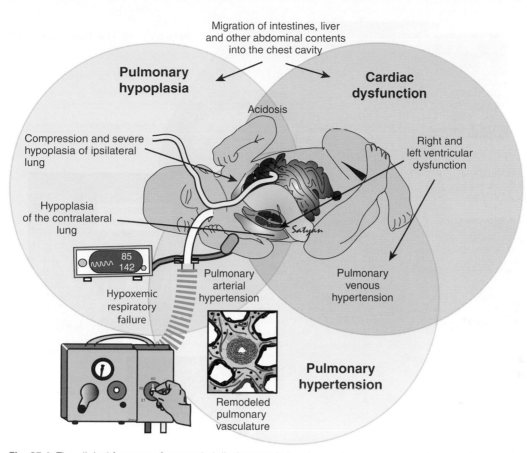

Fig. 35.1 The clinical features of congenital diaphragmatic hernia are characterized by pulmonary hypoplasia, cardiac dysfunction, and pulmonary hypertension. Herniation of abdominal contents into the thoracic cavity (usually the left side) leads to compression and hypoplasia of the ipsilateral lung, mediastinal shift and hypoplasia of the contralateral lung. Pulmonary hypertension with remodeling of pulmonary vasculature and hypoxemic respiratory failure is complicated by pulmonary venous hypertension due to left ventricular dysfunction. (From Satyan Lakshminrusimha, Copyright 2020.)

2. Infants with CDH or suspected CDH who have respiratory distress are intubated soon after birth, and a large-bore (10 French in term infants) Replogle suction tube is placed and connected to low intermittent suction.[19] The length on insertion of the endotracheal tube might be slightly shorter in infants with CDH because of short trachea (Fig. 35.4). To minimize the risk of right main stem intubation, a modified formula with 5.5 + weight in kg is used to determine the length of endotracheal tube at the lip.[20] Bag-mask ventilation should be avoided to prevent stomach and bowel distention. Infants with mild lung hypoplasia because of CDH (defined as gestational age ≥35 weeks, O/E LHR ≥50%, isolated left CDH with liver in the abdomen) without need for positive-pressure ventilation can be treated with nasal cannula oxygen with brief continuous positive airway pressure if needed after placement of an orogastric tube for suction. In a recent study, 40% of infants who met the previous criteria could be managed without intubation during the preoperative period.[21]

3. A preductal pulse oximeter is placed on the right upper extremity as soon as feasible (Fig. 35.5). Oxygen saturation targets are based on neonatal resuscitation program guidelines. Many centers tolerate a lower limit of 80% saturations after the first 5 minutes of life in the delivery room and accept preductal oxygen saturation (SpO_2) of 85% or more in the neonatal intensive care unit (NICU) as long as the baby does not develop significant metabolic acidosis.

4. Inspired oxygen concentration can be started at 21% to 50% and titrated based on preductal pulse oximeter values. In the presence of bradycardia or persistent oxygen saturation under 80% at 5 minutes, consider increasing fraction of inspired oxygen (FiO_2).[23]

5. High airway pressures should be avoided, and ventilation using a T-piece resuscitator, rather than a self-inflating bag, is preferred. Peak inflation pressures (PIPs), preferably 25 cm H_2O or less, are given to avoid lung damage to the hypoplastic lungs. However, if heart rate is low (<60 beats per minute) with inadequate ventilation, it may be appropriate to transiently increase PIP. In a study of respiratory monitoring during resuscitation of CDH patients, the median PIP necessary to achieve adequate tidal volume (V_T) and chest rise was 30 to 33 cm H_2O.[24] It is not uncommon to observe low end-tidal carbon dioxide (CO_2)[24] or a delay in change in color of the colorimetric capnographic device after intubation in infants with CDH with severe pulmonary hypoplasia and ventilation-perfusion mismatch caused by low pulmonary blood flow.[25]

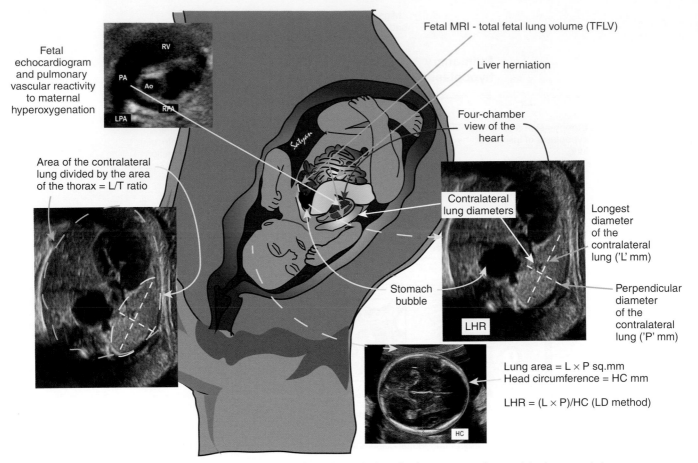

Fig. 35.2 Antenatal assessment of severity of lung hypoplasia and pulmonary vascular reactivity in congenital diaphragmatic hernia. Modified from Chandrasekharan et al.[7] Lung volumes can be measured by ultrasound or magnetic resonance imaging (*MRI*). Lung-to-head ratio (*LHR*) is the ratio of contralateral lung area (at the level of the four-chamber view of the heart) to the head circumference measured by ultrasound. The lung area can be measured by longest diameter (LD method—product of the longest diameter of the lung L mm × perpendicular diameter D mm – shown here), anteroposterior (AP method—AP diameter at the midclavicular line × perpendicular diameter at the midpoint of AP diameter), or trace method (manual tracing of lung circumference). Area of the contralateral lung divided by the thoracic area is referred to as the L/T ratio. Fetal MRI can directly measure the sum of both lung volumes (total fetal lung volume [*TFLV*]). Pulmonary vascular reactivity is assessed by Doppler measurement of pulmonary flow in left and right pulmonary arteries before and after maternal oxygenation with 60% oxygen.[8] Of these measurements, observed-to-expected (O/E) ratios of LHR and TFLV, along with location of the liver, are considered most predictive of outcome. (Based on Canadian Congenital Diaphragmatic Hernia Collaborative: Diagnosis and management of congenital diaphragmatic hernia: a clinical practice guideline. CMAJ 190(4):E103–E12, 2018; and Satyan Lakshminrusimha, Copyright 2020.)

6. Use of lower positive end-expiratory pressure ([PEEP] 2–3 cm H_2O) may be beneficial[26] but has not been studied in the delivery room setting. Limited studies demonstrate benefit with the use of low PEEP after surgery in CDH (Fig. 35.6). It is reasonable to start with a standard PEEP of 4 cm H_2O.

Effective management of CDH in the delivery room leads to prevention of hypoxemia, hypercarbia, and acidosis without inducing excessive lung injury.

TRANSPORT FROM DELIVERY ROOM TO NEONATAL INTENSIVE CARE UNIT

The optimal environment for delivery of the known high-risk CDH fetus is in an experienced center. Ideally, the infant should be moved as few times as possible as even a short transport

from the delivery room to the NICU can have adverse consequences. Careful preparation and execution are necessary. Some centers may be able to deliver the mother within a Children's Hospital proximate to the NICU. Others may have delivery rooms that directly abut the NICU and allow the baby to be immediately moved into their NICU bed for resuscitation and subsequent care. More often, the baby is delivered and resuscitated within the labor and delivery suite and then subsequently transported to the NICU. Continuation of gentle respiratory support and handling during transfer from the resuscitation bed to a transporter and then to the NICU warmer are critical. Endotracheal tubes can be inadvertently dislodged into the esophagus or malpositioned deeper in the airway. Both of these preventable problems can seriously affect gas exchange and hemodynamic stability. "Hand-bagging" should be avoided;

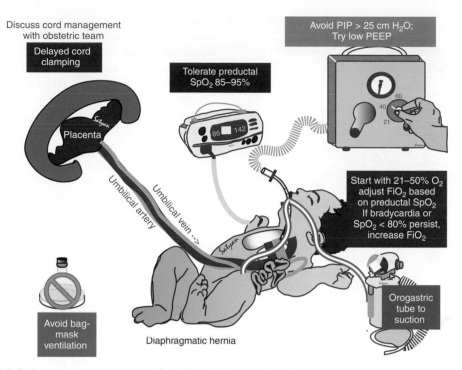

Fig. 35.3 Delivery room management of an infant with congenital diaphragmatic hernia. Prior discussion with the obstetric team regarding cord management is recommended. Placement of an orogastric tube for suction and intubation, if indicated, followed by ventilation to achieve optimal oxygen saturation range of 85% to 95% by 10 minutes after birth while minimizing volutrauma are important steps in the delivery room.[9] *PEEP*, Positive end-expiratory pressure; *PIP*, peak inflation pressure. (From Satyan Lakshminrusimha, Copyright 2020.)

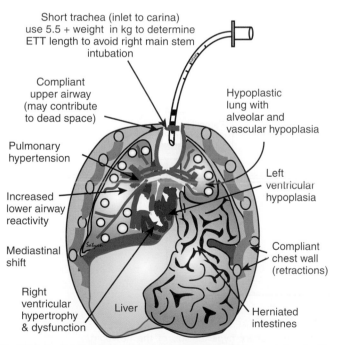

Fig. 35.4 Anatomical abnormalities in congenital diaphragmatic hernia: (1) a short compliant trachea increases the risk of right mainstem intubation and deadspace; (2) pulmonary hypoplasia increases the risk of airleaks and hypercarbia; (3) right ventricular hypertrophy and/or dilation because of pulmonary hypertension leads to dysfunction; (4) left ventricular dysfunction secondary to hypoplasia contributes to pulmonary venous hypertension; (5) compliant chest wall increases retractions; pulmonary hypertension (both arterial and venous) exacerbates hypoxemia. *ETT*, Endotracheal tube. (From Satyan Lakshminrusimha, Copyright 2020.)

instead support should be provided by a transport ventilator or T-piece resuscitator using the lowest pressures needed to achieve visible chest movement and to sustain adequate oxygenation. These challenges are magnified if delivery occurs outside of a specialized referral center necessitating transport of an outborn infant. Skilled neonatal transport teams with experience in moving babies with CDH should be employed. Some centers prefer using high-frequency ventilation during interhospital transport of these infants (Bronchotron Transport, Percussionaire Corp, Sand Point, ID;[27] Life Pulse Jet, Bunnell Inc., Salt Lake City, UT, USA).[28] However, there are no trials to define the optimal ventilatory approach during transport. (See Chapter 24 on high-frequency ventilation.)

INITIAL VENTILATION IN CONGENITAL DIAPHRAGMATIC HERNIA

Recently, general "consensus" guidelines to the management of CDH have emerged, with specific guidelines targeting early ventilator management of hypoplastic lungs.[5,29,30] Adoption of a "gentle ventilation" approach with permissive hypercapnia and tolerable hypoxemia without hypoxia has been associated with reported improvements in morbidity and mortality in CDH.[30,31] However, it remains unclear what the best ventilation mode is to provide "gentle" support. It was hoped that the VICI trial, a large randomized controlled trial (RCT) comparing initial ventilator support with high-frequency oscillation ventilation (HFOV) to pressure-controlled conventional ventilation,

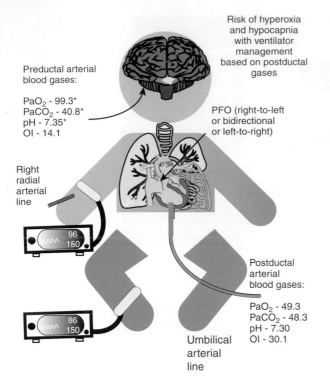

Fig. 35.5 Graphic abstract of Gien et al. emphasizing the importance of monitoring preductal blood gases and oxygen saturation during management of congenital diaphragmatic hernia. If ventilator management is based on umbilical arterial gases, significantly higher preductal partial pressure of oxygen (PaO_2) can potentially cause oxidative stress and significantly lower partial pressure of carbon dioxide ($PaCO_2$) can be associated with cerebral hypoperfusion. Values shown for $PaCO_2$ and PaO_2 are mean values in mm Hg. *PFO,* Patent foramen ovale. (From Gien J, Kinsella JP: Differences in preductal and postductal arterial blood gas measurements in infants with severe congenital diaphragmatic hernia. Arch Dis Childhood Fetal Neonatal Ed 101(4):F314–F318, 2016; and Satyan Lakshminrusimha, Copyright 2020.)

would help provide answers to this question in the CDH population.[32] Findings from this study included no significant difference in the combined outcome of mortality or chronic lung disease between the two ventilation groups for infants with prenatally diagnosed CDH. Of interest, there was a relative benefit with initial use of conventional ventilation, including shorter duration of ventilator support, less inotrope use, and decreased need of ECMO. Methodologically, however, the study was seriously compromised by the use of much higher mean airway pressure (P_{aw}) in the high-frequency group compared with the conventional mechanical ventilation group. Excessive P_{aw} can result in lung overinflation and contribute to direct compression of alveolar vessels, increasing PVR and right-to-left shunting, and limited ventricular preload because of impaired venous return (Fig. 35.5).[3-35] Therefore, the results of the VICI trial must be understood to reflect a comparison of gentle conventional ventilation to a relatively aggressive lung recruitment strategy of HFOV, an approach generally not recommended in the CDH population.

GENTLE VENTILATION IN CONGENITAL DIAPHRAGMATIC HERNIA

Lung protective strategy or "gentle ventilation" was pioneered by Wung et al. in 1985.[30,31] Based on the results of the VICI trial (despite the limitations of this trial—see later), recent published guidelines recommend initiating ventilation with volume targeted conventional ventilation. The recommended initial settings on different modes of ventilators are shown in Table 35.1.

The overall goal of ventilation in CDH is to protect the lung while maintaining acceptable gas exchange and avoiding worsening of PPHN. We recommend targeting preductal

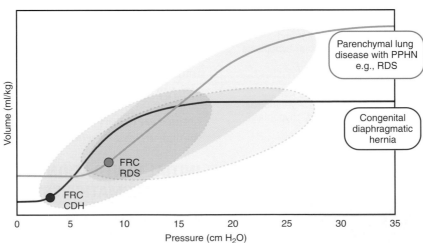

Fig. 35.6 Pressure volume curve of a neonate with persistent pulmonary hypertension of the newborn (*PPHN*) secondary to parenchymal lung disease (such as respiratory distress syndrome [*RDS*]) is shown in the *green line.* Ventilation with a peak inflation pressure (PIP) of approximately 30 cm H_2O and positive end-expiratory pressure (PEEP) of 5 to 7 cm H_2O may be needed to recruit the lung initially in patients with parenchymal lung disease (*green oval*). However, the lungs of infants with congenital diaphragmatic hernia are hypoplastic, and an increase in pressure does not lead to any additional recruitment (*red line*). Use of similar pressures used to recruit neonates with parenchymal lung disease results in baro/volu-trauma and risk of air leaks with a flattened pressure volume curve (*blue oval*). The use of lower PEEP (2–3 cm H_2O) may achieve lower PIP and better compliance (*pink oval*). *CDH,* Congenital diaphragmatic hernia; *FRC,* functional residual capacity. (From Satyan Lakshminrusimha, Copyright 2020.)

TABLE 35.1 **Recommended Initial Ventilator Settings for Neonates with Diaphragmatic Hernia**[4,5,28,29,31,32,36,37]

	HFOV	HFJV	Conventional
ΔP/PIP Max PIP	24–28 (amplitude)	20–25 cm H_2O	V_T 4–5 mL/kg ≤25 cm H_2O
P_{aw}/PEEP Max P_{aw}	10–12 cm H_2O Rarely >16 cm H_2O	10–12/6–8 cm H_2O Rarely >16 cm H_2O	3–5 cm H_2O
Frequency	8–10 Hz	360–420 bpm (6–7 Hz)	40–60 bpm
I:E/I-time	1:2	0.02 sec	0.3 sec
FiO_2	0.40	0.40	0.40
SpO_2 preductal			
First hour	>80%	>80%	>80%
Goal	92%–98%	92%–98%	92%–98%
"Tolerated"	>90%	>90%	>90%
PaO_2 preductal			
Goal	50–70 mm Hg	50–70 mm Hg	50–70 mm Hg
"Tolerated"	≥ 45 mm Hg	≥45 mm Hg	≥45 mm Hg
$PaCO_2$			
Goal	45–55 mm Hg	45–55 mm Hg	45–55 mm Hg
"Tolerated"	<65 mm Hg (if pH is >7.2)	<65 mm Hg (if pH is >7.2)	< 65 mm Hg (if pH is >7.2)
Chest x-ray	8–9 rib inflation contralateral lung	8–9 rib inflation contralateral lung	8–9 rib inflation contralateral lung

bpm, Breaths per minute; *FiO₂*, fraction of inspired oxygen; *HFOV*, high-frequency oscillatory ventilation; *HFJV*, high-frequency jet ventilation; *I:E*, inflation to expiratory ratio; *I-time*, inflation time; *ΔP*, delta pressure (amplitude); *PaCO₂*, partial pressure arterial carbon dioxide; *Paw*, mean airway pressure; *PEEP*, positive end-expiratory pressure; *PIP*, peak inflation pressure; *SpO₂*, oxygen saturation; *VT*, tidal volume.
(Modified from Yoder and Grubb, Mechanical Ventilation: Disease Specific Strategies.)

oxygen saturations between 85% and 95%. Postductal saturations are maintained above 70% as long as perfusion is adequate with urine output greater than 1 mL/kg/h without any lactic acidosis (lactate <2 mM/L). These guidelines are not evidence based and based on expert consensus.[5,29] Oxygen titration should be based on preductal oxygen saturations or blood gases with a goal to maintain partial pressure of arterial oxygen (PaO_2) in the 50 to 70 mm Hg range.[22] Adjusting inspired oxygen concentration based on postductal SpO_2 or postductal PaO_2 might result in excess oxygen exposure (Fig. 35.5).[22] The brain and myocardium are exposed to preductal blood, and therefore, assuming adequate cardiac output, adequate preductal blood gas levels ensure adequate oxygen delivery to these vital organs, regardless of the postductal levels. Arterial PCO_2 is maintained between 45 and 55 mm Hg (<65 mm Hg in some centers, permissive hypercapnia). Postductal (umbilical arterial) gases not only have significantly lower PaO_2 levels but may also have higher partial pressure of arterial carbon dioxide ($PaCO_2$) levels compared with preductal gases.[22] As cerebral

perfusion is based on preductal $PaCO_2$ levels, it is important to avoid preductal hypocapnia (Fig. 35.5).[38]

1. Conventional ventilation: Based on the results from the VICI trial, conventional ventilation may be the preferred mode for initial ventilation in CDH.[39] The PIP limit is usually set at around 25 cm H_2O. Most centers use PEEP of 4 to 5 cm H_2O, but some centers start with a lower PEEP (2–3 cm H_2O) to operate on the steep portion of the pressure-volume loop owing to hypoplasia (Fig. 35.6). If volume-targeted ventilation is used, lower initial V_T values, coupled with higher rate, are often used (~4 mL/kg) to account for the lung hypoplasia and limit the risk of lung injury. Many infants with CDH have airway anomalies and possibly tracheal distention (especially after FETO), contributing to increased anatomical deadspace.[40,41] Rather than selecting an arbitrary V_T, the minimal volume necessary to provide adequate oxygenation and ventilation should be established. Relatively low PEEP is often necessary as pulmonary arterial perfusion is very sensitive to level of PEEP and P_{aw}. Studies in postoperative patients with CDH suggest that use of 2 cm H_2O PEEP results in higher V_T and better compliance (Fig. 35.6). Although the minute ventilation necessary to achieve normocarbia should be the same in CDH as for infants with normal lungs,[36] use of a V_T on the higher end of "normal" (i.e., >5 mL/kg) may initiate lung injury owing to volutrauma as this V_T is distributed to a decreased number of alveoli in these hypoplastic lungs. However, studies by Landolfo[42] and Sharma[36] report relatively normal to high V_T to achieve effective ventilation. It is unclear, whether higher rates (i.e., 60 breaths per minute) and lower V_T (4 mL/kg) or higher V_T (6 mL/kg) at lower rates have an effect on short- or long-term outcomes for lung hypoplasia disorders. As of March 2020, there is an ongoing trial at King's College in London to compare the effectiveness and safety of conventional ventilation using 4, 5, and 6 mL/kg in babies with CDH (ClinicalTrials.gov Identifier: NCT02849054). In this context, it is also important to note that those infants with the greatest degree of lung hypoplasia have increased deadspace-to-V_T ratios, suggesting that more of the applied V_T is "lost" as ineffective deadspace ventilation.[43] We speculate that part of this V_T is lost because of an extremely compliant tracheobronchial tree in patients with CDH (Fig. 35.4). We recommend use V_T of around 4 mL/kg with high rates (60 breaths per minute) to maintain target $PaCO_2$. This may necessitate a shorter inspiratory time than is typical of term infants. Weaning from conventional ventilation should preferentially be by means of decreasing V_T (directly or by lowering PIP) first, followed by a decrease in rate. If $PaCO_2$ cannot be maintained under 65 mm Hg in spite of using a PIP of 25 cm H_2O or more, high-frequency ventilation should be considered. If the infant needs to be ventilated with a T-piece resuscitator or a bag manually during transport, avoid using PIPs over 25 cm H_2O.

2. HFOV: The initial settings are usually a P_{aw} of 10 to 12 cm H_2O, frequency 8 to 10 Hz, and amplitude in the mid-20s cm H_2O depending on the adequacy of chest wall motion and then should be adjusted based on $PaCO_2$ and chest

radiograph. Small changes and frequent reassessment are critical. The target P_{aw} is that needed to achieve adequate oxygenation and is typically 10 to 13 cm H_2O, with an upper limit of 16 cm H_2O. It is optimal to achieve an expansion on the contralateral side of eight to nine ribs with FiO_2 of 0.6 or less. Rarely, some infants will require a 9 to 10 rib expansion on the contralateral side to achieve adequate oxygenation. Excessive P_{aw} should be avoided as it may, in the presence of the abnormal lungs in patients with CDH, lead to air leak, as well as exacerbation of systemic hypotension and worsening PVR. In particular, P_{aw} of 18 cm H_2O or more should be avoided. If an increase in P_{aw} is needed to improve lung aeration, attempts should be made to reduce the P_{aw} back to a lower level again, because once recruited, the lung becomes more compliant (see Chapter 24 on HFOV). Failure to reduce the P_{aw} to a minimum needed to maintain adequate lung volume will aggravate pulmonary hypertension. In some centers, HFOV may be considered as the initial ventilator strategy for infants with CDH, particularly those with the liver in the chest. When switching from conventional ventilation to HFOV for respiratory acidosis, consider starting at the same P_{aw} as on conventional ventilation. The goal is to minimize both under- and overinflation of the lungs (Fig. 35.7). It is important to emphasize that there is no clear evidence that HFOV (using settings described earlier) provides increased benefit (or risk) compared with high-frequency jet ventilation ([HFJV], see later) or conventional mechanical ventilation. Yang et al. evaluated retrospective data contrasting the higher P_{aw} approach as used in the VICI Trial (starting at 13–17 cm H_2O) to a lower P_{aw} approach (starting at 10–12 cm H_2O).[37] Initiating HFOV support at the lower P_{aw}, in association with several other management changes (such as weaning FiO_2 based on preductal gases and SpO_2 and strict guidelines for initiating pulmonary vasodilators), was associated with significantly lower use of inhaled nitric oxide (iNO) and inotropes, as well as decreased need for ECMO and improved survival.

3. HFJV: The use of HFJV as an initial ventilatory approach or rescue therapy, in lieu of HFOV, and the parameters employed have not been well described.[28,44,45] However, there is clinical evidence to suggest that HFJV may use lower P_{aw} with small V_T and be one of the optimal approaches for initial or rescue ventilation of babies with CDH.[45-47] The potential of HFJV to achieve effective ventilation with less impact on pulmonary blood flow needs to be evaluated in a prospective randomized trial. Initial suggested settings for HFJV are shown in Table 35.1.

4. Irrespective of the ventilatory approach used for managing CDH, several key concepts must be kept in mind. First, in patients with CDH, both lungs are small, with a functional residual capacity and total lung capacity that may be considerably less than normal with a compliant tracheobronchial tree that might contribute to deadspace (Fig. 35.4).[42] Given the effects that both atelectasis and hyperinflation have on pulmonary microvasculature and vascular resistance, careful attention must be paid to optimizing lung inflation.[26] In that regard, the P_{aw} needed to achieve optimal lung inflation may be less than that required for a normal-sized lung (Fig. 35.7). Increasing P_{aw} can lead to overdistention of the lung and increase PVR, leading to aggravation of PPHN. It is also considerably more difficult to determine optimal P_{aw} and lung inflation under conditions of lung hypoplasia. Attempting to employ the stepwise increase in P_{aw} as an "open lung recruitment" maneuver as is often done with parenchymal lung disease is not recommended in babies with lung hypoplasia with CDH as it may result in a higher P_{aw} than is necessary, at an increased risk for air leak, and without any identifiable improvement in oxygenation.

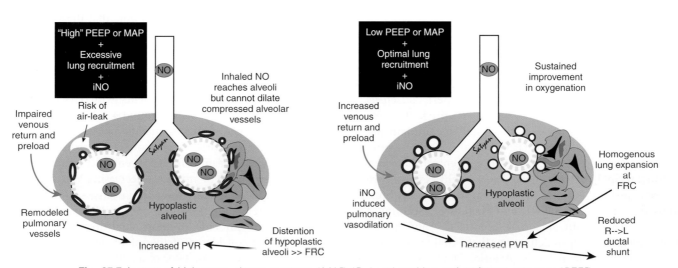

Fig. 35.7 Impact of high mean airway pressure (*MAP*) (*P$_{aw}$*) and positive end-expiratory pressure (*PEEP*) on pulmonary vascular resistance (*PVR*) in congenital diaphragmatic hernia (CDH). The left panel shows compression of alveolar vessels, impaired venous return, and increased risk of airleak with high *P$_{aw}$*. The net effect is increased PVR and right-to-left shunting. Optimal *P$_{aw}$* and PEEP to achieve inflation closer to the lower functional residual capacity (*FRC*) of the CDH lung decreases PVR and improves venous return, optimizing cardiac preload. *iNO,* Inhaled nitric oxide. (From Satyan Lakshminrusimha, Copyright 2020.)

Nonetheless, such an approach has been described by Lista and colleagues.[48] We prefer, however, to start at a lower P_{aw} and gradually adjust upward based on oxygenation, ventilation, perfusion, and radiographic lung inflation.

SUPPORTIVE MEASURES

Patients with CDH need a peripheral (or preferably a central) venous line to allow administration of fluids and medications. There is a common need for vasopressors, and hence, a double-lumen umbilical venous line or a percutaneous intravenous (IV) central catheter is ideal. An arterial line is placed for blood pressure monitoring and to draw arterial blood gases. To avoid delays and unnecessary pain and agitation, an umbilical arterial line should generally be the first choice. Right radial arterial line is preductal and may allow more appropriate weaning of FiO_2 and ventilator as $PaCO_2$ can be lower and PaO_2 higher with preductal gases (Fig. 35.5).[22] Umbilical arterial line, posterior tibial lines, and some left radial lines are postductal and should be used in conjunction with preductal pulse oximetry and end-tidal or transcutaneous CO_2 monitoring. Systemic blood pressure monitoring and management are discussed in Chapter 33, and PPHN, in Chapter 34. Sedation and analgesia are initiated with careful monitoring of blood pressure. Routine use of neuromuscular blocking agents is not recommended. A chest radiograph should be obtained as soon as possible to assess initial condition of the lung and herniated bowel and repeated based on clinical condition and ventilator status.

Surfactant is not indicated[49] unless the infant is premature and/or has evidence of RDS on chest x-ray. Laboratory investigations such as blood gases are performed on admission and repeated as needed. Frequent monitoring of blood gases in the first 12 hours of life as the lung is being recruited and the baby is transitioning may be of value in optimizing ventilator settings. Presence of high $PaCO_2$ despite maximal ventilatory support is associated with a high need for ECMO and/or mortality in CDH.[1] Serum lactate monitoring may be indicated if there is a concern about systemic hypoperfusion. A cranial sonogram at baseline soon after admission is indicated if the patient is sick and has the potential to require ECMO.

Echocardiogram

The timing of the first echocardiogram remains controversial. Some investigators support very early echocardiographic assessment to identify the optimal pulmonary vasodilator therapy,[50,51] while others have noted improved outcomes using a delayed echo approach.[37] Most current guidelines suggest getting an echocardiogram within the first 24 to 48 hours after birth, although again, there is no good evidence as to the optimal timing of initial echocardiography. Repeat echocardiogram can be obtained as needed.[5,29] Indications for repeat echocardiogram include presence of clinical or biochemical signs of hypoperfusion (lactic acidosis, oliguria or lethargy), persistent systemic hypotension (in spite of optimal vasopressor therapy), persistent hypoxemia, and persistent pulmonary hypertension (as evidenced by labile hypoxemia). If patients continue to require supplemental oxygen, weekly echocardiograms to evaluate progress and guide therapy are warranted.

PULMONARY VASODILATOR THERAPY

Pulmonary hypertension is an important contributor to morbidity and mortality in CDH. It is disappointing that there is only one randomized trial published evaluating pulmonary vasodilator therapy in CDH.[52] Two current trials are recruiting patients to evaluate milrinone, sildenafil, and iNO.[2,53] A brief review of all the pulmonary vasodilators evaluated in CDH is given here.[54]

Inhaled Nitric Oxide

If pulmonary hypertension persists on echocardiogram after optimizing ventilator and hemodynamic status, most centers consider pulmonary vasodilator therapy. iNO is often the first therapeutic choice in spite of its association with higher need for ECMO in the NINOS-CDH trial.[52] The most recent Cochrane review on the use of iNO in term and near-term infants with respiratory failure concluded that iNO does not convey an apparent benefit in CDH infants with hypoxic respiratory failure.[55] However, iNO is used in 39% of patients with CDH delivered at 36 weeks' postmenstrual age (PMA) or more in the neonatal research network.[53] Within the CDH registry, 62.3% of patients with CDH received iNO (including 74.2% of CDH with PPHN). Most centers initiate iNO at an oxygenation index (OI) of 20 or higher and/or a pre- and postductal oxygen saturation difference of 10% or more. In many instances, iNO leads to short-term improvement in oxygenation. The usual initial dose of iNO is 20 parts per million. Inhaled NO selectively dilates the pulmonary circulation and is not associated with systemic hypotension and can be effective even in the presence of systemic hypotension by reducing right ventricular (RV) afterload.

Why was iNO associated with higher need for ECMO in the CDH NINOS trial? The patients in this trial had critical hypoxemic respiratory failure (HRF) and on the verge of ECMO with mean OI in the mid-40s.[52] The P_{aw} at randomization was approximately 17 cm H_2O, with over half of the patients being on HFOV in this study (similar strategy to the HFOV arm of the VICI trial). This high P_{aw} might have contributed to the poor response to iNO in this study (Fig. 35.7). Prolonged hyperoxic ventilation (as was the case with many infants in this study) has been shown to reduce the effectiveness of iNO by oxidizing target enzymes of iNO and enhancing Phosphodiesterase (PDE) type 5 activity.[56] In addition, patients with left ventricular dysfunction (common in CDH; see Fig. 35.8) do not respond to inhaled pulmonary vasodilators because of the presence of pulmonary venous hypertension (Fig. 35.9).

We recommend a trial of iNO in CDH if HRF is associated with echocardiographic evidence of pulmonary hypertension and/or RV dysfunction without any evidence of pulmonary venous hypertension because of LV dysfunction and the OI is 20 or more (Fig. 35.9).

Milrinone

Milrinone is a PDE3 inhibitor with inotropic and vasodilator properties. It is commonly used to manage RV dysfunction in the presence of pulmonary hypertension.[57,58] It is also effective in improving left ventricular function and improving pulmonary

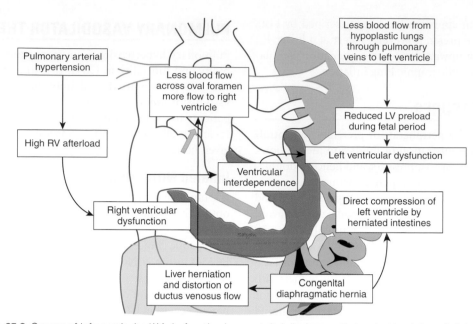

Fig. 35.8 Causes of left ventricular (*LV*) dysfunction in congenital diaphragmatic hernia. Herniation of abdominal contents into the thoracic cavity results in pulmonary hypoplasia, direct compression on the LV, and distortion of the ductus venosus in the liver. Pulmonary hypoplasia is associated with pulmonary hypertension, reduced pulmonary blood flow, and decreased venous return to the left atrium. Reduction in ductus venosus flow leads to reduced blood flow to the right atrium. More right atrial blood flows into the right ventricle (*RV*) instead of crossing over to the left atrium through the oval foramen because of higher left atrial pressure secondary to LV compression. RV dysfunction secondary to pulmonary hypertension can decrease LV preload and function because of septal deviation to the left and ventricular interdependence. (From Satyan Lakshminrusimha, Copyright 2020.)

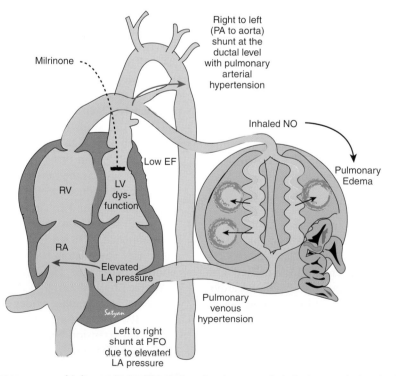

Fig. 35.9 Consequences of left ventricular (*LV*) dysfunction in congenital diaphragmatic hernia. LV dysfunction results in elevated left atrial (*LA*) pressure with pulmonary venous hypertension leading to pulmonary edema. The use of a pulmonary vasodilator such as inhaled nitric oxide (*NO*) can potentially flood the lungs and exacerbate pulmonary edema. The use of milrinone to improve LV function is recommended before using inhaled NO. *EF*, Ejection fraction; *PA*, pulmonary artery; *PFO*, patent foramen ovale; *RA*, right atrium; *RV*, right ventricle. (From Satyan Lakshminrusimha, Copyright 2020.)

venous hypertension (Figs. 35.9 and 35.10). The efficacy of milrinone in the absence of cardiac dysfunction in CDH is not clear.[59] Extreme caution should be exercised in the presence of systemic hypotension, especially with the use of a bolus dose of milrinone or if milrinone is used in conjunction with other IV vasodilators. Blood pressure and echocardiograms should be closely monitored during milrinone infusion. The early use of milrinone infusion in CDH is currently being investigated in an RCT.[53]

Prostaglandin Infusion

If there is insufficient response to iNO, some centers consider the use of IV or inhaled prostacyclin (PGI₂) as an additional pulmonary vasodilator and/or prostaglandin E1 infusion to reduce the RV afterload by maintaining ductal patency (Fig. 35.10).[60] If the echocardiogram demonstrates right-to-left shunting through the patent foramen ovale, the RV may be overloaded, as demonstrated by enlargement of the RV and a leftward shift of the interventricular septum. Bulging of the septum into the left ventricle may compromise left ventricular function and worsen systemic hypotension. Reopening the ductus and maintaining its

patency with IV prostaglandin E1 may protect the RV from excessive afterload and improve left ventricular function.[61] Caution should be exercised as IV milrinone and prostaglandins may be synergistic in reducing systemic blood pressure. Cases of gastric outlet obstruction and aneurysmal dilation of the ductus in CDH related to prostaglandin E1 (PGE1) infusion have been reported,[60,62-64] and some older studies found PGE1 to be less beneficial.[63] Hence, routine use of IV PGE1 is not recommended in CDH. Selective use to reduce RV afterload is preferred when there is evidence of severe RV strain.

Sildenafil

Sildenafil, a PDE5 inhibitor, has been used in the treatment of pulmonary hypertension in case reports in newborn infants with CDH both as a primary vasodilator and as an adjuvant to iNO. The use of IV sildenafil in CDH is currently being investigated in the multicenter CoDiNOS trial.[2] The typical dose of IV sildenafil, 0.4 mg/kg total dose as a 3-hour load (approximately 0.14 mg/kg/h for 3 hours) followed by 1.6 mg/kg/day as a continuous infusion, appears to achieve adequate levels in infants with CDH.[65] Close monitoring of systemic blood pressure is important during

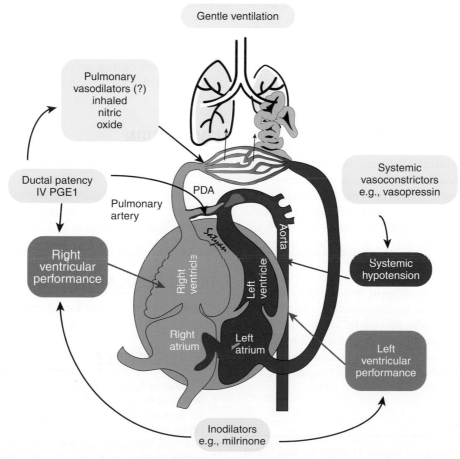

Fig. 35.10 Overview of management of congenital diaphragmatic hernia (CDH). Gentle ventilation, reduction in right ventricular afterload with selective pulmonary vasodilators such as inhaled nitric oxide, maintaining ductal patency with IV PGE1, improving ventricular performance using milrinone, and optimizing systemic blood pressure with a selective systemic vasoconstrictor such as vasopressin are components of persistent pulmonary hypertension of the newborn management in CDH. *PDA*, Patent ductus arteriosus. (From Satyan Lakshminrusimha, Copyright 2020.)

the initiation of IV sildenafil therapy.[66] Caution must be used with simultaneous use of sedation and IV PDE3 (milrinone) and PDE5 inhibitors (sildenafil) owing to an additive effect in reducing systemic blood pressure. During the postoperative period, oral sildenafil is more appropriate for the management of chronic pulmonary hypertension associated with CDH.[67]

Other pulmonary vasodilators such as endothelin antagonists have been used to manage PPHN associated with CDH. Many experts feel that vasodilators such as sildenafil and bosentan (endothelin receptor antagonist) should be used mainly in the chronic phase of pulmonary hypertension in CDH.[4] Selective systemic vasoconstriction with vasopressin might be beneficial during CDH management (Fig. 35.10). Careful monitoring of urine output and serum sodium to avoid hyponatremia is warranted during vasopressin use.[68,69]

EXTRACORPOREAL MEMBRANE OXYGENATION

CDH is the leading indication of neonatal respiratory ECMO.[70] However, the precise role and optimal timing of ECMO are unclear in CDH.[5] In nonrandomized trials, ECMO has been reported to improve survival in infants with CDH only with significant pulmonary hypoplasia (with lowest $PaCO_2$ of ≥ 55 mm Hg in the first 24 hours of postnatal period).[1] The use of ECMO has decreased, and it is now more often used in preoperative stabilization. Reports of stabilization and subsequent repair on ECMO have highlighted the benefit of delaying surgery and performing surgery either on ECMO or after ECMO. The use of ECMO for all infants with CDH with birth weight greater than 2 kg and no lethal anomalies who meet one or more of these criteria in spite of maximal support should be discussed with parents. ECMO criteria in CDH include OI that consistently is 40 or more, inability to maintain preductal saturations over 85% or postductal saturations greater than 70% with FiO_2 of 1.0, increased $PaCO_2$ and respiratory acidosis with pH under 7.15 despite optimization of ventilator management, PIP over 28 cm H_2O or P_{aw} over 17 cm H_2O required to achieve saturations greater than 85% and $PaCO_2$ over 65 mm Hg, inadequate oxygen delivery with metabolic acidosis as measured by elevated lactate 4.5 mEq/L or more and pH under 7.15, or pressor resistant hypotension (systemic hypotension, resistant to fluid and inotropic support, resulting in urine output <0.5 mL/kg/h for at least 12–24 hours). In many centers, a lower OI of around 25 is considered an indication for ECMO because of the imperative of avoiding ventilator-induced lung injury in the face of pulmonary hypoplasia and the recognition that escalating P_{aw} may be counterproductive. In the CDH registry, ECMO use is associated with a 46.9% mortality in CDH.[1]

SURGICAL REPAIR

The optimal timing of surgical repair is controversial. Most centers repair the diaphragmatic defect after physiological stabilization, defined as (1) a preductal oxygen saturation of more than 85% on inspired oxygen under 50%, (2) stable ventilator settings, (3) mean blood pressure normal for gestation, (4) lactate level under 3 mM/L, and (5) urine output of 2 mL/kg/h or

more. In some centers, repair on ECMO may also be considered. The Canadian guidelines also recommend echocardiographic criteria demonstrating estimated pulmonary artery pressures less than systemic pressures.[5] Failure to meet these criteria within 2 weeks should prompt consideration of either attempted repair or a palliative approach.[5] These principles are based on the fact that lower PVR and a relatively low oxygenation index (e.g., <9.4) reduce the risk of respiratory deterioration after surgery.

PULMONARY AND NUTRITIONAL OUTCOME

Infants with CDH are at high risk of chronic lung disease and may require home oxygen therapy. Some infants need bronchodilator therapy. Nutritional morbidity remains a problem in survivors with CDH, particularly gastroesophageal reflux during the first year of life. Some infants suffer from oral aversion and need tube enteral feeding or gastrostomy tube placement.

DISCHARGE AND FOLLOW-UP

Infants with CDH treated with either inhaled, IV, or oral vasodilators during their course in the NICU should be followed up by a cardiology or pulmonary hypertension clinic at least for one visit after discharge. Infants who have evidence of pulmonary hypertension on echocardiogram at the time of discharge and/or being discharged on pulmonary vasodilators need close follow-up with cardiology/pulmonary hypertension services.[71] All infants with CDH should be referred for neurodevelopmental testing.

CONCLUSION

Several advances have been made in the field of CDH ventilation and pulmonary vasodilator therapy. Despite these improvements, the morbidity and mortality with CDH continue to be high. Newer trials to optimize postnatal management are currently enrolling patients and are likely to shed light on evidence-based therapies likely to improve outcome.

ACKNOWLEDGMENT

We thank Dr. Tri Nguyen for his critical review of this chapter.

KEY REFERENCES

1. Jancelewicz T, Langham MR, Jr., Brindle ME, et al: Survival benefit associated with the use of extracorporeal life support for neonates with congenital diaphragmatic hernia. Ann Surg. [Epub ahead of print]
3. Keller RL: Management of the infant with congenital diaphragmatic hernia. In: Bancalari E, Polin RA (eds): The Newborn Lung. 2nd ed. Philadelphia, Elsevier Saunders, 2012, pp. 381–406.
4. Reiss I, Schaible T, van den Hout L, et al: Standardized postnatal management of infants with congenital diaphragmatic hernia in Europe: the CDH EURO Consortium consensus. Neonatology 98(4):354–364, 2010.

5. Canadian Congenital Diaphragmatic Hernia Collaborative: Diagnosis and management of congenital diaphragmatic hernia: a clinical practice guideline. CMAJ 190(4):E103–E12, 2018.

23. Riley JS, Antiel RM, Rintoul NE, et al: Reduced oxygen concentration for the resuscitation of infants with congenital diaphragmatic hernia. J Perinatol 38(7):834–843, 2018.

24. O'Rourke-Potocki A, Ali K, Murthy V, et al: Resuscitation of infants with congenital diaphragmatic hernia. Arch Dis Childhood Fetal Neonatal Ed 102(4):F320–F323, 2017.

26. Guevorkian D, Mur S, Cavatorta E, et al: Lower distending pressure improves respiratory mechanics in congenital diaphragmatic hernia complicated by persistent pulmonary hypertension. J Pediatr 200:38–43, 2018.

31. Wung JT, Sahni R, Moffitt ST, et al: Congenital diaphragmatic hernia: survival treated with very delayed surgery, spontaneous respiration, and no chest tube. J Pediatr Surg 30(3):406–409, 1995.

32. Snoek KG, Capolupo I, van Rosmalen J, et al: Conventional mechanical ventilation versus high-frequency oscillatory ventilation for congenital diaphragmatic hernia: a randomized clinical trial (the VICI-trial). Ann Surg 263(5):867–874, 2016.

36

Management of the Infant With Bronchopulmonary Dysplasia

Huayan Zhang and Nicolas Bamat

KEY POINTS

- Bronchopulmonary dysplasia (BPD) remains a frequent complication of extremely preterm birth, despite all efforts at prevention, in part because of increasing survival of the most immature infants.
- The pathophysiology and lung mechanics of established BPD differ markedly from that of acute respiratory conditions of prematurity and consequently requires a dramatically different approach to mechanical ventilation, which includes lower ventilator rate, longer inspiratory and expiratory time, larger tidal volume, higher end-expiratory pressure, and avoidance of hypoxemia.
- Established BPD does not improve rapidly, and thus, the care of infants with BPD requires a chronic care approach with an emphasis on adequacy of respiratory support and optimal nutrition to facilitate growth and healing, rather than urgency of weaning from mechanical ventilation.
- BPD is associated with many comorbidities, including pulmonary hypertension, developmental delay, oral aversion, gastroesophageal reflux, and airway pathology and consequently requires a multidisciplinary teach approach.

INTRODUCTION

Infant chronic lung disease (CLD), or bronchopulmonary dysplasia (BPD), is a debilitating lung disease that occurs in premature infants. Over the past four decades, advances in neonatal intensive care have led to the survival of smaller and more immature infants born at earlier stages of lung development. As the survival of very premature infants improved, the rate of BPD has increased. Survivors with BPD have serious consequences ranging from chronic cardiopulmonary impairment to growth failure, developmental delay, and impaired social functioning of the patient and family. Lengthy hospitalizations, persistent respiratory illness, pulmonary hypertension (PH), delayed growth and development, and poor long-term neurodevelopmental outcomes are common in this population.[1-3] Currently, there is no definitive treatment or prevention for BPD. Many clinical practices currently used in these infants are inadequately studied to assure safety or efficacy, with potentially serious consequences. The lack of an evidence base has led to large practice variation between different neonatal intensive care units and within individual centers. Therefore, management of infants with BPD, especially those with severe disease, can be extremely challenging. This chapter will provide an overview of the prevention and management of BPD and primarily focus on the respiratory management of patients with established BPD.

EPIDEMIOLOGY, PATHOPHYSIOLOGY, AND DIAGNOSIS OF BRONCHOPULMONARY DYSPLASIA

Despite efforts to reduce premature birth, there were still over 59,000 infants born at less than 32 weeks postmenstrual age (PMA) in 2019 in the United States. Over 51,000 are very low birth weight (VLBW) infants born with a birth weight of less than 1500 g.[4] BPD is the most prevalent chronic complication of preterm birth, affecting 10,000 to 15,000 infants annually in the United States alone.[5] Data from Israeli, Canadian, and Japanese Neonatal Networks report rates of BPD in VLBW infants of 13.7%, 12.3%, and 14.6%, respectively.[6,7]

The etiology of BPD is multifactorial and many potential risk factors for BPD have been identified. Some commonly discussed risk factors for BPD are listed in Box 36.1.[8,9] The most important risk factor for developing BPD is extreme prematurity. The incidence of BPD in VLBW infant ranges between 15% and 65%, and this incidence increases as gestational age (GA) decreases.[5,10] A large cohort study from the California Perinatal Quality Care Collaborative reported that rates of BPD were as high as 80.7% for infants born at under 750 g and 93.8% for those with GA less than 24 weeks, while the overall rate of BPD was 33.1% in the entire cohort of more than 15,000 VLBW infants.[9] A recent study from Turkey found a similar trend in 872 VLBW infants—BPD was present in 73.7% infants born 750 g or less and 63.2% of infants with GA 28 weeks or less. However, unlike other studies, they found no association between chorioamnionitis, antenatal steroids, small for gestation age, early sepsis, or type of birth and BPD.[11] In the current era of widespread availability of noninvasive ventilation (NIV) in the delivery room, low birth weight, intrauterine growth restriction, male gender, surfactant use, blood transfusion, and cumulative duration of oxygen and mechanical ventilation (MV) have been identified as important predictors of moderate BPD/severe BPD (sBPD).[12]

Northway et al. first described BPD in a group of premature infants studied after receiving MV and oxygen therapy for respiratory distress syndrome (RDS) in 1967. This was later described as "classic" or "old BPD" as it occurred mainly in relatively large premature newborns (born at 30–34 weeks' GA) subjected to relatively crude positive pressure ventilation. Those who died exhibited pathological features characterized by extensive heterogeneous lung injury with alternating areas of atelectasis, cystic changes and fibrosis, pulmonary artery muscularization, and severe large airway injury.[13] Over the past 50 years, there have been significant advancements in the care of premature infants including the routine use of surfactant replacement, antenatal steroids, and the introduction of more gentle ventilation modalities. As a result, smaller and more immature infants born at the late canalicular or early saccular stages of lung development are surviving. These infants are born several weeks before alveolarization begins and their lungs are extremely prone to injury. However, with the advance in the clinical care, many of these premature infants have a much milder clinical course and the concept of "new BPD" was proposed in the 1990s.[14,15] The effects of various injuries on the developing lung give rise to a pathological picture characterized by impaired alveolar and

pulmonary vascular development but less heterogeneous lung injury. These injurious stimuli include inflammation, oxidative stress, ventilator-induced lung injury, infection, drugs, and other factors such as maternal smoking.[16] In recent years, BPD has become less common in infants born at 30 or more weeks' GA and much of the discussion has focused on the new BPD. However, with the prolonged survival of the smallest and sickest premature infants, we have also seen a slow increase in the number of infants with extremely sBPD. At autopsy, the lung histology of these infants who die with extremely severe lung disease displays a mixed feature of severely delayed lung development and significant lung injury, features of both the old and the new BPD (Fig. 36.1). BPD in the current era therefore represents the complex interplay between delayed lung development and lung injury/repair in extremely premature infants.

With the evolving pathophysiology and clinical features of BPD, it has been difficult to properly define this disease, and various diagnostic criteria for BPD have been developed over the years. Traditionally, the diagnosis of BPD was based on the presence of a persistent oxygen requirement and abnormal chest radiograph at 1 month of age or at 36 weeks' PMA. For the past 20 years, the two most widely used criteria were the Shennan criteria published in 1988[17] and the severity-based National Institutes of Health (NIH) consensus definition published in 2001.[18] The Shennan criteria use oxygen requirement at 36 weeks' PMA to define BPD. In the NIH consensus definition, the diagnosis of BPD is first based on treatment with more than 21% oxygen for at least 28 cumulative days after birth and then the severity of BPD is based on the degree of oxygen and respiratory support at 36 weeks' PMA. In addition to acknowledging the presence of a spectrum of disease severity, the NIH consensus definition identified more infants with BPD and better predicted oxygen requirement at discharge when compared to the Shennan criteria.[19] However, there had

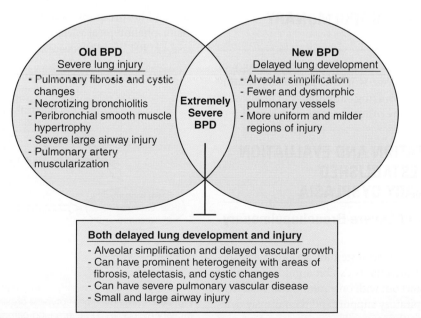

Fig. 36.1 Pathologic feature of "old," "new," and severe bronchopulmonary dysplasia (*BPD*). Severe BPD demonstrates mixed pathological features from both "old" and "new" BPD with arrest of lung development as well as significant lung injury.

been significant center-to-center variability in oxygen use because of the ongoing controversy of appropriate oxygen saturation limits for premature infants. To decrease this variability, Walsh et al. proposed a "physiologic" definition of BPD that uses an oxygen reduction test to determine oxygen dependency at 36 weeks' PMA in infants receiving 30% or less supplemental oxygen.[20] Depending on the diagnostic criteria used, the rate of BPD in extremely premature infants of 22 to 28 weeks' gestation in the Eunice Kennedy Shriver National Institute of Child Health and Human Development (NICHD) Neonatal Research Network centers varies from 68% by NIH consensus definition, to 42% defined as supplemental oxygen use at 36 weeks' PMA, to 40% by the physiologic definition.[5] Aiming to address changes in clinical practice, better categorize disease severity, and prognosticate long term outcomes, several new definitions have been proposed in the recent years. The BPD Collaborative Group proposed subdividing sBPD into type I and type II, with the latter being infants who remain ventilator dependent at 36 weeks' PMA.[21] The NICHD 2016 workshop classified nasal cannula (NC) 3 L/min or more, nasal continuous positive airway pressure (nCPAP), nasal intermittent positive pressure ventilation (NIPPV), and invasive intermittent positive pressure ventilation (IPPV) as grade III BPD and early death between 14 days postnatal age and 36 weeks' PMA because of persistent lung disease as grade III(A) BPD.[22] In contrast to other definitions, Jensen et al. found that diagnostic criteria based on the mode of respiratory support at 36 weeks' PMA, regardless of duration or level of oxygen therapy, best predicted late death, or serious respiratory morbidity through 18 to 26 months' corrected age in very premature infants.[23] However, all of these new definitions still define the disease on the basis of the therapies used to treat it. A pragmatic pathophysiology-based definition that can properly categorize disease severity and predict outcomes is yet to be developed.

PREVENTION OF BRONCHOPULMONARY DYSPLASIA

Given what is currently known about the pathophysiology of BPD, the key to prevent the disease would be promoting healthy lung development while minimizing lung injury. These issues are addressed in detail in many other chapters in this book.

CLINICAL PRESENTATION AND EVALUATION OF INFANTS WITH ESTABLISHED BRONCHOPULMONARY DYSPLASIA

Clinical Presentation of Severe Bronchopulmonary Dysplasia

With the widespread use of antenatal steroids and postnatal surfactant, many small premature infants exhibit a milder course of BPD. These infants often start out with only minimal or mild RDS requiring low levels of respiratory support and then display deterioration in lung function with increased respiratory support and/or oxygen requirements within a few days or weeks after birth. The typical radiographic changes in these patients are usually

mild diffuse haziness that persists over time and the pathologic findings are typical of "new" BPD. With proper nutritional and respiratory support and prevention and control of infection and other interventions, such as control of pulmonary overcirculation from pathologic persistent patent ductus arteriosus (PDA), many of these infants may demonstrate slow but steady improvement in their lung function. After a variable period of time, respiratory and oxygen support can be discontinued.

However, despite all the therapeutic improvements, sBPD remains common. Using data from the NICHD Neonatal Research Network Generic Database, Natarajan et al. found that 537 of 1159 (46%) infants with birth weights of 401 to 1000 g born in 2006 and 2007 still required MV or continuous positive airway pressure (CPAP) or supplemental oxygen with an effective FiO_2 over 30% at 36 weeks' PMA.[24] Many of these infants require high levels of respiratory support and high concentrations of inspired oxygen from the first week of life. Their initial postnatal courses are frequently complicated by severe RDS, pneumothorax, pulmonary interstitial emphysema (PIE), and pulmonary hemorrhage. Some infants may have a milder initial course but deteriorate after infections or other insults, such as spontaneous intestinal perforation or necrotizing enterocolitis, or from pulmonary edema secondary to a large PDA. As described earlier in this chapter, the pathological feature of their lung disease is a combination of delayed lung development and severe injury.

Since the establishment of the Newborn and Infant Chronic Lung Disease (NeoCLD) Program at the Children's Hospital of Philadelphia (CHOP) in September 2010, we have treated over 500 premature infants with sBPD. The majority of these patients are former premature neonates with extremely severe lung disease that results in high rates of mortality and long-term ventilation needs. However, although all have a diagnosis of sBPD, they may have very different clinical presentations. This may be because of the different lung developmental stages at which lung injury occurred and the interaction between injury and host response. Over the years, we have observed three major phenotypical variants: (1) severe lung parenchymal disease, (2) PH, and (3) severe airway disease (Fig. 36.2), each with

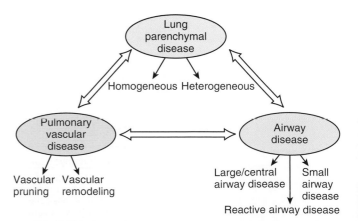

Fig. 36.2 Three main phenotypical presentations of severe bronchopulmonary dysplasia: (1) severe lung parenchymal disease; (2) pulmonary vascular disease; (3) airway disease, as the leading clinical feature. Each phenotype has various subtypes and an individual patient may have overlapping clinical features from different phenotypes.

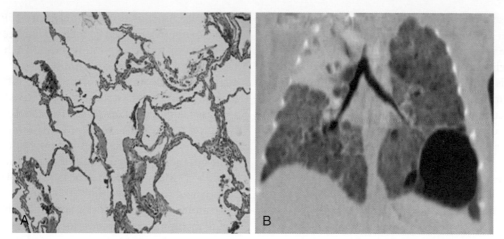

Fig. 36.3 Homogenous or heterogeneous lung disease in patients with severe lung parenchymal disease. (A) Lung biopsy sample demonstrating homogenous alveolar simplification at 50 weeks postmenstrual age. (B) Chest computed tomography scan of an infant with heterogeneous lung disease demonstrating areas of opacification and cystic changes.

various subtypes. In an evaluation of disease phenotypes among a subset of sBPD infants followed by the NeoCLD program at CHOP, Wu et al. found the presence of all three phenotypes to be the most common combination (32%), whereas the presence of a single predominant phenotype occurred in only 27% of patients. The presence of multiple phenotypic components was associated with an incremental increase in the risk for the composite outcome of death before discharge, tracheostomy, or home pulmonary vasodilator use.[25]

Severe Lung Parenchymal Disease as the Leading Feature of Severe Bronchopulmonary Dysplasia

The underlying pathologic changes in these patients may range from homogenous alveolar simplification (Fig. 36.3A) to heterogeneous microcystic/macrocystic changes with areas of fibrosis and/or atelectasis. The radiographic appearance therefore varies from generalized parenchymal opacification to bubble-like patterns to mixed areas of hyperinflation, cystic changes, and opacifications (Fig. 36.3B).

Pulmonary Hypertension as the Leading Feature of Severe Bronchopulmonary Dysplasia

PH often complicates the course of BPD and contributes to late morbidity and mortality during infancy.[26] Some patients with relatively mild lung disease develop PH, while other infants with severe lung disease may not. Nonetheless, this group of patients presents with significant or worsening PH as their key clinical feature in addition to various degrees of lung parenchymal disease. The pulmonary vasculature of these patients not only is underdeveloped and hyperreactive but also undergoes remodeling.[27] Clinically, these infants often present with chronic respiratory insufficiency with oxygen dependency, intermittent cyanotic or life-threatening episodes ("BPD spells") when agitated, and poor growth. These symptoms are typically not seen until 3 to 4 months after birth when the patient starts to "outgrow" his/her own pulmonary vascular supply. Significant pulmonary vascular "pruning" can be seen in these patients. Of the three

common clinical phenotypes of sBPD, PH was the strongest predictor of mortality before discharge in the study by Wu et al.[25] Other studies have also shown that PH is closely associated with increased mortality and morbidity in infants with BPD,[28,29] highlighting the importance of early identification and management.

Airway Disease as the Leading Feature of Severe Bronchopulmonary Dysplasia

These patients have striking airway abnormalities in addition to varying degrees of lung disease. The upper and central airway abnormalities, for example, glottic/subglottic stenosis and tracheal stenosis, are well-known complications of tracheal intubation and prolonged MV. However, the importance of tracheobronchomalacia and acquired tracheomegaly is less recognized. The so-called "BPD spells" in some patients are caused by airway collapse rather than PH crises, and therefore, the management strategy is different from that of PH. In addition, patients with BPD often have asthma-like symptoms associated with increased small airway reactivity. However, chronic wheezing in some patients may be associated with airway obstruction owing to malacia and therefore unresponsive to bronchodilator therapy.

Evaluation of Infants With Severe Bronchopulmonary Dysplasia

With multifactorial etiologies and complex pathophysiology, the clinical course and phenotype of infants with BPD are often different. In addition, most infants with BPD have other complications of prematurity. Multisystem problems, including but not limited to nutritional problems, PDA and other cardiac complications, infection, microaspiration, retinopathy of prematurity (ROP), hearing deficits, and neurodevelopmental issues, are common in these infants. These multisystem problems interact with pulmonary insufficiency, influencing the trajectory of the individual problems and together affecting long-term cardiopulmonary and neurodevelopmental outcomes. Therefore, a comprehensive multisystem evaluation with ongoing reassessments is crucial to the selection of adequate management strategies. Of all evaluation tools, a thorough review of the medical history and careful observation of the infant's daily clinical status can be the most informative. An overview of this subject can be found in a recent review by Bamat et al.[30] In brief, periodic reevaluation of the following aspects should be considered:

1. Severity of lung disease and pulmonary mechanics
2. Existence and severity of PH and pulmonary vascular disease
3. Presence of large and/or small airway disease
4. Growth and adequacy of interval growth
5. Developmental stages in relation to corrected age
6. Existence and impact of gastroesophageal reflux (GER)
7. Bone health
8. Ongoing infection
9. Uncommon causes of chronic respiratory insufficiency in an infant with atypical course of BPD

PHYSIOLOGIC BASIS FOR RESPIRATORY SUPPORT IN INFANTS WITH ESTABLISHED BRONCHOPULMONARY DYSPLASIA

Ventilatory Control in Infants With Bronchopulmonary Dysplasia

Carotid body function plays an important role in the normal ventilatory response to hypoxia or hyperoxia. Perinatal environment has been shown to affect the development of normal carotid body morphometry and function. Supplemental oxygen at birth blunts future carotid body development. In rodent BPD models, perinatal hyperoxia causes impaired oxygen sensitivity, carotid body hypoplasia, and decreased total afferent neuron number.[31] Infants with BPD have been shown to have decreased response to both hypoxia-induced increase in ventilation[32] and hyperoxic ventilator depression as compared to premature infants who did not receive MV or supplemental oxygen.[33] In infants with BPD, ventilation control dysfunction, in combination with decreased efficiency of gas exchange, muscle immaturity, and increased work of breathing, may contribute to difficulties with oral feeding[34] and disordered breathing during sleep with more central and obstructive apnea.[35] Because these infants have been exposed to prolonged hypercarbia, the control of PCO_2 is reset and they can appear comfortable at high PCO_2 levels, in large measure because of adequate renal compensation. This tolerance of compensated respiratory acidosis reflects the fact that the primary driver of ventilation is pH, not PCO_2. It is unknown what degree of hypercarbia is safe in these infants, particularly in the context of pH.

Pulmonary Mechanics in Infants With Bronchopulmonary Dysplasia

Many methods have been used to evaluate pulmonary mechanics in infants with established BPD. For example, resistance and compliance can be measured using an esophageal pressure catheter, or the single-breath occlusion method; plethysmography or nitrogen washout and gas dilution methods can be used to measure functional residual capacity (FRC); and the rapid thoracic compression (RTC) method has been used in the measurements of forced expiratory flows. Each of these methods has its own advantages and limitations,[36] and accurate measurements in the unstable infant can be difficult to achieve. In general, infants with established BPD have been found to have decreased compliance, increased resistance with decreased conductance, reduced FRC, and reduced forced expiratory flows. These abnormalities may improve over time in the first 3 years of life but many persist until adolescence and even young adulthood.[14,37,38] Many modern ventilators display resistance, compliance, and pressure-volume (P-V) loops. Although the resistance and compliance values may not be absolute, they can be useful in monitoring trends in a patient over time. Noting changes in resistance and compliance while adjusting ventilator settings at the bedside can be a valuable tool if the infant remains in a calm, consistent behavioral state. Changes in respiratory drive, sleep–wake state, activity, and agitation impact the observed mechanics. Of note, the spontaneous respiratory effort of the infant is not measured, thus often overestimating true compliance and underestimating resistance in a spontaneously breathing baby.

The ventilation pattern and pulmonary mechanics of a premature lung evolve over time from RDS to BPD. The characteristic pulmonary mechanics in an infant with RDS are those of a "stiff lung." With low compliance, high elastance, and relatively normal airway resistance, the alveoli of the RDS lungs inflate quickly and collapse easily. In many patients with sBPD, there are heterogeneous cystic changes with areas of atelectasis in the lung. Ventilation in these patients is not uniform throughout the lung fields and time constants vary in different parts of lung. The respiratory system mechanics in these patients are therefore often better explained by a two-compartment (fast and slow) model, rather than a linear one-compartment model.[39] When compliance is similar, the slow compartment has higher resistance and a longer time constant than the fast compartment. The utility of the two-compartment model in sBPD has been explained in detail by Castile and Nelin.[40] In addition, many infants with established BPD have obstructive rather than restrictive disease, with small airways as the primary contributor to the obstruction.[41] Follow-up studies have demonstrated that this obstructive airway disease with air trapping persists despite increases in total lung capacity (TLC) over the first 2 years of life.[42] These changes in lung mechanics need to be considered when selecting respiratory support strategies.

MANAGEMENT OF INFANTS WITH ESTABLISHED BRONCHOPULMONARY DYSPLASIA

Keys to Successful Bronchopulmonary Dysplasia Management

Because BPD is a pulmonary disease defined by the use of respiratory support and/or oxygen supplementation, some clinicians may focus their therapeutic efforts on weaning respiratory support and oxygen supplementation as a sign of clinical progress.

However, a perspective that considers the chronic nature of BPD and the long-term goals of the infant and family should guide management. Lung growth and injury repair are slow processes, occurring over months to years. The ultimate goal of BPD management should be to promote healthy development, not to simply remove pulmonary support. We suggest that clinicians allow the following key concepts to guide the management of infants with BPD:

1. Consider management from a chronic rather than an acute care model; and

2. Treat the whole infant, with a goal of supporting growth, development, and long-term quality of life for the infant and family.

Respiratory Management in Infants With Established Bronchopulmonary Dysplasia

Ventilatory strategies to prevent BPD are modestly effective. Major changes in respiratory support strategies include an attempt to redefine the goals for "adequate gas exchange" allowing for permissive hypercapnia[43,44] and permissive hypoxemia;[45] and the widespread increased use of NIV.[46,47] These strategies all aim to minimize exposure to MV. However, in infants with established sBPD, the focus of respiratory support is no longer to minimize the acute injury that contributes to BPD, but rather to provide adequate support to promote lung growth while minimizing further lung injury.

Noninvasive Ventilation

Preferential use of noninvasive respiratory support in the early postnatal period has been shown to reduce the risk of BPD.[48-50] These data have been quickly extrapolated to older populations beyond the immediate neonatal period. In infants with typical "new" BPD with mild respiratory insufficiency, noninvasive support may be able to provide adequate support until maturation and stability allow gradual discontinuation of respiratory support. Unfortunately, in some infants with evolving or established BPD, prolonged periods of inadequate support may have severe consequences, including poor growth (both somatic and alveolar/pulmonary vascular growth), and persistent V/Q mismatch contributing to lung injury and the development of PH. Although recent studies have questioned the safety and efficacy of permissive hypercarbia,[51-54] and despite a lack of data demonstrating the efficacy of noninvasive respiratory support modalities in infants with evolving or established BPD, a reluctance to intubate infants with chronic respiratory insufficiency in favor of continued high levels of noninvasive support is often observed. Fig. 36.4 shows the CT scan of a 6-month infant born at 26 weeks' GA. She received 6 weeks of MV followed by 4 months of noninvasive support. Despite chronic respiratory failure with PCO_2 values between 80 and 100 mm Hg, she was maintained on noninvasive support with chronic diuretics and systemic steroids. Her providers were reluctant to transition from 7 L per minute (LPM) of HFNC with 100% FiO_2 to MV despite an inability to maintain oxygen saturation above 70%, PCO_2 values over 110 mm Hg, persistent tachycardia, evidence of PH, and severe growth failure at 52 weeks' PMA. Although an extreme example, this case reflects a current practice of

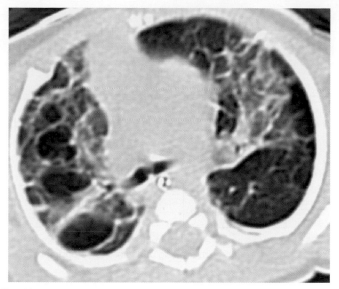

Fig. 36.4 Chest computed tomography of an infant after 4 months of noninvasive ventilation. Born at 26 weeks' gestational age, the infant received mechanical ventilation for 6 weeks after birth followed by prolonged noninvasive ventilation. She was maintained on 7 L/min high-flow nasal cannula at 52 weeks postmenstrual age despite chronic respiratory failure, progressively worsening pulmonary hypertension and severe growth failure.

overreliance on preferential noninvasive support and avoidance of MV at all costs. Over the past 10 years, nearly half of infants transferred to the CHOP NeoCLD program for sBPD management at term or beyond term corrected age were on noninvasive support, and we have observed a trend toward higher levels of noninvasive support (NCPAP >10 cm H_2O, HFNC >8 LPM) at transfer. Some providers may feel that weaning the patient to lower respiratory support modalities (i.e., CPAP or HFNC) is a marker of clinical progress. However, this may not be true in this group of patients. Maintaining high levels of noninvasive support may not best support the long-term goals of these patients.

The goal of noninvasive support in infants with established BPD is to provide adequate support to minimize V/Q mismatch and promote growth, rather than to simply avoid intubation. Although there is no evidence-based consensus on the best approach to titrate the noninvasive support[55] or determining when noninvasive support has failed, the practice of "avoiding intubation at all costs" may cause more harm than benefit in some infants with BPD. For patients with evolving or established BPD on noninvasive support, we recommend that cardiorespiratory status, tolerance of developmental therapies, and growth be closely monitored and considered when assessing the adequacy of noninvasive support. In patients who are not adequately supported, MV via endotracheal tube (ETT) or tracheostomy should be considered (Fig. 36.5).

Mechanical Ventilation

Despite advancements in respiratory care, a subset of infants with sBPD requires prolonged MV. Severe ventilator-dependent BPD

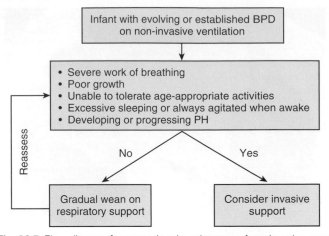

Fig. 36.5 Flow diagram for assessing the adequacy of noninvasive respiratory support for infants with evolving or established bronchopulmonary dysplasia (*BPD*).

may be uncommon in most delivery centers but is common in many referral centers that focus on the care of infants with BPD. A report of data from eight US academic centers, members of the BPD Collaborative, showed that 28% of infants with sBPD were on invasive MV at a mean (range) PMA of 47 (36–86) weeks.[56] There is a dearth of evidence from clinical trials to guide the optimal ventilator management in established BPD. As with noninvasive support, the goal of MV should be to improve V/Q matching and promote optimal growth. MV strategies should be based on the lung physiological and pathological changes of each patient. Identification of the predominant phenotype and determining the underlying lung pathology is therefore an important first step.

Conventional Mechanical Ventilation. Intermittent mandatory ventilation with time-cycled, pressure-limited ventilation has been the main mode of conventional MV (CMV) in neonates. A variety of patient-triggered synchronized modes are available, including synchronized intermittent mandatory ventilation (SIMV), assist-control (AC) ventilation, and pressure support (flow-cycled) ventilation (PSV). In addition, real-time graphics displayed on newer ventilators now enable clinicians to monitor respiratory mechanics breath-to-breath. Recent advances in ventilation techniques include volume-targeted ventilation (VTV) and neurally adjusted ventilatory assist (NAVA). Unfortunately, most clinical trials in premature infants focus on the early postnatal period and there is no high-level evidence from randomized trials for optimal ventilatory strategies in infants with established BPD. We summarize here the three guiding principles for managing ventilatory support in sBPD, based on our clinical experience and the collective experience of the BPD Collaborative:

i. Focus on providing sufficient support to meet patient needs, over a focus on weaning;
ii. Ensure adequate lung recruitment; that is, use an open lung strategy;
iii. Ensure adequate expiration, to minimize air trapping.

We describe here the application of these guiding principles, using SIMV + PSV mode as an example. The main parameters to adjust in this mode include tidal volume (V_T) or peak inflation pressure (PIP) to achieve the targeted V_T, mandatory ventilator rate, inspiration time (i-time), positive end-expiratory pressure (PEEP), and pressure support (PS). Flow rate may need to be adjusted in some ventilators/modes without auto/variable flow. The targets and strategies used to set the ventilator parameters are summarized in Table 36.1. Other ventilator modes can be used successfully, following the same guiding principles.

When adjusting the ventilator parameters to achieve these targets, it is important to consider the interplay of the targets. Adjusting one or two parameters may produce profound impact in one area but may not result in overall improvement. In the following paragraphs, we will discuss each key parameter in more detail.

1. Setting the target V_T

Because volutrauma is associated with lung injury, VTV has been advocated in neonatal MV in recent years.[57,58] In the early postnatal period, reported benefits of VTV included reduced variation in V_T values and carbon dioxide levels, less air leak, fewer days of ventilation, less severe intraventricular hemorrhage, and most importantly, decreased death or BPD.[59-61] Patients with sBPD often have marked variability in compliance and resistance over time, therefore, they may benefit from volume-targeted or patient-initiated pressure regulated and volume-controlled ventilation to ensure delivery of adequate V_T. Unfortunately, there is a lack of research evidence to guide the use of VTV in patients with sBPD. In our experience, these patients may benefit from

TABLE 36.1 Targets and Strategies When Setting Ventilator Support Under the SIMV + PSV Mode	
Target	**Strategies**
Establish optimal lung volume	• May need higher V_T of 8–12 mL/kg • Provide adequate PEEP (may need PEEP >10–15 cm H_2O) • Adequate PS to support spontaneous breath (maybe as high as the PIP needed on the mandatory vent breath)
Promote even distribution of ventilation	• Long i-time and expiration time (e-time) to adequately ventilate the slow compartments (i-time may be >0.5–0.8 seconds) • Low set vent rate (10-20/min) to ensure long enough e-time • Adequate PS to help maintain minute ventilation and achieve overall low respiratory rate
Maintain open airway	• Inspiration phase: enough pressure from both vent breath PIP and PS • Exhalation phase: adequate PEEP

PEEP, Positive end-expiratory pressure; *PIP,* peak inflation pressure; *PS,* pressure support.

much higher V_T values (8–12 mL/kg) than used in younger premature infants. The recommendation for larger V_T is based not only on extensive experience but also on pathophysiologic considerations. The high airway resistance with long time constants dictates slow ventilator rate to allow complete exhalation of the slow compartments (see later). With the usual set ventilator rate of 20 or less breaths per minute, adequate minute ventilation can be achieved only with a larger V_T. The heterogeneous inflation and frequent air-trapping increase alveolar dead space, leading to wasted ventilation and a need for larger V_T to maintain adequate alveolar minute ventilation, as does acquired tracheomegaly (distention over time of the large airways owing to cyclic stretch with prolonged MV) that results in increased anatomical dead space. High V_T, in conjunction with adequate support during spontaneous breaths, ensures adequate alveolar minute ventilation and improves a patient's comfort, which in turn will decrease work of breathing and tachypnea, thereby reducing energy expenditure.

Because of high airway resistance and tracheal distension from prolonged intubation and positive pressure ventilation, many infants with sBPD have significant ETT leak. The leak can be greater than 50% of the inflation and vary with each inflation. This challenges effective volume-controlled ventilation. In the presence of an ETT leak, the expired volume best represents the effective V_T delivered to the patient and can be targeted when adjusting settings. Many newer ventilators now have the flow sensor at the "Y" connector and are able to measure and display the V_T going in and out of the baby without distortion by circuit compliance. This improvement enables the ventilator to be operated effectively in a volume-targeted mode, such as Volume Guarantee. These modalities are pressure-controlled (PC) modes with volume targeting (see Chapter 22) and provide excellent leak compensation. Thus, clinicians are able to achieve tighter control of the delivered V_T and better intrapulmonary gas distribution as PC delivers the bulk of the V_T earlier in each cycle. However, in cases of severe leak and when the newer ventilators are not available, volume ventilation may not be feasible. In these cases, patients may need high PIP settings in the 30 to 40 cm H_2O range or higher to achieve adequate V_T in the setting of poor lung compliance. The PIP needed to achieve similar V_T with pressure-controlled vs volume-controlled or targeted ventilation is roughly equal and the focus in these infants is the delivery of adequate V_T using whatever pressure is necessary to achieve that goal.

2. Finding appropriate rate and inspiration time

Most patients with sBPD have heterogeneous lung disease (see Fig. 36.3B) with both collapsed and overinflated areas causing significant maldistribution of ventilation. As discussed earlier, the lung mechanics of these patients are better explained by a two-compartment model with differing time constants. To ensure adequate gas exchange and emptying of the slower compartment, a low rate with long inspiratory time strategy may be more appropriate. This strategy has been used successfully in several centers with programs for infants with sBPD.[40] Spontaneous breathing in these patients is often rapid, with a short inspiration time. Setting a long i-time during mandatory ventilator inflations helps ensure ventilation of the slow compartments. However, these slow compartments also need long expiration times (e-time) for alveolar pressure to equilibrate with the upper airway pressure. Therefore, a slow rate allowing enough time for expiration and emptying of the slow compartments is critical in minimizing gas trapping. To ensure an overall slow respiratory rate and an adequate inspiratory-to-expiratory (I:E) ratio, we advocate using a slow ventilator rate (10–20 per minute) along with adequate V_T and PS. The adequacy of inspiratory and expiratory time in an individual patient is best determined by observing the flow waveform on the ventilator display and ensuring that inspiratory and expiratory flow is completed within the set parameters (see Chapter 12). Adding an adequate PS of spontaneous breaths will help prevent underventilation of the fast compartment. The combined effort of improving ventilation in both the slow and fast compartments can result in improved minute ventilation and patient comfort, which in turn helps slow the breathing rate and decrease air trapping. The resting respiratory rate can help identify adequate respiratory support; a tachypneic infant with increased work of breathing is not adequately supported, even if the blood gas values are acceptable.

A slow rate, long inspiration time with adequate PS strategy is often effective in infants with sBPD. However, in the minority of patients with uniform lung disease (see Fig. 36.3A) who have a homogeneous hazy chest radiographic appearance and underlying pathological feature of generalized alveolar simplification, respiratory insufficiency may be more reflective of decreased alveolar surface area, rather than maldistribution of ventilation. Lung compliance tends to be more consistent throughout the lung fields and the time constant is relatively short. These patients may benefit from a faster rate and a shorter inspiration time.

3. Setting optimal PEEP

Setting an appropriate PEEP is an important component of ventilatory management. Appropriate PEEP levels can maintain FRC, promote alveolar recruitment, reduce work of breathing, reduce small and large airway collapse, and improve V/Q matching.[62,63] Animal studies have suggested that low PEEP will lead to impaired gas exchange and increased risk of lung injury,[64,65] while open lung ventilation improves gas exchange and attenuates secondary lung injury.[66] Concerns about high PEEP levels are that they may decrease tidal and minute ventilation, impair expiration and cause gas trapping, and decrease cardiac output through impaired venous return.[67,68] Randomized clinical trials comparing different PEEP levels have been performed in both adults and neonates with acute RDS, but not in infants with BPD.[69,70] Our clinical observations suggest that high levels of PEEP are often necessary and well tolerated in infants with sBPD.

Paradoxically, increased PEEP may be indicated when the lungs appear overexpanded. Although contrary to common practice, this is based on sound pathophysiologic principles.

As described earlier, infants with established BPD may have decreased lung compliance, increased resistance, and an obstructive lung disease pattern. In addition, many patients with sBPD have tracheobronchomalacia with dynamic airway collapse. These characteristics increase the risk of developing inadvertent or intrinsic PEEP (PEEPi). When the set ventilator PEEP is less than PEEPi, the nonparalyzed infant's spontaneous breathing effort must overcome the imposed elastic load of the PEEPi before inspiratory flow is generated and PS is triggered. An inability to achieve this extra load results in ineffective inspiratory efforts, loss of patient-ventilator synchrony, air hunger, and excessive respiratory work.[71,72] This may also be the source of some "BPD" spells (desaturation episodes), as the infant's ineffective efforts lead to air hunger, agitation, increased oxygen consumption, and hypoxemia. The floppy small airways of infants with sBPD are also susceptible to collapse in exhalation as lung volume decreases, especially in the setting of agitation.

It is imperative that PEEP levels be individualized between patients and within patients over time as the lung disease changes. The optimal PEEP is determined by the interplay between the severity of airway collapse, or tracheobronchomalacia, and severity of parenchymal lung disease. Finding this optimal PEEP may help break the cycle of alveolar collapse and airway instability. Several methods may be used to help identify individual optimal PEEP: (1) identifying lung hyperinflation and/or atelectasis on chest x-ray; (2) observing patient-ventilator synchrony at the bedside; (3) utilizing ventilator graphics, for example, P-V loop,[73] flow-volume (F-V) loop, and flow-time curve; (4) documenting airway malacia using full-inflation and end-exhalation controlled-ventilation chest CT or bedside flexible bronchoscopy[74-76]; and (5) titrating PEEP levels at the bedside with the use of bronchoscopy, by applying a stepwise increase/decrease in PEEP and directly visualizing to determine the effect of PEEP changes on airways collapse. Fig. 36.6A shows the admission chest radiograph of an infant with sBPD. She was transferred to our center because of persistent lung hyperinflation

despite decreasing PEEP to 3 cm H_2O and had requirement 100% supplemental oxygen for several weeks before transfer. She was unable to trigger the ventilator despite setting a minimal trigger threshold. We observed changes in the P-V and F-V loops with different levels of PEEP, which suggested the patient would benefit from a PEEP of 14 to 15 cm H_2O (Fig. 36.6B). A bedside bronchoscopy demonstrated collapse of the mainstem bronchi when PEEP was decreased below 8 cm H_2O. Her oxygenation improved dramatically and the lung hyperinflation gradually decreased despite higher PEEP levels.

We have also used bedside PEEP grids to help identify optimal PEEP levels in individual patients. Fig. 36.7 demonstrates the identification of peak and plateau pressure, peak flow, and volume under PEEP of 12 cm H_2O during a PEEP grid testing. Compliance and resistance at different PEEP levels (5–18 cm H_2O) were calculated based on the identified values. In addition, PEEPi can be detected by simultaneously measuring esophageal pressure and airflow at the airway opening in a spontaneously breathing patient, as described by Napolitano et al.[77] There are several challenges to using these methods: (1) they are often time consuming; (2) a calm, sleeping, or sedated behavioral state is often needed to obtain accurate values; and (3) PEEP requirements are dynamic and may vary day to day, during agitation or with evolution of the underlying lung disease.

Transition from the high ventilator rate, short inspiratory time, and low V_T approach appropriate early in the postnatal course of premature infants needs to occur as the lung disease evolves from the relatively homogeneous atelectasis-prone neonatal disease with short time constants to an approach that addresses the complex interaction between small and large airways disease as well as heterogeneity of lung parenchymal disease in established BPD. This transition needs to occur gradually as the disease evolves. The rate at which this transition should be individualized based on radiographic and clinical evolution and informed by periodic analysis of ventilator waveforms. Although high-quality evidence from randomized trials is lacking, the low rate, long

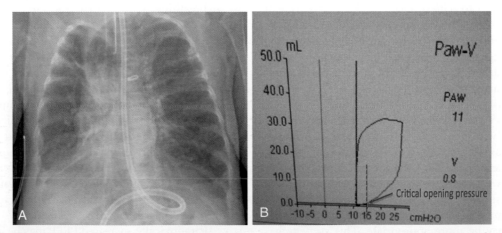

Fig. 36.6 Chest radiograph and pressure-volume curve of a patient with severe lung hyperinflation. (A) Chest radiograph showing severe lung hyperinflation on positive end-expiratory pressure of 3 cm H_2O. (B) Pressure-volume loop of same patient suggesting a critical opening pressure about 15 cm H_2O.

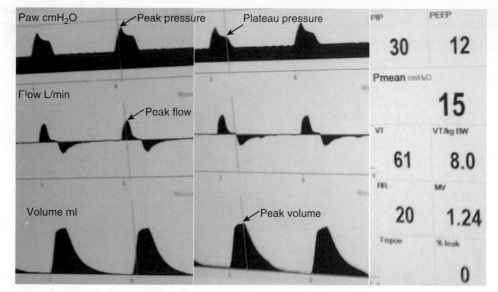

Fig. 36.7 Identifying optimal positive end-expiratory pressure (*PEEP*) with PEEP grid. PEEP grid was done on Dräger V500 ventilator under Pediatric volume mode and with fixed flow rate. Peak and plateau pressure and peak volume were measured under different PEEP levels. Compliance and resistance were calculated and optimal PEEP was selected based on the PEEP level that produced the best compliance and lowest resistance.

inspiratory time, large V_T, adequate PEEP, and PS strategy is based on sound physiologic principles and validated by extensive clinical experience. This approach allows for more effective respiratory support and often results in significant improvements in gas exchange, improved patient comfort, better growth, and clinical stability.

High-Frequency Ventilation. Although some studies suggest early high-frequency oscillatory ventilation (HFOV) use in the course of RDS may reduce the incidence of BPD,[78,79] there is currently no high-quality evidence supporting the use of HFOV in infants with established BPD. There is concern that the active exhalation and relatively high I:E ratio (1:2) of HFOV may promote airway collapse and air trapping in BPD infants with heterogeneous lung disease and floppy airways. In contrast, the much lower I:E ratio of high-frequency jet ventilation (HFJV) (1·7–1·11) may minimize gas trapping and improve gas exchange in such patients. In one retrospective study, Friedlich et al.[80] reported that HFJV improved hypoxemic respiratory failure unresponsive to HFOV in premature infants who required MV for at least 4 weeks. In a small prospective pilot trial, Plavka et al.[81] demonstrated that HFJV improved gas exchange and facilitated weaning from MV in premature infants with evolving BPD. Lower jet rates in the range of 260 to 320 are suggested for infants with established BPD, with a goal of lengthening expiration time and allowing adequate time for passive exhalation. However, the efficacy of this strategy again is based on physiologic principles, not hard data.

In recent years, nasal HFOV (nHFOV) has been proposed as an alternative NIV method for respiratory support in the early postnatal days. A meta-analysis by Li et al. included eight RCTs of 463 patients. They reported that nHFOV, compared with NCPAP, may be more effective in CO_2 elimination (weighted mean difference, –4.61; 95% confidence interval [CI], –7.94 to –1.28) and reducing the risk of intubation (relative risk [RR],

0.50; 95% CI, 0.36–0.7).[82] However, these trials, with small sample sizes and moderate to high risk of bias, are not sufficient to provide enough information regarding appropriate nHFOV parameters, safety in the extremely premature infants, or efficacy in BPD prevention or treatment.

The mechanism of gas transport during high-frequency ventilation (HFV) may facilitate diffusion and gas exchange in compartments with differing time constants and therefore may be beneficial in infants with established BPD. However, the specific mode of HFV, the optimal timing and settings of HFV, as well as the impact on long-term outcomes in this population need further investigation.

ADJUNCTIVE RESPIRATORY SUPPORT THERAPIES IN INFANTS WITH ESTABLISHED BRONCHOPULMONARY DYSPLASIA

Heliox

Heliox, a helium-oxygen gas mixture with less density than atmospheric air, may improve gas flow in the airways and increase oxygen and carbon dioxide diffusion in the alveoli by reducing turbulence. Given this property, it has been hypothesized to be of potential benefit in BPD infants with an obstructive lung disease pattern. Decreased pulmonary resistance, reduced work of breathing, improvement in V_T, and oxygenation have been reported in BPD infants both on noninvasive respiratory support[83] and on MV.[84] However, although heliox was well tolerated in small studies (12–15 patients), poor tolerance with changes in behavior, a decrease in skin temperature, and hypoxia have been observed in others.[85,86] Szczapa et al.[84] suggest heliox should be used in BPD patients during exacerbations to minimize further lung injury associated with MV, and stopped when lung function improves. However, conclusions cannot be

TABLE 36.2   Frequently Used Medications in Infants With Severe Bronchopulmonary Dysplasia

Class of Therapy	Potential Benefits	Concerns
Methylxanthines • Caffeine • Theophylline	Central respiratory stimulant, decreases diaphragmatic fatigability, weak bronchodilator and diuretic	Decrease incidence of BPD[91] but no data in established BPD
Diuretics • Furosemide • Spironolactone • Thiazides	Improve lung mechanics, may improve gas exchange, decrease extubation failure[92]	• Electrolyte and acid–base imbalance; osteopenia and/or nephrocalcinosis; endocrine and metabolic effect of spironolactone • Few RCTs with small number of patients • No evidence to support benefit in nonintubated patients[92] • Generalizability of existing data to modern clinical care may be limited.
Systemic steroids	• Antiinflammatory • Facilitate weaning down or off mechanical ventilation	• Variable dosing, duration and timing • Concerns for adverse neurodevelopmental outcomes[93] • Benefits likely outweigh risks when risk of BPD is high[94]
Inhaled steroids	• Decrease pulmonary inflammation • Trend toward reduced use of systemic steroids[95]	• Low number of patients in RCTs • Unclear efficacy • Paucity of data on adverse effects
Beta agonists	• Bronchodilation and decrease airway resistance • Improve dynamic compliance	Limited RCT data of efficacy or adverse effects[96]
Anticholinergics	• Often used with beta agonists • Bronchodilation, decrease respiratory resistance, and increase compliance[97,98]	Limited data of efficacy or adverse effects

BPD, Bronchopulmonary dysplasia; *RCT*, randomized controlled trial; *sBPD*, severe bronchopulmonary dysplasia.

drawn regarding the efficacy, safety, dose, timing, and duration of heliox use based on current available data.

Pharmacotherapies

Infants with established BPD are exposed to many medications.[87] Medical therapies such as corticosteroids, bronchodilators, and diuretics are frequently used in conjunction with respiratory support modalities in infants with BPD. These commonly used drug therapies are summarized in Table 36.2. Unfortunately, randomized controlled trials in this population are rare and definitive evidence of efficacy and/or safety for these drugs is lacking. Data on other potentially beneficial medications such as superoxide dismutase, leukotriene receptor antagonist, citrulline, and inositol are also very limited. This lack of evidence likely contributes to the observed significant variation in medication use in infants with sBPD.[56,88] When exposing an infant to a medication, clinicians should consider the underlying pathophysiology being targeted, the expected treatment response, and the duration of therapy needed to observe the response. Ideally, this response can be measured and assessed before continuing therapy. The effectiveness of most pharmacotherapies likely depends on appropriate patient selection. For example, a recent study by Shepherd and colleagues found bronchodilator responsiveness in 74% of infants with primarily obstructive disease, but only 25% of infants with restrictive disease.[89] When selecting medication dose and frequency, it is important to consider the postmenstrual and postnatal age, as well as the infant's hepatic and renal health. Developmental pharmacology is dynamic in the period between preterm birth and classification with BPD at 36 weeks' PMA, and dosage regimens intended for younger premature infants may not be appropriate in this older neonatal intensive care unit (NICU) population. Lastly, clinicians need to carefully weigh any potential benefit against possible adverse effects of the medications. Well-designed clinical studies examining the efficacy, safety, and long-term effects of these medications are urgently needed. Additional information on the pharmacologic management of infants with sBPD can be found in a recent review by Truog and colleagues[90] and also in Chapter 32.

Management of Pulmonary Hypertension

PH often contributes to morbidity and mortality in infants with BPD.[99,100] The reported incidence ranges from 16% in a prospective study screening all extremely premature infants[100] to 25% in a retrospective study of infants with BPD.[101] However, the optimal timing and methods to diagnose and monitor the progression of PH remain unclear. Although cardiac catheterization remains the gold standard for the diagnosis of PH, it is invasive and not widely available. Transthoracic echocardiography, being noninvasive and readily available, is the most commonly used diagnostic method. However, echocardiography can be especially challenging in infants with BPD because of lung hyperinflation, expansion of thoracic cage, and heart rotation. In a retrospective study of infants with CLD, Mourani et al. found that echocardiography was able to detect a measurable tricuspid regurgitant jet velocity (TRJV) in only 61% of subjects. When compared to subsequent cardiac catheterization, echocardiography was able to correctly determine the severity of PH in only 47% of cases, even in the presence of a measurable TRJV. In addition, it failed to diagnose PH in 11% and inaccurately diagnosed PH in another 11%.[102] Nonetheless, several studies have demonstrated good interrater and intrarater agreement for echocardiographic diagnosis of PH in at-risk premature infants, especially at 36 weeks' PMA and in the presence of a standardized protocol for interpretation.[103,104]

A current common practice recommended by the Pediatric Pulmonary Hypertension Network (PPHNet) is to perform comprehensive echocardiogram at 36 weeks' PMA for PH screening in infants with moderate BPD or sBPD or those with mild disease that is failing to improve or clinically worsening.[105] Box 36.2 lists the suggested parameters for inclusion in a comprehensive echocardiogram evaluation, as well as other parameters that are increasingly used to diagnose and monitor PH. Similarly, the BPD Collaborative group suggested that screening echocardiogram should be performed in all infants with sBPD. Although lacking high-quality evidence, such consensus-based recommendations do provide a practical guide to clinicians and may help reduce practice variation. Of note, these recommendations call for echocardiogram screening in a subset of infants with BPD who are at high risk of BPD associated PH, not all infants with BPD.

Brain-type natriuretic peptide (BNP) or N-terminal pro-BNP (NT-proBNP) has been used as an adjunct for the screening and follow-up of BPD-associated PH. BNP and NT-proBNP have been shown to correlate with mean pulmonary artery pressure, pulmonary vascular resistance, and right atrial pressure in both adults and pediatric populations.[106,107] Higher BNP levels have been found at 36 weeks' PMA and at discharge in premature infants with BPD compared to those without BPD and also correlate with BPD disease severity.[108] However, elevated BNP in BPD can reflect PH, left ventricular dysfunction, or chronic pulmonary disease itself. In a retrospective cohort study, a BNP cut-point of 130 pg/mL correctly classified the presence or absence of PH in 70% of 128 infants with sBPD, with 92% specificity but only 50% sensitivity.[109] In another study, a BNP value of 220 pg/mL was found to have 65% specificity and 90% sensitivity in predicting mortality in infants with BPD-associated PH.[110] Serial BNP or NT-proBNP levels may therefore be useful biomarkers for augmenting clinical decision making and decreasing the number of echocardiograms. However, these data highlight limitations, and they should not replace the use of echocardiogram or cardiac catheterization for PH assessment. In infants whose echocardiographic measures of PH and BNP fail to improve, cardiac catheterization in an experienced center should be considered to assess PH more accurately and evaluate comorbidities such as pulmonary vein stenosis (PVS) and shunts. A positive response to vasodilation (i.e., positive acute vasoreactivity testing [AVT] during cardiac catheterization) may help guide further treatment.[111]

Currently, treatment of PH in BPD mainly focuses on pharmacologic treatment with vasodilators such as inhaled nitric oxide (iNO) and sildenafil.[112] However, PH that complicates BPD is often multifactorial, and pursuing vasodilation without understanding the underlying pathophysiology may not achieve the therapeutic goals, or be detrimental. Fig. 36.8 shows a chest radiograph of an infant with severe PH. He had severely increased work of breathing with frequent desaturation episodes, poor growth, and signs of right heart failure on noninvasive respiratory support. His PH and right heart failure improved dramatically after intubation and MV. Further examination by bronchoscopy found severe tracheobronchomalacia with frequent airway collapse despite high noninvasive distending pressures. The key intervention in this patient was adequate respiratory support, rather than PH medications.

Both hypoxemia and hyperoxia can lead to pulmonary vascular constriction and remodeling. However, vasodilators only dilate existing vessels, and vasodilation in poorly ventilated areas may worsen V/Q mismatch and exacerbate hypoxemia. Therefore, an important aspect of PH management in BPD is adequate respiratory support and oxygen therapy. Well-supported infants may have improved lung growth and gas exchange with less agitation and intermittent hypoxia, which will facilitate lung vascular growth and decrease pulmonary vasoconstriction. Aggressively weaning patients off supplemental oxygen may have detrimental effects, as previous studies have

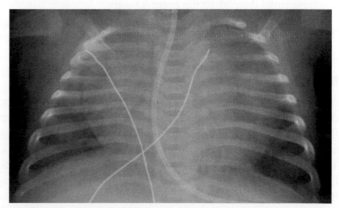

Fig. 36.8 Chest radiograph of an infant with severe pulmonary hypertension (PH). He was found to have severe tracheobronchomalacia. A high level of nasal intermittent positive pressure ventilation (peak inflation pressure of 28 and positive end-expiratory pressure [PEEP] of 14) was unable to maintain an open airway in this patient. His PH quickly improved after intubation and appropriate ventilation and he was eventually discharged home on room air with PEEP/pressure support via tracheostomy.

shown that pulmonary vascular resistance in BPD is responsive to oxygen.[113,114] Currently, both the BPD collaborative group and PPHnet advocate maintaining oxygen saturation in the range of 92% to 95%.[21,105] However, the optimal oxygen saturation target in this population remains unknown. Similarly, the optimal PCO_2 level in patients with BPD and BPD associated PH is also not known. There are conflicting data, with some suggesting hypercapnia to be beneficial and others detrimental to the lungs and pulmonary vasculature.[115]

In summary, high-quality evidence to guide the management of BPD associate PH is lacking. Currently recommended strategies by expert groups include the following:

1. Diagnosis and monitoring
   a. PH screening by echocardiography at 36 weeks' PMA in infants with moderate to sBPD or whenever PH is suspected;
   b. In infants with sBPD whose initial echocardiogram was normal, rescreen or follow-up echocardiography every 1 to 2 months until respiratory status significantly improved;
   c. In infants with improved echocardiographic PH measurements, repeat evaluation every 2 to 4 months until the infant no longer requires oxygen therapy;
   d. Trending BNP or NT-proBNP may be useful in conjunction with echocardiography;
   e. Consider cardiac catheterization before the initiation of long-term therapy or combination therapy.

2. Treatment of BPD-associated PH
   a. Provide adequate respiratory support, with a goal of supporting pulmonary vascular growth and avoiding hypoxemia; this should be considered the key therapy for BPD-associated PH;
   b. Maintain oxygen saturation between 92% and 95% when possible;
   c. Use iNO in acute PH crisis and wean after stabilization
   d. If prolonged vasodilator therapy is deemed necessary, transition iNO to sildenafil starting with a low dose of 0.25 mg/kg per dose every 8 hours and gradually advancing to 2 mg/kg per dose every 8 hours as tolerated, without exceeding a maximal dose of 10 mg every 8 hours;
   d. Consider adding a second agent (such as endothelin receptor antagonists or prostacyclin analogs) if unable to wean off iNO.

Management of Persistent Ductus Arteriosus

A PDA is very common in premature infants. Although the open ductus protects the fetal pulmonary circulation from unnecessary flow, PDA after birth has multiple effects on the developing lung and can contribute to the development or worsening of BPD. These may include (1) excessive blood flow that negatively affects the development of the pulmonary vasculature and induce endothelial injury;[116-118] (2) increased levels of inflammatory cytokines such as tumor necrosis factor-α, platelet-activating factor, and activated neutrophils;[119-121] (3) increased vascular resistance and decreased dynamic lung compliance, which may result in higher levels and longer duration of ventilatory support;[122,123] and (4) inhibition of alveolarization.[124,125] Consistent with experimental evidence, several clinical studies have found an association between symptomatic PDA, particularly when present for over

2 weeks, and an increased risk of BPD.[126-128] However, data from prospective clinical trials suggest an uncertain causative relationship. Clinical trials have failed to demonstrate a meaningful long-term benefit of PDA closure[129-131] and several studies have suggested that early surgical PDA ligation is an independent risk factor for the development of BPD.[132,133] With the ongoing controversy regarding the efficacy and safety of PDA treatment, we have seen a shift in clinical practice from early aggressive therapy to selective treatment of hemodynamically significant PDA (hsPDA).[134] Unfortunately, there are currently no high-quality data to guide the diagnosis, timing, and methods of treatment of hsPDA at older postnatal ages. Although closure of the ductus may result in significant clinical improvement in some patients with established sBPD, it is hard to determine which PDA contributes to worsening pulmonary mechanics and the development of severe PH. In addition, when severe PH with significant right-to-left shunting and RV dysfunction is present, closing the ductus may severely increase RV pressure by eliminating the ductus as a pressure "pop-off." Thus, clinicians need to carefully evaluate the risks and benefits of ductal closure in these infants. In older infants with sBPD, using cardiac catheterization to first evaluate pulmonary hemodynamics followed by transcatheter closure of the ductus in select patients may be a safe and effective alternative to surgical ligation, but further study is needed to identify ideal patients. In our experience, these patients typically have a favorable clinical response to ductal closure and an uncomplicated recovery from the procedure, although this response is not uniform. This method is also not feasible in smaller centers, and the role of cardiac catheterization in the management of PH complicating BPD needs further study.

Nutritional Support

Infants with sBPD face nutritional challenges because of increased energy expenditure from increased respiratory demands and generalized growth suppression from chronic stress, inflammation, and medication use.[135,136] Data from the Children's Hospital Neonatal Database reported that more than half of infants with sBPD had postnatal growth failure at 36 weeks' PMA, and rates continued to increase in those hospitalized beyond 36 weeks' PMA.[136] Infants with sBPD have also been reported to have a high incidence of metabolic bone disease.[137] Several important impacts of poor nutrition on the outcomes of infants with BPD have been identified: (1) adverse effects on both somatic and lung growth, possibly through limiting vital pulmonary cell signaling in cell multiplication, differentiation, growth, and extracellular matrix protein deposition;[138-141] (2) adverse effects on lung function through the breakdown of connective tissues fibers, possibly contributing to emphysema, and inadequate ossification of the bony skeleton supporting the stability of the thoracic cage;[142,143] (3) decreased antioxidant enzymes and increased susceptibility to hyperoxic injury;[144,145] (4) dysregulation of alveolar fluid balance leading to pulmonary edema;[146,147] (5) increased susceptibility to infection and predisposition to pulmonary infection;[148] and (6) poor linear growth, associated with reduced lean body mass accretion and poor brain growth and development.[149] In light of this, the focus of nutritional management in infants with BPD should be

TABLE 36.3	Nutritional Interventions in Infants With Bronchopulmonary Dysplasia	
	Suggestions	**Rationale**
Goal of nutritional management	• Delivery of adequate nutritional constituents to match each patient's specific needs over time • Seeking balanced proportional growth with an ideal weight for length target of ~50%	• Nutritional needs change with time in infants with sBPD. • Linear growth is regarded as a good reflection of lean body mass accretion and organ growth and development.
Nutritional assessment	• Include a thorough review of medical history, medication exposure, clinical status and growth parameters. • Plot and follow an infant's growth chart to assess changes in growth trajectories.	• Comprehensive review and periodic reevaluation help to determine an infant's nutritional status and needs. • Excessive weight gain at a rate that crosses growth chart percentiles without the same growth pattern in linear growth warrants a reevaluation of energy intake and changes in the clinical status.
Caloric intake (Kcal/kg/d)	Unstable BPD: >130 Recovery phase: 100–120 Older stable BPD: 80–100	Energy requirement changes depending on the level of energy expenditure: severe disease (e.g., sepsis), severe work of breathing, and high physical activity result in catabolic or hypermetabolic states with increased energy expenditure.
Fluid intake	Usually in the range of 130–160 ml/kg/day	Although infants with BPD may be prone to interstitial pulmonary edema, excessive fluid restriction will result in inadequate delivery of nutrients not meeting nutritional requirements, as well as severe constipation.
Protein	• Providing adequate protein for corrected GA • Consider aiming toward the higher range when protein turnover is high.	• Improved linear growth, lean tissue accretion and bone mass in BPD infants with higher protein intake • Protein need is increased during catabolic or hypermetabolic states when protein turnover is high.
Carbohydrate and fat	Avoid dietary imbalance of high carbohydrate to low fat.	Excessive calories from carbohydrate may increase CO_2 production and therefore increase respiratory burden.
Minerals and vitamins	Provide adequate calcium, phosphorous, iron, and Vitamin D.	Infants with BPD are at high risk for metabolic bone disease because of low calcium and phosphorus accumulation prenatally from prematurity and postnatally from poor nutritional supplementation, physical inactivity and multiple medication use that affects bone health.

BPD, Bronchopulmonary dysplasia; *GA*, gestational age; *sBPD*, severe bronchopulmonary dysplasia.

the delivery of adequate and titrated nutrition that meets individual patient needs. The concept of achieving a "pro-growth" state with balanced weight gain and linear growth has been proposed by the BPD Collaborative group.[21] To achieve this "pro-growth" state, care needs to be individualized and tailored to the different nutritional requirements at different stages of growth and illness. Table 36.3 provides some basic guiding principles, but there is a lack of evidence-based data to guide optimal nutritional interventions. In addition to providing balanced nutrition, attention should be given to ways of decreasing energy expenditure and facilitating physical activities. Providing adequate respiratory support should therefore be viewed as "nutrition" for infants with BPD. Rather than focusing on achieving "acceptable" PCO_2 and SPO_2 levels, respiratory support in an infant with sBPD should aim to avoid frequent hypoxia, reduce energy expenditure from excessive work of breathing, and minimize stress from respiratory insufficiency. Meeting these goals will help promote good proportional growth.

Minimizing Pulmonary Micro-Aspiration

Pulmonary aspiration may exacerbate lung disease in infants with BPD.[150] Potential sources of aspiration are aspiration during oral feeding, GER, or aspiration of oral secretions. GER is common in premature infants, especially infants with BPD.

Increased work of breathing and frequent transient increases in intra-abdominal pressure because of coughing, agitation, and air flow obstruction in infants with BPD can decrease lower esophageal sphincter (LES) tone, potentially increasing the risk of GER.[151] Recent studies have reported increased frequencies of GER events (especially acid reflux related events), longer acid clearance time, and higher symptom sensitivity index (SSI) scores in infants with BPD as compared to infants without BPD. In addition, Jadcherla et al. reported that acid reflux events in the pharynx were associated with increased symptom occurrence and delayed symptom clearance.[152-154] Improvement in respiratory status has been reported in infants with BPD after medical or surgical antireflux therapy.[137,152,153,155] However, there are increasing concerns about the safety and efficacy of antireflux and acid suppressive medications among premature infants and there are currently no reliable diagnostic or clinical criteria to guide antireflux treatment.

A trial of postpyloric feeds in select infants with sBPD may be warranted. In our clinical experience, some infants demonstrate significant clinical improvement, with decreased respiratory distress, less agitation, and improved oxygenation. Most patients are able to transition back to gastric feeds after their respiratory status improves. Patients who show clinical worsening upon returning to gastric feeds may be considered for antireflux surgery. The majority of our patients undergo laparoscopic fundoplication with gastric tube placement, and our data indicated that the procedure could be safely performed in infants with sBPD.[137] Considering the current deficiency in reliable diagnostic tools and the risk of treatment, multicenter coordinated studies on the optimal management of GER in infants with sBPD are needed before definitive recommendations can be made.

As previously discussed, chemoreceptor hypersensitivity may contribute to feeding difficulties in infants with BPD. In addition, infants with sBPD have decreased opportunity to develop oral motor and swallowing skills and have lower tolerance for breathing pauses during sucking and swallowing. All of these factors place them at higher risk for aspiration during oral feeding. Therefore, safety of oral feeding needs to be established and frequently reevaluated when trying to promote oral feedings. This is best achieved through a multidisciplinary coordinated approach.[156]

Role of Tracheostomy in Infants Requiring Long-Term Support

BPD is an independent risk factor for neurodevelopmental impairment in preterm infants.[157] Furthermore, a protracted course of MV is associated with increased mortality and neurodevelopmental disability.[158] BPD requiring long-term MV has been reported as the most common reason for tracheostomy in premature infants.[159] Although tracheostomy is commonly viewed as an undesirable outcome, it may be a valuable therapeutic strategy in some infants with sBPD. Removal of the ETT allows for better development of oral motor skills and may reduce oral aversion. We have observed that tracheostomy placement in infants with sBPD may be associated with better proportional growth, less need for sedation, and increased ability to participate in age-appropriate developmental activities.[160] This is consistent with data from DeMauro et al., who found an association between earlier (<120 days) rather than later tracheostomy and better neurodevelopmental outcomes.[161] Although tracheostomy does not treat lung disease, it provides a stable airway that allows clinicians to transition their treatment focus from weaning off ventilator support to providing adequate support and developmental enrichment. In our experience, and also reported by Mandy et al., tracheostomy placement is safe even in infants requiring high ventilator support. Mandy et al. have suggested that chronically ventilated infants should be evaluated for tracheostomy placement at around or shortly after 40 weeks corrected gestation.[162] When clinicians and parents consider whether or not to pursue tracheostomy, the therapeutic advantages, particularly the benefits on growth and development, should be balanced against the risks and caregiver burden of tracheostomy.

PULMONARY OUTCOMES IN INFANTS WITH BRONCHOPULMONARY DYSPLASIA

Current reports suggest that infants with BPD often have significant pulmonary sequelae during childhood and adolescence. These include persistence of respiratory symptoms with increased rehospitalization for respiratory illness, decreased pulmonary function, persistent small and large airway dysfunction, and decreased respiratory reserve. However, the frequency of respiratory symptoms and rehospitalization decreases over the first few years, and pulmonary mechanics and lung volumes improve over time.[163] Although these data suggest that with proper management infants with BPD may have encouraging long-term outcomes, continued surveillance of young adults with BPD is critical. The reader is referred to Chapter 44 for a more complete discussion of pulmonary outcomes of ventilated neonates. Transition to home care for these complex, technology-dependent patients is discussed in Chapter 42.

CONCLUSION

In infants with established BPD, treatment should focus on promoting growth while minimizing further lung injury. To achieve this goal, it is important to understand the underlying pathophysiology and clinical presentation of each individual patient and provide adequate respiratory and multisystem support accordingly. An interdisciplinary approach that provides comprehensive support is important for these patients. High-quality, multicenter research data are urgently needed to guide the optimal care strategies in this patient population. In addition, long-term airway, pulmonary, and neurodevelopmental follow-up is critical in ensuring the best possible long-term outcomes and provide prognostic information for this special patient population.

SELECTED READINGS

5. Stoll BJ, Hansen NI, Bell EF, et al: Neonatal outcomes of extremely preterm infants from the NICHD Neonatal Research Network. Pediatrics 126(3):443–456, 2010.

18. Jobe AH, Bancalari E: Bronchopulmonary dysplasia. Am J Respir Crit Care Med 163(7):1723–1729, 2001.

21. Abman SH, Collaco JM, Shepherd EG, et al: Interdisciplinary care of children with severe bronchopulmonary dysplasia. J Pediatr 181:12–28 e11, 2017.

23. Jensen EA, Dysart K, Gantz MG, et al: The diagnosis of bronchopulmonary dysplasia in very preterm infants. An evidence-based approach. Am J Respir Crit Care Med 200(6):751–759, 2019.

28. Lagatta JM, Hysinger EB, Zaniletti I, et al: The impact of pulmonary hypertension in preterm infants with severe bronchopulmonary dysplasia through 1 year. J Pediatr 203:218–224 e213, 2018.

87. Bamat NA, Kirpalani H, Feudtner C, et al: Medication use in infants with severe bronchopulmonary dysplasia admitted to United States children's hospitals. J Perinatol 39(9):1291–1299, 2019.

105. Krishnan U, Feinstein JA, Adatia I, et al: Evaluation and management of pulmonary hypertension in children with bronchopulmonary dysplasia. J Pediatr 188:24–34 e21, 2017.

114. Mourani PM, Ivy DD, Gao D, Abman SH: Pulmonary vascular effects of inhaled nitric oxide and oxygen tension in bronchopulmonary dysplasia. Am J Respir Crit Care Med 170(9):1006–1013, 2004.

158. Walsh MC, Morris BH, Wrage LA, et al: Extremely low birthweight neonates with protracted ventilation: mortality and 18-month neurodevelopmental outcomes. J Pediatr 146(6):798–804, 2005.

160. Luo J, Shepard S, Nilan K, et al: Improved growth and developmental activity post tracheostomy in preterm infants with severe BPD. Pediatr Pulmonol 53(9):1237–1244, 2018.

37

Medical and Surgical Interventions for Respiratory Distress and Airway Management

Nathaniel Koo, Thomas Sims, Robert M. Arensman, Nishant Srinivasan,
Saurabhkumar Patel, Akhil Maheshwari, and Namasivayam Ambalavanan

KEY POINTS

- The neonatal airway is distinctly different from the adult airway, and the lower airway in the premature infant is significantly narrower compared to that of older children and adults
- Multiple congenital or acquired disorders of the airway or lungs may cause respiratory distress, requiring urgent evaluation by a multidisciplinary team
- The medical and surgical management of conditions involving the neonatal airway may be complex and depends upon the anatomic and pathophysiologic nature of the condition, the established therapies for such conditions, and the clinical status including other comorbidities in the infant.

INTRODUCTION

The advent of the specialty of neonatal-perinatal medicine has improved the care and survival of ever-increasing numbers of very preterm and critically ill term newborns. These infants have a whole host of complex anatomic problems. Consequently, neonatologists and pediatric surgeons face vast challenges in the management of problems with the airway and lungs. In this chapter, we look first at medical management of the neonatal airway and then progress to the supporting role of pediatric surgeons and otolaryngologists in the diagnosis and management of complex airway problems.

MEDICAL MANAGEMENT OF THE NEONATAL AIRWAY

Maintenance of the airway in sick neonates is critical for ensuring their survival. A compromised airway such as a partial obstruction could potentially lead to gas trapping and ventilatory problems. This in turn can lead to hypoxia, hypercarbia, and serious hemodynamic disturbances. Successful airway management in neonates requires accurate and frequent assessments of the patient by a team of skilled care providers. Adequate preparation before performing airway securing procedures is vital to avoid complications associated with artificial airway maintenance. Adequate preparation includes checking all required equipment for availability and full functionality, judicious utilization of resources available in the neonatal intensive care unit (NICU) such as nurses and respiratory therapists, and last, but not least, due diligence on the part of the neonatologist to anticipate and prepare for complications (see Chapter 29).

Typically, the neonatal airway is managed by a team of neonatologists, respiratory therapists, and nurses in the NICU. The NICU has developed into a unit that provides care not only for premature infants but also for infants with surgical or cardiac problems. Airway needs and indications for interventions may be completely different in such situations and may require the intervention of airway experts such as otolaryngologists and pediatric surgeons. In this section, we will discuss the challenges involved in management of the neonatal airway and the medical interventions performed for airway maintenance before seeking surgical support.

ANATOMIC DISADVANTAGES OF THE NEONATAL AIRWAY

The neonatal airway is distinctly different from the adult airway. The anatomic disadvantages begin with the shape of the head in neonates, who have a larger occiput. The larger occiput in a supine posture naturally places the infant's neck in a flexed position that may cause kinking of the airway, potentially leading to obstruction. This may also obscure visualization of the larynx during intubation, which may require a shoulder roll to reduce neck flexion. A "sniffing posture" with slight extension of the neck when the infant is supine is often required to align the airway axis to achieve unobstructed air entry.

Neonates are obligate nasal breathers, which makes their nasopharynx a vital conduit for ventilation. Secretions and mucosal edema causing impediment to airflow at the level of the nasopharynx can significantly compromise the neonate's airway. Therefore, care providers managing the airway of neonates should not only be proactive about clearing secretions but also be cognizant and use extreme caution to avoid iatrogenic nasal mucosal edema.

Hypopharyngeal structures such as the vallecula, the epiglottis, and the laryngeal structures such as arytenoids that commonly serve as landmarks during laryngoscopy and intubation also differ in neonates. The epiglottis is omega shaped and is generally longer, larger, and less flexible in infants, making this structure more susceptible to injury during intubation and suctioning. Abnormalities of the epiglottis and trauma could pose a challenge during endotracheal intubation. The soft tissue structures of the hypopharynx and larynx follow the physical principles of Bernoulli and the Venturi effect and collapse easily. Bernoulli's principle states that, when these structures are subjected to fast airflow, a low pressure is exerted on the walls of the tube. The Venturi effect is seen during inspiration when these low-pressure walls collapse. Conditions such as laryngomalacia may exaggerate these effects and compromise the airway further.

The lower airway in the premature infant is significantly narrower compared to that of older children and adults. In 1982, Wailoo and Emery described the normal development of the trachea from 28 weeks to 14 years of age based on postmortem quantitative assessment of the trachea.[1] It was observed that the trachea is funnel shaped, with the upper end wider than the lower end in the neonatal period. It becomes cylindrical with increasing age. This discrepancy was also found to be inversely proportional to the gestational age of the infant.[1] The narrowest part of the infant's trachea is considered to be at the level of the cricoid cartilage, whereas in adults, it is at the level of the epiglottis.[1] The unique funnel-shaped trachea with a natural subglottic narrowing places neonates at a certain disadvantage and at higher risk for further airway compromise, especially with development of mucosal edema following prolonged intubations. The cricoid cartilage is composed of two parts: a posterior plate-like portion that forms the posterior wall of the larynx and an inferior ring. In neonates, the plate is inclined posteriorly, with the narrowest part of the funneled trachea at the level of the cricoid ring.

As the infant grows, the cricoid plate becomes vertical, the ring enlarges, and the point of narrowing at the funnel spout disappears. In addition to the anatomic orientation of the trachea, the susceptibility of the subglottic area to mucosal edema is related to the difference in cellular lining. The lining above the cords is resilient squamous epithelium, whereas below the cords, it is ciliated columnar epithelium that is loosely attached to the submucosal tissue and can be easily infiltrated by fluid to form edema. This alters the internal diameter of the already narrow subglottic trachea. As explained by Poiseuille's law, the resistance to airflow is inversely proportional to the fourth power of the radius of the airway during laminar airflow and to the fifth power during turbulent flow. When the internal diameter of the neonatal airway is decreased to 50% in conditions such as mucosal edema, the resistance to airflow is increased 16-fold.[2] This highlights the importance of timely assessments of airway status and suitable interventions to prevent obstruction to airflow.

Infants with airway narrowing or obstruction may require immediate airway assistance. Interventions are aimed at splinting the airway open for unobstructed airflow. Use of nasal continuous positive airway pressure (CPAP) has gained popularity among neonatologists as a noninvasive pneumatic splint of the upper airway, especially in premature infants. Nasopharyngeal airways or nasal trumpets are effective in maintaining temporary patency of the airway in infants with upper airway abnormalities. However, when these interventions fail to establish adequate ventilation, tracheal intubation with an endotracheal tube (ETT) becomes necessary.

Traditionally, the adequacy of ventilation has been assessed using vital sign parameters and blood gases. However, the disadvantage of heavy reliance on these measures to plan interventions could result in missing smaller inadequacies in oxygenation and ventilation, which over time may have a larger impact on the infant's outcomes. Use of newer technologies such as pulse oximetry histograms to evaluate precise amounts of time patient spent below certain saturations levels provides the ability to develop longitudinal and comparative analyses. This also gives providers a broader picture of the infant's ventilatory status, which in turn can help better plan management of the airway and ventilation. Polysomnography studies, when available, are also used in the evaluation of ventilation adequacy in infants with airway problems. However, further studies are needed to strengthen evidence supporting the role of polysomnography in the evaluation and management of upper airway obstruction.[3]

MEDICAL MANAGEMENT OF NEONATES WITH COMMON RESPIRATORY DISORDERS REQUIRING SURGICAL INTERVENTION

With increasing emphasis on prenatal care and availability of fetal ultrasonography, a large number of congenital respiratory disorders are being detected during fetal life. The availability of early diagnosis provides ample opportunity to plan the early neonatal and preoperative management to reduce the risk of surgical complications and improve postoperative outcomes. Planning often involves availability of medical personnel, which includes neonatologists, respiratory therapists, skilled nurses, pediatric surgeons, otolaryngologists, and bronchoscopists; availability of all required equipment and infrastructure, which includes operating rooms, bronchoscope, and tertiary-level NICU; and ability to perform extracorporeal membrane oxygenation (ECMO) or rapidly transfer the baby to a center with such capabilities. However, a lack of prenatal diagnosis may result in quick decompensation of the neonate, which in turn might create challenges in the surgical management and long-term outcomes of the infant. Most of these neonatal conditions may require specific corrective or palliative interventions. However, the overall management of the infant before surgery often follows common principles.

Congenital Airway Disorders

Congenital respiratory or airway disorders such as laryngomalacia, macroglossia, retrognathia or micrognathia, neck masses, hydrops fetalis with neck swelling, congenital diaphragmatic hernia, cystic adenomatoid malformation, congenital lobar emphysema, and similar anomalies can lead to rapid respiratory failure and hemodynamic instability in infants. Stabilization of the infant in the delivery room and a well-planned and well-executed initial management in the NICU may minimize further complications. The airway should be assessed immediately upon delivery for patency. Secretions should be cleared using bulb suction or other suction devices if needed. Studies by Kelleher et al. have shown that wiping could be as effective as suctioning in certain cases.[4] In many circumstances, infants with congenital respiratory disorders will require assisted forms of ventilation, and each infant should be individually assessed and managed. In less severe cases, use of nasopharyngeal airways and noninvasive ventilation such as nasal

CPAP or nasal intermittent mandatory ventilation may be adequate to achieve target oxygenation and ventilation parameters. In infants with critical airway obstruction, tracheal intubation through oral or sometimes even nasal routes may be necessary. However, overcoming anatomic anomalies such as micrognathia/retrognathia may be challenging and often leads to unsuccessful attempts at endotracheal intubation. Use of laryngeal mask airways (LMAs) and fiber-optic approaches, if available, could be helpful during an emergency.

Persistent hypoxemia or hypercarbia as a result of inadequate ventilation can result in failure of the infant to transition from the fetal to the neonatal circulation, resulting in persistent pulmonary hypertension of the newborn (PPHN). It is important to closely monitor arterial or transcutaneous blood gases and chest x-ray to optimize ventilation. Certain airway disorders lead to persistent hypoxia that in turn can activate various pathways in the lung that result in airway and pulmonary vascular remodeling. These infants may require alternate modes of oxygenation such as ECMO. Ideally, infants should be adequately ventilated and oxygenated (although with caution in premature infants to minimize risks of oxygen toxicity) to avoid complications such as persistent hypoxia, acidosis, or PPHN. At the same time, extreme caution should be taken to avoid volutrauma, oxytrauma, and barotrauma, which are commonly associated with assisted invasive ventilation. This can be achieved by adopting gentle ventilation strategies and permissive hypercarbia.

Once the infant is stabilized, a formal consultation with the surgical specialty should be arranged and appropriate imaging studies ordered to confirm the diagnosis. Frequently, chest X-ray is the initial study of choice to assess lung expansion and extent of abnormality. Other studies that are commonly used are chest ultrasonography, direct laryngoscopy, direct bronchoscopy, polysomnography, computed tomography (CT), and magnetic resonance imaging (MRI). Infants should always be accompanied to these studies by a provider capable of intubation and resuscitation. Sedation for long procedures is commonly done by the neonatologist or anesthesiologist. In recent times, infant immobilizing devices have been used as a safer alternative to sedation for imaging procedures.[5]

Nutrition plays a major role in preparing these infants for surgery. Although the caloric requirement is better met with enteral feeding, in some infants with respiratory disorders requiring ventilatory support, enteral feeding may not be feasible. Parenteral forms of nutrition are preferred in such infants and instituted early, typically within 24 hours of birth, to provide necessary proteins and lipids that could contribute to growth and body building. Lower total body fat mass and acute and chronic malnourishment are associated with worse clinical outcomes in children undergoing major surgeries.

Acquired Airway Disorders

Acquired airway disorders commonly seen in neonates are often secondary to traumatic laryngoscopic procedures, prolonged intubation, and chronic irritation from a hard-nasal cannula. The most vulnerable site for problems in the neonatal airway appears to be the subglottic portion of the trachea at the level of the cricoid ring because of the previously mentioned anatomy and physiologic mechanisms. These complications can be avoided by using gentle techniques during naso-oropharyngeal suctioning and endotracheal intubation. Longer duration of intubation and multiple reintubations increase the risk of subglottic stenosis, which makes it more challenging to extubate. Infants who require prolonged ventilation should be intubated only with uncuffed ETTs. This could potentially minimize an inflammatory response in the wall of the subglottic trachea. However, with prolonged duration of intubation, these changes might become inevitable. These neonates should be evaluated at regular intervals for signs of obstruction or airway edema. Currently used ventilators provide information on ETT leak and tidal volume. Infants with significant airway edema tend to have minimal to no leak around the ETT. In some cases, altered breath sounds such as stridor, crowing, or dysphonic or raspy cry in association with respiratory distress, which are signs of airway edema, are identified only post extubation. The goal, however, should be to identify infants at risk for development of airway edema before extubation. Cautiously planned and timely efforts to extubate infants to a noninvasive form of ventilation are needed. The provision of positive end-expiratory pressure in some form (CPAP, high-flow nasal cannula, noninvasive ventilation) is often helpful in avoiding extubation failure. Use of a short course of dexamethasone in high-risk cases is sometimes recommended before extubation to reduce airway edema and risk of reintubation.[6] Racemic epinephrine may be used with caution to decrease the vascular congestion in the trachea and improve stridor postextubation, although there is limited evidence supporting this practice.[7] Reflux precautions in these infants can also be helpful in preventing caustic damage to the airway by stomach acid. However, use of antireflux medications generally should be avoided because of adverse effects in the neonatal population and reserved for infants with unique anatomic problems such as tracheoesophageal fistula. Unfortunately, some infants are exceedingly dependent on artificial airways and may eventually require surgical interventions such as a tracheostomy as a long-term solution.

SURGICAL MANAGEMENT OF THE NEONATAL AIRWAY

Respiratory distress in the neonate has a variety of causes (Box 37.1), and pediatric surgeons and otolaryngologists are increasingly becoming involved in the care of these patients. The ability to intubate, mechanically ventilate, and thereby

---

BOX 37.1　Indications for Neonatal Bronchoscopy

- Prolonged intubation (6-8 weeks)
- Repetitive failure of extubations
- Inability to aerate all lobes of the lung (persistent atelectasis)
- Clinical need for cultures or bronchial washings
- Suspicion of necrotizing tracheobronchitis
- Evaluation of stridor

BOX 37.2   Differential Diagnosis of Neonatal Stridor (Anatomic Approach)

Nasopharynx
  Choanal atresia
Tongue
  Idiopathic
  Beckwith-Wiedemann syndrome
  Metabolic disorders
      Hypothyroidism/lingual thyroid
      Glycogen storage disease
  Down syndrome
Oropharynx (micrognathia and glossoptosis)
  Pierre Robin sequence
  Treacher Collins syndrome
  Hallermann-Streiff syndrome
  Möbius syndrome
  Freeman-Sheldon syndrome
  Nager syndrome
Larynx
  Laryngeal atresia
  Laryngeal web
  Vocal cord paralysis
  Laryngomalacia
  Subglottic stenosis
      Congenital/traumatic
  Laryngocele
  Laryngeal cleft
  Subglottic hemangioma
Trachea
  Intrinsic compression
      Tracheomalacia
      Tracheal stenosis
      Necrotizing tracheobronchitis
  Extrinsic compression
      Cystic hygroma
      Vascular rings

Developmental Abnormalities of the Airway
Nasopharyngeal Obstruction

Stridor signals a need for urgent diagnosis and possible intervention because of the narrow size of the infant airway and the ease at which it can reach critical narrowing. The severity of neonatal stridor can vary. Some cases may be managed medically, whereas other cases may represent impending total obstruction; therefore, the approach to diagnosis is deliberate (Fig. 37.1).

A differential diagnosis for neonatal upper airway obstruction can be formulated by approaching the subject anatomically, beginning in the nasopharynx and oropharynx and progressing down through the respiratory tract.

Choanal Atresia

Choanal atresia, a rare anomaly, with a reported incidence of 1 in 8000 births, involves occlusion of the posterior nares by a membranous (10%) or bony (90%) septum (Fig. 37.2). Unilateral lesions can be asymptomatic, but bilateral lesions may cause total airway obstruction because neonates are preferential nasal breathers. Symptoms are most evident when a baby is at rest, because when agitated and crying, the infant breathes via the open mouth and oropharynx. Associated anomalies include esophageal atresia, congenital cardiac lesions, colobomata, and Treacher Collins syndrome, among a large number of rarer associations.[8,9] Diagnosis is suspected by the inability to pass a catheter through the nostrils into the oropharynx. Diagnosis is made by the combination of nasofiberscopy or nasal rigid endoscopy and CT imaging. Management ranges from simple

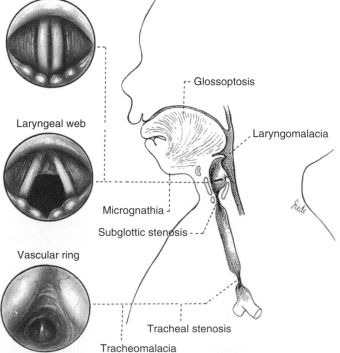

prolong the lives of children with neonatal asphyxia, congenital anomalies, or other causes of respiratory distress redefines the role of the surgeon as part of the neonatal management team.

The role of the surgeon is twofold: (1) as a diagnostician and therapist for those infants who manifest respiratory distress from an anatomic problem or who present with congenital airway obstruction (i.e., congenital stridor; Box 37.2) and (2) as a consultant for neonates undergoing medical treatment requiring long-term intubation of their airways.

THE PEDIATRIC SURGEON/ OTOLARYNGOLOGIST AS DIAGNOSTICIAN AND THERAPIST

The anatomic abnormalities present often determine the role of the pediatric surgeon/otolaryngologist in the care of the infant. Consequently, the material presented here is organized into developmental abnormalities of (1) the airway, (2) the lung, (3) the diaphragm, and (4) the skeleton.

Fig. 37.1 Composite diagram of some of the lesions that result in neonatal stridor (proceeding downward through the respiratory passages).

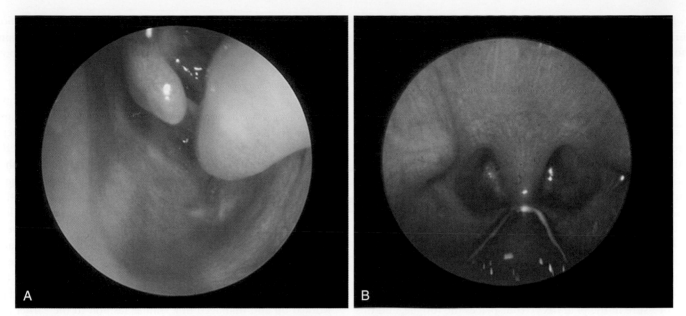

Fig. 37.2 Choanal atresia. **(A)** Endoscopic view. **(B)** Nasopharyngeal view.

placement of an oropharyngeal airway to operative opening of the occlusion with or without placement of stents.[10,11] Transnasal endoscopic repair is the preferred technique for repair with transpalatal approach reserved for patients in whom transnasal repair would be impossible.[11,12]

Oropharyngeal Obstruction

Macroglossia. An enlarged tongue often causes obstruction. Stridor in a neonate can occur if the tongue is disproportionately larger than the infant's oropharynx. Physical examination confirms the diagnosis. Insertion of an oral airway is usually successful in treating the airway obstruction. Several well-known syndromes include macroglossia as a component.

Beckwith-Wiedemann syndrome. Severe hypoglycemia, in many cases secondary to hyperinsulinemia, initially brought these examples of infantile gigantism to medical attention. Macroglossia secondary to muscular hypertrophy is the most common feature present in this syndrome. Visceromegaly, and a series of umbilical abnormalities ranging from congenital umbilical hernia to omphalocele, also compose this syndrome.[13] Affected infants may also demonstrate a facial nevus flammeus, renal medullary dysplasia, and a characteristic pit on the tragus of the ear. These babies are typically large for gestational age. The congenital stridor resulting from the enlarged tongue usually resolves rapidly with the insertion of an oropharyngeal airway. Little further diagnostic workup of the airway is necessary if the child is identified as having this syndrome. Some authors are now advocating for earlier partial glossectomy during infancy to prevent dental and mandibular deformity, improve speech development, enhance oral feeding, and treat sleep-disordered breathing, including obstructive sleep apnea,[14-18] but this is rarely necessary in the neonatal period.

Metabolic disorders. Several neonatal metabolic disorders cause macroglossia and result in congenital stridor, the best known of which are hypothyroidism and glycogen storage disease. The large tongue, high nature of the airway obstruction and findings consistent with the underlying condition should suggest the diagnosis and appropriate workup early in the course of the disease. The stridor in these babies is generally mild, usually successfully treated with an oropharyngeal airway, and disappears shortly after birth as the underlying condition is successfully treated. Diagnostic evaluation in these patients should be directed at the underlying metabolic disorder; little additional diagnostic work is needed for the tracheobronchial tree.

Trisomy 21 (Down syndrome). Children affected by Trisomy 21 are easily identified by their constellation of abnormalities. Their relative macroglossia may result in a mild congenital stridor. Because of the reported association between Trisomy 21 and airway malacia, as well as congenital subglottic stenosis, endoscopy may be necessary to establish the cause of the stridor.[19,20]

Severe bronchopulmonary dysplasia. Although not generally reported or appreciated, macroglossia can develop in infants with severe bronchopulmonary dysplasia and worsen the chronic pulmonary compromise. Chronic hypoxia leads to this condition (similar to clubbing of the fingernails) and often heralds a poor outcome. The obstruction is best treated by tracheostomy as opposed to surgical reduction of the tongue. These patients benefit from a multidisciplinary approach, and a capping trial with polysomnography should be considered before decannulation.[21,22]

Lingual thyroid. Although rare, lingual thyroid can be a cause of oropharyngeal obstruction.[23,24] Stertor in the presence of hypothyroidism, detected by persistent elevation of thyroid-stimulating hormone on routine neonatal screening, raises the suspicion of lingual thyroid, although other lesions are more commonly responsible. This condition occurs in just over 1 in 10,000 births.

Laryngoscopy identifies a mass at the base of the tongue. Further characterization by CT scan and thyroid scintigraphy should be performed. Of note, the thyroid may continue to hypertrophy during early infancy and childhood. Respiratory complications associated with hypothyroidism, such as respiratory depression, may not occur until later.

Craniofacial dysmorphology syndromes. The craniofacial dysmorphology syndromes range from unusual to extremely rare. All result in an obstruction located in the oropharynx. This is secondary to micrognathia with glossoptosis.[25] Stridor varies from mild to severe, and it is important to identify the underlying problem, which is often genetic. More complete descriptions of these conditions can be found in texts on congenital malformations.

Pierre Robin sequence. Pierre Robin sequence[26,27] represents the most common craniofacial dysmorphology with the clinical triad of micrognathia, glossoptosis, and airway compromise, with variable inclusion of cleft palate. During inspiration, negative pressure in the pharynx retrodisplaces the tongue, and this increases the degree of pharyngeal obstruction. Stridor consequently results. The airway obstruction is usually resolved with insertion of an oropharyngeal airway or nasopharyngeal stent, and these patients tend to breathe more comfortably in a prone position. CPAP may also be useful. Feeding may create further problems for these babies and necessitate special nipples or gavage nutrition.

Work-up should include polysomnography, nasoendoscopy, and bronchoscopy. Tracheostomies are rarely necessary in these cases and are to be avoided if at all possible because of the risks of airway occlusion and death. Mandibular distraction osteogenesis or tongue-lip adhesion are preferred when operative intervention is indicated.[28] The first few months of life are critical in determining the severity of a particular infant's anomaly and its importance in the overall prognosis.

Treacher Collins syndrome. Treacher Collins syndrome,[29,30] also known as *mandibulofacial dysostosis*, is an autosomal dominant disorder with variable penetrance, causing a variable and diffuse group of craniofacial anomalies. The presumed genetic defect is autosomal dominant, with mutation in the *TCOF1* gene or *POLR1D* gene, or biallelic (autosomal recessive) pathogenic variants in *POLR1C* or *POLR1D* genes. This syndrome is characterized by downward-sloping palpebral fissures, canthal dystopia, coloboma, mandibulomaxillary hypoplasia, hairline displacement, microtia, and blind fistulae on an angle between the mouth and the ears (Fig. 37.3). Deafness is common, and micrognathia/retrognathia and cleft anomalies may be present.

Pierre Robin sequence contributes to the obstruction in the hypopharynx. These cases of stridor and obstruction should be worked up and managed in a similar fashion to the earlier description for Pierre Robin sequence.[31]

Hallermann-Streiff syndrome. The Hallermann-Streiff syndrome[32] is a rare syndrome that consists of microphthalmia, cataracts, blue sclerae, and nystagmus. Associated anomalies include a pinched nose, micrognathia, and hypertrichosis of the scalp, eyebrows, and eyelashes (Fig. 37.4). The molecular basis is still unknown.[33] Congenital stridor in these infants arises from micrognathia with relative glossoptosis, and treatment is similar to that outlined for Pierre Robin or Treacher Collins syndrome.[34]

Möbius syndrome. Infants with the Möbius syndrome[35] have a characteristic absence or maldevelopment of various

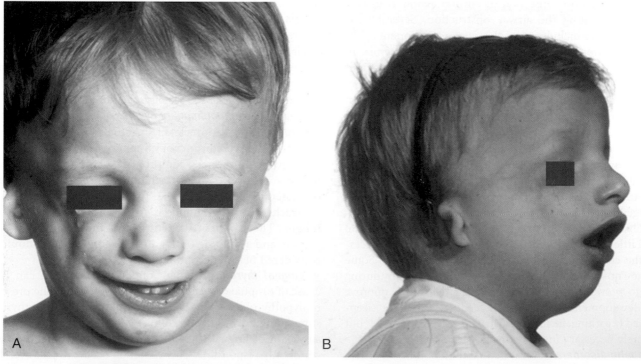

Fig. 37.3 Example of a child with Treacher Collins syndrome demonstrating sunken cheek bones, downward sloping palpebral fissures, and micrognathia.

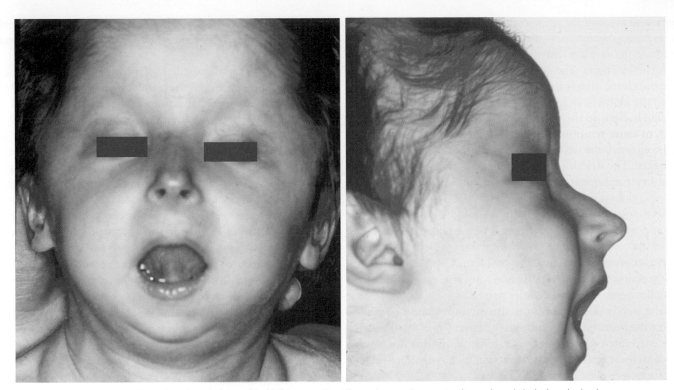

Fig. 37.4 Example of an infant with Hallermann-Streiff syndrome demonstrating microphthalmia, pinched nose, micrognathia, and hypertrichosis of the scalp.

cranial nerve nuclei. Cranial nerves VII (facial nerve) and VI (abducens) are most commonly affected. Common findings include facial paralysis, ptosis, ophthalmoplegia, clubbed feet, and syndactyly. Mutations in the MBS1, MBS2, and MBS3 gene loci; HOX family genes; and others have been linked to this syndrome.[36]

Paralysis of the facial nerve is the cause of upper airway obstruction as well as difficulties with mastication and deglutition. Both inspiratory and expiratory components of stridor result from the relatively fixed nature of the obstruction. Tracheostomy may be required in severe cases. Many children, however, can be successfully treated by careful feeding techniques.

Freeman-Sheldon syndrome. Freeman-Sheldon syndrome (also called Freeman-Burian syndrome or craniocarpotarsal dystrophy or whistling face syndrome or distal arthrogyrposis type 2A)[37] has hypoplastic alae nasi, clubbed feet, and mask-like whistling facies. Patients' eyes are deep set with blepharophimosis, ptosis, and strabismus. Transmission is autosomal dominant with some variations that transmit as autosomal recessive.

Stridor in these children is the result of air passage through a narrow channel. Although the sound may be alarming, it usually does not require intervention but rarely requires tracheostomy.[38] Of note, patients with microstomia have been linked with malignant hyperthermia.

Nager syndrome. Nager syndrome[39,40] is a rare acrofacial dysostosis that presents with upper limb malformation, mandibular and malar hypoplasia, downward-slanting palpebral fissures, absent eyelashes in the medial third of the lower lids, dysplastic ears with conductive deafness, and palate anomalies. It is sometimes mistaken for Treacher Collins syndrome. Nager

syndrome is associated with chromosome 9 defects. Posterior tongue displacement from hypoplasia of the mandible can cause airway obstruction. Acute management may require early tracheostomy and subsequent mandibular distraction.

Laryngeal Anomalies

Laryngeal anomalies account for the majority of cases of stridor in newborns. Congenital high airway obstruction syndrome (CHAOS) results from complete obstruction because of laryngeal atresia, stenosis, web, or cyst. In utero, fluid builds up in the lungs and tracheobronchial tree, expanding these structures, and sometimes leads to ascites. Neonates born with CHAOS cannot survive without fetal or immediate perinatal intervention.[41]

Laryngeal atresia. The most extreme form of obstruction at this level, laryngeal atresia, results in a desperate emergency during the first few moments after birth. This lesion was originally described in 1826, but only 51 cases were reported in the subsequent 160 years. Without surgical intervention to secure a definitive airway within 2 to 5 minutes of clamping of the umbilical cord, the infant will not survive.[42,43]

The most dramatic physical finding is that the child is aphonic, with absence of any cry or gasp at birth. If the lesion is immediately recognized on direct laryngoscopy, an emergency cricothyroidotomy should be performed. Although difficult, diagnosis of laryngeal atresia can be made prenatally[44] and clinicians may be able to prepare for emergent airway management at birth or schedule the child for an ex utero intrapartum treatment (EXIT) procedure to obtain an emergent airway while the child is still supported through the umbilical cord.

Laryngeal web. Laryngeal webs arise about the 10th week of gestation, probably as an arrest of the development of the larynx, and account for approximately 5% of laryngeal anomalies (Fig. 37.5). Some 75% of these lesions occur at the level of the cords; the rest are distributed between subglottic and supraglottic locations. The web generally occurs anteriorly. Because the glottic area is triangular, these anteriorly placed webs reduce the glottic area by only 15% to 20%, and if they extend less than halfway to the posterior wall, they are usually not sufficient to cause symptoms.

In contrast, if the web extends posteriorly, the symptoms may be marked. The stridor is primarily inspiratory but often has an expiratory component. The affected infant's cry is hoarse and weak; the child is rarely aphonic and often is dyspneic at rest.

Laryngoscopy and bronchoscopy should be performed as soon as possible. If a thin, transparent web is encountered at the level of the cords, it may be easily swept away with the bronchoscope, completely correcting the problem. Completion of the bronchoscopy should be performed to rule out associated anomalies beneath the area of the web.

If the web is thick and fibrous, no attempt should be made to force the bronchoscope through the area. This kind of web is often encountered in the subglottic region. Endoscopic laser lysis of webs or open surgical correction by laryngotracheal reconstruction may be needed.[45,46]

Congenital vocal cord paralysis. Congenital vocal cord paralysis is the second most common cause of congenital stridor.[47] Birth trauma was frequently implicated but now appears to be a declining cause. Intracranial lesions and the possibility of congenital cardiac lesions, especially one impinging on the recurrent laryngeal nerve, must be considered.

Fortunately, paralysis is unilateral in 70% to 80% of cases. Some studies report that both sides are equally involved, but left-sided paralysis is typically associated with underlying congenital cardiac anomalies. These infants have a hoarse weak cry, and if the paralysis is bilateral, it may result in aphonia. The

inspiratory stridor is obviously worse in bilateral paralysis. Marked suprasternal and intercostal retractions may be present in these children.

Diagnosis is rapidly made by laryngoscopy, and treatment depends on the severity of the problem. In a unilateral paralysis with minimal or no dyspnea, simple observation is appropriate. Generally associated with severe symptoms, bilateral paralysis necessitates tracheostomy.[48] Once the airway is adequately secured, the cause of the paralysis can be explored. If the causal lesion can be identified and corrected, the stridor may improve. If no lesion can be found or if it cannot be safely corrected, later fixation of the arytenoids with the vocal cord in abduction may result in satisfactory control of the stridor and decannulation.

Laryngomalacia. Laryngomalacia is the most common cause of congenital stridor, accounting for 60% to 75% of cases of stridor in newborns[49] and three-fourths of the congenital laryngeal abnormalities. The pathophysiology of this condition involves an immature, floppy larynx that collapses during each inspiration (Fig. 37.6), producing an inspiratory stridor of varying severity that is often much worse when the baby is agitated or crying.

Laryngomalacia occurs with a 2:1 male-to-female predominance and is usually evident at birth, but the first symptoms may not appear immediately. Many cases are reported to have micrognathia, and some may be confused with Pierre Robin sequence.

Diagnosis is made easily on laryngoscopy, which shows a soft, enfolded epiglottis. The larynx is often difficult to expose, sitting high under the tongue. Bronchoscopy should accompany laryngoscopy to rule out associated anomalies or extensive malacia, such as tracheomalacia and/or bronchomalacia.

Maturation of the epiglottis usually results in resolution of the stridor by the age of 18 to 24 months. Accordingly, tracheostomy is rarely necessary, but about 10% of laryngomalacia patients require supraglottoplasty, which is generally performed endoscopically with a good success rate.[49]

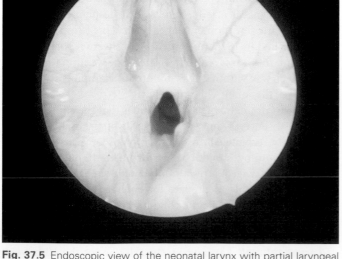

Fig. 37.5 Endoscopic view of the neonatal larynx with partial laryngeal atresia and a laryngeal web partially obstructing the laryngeal orifice.

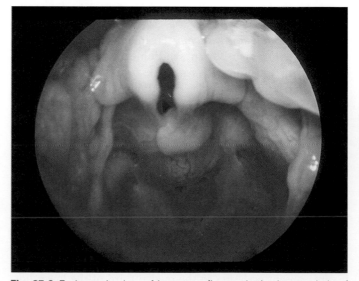

Fig. 37.6 Endoscopic view of immature floppy glottis characteristic of laryngomalacia. Dynamic examination demonstrates downward placement of glottis into larynx with inspiration.

Congenital subglottic stenosis. The incidence of congenital subglottic stenosis is unknown because many such cases remain undiagnosed. In the full-term neonate, subglottic stenosis is defined as a lumen 4 mm or smaller in diameter at the level of the cricoid.[50] The proposed cause of the congenital group is failure of complete recanalization of the laryngeal lumen in embryonic life, from the cricoid cartilage, which is a derivative of the sixth branchial arch.

The stridor, if present at all, is usually biphasic and sometimes arises during the first or second month of life. Respiratory distress after an upper respiratory tract infection is typically the presenting symptom. These patients are generally unable to clear the resultant increased secretions found in association with infection. Affected children are often treated for recurrent pneumonias or prolonged tracheobronchitis. Many cases are not discovered until a severe episode of croup or epiglottitis results in emergency intubation or tracheostomy.

Mild lesions should be observed, and antibiotic therapy should be added during periods of upper respiratory tract infection. A range of endoscopic and open procedures are currently used in the management of subglottic stenosis with good outcomes.[50] Tracheostomy is frequently necessary in children with severe stenosis, followed by serial monthly dilation done gently to prevent further damage or fibrosis of the subglottic region.

Acquired subglottic stenosis. Acquired subglottic stenosis is most often caused by prolonged endotracheal intubation. Because of the increased survival of neonates with respiratory difficulties requiring intubation (especially extremely low birth weight infants), this lesion is increasing in frequency as a cause of stridor. In its mildest form, the stenosis consists of laryngeal edema and has been reported in 30% of infants immediately after intubation. Stridor in these patients is inspiratory and presents soon after tube removal. This usually resolves within 72 hours. During this 3-day period, the mild form of this disorder is treated with head elevation, humidified air, racemic epinephrine, nasal CPAP or noninvasive nasal ventilation, and occasionally systemic steroids.

In its most severe form, acquired stenosis is a dense scar of well-organized fibrous tissue. This lesion may require tracheostomy before the actual stenosis can safely be manipulated. Initial treatment includes graded, gentle dilation with or without intralesional steroids. As many as half of the stenotic scars will improve and often stabilize after four to six treatments. Failure to achieve significant improvement by then indicates the need for more aggressive treatment such as cryosurgery, laser ablation, cricoid split procedure, or resection and reconstruction with stents. There have been reasonable results with the cricoid split procedure, and this alternative should always be considered.

Laryngeal cleft. Although laryngeal clefts were once considered extremely rare lesions, they have frequently been reported in recent decades.[51] This is probably a result of enhanced endoscopy techniques and improved ability to make the diagnosis in the antemortem period. The lesion forms owing to a failure of dorsal fusion during the chondrification of the cricoid cartilage. This results in a posterior midline cleft that extends down between the arytenoids into the upper portion of the esophagus and trachea. Severe stridor is a frequent finding in affected children, and inadequate resuscitation can lead to death. In addition to their respiratory difficulties, these patients are at risk for aspiration and pneumonitis if they are fed without regard for their clefts. Therefore, recognition of the lesion is imperative, with subsequent intubation and stabilization. Stable enteral access is often created with a feeding gastrostomy and possible fundoplication until definitive repair can be performed. After extubation, the patient should be carefully monitored for continuous passage of upper airway secretions into the lungs. This may be a cause of recurrent pneumonia and respiratory distress, which could be an indication for the placement of a tracheostomy until surgical closure of the cleft can be completed.

Subglottic hemangioma. Another potential source of congenital subglottic obstruction is a hemangioma. Symptoms are related to the growth and development of the lesions, so their onset is variable. Hemangiomas begin as small lesions and may have a period of rapid growth, followed by a prolonged plateau and slow involution. Time to presentation for these patients will depend on when the hemangioma develops. In those for whom the hemangioma develops in fetal life, symptoms will appear when the patient is younger. Alternatively, if the subglottic hemangioma develops after birth, symptoms may not present for several months. Hemangiomas on other parts of the body may be an indication of the presence of a subglottic hemangioma. Laryngoscopic and bronchoscopic examination provides a definitive diagnosis.

The finding of a red or purple mass just below the vocal cords on bronchoscopy is generally considered diagnostic. A biopsy of this vascular mass introduces the risk of significant hemorrhage that may necessitate emergent surgery. And for that reason, it is generally not recommended. Once the diagnosis is confirmed, the appropriate treatment options are selected based on symptom severity. In a stable child with normal blood gas values at rest, observation is satisfactory. If the obstruction caused by the subglottic hemangioma results in dyspnea, severe stridor, and possibly abnormal blood gas values, consideration should be given to a tracheostomy below the lesion. Before surgical intervention, it is important to take the possibility of platelet trapping (Kasabach-Merritt syndrome) into account.

Beta-blockers, such as propranolol, sometimes combined with prednisone, are quite beneficial if the hemangioma is growing quickly and causing thrombocytopenia.[52] Some infants may require intralesional steroids, laser resection, or open surgical excision.

Tracheal Anomalies

Intrinsic tracheal compression.

Tracheomalacia. Tracheomalacia results from inadequate support of the round shape of the normal trachea from the cartilaginous rings. The hypoplastic cartilages allow the trachea to collapse, which is most pronounced during expiration (Fig. 37.7). Although tracheomalacia is commonly noted in babies and children undergoing bronchoscopic evaluation, it is only incidentally responsible for stridor in a moderate number of them. The stridor is heard upon expiration, which is when the collapse of the

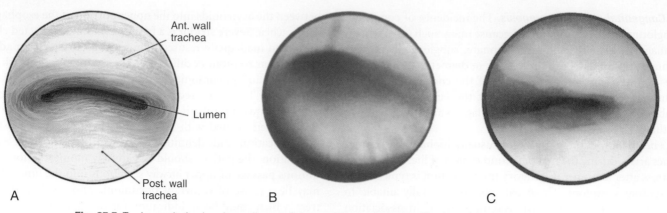

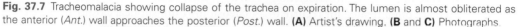

Ant. wall
trachea

Lumen

Post. wall
trachea

A   B   C

Fig. 37.7 Tracheomalacia showing collapse of the trachea on expiration. The lumen is almost obliterated as the anterior (*Ant.*) wall approaches the posterior (*Post.*) wall. **(A)** Artist's drawing. **(B and C)** Photographs.

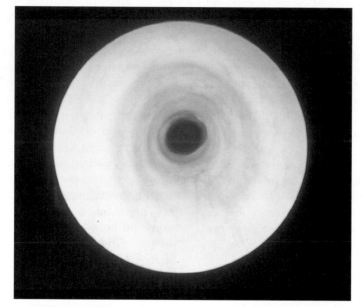

Fig. 37.8 Endoscopic view of tracheal stenosis as a result of complete tracheal rings tapering to a narrow lumen.

trachea causes obstruction of the airway. This is typically seen as a diffuse condition that involves the length of the trachea.

Bronchoscopy provides the diagnosis. Once past the vocal cords, the trachea is seen to have a transverse or ovoid appearance, which is accentuated as expiration takes place. Often, visualization of the carina will be difficult because of the anterior tracheal wall collapse. Although the findings can appear impressive in some children, tracheomalacia rarely necessitates any treatment, and it commonly resolves with growth and maturation. Rarely, such as in infants with bronchopulmonary dysplasia and associated severe tracheomalacia who require prolonged mechanical ventilation for months, tracheostomy may be needed.

Tracheal stenosis. Tracheal stenosis can involve either a short stenotic segment in an otherwise normal trachea or a long segment with a cylindrical tapering from the subglottic region (Fig. 37.8). Either form may demonstrate a fixed obstruction resulting in inspiratory and expiratory stridor. Tracheal cartilages are often absent when this occurs, and instability of the tracheal lumen is not uncommon.

Depending on the severity of the stenosis and its length, affected children may have severe respiratory distress with cyanosis. Respiratory sounds may be weak, and the danger of sudden and acute obstruction is quite possible. Bronchoscopy is the best study to confirm the diagnosis. Slide tracheoplasty or other surgery may be required,[53] although less severely affected infants may be managed conservatively.[54]

Necrotizing tracheobronchitis. The necrotizing tracheobronchitis lesion is mainly of historical interest after having been reported in the 1980s in preterm infants receiving high frequency ventilation. It is a necrotizing process that results in sloughing of the tracheal mucosa. Although the cause is unknown, it seems to be associated with hypoperfusion (such as a difficult birth requiring extensive resuscitation) and the use of high-frequency ventilators.[55,56] With improvement of ventilator humidification, very few cases have since been reported.

Clinical presentation primarily involves deterioration of respiratory status. Affected babies generally manifest sudden carbon dioxide retention that fails to respond to changes in ventilator settings, change of ETT, or intratracheal suctioning. Pulmonary graphics show evidence of severely increased airway resistance. Mortality is high unless suspicion of the lesion leads to bronchoscopy and mechanical clearing of the airway. Moreover, even if a child is able to recover from an acute episode, chronic strictures may result.

Extrinsic tracheal compression.

Cystic hygroma. Cystic hygromas are developmental abnormalities of the lymphoid system and frequently occur in the neck.[57] They have been reported to reach sufficient size and extension to result in compression of the trachea, thus resulting in stridor. When these lesions are severe enough to result in stridor, they almost always produce respiratory distress and require surgical intervention. The goal of the initial treatment is to relieve the compression, which may be attempted by simple aspiration of fluid from the cyst. This can be followed by bronchoscopy to rule out the possibility of associated laryngotracheal anomaly and by surgical extirpation of the cyst. Cystic hygromas are benign lesions, and as such, critical structures must be preserved during resection whenever possible.

Vascular rings. Vascular rings arise from anomalous formation of the great vessels that cross over or encircle the trachea and the esophagus.[58,59] The variety of anomalies is quite extensive, but the few categories that commonly occur and lead to problems can be classified under four to six headings. Those structures usually responsible for congenital stridor are the double aortic arch, the right aortic arch with left ductus arteriosus or ligamentum arteriosum, and the anomalous innominate artery. More rarely, an anomalous right subclavian artery (Fig. 37.9), an anomalous left pulmonary artery sling, or an anomalous left common carotid artery may give rise to symptoms. For technical accuracy, only a few of these conditions should be considered true vascular rings that are complete encirclement of the trachea and esophagus by vascular structures. Specifically, these lesions include the double aortic arch and the right aortic arch with left ductus. The others are more correctly referred to as *slings* because they pass around the trachea or esophagus and compress one or the other but do not completely encircle them. Stridor in affected neonates is present at birth or by 1 to 2 months of age. With the fixed nature of the obstruction, stridor is both inspiratory and expiratory. Afflicted infants have a brassy, barking cough. If the compression of the vascular anomaly affects the esophagus, as it does in a few cases, the neonate may have associated problems with deglutition, such as regurgitation, vomiting, and aspiration.

Evaluation of these infants by barium swallow usually shows a single or double oblique indentation on the esophagus. Subsequent bronchoscopy often reveals the pulsatile compressing mass passing over the anterior portion of the trachea on either the right or the left side. Depending on the location of the indentation, a presumptive diagnosis can be made. Also, one can occasionally compress the pulsatile area to check for disappearance of pulses to suggest which of the vascular anomalies is present. Frequently, echocardiography may identify the abnormal course of the vascular structures. In most of these cases, CT or MRI with contrast materials will give an excellent view of the exact anatomy.

Treatment of these lesions is essentially surgical division of the ring when one is present. In cases of double aortic arch or right arch with left ductus arteriosus, division of the ring at its narrowest portion or ductal ligation and division usually result in considerable improvement. In the case of sling lesions, the offending vessel may be divided (as in treatment of the anomalous right subclavian artery) with or without reanastomosis. If transection alone does not relieve the obstruction, dissection of the trachea and esophagus with vessel suspension to the anterior chest wall has been performed with considerable improvement of symptoms.

The outcomes of surgical intervention are generally good. The anomalous left pulmonary artery sling is fortunately one of the rarest of the vascular slings and is more difficult to handle surgically. Families must be warned that a residual tracheal deformity and tracheomalacia will persist after surgery and that stridor may not abate for 6 to 24 months.

Developmental Abnormalities of the Lung
Pulmonary and Lobar Agenesis

During intrauterine development, an entire lung or a portion of a lung may fail to form. The etiology for this is not definitively known. Reported cases of lobar agenesis in neonates have documented little clinical effect. On the other hand, a right or left pulmonary agenesis generally creates respiratory distress and has a significant mortality. Interestingly, mortality seems to be greatest when the lung missing is the right lung. Numerous associated anomalies have been reported in all the organ systems.

A neonate born with this problem generally requires immediate intubation. An opaque hemithorax with narrowed rib spaces and variable mediastinal shift is seen on chest radiograph. It may even be possible to see the absence of a carina or a blind-ended bronchial stump if the chest radiograph has been sufficiently penetrating.

Once the neonate has stabilized after intubation, attempts are made to wean from ventilator support. In the event of success and survival, the neonate is at risk for recurrent pulmonary infection.

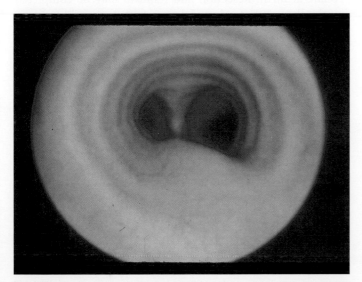

Fig. 37.9 Endoscopic view of anomalous right subclavian artery with impingement on the tracheal membrane.

Pulmonary Hypoplasia

Pulmonary hypoplasia is discussed elsewhere in this text in terms of ventilatory management (see Chapters 24 and 25). However, there are several lesions that are well known to produce pulmonary hypoplasia from lung compression. The most recognized is the diaphragmatic hernia, but large intrauterine tumors such as tonsillar or head/neck teratomas can produce the same result. In cases such as diaphragmatic hernia, surgical intervention may be necessary, but the airway is usually not involved.

Congenital Lobar Emphysema

Congenital lobar emphysema,[60] frequently referred to as CLE, is extremely rare, usually present at birth or apparent within the first 6 months, and is of unknown etiology. The mechanism of development is a ball–valve obstruction leading to overinflation of a lung lobe. This obstruction is attributed to deficient cartilage formation in the bronchi accompanied by bronchomalacia. However, fully half of the lungs removed as therapy fail to show any significant anatomic abnormality other than hyperinflation. Most series report a male preponderance of 2:1.

The affected lobes are, in order, the left upper lobe (40%-45% of cases), then the right middle lobe (30%-35% of cases), and finally the right upper lobe (20%-25% of cases). Rarely, two lobes are affected at the same time, and a few reports of metachronous involvement of two lobes have been described.

The presenting symptom is respiratory distress, possible with cyanosis. Intubation may stabilize the situation, especially if the intubation is bronchial in the unaffected lung. In fact, contralateral bronchial intubation may result in resolution of hyperinflation that fails to return when the endobronchial tube is removed. Mild cases may be observed, but severe distress requires lobectomy.[61] Chest x-ray alone is often sufficient for the diagnosis, based on hyperinflation, widened rib space, mediastinal shift, and collapse of the other lung. CT and ventilation-perfusion scanning have been advocated to confirm the diagnosis and add anatomic information, but in most cases, these modalities are not necessary.

Congenital Pulmonary Airway Malformation

Congenital pulmonary airway malformation (CPAM),[60,62] previously referred to as congenital cystic adenomatoid malformation (CCAM) is, again, a rare pulmonary malformation that can affect any lobe, affects both sexes equally and produces nonfunctional pulmonary tissue that has cysts, increased amounts of cellular elements, and abnormalities of cartilage, elastin, and other tissues. The cystic component may be microcystic or macrocystic. The respiratory compromise is caused by space occupation with nonfunctioning pulmonary tissue that produces respiratory distress and a predilection for infection (Fig. 37.10).

Maternal polyhydramnios is common, and one in four neonates affected will die from nonimmune hydrops. On the other hand, many antenatally diagnosed cases of CPAM spontaneously regress before birth. The clinical presentation of these patients is quite variable. Some neonates have no symptoms at

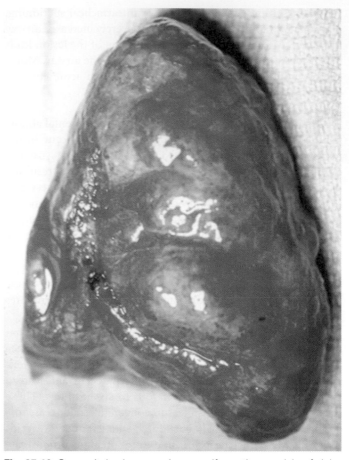

Fig. 37.10 Congenital pulmonary airway malformation—red, beefy lobe from lung with increased terminal alveolar tissue.

birth; others are severely compromised. Many of these infants are now diagnosed with prenatal ultrasound, so planning can be done to support the newborn at birth in case respiratory compromise is severe.

Space occupation and mediastinal shift may compromise a neonate at birth. Resection and removal may be completely curative therapy, but many of these infants have mild or severe pulmonary hypoplasia and pulmonary hypertension. Surgery will not solve these problems, so recourse to extracorporeal life support (ECMO), long-term ventilation, and all the various modalities of ventilation and pharmacologic therapies may be necessary. Despite this gamut of therapies, some children have inadequate lung volume for survival (particularly those with severe mediastinal shift and marked polyhydramnios in utero).

Sequestration

Sequestrations[60,63,64] are masses of pulmonary tissue that do not attach to the bronchopulmonary tree. In other words, they are sequestered segments of mesoderm that should have contributed to the alveolar mass of the lung on the side where they are found. The exact etiology is unknown, but this lesion seems to affect males three or four to one over females, involves the lower lobes more frequently than the upper, has a systemic arterial blood supply, and often has an anomalous venous drainage system.

Symptoms occur when these sequestrations become infected or attain a size that results in significant space occupation (often because they have become a huge intrathoracic abscess). Antibiotic therapy and fluid resuscitation may be the initial treatment, but surgical resection is eventually necessary.

Sequestrations are often divided into two groups depending on the proximity of the sequestered mass to the actual lung. Those immediately adjacent or within a lobe are called *intralobar* (Fig. 37.11). Those more remote and often with a complete pleura covering are called *extralobar*. The latter group is often seen with other anomalies; about half of the extralobar type occur around the opening of a diaphragmatic hernia.

These lesions have a systemic arterial blood supply. Often, this systemic arterial supply originates from the thoracic aorta and traverses the diaphragm. This is also frequently seen with CPAM, and the similarity of some of these characteristics has led to the suggestion that these lesions may represent a spectrum of developmental lung pathology.

Pulmonary Cystic Lesions

Pulmonary cystic lesions[60,64] may be developmental or acquired. Within the first group are the bronchogenic cysts and the duplication cysts. In all these lesions, sequestration or maldevelopment of some portion of the tracheobronchial tree or foregut results in the development of a cystic lesion that may grow over time, especially if there is a secretory lining. Within the group of acquired lesions are the cysts that result from barotrauma secondary to prolonged intubation, ventilation, suctioning, and recurrent infection. These often appear later in the neonatal course, having not been evident on x-ray at birth, and are often referred to as pneumatoceles.

Size can vary from small to enormous, and these can essentially replace an entire lung. Symptoms result from space occupation or infection. Often infection creates the increase in size (abscess) that finally leads to the diagnosis of the lesion. Plain radiography is generally sufficient to make this diagnosis, but barium swallow, CT, and MRI may all occasionally be needed.

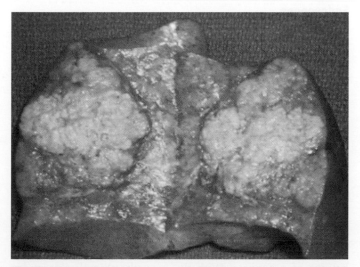

Fig. 37.11 Intralobar pulmonary sequestration treated by pulmonary lobectomy.

Generally, surgical resection is the best solution because it eliminates the chance of infection and prevents any further enlargement and anatomic displacement. If the baby is ventilator dependent on high settings, a ventilation strategy such as low-volume high-frequency ventilation may be necessary to prevent a recurrence in other areas of the lung postoperatively.

Developmental Abnormalities of the Diaphragm

Only three conditions need be considered here: diaphragmatic hernia, diaphragmatic paralysis, and diaphragmatic eventration. Concerning diaphragmatic hernias, only the congenital diaphragmatic hernia of Bochdalek is of concern clinically because the other hernias are rare, and seldom do any of them create major respiratory problems in the neonatal period.

Diaphragmatic Hernia of Bochdalek

The posterolateral diaphragmatic hernia, most common on the left as described by Bochdalek, occurs in approximately 1 in 2500 live births.[65,66] The etiology is unclear, but we now have a rat model in which the diaphragmatic defect and the pulmonary hypoplasia can be induced by maternal ingestion of the teratogen nitrofen (2,4-dichlorophenyl-*p*-nitrophenyl ether; a herbicide withdrawn from the market). The diaphragmatic hernia is complicated by serious pulmonary hypoplasia that exists not only on the side of the diaphragmatic defect but also in the contralateral lung.

Many neonates afflicted with this problem have associated anomalies and die in utero. Those who survive to term are generally fairly large and surprisingly free of other problems. Males comprise about two-thirds of the reported cases.

Many of these cases are now diagnosed prenatally, and sufficient data are now available to prognosticate on ultimate outcome in a general fashion. Neonates who have a small chest consistent with pulmonary hypoplasia; large amounts of abdominal viscera within the chest, particularly the left lobe of the liver; and marked mediastinal shift can be expected to have severe problems at the time of birth and often are nonsurvivors. In marked contrast are the babies born without symptoms or babies who are not diagnosed until 1 to 2 months of age. Virtually all of these children are survivors.

Presentation is generally some degree of respiratory distress that requires intubation at birth or shortly thereafter. Those who are tolerating the lesions without problems or who have minimal symptoms are brought to elective repair when other anomalies have been excluded and pulmonary hypertension has had a chance to abate. For those who require immediate intubation, a large number of lung protective ventilation strategies have proven quite successful, although inhaled nitric oxide has only a limited role in the acute phase.[67]

Those who fail these modalities can be taken to ECMO with ultimate repair on the pump or after successful decannulation (see Chapter 28), although the latter approach may have advantages of diminished hemorrhage after completion of anticoagulation. Use of all the modalities has produced survival rates that are near 80% today compared with historical reports of 40% survival. (See also Chapter 35.)

Diaphragmatic Paralysis/Eventration

Diaphragmatic paralysis and eventration can be lumped together because it is virtually impossible to distinguish them from each other. They look alike and act in a similar fashion. If a neonate has had a traumatic birth and has other neurologic deficits or if the baby has undergone intrathoracic surgery, it is reasonable to assume that the child has paralysis. If those conditions are not met, it is just as likely to be one lesion as the other.

In both conditions, one or both diaphragms assume a high position on chest X-ray and may compromise function of the lung owing to compression. Fluoroscopy or sonographic evaluation for paradoxical motion suggests paralysis, but a thin, attenuated muscle may give very similar results. In addition to the space problems, the paradoxical motion creates increased work of breathing, tires the baby, and makes effective spontaneous ventilation difficult.

If either of these conditions is present but asymptomatic, the situation can be observed. Obviously, if the baby needs ventilation, some future action may be needed. The literature is replete with recommendations, none based on any good objective data, that suggest diaphragmatic plication be done in 3 to 6 weeks if the neonate cannot be weaned from ventilation. These recommendations do not seem unreasonable because intubation and ventilation are not without their own risks and complications. The folding and suturing of the diaphragm create a stable platform against which the other diaphragm can effectively achieve normal or near-normal breathing.

Developmental Abnormalities of the Skeleton

There are a host of skeletal anomalies that result in thoracic asphyxiation at the time of birth or shortly thereafter. These are beyond the scope of this chapter, but the reader should be aware that there are some surgical expansion procedures offered in a limited number of institutions in the United States that can increase thoracic volume and hold some small promise for some of these children.

THE PEDIATRIC SURGEON/ OTOLARYNGOLOGIST AS CONSULTANT

Neonatal Bronchoscopy

The increased frequency of long-term neonatal intubation and the survival of children with severe respiratory difficulties have been associated with increased airway complications. The pediatric surgeon has an important role in the evaluation of congenital stridor, persistent atelectasis, ETT position, or patency and as an aid in difficult intubations.

Anatomic Considerations

A neonate's air passages are obviously smaller than those of an adult or a larger child, and this increases vulnerability to obstruction. Care must be observed during neonatal bronchoscopy because the mucosa of these patients is softer, looser, and more fragile. The location of the epiglottis and larynx of the neonate's airway is more cephalad and anterior than in an adult. Generally, the cricoid cartilage is the narrowest point in an infant's upper airway. This feature not only obviates the use of a cuffed ETT

but also increases the risk of subglottic stenosis from pressure during prolonged intubation. Furthermore, at an infant's carina, the main stem bronchi angulate almost symmetrically, unlike the anatomy in older children and adults.

Pathophysiology

Edema is the minimum adverse effect of endotracheal intubation. If intubation continues for longer than a few hours, acute inflammation becomes superimposed on edema. This proceeds over days and weeks to mucosal ulceration, submucosal inflammation, chondritis, cartilage fragmentation, and tracheomalacia. The body's reparative response to these changes is fibrosis and scarring that, if severe, results in laryngotracheal stenosis.

To minimize this cycle of destruction when intubation is mandatory, an ETT of appropriate size must be used. Furthermore, the ETT should be fixed in position to minimize lateral or horizontal motion. Finally, every attempt should be made to shorten the time necessary for intubation. Some clinicians advocate nasotracheal intubation and fixation for prolonged intubation, but this technique has the same serious adverse sequelae associated with orotracheal intubation and has the added risk of nasopharyngeal trauma and potential for sinusitis.

Evaluation of Intubation

Because the majority of patients admitted to most NICUs for intubation and ventilatory support are treated medically, the role of the surgeon is primarily one of consultation. Improved techniques for orotracheal and nasotracheal intubation and the use of noninvasive ventilation and nasal CPAP have shortened the time of intubation in most units. The development of better neonatal ventilators makes it quite possible to maintain most infants safely on respiratory support for 6 to 8 weeks with minimal concern for permanent pressure damage to the airway. After 6 to 8 weeks of endotracheal intubation, one should consider bronchoscopic evaluation to determine whether damage has occurred and whether continued intubation is appropriate management (see "Tracheostomy"). For a list of other indications for diagnostic bronchoscopy, see Box 37.1.

Endoscopes

Excellent rigid and flexible endoscopes are now available for examination of the neonatal airway. In addition, ultrathin flexible bronchoscopes are available that allow examination of the tracheobronchial tree through ETTs. The scopes are available in diameters from 1.3 to 2.7 mm.[68,69] They allow bronchoscopic examination without major disruption to positive-pressure ventilation when a Y-adaptor (Vigo, France) is used between the ETT and the ventilator. These scopes are easy to maneuver, and serious complications such as perforation are unlikely. As such, these procedures are as safe to perform in the NICU as in the operative theater. Unfortunately, the majority of these scopes do not provide capabilities for significant lavage or suction, and their resolution is somewhat limited. Furthermore, scopes of sizes smaller than 2.7 mm do not have flexible tips.

One role for flexible bronchoscopy is aiding in difficult intubations of a neonate. With the new ultrathin flexible endoscopes, it is possible to place an ETT under direct vision by passing the tube over the bronchoscope. This can be particularly useful in neonates with congenital airway obstruction or craniofacial anomalies. The flexible endoscopes can also rapidly provide information about ETT position and patency. For major diagnostic and all therapeutic procedures, however, rigid bronchoscopy performed by an experienced bronchoscopist provides the maximum yield. Performed with appropriate anesthesia, lighting, and suction, rigid bronchoscopy is associated with minimal morbidity and mortality.

Rigid scopes, such as those provided by Storz equipped with Hopkins telescopes, are available for neonates in sizes from 2.5 to 4.0 mm. These provide superb illumination and magnification for inspection as well as an adequate lumen through which to insert tubes or instruments. A technique for using the Hopkins telescope without the sheath but instead inserting it directly through an ETT via a Y-adapter has also been described and allows continuation of endotracheal intubation and positive-pressure ventilation throughout the procedure.[70]

Both flexible and rigid scopes can easily be used in the NICU when the condition of a baby precludes moving him or her to the operating room; consequently, it is rare for an infant to be denied an endoscopic examination when diagnostic or therapeutic benefits are likely.

If an ETT has been in place for several weeks, mucosal edema, petechiae, and erythema are inevitable. The finding of worse sequelae of intubation indicates that these patients should undergo tracheostomy. Mucosal erosion, granulation and early fibrosis, and ultimately stricture are ominous signs and will probably progress if irritation from the ETT continues.

Tracheostomy

Although physicians at some centers continue endotracheal intubation if no damage is encountered on evaluation of the airway, many clinicians proceed with neonatal tracheostomy after prolonged periods of continuous intubation (generally 6-8 weeks).[71] Such a procedure helps respiratory function by decreasing the work of breathing and reducing dead space and makes oral motor activity possible for the baby. Tracheostomy should also be seriously considered for infants who manifest central nervous system failure, severe bronchopulmonary dysplasia, complex cardiovascular disease, or in whom an ETT is inadequate for maintaining pulmonary toilet.

The specific technique of neonatal tracheostomy varies little from a well-performed tracheostomy at any age. Except in dire emergency, when a needle cricothyroidotomy is the preferred approach, neonatal tracheostomy should be performed under operating room conditions (which can be replicated in a good NICU), and the infant should be intubated before the surgical procedure begins.

Procedure

After the landmarks of the anterior triangle of the neck are well established, a transverse or midline skin incision can be made (Fig. 37.12). The choice of skin incision used appears to make little difference in the overall outcome and should reflect the preference and experience of the operating surgeon. Once the skin

and subcutaneous tissues have been opened, midline dissection is mandatory to prevent damage to vascular or neural structures. Division of the thyroid isthmus may occasionally be necessary and can easily be performed with electrocautery (Fig. 37.13). Either a simple transverse[72] or a T-type tracheal incision is performed in neonatal cases (Fig. 37.14). Stay sutures, often called *trapdoor* sutures, are placed through the cartilages of the tracheostomy site at the time the initial incision into the trachea is made. If reintubation in the early postoperative period is necessary, these sutures aid the replacement, decrease the trauma of replacement, and may prevent placement into subcutaneous tissues. At no time should cartilaginous rings or portions of them be removed, because this almost inevitably results in stricture formation if decannulation is successful in the future.

Because a neonatal tracheostomy is performed over an ETT (almost without exception), the ETT is removed under direct vision as the tracheostomy tube is inserted (Fig. 37.15). This ensures control of the neonatal airway throughout the entire procedure. Finally, fixation of the tube is critical, because dislodgment in the postoperative period can be fatal if experienced

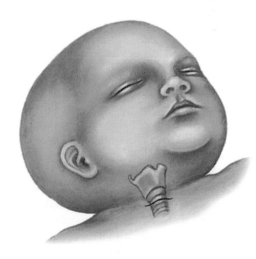

Fig. 37.12 Transverse skin incision over tracheal rings (1 to 3)

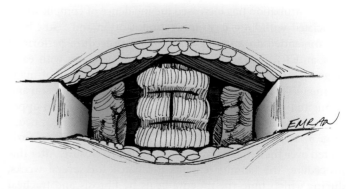

Fig. 37.13 Platysma and strap muscles retracted laterally to allow midline dissection to the trachea. The thyroid isthmus is retracted or cut as necessary.

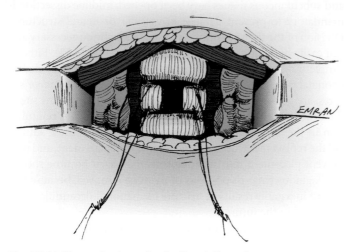

Fig. 37.14 The tracheal opening is dilated. Retention sutures are sewn through the cartilages to aid postoperative reinsertion if necessary. No tracheal cartilage is removed at any time.

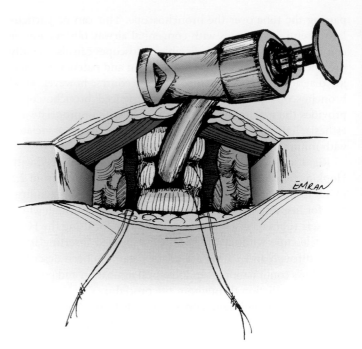

Fig. 37.15 A tracheostomy tube is inserted following slow withdrawal of the endotracheal tube under direct vision.

personnel are unable to reinsert the tube immediately. Consequently, the tube must be tied securely by those familiar with this technique; alternatively, the tube may be sutured directly to the lateral aspects of the neck (Fig. 37.16).

Despite all efforts to prevent tracheostomy dislodgment, these events still occur. If the tracheostomy becomes dislodged in the perioperative period before maturation of the tracheostomy tract, replacement of the tracheostomy tube can be quite difficult despite the presence of stay sutures. Recannulation of the trachea through the neck wound can be attempted and if successful resolves the problem. It should be noted, though, that if recannulation through the neck wound is unsuccessful, then definitive airway control should be obtained through orotracheal intubation. In the meantime, until definitive airway control is obtained, patients can be bag–valve ventilated as a sufficient temporizing measure with simple digital occlusion of the neck wound/tracheotomy to prevent loss of the tidal volumes through the neck wound.

Anterior Cricoid Split Procedure

The improved survival of premature infants who require prolonged intubation has increased the incidence of complications associated with long-term intubation. Cotton and Seid[73] have recommended an anterior cricoid split procedure performed over an ETT, instead of tracheostomy in neonates with early stages of subglottic stenosis, as an alternative method of management. This procedure involves a transverse skin incision and a longitudinal incision through the cricoid cartilage and upper two tracheal rings as well as through the underlying mucosa (Fig. 37.17). The soft tissues of the neck are then reapproximated over the defect via a single-layer (skin) closure. After this procedure, the patient remains intubated for several weeks, during which time the mucosa heals by fibrosis and tracheal stability is reestablished (Fig. 37.18). Finally, extubation is attempted when the trachea is healed.

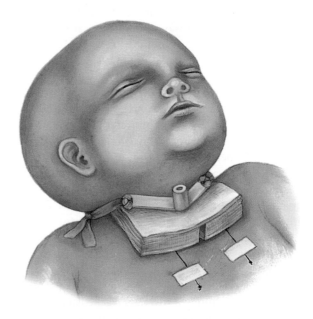

Fig. 37.16 Completed tracheostomy with dressing and tapes in place.

Experience with this technique has shown it to be a reasonable alternative to tracheostomy in the treatment of subglottic stenosis. Its use results in about a 75% rate of successful extubation. Unfortunately, reintubation and positive-pressure ventilation put the patient at risk of potential aerocele or fistulas if he or she subsequently undergoes respiratory failure once again.[74,75] Therefore, these patients should be carefully selected for the anterior cricoid split procedure. Tracheostomy should remain

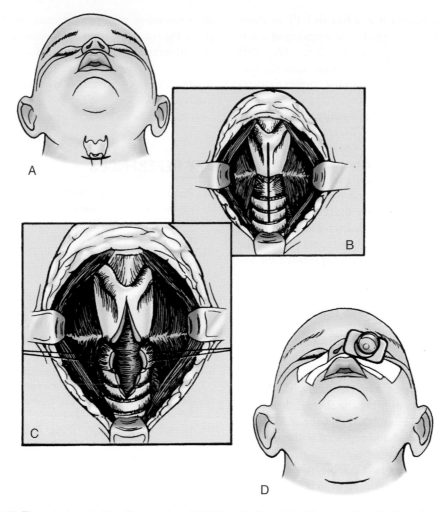

Fig. 37.17 The anterior cricoid split procedure. **(A)** Make a horizontal incision over the cricoid cartilage. **(B)** Use a combination of sharp and blunt dissection to expose the larynx and upper trachea. **(C)** Split the lower portion of the thyroid cartilage, the cricoid cartilage, and upper tracheal rings. **(D)** Close the wound loosely over a drain with the airway stented by a nasotracheal tube. (Adapted from Othersen HB Jr, editor. The Pediatric Airway. Philadelphia: WB Saunders; 1991.)

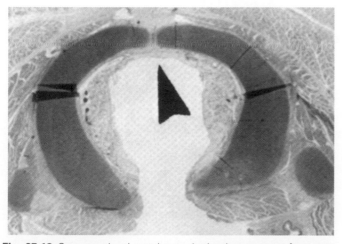

Fig. 37.18 Cross-sectional specimen obtained at autopsy from a patient who had previously undergone an anterior cricoid split. The *arrowhead* indicates the site of the cricoid split (the posterior opening was created by the pathologist during autopsy). (From Cotton RT, Seid AB: Management of the extubation problem in the premature child: anterior cricoid split as an alternative to tracheostomy. Ann Otol Rhinol Laryngol 89:510, 1980.)

the gold standard of treatment for the majority of neonates with complications associated with prolonged endotracheal intubation.

Tracheostomy Tubes

The choice of an appropriate tracheostomy tube is as important as the correct technique of tracheostomy placement. The soft, pliable, polyvinyl chloride tubes manufactured under the Shiley and Portex trade names are best suited to the neonatal airway. The Aberdeen tube, a silicone elastomer tube, is also an excellent alternative but is available in fewer sizes. These tubes remain pliable at physiologic body temperature and conform well to individual anatomy. Additionally, the balloons associated with cuffed tracheostomy tubes are designed to exert less pressure on the tracheal walls. These factors reduce trauma and the risk of subsequent stricture formation in cases of prolonged mechanical ventilation. Additionally, the softer tubes are more comfortable for a patient and reduce the chances of cervical skin irritation or abrasions from sharp metal edges. Rigid metal tracheostomy tubes are contraindicated in this population.

If a patient undergoing tracheostomy has an ETT in place, the size of the ETT can be used to guide the selection of a tracheostomy tube of appropriate size. A reasonably reliable rule is that the tracheostomy tube can be 0.5 mm larger than the correct orotracheal tube or 1.0 mm larger than the correct nasotracheal tube.

Choosing a tube of proper length is usually more difficult than finding the proper diameter. At birth, tracheal length for the normal term birth weight infants is a maximum of 5 to 6 cm. Even a very short tracheostomy tube may lie dangerously close to the carina and risk right or left main stem bronchus intubation with subsequent exclusion of the other bronchus and lung. Alternatively, if the tube is too short and lies high in the neck, the chance of dislodgment is increased. Generally, pediatric tubes are 3 to 6 mm longer than neonatal tubes of the same diameter and can be used if the neonatal tube of the appropriate width is too short. Today, all the manufacturers will provide custom-constructed tubes, usually with only a 2- to 3-day delay in delivery. Consequently, it is possible to request the appropriately sized tube for any infant.

Once a tracheostomy is in place with adequate tract formation, daily changing of the dressing and weekly changing of the tube seem adequate when coupled with fastidious tracheostomy care provided by the nursing staff. Generally, it is best to have the surgeon or surgical team make the first tracheostomy tube change. Once it has been established that the tract is well healed and tubes can be removed and replaced without major problems, the nurse and family members may assume this task. An alternative tube should always be available at the bedside. This is cleansed with soap and water, stored in a clean container, and used in the event that sudden replacement is necessary. Suctioning is performed as necessary to keep the airway clear of secretions to maintain adequate pulmonary hygiene and decrease the risk of pulmonary infectious complications, and details of suctioning are similar to those for ETTs (see Chapter 29).

A complete reference list is available at https://expertconsult. inkling.com/.

KEY REFERENCES

8. Rajan R, Tunkel DE: Choanal atresia and other neonatal nasal anomalies. Clin Perinatol 45(4):751-767, 2018.
26. Hsieh ST, Woo AS: Pierre Robin sequence. Clin Plast Surg 46(2):249-259, 2019.
31. Cobb AR, Green B, Gill D, et al: The surgical management of Treacher Collins syndrome. Br J Oral Maxillofac Surg 52(7): 581-589, 2014.
41. Ryan G, Somme S, Crombleholme TM: Airway compromise in the fetus and neonate: Prenatal assessment and perinatal management. Semin Fetal Neonatal Med 21(4):230-239, 2016.
49. Bedwell J, Zalzal G: Laryngomalacia. Semin Pediatr Surg 25(3):119-122, 2016.
57. Gallagher PG, Mahoney MJ, Gosche JR: Cystic hygroma in the fetus and newborn. Semin Perinatol 23(4):341-356, 1999.
60. Zobel M, Gologorsky R, Lee H, et al: Congenital lung lesions. Semin Pediatr Surg 28(4):150821, 2019.
62. Wong KKY, Flake AW, Tibboel D, et al: Congenital pulmonary airway malformation: advances and controversies. Lancet Child Adolesc Health 2(4):290-297, 2018.
64. Durell J, Lakhoo K: Congenital cystic lesions of the lung. Early Hum Dev 90(12):935-939, 2014.
71. Walsh J, Rastatter J: Neonatal tracheostomy. Clin Perinatol 45(4):805-816, 2018.

38

Intraoperative Management of the Neonate

Christopher E. Colby, Raymond C. Stetson, and Malinda N. Harris

The neonatal patient requiring surgery presents a unique challenge in the delivery of safe and effective airway management, ventilation, sedation, and anesthesia. The physiology of the neonate is unique and cannot simply be extrapolated from experiences with the older pediatric surgical patient. This chapter will begin with a review of fetal lung development, transitional physiology, and congenital anomalies as they pertain to the development of operative ventilation strategies. The remainder of the chapter will explore the procedural components that may improve patient safety and outcomes such as a risk and facilities assessment to determine if the patient is best served by undergoing the operation in the intensive care unit or the standard operating theater.

When considering operative intervention for the neonate, a multidisciplinary preoperative review of clinical status, with consideration given to anatomic complexities, current modality and degree of respiratory support, medications, and recent laboratory and radiographic data, should be performed. In preparation for the operation, a thoughtful approach to premedication for intubation and selection of the appropriate endotracheal tube is recommended. The use of a standardized checklist in the perioperative period may facilitate enhancing the situational awareness of the patient's condition during these important transitions of care (Table 38.1). During the operation, ventilation of the patient may be performed successfully using vigilant monitoring of the vital signs, end-tidal or transcutaneous carbon dioxide, and blood gas parameters.

"Children are not simply small adults" is a tenet within pediatrics. An accurate reinterpretation of this maxim could be "Neonates are not simply small children." The acutely ill newborn population is often cohorted in the neonatal intensive care unit (NICU) until the first discharge from the hospital. Despite the commonality of location, the physiology and developmental status of the pulmonary system for patients within the NICU are heterogeneous. A fetus delivered at a gestational age considered at the margin of viability will have lungs with marked developmental immaturities. The pulmonary system of this patient may be in the canalicular stage of development, reliant on newly formed acini as the basic structure for gas exchange with a paucity of both alveolar development and surfactant production by type II pneumocytes. Unique physiology is also encountered in the NICU. The transition from fetal to extrauterine circulation may occur without interruption after birth or may present ongoing management challenges for the patient who requires surgery during the first several days of life. Concerns for pulmonary hypertension may persist for some neonates as a sequela of ventilator dependence, birth depression, prematurity, or congenital anomalies. Finally, congenital anomalies requiring surgical intervention necessitate a disease- and patient-specific management plan to account for challenges that may be encountered during the operation.

TRANSITIONAL PHYSIOLOGY AND PULMONARY HYPERTENSION

During pregnancy, the fetus is dependent on gas exchange, which occurs at the level of the placenta. For centuries, the uterus had been referred to as the uterine lung.[1] This description is appropriate, as development of the fetus requires oxygen delivery and elimination of carbon dioxide through the placenta. Both maternal and fetal blood flow to the placenta increases throughout gestation. Oxygenated blood is supplied to the fetus through the umbilical vein and returns to the placenta through the umbilical arteries. This unique circulation results in an oxygen saturation of approximately 60% in the term fetus before delivery.[2]

Once the infant is delivered and the umbilical cord is clamped, the newborn is dependent on ventilation occurring at the level of the alveolar capillary interface. With spontaneous breathing, the lungs become inflated and stretch receptors are activated, which promote pulmonary vasodilation. Inspired oxygen and the newborn's production of endogenous nitric oxide result in a decrease in pulmonary vascular resistance. Shunts at the level of the foramen ovale and ductus arteriosus, which had previously been very important in fetal development, close. The transition from fetal to extrauterine circulation is clinically apparent within the first 10 minutes of life. The immediate newborn oxygen saturation level will reflect the native fetal oxygen saturation of approximately 60%, but by 10 minutes of life, the preductal oxygen saturation should increase to greater than 90%.[3]

This transition to extrauterine circulation can be delayed in some newborns. The diagnosis of persistent pulmonary hypertension, historically referred to as persistent fetal circulation,

TABLE 38.1 Perioperative Checklist to Facilitate Transitions of Care	
Presurgical	**Postsurgical**
Gestational age	Estimated blood loss
Pertinent medical history	Modifications to preoperative mode of ventilation
Current mode of ventilation	
Review of recent labs and radiographs	Description of intraoperative patient stability
Medication list and dosing	Medications and intravenous fluids administered during operation
Current nutritional support and intravenous fluids	
	Intraoperative blood gas review
Airway status including type and depth of artificial airway	Challenges or complications that occurred intraoperatively
Confirm consent has been obtained	Operation performed
	Status of parental postoperative update

TABLE 38.2 Differential Diagnosis of Pulmonary Hypertension	
Persistent pulmonary hypertension (idiopathic)	Respiratory distress syndrome
	Hypothermia
Meconium aspiration	Chronic lung disease
Blood aspiration	Maternal medications
Pulmonary hypoplasia	• Nonsteroidal antiinflammatories
Congenital diaphragmatic hernia	• Selective serotonin reuptake inhibitors
Pneumonia/sepsis	

should be suspected in infants requiring supplemental oxygen to maintain ideal oxygen saturations who lack primary lung disease such as surfactant deficiency. In infants with a patent ductus arteriosus (PDA) and pulmonary hypertension, there is often significant difference in oximetry measured in the preductal, right upper extremity, and postductal location, either lower extremity. This difference in preductal and postductal saturations is attributed to right-to-left shunting from the pulmonary artery through the PDA to the descending aorta. The lack of a preductal and postductal saturation differential does not exclude pulmonary hypertension. Infants with a closed ductus arteriosus and pulmonary hypertension can still have significant intracardiac shunting through atrial level shunts. The differential diagnosis for persistent pulmonary hypertension of the newborn (PPHN) is found in Table 38.2 and further discussed in Chapter 34. Pulmonary vascular resistance will normally decrease throughout the first several days of life. This can be assessed through serial echocardiography, the difference in preductal and postductal saturation levels, and a bedside evaluation of the fraction of inspired oxygen required to maintain ideal preductal saturations.

This is clinically relevant for the anesthetist when surgery is considered in the first postnatal days for an infant diagnosed with primary pulmonary disease with or without PPHN. If the infant is improving from the perspective of pulmonary hypertension, waiting to perform a nonemergent procedure may allow a greater margin for safety and effective ventilation during the case. Preoperative identification of a patient with a history of PPHN or lung disease who may develop PPHN intraoperatively allows the anesthetist to predict risk for rebound pulmonary hypertension and be prepared to recognize and initiate appropriate therapies.

The diagnosis of pulmonary hypertension may also become clinically relevant in the former premature infant with bronchopulmonary dysplasia (BPD). Premature infants with BPD are at risk for concomitant pulmonary hypertension, although it remains unclear which of the two is the principal diagnosis.[4-6] In most cases, infants with BPD and associated pulmonary hypertension will continue to require oxygen for several months after birth. In severe cases, systemic medications such as sildenafil, treprostinil, bosentan, or ambrisentan may also be prescribed. These infants may present to the anesthetist just before discharge from the initial hospitalization for procedures including tracheostomy, gastrostomy tube placement, inguinal herniorrhaphy, and intervention for progressive retinopathy of prematurity.

There are special considerations for the surgical patient with pulmonary hypertension. Ventilation strategies that were being used in the NICU before the operation may continue to be effective during the operation. These strategies typically include avoidance of hypoxemia and acidosis. Hypoxemia and acidosis increase pulmonary vascular resistance, worsening pulmonary hypertension and placing increased strain on the right ventricle. Pharmacologic and nonpharmacologic interventions to decrease pain and agitation are indicated. Inhaled nitric oxide, a selective pulmonary vasodilator, may be a component of the ventilation strategy used in the NICU and should be continued throughout the operation. Alternatively, it may be considered as an intraoperative rescue strategy through the mechanical ventilation circuit. Additional therapies considered in the treatment of pulmonary hypertension include milrinone or vasopressin as adjunctive intravenous (IV) infusions that may provide additional pulmonary vasodilatory effects. Milrinone may also affect systemic vascular resistance, necessitating vigilant blood pressure monitoring.

KEY POINTS

- Common causes of pulmonary hypertension in the infant are delayed transition to extrauterine life, prematurity, and primary pulmonary disease.
- Suspect pulmonary hypertension if there is a significant difference in preductal and postductal oxygen saturation and an increased oxygen requirement.
- Intraoperative treatment strategies for patients with PPHN include avoidance of hypoxemia and acidosis, adequate sedation, and utilization of inhaled nitric oxide.

PULMONARY DEVELOPMENT AND LUNG INJURY

The diversity of size of patients within the NICU is remarkable. There may be more than a 10-fold difference in the weight of the smallest to the largest patient. Beyond the marked variation in the birth weight of this population, the individual patients are at different stages of the lung development continuum. The smallest and often most premature babies are dependent on primordial gas exchange units within the lungs, whereas the largest patients may have progressed toward a fully developed alveolar capillary interface. Additionally, a patient who began life as a fragile extremely low birth weight newborn may have developed BPD during their extrauterine development while hospitalized. Despite the appearance of a now robust infant approaching or past the estimated due date, the pulmonary system of the former premature patient may be markedly abnormal. Recognition of normal lung development stages and potential abnormal pathophysiology will allow the anesthetist to develop a ventilation strategy appropriate for the individual patient.

The respiratory system of many premature babies in the NICU may be at the canalicular stage, which typically occurs between 16 and 25 weeks of gestation. Characteristics of this stage of lung development include the formation of the earliest gas exchange units and early evidence of surfactant production by the type II pneumocytes. The lungs begin to develop both respiratory and nonrespiratory bronchioli. During this developmental stage, an extensive capillary network becomes progressively approximated to the epithelium of the developing airspaces.

Beyond 25 weeks, the lung enters into the terminal sac stage of development. The appearance of immature alveoli may be seen as early as 28 weeks' gestation. Lung volume and surface area increase throughout this stage to allow for sufficient gas exchange.

Premature infants are at risk for the development of BPD, a disease in which there is arrest of lung maturation[7] (see Chapter 36). A multitude of factors may contribute to this pathology including the administration of exogenous corticosteroids, exposure to prolonged mechanical ventilation, and inadequate postnatal nutrition. Following the initial injury, further exposure to excessive oxygen delivered to the developing airway, mechanical ventilation, and baro/volutrauma may activate release of cytokines, thus contributing to continued airway inflammation. BPD is characterized by reduced lung compliance and increased airway resistance. Radiographically, a heterogeneous appearance to the lung, with areas of atelectasis and hyperinflation, may be observed.

The patient may have a chronic supplemental oxygen requirement to achieve target oxygen saturations. Often, the blood gas of infants with BPD demonstrates a markedly compensated respiratory acidosis, with serum bicarbonate levels significantly above normative values. Blood gases in the operating room will reflect this long-standing compensated hypercarbic baseline. Operative ventilation strategies should support adequate gas exchange while minimizing risks to the developing lung.

Intraoperative homeostasis for a chronic BPD patient may be to replicate the compensated respiratory acidosis from the preoperative state rather than the achievement of "normal" blood gases.

ANATOMIC CONSIDERATIONS

A variety of congenital anomalies requiring operative intervention shortly after birth are commonly encountered in the NICU. In the case of a thoracic anomaly, the lungs may be smaller and abnormally developed compared to those of an equivalently aged healthy infant.[8] Alternately, infants born with abdominal wall defects may have healthy lungs equivalent to those of healthy newborns, but the operation to repair the defect may cause a temporary reduction in total lung capacity and loss of functional residual capacity (FRC) owing to displacement of the diaphragm cephalad after restoration of the contents to an intra-abdominal position (Fig. 38.1).

Intrathoracic Masses

Infants with a prenatally diagnosed intrathoracic mass, such as a congenital diaphragmatic hernia (CDH) or a congenital pulmonary adenomatous malformation, are at high risk for pulmonary hypoplasia owing to abnormal fetal lung development. Pulmonary hypoplasia is most typically encountered in the lung ipsilateral to the mass, but in severe cases, both lungs may be significantly hypoplastic. In addition to pulmonary hypoplasia, a patient with CDH may have marked developmental abnormalities of the smooth muscle of the pulmonary vasculature leading to a severe form of PPHN. When viewed microscopically, the lungs of infants with CDH have fewer alveoli, increased interstitial tissue, thickened alveolar walls,[9] and pulmonary arteries with increased medial and adventitial tissue present.[10] These findings and altered autonomic regulation are likely to unite to create higher pulmonary pressures, which are often "fixed," or not responsive to typical pulmonary vasodilators like inhaled nitric oxide.[11,12] In fact, the largest study as of this writing investigating the role of inhaled nitric oxide in patients with CDH

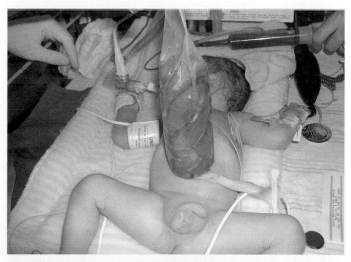

Fig. 38.1 Newborn with gastroschisis. Compare the amount of intestine in the silo to the small abdominal cavity.

KEY POINTS

- Postnatally, premature infants continue to develop sufficient gas exchange by maturation of the alveolar capillary interface.
- Premature infants are at risk for BPD and require lung-protective ventilatory strategies such as lower tidal volumes and oxygen saturation limits to prevent exposure to barotraumas and excess oxygen exposure.
- Infants with BPD have reduced lung compliance and increased airway resistance; they may require supplemental oxygen and unique ventilator strategies intraoperatively.

demonstrated immediate short-term improvements in oxygenation in some treated infants but no reduction in the need for ECMO or death.[13]

Following delivery, infants with CDH are often ventilated over several days with a lung-protective strategy, minimizing exposure to barotrauma,[14] until pulmonary vascular resistance has decreased before operative interventions.[15-17] High-frequency ventilation with a high-frequency oscillator or jet ventilation may be considered. It is appropriate during the surgical repair of CDH to continue a lung-protective strategy while being mindful of recurrence of pulmonary hypertension. Although the entirety of the pulmonary hypertension in these patients may not be responsive to acute modulation, avoidance of hypoxemia and acidosis is recommended while monitoring for acute pulmonary vasculature hyperreactivity. Pulmonary hypertension in the setting of operative stress or alterations in pH and carbon dioxide levels may be recognized by continuous intraoperative monitoring of preductal and postductal saturations as well as continuous end-tidal or transcutaneous Pco_2 levels. An increasing difference between preductal and postductal saturations during the case suggests a right-to-left shunting of deoxygenated blood through the PDA. At the time of hernia reduction, it is also important to maintain awareness of thoracic anatomy and recognize that as the tracheobronchial tree shifts toward midline, tube displacement may occur, resulting in the tip of the endotracheal tube becoming located within the right main stem bronchus. This scenario should be considered if the patient develops worsening respiratory stability after the bowel has been reduced and the hernia repaired. Following the reduction of intestine and repair of the hernia, a "potential" space within the thoracic cavity remains on the affected side. In concept, this can be considered a pneumothorax ex vacuo, and this space will fill with fluid postoperatively. The decision to leave a chest tube in place at the end of the operation is dependent more on the surgeon's preference than evidence. Chest tube placement is associated with lower rates of pleural complications such as pneumothorax.[18] Foregoing chest tube placement may prevent potential exposure of the hypoplastic lung to excess distention by allowing some fluid to accumulate in the intrapleural space.[19]

Abdominal Wall Defects

Infants with omphalocele and gastroschisis often have normal fetal lung development; however, infants with giant omphaloceles are at risk for pulmonary hypoplasia.[20] This is likely because of abnormal thoracic cage development related to liver displacement.[21,22] Most often, infants with abdominal wall defects are born at term, require no significant respiratory intervention at the time of birth, and remain without respiratory support until the time of surgery.

Some lesions, depending on the amount of displaced bowel content, can be replaced intra-abdominally in the first few hours of life. Larger lesions often require a staged approach to avoid the development of abdominal compartment syndrome. Over the first days to week of life, attempts are made to reduce the bowel slowly into the relatively hypoplastic abdominal cavity through a silastic silo created soon after birth.[23] When the surgeon determines that bowel reduction from the silastic silo into the peritoneum is adequate, complete operative reduction and abdominal wall closure occur. Once the abdominal contents are reduced, intraperitoneal pressure increases, resulting in a reduction of total lung capacity and FRC. With a reduction in FRC, lung compliance decreases and the infant may require increased peak inflation pressures to maintain adequate minute ventilation. Positive end-expiratory pressure (PEEP) may need to be increased once the bowel has been reduced to preserve FRC. Maintaining appropriate minute ventilation may also be addressed by increasing the mandatory rate or through high-frequency ventilation. Postoperatively the use of pulmonary function studies may help guide ventilator management.

KEY POINTS

- Intraoperative ventilation strategies for the patient with congenital anomalies should include consideration of how the anatomy may influence respiratory mechanics.
- Infants with thoracic anomalies are at high risk for pulmonary hypoplasia and require a lung-protective ventilatory strategy that minimizes barotrauma.
- Infants with abdominal wall defects can develop reduced total lung capacity following surgery and may require a ventilatory strategy that focuses on maintaining minute ventilation. This can be accomplished by an increased ventilation rate and lung recruitment through increased PEEP.
- An operative ventilatory strategy should include close monitoring for pulmonary vascular hyperreactivity for infants with pulmonary hypoplasia who are at high risk for pulmonary hypertension.

LOCATION OF OPERATION

Performing neonatal surgery in the intensive care unit is well described.[24-26] One of the primary incentives for operating at the patient's bedside is the inherent risk associated with transporting the unstable neonatal patient between the intensive care unit and the operating room. In addition to central line placement, the two most common neonatal surgeries that occur at the patient bedside are ligation of the PDA and laparotomy or peritoneal drain placement for necrotizing enterocolitis.[27,28] Other surgeries frequently performed at the bedside include reservoir placement for posthemorrhagic hydrocephalus and surgeries associated with extracorporeal membrane oxygenation including cannulation and decannulation. Although it may seem desirable to bring the surgeon to the infant's bedside, there is concern for and increased risk for infection and, of most concern, inadequate lighting in the operative field. At centers with experience bringing the operating team and requisite equipment to the intensive care unit, these interventions have been performed safely and with outcomes at least equivalent to, if not better than, transporting the patient to the operating room.[29] The provider who will direct the ventilation during the operation will need to become familiar with mechanical ventilators that may not be commonly used in the operating room, such as high frequency oscillator ventilators or high frequency jet ventilators. This can be achieved by performing a presurgical briefing between the anesthesia team that will be managing the case and the neonatology team that has been providing care for the patient preoperatively. The mode of ventilation and recent blood gases should be discussed collaboratively to determine if change is necessary and anticipated before surgery. Once the operation has finished, a similar postsurgical debriefing should occur between teams to ensure a safe transition of care.

Premedication for Intubation

Neonatal tracheal intubation and mechanical ventilation support are usually necessary for the operative procedure. Recent position statements recognize that intubation may need to proceed without premedication during an emergent resuscitation or in certain neonates with airway anomalies.[30,31] However, most presurgical neonatal intubations present an opportunity to provide premedication before insertion of the endotracheal tube. This painful procedure is known to induce apnea, hypoxemia, and bradycardia while causing increases in systemic and intracranial pressure.[32,33] Along with the technical skill required to successfully intubate, an evidence-based approach to selection of analgesia, sedation, vagolytics, and muscle relaxants is essential to optimize the quality of this procedure.

Providing adequate analgesia for this invasive procedure is indicated to provide patient comfort, avoid hypertension, and optimize intubation conditions. The ideal analgesic would be fast acting, with a short half-life and minimal side effects.

The opioids most commonly considered for neonatal premedication include natural (morphine) as well as synthetic (fentanyl and remifentanil) opioids. Administration of IV morphine results in peak analgesia in 15 minutes.[34] The clearance of morphine is gestational age dependent, with a longer half-life observed in premature infants compared to term.[35] Systemic hypotension as a result of histamine release is a potential side effect of morphine administration.[36] Fentanyl has a rapid onset of action within 2 to 3 minutes and a short duration of action of 60 minutes.[37] Clearance of fentanyl is also positively correlated with gestational age and birth weight.[38] Remifentanil has an immediate onset of action, has a half-life of less than 5 minutes, and has been used in the term and preterm populations.[39-41] Benzodiazepines and barbiturates have been investigated as classes of medications that may be used for premedication because of their sedative effects. Midazolam is the most widely used benzodiazepine for premedication for endotracheal intubation. Pharmacokinetics varies among individual neonates, and clearance appears to be positively correlated with gestational age.[42] Propofol is an amnestic sedative that appears to have several mechanisms of action including activation of γ-aminobutyric acid receptors, inhibition of N-methyl-d-aspartate receptors, modulation of calcium influx through slow calcium ion channel activity, and sodium channel blockade.[43,44] Early reports of the use of propofol as an induction agent for endotracheal intubation in preterm infants with gestational ages of 25 to 30 weeks suggested a reassuring safety profile.[45] However, more recent data suggest that propofol use for this indication in this population should be approached with caution owing to its significant cardiovascular side effects.[46,47]

Vagolytic agents have been investigated as medications to be used for premedication because of the ability to reduce vagal-induced bradycardia and to decrease oral secretions. Both atropine and glycopyrrolate have been shown to be effective in preventing vagal bradycardia during endotracheal intubation in neonates.[48,49]

Muscle relaxation is another component of optimizing intubation conditions. The intended effect is primarily to decrease patient movement, allowing the provider to have a more controlled field for visualization. The secondary effect of neuromuscular blockade is a decrease in intracranial pressure.[50,51] These medications act at the end plate of the neuromuscular junction to block transmission between motor nerve endings, causing paralysis of the skeletal muscles to facilitate endotracheal intubation. Neuromuscular blockers can be classified as nondepolarizing (atracurium, mivacurium, vecuronium, rocuronium, and pancuronium) and depolarizing (succinylcholine). Succinylcholine should be approached with caution in patients with hyperkalemia or a family history of malignant hyperthermia.

It is recommended to use premedication for nonurgent neonatal intubations, including analgesic agents or an anesthetic dose of hypnotic drugs. Vagolytic agents and rapid-onset muscle relaxants should be considered. Use of sedatives alone such as benzodiazepines without analgesics should be avoided, and muscle relaxants should be given only after an analgesic agent has been used (Table 38.3).

Selection and Placement of the Endotracheal Tube

The anatomy and dimensions of the neonatal airway differ from those of the adult. Historically, the neonatal airway has been described as being conical in the anterior-posterior (AP) dimension, with the cricoid ring being the narrowest portion of the airway and circular in the transverse dimension. More recent studies utilizing advanced airway imaging such as magnetic resonance and computed tomography in sedated as well as spontaneously breathing subjects have found that the airway of a neonate is in fact elliptical in the transverse dimension, with the larynx most closely resembling a cylinder in the AP dimension. The smallest part of the airway is at the level of the vocal cords and subvocal cords.[52,53] These differences raise legitimate questions regarding our choices of endotracheal tubes that are used during an operation. An appropriately sized uncuffed endotracheal tube will have a leak as the circular tube is inserted into an elliptical airway. It is likely, given the anatomy of the airway, that a tube with no leak may be placing excess pressure on the lateral walls of the airway.

This problem is not fully solved with the use of a cuffed tube, as a cuffed tube may still not prevent an air leak from occurring, although the pressure exerted on the lateral walls may be lessened. Advantages to using a cuffed endotracheal tube include more consistent sealing of the airway, thus providing (1) accuracy in quantitative measurements of ventilation, (2) prevention of aspiration of gastric contents into the lungs, and (3) accurate end-tidal carbon dioxide monitoring.[48] However, hesitation occurs frequently on the part of the neonatal provider in utilizing a cuffed endotracheal tube owing to concerns

TABLE 38.3 Medications for Elective Intubation

Drug	Dose (IV)	Onset of Action	Common Adverse Effects
Analgesic			
Fentanyl	1–4 μg/kg	Almost immediate	Apnea, hypotension, CNS depression, chest wall rigidity—give slowly
Remifentanil	1–3 μg/kg	Almost immediate	Apnea, hypotension, CNS depression, chest wall rigidity
Morphine	0.05–0.1 mg/kg	5–15 minutes	Apnea, hypotension, CNS depression
Hypnotic/Sedative			
Midazolam	0.05–0.1 mg/kg	5–10 minutes	Apnea, hypotension, CNS depression
Propofol	2.5 mg/kg	30 seconds to 10 minutes	Histamine release Apnea Bronchospasm Bradycardia
Muscle Relaxant			
Pancuronium	0.05–0.1 mg/kg	1–3 minutes	Hypertension Tachycardia Bronchospasm Salivation
Vecuronium	0.1 mg/kg	2–3 minutes	Hypertension/ hypotension Tachycardia Bronchospasm Arrhythmias
Rocuronium	0.6–1.2 mg/kg	1–2 minutes	Hypertension/ hypotension Tachycardia Bronchospasm Arrhythmias
Vagolytic			
Atropine	0.02 mg/kg	1–2 minutes	Dry hot skin Tachycardia
Glycopyrrolate	4–10 μg/kg	1–10 minutes	Dry hot skin Tachycardia

CNS, Central nervous system; *IV*, intravenous.

including excess cuff pressure placed on the developing airway, as well as the size of the tube, as a smaller tube may inhibit suctioning and increase airway resistance. Studies of cuffed versus uncuffed endotracheal tubes have not demonstrated increased postextubation stridor in subjects with a cuffed endotracheal tube.[54,55] The elliptical anatomy suggests that pressure exerted on the airway is likely to be higher in those who are intubated with an uncuffed endotracheal tube.

A cuffed endotracheal tube may be considered in larger newborns, as there is less impact on ventilation and oxygenation from airway resistance related to tube size in infants of term or near-term size. However, in growth-restricted infants or infants born prematurely, a cuffed tube may be too large for the airway. In the case of premature infants, an uncuffed tube may be used

while recognizing that ventilation and oxygenation may be a challenge and quantitative end-tidal carbon dioxide monitoring is inaccurate in the setting of substantial air leak. This strategy may require transcutaneous or blood gas measurement of carbon dioxide.

Identification of the correct depth of insertion of the endotracheal tube can also be a challenge. The "7-8-9 rule" is widely used within neonatology and endorsed by the American Academy of Pediatrics and the Neonatal Resuscitation Program. This rule entails adding the infant's weight in kilograms to 6, resulting in the appropriate depth in centimeters from the tip of the tube to the vermilion border of the lips. This formula has been found to be particularly inaccurate in infants weighing under 750 g, although the accuracy improves as birth weight increases.[56] The risks of inappropriate tube depth include accidental extubation if too shallow, as well as barotrauma/volutrauma, pneumothorax, and poor ventilation if too deep. Methods of assessing adequate depth, such as auscultating bilateral breath sounds, have been found to be inaccurate in 30% of subjects, the majority of which were infants and children.[57] Alternative approaches have been suggested, and one that has been successful has been utilizing the distance between the base of the nasal septum and the tip of the tragus to estimate tube depth. In this method the appropriate depth of the tube when secured at the lip is equivalent to the nasal-tragus length +1.[58-60] When used in the study setting, this method was more than 90% accurate. We recommend that consideration be given to utilizing nasal-tragus length as a method of estimating tube depth, particularly in those infants of under 750 g in which the "7-8-9 rule" may not be as accurate (Fig. 38.2). Some institutions intubate surgical babies in the NICU and confirm placement with a chest x-ray before transport to the operating room. This strategy may improve safety and efficiency once the final confirmation of the surgical case has occurred.

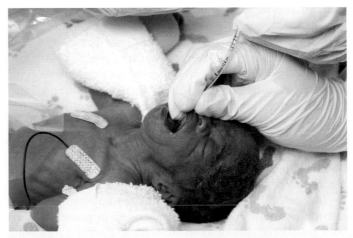

Fig. 38.2 Recently intubated newborn. Note the delicate handling of the patient and the endotracheal tube. While waiting for the endotracheal tube to be secured, the proceduralist holds the endotracheal tube against the patient's hard palate. This will reduce the likelihood of tube displacement.

OPERATIVE MANAGEMENT

The ventilator aspects of operative management of a neonate can be subdivided into three distinct domains. The first is selection of appropriate mode of ventilation. The second is that of vital sign monitoring, including respiratory rate, heart rate, blood pressure, and oxygen saturation as well as periodic measurements of blood pH and carbon dioxide levels. Finally, consideration must be given to ongoing operative ventilation management and troubleshooting.

Ventilator Mode

A myriad of ventilator modes are available. This is another opportunity to resist the temptation to simply apply adult principles to newborns. Effective intraoperative ventilator management is optimal when the neonatal patient is recognized as requiring specific strategies to safely support the patient through the operation but also reduces the risk of ventilator- or oxygen-associated lung injury. Historically, pressure-controlled ventilation was used in NICUs because it was the only type of ventilation available. As ventilators evolved, volume-targeted, pressure-controlled ventilation was demonstrated to decrease morbidities such as pneumothorax and intracranial hemorrhage among premature neonates.[61,62] This technology has become widely used within the NICU.

For most commercially available patient ventilators, the lowest set tidal volume is 2.5 to 3 mL. If these target tidal volumes are used for our smallest patients (e.g., <500 g), the patient may be exposed to volutrauma as the milliliters per kilogram per breath may exceed the typical target of 4 to 6 mL/kg for infants with respiratory distress syndrome. The performance characteristics of many ventilators may make volume-targeted, pressure-controlled ventilation a challenge in patients who weigh less than 500 g. Additionally, these ventilators may be found only in the NICU and not be available in the operating room. This reason alone may lead to performing a procedure in the NICU rather than the operating theater or bringing the mechanical ventilator from the NICU to the operating room.

If volume-targeted, pressure-controlled ventilation cannot be used, pressure-controlled ventilation may be used while monitoring "in-line" exhaled tidal volumes and adjusting both the PEEP and the peak inflation pressure to deliver 4- to 6-mL/kg tidal volumes where appropriate. Hyperventilation from excess minute ventilation may result in hypocarbia, a risk factor for white matter injury and neurodevelopmental impairment, especially in

very low birth weight (VLBW) infants.[63,64] Providing prolonged manual ventilation ("hand bagging") of the neonate should be avoided owing to the great variability in rate, peak inspiratory pressure, PEEP, and tidal volumes delivered.

There has been increasing suggestion that neonates may not need to be intubated and mechanically ventilated for all procedures. A prime example of this is the performance of laser surgery for retinopathy of prematurity while maintaining neonates on continuous positive airway pressure only or with the use of a laryngeal mask airway. Although there is appeal in the less invasive nature of this approach to decrease ventilator-induced lung injury, there is insufficient evidence to recommend this strategy routinely. However, in time, noninvasive ventilatory support during less complex operative procedures may become more common.

Vital Signs

The set mandatory rate of mechanical breaths for a sedated and paralyzed neonate may range anywhere from 35 to 75 inflations per minute, depending on severity and type of lung disease, degree of pulmonary insufficiency, and gestational age. The preoperative briefing and evaluation are vital for determining the infant's respiratory support requirements.

The patient's heart rate and blood pressure parameters require frequent monitoring throughout the case. Although both may vary because of the ongoing operation, changes in oxygenation and ventilation status may affect each other as well. Blood pressures may trend downward if the ventilator mean airway pressures remain too high, thus limiting venous return to the heart. Systemic vasodilation and hypotension may also occur as a side effect of anesthetic medications. The heart rate may become quite elevated if the patient is uncomfortable because of inadequate analgesia, sedation, or ventilation.

Of particular importance in the premature neonate is recognition of hyperoxia and the adverse effects of prolonged exposure to hyperoxia. Neonatologists have long recognized that newborn infants exposed to excess oxygen are at higher risk for retinopathy of prematurity (the leading cause of blindness in the premature population) and chronic lung disease. Prolonged exposure of the developing neonatal lungs, brain, and eyes to oxygen free radicals may result in damage to the developing vasculature and tissue of the respective organ systems. The field of neonatology has focused on identifying the optimal amount of oxygen to provide adequate oxygen delivery in premature neonates while recognizing a higher risk of morbidity related to excess oxygen exposure. Evidence suggesting that consistent exposure to higher oxygen saturations led to an increased risk of retinopathy of prematurity[60] resulted in the adoption of lower oxygen saturation limits (i.e., 85%–92%) in many NICUs. However, a meta-analysis of three international trials (Surfactant, Positive Pressure, and Pulse Oximetry Randomized Trial [SUPPORT], Benefits of Oxygen Saturation Targeting [BOOST II], and Canadian Oxygen Trial [COT]) concluded that, while targeting a lower oxygen saturation limit did reduce the risk of retinopathy of prematurity, it increased the risk of necrotizing enterocolitis and death. The authors concluded that a target oxygen saturation of 90% to 95% should be used.[65] This sentiment has been supported by expert opinion.[66,67] It would stand to reason that these saturation targets would be equally appropriate during operative interventions in an effort to avoid prolonged periods of hyperoxia while delivering adequate oxygen content to the developing tissues. Because of this, it is of utmost importance that an oxygen blender is available in the operating room as well as in transport to and from that location. The preoperative briefing should include the oxygen saturation range goal used in the NICU, and that goal range should be maintained throughout the procedure, promoting consistency in care between the NICU and the operating room. Exposure to hyperoxia during surgery may have little recognized morbidity in older patients, but in neonates, it may contribute to an already higher risk of long-term morbidity.

In an attempt to mitigate morbidities such as BPD, permissive hypercarbia increases the efficiency of carbon dioxide removal,[68] improves ventilation-perfusion matching in the lung,[69] and potentially increases respiratory drive, resulting in less apnea,[70] of which premature infants already have a higher risk. Previous studies in neonates have indicated that this strategy may reduce the risk of death or BPD and reduce mechanical ventilation days overall.[71-74] This strategy tolerates higher serum carbon dioxide values and lower serum pH values to reduce exposure of the neonatal lung to barotrauma/volutrauma as a result of aggressive mechanical ventilation.[68] The details of ranges tolerated may be unit specific but may incorporate tolerating arterial CO_2 levels of up to 65 mm Hg and pH of 7.25 to 7.35 (see Chapter 21).

End-tidal carbon dioxide measurements may be inaccurate in premature infants, particularly those with an uncuffed endotracheal tube and air leaks. The anesthetist may wish to trial the use of an end-tidal or transcutaneous carbon dioxide detector, but correlation should be made with arterial or capillary values, particularly when the PCO_2 value shown appears out of target range or appears to be varying considerably throughout the procedure. End-tidal carbon dioxide detectors also add additional dead space to the ventilator circuit, which may hamper effective ventilation of premature infants. Hypocarbia (CO_2 values <35 mm Hg) during the operation should also be avoided as prolonged exposure to hypocarbia can result in cerebral vasoconstriction and has been shown to have an impact on the risk of neurodevelopmental impairments such as cerebral palsy, especially in VLBW infants.[63,64]

Intraoperative Fluid Management and Electrolyte Management

Appropriate IV fluid administration among ill neonates, particularly those who are premature, is a key management tactic that influences all other areas of management. Exposing critically ill neonates to excess fluid can result in volume overload, which causes significant capillary leak, particularly in the lungs, and in worsening of respiratory distress. Providing too little IV fluid can result in hypovolemia, manifested as tachycardia, poor urine output, acute kidney injury, acidosis, and hypotension. Several factors are taken into consideration when selecting the typical daily IV fluid prescription for each neonate. These factors include gestational age,

postnatal day, current weight, postnatal growth, urine output, vital sign parameters, ventilatory requirements, and oxygen requirements. In an otherwise well infant undergoing a routine procedure (i.e., herniorrhaphy, etc.) during which fluid resuscitation is not expected, it could be considered prudent of the anesthetist to leave the neonate on the IV fluids prescribed by the neonatologist, as that volume is probably adequate for needs. If the infant does require a fluid bolus (e.g., because of hypotension as a result of anesthesia induction) a small (10 mL/kg) bolus of normal saline or lactated Ringer solution could be given. This can be repeated if no improvement is seen. In preterm infants in the first week of life, rapid infusion of IV fluid should be avoided because a rapid increase in blood pressure may increase the risk of intracranial hemorrhage. Care should also be taken not to expose the neonate to excess IV fluid when unneeded. Placing a peripheral IV tube and running TKO ("to keep open") fluids at 2 mL/h may be common in older children, but that rate of fluid can add up to a great deal of fluids in proportion to a neonate's body mass. Depending on institutional practice, peripheral IVs may be saline-locked when not in use or run at a lower rate (e.g., 1 mL/h).

In a more critically ill neonate, undergoing a procedure such as an abdominal laparotomy or cardiac surgery, during which consistent fluid resuscitation is expected, it may be indicated to continue the IV fluids with which the patient arrives at the operating room. However, through the course of the operation, events may arise that require discontinuation of fluids owing to their content (i.e., potassium-containing maintenance IV fluids or total parenteral nutrition). In this event, it is imperative that the anesthesia team recognize that any new fluids used must contain an adequate amount of dextrose to maintain euglycemia. If dextrose concentration is changed during the procedure, the anesthetist should regularly check blood glucose values so that unrecognized hypoglycemia does not occur.

There are several electrolyte abnormalities that may be observed in neonates in the intensive care and operating room setting. The provider may correctly anticipate these findings based on risk factor assessment and respond appropriately (Table 38.4).

KEY POINTS

- Volume-targeted, pressure-controlled ventilation is preferable when the weight of the patient allows for accurate volume delivery.
- Operative ventilatory strategy for premature neonates should include strict avoidance of hyperoxia and hypocarbia and may incorporate permissive hypercarbia.
- End-tidal carbon dioxide measurements should be correlated with arterial or capillary values in neonates with uncuffed endotracheal tubes.
- Intraoperative ventilation of the neonate is best provided by a mechanical ventilator for consistent and accurate volume delivery.
- IV fluids should be provided cautiously and with recognition of the risk of fluid overload in neonates.

TABLE 38.4 Electrolyte Imbalances

	Risk Factor(s)	Intervention
Glucose		
Hypoglycemia	Infant of a diabetic mother	200 mg/kg (2 mL/kg D10W) infusion and increase basal glucose infusion rate
	Small for gestational age	
	Sepsis	
	Insufficient glucose infusion rate in maintenance fluids	
Hyperglycemia	Surgical stress	Examine current glucose infusion rate to determine if it could be decreased. If glucose infusion rate is ≤4 mg/kg/min, consider insulin infusion
	Corticosteroid therapy	
Calcium		
Hypocalcemia	Prematurity	Calcium chloride (10–20 mg/kg) or calcium gluconate (100–200 mg/kg)
	Small or large for gestational age	
	DiGeorge syndrome	Note: Should be given through central venous access[a]
Sodium		
Hyponatremia	Excess free water administration	Examine current fluid infusion rate. Determine if maintenance fluid rate could be decreased
Hypernatremia	Dehydration	Examine current fluid infusion rate. Determine if maintenance fluid rate could be increased
Potassium		
Hypokalemia	Furosemide	Consider potassium chloride infusion (1 mEq/kg)
Hyperkalemia	Prematurity	Examine intravenous fluid composition and remove potassium. Consider calcium (above), sodium bicarbonate (1 mEq/kg), and insulin infusion if hyperkalemia persists

[a]D10W, 10% dextrose water.

TABLE 38.5 Hypothermia

Causes	Treatment Considerations
Cold exposure	Maintain operating room temperature between 27° C and 29° C
	Warm blankets
	Radiant heaters
	Warming mattresses
	Forced-air patient warming devices (e.g., 3M Bair Hugger)
	Frequent intraoperative core temperature monitoring (bladder, esophageal, rectal)
Skin preparation with cold solutions	Consider warming antiseptic solutions before application
Infusion of cold intravenous solutions	Warm intravenous fluids
Irrigation of wounds with cold solution	Warm irrigation fluids before instillation
Dry gases through mechanical ventilation circuit	Heated and humidified gases

ADDITIONAL OPERATIVE CONSIDERATIONS

Troubleshooting

Sudden, unexplained decompensation of the neonatal patient during surgery should lead the anesthetist to the DOPE mnemonic. Tube **d**isplacement is the most likely complication in this situation. Given the small length of airway available in the neonate, it would take a minimal change in depth to cause either a main stem intubation or extubation. In a surgery such as CDH repair, in which tracheal position may change throughout the procedure, this potential complication may arise. Tube depth should be evaluated as well as capnography and potentially direct visualization via laryngoscopy. Tube **o**bstruction is a potential problem given the small size of endotracheal tube often used in neonates, particularly those preterm. The tube should be suctioned carefully to evaluate for excessive secretions or plugging. An acute **p**neumothorax is less likely but certainly a potential problem if the patient has had a main stem intubation or has been requiring higher peak inflation pressures during the procedure (an indication intraoperatively that the tube may have been at the carina). Finally, faulty **e**quipment should be evaluated by removing the infant from the ventilator and hand bagging. Again, care should be taken not to expose the infant to excess pressure or volume during manual ventilation.

Temperature Regulation

Neonates are prone to heat loss because of their large body surface area-to-mass ratio and limited subcutaneous fat. They lose heat by radiation, conduction, convection, and evaporation. The operating room environment may also increase convection heat loss as room air exchange rates are typically greater than in the NICU setting. Anesthetic medication administration also reduces the threshold for vasoconstriction and further exacerbates risk of hypothermia.[75] Hypothermia leads to increased oxygen and glucose consumption, inadequate oxygen delivery, hypoventilation, apnea, acidosis, and, if untreated, cardiovascular collapse. Sources of cold stress and management considerations are noted in Table 38.5.

Neonate Pain Perception

Although an extensive presentation of intraoperative anesthetic management is beyond the scope of this textbook, commonly used medications are listed in Table 38.6. Providers should be mindful that any neonate who will undergo surgical intervention is capable of feeling pain irrespective of gestational age. Poor pain control may lead to an increase in morbidity and mortality as well as potentially life-altering longitudinal complications for the newborn, including intraventricular hemorrhage and subsequent sequelae. Operative management may be complicated by inadequate pain control including acute onset of pulmonary hypertension, systemic hypertension, and exaggerated stress responses. Validated and standardized pain assessment tools are widely available.[76-78] Each institution should select one instrument to

TABLE 38.6 Intravenous Anesthetic Drugs for the Neonate: Dosages

Anesthetic Agents	Premedication (mg/kg)	Induction (mg/kg)	Maintenance (μg/kg)	Intubation (mg/kg)	Reversal (mg/kg)
Anticholinergics					
Atropine	0.01–0.02				
Glycopyrrolate	0.005–0.01				
Hypnotics					
Propofol		2.5–3.0			
Thiopental		4–6			
Ketamine		0.5–2.0			
Midazolam		0.02–0.05			
Opioids					
Fentanyl		0.005–0.010	1–2 μg/kg/h		
Morphine		0.05–0.1	10–50 μg/kg/h		
Sufentanil		0.0001–0.0002	0.05–0.1 μg/kg/h		
Remifentanil		0.0001	1.5–3 μg/kg/min		
Muscle Relaxants					
Succinylcholine				1–2	
Pancuronium				0.05–0.1	
Vecuronium				0.1–0.15	
Rocuronium				0.8–1.2	
Anticholinesterases					
Neostigmine					0.05–0.08
Pyridostigmine					0.02–0.03
Narcotic Antagonist					
Naloxone					0.005–0.01

facilitate appropriate evaluation and management of intraoperative and postoperative pain.

CONCLUSION

Delivering safe and effective mechanical ventilation for neonates requiring surgery is an important aspect of operative care. It is important to understand the unique physiology, stages of lung development, and anatomic considerations for neonatal patients. Use of neonatal-specific devices and application of lung-protective strategies intraoperatively will help providers achieve optimal outcomes.

A complete reference list is available at https://expertconsult. inkling.com/.

KEY REFERENCES

3. Wyckoff MH, Aziz K, Escobedo MB, et al: Part 13: neonatal resuscitation: 2015 American Heart Association guidelines update for cardiopulmonary resuscitation and emergency cardiovascular care. Circulation 132:S543–S560, 2015.

5. Mirza H, Ziegler J, Ford S, et al: Pulmonary hypertension in preterm infants: prevalence and association with bronchopulmonary dysplasia. J Pediatr 165:909–914.e1, 2014.

8. Ameis D, Khoshgoo N, Keijzer R, et al: Abnormal lung development in congenital diaphragmatic hernia. Semin Pediatr Surg 26(3): 123–128, 2017.

27. Mallick MS, Jado AM, Al-Bassam AR: Surgical procedures performed in the neonatal intensive care unit on critically ill neonates: feasibility and safety. Ann Saudi Med 28:105–108, 2008.

29. Lee LK, Woodfin MY, Vardi MG, et al: A comparison of postoperative outcomes with PDA ligation in the OR versus the NICU: a retrospective cohort study on the risks of transport. BMC Anesthesiol 18:199, 2018.

31. Kumar P, Denson SE, Mancuso TJ: Premedication for nonemergency endotracheal intubation in the neonate. Pediatrics 125: 608–615, 2010.

38. Saarenmaa E, Neuvonen PJ, Fellman V: Gestational age and birth weight effects on plasma clearance of fentanyl in newborn infants. J Pediatr 136:767–770, 2000.

61. Peng W, Zhu H, Shi H, et al: Volume-targeted ventilation is more suitable than pressure-limited ventilation for preterm infants: a systematic review and meta-analysis. Arch Dis Child Fetal Neonatal Ed 99:F158–F165, 2014.

70. Sinclair SE, Kregenow DA, Starr I, et al: Therapeutic hypercapnia and ventilation-perfusion matching in acute lung injury: low minute ventilation vs inspired CO_2. Chest 130:85–92, 2006.

76. Sessler D: Perioperative thermoregulation and heat balance. Lancet 387(10038):2655–2664, 2016.

Complications of Respiratory Support

Lakshmi Katakam

KEY POINTS

- Many forms of invasive and noninvasive ventilatory strategies are commonly used to support critically ill neonates in the neonatal intensive care unit. Although life saving, many of these strategies have important complications associated with them.
- The benefits of mechanical ventilation such as improvement in gas exchange are often immediately evident to the clinician. However, lung injury and other adverse effects (including adverse effects on nonrespiratory organs) resulting from mechanical ventilation and other forms of respiratory support are not as easily evident and often not detected by bedside monitoring methods.
- In providing respiratory support to neonatal patients, clinicians should not only ensure optimal gas exchange and oxygen delivery to the tissues but also minimize and eliminate preventable complications of respiratory support.
- In general, complications of respiratory support and lung injury can be decreased by using less invasive forms of respiratory support, use of the lowest possible settings on mechanical ventilation ("gentle ventilation"), early extubation, high compliance with known preventive measures, close monitoring for complications, and early intervention when complications are detected.

COMPLICATIONS OF RESPIRATORY SUPPORT

Neonates requiring intensive care often require respiratory support in varying forms throughout their hospitalization. Although a number of different invasive and noninvasive modes of respiratory support are commonly used in the neonatal intensive care unit (NICU) as life-saving therapies, each modality has benefits and complications associated with it that need careful consideration (Table 39.1).

MECHANICAL VENTILATION

Mechanical ventilation continues to be an essential therapy in the respiratory care of critically ill neonates. Although the benefits of mechanical ventilation such as decreased mortality and improvement in gas exchange are easily evident, the associated complications, such as lung injury and development of bronchopulmonary

dysplasia (BPD), and the subsequent impact on neurodevelopmental outcomes are not immediately evident.

ENDOTRACHEAL INTUBATION

Mechanical ventilation is often provided via placement of an endotracheal tube in neonates. The procedure of endotracheal intubation itself is associated with several complications. Single-center observational studies have reported adverse event rates ranging from 22% to 39% among infants undergoing endotracheal intubation in the NICU.[1,2] Most commonly reported events include oxygen desaturation, misplacement of the endotracheal tube, and airway trauma or bleeding.[2] Although endotracheal intubation is considered a complex task with interplay between provider technical skills, team behavioral skills, and patient characteristics, adverse events related to the procedure have been minimized through quality improvement initiatives.[3] Premedication with neuromuscular blocking drugs is associated with a decrease in adverse events such as bradycardia and desaturations and increase in intubation success rate.[4] Use of video laryngoscope is associated with higher intubation success rate but does not impact adverse events such as bradycardia and desaturations.[5,6] Larger clinical trials could inform on the role of premedication and video laryngoscopy in improving intubation safety in neonates. Stylet use is common among providers in United States and thought to be associated with complications such as airway bleeding, tracheal perforation, and dislodgement of the tube but no clear evidence on the frequency of these adverse events and the strength of association.[7] In general, the risk of adverse events seems to increase with increasing number of intubation attempts and with emergent intubations rather than elective intubations.[2]

UNPLANNED EXTUBATION

Unplanned extubation (UE) is commonly defined as an unintentional dislodgement or removal of endotracheal tube from the trachea of an intubated patient. Among the pediatric population, these unplanned events have been associated with significant patient harm, including cardiac arrest and increase in length of hospitalization and health care costs. The event frequency is typically measured per 100 ventilator days and reported to range from 0.6 to 4.5 UEs per 100 ventilator days among NICU patients.[8]

Neonates are thought to be particularly vulnerable to UEs compared with older pediatric patients because of challenges related to airway securement, longer duration of mechanical ventilation, lack of routine use of sedatives for intubated patients, and nature of NICU care that involves transfer of patient in and out of bed for procedures and kangaroo care.[8] However, despite these unique challenges related to patients in the NICU, many centers report reductions in UE rates with use of quality improvement methodology and creation of standardized bundles of respiratory care practices aimed at safe airway maintenance in intubated patients.[8-11]

VENTILATOR-INDUCED LUNG INJURY

Although mechanical ventilation is often a life-saving therapy in preterm and term infants with respiratory failure, use of ventilators has also been associated with important adverse effects on a number of organ systems including the brain and lungs. Complications such as air leak syndromes from ventilator-related trauma still occur in the postsurfactant era.[12] The deleterious effects of mechanical ventilation on healthy and diseased lungs were recognized first when specific patterns of lung pathology were seen on postmortem evaluation of mechanically ventilated adult patients.[13] Ventilator-induced lung injury (VILI) has been identified in adults with acute respiratory distress syndrome (ARDS) after recognizing a decrease in mortality associated with have decrease risk of mortality when strategies to minimize lung injury were employed.[13] More recently, the significance of VILI among preterm infants is gaining awareness and is being taken into consideration when determining optimal ventilatory strategies for this vulnerable population.[14-17]

The most commonly recognized mechanisms of VILI include volutrauma, barotrauma, atelectotrauma, and biotrauma.[13,14] Volutrauma is injury that results from overdistension of the lungs because of delivering excessive tidal volume, while barotrauma is injury that results from delivery of excessive pressure and corresponding high lung volumes, and atelectotrauma is caused by shear stress from repeated alveolar collapse and reexpansion. Disruption of alveolar lining that results from this type of stretching of lung tissue in turn initiates an inflammatory cascade that results in activation of macrophages and neutrophils, causing the type of injury referred to as biotrauma.[13] Although they may seem to be distinct mechanisms, lung injury is multifactorial and has varying degrees of contributions from each of these types of VILI.

The best way to prevent VILI is to reduce the use of invasive ventilation when possible, use volume-targeted ventilation with small tidal volumes, and wean promptly from the ventilator. Because mechanical ventilation continues to be a frequently used therapy for many preterm infants, steps can be taken to minimize VILI by using specific ventilatory strategies aimed to reduce lung injury. Although many modes of ventilation are

available for use in the NICU, volume-targeted ventilation may be a gentler mode of ventilation for preterm infants if low tidal volumes are used.[14] In volume-targeted ventilation, the ventilator adjusts inflation pressure as needed based on lung compliance to deliver a prespecified tidal volume. Therefore, a lower inflation pressure is delivered to the infant when lung compliance improves to achieve targeted tidal volume and minute ventilation. By automatically adjusting the pressure delivered to maintain tidal volume in a safe range, inadvertent over distension and under expansion of the lungs can be avoided, minimizing risk of volutrauma, barotrauma, and atelectotrauma. A meta-analysis of 21 randomized controlled trials reported benefits including lower rates of BPD, severe intraventricular hemorrhage (IVH), periventricular leukomalacia, and pneumothorax as well as shorter duration of mechanical ventilation.[18] Although volume-targeted ventilation may be beneficial for many preterm infants, experts in neonatal respiratory care recommend choosing modalities of respiratory support based on each patient's underlying lung pathophysiology while being cognizant of the risk benefit balance between adequate gas exchange and lung injury.[19]

VENTILATOR-ASSOCIATED PNEUMONIA

Mechanically ventilated neonates are at increased risk for acquiring healthcare associated infections such as ventilator-associated pneumonia (VAP) because an endotracheal tube can serve as a portal of entry for pathogens colonizing the airway. VAP is a common complication in the intensive care setting and has been frequently studied and reported in adult and pediatric populations. However, the definition, incidence, and significance of this morbidity still remain unclear for the neonatal population. Most of the available evidence regarding VAPs in the NICU over the past decade is derived from observational studies and single-center experiences that are mostly from outside of United States.[20,21] In general, prematurity, low birth weight, and longer duration of mechanical ventilation are reported to be the most common risk factors for VAP in neonates.[22] It is difficult to estimate the true incidence of VAP in the NICU as a wide range of rates have been reported in literature. As expected, rates of suspected VAPs are higher than the rates of confirmed VAPs among neonates owing to the lack of standardized definition and unreliable diagnostic tools.[22] In the absence of neonatal-specific consensus definition and because of confounding factors such as chronic lung disease and atelectasis, using chest radiographs to diagnose VAP can be challenging. The role of diagnostic tools other than chest radiographs has been explored recently, and early results show the potential utility of lung ultrasound in diagnosing VAP.[23] However, it is necessary to estimate the sensitivity and specificity of this tool before a recommendation can be made regarding its role in the diagnosis of VAP. Despite these challenges, implementation of quality improvement methods and standardized protocols has been associated with a decrease in the incidence of VAP and the use of antimicrobials for treatment of VAP in the NICU setting.[22,23]

VENTILATOR-ASSOCIATED EVENTS AND VENTILATOR-ASSOCIATED CONDITIONS

Because of the challenges with reliably diagnosing ventilator associated pneumonia in patients of all age groups (complexity, subjectivity, limited correlation with outcomes, and incomplete capture of many important and morbid complications of mechanical ventilation), in recent years, expert panels have coined the terms ventilator-associated events (VAEs) and ventilator-associated conditions (VACs). In 2013, the US Centers for Disease Control and Prevention (CDC) started using the term *ventilator-associated event* instead of VAP for monitoring quality of care in ventilated adult patients. The definition for VAE was designed to overcome many of the limitations of VAP definitions. VAE definitions broadened the focus of surveillance from pneumonia alone to the syndrome of nosocomial complications in ventilated patients, as marked by sustained increases in ventilator settings after a period of stable or decreasing ventilator settings. VAE was defined by an increase in support (fraction of inspired oxygen or positive end expiratory pressure) in a mechanically ventilated patient who had been previously stable or improving, and was purposefully meant to be a more general and more objective measure of ventilator-associated complications than VAP. Most VAEs are caused by pneumonia, fluid overload, ARDS, and atelectasis. Not all clinically diagnosed VAPs meet VAE criteria. VAEs are associated in adult patients with a doubling of the risk of death compared to patients without VAEs and compared to patients who meet traditional VAP criteria. In neonates too, there is lack of a clear definition and diagnostic test for VAP in newborns. A definition specific to neonates that recognized their unique characteristics and the complexities of prematurity is not available. Diagnostic criteria promulgated by the CDC for infants under 1 year of age were also applied to neonates. After the CDC's National Healthcare Safety Network (NHSN) replaced surveillance for VAP in adult inpatient locations with surveillance for VAEs, it also stopped VAP surveillance in neonatal locations, leaving VAP surveillance only in pediatric areas. In 2019, NHSN implemented surveillance for pediatric VAEs, with a definition based on an increase in oxygen need or mean airway pressure that had been validated in both pediatric and neonatal patients.[8] Like its adult counterpart, the pediatric VAE measure was designed to capture infectious and noninfectious complications with more precision and objectivity than the previous VAP measure. Further research is required to develop reliable and useful definitions of VAE for neonatal patients for the purpose of surveillance, and definitions of VAP for clinical practice.

NONINVASIVE RESPIRATORY SUPPORT

Over the past three decades, there have been numerous efforts to decrease the rate of BPD by minimizing exposure to mechanical ventilation and using noninvasive respiratory support. With a significant increase in the use of noninvasive respiratory support[24] came an increased recognition of complications resulting from it, such as nasal injury, gastric distension, and air leak syndromes.[25]

Continuous Positive Airway Pressure

Continuous positive airway pressure (CPAP) is used as primary mode of respiratory support for many preterm infants, initiated in the delivery room during resuscitation, and continued in the NICU for maintenance of functional residual capacity (FRC).[26,27] CPAP is an effective alternative to intubation and surfactant administration in preterm infants and is associated with a decrease in the composite outcome of chronic lung disease or death.[28] However, nasal trauma or injury is one of the complications of noninvasive respiratory support and seems to be primarily related to the interface used to deliver pressure. Many interfaces to deliver CPAP are available, and they have variable degrees of effectiveness in delivering positive pressure.[29] It is unclear at this time how the various interfaces compare to each other in terms of causing or preventing nasal injury. The majority of interfaces used to delivery CPAP in the NICU can be divided into two general categories, binasal prongs and nasal masks. Multiple meta-analyses have compared the safety and effectiveness of these two categories of interfaces and found the risk of nasal injury to be lower when CPAP is delivered via nasal mask compared to binasal prongs.[30,31] In addition, CPAP delivered via nasal mask has also been associated with lower rates of nasal injury when compared to the strategy of rotating interfaces in a randomized clinical trial.[32] When bubble CPAP was compared with other forms of CPAP, a higher rate of nasal injury was noted in a meta-analysis that assessed data from nine studies.[33]

Although CPAP has been associated with increase in risk of pneumothorax, CPAP use in the delivery room has not resulted in an increased risk of air leak syndromes when compared to intubation and prophylactic surfactant delivery in preterm infants.[28] However, delivery room practices have evolved over time to increasing utilization of CPAP not only among preterm infants but also in term and near term infants.[34] The complication profile may be different in these larger infants based on limited evidence from observational studies, noting an increase in risk of pneumothorax.[34,35]

High-Flow Nasal Cannula

High-flow nasal cannula (HFNC) is also a commonly used mode of noninvasive respiratory support for preterm infants and has been compared to CPAP for effectiveness and safety. In a recent meta-analysis of 21 randomized controlled trials and 2886 patients, HFNC has been associated with significantly lower rates of nasal trauma and pneumothorax when compared to CPAP for primary respiratory support or postextubation respiratory support in preterm infants.[36] However, randomized controlled trials have shown that HFNC is inferior to CPAP in avoiding escalation of respiratory support when used for treatment of respiratory treatment in preterm infants.[37,38]

Positive Pressure Ventilation

Providing effective positive pressure ventilation (PPV) is one of the key tenants of neonatal resuscitation. Although it is common to use PPV in the delivery room to establish FRC, there are some important complications to take into consideration. Providers underestimate tidal volumes and pressure delivered during bag mask ventilation.[39] Tidal volumes larger than 6 mL/kg inadvertently used for resuscitation increase the risk of IVH and severe IVH.[40] Furthermore, even a few large volume breaths given in the delivery room result in an inflammatory cascade of lung injury that can lead to BPD.[15,41]

Nasal Intermittent Positive Pressure Ventilation

Nasal intermittent PPV (NIPPV) has gained increased acceptance as a tool for providing noninvasive respiratory support and as a strategy for preventing need for mechanical ventilation in preterm infants. In a large randomized controlled trial, the rate of survival to 36 weeks of postmenstrual age without BPD is not different in extremely low birth weight infants treated with NIPPV versus those treated with CPAP as the type of noninvasive support in the first 4 weeks of life.[42] However, when used as postextubation support, NIPPV reduces extubation failure and the subsequent need for intubation in comparison to CPAP.[43] Although there have been reports of increased incidence of gastric distension, feeding intolerance, and intestinal perforations, meta-analyses do not show evidence of gastrointestinal side effects associated with postextubation use of NIPPV when compared to CPAP.[43] NIPPV during the first few days of birth reduces the need for intubation when compared to CPAP, without any increase in incidence of gastrointestinal complications such as necrotizing enterocolitis.[44]

Less Invasive Surfactant Administration

In an attempt to minimize side effects of intubation and mechanical ventilation, less invasive strategies for delivering surfactant for preterm infants with respiratory distress syndrome have been studied. There are numerous different techniques and types of catheters being studied to deliver surfactant to spontaneous breathing infants without using positive pressure breaths. Many of these techniques have been compared to the more traditional mechanisms of surfactant delivery via intubation and endotracheal tube placement. The evidence for efficacy of these less invasive techniques has been fast accruing and seems to be promising for benefits such as lower incidence of BPD and IVH and reduced

need for mechanical ventilation but is notable for short-term, transient side effects such as bradycardia, desaturations, and need for manual ventilation related to the procedure.[45,46] The use of less invasive surfactant administration (LISA) is widespread in Europe, Australia, and other countries and is increasing in the United States. Current ongoing clinical trials of LISA and other forms of noninvasive respiratory support should provide estimates of efficacy and safety upon which strong recommendations for clinical practice may eventually be made.

SUGGESTED READINGS

1. Foglia EE, et al: Factors associated with adverse events during tracheal intubation in the NICU. Neonatology 108(1):23–29, 2015.
2. Slutsky AS, Ranieri VM: Ventilator-induced lung injury. N Engl J Med 369(22):2126–2136, 2013.
3. Keszler M: Mechanical ventilation strategies. Semin Fetal Neonatal Med, 2017. 22(4):267–274.
4. Wiswell TE: Resuscitation in the delivery room: lung protection from the first breath. Respir Care 56(9):1360-1367, 2011. Discussion 1367–1368.
5. Dunn MS, et al: Randomized trial comparing 3 approaches to the initial respiratory management of preterm neonates. Pediatrics 128(5):e1069–e1076, 2011.
6. Finer NN, et al: Early CPAP versus surfactant in extremely preterm infants. N Engl J Med 362(21):1970–1979, 2010.
7. Klingenberg C, et al: Volume-targeted versus pressure-limited ventilation in neonates. Cochrane Database Syst Rev 10(10):CD003666, 2017.
8. Keszler M: Volume-targeted ventilation: one size does not fit all. Evidence-based recommendations for successful use. Arch Dis Child Fetal Neonatal Ed 104(1):F108–F112, 2019.
9. Björklund LJ, et al: Manual ventilation with a few large breaths at birth compromises the therapeutic effect of subsequent surfactant replacement in immature lambs. Pediatr Res 42(3): 348–355, 1997.
10. Kirpalani H, et al: A trial comparing noninvasive ventilation strategies in preterm infants. N Engl J Med 369(7):611–620, 2013.

Neonatal Respiratory Care in Resource-Limited Countries

Amuchou Soraisham and Nalini Singhal

KEY POINTS

- Neonatal respiratory care should be a comprehensive program based on local needs.
- The program should be built on the level of local expertise.
- There should be ongoing quality improvement activities based on local data and audits.
- Babies that require respiratory care should have long-term follow-up.

INTRODUCTION

The first chapter in this book describes the historical background of the development of neonatal ventilation in the Western world. Despite rapid growth in the developed countries, neonatal intensive care units (NICUs) have evolved more slowly in resource-limited countries during the last four decades. Multiple factors such as poor economy, lack of skilled personnel, lack of equipment, and failure to develop structured programs have been responsible for the delayed progress. Furthermore, countries with high infant and neonatal mortality rates (NMRs) have rightfully focused more on prevention of common public health issues, simple programs for resuscitation, and essential care of the newborn rather than establishing expensive NICUs with ventilator care facilities. However, in recent years, globalization has increased access to new medical knowledge and technology for many developing countries.[1] The twenty-first century will see rapid progression of neonatal ventilator care support in neonatal units around the world, although progress will be uneven. The Every Newborn Action Plan calls for an end to preventable newborn deaths.[2] To accomplish this goal, some babies will need the assistance of more advanced respiratory care including continuous positive airway pressure (CPAP) and ventilators.

In this chapter, we review the current status of NICUs in resource-limited countries, barriers to the development of respiratory care programs, and possible strategies to overcome these barriers and develop a functional respiratory care program appropriate to the region.

SCOPE OF THE NEED

High infant mortality rates (IMRs) and NMRs constitute major health problems in low- and middle-income countries. According to World Bank classification system in 2019, a country with a gross national income per capita of less than $1026 is classified as a low-income country and those with between $1026 and $3995 are considered as lower–middle-income countries.[3]

Globally, nearly 2.5 million babies die in the neonatal period (first month of life) and about 1 million newborns die within the first 24 hours.[4] Stillbirth accounted for another 2.5 million deaths yearly.[5] Most newborn deaths occur in low- and middle-income countries. Three causes accounted for more than 75% of neonatal mortality: complications of prematurity, intrapartum-related neonatal deaths (including birth asphyxia), and neonatal infections.

Complications of prematurity are the leading cause of all deaths under 5 years. Newborn resuscitation programs such as Helping Babies Breathe[6] have demonstrated a reduction in neonatal mortality.[7] Resuscitation training in resource-limited facilities can reduce intrapartum-related neonatal death by 30% and early neonatal death by 38%.[8] However, after newborn resuscitation, some newborns may require CPAP or assisted ventilation. An estimated 21% of babies presenting with illness in the first 6 days of life have respiratory symptoms that may require respiratory support.[9] In low- and lower middle-income countries, there is a need for neonatal programs equipped with proper respiratory equipment and trained personnel. Facilities need tools such as oxygen, bags and masks, and possibly CPAP to provide basic respiratory support. The higher-level care hospitals should have the capabilities of CPAP and mechanical ventilation. To provide CPAP and assisted ventilation, the health care facilities must be staffed by well-trained medical and nursing personnel.

Information about level II and III units in resource-limited countries is scanty. As expected, these countries have the highest IMRs and NMRs, and therefore, they have the greatest needs. For example, India, a country with an NMR of 23/1000 live births (2018)[10] and 25 million births/year, would require hundreds of level III and perhaps thousands of level II NICUs. It is estimated that in India, with approximately 1.35 billion people, one level III NICU with 30 beds is required for every 1 million population,[11] with additional level II health facilities. Ideally, to be effective, there should be a coordinated regional perinatal program that is responsible for the coordination of clinical activities, education, resource use, quality improvement, and development of evidence-based clinical pathways for best practices. Local data are necessary to plan effectively as demonstrated by variations in neonatal mortality in India that were mapped on a geospatial 5 km × 5 km grid.[12]

A parallel improvement in hospital-based prenatal and neonatal care is required for further reduction in NMR. Because respiratory compromise is common in all three important causes of neonatal mortality (prematurity, birth asphyxia, and neonatal infections), effective programs for managing respiratory distress could have major impacts.[13]

LIMITING FACTORS

The major barriers to developing regional respiratory care programs in resource-limited countries include limited infrastructure and availability of equipment, properly trained staff, quality improvement programs, and the absence of coordinated systems.[14-17] Health facilities in many resource-limited countries do not meet the basic needs of newborn care, such as provision of warmth, a clean environment, and breast milk. Yet ironically, some of these countries are beginning to open level III units in their district hospitals.[18] Some district-level hospitals are equipped with oxygen and suction; however, resuscitation bags and radiant warmers are often not present, and oxygen hoods are infrequently available.[19] Even when resuscitation bags are available, there is no system in place to clean and store them in an appropriate space. The primary health centers, each of which serve a population of 20,000 to 30,000 and provide basic maternity services, have practically no equipment. There is an urgent need to improve these deficiencies. Respiratory support is either limited to very few hospitals or is only available in the private sector and hence not accessible to most babies. There are several barriers to developing respiratory care services at all levels in resource-limited countries.[16,17] Some of these barriers are described here.

1. Respiratory care program barrier: There is a lack of structured comprehensive respiratory care programs with quality improvement. There are few or no policies or guidelines either for clinical care or maintenance of equipment. Even if equipment is said to be available, it is either not functioning or locked away.
2. Infrastructure: Appropriate physical infrastructure is lacking. The hospitals do not have properly designed intensive care units for adults, much less for newborns. Even in district and teaching hospitals, the space for the management of high-risk infants is arbitrarily allocated and may lack the basic requirements of running water, a consistent supply of electricity, and controlled environment with infection control. There are problems with maintaining a consistent supply of oxygen and/or compressed air. Some units depend on cylinders for air and oxygen. Maintenance of equipment is irregular at the best hospitals and nonexistent in most units.
3. Skilled health care personnel: There is a shortage of skilled medical and nursing staff in resource-limited countries. These limitations put constraints on patient care. Even if nurses are trained, they are assigned to different units, resulting in a constant turnover of staff. Physicians have to assume many responsibilities for which they are ill equipped; such as care of the ventilator. Most general pediatricians are not familiar with ventilator management. A few are able to manage mild cases

of respiratory distress with oxygen. For the most part, physicians are not trained to provide CPAP, endotracheal tube placement, or ventilation. Most NICUs are managed by general pediatricians who have a special interest or have had previous experience in assisted ventilation. Nurses and pediatricians in most resource-limited countries do not have similar degrees of training and proficiency in managing neonatal respiratory support as in developed countries.

Developing countries also face shortages of doctors and nursing staff because of widespread emigration of skilled health care personnel to the developed world, known euphemistically as the "Brain Drain."[20] Innovative programs are needed to retain skilled manpower in resource-limited countries.

4. Support equipment: Ancillary services such as blood gas machines, portable radiology machines, microchemistry laboratories, oxygen saturation monitors, and heart rate monitors are not available in most of the NICUs.

CURRENT STATUS

During the last quarter of the twentieth century, many resource-limited countries successfully developed a few model NICUs with outcomes comparable to that of the developed world. These unique programs were developed mainly through the efforts of committed individuals and concerted efforts of professional organizations. NICU development was complemented by the phenomenon of "globalization and diffusion of technology" during the last three decades.[1] It is recognized that the widespread implementation of low-cost, robust respiratory technologies (e.g., oxygen concentrators, oxygen saturation monitoring, bubble CPAP) could save the lives of many newborns admitted to facilities in resource-limited nations.[13] The evolution of neonatal intensive care and specifically respiratory care is described here in a few select regions of the world.

Asia
India

The development of neonatal intensive care in India has been slow because of constraints[21] such as the availability of required technology and skilled personnel. Economic constraints prevent the development of expensive high-technology NICUs in the country. Faced with high IMR and NMR, policymakers thought it prudent to invest in improving overall health rather than in high-technology medicine. The concept of providing good level II care for premature infants and low birth weight infants was well in place as early as the 1950s. Respiratory support was limited to providing oxygen in addition to providing thermal care and intravenous fluids. It was not until the mid-1970s and early 1980s that NICUs in India began to provide ventilator support. Even today, there are limited numbers of trained neonatologists and respiratory care is provided mostly by general pediatricians and family physicians.

A major impetus to the nationwide growth of neonatal intensive care and, therefore, neonatal ventilation in India came from the professional organization National Neonatology Forum (NNF) which was established in 1980.[22] NNF focused on developing policy guidelines and standardization of care (bedside monitoring, equipment use, evidence-based guidelines and assisted ventilation), designation of levels of care, and an accreditation process for neonatal and perinatal care in the country. The organization also placed a great emphasis on the education and training of pediatricians and nurses. Surveys by NNF demonstrated a gradual improvement in availability of equipment and trained staff.[21,23,24]

Over the past two decades, several neonatal units providing complete care with ventilatory capabilities have evolved, primarily in private settings. The results in these units managed by highly qualified staff are comparable to Western units at almost all birth weight groups (Table 40.1). In a recent survey of 70 neonatal units in India, there was significant progress in infrastructure, availability of equipment and trained manpower, supporting staff, and services.[25] The units had mechanical ventilators but very few had blood gas machines, in-house x-ray facilities, invasive blood pressure monitoring, and ophthalmology support. High-frequency ventilation to provide respiratory support is limited to a few centers. The progress in neonatal ventilation can be indirectly assessed by the number of ventilators purchased in the country. The number of ventilator purchases in India has been increasing at a steady rate of 3% to 4% per year. Based on the large number of births, high rates of birth asphyxia, low birth weight, and prematurely born infants (estimated 7% of births or 1.75 million/year), there is a greater need for further development of NICUs across the country. With nearly 548 special care newborn units in district hospitals, 1810 newborn stabilization units at subdistrict hospitals, and 0.9 million Accredited Social Health Activist workers in the community, the country is gearing up to face the enormous task of providing health care to 26 million neonates born each year.[26] Low-cost and innovative methods to provide respiratory support (such as bubble CPAP) short of mechanical ventilation at subdistrict and district hospitals are also being considered.[27] Recent reports suggest that CPAP is used commonly in neonatal units across government hospitals in India. About 68% of medical college hospitals and 36% of district hospitals used CPAP in neonates.[28] However, air-oxygen blenders were available in half of the units and staff trained in the use of CPAP were present in more than half of these units.

Some privately run NICUs in India meet all the international standards in space, equipment, and skilled medical and nursing staff. A few of these hospitals in the developing countries have been accredited by The Joint Commission.[29] The high cost of care in these hospitals precludes access by the majority of the country's population.

Other Countries

Bhutta et al.[30] reported an encouraging experience in Pakistan. The provision of ventilator support to infants with respiratory distress syndrome (RDS) in Pakistan resulted in increased survival, specifically in infants weighing more than 1000 g. The authors concluded that respiratory care can be developed in selected hospitals to successfully manage neonates with RDS. A recent study from Pakistan reported successful use of bubble CPAP for the management of RDS in preterm neonates with 64% success. Birth weight under 1500 g and typical finding of RDS on x-ray were associated with CPAP failure and required mechanical ventilation.[31]

With the establishment of NICUs, Ho and Chang[32] from Malaysia reported that the survival of all very low birth weight (VLBW) infants improved from 69% in year 1993 to 81% in year 2003; among ventilated infants, survival improved from 53% to 93%. Interestingly, there was no significant improvement in nonventilated babies, suggesting that neonatal ventilation significantly contributed to increased survival among VLBW infants.

Africa

Malawi has the highest rate of preterm births in the world: 18.1% of all newborns in Malawi are born prematurely, with high NMR.[33] The current standard of care in Malawi for babies with any type of respiratory difficulty is nasal oxygen therapy. However, the use of bubble CPAP to treat babies with RDS resulted in 27% absolute improvement in survival to discharge.[34] Only 24% of neonates with RDS treated with nasal oxygen survived to discharge as compared to 65% receiving bubble CPAP. Introduction of CPAP in Fiji was associated with a 50% reduction in need for mechanical ventilation, thereby demonstrating that CPAP for resource-limited settings may be a viable option to decrease neonatal mortality.[35] Moreover, the staff nurses were able to safely apply bubble CPAP after 1–2 months of training.[36]

Latin America

Latin America has high IMR and NMR, with significant disparities among the countries. In some Latin American countries

TABLE 40.1 Neonatal Survival Rates by Birth Weight Category in 1990, 1995, 2010, 2014, and 2019 at All India Institute of Medical Sciences, New Delhi

Birth Weight (g)	1990 (n = 444) (%)	1995 (n = 1672) (%)	2010 (n = 2191) (%)	2014 (n = 2631) (%)	2019 (n = 2423) (%)
<750	0	0	38.5	43.5	23.5
750–999	50	73.3	69.0	80.6	75.0
1000–1249	36.4	77.8	78.9	84.4	90.0
1250–1499	53.8	95.5	97.8	90.9	86.8
1500–1749	94.2	85.3	93.9	97	94.5
1750–1999	97.9	96.2	94.6	95.7	99.0
2000–2499	97.6	98.4	97.8	98.6	99.8
2500–2999	99.9	99.3	99.9	99.4	99.3
3000–3999	99.9	100	99.1	99.5	99.7
4000 or more	93.4	100	100	100	100

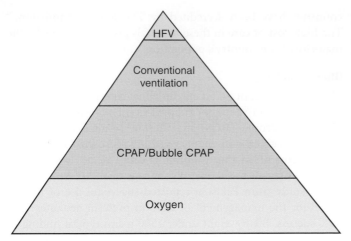

Fig. 40.1 Projected need for respiratory support to save lives in resource-limited countries. *CPAP*, Continuous positive airway pressure; *HFV*, high-frequency ventilation.

(e.g., Argentina, Cuba, Chile, Costa Rica), the NMR ranges from 4 to 9/1000 births, whereas other countries (e.g., Bolivia, Dominican Republic, Guyana, Haiti) report NMRs as high as 24 to 50/1000 births in year 2018.[10] Similar to other resource-limited countries in the world, the major cause of neonatal mortality is respiratory diseases. Most newborns die within days after birth, mostly from inadequate resuscitation at birth and lack of respiratory support after admission. In 1980, Ventura-Junca et al. showed the effectiveness of NICU care in reducing neonatal mortality in Chile.[37] However, such facilities are available mainly in private hospitals. Argentina reported in 1995 that 70% of neonates died less than 48 hours after birth in public hospitals.[38] The majority of these deaths could have been prevented with the development of facilities that provide adequate resuscitation and respiratory support. Making improvements in neonatal respiratory care is an effective way to decrease neonatal and infant mortality in emerging nations, and it requires organization, education, and rationing of resources.[38]

On the basis of reported national NMR, Paul and Singh proposed a stepwise approach to neonatal health care strategies in developing countries.[39] For countries with neonatal mortality of more than 25 per 1000 live births, the focus should be on community-based care. Once the mortality is less than 25 per 1000 live births, perinatal care should be provided by a network of facilities close to the community and managed by midwifes, nurses, and physicians. At this stage, widespread implementation of low-cost, robust respiratory technologies (e.g., oxygen concentrators, oxygen saturation monitoring, bubble CPAP) could save the lives of many newborn infants admitted to the facilities.[13] The projected need for respiratory support to save lives in resource-limited countries is presented in Fig. 40.1.

ESTABLISHING RESPIRATORY CARE PROGRAMS

There is interest among pediatricians and neonatologists in resource-limited countries to establish respiratory care programs

for critically ill newborns and save many more babies. However, establishing a respiratory care unit requires a major commitment of funds, resources, personnel, and time that would have to be diverted away from other health care needs. A one-time capital investment for the purchase of equipment would seem reasonable. However, it should be understood that establishing a respiratory care program requires equipment, clinical care pathways, maintenance of the equipment, ability to obtain replacement parts, ongoing professional development programs for all levels of providers, full-fledged ancillary support systems (e.g., laboratory, radiology), and a regional system of referral that promotes centralized ventilator care. To be cost effective, regional centers that serve large populations should develop assisted ventilation support systems. A regionalized perinatal center requires a well-developed and efficient transport system for in utero transport as well as newborn emergency transport.

Fernandez and Mondkar[11] suggest establishing one tertiary care NICU providing assisted ventilation per 1 million population in resource-limited countries. However, the introduction of CPAP/bubble CPAP may be appropriate for level II centers in these settings. To establish a strong respiratory care program, the following components are necessary (Fig. 40.2).

1. Leadership and partnership: In the past, leadership has consisted of a small group of technical experts or champions. There is a need for engagement of active stakeholders at all levels of the government. They can advocate and set a course of action that is supported at national and local levels. In addition, families are an important partner that can assist with taking care of their baby, recognizing that respiratory care saves lives and increasing the demand for these services. Governments respond to an increase in demand, and it will be easier to develop regionalized services with families as partners.

2. Implementation: Implementation of respiratory service needs adequate infrastructure, resources (equipment and people), clinical care monitoring systems, and ongoing quality improvement programs. Policies have to be developed based on local evidence. Proper infrastructure should be made available depending on the size of the unit. In addition, medications such as antibiotics and surfactant should be readily available.

   Infrastructure: It is the ultimate goal of pediatricians and neonatologists around the world to be able to establish a NICU that provides ventilator care. To be successful and cost effective, the planners must consider certain criteria before attempting to establish a neonatal respiratory care program. Box 40.1 lists some basic requirements for establishing a respiratory care program in the hospital. It describes the operational needs, cost of the ventilator, and criteria for choosing a ventilator. In addition to the provision of basic needs such as space and an uninterrupted supply of power, water, and gases, the availability of appropriate equipment and skilled staff are critical to the successful operation of a respiratory care program.

   Resources: Health care personnel: Critical to the success of improving neonatal respiratory care in resource-limited countries is training of bedside health care personnel in early recognition of, and ability to manage, respiratory distress.

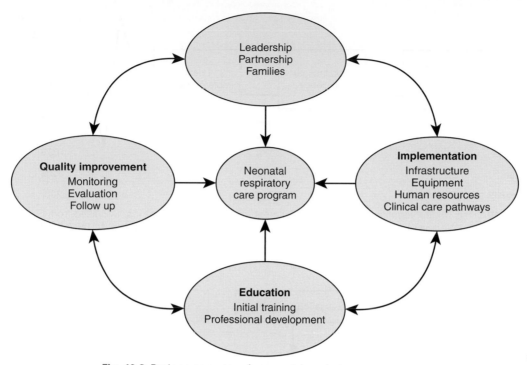

Fig. 40.2 Basic components of a neonatal respiratory care program.

BOX 40.1 Guideline for Setting Up a Respiratory Care Program

A. Operational considerations
- Availability of adequate space
- Uninterrupted availability of power and running water
- Continuous availability of a pediatrician trained in ventilator care
- Availability of sufficient nursing staff trained in ventilator care in the ratio of one nurse to two or three patients
- Availability of maintenance staff trained in ventilator repair
- Continuing education of staff
- Acquisition, review, and analysis of data for quality improvement

B. Typical cost in US dollars of a ventilator in a resource-limited country (approximate cost)
- Cost of ventilator: $30,000–$40,000
- Cost of disposables/year: $300–$350
- Cost of service contract: $200–$300
- First year cost: $30,500–$40,650
- Recurrent yearly cost: $450

C. Choosing a ventilator
- Simplicity of operation
- Cost considerations
- Ease of maintenance, availability of replacement parts
- Brand name
- Lower overall cost of ownership and life cycle cost

Because most of the facilities have minimal or no equipment, health care personnel must be trained in clinical skills that help identify infants at risk who require immediate respiratory support, that is, resuscitation and stabilization until the infant can be transferred to a higher level of care. Transport facilities for sick neonates requiring a higher level of care must be developed.

Worldwide, there is an acute shortage of trained health care personnel, particularly in resource-limited countries.[16,17] Establishment of a neonatal respiratory care program requires innovative methods to overcome this problem. Sen et al.[27] described how a rural district hospital under the government auspices was transformed into a functioning regional center for neonatal intensive care including respiratory care by improving physical facilities and training locally available human resources (health care workers) to provide care for infants admitted to the NICU. Over a 2-year period, they were able to demonstrate a significant decrease in neonatal mortality in a cost-effective manner. Many of the traditional roles of medical providers were modified in what has become known as the Purulia Model. This experience may serve as a model for others contemplating improvement of their programs.

In 2003, the International Liaison Committee on Resuscitation published an Advisory Statement on Education and Resuscitation, conceptualizing a hypothetical "formula of survival" (Fig. 40.3).[40,41] The "formula for survival" materialized in relation to cardiac arrest patients and stipulates that patient outcome is a product of three interactive factors: medical science (guideline quality), educational efficiency (knowledge translation to patient caregivers), and local implementation (actual delivery of health care) (Fig. 40.4).[42] We have good guidelines; however, both the educational efficiency and local implementation at all levels require further planning, support, and evaluation. This formula is as applicable to respiratory care as it is to resuscitation.[41]

Equipment for respiratory care programs: The basic principles of management of an "at-risk" infant include providing warmth and nutritional support. The basic equipment for setting up respiratory care service includes availability of

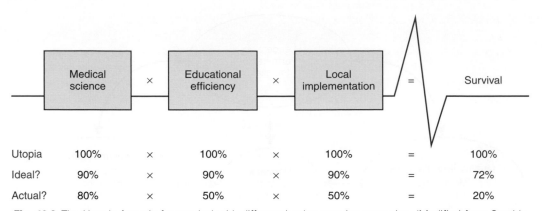

	Medical science	×	Educational efficiency	×	Local implementation	=	Survival
Utopia	100%	×	100%	×	100%	=	100%
Ideal?	90%	×	90%	×	90%	=	72%
Actual?	80%	×	50%	×	50%	=	20%

Fig. 40.3 The Utstein formula for survival with different implementation scenarios. (Modified from Søreide E, Morrison L, Hillman K, et al: The formula for survival in resuscitation. Resuscitation 84:1487–1493, 2013. With permission.)

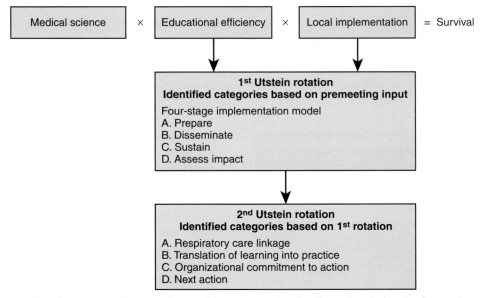

Fig. 40.4 The four-stage implementation model and categories for discussion during the first and second Utstein rotations related to the Utstein formula for survival. (A) Prepare: partners and strategic planning; (B) Disseminate: education and systems for delivery of training; (C) Sustain: maintenance and implementation with quality improvement; (D) Assess Impact: monitoring, evaluation, and feedback to strategic planning. (Modified from Søreide E, Morrison L, Hillman K, et al: The formula for survival in resuscitation. Resuscitation 84:1487–1493, 2013. With permission.)

oxygen, compressed air, blenders, suction devices, bags and masks, oxygen hoods, nasal cannulas, nasal prongs, face masks, CPAP devices, ventilators, pulse oximeters, cardiorespiratory monitoring devices, disposable gas and suction circuits, other noninvasive monitoring devices, and possibly oxygen analyzers. Lack of essential equipment may allow for the delivery of oxygen without appropriate monitoring and result in significant complications or death.

With globalization and increasing diffusion of technology today, the resource-poor countries have some access to incubators, electronic monitoring systems, pulse oximetry, IV fluids, CPAP devices, and neonatal ventilators.[1] On the other hand, these same countries experience difficulty in obtaining consumable commodities such as oxygen and

have difficulty in maintaining equipment that is in working order, both of which are vital to the management of infants in respiratory distress. The lack of readily available oxygen has been reported as a major cause of death in Africa and other developing countries.[43]

In developed countries, oxygen is stored at -183°C and is supplied via wall outlets. This requires highly sophisticated cryotechnology. In resource-limited countries, oxygen is supplied in pressurized tanks. This is an expensive method and has no reliability of constant supply in remote health facilities with poor transport systems.

There is a lack of appropriate methods for administering oxygen. Oxygen is administered in the nursery by different techniques, commonly by an oxygen hood (tent). However, the oxygen hood cannot ensure the delivery of an intended concentration of oxygen, especially when there is no oxygen analyzer. It is difficult to achieve concentrations more than 40% unless the hood is leak proof. There is also a great wastage of oxygen, which adds to the cost. Delivery of oxygen by nasal cannula minimizes loss of oxygen and ensures direct delivery even at low flow rates. In the absence of nasal cannula, oxygen can be delivered by using a face mask. Commercially available face masks, infrequently used in NICUs in the developed world, come in different sizes for term and premature infants.

Physicians and health care workers can use the commercially available equipment (nasal cannula, oxygen hoods, and CPAP devices) where feasible and affordable or develop innovative methods using basic principles of physics and physiology combined with ingenuity.

Neonatal equipment such as incubators, warmers, and bubble CPAP, made by local companies in the low- and middle-income countries, constitute about one-tenth the cost of imported equipment. A simple bubble CPAP may be assembled using old ventilator tubing for as little as US $5.[44,45] Nasal prongs are simple to use and ensure effective oxygen delivery. Sahni and Wung have demonstrated that CPAP devices are important tools in the management of RDS.[46] The techniques of oxygen delivery and application of CPAP are well described elsewhere in this book. Judicious application of CPAP in infants in respiratory distress has been shown to be very effective in managing infants with RDS in resource-poor countries.[47,48]

Bubble CPAP: Bubble CPAP for resource-limited areas of the world is an attractive device for treating neonates with respiratory distress because of its simple design, low cost, and potential to improve survival rates in settings where there is no mechanical ventilation. Bubble CPAP is based on a simple system where expiration occurs against a pressure generated by bubbling gas underwater.[47] The airway distending pressure is determined by the depth at which the expiratory limb is placed, that is, 5 cm of water pressure is produced by placing the expiratory tubing of the breathing circuit 5 cm under water. The components of a CPAP circuit are a gas flow source (oxygen and air), a mechanism to control oxygen concentrations, a humidifier, nasal prongs or mask as the patient interface, connecting tubing, and a vessel of water into which the expiratory tubing is submerged.

Published reports of neonates treated with bubble CPAP in low- and middle-income countries are limited and heterogeneous.[34,35,47-56] Two systematic reviews in 2014 and 2016 concluded that bubble CPAP is safe and reduced the need for mechanical ventilation in neonates with respiratory distress in tertiary referral hospitals in low- and middle-income counties.[47,48] The pooled analysis of four observational studies showed 66% reduction in in-hospital mortality following CPAP in preterm neonates (odds ratio, 0.34; 95% confidence interval [CI], 0.14–0.82).[48] In a study from eastern Uganda in 2019, introduction of bubble CPAP to treat RDS in VLBW neonates resulted in significant improvement in their survival from 61% to 73.5%.[56] Introduction of CPAP in a level II unit significantly reduced (from 74% to 37%) the

need for transferring of infants to tertiary care units in India.[57] A recent randomized trial from India showed that infant with meconium aspiration syndrome treated with bubble CPAP reduced the need for mechanical ventilation in the first 7 days of age as compared to standard care.[58]

Bubble CPAP can be effectively applied by nurses and other health care workers after a short training period to improve neonatal survival and quality of neonatal care in these settings.[47,48,55] Hence, in resource-limited countries, starting bubble CPAP services in special care newborn units with good level II care may be a better option than mechanical ventilation and parallels recent thinking in developed regions of the world where mechanical ventilators are freely available but attempts are being made to reduce ventilator-induced lung injury by using CPAP.

There are a number of commercially available CPAP devices manufactured in the United States and United Kingdom that are available in the markets of resource-limited countries. However, the cost of commercially available CPAP devices and circuits could be as high as 7 times that of indigenously made CPAP devices. The cost of bubble CPAP ranges from as little as US $10 for simple devices to US $6000 for commercial units. Bubble CPAP is cheaper, less invasive, and more accessible and requires less technical skill for application than currently available commercial ventilators.[48]

Ventilator: The purchase of ventilators is a major investment for hospitals in resource-limited countries. The initial cost is a major determining factor in establishing a respiratory care program. The typical costs of ventilator and supplies are shown in Box 40.1. Often, physicians and hospital administrators are pressured into buying expensive equipment based on its brand name recognition. Health professionals and administrators must consider some basic guidelines shown in Box 40.1 in selecting a particular brand of ventilator. Besides a well-recognized brand name, simplicity of operation, ease of maintenance, and availability of spare parts should be the important considerations in selecting a specific ventilator. Because of limited funding, ventilators that can serve different age groups may be more economical. The ventilator should have an overall low life-cycle cost.

In addition to the purchase of the ventilator, the purchase of disposables and service contracts are to be taken into consideration to maintain a functioning program. Most programs fail to maintain service contracts because of yearly budget constraints, a major barrier faced in all low- and middle-income countries. Once purchased, the unit should designate a professional (doctor/nurse) in the unit with the responsibility of maintenance and ordering of disposable supplies. Regular maintenance check-ups of the ventilators are essential.

Even though newer ventilators are being developed that have enhanced functions, the best outcomes are in units where staff are more familiar with how to use the ventilator in their units. It is recommended that only a few different types of ventilators be used in any one unit so that all care providers are well familiar with the functions of the ventilator and have experience using the device. Even though ventilation is a science, there is an art of ventilating babies.

Clinical care pathways: Pathways for clinical management, including management of babies on CPAP or assisted ventilation, skin-to-skin care, and monitoring for ventilator-associated infections, nosocomial infections, blood gases, and nutritional support, are essential parts of establishing respiratory care programs. Standardizing care and developing clinical care pathways can be helpful in day-to-day management. An increase in the use of evidence-based practices has been associated with an increase in survival.[59] As the babies will need continuous support and the most senior person is not at the bedside at all times, having clinical care pathways that are evidence based helps the bedside provider manage the patient. Indian nurses report having to manage respiratory problems with very little support at night in some hospitals.[60]

Clinical monitoring: Monitoring of critically ill infants in resource-poor countries is based mainly on clinical observation because very few electronic monitors are available. Several investigators have adopted different methods to train health care personnel in assessing clinical hypoxemia. Bang et al.[61] have shown that lay village workers can be trained to recognize infants in respiratory distress in the community. However, no such studies have been done in the immediate neonatal period.

Downes et al.[62] published a clinical scoring system, the "RDS" score, which correlated with blood gas measurements. The original Downes score consists of hourly assessment for five clinical signs: respiratory rate, grunting, color, retractions, and breath sounds on auscultation. Later, it was modified by including gestational age and oxygen requirement in Acute Care of at Risk Newborns Respiratory score[63] (Table 40.2). The score is simple and can be learned by almost any health professional; it requires no electronic or biochemical monitoring and provides a trend of changing clinical status to initiate interventions when required. Based on total score, respiratory distress can be divided into mild, moderate, and severe if the score is under 5, 5 to 8, or over 8, respectively. Babies with a respiratory score of less than 5 in the first 4 hours need close observation and possible oxygen supplementation. Babies with moderate respiratory distress (i.e., score of 5–8) may need some degree of respiratory support such as CPAP, and sometimes mechanical ventilation to prevent progression into severe respiratory distress and respiratory failure. Babies with severe respiratory distress (score >8) require immediate intubation and assisted ventilation. A modified Downes score has been adopted in several resource-poor countries including Indonesia and the Russian Federation-States.[64] The respiratory score is used to clinically evaluate hypoxemia in neonates with respiratory distress in resource-poor countries where pulse oximetry and blood gas analysis are not available.

3. Education: To sustain respiratory care services, there should be a program for training all health care staff. Nurses require orientation to care of the newborn[60] and then require ongoing support from the medical staff to care for these fragile babies. The training should be done with the initial orientation to the unit. Ongoing educational programs and professional development training programs should be available to enhance the skill and knowledge of health care workers and implementation of evidence-based practices.

4. Quality improvement: An ongoing quality improvement program is necessary to evaluate the success of respiratory care. One example is the Evidence-based practice for Improving Quality (EPIQ) program, launched in 2003 within the Canadian Neonatal Network. It was a collaborative, multifaceted quality improvement approach that combined iterative learning techniques using the plan-do-study-act (PDSA) cycles of rapid change with a process to facilitate quality improvement through benchmarking, best-practice consensus, engagement of frontline staff and mutual learning via networking. The EPIQ program in Canada has led to increases in survival without major morbidity (from 56.7% to 70.9%) among infants born preterm, alongside the provision of improved care practices.[65]

Retinopathy of prematurity (ROP) is emerging as a commonest cause of avoidable blindness in children in the low- and middle-income countries of Latin American and Asia where neonatal intensive care services have improved the survival of high-risk neonates.[66-69] Approximately 32,300 preterm infants are becoming visually impaired or blind every year in 2010.[69] Unfortunately, a significant number of infants with stage 5 ROP are presenting late to tertiary eye care departments when it is too late to restore visual function.[69] About 65% of those visually impaired from ROP were born in resource-limited countries.[70] Approximately 6% of all ROP visually impaired infants were born at under 32 weeks' gestation.

It appears that the overzealous administrations of oxygen without appropriate monitoring in addition to the survival

TABLE 40.2 Acute Care of at Risk Newborns Respiratory Distress Score System

Score	0	1	2
Respiratory rate	40–60/minutes	60–80/minutes	>80/minutes
Oxygen requirement[a]	None	≤50%	>50%
Retractions	None	Mild to moderate	Severe
Grunting	None	With stimulation	Continuous at rest
Breath sounds on auscultation	Easily heard throughout	Decreased	Barely heard
Prematurity	>34 weeks	30–34 weeks	<30 weeks

[a]A baby receiving oxygen prior to set up of oxygen analyzer should be assigned a score of 1.
(Modified from Downes JJ, Vidyasagar D, Boggs TR Jr, et al: Respiratory distress syndrome of newborn infants. I. New clinical scoring system (RDS score) with acid-base and blood gas correlations. Clin Pediatr 1970; 9(6):325–331.)

of more VLBW infants are responsible for this phenomenon. Therefore, improved oxygen delivery and monitoring, along with locally adapted screening/treatment programs, are necessary when considering respiratory care services. To rapidly increase ROP screening coverage, it may be necessary to consider a paradigm shift of the owners and operators of the screening program. A tele-ROP program, called KIDROP (Karnataka Internet Assisted Diagnosis of ROP), has been providing ROP screening and subsequent treatment using an indigenously developed telemedicine network in India.[71] In this program, trained and accredited technicians capture, analyze, and report images of "at-risk" infants in rural outreach centers by using a portable, wide-field, digital, ocular, imaging camera, namely, the Retcam Shuttle (Clarity MSI, Pleasanton, CA, USA). Remote city ROP specialists review the images and provide diagnosis and treatment.[72]

Health care–associated infection and ventilator-associated pneumonia (VAP) are common and serious problems among mechanically ventilated neonates. The incidence of VAP is reported to be 17.3% to 57.1% in resource-limited countries.[73-76] Factors such as prolonged NICU stay, reintubation, parenteral nutrition, and blood transfusion are additional risk factors for VAP.[77] VAP care bundle implementation with education prepared according to evidence-based guidelines decreased VAP rates.[78,79]

There is an urgent need for quality improvement initiatives to monitor and decrease important morbidities such as health care associated infections, VAP, ROP, and chronic lung disease (CLD).

Evaluation: The respiratory care units should also develop database systems for frequent auditing, maintaining quality control, and addressing ongoing quality improvement of services provided. Clinical care teams at health facilities need to be trained in monitoring and improving quality of care by conducting PDSA cycles. Ongoing evaluation should consist of data collection, monitoring systems for implementing change, and follow-up.

OUTCOMES OF NEONATAL VENTILATION

The outcomes of infants treated with neonatal ventilation in resource-limited countries have been published in recent years. Investigators of the National Neonatal-Perinatal Database (NNPD) from India reported that 45% of outborn babies admitted to the NICU required oxygen therapy, and 16% required assisted ventilation.[80] The survival rate of ventilated infants in resource-limited countries ranges from 46% to 58%.[81-85] Increasing gestational age and birth weight were significantly associated with improved survival rates. A study from China reported that the incidences of cerebral palsy (CP) at 18 months among ventilated preterm infants were 17%, 5%, and 2% in infants less than 28 weeks' gestation, 28 to 30 weeks, and 30 to 32 weeks, respectively.[86] The incidences of Mental Developmental Index (MDI) scores less than 70 were 49%, 24%, and 13% in infants less than 28 weeks' gestation, 28 to 30 weeks, and 30 to 32 weeks, respectively. Infants ventilated by conventional mode had significantly higher incidences of CP and cognitive delay as compared to those

ventilated on high-frequency oscillatory ventilation. Longer duration of mechanical ventilation and blood transfusions were associated with an increased risk of having an MDI under 70 or CP.

A report from Ghana showed that the establishment of a ventilator support program in the NICU at a teaching hospital led to a dramatic decrease in mortality of infants admitted to the unit.[87] The significant finding of this report was that the major single intervention in an already existing NICU was the addition of ventilators and improved physical facilities. This was a one-time capital budget commitment. No new nurses were added; however, the existing staff was given on-site additional training in ventilator care. These observations suggest that it is possible to develop NICUs with ventilatory support even in developing countries with minimum investments.

Initiating ventilator support is associated with emergence of new morbidities, specifically CLD and ROP. Improved survival of VLBW infants was associated with an increase in CLD.[88,89] Similarly, there are reports of increasing occurrence of ROP in survivors after ventilation in resource-poor countries.[67-70] However, the programs in these resource-poor countries lack the required pediatric ophthalmologic services. Considering these limitations, one should take a cautious approach in developing ventilator care programs in resource-limited countries. especially for extremely preterm infants.

PROJECTED GROWTH IN NEONATAL VENTILATION: A GLOBAL PERSPECTIVE

It is interesting to note that in spite of the aforementioned difficulties, there is steady growth in the neonatal ventilator market worldwide. There is increasing awareness and interest in the purchase and use of ventilator support for adults and newborns around the world. There has been a rapid and progressive increase in ventilator purchases in low- and middle-income countries, especially China, Latin America, and India. The total world market sales for mechanical ventilators (adults and neonates), as well as associated disposable and maintenance services, have increased significantly in the past two decades. The neonatal ventilator market is also expected to grow steadily. The United States is the largest market, whereas India is the fastest growing, followed by Latin America.

Globally, neonatal ventilators account for about 10% to 11% of all ventilators sold. Sales of high-frequency ventilator units are expected to grow at a rate of 1.3% per year. The Americas have the largest market share, followed by Europe, and then the Asia Pacific countries.

Even though neonatal ventilator purchases are increasing in resource-limited countries, these acquisitions are far fewer than these countries need. With the current projected rate, India will have one ventilator per 80,000 live born babies; China will have one ventilator per 30,000 live births as compared to one ventilator per 500 births in the United States. Considering higher neonatal morbidity from prematurity and birth asphyxia rates in India and China, the requirements of ventilators are many times higher than the previous estimates. The current estimated rate of purchases of 100 ventilators per year in each country is insufficient to meet current and future needs.

ETHICAL DILEMMAS

The introduction of neonatal and critical care services poses several economic and ethical dilemmas. In a national study in India, NNF found that 7.5% of infants from the NICU were discharged against physician advice.[80] These discharges were most likely attributed to economic, social, and family reasons. Moazam and Lakhani discussed the dilemmas of providing neonatal intensive care in a resource-limited country.[90] Their concerns were related to the high cost of NICU care. Narang et al.[91] reported that the average total cost of care for a baby less than 1000 g in India was Rs. 168,000 (US $3800), Rs. 88,300 (US $2000) for babies 1000 g to 1250 g, and Rs. 41,700 (US $950) for those between 1250 and 1500 g. In addition, one needs to consider the associated disease burden secondary to associated morbidities of CLD, ROP, and neurodevelopmental disabilities in resource-limited countries. The ethical question is "Is it justifiable to invest a country's meager health care resources to benefit a few sick infants?" With increasing awareness of available technologies to save critically ill infants, parents have higher expectations. But daily expenses incurred for the care given in the NICU challenge parental support. The mounting daily hospital costs may exceed the capabilities of the family. Therefore, every attempt should be made to honor distributive justice.

Physicians and health care administrators in these regions should define a priority and decide the level of care based on the resources available. All babies must be given the basic care available in the country. Decisions to offer ventilator care should be based not only on immediate clinical needs but also on the implications of long-term needs of health care and the availability of support systems in the community once the infant recovers from the acute illness.[92] In an article on ethical and social issues in the care of the newborn, Singh offers some suggestions regarding the ethical issues faced by pediatric and neonatal practitioners in resource-limited countries (Box 40.2).[92] Clearly, each society must develop guidelines based on its local values, cultural variations, and resources.

CONCLUSION

It is clear that resource-limited countries have the highest neonatal and infant mortality from respiratory problems and that there is a great unmet need for respiratory care and ventilatory support. Yet these are the same countries that lack the most essential minimum equipment such as bags and masks for resuscitation, continuous supplies of oxygen, and oxygen delivery devices. It is suggested that the World Health Organization (WHO) designate this life-saving equipment as part of essential equipment, similar to the WHO Essential Drug List.[93] Such policies would make a major impact on neonatal survival internationally. Health care workers at primary health care centers and hospitals should be trained in providing basic respiratory care, that is, clinical assessment using the RDS score, basic principles of care including clearing the airway, bag and mask ventilation, and proper oxygen therapy. The staff at level II units must be routinely trained in providing oxygen therapy and applying CPAP. Staff in level III units should be capable of providing ventilatory support using mechanical ventilation.

Countries with high birth rates and high NMR require the establishment of regional NICUs with ventilatory support. These centers of excellence must provide nationwide training of health care personnel in providing basic resuscitation, stabilization with nasal CPAP, and triage and transport to hospitals that can provide higher levels of respiratory care. The market research data also show that developing countries are rapidly acquiring neonatal ventilators; however, there is a lack of concurrent development of respiratory care programs. The NNF of India provides a model in which a professional physician organization has started a major initiative to improve newborn care in the country. Other countries have developed individual units. A combination of the models may work well for other resource-limited countries.

Because of the large global need, it is important that professionals, organizations, institutions, and government agencies in developed countries extend their services and participate in global programs to accelerate the transfer of knowledge and skills of respiratory care to resource-limited countries. These goals can be achieved through bilateral exchange of medical faculty and nurses between institutions in resource-limited and developed countries. In our own experience, these approaches have made an enormous impact in several countries.

ACKNOWLEDGMENT

We would like to acknowledge Dr Ramesh Agarwal for his contributions for the AIIMS data.

> ### BOX 40.2 Ethical Questions to Consider in Resource-Limited Countries
>
> - Should the best interest of the baby or the global interest of the family determine the care given?
> - Should each country decide a cut-off weight below which no NICU care is given?
> - Should NICU ventilator care be denied to those who cannot afford to pay?
> - Can therapy be stopped when a family cannot afford to pay for further care?
> - Should expensive NICU care be given to extremely or very low-birth-weight infants of parents who do not have basic amenities at home and where social support from the government is not available?

NICU, Neonatal intensive care unit.

KEY REFERENCES

7. Versantvoort JMD, Kleinhout MY, Ockhuijsen HDL, et al: Helping Babies Breathe and its effects on intrapartum-related stillbirths and neonatal mortality in low-resource settings: a systematic review. Arch Dis Child 105:127–133, 2020.

8. Lee AC, Cousens S, Wall SN, et al: Neonatal resuscitation and immediate newborn assessment and stimulation for the prevention of neonatal deaths: a systematic review, meta-analysis and Delphi estimation of mortality effect. BMC Public Health 11(suppl 3):S12, 2011.

16. Kinshella MW, Walker CR, Hiwa T, et al: Barriers and facilitators to implementing bubble CPAP to improve neonatal health in sub-Saharan Africa: a systematic review. Public Health Rev 41:6, 2020

17. Inglis R, Ayebale E, Schultz MJ: Optimizing respiratory management in resource-limited settings. Curr Opin Crit Care 25(1):45–53, 2019.

44. Sivanandan S, Agarwal R, Sethi A: Respiratory distress in term neonates in low-resource settings. Semin Fetal Neonatal Med 22(4):260–226, 2017.

47. Martin S, Duke T, Davis P: Efficacy and safety of bubble CPAP in neonatal care in low and middle income countries: a systematic review. Arch Dis Child Fetal Neonatal Ed 99(6): F495–F504, 2014.

48. Thukral A, Sankar MJ, Chandrasekaran A, et al: Efficacy and safety of CPAP in low- and middle-income countries. J Perinatol 36(suppl 1):S21–S28, 2016.

72. Vinekar A, Jayadev C, Mangalesh S, et al: Role of tele-medicine in retinopathy of prematurity screening in rural outreach centers in India – a report of 20,214 imaging sessions in the KIDROP program. Semin Fetal Neonatal Med 20:335–45, 2015.

77. Tan B, Zhang F, Zhang X, et al: Risk factors for ventilator-associated pneumonia in the neonatal intensive care unit: a meta-analysis of observational studies. Eur J Pediatr 173(4):427–434, 2014.

41

Transport of the Ventilated Infant

Robert M. Insoft

KEY POINTS

- Regional perinatal and interhospital transport teams for critically ill newborns and infants contribute to decreased morbidity and mortality.
- Transport team composition depends on institutional preferences, skill levels, and team demands.
- Continued education and skills training for team members should highlight real neonatal intensive care unit and transport clinical situations.
- Competence in basic aviation physiology should be required for all air transport team members.
- Transport systems have now been specifically designed to incorporate all of the critical life support systems and technology in a single mobile unit.
- The role of the transport team has expanded as technology has advanced and has made it possible to deliver sophisticated respiratory and medical therapies to infants out in the field.

IMPORTANT ROLE OF THE TRANSPORT TEAM

The widespread development of both regional perinatal centers and interhospital transport services for critically ill newborns and infants has been an important factor in decreasing perinatal morbidity and mortality. Starting in the 1970s, the growing recognition that regionalization of care improved patient outcomes resulted in the formation of regionalized centers for perinatal and neonatal care. With this development of regionalized care, the need for skilled transport teams was realized. Today, as advanced technologies have become more available and portable, the transport team has become an extension of the intensive care unit, and transport teams now initiate the comprehensive specialized care in the referral hospital that will be continued in the tertiary care center. Transport teams bring the intensive care environment to the infant, even starting care in the referring hospital's delivery room, stabilizing the infant to ensure a safe and effective transfer.

As advanced technologies have been approved and adopted, sophisticated treatments such as high-frequency ventilation (HFV) and inhaled nitric oxide (iNO) are now frequently initiated in many level 3 and 4 units. When these therapies fail to stabilize the infant in intensive care units that do not offer extracorporeal membrane oxygenation (ECMO), transport to a quaternary neonatal care unit is often necessary. Transfer of these highly complex neonates requires a sophisticated and skilled transport team and may be aided by real-time audio and video cell phone capabilities and wireless electronic medical records.

The modern transport team has adapted to meet the needs of these complex infants. Teams now have the ability to provide intensive therapies such as surfactant therapy, HFV, iNO, passive or active therapeutic hypothermia, and even mobile ECMO in some cases. Team members competent in the critical care of an ill newborn must be able to provide a rapid response to the referral hospitals who request their services. They must provide appropriate stabilization for transport in an expedient and safe manner. Importantly, as the skills and technologies of transport teams continue to change and develop, it is becoming evident that comprehensive care and therapies initiated during transport can improve patient outcomes.

REGIONALIZED CARE

More than 50 years ago, clinicians recognized that neonates treated at tertiary centers had improved outcomes, and the push for regionalized care began. Usher[1] demonstrated a 50% reduction in mortality for critically ill newborns that received care at tertiary centers. Other studies confirmed these results and also showed improved mortality rates for infants transported to regional care centers.[2,3]

Although the previous studies supported the early transfer of high-risk mothers and fetuses to tertiary centers, the birth of high-risk infants in nontertiary centers has continued to occur, and data suggest that 14% to 25% of very low birth weight (VLBW) infants are delivered in nontertiary hospitals.[4-6] Studies of such infants further support the fact that outborn infants experience significantly higher morbidity and mortality when compared with infants delivered at tertiary perinatal centers. Chien et al.[7] found that outborn infants were at higher risk of death, severe intraventricular hemorrhage (IVH), patent ductus arteriosus, respiratory distress syndrome (RDS), and nosocomial infections, even after adjusting for perinatal risks and illness severity.

Lui et al.[8] performed an interesting study comparing inborn and outborn infants born between 23 and 28 weeks 6 days of gestation before and after the development of regionalized care. They compared outcomes for infants born from 1992 to 1995 to those born from 1997 to 2002. They showed that optimization of in utero transfers resulted in 25% fewer nontertiary hospital births and that with provision of perinatal consults, increased provision of antenatal steroids, and centralization of the neonatal retrieval system, outborn mortality rates decreased significantly from 39.4% to 25.1%. Rates of severe IVH and necrotizing enterocolitis (NEC) also decreased in outborn infants between the two periods after interventions were started. Importantly, however, morbidity for outborn infants continued to be significantly higher than that for inborn infants, especially with regard to severe (grade 3 or 4) IVH (19.4% outborn vs. 10% inborn, $P < 0.002$) and radiologically or surgically proven NEC (7.2% outborn vs. 1.7% inborn, $P < 0.001$). These data demonstrate that implementation of a coordinated system to provide perinatal consults and appropriate neonatal transport improves outcomes, but outborn infants continue to face higher morbidity despite these interventions. Thus in utero transfer of high-risk pregnancies to a tertiary center still remains the best option. When maternal transfer cannot be accomplished because of rapid labor progression, pending delivery, or fetal or maternal compromise, the specialized services offered by the neonatal transport team play an important role in optimizing outborn infant care. Many teams will even now offer to attend unexpected high risk deliveries in community settings if a maternal transport is prohibited.

TRANSPORT TEAM COMPOSITION

Multiple approaches have been used when determining the make-up of the ideal transport team. Each institution must determine the most appropriate model for their facility based on the volume, types of transports (ground vs. rotor-wing vs. fixed wing), travel times, the skills required for efficient and safe transfers, the availability of team members, and the overall costs. The American Academy of Pediatrics (AAP) has recommended that transport teams consist of at least two providers, with one member being a nurse who has 5 years or more of nursing experience.[9] Team members can include emergency or intensive care nurses, nurse practitioners, pediatric respiratory therapists (RTs), paramedics, and physicians, including attending staff, fellows, or residents in training. Most commonly teams are made up of RT-nurse pairs or nurse-nurse pairs with paramedic support. Given the significant number of neonatal transports requiring respiratory interventions, many teams find the skills of an RT helpful and often necessary. However, all transport team members should be cross-trained and capable of supporting all transport procedures and interventions.

Karlsen et al.[10] have studied transport volume, different team models, and their effect on patient care outcomes. Karlsen's survey found wide variation in many aspects of team organization, including team configuration, staff orientation, use of protocols, as well as quality improvement methodologies. Consistent with previous work, Karlsen found no difference in patient care outcomes when comparing variations in team members, including registered nurse (RN)/RT, nurse practitioner (NP)/RT and medical doctor (MD)/RN/RT. The presence of a physician did not alter patient outcomes in this study.

Multiple other studies have supported the idea that nonphysician teams are capable of providing care that is effective, and potentially timelier, than teams accompanied by a physician. Beyer et al.[11] demonstrated that nonphysician teams were able to provide care and transport intubated neonates without problems.

In their cohort, 20% of infants were intubated by a transport nurse or RT at the referring facility. They concluded that there was a low incidence of complications in intubated neonates when transported by personnel trained in intubation and neonatal resuscitation. Leslie and Stephenson[12] found that transports directed by advanced neonatal nurse practitioners were as effective as those directed by physicians, and King et al.[13] found that there was no change in mortality or complications when teams were converted from nurse-physician teams to nurse-nurse teams, but that response time did improve. Voluntary reporting by pediatric and neonatal transport teams to the AAP Section of Transport Medicine team database indicates that almost half of the teams providing information (37 of 82 teams) do not include physicians on transport.[14] Thus, with a well-trained, experienced transport team, availability of a medical control physician by telephone may be all that is required.

Regardless of the model chosen, however, team members should be specialists in neonatal and pediatric care because specialized teams have been shown to make a significant difference in outcome. Early studies demonstrated that dedicated neonatal transport teams reduced both morbidity and mortality in VLBW infants that required transfer to a tertiary center[15,16] and that outborn infants who were not transferred by a specialized transport team experienced a 60% greater mortality rate.[17]

More recent studies confirm that the incidence of transport-related morbidity increases when personnel without specific pediatric training transport critically ill children. A study by Edge et al.[18] demonstrated that adverse events during interhospital transport, such as accidental extubation or intravenous (IV) access problems, were significantly higher in transports performed by a nonspecialized team (20%) compared with transports performed by a specialized pediatric team (2%). Similarly, Macnab[19] demonstrated a higher rate of secondary complications in infants transported by nonspecialized transport teams when compared with pediatric transport teams.

High-volume transport programs have the advantage of being able to develop full-time transport teams dedicated solely to neonatal transport, where experience is greater and skills are more easily maintained. Smaller services that use team members on a more infrequent basis must invest significantly in continuing education to maintain their knowledge base and technical skills to provide specialized services. Data from the ongoing AAP voluntary registration of transport teams suggest that the majority of teams provide combined pediatric and neonatal transport services.[14] Although this is often necessary and allows the maintenance of a dedicated team, team members should track the number of neonatal transports they perform to be sure they are maintaining adequate exposure to the unique circumstances involved in neonatal resuscitation and transport. A lack of exposure should be offset by continuing education including in unit training and simulation.

Transport teams are frequently called to attend and participate in the delivery of high-risk preterm infants that occur outside of the tertiary center. Although all delivery hospitals should have at least one attendant certified in neonatal resuscitation available at all times, transport personnel may be asked to support referral staff or, in some cases, may be the primary resuscitator at a preterm delivery. Although this is often a stressful situation, the presence of a dedicated neonatal retrieval team can improve delivery room resuscitation of these outborn premature infants.[6] In this study, neonates that were resuscitated by a specialized transport team were intubated more promptly with fewer attempts, had fewer accidental extubations, and were more likely to receive surfactant therapy in a timely manner.

Neonates cared for only by the referring hospital team had higher rates of hypothermia, lack of vascular access, and more extensive resuscitation. Despite having the same average gestational age, infants resuscitated by the referral team received longer chest compressions (6 vs. 0.5 minutes), longer bag-mask ventilation (13.5 vs. 7 minutes), and longer continuous positive airway pressure (CPAP) (14 vs. 2 minutes), all of which may reflect a delay in intubation by the referral team. These differences are not surprising, because referral hospitals that appropriately transfer high-risk mothers and fetuses lack a critical mass of preterm births and experience in resuscitation of extremely low birth weight (ELBW) and VLBW preterm infants.

Dedicated teams with specialized training and increased experience can provide better specialized care and resuscitation. Given the evidence that the first few minutes of resuscitation and early oxygen exposure can influence long-term outcome, the need to optimize resuscitation is evident.[20-22] These studies reinforce the fact that transport teams should be made up of clinicians with specific training in comprehensive neonatal care and resuscitation and also suggest that the use of the transport team as a neonatal resuscitation team for outborn infants may be optimal.

TRANSPORT EDUCATION

The need for extensive education of team members who transport neonates is obvious because team members are expected to recognize and treat a wide array of disorders. They must be able to resuscitate and stabilize neonates in critical condition and ensure their safe transport, often under conditions that may be suboptimal. Although no standard curriculum exists, guidelines for team education have been published by the AAP Section on Transport Medicine.[23] Education of transport team members includes a requirement for resuscitation training through the Neonatal Resuscitation Program (AAP and American Heart Association provider course) or a similar program, as well as continuing education in neonatal pathology and disease. Continuing medical education (CME) and transport review conferences ensure that team members maintain their skills in neonatal stabilization and expose them to new topics in neonatal care. CME opportunities should include skills lab, with stations focusing on skilled intubation, effective bag-mask ventilation, handling of the difficult airway, chest tube placement, and vascular access, including IV line placement, umbilical line placement, and intraosseous line placement. In addition, simulation-based exercises should be employed when possible.

Unique to transport team education are the requirements for basic knowledge about flight physiology and its contribution to disease states, the physical and mental stresses of transport, and the need for a significant focus on safety that includes both team and patient safety. Given the many unique challenges encountered during transport (excessive noise, vibration and rotation forces, low-level lighting, variable ambient temperatures/humidity, and the need for specific safety measures), team members should receive extensive supervised orientation and then must participate in transports with sufficient regularity to maintain their skills in all transport settings. Team members may also benefit from training on ethical and legal issues such as the withdrawal of support because they may be involved in situations where support is stopped after resuscitation or where infants are deemed appropriate for withdrawal of care at the referring facility, where the family can participate, rather than transport to a distant facility. Training should also be given regarding the social aspects of transport to help team members work more compassionately with families and help raise team awareness of the many emotional issues that are faced by parents and family members during the crisis precipitated by a neonatal transport.

TRANSPORT PHYSIOLOGY

The effect of altitude and the stresses of flight can have a significant impact on the neonate during fixed-wing or helicopter transport, especially in the already compromised infant. The transport environment itself, including ground transport, introduces unique stressors such as noise, vibration, and temperature variation. Transport team members must understand altitude physiology and the physiologic stresses of neonatal transport to anticipate and properly treat problems that may occur during transport. Each of these factors can affect team members as well. The most significant concerns include the following:

1. Hypoxia
2. Air expansion
3. Noise and vibration
4. Thermoregulation

Hypoxia

As an aircraft ascends, the partial pressure of gas decreases. As the altitude above sea level increases, the barometric pressure falls, and the partial pressure of ambient oxygen and thus the alveolar oxygen partial pressure decrease. During this time, infants may develop hypoxia. This is demonstrated using the simplified alveolar gas equation, $PaO_2 = (P_B - 47) \times FiO_2 - PaCO_2/0.8$, where PaO_2 is the partial pressure of alveolar oxygen, P_B is the barometric pressure, 47 is the partial pressure of water vapor, FiO_2 is the inspired oxygen concentration, $PaCO_2$ is the partial pressure of arterial carbon dioxide (CO_2), and 0.8 is the respiratory quotient. If an infant receiving 50% inspired oxygen with a $PaCO_2$ of 50 is transported from sea level (barometric pressure = 760) in a nonpressurized aircraft that must achieve 8000 feet for the transfer (barometric pressure = 570), then the alveolar oxygen partial pressure will drop from 294 at sea level to 199 at altitude, if you assume no change in minute ventilation, FiO_2, or $PaCO_2$. In reality, the partial pressure of arterial CO_2 and water vapor will decrease at altitude as well, making the alveolar oxygen partial pressure slightly greater than that calculated by the equation.

$$P_AO_2 \text{ (sea level)} = (760 - 47)$$
$$\times\ 0.5 - 50/0.8 = 294 \qquad \textbf{(Eq. 41.1)}$$

$$P_AO_2 \text{ (8000 ft)} = (570 - 47)$$
$$\times\ 0.5 - 50/0.8 = 199 \qquad \textbf{(Eq. 41.2)}$$

Preterm infants, infants with respiratory diseases, and infants with high oxygen demands (sepsis, shock) are at particular risk of developing hypoxia. Careful monitoring of oxygen saturations helps with identification of infants experiencing hypoxia, who usually respond to increased FiO_2 levels or increased positive end-expiratory pressure (PEEP). For infants already receiving oxygen before transport, the need for increased oxygen during flight should be anticipated. The anticipated adjustment in oxygen administration can be calculated using Eq. 41.3

$$\text{Adjusted } FiO_2 = (FiO_2 \times P_{B1})/P_{B2} \qquad \textbf{(Eq. 41.3)}$$

where FiO_2 represents the current FiO_2 being administered, P_{B1} is the current barometric pressure, and P_{B2} is the barometric pressure at the highest anticipated altitude during transport.

Air Expansion

As an aircraft ascends and barometric pressure falls, the volume of gas within a closed space expands. Gas in an enclosed space at sea level (i.e., a pneumothorax) will expand by a factor of 1.5 at 10,000 feet. This is most significant for the infant with a pneumothorax or a pneumopericardium, although it may influence the status of the newborn or infant with a pneumoperitoneum or pneumatosis as well. Ideally, air leaks are treated before flight because of the concern of further expansion at higher altitudes.

Noise and Vibration

Noise and vibration are significant problems encountered during both air and ground transports. Studies have shown that neonates are exposed to very high levels of sound during transport and that mean sound levels for all modes of transport exceed the recommended levels for neonatal intensive care.[24,25] Similarly, neonates experience high vibration accelerations within the transport incubator.[25] Configuration of the transport unit should be optimized to reduce vibration, and ear protection should be considered for neonates during transport, particularly during air transport, where sound exposure is greatest.

Thermoregulation

Ambient temperatures change significantly with altitude variation and with seasonal variation during ground transport. Proper thermoregulation has been shown to be critical for the intact survival of VLBW infants,[26,27] whereas hyperthermia can be detrimental to infants with perinatal acidosis and hypoxic-ischemic encephalopathy.[28,29] Temperature variation will also increase metabolic and oxygen demands, which can cause further compromise in the hypoxic or septic patient. Transport members must be thoughtful about optimizing the thermal factors they can control. Conductive heat loss can be minimized by preheating the transport incubator and blankets and using a chemical heating mattress. Evaporative heat losses are minimized by keeping the skin surface dry, using a polyethylene bag

for ELBW/VLBW infants, and heating and humidifying inspired gases. Additional efforts to control cabin temperature may be required during specific seasons.

STABILIZATION

The goal of the transport team is to initiate definitive care for the ill neonate and to bring the resources of the tertiary center to the infant. Ideally, neonates should be transported when they are stable, so that transport can occur in a safe and controlled manner. This means that the ill neonate should be stabilized as much as possible in the referring hospital environment, which offers the advantages of space; easy access to the infant; better lighting and visibility; access to personnel, equipment, and support (laboratory and radiology); thermal stability for the infant; and ease of communication with the tertiary center neonatologist. Stabilization involves identifying and treating factors that could lead to deterioration of the infant's condition. Procedures or interventions that are needed, such as intubation, chest tube placement, or vascular access, should be anticipated as much as possible and performed before transport. Given the limitations of the transport space, and the complexity added to the transport environment by vibration and noise, only rarely should a major intervention such as intubation need to be performed during the course of transport itself. Despite the inherent desire to expedite the transport process, time spent stabilizing an infant at the referring facility is an important investment to ensure a safe and effective transport. There are rare situations (e.g., transposition of the great vessels with intact ventricular septum) where definitive treatment can be offered only at the tertiary institution and the benefit of rapid transport outweighs the risk of transporting an unstable infant.

CLINICAL ISSUES

The members of a specialized transport team must recognize and treat a wide array of neonatal disorders. Although each transport is different, there are a standard set of broad issues that must be addressed in every neonatal transport. These include the following:

1. Respiratory support and airway issues
2. Cardiovascular support
3. Vascular access
4. Glucose stability
5. Thermal regulation
6. Infection risks and treatment

The most common problem encountered by neonatal transport personnel is respiratory distress. Key studies[30] have found that over 85% of neonates that are transported received some form of assisted ventilation, and transport teams performed intubation as well as initiated ventilation in a vast majority of transported infants. Newborns most commonly present with respiratory diseases, so it is not surprising that airway interventions (intubation, mechanical ventilation including CPAP) are the most common interventions performed by the transport team.[30,31] Transport personnel must be skilled in establishing and maintaining an airway in a neonate. Airway skills should include not only intubation but also appropriate bag-valve mask ventilation and T-piece resuscitator, use of nasal and oral airways, placement of CPAP prongs, use of a laryngeal mask airway (LMA), and options for handling a difficult airway. Skills in basic chest x-ray interpretation are needed for diagnosis and optimal management of respiratory diseases.

Transport personnel must also understand the concepts of mechanical ventilation. They should be able to recognize and treat complications encountered with the use of positive pressure and an endotracheal tube because endotracheal tube or ventilator problems occur in almost 10% of transports.[32] Priority must be given to properly securing the endotracheal tube to avoid accidental extubation in transit. Team members should be able to recognize and treat pulmonary air leaks of various forms and need to have experience in needle thoracentesis or chest tube placement. Optimization of ventilation and oxygenation before and during transport is important for maintaining stabilization and for achieving the goal of providing comprehensive care. There is room for improvement in transport ventilator management; recent studies have shown that 15% to 25% of transported infants have suboptimal pH or PCO_2 levels at tertiary center arrival.[33,34]

From a cardiovascular standpoint, transport personnel must be able to recognize and appropriately stabilize infants with congenital heart disease. Differentiating severe pulmonary disease from cyanotic congenital heart disease can be difficult, but proper recognition and initiation of prostaglandin can significantly influence outcome. Team members must be well versed in the use of prostaglandin and its complications. Teams in communication with medical control must make a decision about intubation of infants on prostaglandin E_1 (PGE_1) based on the stability of the infant, the dose of medication being used, and the length and mode of transport. Limited evidence exists regarding the need for intubation of infants on PGE_1 before transport. Apnea has been reported to occur in 12% to 30% of infants treated with PGE_1, but the incidence can be as high as 42% in infants weighing less than 2 kg.[35] Browning Carmo et al.[36] evaluated 93 of 300 infants with congenital heart disease undergoing transport that did not have mechanical ventilation initiated at the beginning of the PGE_1 infusion. Of these infants, 17% went on to require intubation for apnea within 1 hour of PGE_1 initiation, and 2.6% of the remaining infants developed apnea during transport. Overall, 25% of infants were able to be successfully transported without intubation, but these infants were receiving very low doses of PGE_1 at less than 0.015 µg/kg/min. Although each situation must be individually assessed, in general, term infants who are receiving standard PGE_1 doses may be transported short distances safely without intubation. Transport teams also have the ability to supply nitrogen or CO_2 to unstable infants with hypoplastic left heart physiology during transport, but extensive education is needed before this approach is implemented.

The ability to establish vascular access is a critical skill for transport team members to possess. Team personnel must be able to place an umbilical venous line emergently during resuscitation for the purpose of administering epinephrine and volume, as well as nonemergently for administration of IV fluids, medications, or blood products. Some centers expect that transport personnel will be able to place umbilical arterial lines as well; however, the time necessary for umbilical arterial line placement should be weighed against earlier transport to the tertiary center where the procedure can be done under more ideal circumstances. Only if central blood pressure and/or arterial blood gas (ABG) monitoring are needed on transport, this procedure is typically deferred to the tertiary center. Team members also should have the training and skills required for intraosseous line placement for emergent situations.

Maintenance of normal glucose levels and maintenance of thermal stability have both been shown to be critical for neonatal morbidity and mortality prevention.[26,28,37] Transport team members must recognize the importance of glucose stability and thermal stability in neonates and should have protocols that address these two key issues for every transport. Although glucose and temperature alterations are problems that are usually easily treated or controlled, they are also easily overlooked. Several studies evaluating optimization during transport have shown that approximately 10% of neonates have hypothermia and 10% of neonates have hypoglycemia on arrival following transport.[32,34]

Ongoing quality improvement is an essential piece to transport management. Lee et al.[33] first validated a physiology-based scoring system for assessment of neonatal transport. The Transport Risk Index of Physiologic Stability (TRIPS) allows for prediction of 7-day mortality following transport, neonatal intensive care unit (NICU) mortality, and severe IVH. Recently, Schwartz et al.[38] and Lee[39] have demonstrated widespread agreement on the basic key quality metrics to ensure for the success of a high-reliability program. His studies showed that transport metrics can be grouped into the following five basic categories: (1) effectiveness (intubation success rates); (2) safety metrics (medication administration errors); (3) efficiency (standardized patient hand off); (4) family/patient centeredness (family members on transport); and (5) timeliness (mobilization times). In addition, these investigators demonstrate that patient acuity scoring is relatively new to this field and has shown mixed benefit in clinical practice compared with the NICU or pediatric intensive care unit.

Finally, the suspicion for or true incidence of infection in newborn infants is high, and transport teams must consider these risks to perform appropriate evaluations and testing and initiate antibacterial or antiviral therapy in a timely manner.

EQUIPMENT

The equipment carried by the transport team must be lightweight, durable, compact, and easily secured, but most of all it must be complete to meet the safe needs of transport. The assumption should be made that the referring hospital will not have equipment needed to stabilize the neonate before transport. Medications and basic support supplies for interhospital transport are listed in Boxes 41.1 and 41.2. A variety of durable equipment bags exist for organizing consumable supplies and medications. Supply bags should be checked and replenished after every transport.

BOX 41.1 Suggested Medications for Interhospital Transport

Adenosine 6 mg/2 mL	Gentamicin 10 mg/mL
Albumin 5%	Heparinized saline
Alprostadil (PGE1) 500 µg/mL	Lacri-lube
Ampicillin 100 mg/mL	Lidocaine 1% 10 mg/mL
Atropine 0.1 mg/mL	Lorazepam (Ativan) 2 mg/mL
Calcium chloride 10% 100 mg/mL	Magnesium sulfate 1 g/2 mL
Calcium gluconate 10% 100 mg/mL	Midazolam (Versed) 1 mg/mL
Cefotaxime 100 mg/mL	Morphine 2 mg/mL
Clindamycin 150 mg/mL	Naloxone (Narcan) 1 mg/mL
D10W 250 mL	Nipride 50 mg/2 mL
Digoxin 100 µg/mL	Normal saline
Dobutamine 250 mg/20 mL	Phenobarbital 65 mg/mL
Dopamine 400 mg/5 mL	Rocuronium 10 mg/mL
Epinephrine 1:1000	Sodium bicarbonate 4.2%
Epinephrine 1:10,000	Sodium chloride, 3 mEq/mL
Fentanyl 0.05 mg/mL	Sterile water
Flumazenil 0.5 mg/5 mL	Surfactant
Fosphenytoin 100 mg/2 mL	Vecuronium 1 mg/mL
Furosemide (Lasix) 10 mg/mL	

BOX 41.2 Suggested Supplies for Interhospital Transport

Intravenous Supplies	Airway Supplies
Alcohol and Betadine swabs	Resuscitation masks (various sizes)
Chlorhexidine prep	Anesthesia bag
Gauze (2 × 2 and 4 × 4)	Endotracheal tubes (2.5, 3.0, 3.5, and 4.0)
Cotton balls	Stylet
Band-Aids	Skin protector (DuoDERM)
Label tape	Adhesive and adhesive remover
Clear tape (½ inch, 1 inch)	Adhesive tape
Self-adherent wrap (1 inch)	CO_2 detector
Tegaderm, small and large	Suction catheters (6, 8, and 10 Fr)
Needles (23 gauge, 19 gauge)	Laryngoscope and blades (00, 0, and 1)
IO needles (18 gauge)	Spare laryngoscope bulb and batteries
IV catheters (14, 16, 18, and 24 gauge)	Magill forceps
Butterfly needle (19, 23, and 25 gauge)	Nasal CPAP prongs (10.5, 12, and 15 Fr)
Syringes (blood gas, 1, 3, 5, 10, and 30 mL)	Endotracheal tube bridge
Arm board	Laryngeal mask airway (1 and 1.5)
IV extension tubing	Nasal trumpet
Y-adapter and T-connector	Oral airway (00, 0, 1, and 2)
IV pump tubing	Thoracostomy tubes (8, 10, and 12 Fr)
Three-way stopcock	Thoracostomy tray
Heparin lock	Heimlich valve
Catheter adapters (18, 20, and 21)	5-to-1 (Christmas tree) adapter
Umbilical line supplies	Vaseline gauze
Catheters (3.5 and 5 Fr with double lumen 5 Fr)	Nasal cannula
Umbilical tape	Normal saline bullets
Umbilical line tray	Bulb syringe
Suture	Meconium aspirator
Umbilical line bridges	GI supplies
Phlebotomy supplies	Replogle catheters (6, 8, 10, and 12 Fr)
Lancets	Feeding tubes (5, 6.5, and 8 Fr)
Capillary tubes	Sterile specimen (bowel) bag
Heparin tubes	Other
Tourniquet	Soft restraints
Blood culture bottles	Stockinette cap
Chemstrips	Safety pins
Chemical warmers, small	Rubber bands
Monitoring Supplies	Scissors
ECG leads	Hemostats
Oximeter probe	Penlight
BP cuff (1, 2, 3, and 4)	Flashlight
Thermometer	Sterile gloves

BP, Blood pressure; *CPAP*, continuous positive airway pressure; *ECG*, electrocardiogram; *GI*, gastrointestinal; *IO*, intraosseous; *IV*, intravenous.

Transport systems have now been specifically designed to incorporate all of the critical life support systems and technology in a single mobile unit, including the transport incubator, ventilator, monitoring systems, suction apparatus, and infusion pumps. Medical gas tanks are usually stowed on the bottom of the transport sled to provide compact storage but easy accessibility. Equipment used during transport can be run via an AC/DC power source or via internal battery if necessary. Transport ventilators may be powered pneumatically or by AC/DC power with battery backup. These complete systems have been designed to promote ease of movement, security within the transport vehicle to minimize the effect of vibration and motion, clear visualization of both monitors and the baby, and easy access to the infant.

Monitoring during transport of the ventilated infant has become significantly easier with the development of the pulse oximeter. Current models available provide adequate readouts despite the vibration contributed by the transport environment. Monitoring with pulse oximetry and electrocardiograph leads is standard during all transports. Target ranges for oxygen saturation should be adhered to during transport, especially for the ELBW infant. Several teams have also used noninvasive end-tidal CO_2 detectors or transcutaneous CO_2 monitors for evaluation during transport and found them to be effective, although some have noted problems with specific monitors being cumbersome and difficult to secure during transport.[40-42] Tingay et al.,[43] however, found that end-tidal CO_2 monitoring underestimated arterial CO_2 levels and did not trend reliably over time. Transport teams must still evaluate these adjuncts individually to determine their benefit, because no single standard has been adopted. Colorimetric CO_2 monitors that are placed briefly on the end of the endotracheal tube have been more universally adopted and have proven useful for confirming initial endotracheal intubation and for confirming continued intubation after

movement from the incubator to warmer and back during transport.[42]

Quality of care and efficiency during transport have been greatly improved by the use of point-of-care devices that allow point-of-care analysis of blood gases, hematocrit, glucose, electrolytes, and ionized calcium on a small amount of blood (0.3 mL). Compact and easy to use, this handheld instrument is easily carried in the equipment pack and provides rapid analysis at outlying hospitals, where blood gas measurements may be difficult to obtain in a timely manner and a small blood sample. Macnab et al.[44] demonstrated that there is significant cost efficacy with the use of this technology and that use of point-of-care testing can reduce stabilization times and improve quality of care.

One piece of equipment not carried by all transport teams is the LMA. The laryngeal mask is a supraglottic airway device that fits over the laryngeal inlet to provide a means for positive pressure ventilation. The deflated mask is inserted into the mouth of the infant using two fingers and is guided blindly along the hard palate without laryngoscopy or instrumentation. Once resistance is met, the mask is seated by inflating the rim with 2 to 4 mL of air, occluding the esophagus while covering the laryngeal opening. The most frequently reported use of laryngeal masks in neonates is for airway rescue when facemask ventilation and endotracheal intubation have failed. Multiple single case reports or small retrospective series have described successful use of a laryngeal mask as a lifesaving maneuver during management of a difficult airway. In a meta-analysis, Mora and Weiner[45] concluded that a fairly strong recommendation could be made to attempt laryngeal mask ventilation during resuscitation when other methods fail, based on the fact that placement of the laryngeal mask is fairly noninvasive, is easily placed by most providers, has a relatively low incidence of reported complications, and may be life-saving.

There are several case reports on the use of the LMA during transport. These case reports have documented the use of the LMA to resuscitate, and in some cases transport, infants with congenital anomalies and difficult airways, including descriptions of its successful use for choanal atresia,[46] severe micrognathia,[46] and laryngotracheoesophageal clefts.[47] The International Guidelines for Neonatal Resuscitation state that the LMA may be an effective alternative for establishing an airway if bag-mask ventilation is ineffective or attempts at intubation have failed, but routine use of the LMA is not currently recommended.[48] Given the unpredictable nature of difficult airway presentations and the challenge of providing optimal resuscitation in sometimes suboptimal conditions, transport teams may consider including an LMA in their equipment box and providing training to personnel in the use of the LMA. The smallest size LMA (size 1) is appropriate for most term and larger preterm neonates but is too large for infants weighing less than 1500 g.

Transport Ventilators

The Bio-Med MVP-10 ventilator has been the prototypic ventilator used for transport for some time and was, for many years, the "workhorse" ventilator used by many transport teams and is configured into many modular transport incubators (Bio-Med Devices Inc., Guilford, CT, USA). The MVP-10 is a pneumatically powered ventilator that provides time-cycled pressure-limited ventilation. It is capable of meeting standard ventilation needs and provides intermittent mandatory ventilation (IMV), PEEP, and CPAP. However, it lacks the ability to synchronize with the patient respiratory effort or to measure tidal volume.

Modern transport ventilators are capable of pressure or volume ventilation with assist control, synchronized IMV, PEEP, CPAP, and pressure support modes. Patient-triggered systems that respond to pressure or flow are also available and tidal volume measurement is now routine. Ventilators may be pneumatically powered or have AC/DC operation with internal battery backup.

During transport, it is essential to be able to deliver oxygen concentrations between 21% and 100% to limit oxygen exposure for preterm infants and infants with congenital heart disease yet provide high oxygen concentrations for infants with pulmonary hypertension and hypoxic respiratory failure. Air-oxygen blenders are available and should be used to adjust oxygen delivery. Medical gases for the ventilator are provided by cylinders mounted on the transport system frame during transfer or by larger cylinders that are part of the ambulance or aircraft configuration during transport itself. Table 41.1 lists the characteristics and expected life of various gas cylinders at differing flow rates. Team members should be familiar with cylinder capacity and the number of hours of flow provided, particularly for long transports or for infants requiring high concentrations and high flows of inspired oxygen.

High-Frequency Ventilation

HFV has been shown to be useful for the treatment of many respiratory disorders, including RDS, air leaks, meconium aspiration syndrome, and persistent pulmonary hypertension.[49-51] Many intensive care nurseries use HFV for infants who have failed conventional management, whereas others use it as their primary ventilator strategy for preterm infants at risk for chronic lung injury (see Chapter 24). Delivery of iNO has been shown to be more effective with high-frequency oscillatory ventilation (HFOV) for infants with hypoxic respiratory failure and severe parenchymal lung disease,[52] and it is this scenario that can pose difficulties for transport, when an unstable infant must be converted from HFV to conventional ventilation for transfer. Risks associated with such a conversion include loss of lung recruitment, atelectasis, and subsequent hypoxic respiratory failure. To maintain stability for infants already being treated with HFV at the outlying institution, as well as to extend a standard tertiary resource out to the transport environment, HFVs providing high-frequency jet ventilation (HFJV) or high-frequency flow interruption are now available for use on transport.

Although HFVs are now available, few studies have been performed to evaluate the risks and benefits of transport HFV. In a retrospective study, Mainali et al.[53] compared the use of HFJV, with or without iNO, to that of conventional ventilation. Twelve infants were transported on HFJV alone, 17 on HFJV with iNO, and 9 infants were transported on conventional ventilation with iNO. The infants transported on HFJV, regardless of the use of nitric oxide, demonstrated significant improvement in ventilation during transport after conversion to HFJV without an escalation in support. This included infants converted from conventional ventilation and HFOV. Infants on HFJV also demonstrated a trend toward improved oxygenation and oxygen index, but this did not reach statistical significance. It is important to note, however, that there was an increased incidence of pneumothorax both pre- and posttransport in the infants that received HFV when compared with those receiving conventional ventilation (7/29 HFJV vs. 1/9 conventional

TABLE 41.1 Characteristics of Portable Gas Cylinders

SPECIFICATIONS OF OXYGEN CYLINDERS (E, M, H TYPE)

Cylinder Type	CAPACITY (cu ft)	(gal)	(L)	Height (in)	Diameter (in)	Weight of Full Tank (lb)
E	22	165	620	20	4¼	15
M	122	900	3450	46	7⅛	86
H	244	1800	6900	55	9	130

VOLUME AND FLOW DURATION OF OXYGEN IN THREE CYLINDER SIZES

	FULL			¾			½			¼		
Cylinder Type	E	M	H	E	M	H	E	M	H	E	M	H
Contents (cu ft)	22	107	244	16.5	80.2	193	11	53.5	122	5.5	26.8	6
Liters	622	3028	6900	466.5	2271	5175	311	1514	3450	155.5	757	172
Pressure (psi)		2000			1500			1000			500	

APPROXIMATE NUMBER OF HOURS OF FLOW IN THREE CYLINDER SIZES

	FULL			¾			½			¼		
Cylinder Type	E	M	H	E	M	H	E	M	H	E	M	H
Flow rate (L/min)												
2	5.1	25	56	3.8	18.5	42	2.5	12.5	28	1.3	6	14
4	2.5	12.6	28	1.8	10.4	21	1.2	6.3	14	0.6	3.1	7
6	1.7	8.4	18.5	1.3	6.3	13.7	0.9	4.2	9.2	0.4	2.1	4.5
8	1.2	6.3	14	0.9	4.6	10.5	0.6	3.1	7	0.3	1.5	3.5
10	1	5	11	0.7	3.7	8.2	0.5	2.5	5.5	0.2	1.2	2.7
12	0.8	4.2	9.2	0.6	3	6.7	0.4	2.1	4.5	0.2	1	2.2
15	0.6	3.4	7.2	0.4	2.5	5.5	0.3	1.7	3.5	0.1	0.8	1.7

pretransport and 3/29 HFJV and 0/9 conventional posttransport), although the presence of a pneumothorax pretransport may have biased decision making toward the use of HFJV. The authors concluded that HFJV with or without iNO is safe and efficacious during transport and may even be preferred to conventional ventilation.

Honey et al.[54] recently reported their experience transporting 134 infants using with the Duotron high-frequency flow interruptor. Sixty percent of the infants were less than 37 weeks, and 16% were less than 28 weeks gestational age. Infants were successfully transported on HFV 96% of the time. Reassuringly, there were no pneumothoraces in any of the transported infants. For the small number of infants that had pre- and posttransport blood gases available ($n = 24$), pH improved significantly after the initiation of HFV, whereas oxygenation and ventilation remained stable. Insights that were provided by the study include the fact that extensive training and education are needed for implementation of HFV on transport, and that there is a steep learning curve with its use. Differences in ventilator readouts and the need for fine-tuning of ventilator settings further complicate training, even for those with prior experience using HFV. Finally, point-of-care testing for blood gas analysis and complete monitoring with cardiorespiratory, oxygen (O_2) saturation, and CO_2 monitoring are necessary for optimal management of an infant on transport HFV. The Children's Mercy Hospital, Kansas City, MO, transport team found frequent blood gas analysis to be essential, with overventilation being a common problem encountered during the use of HFV (personal communication). Despite these limitations,

the Bronchotron, a successor of the Duotron (Percussionaire Corporation in Sandpoint, ID), remains the most widely used high-frequency transport ventilator. The recently released smaller, lighter high-frequency jet ventilator (Bunnell LifePulse model 204, Salt Lake City, UT) will likely lead to increased interest in HFJV during transport.

Continuous Positive Airway Pressure

The increasing use of CPAP for the respiratory support of newborn infants has necessitated that transport teams become more familiar and facile with its use. Despite a large body of evidence supporting the use of CPAP in the delivery room and intensive care unit, there is a paucity of data regarding its use during transport. The few studies that have been done suggest that CPAP can be delivered safely and effectively in appropriately selected infants during transport. Simpson et al.[55] reported their experience with seven preterm neonates and reported no complications during transport. Bomont et al.[56] reviewed their experience with 100 infants transferred on CPAP. Infants required minimal intervention during transport and were safely transported on CPAP with adequate blood gases on arrival. Five out of 100 infants required stimulation or prong repositioning for apnea, bradycardia, and desaturation, but no major intervention was needed.

Several limitations of the transport environment make the use of CPAP more difficult, however. Visual and auditory assessment is limited in the transport environment, and it can be difficult to achieve proper infant positioning in the transport incubator for adequate CPAP delivery. The use of more extensive transcutaneous CO_2 monitoring may facilitate the evaluation of the infant on transport CPAP. Because of these limitations, however, careful consideration must be given to the safety and stability of an infant being transported on CPAP, and factors such as the length of transport, mode of transport, and the gestational and chronologic age of the infant may all influence decision making regarding the appropriateness of CPAP in transport. Given the increasing use of CPAP in the delivery room for preterm infants, further study of the safety and efficacy of CPAP on transport should be undertaken.

Surfactant Administration

The administration of surfactant to infants with surfactant deficiency has had a significant impact on the morbidity and mortality of infants with RDS.[57,58] Experience with surfactant replacement in the transport environment has been adopted as part of the standard care offered by most transport teams. Costakos et al.[59] found that surfactant could be administered safely before the interhospital transport of preterm infants but were unable to identify significant benefits in terms of ventilator days, time to discharge, or incidence of bronchopulmonary dysplasia for infants who received surfactant before transport.[59] Endotracheal administration of surfactant is associated with the risk of respiratory compromise (desaturation, hypoxemia, bradycardia)[60] and should be performed by personnel with adequate experience in administration. Moreover, the change in lung compliance that usually follows surfactant administration should be carefully monitored by the transport team by monitoring changes in measured tidal volume; chest wall movement may be difficult to discern in a transport vehicle.

Inhaled Nitric Oxide

iNO has been shown to improve oxygenation and reduce the need for ECMO in near-term and term infants with persistent pulmonary hypertension (PPHN) and hypoxemic respiratory failure.[52,61,62] Since the US Food and Drug Administration (FDA) approved the use of iNO for respiratory failure, iNO has become available at most level III NICUs. Although this benefits most infants, 30% to 40% of infants fail to show a sustained response to iNO and may require transport to an ECMO center.[63] Further, rapid withdrawal of iNO can precipitate rebound hypoxemia, thereby further compromising an already unstable infant.[64] The need to continue iNO initiated at the outlying institution has prompted most transport teams to become capable of delivering iNO during transfer.

Several studies have evaluated the use of iNO during transport.[63,65-67] Kinsella et al.[65] and Goldman et al.[66] first demonstrated that critically ill infants with hypoxemic respiratory failure could be safely transported on iNO and that ambient levels of the gas were maintained well below levels of risk in a closed transport vehicle. Since that time, all studies have demonstrated safe transfer of infants on iNO. Kinsella et al.[65] were able to show that inhaled iNO acutely improved oxygenation in hypoxemic infants and that the effect was sustained during transport. iNO was also used to support the conversion from HFOV to conventional ventilation because it minimized the pulmonary vasoreactivity associated with the change and decreased the lability associated with PPHN.

These results were confirmed by Westrope et al.,[67] who retrospectively reviewed their experience in transporting 55 patients on iNO to a tertiary center for ECMO consideration. They found that oxygenation improved after the initiation of iNO, as demonstrated by significant improvement in both PaO_2 and oxygen saturations, and that iNO delivered in transport maintained the stability of patients previously on iNO.

Therapies should be initiated on transport with the goal of providing appropriate stabilization for safe transport, but ultimately with the goal of improving patient outcome. With this in mind, Lowe et al.[68] evaluated whether iNO initiated during transport showed benefit when compared with iNO initiated at arrival at the receiving facility. Although they found no difference in mortality rates or the need for ECMO for infants who received iNO before transfer, they did find a significantly shorter hospital stay for survivors who had iNO initiated in the field, suggesting that iNO initiated in transport may be cost saving.

For teams that decide to offer iNO, two FDA-approved delivery systems are commercially available—the AeroNOx device (Pulmonox Medical Inc., Tofield, Alberta, Canada) and the INOvent device (Datex-Ohmeda, Madison, WI). Safety during transport is of the utmost importance, and teams must be careful when transporting with a hazardous gas. Kinsella et al.[63] have shown that in a "worst-case scenario," where a full "D" cylinder of nitric oxide is completely released, maximum concentrations of nitric oxide would be 25.3 parts per million (ppm), 34 ppm, and 94 ppm in a fixed-wing jet, ambulance, and helicopter, respectively. Maximum allowable transient exposures are 25 to 100 ppm, and in a helicopter, completely released levels approach Occupational Safety and Health and National Institute for Occupational Safety and Health levels that pose an immediate danger to life or health.[69] Transport teams should develop a system in which the choice to carry nitric oxide can be made during the preparation for the transport run, to avoid carrying a hazardous gas unnecessarily for all neonatal transports.

Extracorporeal Membrane Oxygenation

Uncommonly, a neonate may require transport while receiving ECMO. This occurs most often when an infant is unable to be weaned off ECMO but requires specialized services at another institution. It also may occur in an infant too unstable to survive transport, necessitating cannulation at the referring facility before transport. As of this writing, 12 centers in the United States offer transport ECMO. Wilford Hall Medical Center provides global transport ECMO and has reported their 22-year experience with 68 children transported on ECMO by ground or fixed-wing aircraft.[70] All children survived transport. Survival to discharge was 65% for transported ECMO infants, which was equivalent to a survival rate of 70% for in-house patients receiving ECMO. Given the increasing use of extracorporeal cardiopulmonary resuscitation,[71,72] the need for transport ECMO may increase in the future but will likely continue to be a specialized service offered by only a few institutions with specialized training.

Hypothermia for Hypoxic Ischemic Encephalopathy

Therapeutic hypothermia (either by whole body or selective head cooling methods) is now standard of care for selected newborn infants with moderate to severe hypoxic ischemic encephalopathy (HIE). Multiple studies have shown that efficacy of treatment is enhanced by meeting early inclusion criteria and starting cooling before 6 hours of life. Therefore, starting cooling before and on transport is a natural extension, because in many cases, the appropriate window to commence treatment may already pass before a neonate is transported and admitted to a tertiary center. There are limited data suggesting how to perform cooling during transport, either passively or by certain manufactured or home-built cooling methods. Programs should work in close connection with their neurologists and intensivists to arrive at an agreed-on method, and appropriate training should be documented for all team personnel.[73] Through outreach education, referring centers should be aware of uniform inclusion criteria and delivery methods. The largest study published in 2013 by the California Perinatal Quality Care Collaborative confirmed earlier observations that there is variability in delivery methods and that most patients do not achieve target temperature by the time of arrival at the accepting cooling center. Manufactured cooling devices and not passive cooling methods is the recommended mode on transport. Outcome studies now show clearly that infants with moderate HIE may benefit more than those with severe HIE.[31,73]

FUTURE DIRECTIONS

The neonatal transport team plays a critical role in providing optimal care to the ill outborn neonate. The role of the transport team has expanded as technology has advanced and has made it possible to deliver sophisticated therapies to infants out in the field. The integration of wireless web-based cellular technology and telemedicine allows tertiary centers to observe and interact in real time with the transport team. We have now begun to consider that earlier initiation of specific therapies, beginning in transport, may influence long-term outcomes. Although it is more difficult to conduct studies in the transport arena, prospective studies are possible and are now being done. The transport environment will continue to change as new technology and therapies develop. The expanding use of clinical simulators should be useful for transport team education and should be used to promote technical and clinical skill maintenance for team members. The emerging use of telemedicine, and its use on transport, may significantly change interactions with outlying practitioners and team communication with medical control. As changes come, the neonatal transport team will continue to play a vital role in stabilizing and transferring infants who require specialized care.

KEY REFERENCES

6. McNamara PJ, Mak W, Whyte HE: Dedicated neonatal retrieval teams improve delivery room resuscitation of outborn premature infants. J Perinat 25:309–314, 2005.

9. Woodward GE, Insoft RM, Pearson-Shaver AL, et al: The state of pediatric interfacility transport: consensus of the Second National Pediatric and Neonatal Interfacility Transport Medicine Leadership Conference. Ped Emerg Care 18:38–43, 2002.

10. Karlsen KA, Trautman M, Price-Douglas W, et al: National survey of neonatal transport teams in the United States. Pediatrics 128:685–691, 2011.

23. American Academy of Pediatrics: Section on transport medicine. In Insoft RM, Schwartz H (eds): Guidelines for Air and Ground Transport of Neonatal and Pediatric Patients. 4th ed. Elk Grove Village, IL, American Academy of Pediatrics, 2015, pp. 33–55.

24. American Academy of Pediatrics: Section on transport medicine. In Meyer K, Fernandes C (eds): Field Guide for Air and Ground Transport of Neonatal and Pediatric Patients. 1st ed. Elk Grove Village, IL, American Academy of Pediatrics, 2019, pp. 36–38.

34. Schwartz H, Bigham M, Schoettker P, et al: Quality metrics in neonatal and pediatric critical care transport: a national Delphi project. Pediatr Crit Care 16:711–717, 2015.

39. Singh S, Allen WD, Venkataraman S, et al: Utility of a novel quantitative handheld microstream capnometer during transport of critically ill children. Am J Emerg Med 24:302–307, 2006.

48. Courtney SE, Durand DJ, Asselin JM, et al: High-frequency oscillatory ventilation versus conventional mechanical ventilation for very-low-birth-weight infants. N Engl J Med 347:643–652, 2002.

72. Akula VP, Gould JB, Hackel A, Oehlert A, Van Meurs KP. Therapeutic hypothermia during neonatal transport: data from the California Perinatal Quality Care Collaborative and California Perinatal Transport System for 2010. J Perinatol 33: 194–197, 2013.

42

Discharge and Transition to Home Care

Lawrence Rhein

The discharge readiness of infants is usually determined by the demonstration of achieving several minimum functional competencies. These competencies include (1) thermoregulation; (2) control of breathing without apnea, bradycardia, or desaturation; (3) respiratory stability with adequate oxygen saturation and ventilation; and (4) sustained weight gain.[1,2] With improvements in neonatal intensive care leading to increased survival of very preterm and very ill infants, a growing number of infants may not achieve these minimum competencies, especially those involving adequate respiratory function, in a reasonable time frame without requiring especially prolonged hospitalization or without use of technology.[3-8]

Prolonged use of technology to support respiration results in difficult choices about disposition. Simply extending hospitalization allows continuity of care. However, prolonging inpatient hospitalization has several significant disadvantages. These include the following:

1. Increasing the period of separation of infants from their families. Several studies have shown that decreased visitation by parents during the neonatal intensive care unit (NICU) hospitalization results in decreased bonding.[9-14]
2. Increasing the exposure to risks of hospital-acquired morbidities, such as hospital-acquired infections.[15]
3. Decreased availability of required developmental therapies. Most infants who require technology to support breathing are in acute care facilities. Such facilities tend to dedicate fewer resources to rehabilitation services (occupational therapy, physical therapy, etc.) that growing infants often require to optimize neurodevelopment.

Depending on the capabilities of home caretakers and the resources in the community, pediatric home ventilation may be a feasible option in certain situations because of improvements in ventilator technology and increased prevalence of outpatient follow-up support.[16-19] However, to minimize risks, careful planning is required.

The goal of this chapter is to review the factors to consider when deciding to discharge a technology-dependent infant to home, as well as to provide guidelines to accomplish a safe transition.

FACTORS TO CONSIDER WHEN DETERMINING READINESS FOR DISCHARGE

Determining the appropriate timing to safely discharge a technology-dependent infant from the hospital after a stay in the NICU can be complicated. This decision is made primarily based on the infant's medical status but requires consideration of several additional factors (Box 42.1). These factors include:

1. Medical stability of the child.

    Infants need to be clinically stable for a minimum of 2 to 4 weeks. Clinically stable means no major diagnostic or therapeutic changes in the management, with stable ventilator settings and oxygen requirement.[20] There is no absolute maximum level of support that precludes discharge,[21] but typically, the oxygen requirement includes FIO_2 of 40% or less and peak inspiratory pressure (PIP) under 40 cm H_2O for pressure-limited ventilation. For all parameters (PIP, oxygen concentration, etc.), there needs to be an ability to increase levels at home without automatically requiring visit to the emergency department. In addition, the infant needs to be able to tolerate a nutritional regimen that allows adequate growth.

2. Availability of care providers.

    The level of care/support required at home varies with each child. Most providers for the care of pediatric home ventilator patients recommend that two caregivers should be trained to discharge a child home safely.[20] Patients should spend at least 24 to 48 hours on their personal home ventilator before discharge home, and caregivers should spend this same 24 to 48 hours doing independent caregiving for the child while he or she is in the hospital before discharge. Families of technology-dependent children qualify for home nursing support, but the number of hours filled

BOX 42.1 Discharge Criteria

Medical Stability

Treatment plan for all medical conditions is in place, will not require frequent changes, and can be implemented at home

Adequate nutritional plan in place

Respiratory Stability

Safe and secure airway: tracheostomy with sufficient mature stoma to allow tube changes or stabilized on regimen of NIV with minimal risk for aspiration

Able to clear secretions, spontaneously or with assistance

Oxygenation stable including during suctioning and repositioning

Stable $FiO_2 \leq 0.4$ with PEEP ≤ 8 cm H_2O

Stable ventilator settings with PIP ≤ 30 cm

Stability criteria met for 2–4 weeks

Home Stability

Stable home and family setting

Willing and able caregivers identified and trained before discharge

Adequate financial resources and mechanisms for reimbursement identified before discharge

NIV, Noninvasive ventilation; *PEEP*, positive end-expiratory pressure; *PIP*, peak inspiratory pressure.

often falls short of those eligible or those deemed necessary.[22,23] Especially in households with other siblings, the increased care needs of the technology-dependent child often require a caregiver without other distracting responsibilities.

3. Seasonal factors.

Although technology-dependent infants can be discharged in any season, the risk of rehospitalization owing to viral infection is increased in the fall and winter months. If available, transition to a rehabilitation facility during the peak viral season may be desirable to both minimize infectious risk and allow additional training and potential improvement in medical stability.

Most importantly, the decision to initiate transfer of a ventilated patient to home (instead of extension of hospitalization in an acute-care facility or transfer to a rehabilitation facility) requires confirmation that the patient's needs can be balanced with resources at home. The needs to be considered include physician availability and care (including pulmonary subspecialist care), appropriate equipment, and personnel (nursing care, respiratory care, personal care attendants and family members). The remainder of this chapter will describe guidelines to facilitate a successful transition to home and will also provide guidance regarding discharge of infants on home oxygen therapy (HOT).

DISCHARGE TEAM

Discharge of the ventilator-dependent child requires a multidisciplinary approach.[19,24-27] The team needs to include hospital and community-based personnel, including those who will continue to monitor the patient in the outpatient setting. Although there is no standard method for coordinating the discharge, we recommend a collaborative team approach that includes the following components:

Family caregivers: Clearly, the most important decision makers in the process of discharging ventilated patients are the family members themselves, who need to be involved in all aspects and need to fully be able to medically care for the patient.

Medical discharge coordinator: Hospital discharge planners have specific expertise with reimbursement-related issues; specifically, the financial issues include coverage of durable medical equipment (DME) by health care benefits, and coverage of nursing personnel. Discharge planners assist families in the identification of all health care benefits covered by third party insurers, entitlements, and assistance from federal, state, or local agencies.

Bedside clinical nursing staff: Before discharge, the bedside nursing team needs to identify all potential physician subspecialist caregivers (potentially pulmonologist, otolaryngologist, and certainly the primary care pediatrician) to confirm that all discharge criteria for each specialty have been met and to arrange appropriate follow-up visit schedules. In addition, bedside nursing is often responsible for the direct teaching of basic nursing care skills to the home caregivers.

Respiratory care clinicians: Although the bedside nursing staff is responsible for teaching nursing cares, the respiratory care therapist provides the specific teaching regarding the operation and use of the ventilator and tracheostomy care.

DME provider: DME providers are responsible for providing the ventilators and associated supplies to patients on long-term ventilation.

Primary outpatient physician: For most patients, even those with complex medical needs, the primary leader of the outpatient team is the primary care pediatrician. For ventilator-dependent patients, a specialist (pulmonologist or home ventilator team clinician) should be included as a primary consultant for families.

PREDISCHARGE NEEDS ASSESSMENT

Before discharge home, all infants require a thorough assessment to ensure that they are in fact ready for discharge. The components of a comprehensive assessment include the home environment, the availability of necessary equipment, and the availability of personnel resources to allow safe care. The level of support required at home will vary with each child and family. Factors to consider include level of medical care required, including (1) the time the child is dependent on the ventilator; (2) the amount of "reserve" in the event of ventilator failure or disconnection, or airway obstruction; (3) other care needs related to feeding issues; and (4) other demands on the family's time, particularly the presence of other children and work commitments. Especially when siblings who attend daycare or school are present, discharges in the peak of viral season, when infectious risks are highest, may be deferred. Finally, the availability of nonfamily assistance (home nursing) must be a primary consideration.

HOME ENVIRONMENT

The home environment needs to include sufficient space for all of the medical equipment and supplies, including the ventilator. The home environment needs to have appropriate power supplies for all the equipment and accessibility to emergency medical services needs to be ensured through the presence of a working telephone. Power companies should be notified of the electrical requirements and location of persons who require mechanical ventilation.

EQUIPMENT AND SUPPLIES

All children should be trialed on the equipment designated for home use while still in the hospital. Of note, most ventilators are not approved for use in infants below a minimum weight of 5 kg, so discharge may need to be deferred until an infant has achieved this minimal weight.

In addition to the ventilator, an itemized equipment list should be prepared and checked by the team (Box 42.2). A monthly estimate of disposable supplies and consumables also needs to be provided.

A second ventilator is required for any child who is unable to cope for 6 hours without ventilator support. In the event of power failure, it is critical to have an alternative power source available, in the form of either batteries or a generator. Some

---

BOX 42.2 Checklist of Equipment and Supplies to be Considered for Ventilator-Assisted Patients

Mechanical ventilator (also need back-up)
Exhalation valve
Tracheotomy tube adapter/connector
Humidifier and heater
Humidifier bracket
Heat and moisture exchanger
Manual resuscitator
Oxygen supply system (stationary and portable)
Oxygen bleed-in adapter to ventilator
Noninvasive patient interfaces
Face mask
Nasal mask or nasal pillows
Suction machine (stationary and portable)
Suction catheters
Connecting tubing
Suction collection container
Gloves
Other secretion clearance aids such as cough inex-sufflator
Spare tracheostomy tube (including next smaller size)
10-mL syringe used only to inflate or deflate cuff (for cuffed tracheostomy tubes)
Velcro trach tube strap
Tracheostomy tape
Sterile saline solution
Antibiotic ointment
Cotton-tipped applicators
Compressor for aerosolized medications

---

home ventilators have internal battery life of 12 hours or more when fully charged, but backup is still desirable.

PERSONNEL RESOURCES

DME providers should have personnel trained to manage ventilator-assisted patients in the home.

In combination with the hospital-based respiratory therapist and bedside nursing staff, DME providers assist in training the family regarding the use and maintenance of the ventilator, as well as in some of the care techniques, such as suctioning and tracheostomy care. The DME provider should always have backup equipment ready to handle emergencies. The DME provider should also have a clearly defined emergency response time.

HOME NURSING

The agency selected to provide home health care should have adequate staff available and have a nurse case manager to follow the patient and the nursing care and staffing provided. Families may also contract with private-duty nursing, but this also requires coordination with the discharge planners.

EMERGENCY PLANNING

Parents or caregivers need to be instructed on common potential scenarios that require urgent intervention. They should be able to recognize early signs and symptoms of illness and know how to respond. Local rescue and ambulance service should be informed that a technology-dependent child is in their region, so they can be prepared to provide emergency treatment or transport. In many cases, the closest hospital to a patient's home may not have pediatric expertise. Still, the local hospital must be notified of potential emergency needs, because in many cases, transport to the local hospital is necessary, with subsequent transport to a more specialized pediatric facility via a trained pediatric transport team.

The discharging facility should provide parents with a printed summary of medical issues, ventilator settings, and medications to provide to emergency responders.[28,29] If limits to resuscitation have been discussed, these also should be documented to avoid unwanted interventions.

POSTDISCHARGE FOLLOW-UP

A primary responsible caregiver needs to be clearly identified to assist in the ongoing management of the technology-dependent child. This may be the child's primary care pediatrician, pulmonary specialist, or another pediatric specialist. The parents/guardians must be able to identify the individual whom they can contact to seek advice, both during normal working hours and after hours, and should be able to identify indications for seeking help (see Box 42.3). Ongoing follow-up to monitor growth,[30] stability of respiratory status, and neurodevelopment are critical.

In summary, transition of the ventilator-dependent infant from hospital to home requires advance planning, teaching

BOX 42.3 Indications for Seeking Additional Assistance

Persistent symptoms of respiratory distress (tachypnea, grunting/flaring/retractions)
Oxygen desaturation
Ventilator alarms (low-minute ventilation, apnea, etc.)
Fever
Lethargy
Feeding intolerance
Pallor/cyanosis
Tachycardia or bradycardia

resources, and a collaborative team willing to partner with families. This chapter highlights some of the considerations required to ensure optimal outcomes and help infants to thrive in their home environment.

TRACHEOSTOMY CARE

Most infants who require ventilator support at home have tracheostomies, although noninvasive ventilation (bilevel positive airway pressure [BiPAP]) may be effective in rare select cases in infants without significant lung disease who do not require ventilation support when awake.[31]

Optimal care of a tracheostomy requires effective suctioning technique at appropriate frequency, as well as appropriate tracheostomy changes.

CHANGING TRACHEOSTOMY TUBES

Frequency of tracheostomy changes is determined by physician preference and availability of tubes. Increased frequency of changes may decrease infection risk but may also cause increased granuloma formation.

Ideally, elective trach changes should occur before feeds to minimize possibility of emesis. Emergency trach change may need to occur if:
- The trach tube is blocked;
- The trach tube slips out of the trachea;
- A suction catheter is unable to pass through the trach tube;
- The trach tube/cuff is not able to stay inflated; and/or
- There are symptoms of respiratory distress, including pallor or cyanosis, retractions, nasal flaring, or ineffective chest wall rise.

Before changing the trach, caregivers must prepare the following supplies:
- Oximeter
- Self-inflating bag with pop-off/mask
- Oxygen
- Suction with appropriate catheter
- Two trach tubes: one that is the current size and one that is a size smaller
- Trach tie
- Stoma dressing
- Syringe (10 mL)
- Water soluble lubricant

- Scissors
- Clean moistened gauze

To change the tracheostomy tube, caregivers should follow the following steps:
1. Suction if secretions are present.
2. Check new tube with cuff inflation (if applicable).
3. Remeasure suction depth with sterile catheter, adding 1 cm to the measured length.
4. Prepare the trach tie and stoma dressing.
5. Attach a tie to the new trach.
6. Apply water-soluble lubricant to the end of the tube and obturator.
7. Position your child with the stoma exposed by putting a rolled towel under the child's shoulders to access the site.
8. Unfasten the trach tie while holding the tube in place.
9. Deflate the cuff (if applicable).
10. Remove the trach tube.
11. Wipe the stoma with moistened gauze.
12. Check the stoma site for any areas that may look abnormal.
13. Place the new tube with an obturator in the stoma following the curve of the airway.
14. Immediately remove the obturator while holding the trach in place.
15. Place the child back on support, such as ventilator, oxygen, etc.
16. Inflate the cuff (if applicable).

Optimal outpatient management includes follow-up with a multidisciplinary team, including pulmonary specialists, respiratory therapists, and otorhinolaryngology surgeons.[32]

OUTPATIENT MANAGEMENT OF SUPPLEMENTAL OXYGEN THERAPY

A subset of infants with bronchopulmonary dysplasia (BPD) meet all other discharge criteria but remain hypoxemic, requiring supplemental oxygen to maintain adequate saturations. For many such infants, the decision to use HOT is an acceptable and desirable option. HOT has been shown to decrease health care costs[33-38] and to improve patient satisfaction compared to prolonged hospitalization.[35,39]

INDICATIONS FOR HOME OXYGEN THERAPY

Hypoxemia

The most common indication for HOT is persistent hypoxemia resulting from diffusion abnormality or parenchymal lung disease. It is important to note that not all causes of hypoxemia are treated with oxygen therapy. Specifically, infants with hypoventilation as a primary cause for their hypoxemia may be harmed by supplemental oxygen because of impairment of respiratory drive, which may worsen hypoxemia.

No randomized controlled trials have been performed to determine what pulse oximeter saturation (SpO_2) criteria should be used for the initiation and management of HOT for BPD. As a result, there is little consensus regarding specific indications for its use.[40-43]

Most reviews suggest that HOT should be considered in infants whose room air SpO_2 is under 92% to 95%, with target saturations over 94%.[42-45] When considering these targets, it may be reasonable to consider adjusting the target based on whether the infant still has either pulmonary hypertension or retinopathy of prematurity. Target saturations in infants with pulmonary hypertension should be slightly higher in infants with BPD not complicated by pulmonary hypertension. In contrast, use of oxygen may need to be more restrictive, with lower tolerable target SPO_2 in infants whose eyes are not yet mature.

Growth Failure

Several studies have shown that HOT improves weight gain.

Groothuis and Rosenberg found that when parents prematurely discontinued supplemental oxygen against medical advice, mean daily weight gain fell significantly and improved once HOT was resumed. Other studies have replicated this finding.[46-48]

Intermittent Hypoxemia and Pulmonary Hypertension

Oxygen supplementation has been shown to decrease episodes of intermittent desaturation,[49] which are known to be extremely common even in otherwise "healthy" preterm infants.[50]

Oxygen is also a potent pulmonary vasodilator. Several studies have shown that supplemental oxygen can decrease pulmonary artery pressure in infants with severe BPD.[51,52]

OXYGEN DELIVERY SYSTEMS FOR HOME OXYGEN THERAPY

There are three basic home oxygen delivery systems: (1) oxygen concentrators, (2) liquid oxygen units, and (3) high-pressure cylinders.

Oxygen Concentrator

A concentrator is a device that separates oxygen from room air. It is small, reliable, and relatively inexpensive. Maximum flow rate is normally 5 to 6 L per minute. Concentrators have a unique advantage in that they are the only approved device for air travel for commercial flights.

Liquid Oxygen

Liquid oxygen is the most highly efficient means of transporting oxygen. One liter of liquid oxygen equals 860 gaseous liters. Liquid oxygen is approximately −297° F and when kept under pressure of 18 to 22 psi will remain in a liquid state. Conventional liquid oxygen vessels require no power source to operate, making it an appropriate choice for patients in areas with frequent power outages. Conventional liquid oxygen systems are quiet and have no major moving parts. Unfortunately, liquid oxygen is significantly more expensive than other oxygen delivery options.

Compressed Gas System

Cylinders of varying sizes are available. Such systems take up significantly more space, and larger cylinders can be very heavy.

Smaller cylinders allow more portability, but drain more quickly, and so require more frequent replacement.

STRATEGIES FOR DISCONTINUATION OF HOME OXYGEN THERAPY

Blending oxygen with room air allows delivery of a wider range of oxygen concentrations but requires blending of varying ratios of 100% oxygen with 21% oxygen. This is impractical in the home setting, so only 100% oxygen is delivered in the outpatient setting. Therefore, the primary variable that influences "effective" oxygen delivery, or the concentration of oxygen seen by the lungs, is the flow rate. Home oxygen is typically delivered via nasal cannula in the pediatric population. The delivered FiO_2 is dependent on the flow through the prongs, the level of entrainment, and the child's tidal volume, with the delivered FiO_2 ranging from 0.22 to 0.95 at a maximum flow of 2 L/min.[53] Cannula should be appropriately secured to the face to prevent skin breakdown and should be replaced as often as weekly if required. The prescribers should be proactive in delineating the appropriate oxygen delivery interface to minimize the risk of equipment-related complications, with special attention to maintaining skin integrity. Older patients or those not tolerating nasal cannulas with a higher oxygen flow rates may opt for the use of an appropriate oxygen mask, although more variability in FiO_2 based on mask positioning and patient tidal volume may be present. Few studies have been performed to determine the appropriate flow rate from which oxygen can be safely discontinued. In a small prospective study, Simoes et al. demonstrated that infants on 20 mL/kg or less of oxygen were more successful.[54] Other studies have suggested that 24% oxygen is the appropriate amount of oxygen from which oxygen weaning can safely be started. Finer et al. evaluated the effective oxygen concentration in infants of different sizes with variable oxygen delivery flow rates.[55] For infants of minimum size for outpatient care (2 kg), a flow rate of 125 mL/min achieves an effective oxygen delivery less than 24%, so this flow rate is an appropriate rate from which to begin a discontinuation plan.

Once a patient is considered ready for discontinuation of nighttime HOT altogether, then an in-home, room air, nocturnal pulse oximetry study should be performed using appropriate pediatric equipment and reference ranges as outlined in this document. Health care providers should encourage families to maintain accessibility to HOT for several months after discontinuation, particularly through the winter season, when viral illnesses are prevalent. This allows for ample opportunity to determine whether the withdrawal of HOT was well timed, in addition to how well respiratory illnesses are tolerated without supplemental oxygen.

As suggested when assessing for patient readiness to wean HOT, it is necessary to monitor responses to each change repeatedly. Given the chronicity of these respiratory conditions, changes should be made on a weeks to months basis, as opposed to more quickly, so that subtle deterioration is not missed, and suboptimal therapy is promptly reversed. The factors to monitor reflect those assessed when considering patient readiness and include patient growth, development, cardiorespiratory status, and stability of health (e.g., handling of respiratory illnesses, travel to altitude).

Simoes et al. suggested that a 40-minute room air trial predicted successful discontinuation of oxygen.[54] In our clinic, we initiate "sprints" off oxygen in increments of 1–2 hours and allow extension of sprints every 3 to 4 days. During the sprints to room air, infants should stay on an oximeter to confirm their ability to maintain saturations above 93%. Assuming uninterrupted successful biweekly extensions of the sprints, infants should be able to remain off oxygen for 12 hours during the day within 3 weeks of starting the sprints. Once this is achieved, we perform a recorded oximetry study off oxygen to confirm that the infants can maintain acceptable saturations greater than 93% off oxygen for a minimum of 8 hours. This is consistent with many other institutions in the United States.[56] If infants can maintain saturations greater than 93% for more than 95% of the recorded time, then the oxygen is discontinued. However, if growth is not maintained, then nocturnal oxygen use may be extended. It is important to note that not only oxygen saturation, but also adequate somatic growth and normalization of pulmonary pressures are important outcomes to consider before discontinuing supplemental oxygen therapy.

Newer technology now allows for more convenient long-term recording of patient oxygen saturations. Studies are underway to determine if such data may improve outpatient weaning protocols.

In summary, for many infants with BPD, safe outpatient use of supplemental oxygen can allow infants to continue to progress in the home environment rather than in the NICU. Further research is needed to determine optimal weaning strategies, but recent published case series can provide guidance until more definitive studies are completed.

KEY REFERENCES

1. Committee on Fetus and Newborn: Hospital discharge of the high-risk neonate: proposed guidelines. Pediatrics 102:411–417, 1998.
6. McDougall CM, Adderley RJ, Wensley DF, et al: Long-term ventilation in children: longitudinal trends and outcomes. Arch Dis Child 98(9):660–665, 2013.
19. Sterni LM, Collaco JM, Baker CD, et al, ATS Pediatric Chronic Home Ventilation Workgroup: An official American Thoracic Society Clinical Practice Guideline: pediatric chronic home invasive ventilation. Am J Respir Crit Care Med 193:e16–e35, 2016.
29. Baker CD, Martin S, Thrasher J, et al: A standardized discharge process decreases length of stay for ventilator-dependent children. Pediatrics 137:e20150637, 2016.
32. Gien J, Kinsella J, Thrasher J, et al: Retrospective analysis of an interdisciplinary ventilator care program intervention on survival of infants with ventilator-dependent bronchopulmonary dysplasia. Am J Perinatol 34:155–163, 2017.
35. Hallam L, Rudbeck B, Bradley M: Resource use and costs of caring for oxygen-dependent children: a comparison of hospital and home-based care. J Neonatal Nurs 2:25–30, 1996.
39. Hayes D Jr, Wilson KC, Krivchenia K, et al: Hayes home oxygen therapy for children. An official American Thoracic Society Clinical Practice Guideline. Am J Respir Crit Care Med 199(3):e5–e23, 2019.
43. Kotecha S, Allen J: Oxygen therapy for infants with chronic lung disease. Arch Dis Child Fetal Neonatal Ed 87:F11–F14, 2002.
48. Moyer-Mileur LJ, Nielson DW, Pfeffer KD, et al: Eliminating sleep-associated hypoxemia improves growth in infants with bronchopulmonary dysplasia. Pediatrics 98:779–783, 1996.
50. Rhein L, Simoneau T, Davis J, et al: Reference values of nocturnal oxygenation for use in outpatient oxygen weaning protocols in premature infants. Pediatr Pulmonol 47(5):453–459, 2012.

43

Neurologic Effects of Respiratory Support in the Neonatal Intensive Care Unit

Vivien Yap and Jeffrey M. Perlman

KEY POINTS

- Neonatal respiratory conditions, such as respiratory distress syndrome and bronchopulmonary dysplasia, and the interventions used to treat these conditions are strongly linked to brain injury in newborns, especially in preterm infants.
- The most common forms of brain injury in the premature infant are periventricular–intraventricular hemorrhage (IVH) and periventricular leukomalacia, which occur in the most underdeveloped brains.
- Perturbations of cerebral blood flow that lead to hemorrhage and/or hypoxia-ischemia in the brain are linked to the primary respiratory disease processes as well as the interventions used to treat them.

INTRODUCTION

The use of respiratory support in the neonatal intensive care unit (NICU) to treat a variety of newborn respiratory conditions (e.g., respiratory distress syndrome [RDS] and chronic lung disease) is common. Both the respiratory pathologies and the interventions used to treat these conditions have been linked to brain injury in preterm and term neonates. This chapter reviews (1) the basic physiology of cerebral blood flow in the neonate; (2) the common causes of neonatal brain injury, including their pathophysiology; (3) how carbon dioxide and oxygen influence brain injury; (4) how mechanical aspects distinct to the mode of ventilation affect brain injury; and (5) how medications used in respiratory management can modulate brain injury. The focus will be on preterm infants because this is the population at the highest risk for permanent brain injury.

CEREBRAL BLOOD FLOW IN THE NEONATE

Cerebral blood flow (CBF) is tightly linked to cerebral metabolic demands in the normal brain.[1-3] CBF is low in the newborn infant, which reflects low neuronal activity in this population.[4] Various methods of evaluation, including positron emission tomography, xenon clearance technique, ultrasound flowmetry, magnetic resonance imaging, and near-infrared spectroscopy (NIRS), indicate a wide range of CBF values of between 5 and 20 mL/100 g/min.[5-10] These values are approximately one-third of the value for a healthy adult brain.[1,8,11] A low CBF value in this population does not imply poor outcome because the lower threshold required to maintain neuronal

viability remains unknown.[8,12] On the first day of life, CBF in preterm infants can be lower than the minimal CBF necessary to preserve viability and metabolism in the adult brain.[13]

CBF is controlled by a pressure gradient across the cerebral vascular bed and is a function of cerebral perfusion pressure (CPP) and cerebrovascular resistance (CVR) as follows: CBF = CPP/CVR.[2,3] Total and regional CBF, coupled with cerebral oxygen consumption, increases with postconceptual and postnatal age corresponding to increases in cerebral metabolic rates and energy demands.[2,14] This increase is most prominent in the first day of life and likely represents a normal adaptive response of the cerebral circulation to postnatal life.[7,12] Regional differences in CBF also reflect varying metabolic demands. For instance, blood flow to parasagittal and periventricular white matter is lower relative to that of other regions such as the cerebellum and basal ganglia.[2]

Cerebral Autoregulation and Pressure-Passive Circulation

Cerebral autoregulation is the intrinsic ability of the cerebral blood vessels to maintain a relatively constant CBF over a range of mean arterial blood pressures (MABPs) (Fig. 43.1). As CPP decreases, CVR also decreases by alterations in the diameter of the precapillary arterioles, thus maintaining CBF.[1,3,4,15] This adaptive ability has a limited capacity and will result in a decrease in CBF when the blood pressure falls below a certain threshold and, conversely, will increase when blood pressure reaches an upper threshold.[16] This is referred to as a loss of autoregulation, or a pressure-passive state.[3,16]

Cerebral autoregulation appears to be intact in fetal and neonatal animal models.[2,3,15] It also appears to be intact in the stable human preterm infant.[3,17,18] In a study of extremely preterm infants with median gestational age of 24 weeks, CBF was found to be low (range of 4.4 to 11 mL/100 g/min), with no relationship of CBF to systemic blood pressure, suggesting intact autoregulation.[12] In another study of preterm infants with a mean gestational age of 26 weeks, normotensive infants (MABP 37 ± 2 mm Hg) were shown to have intact autoregulation, although there was a loss of autoregulation in those who became hypotensive (MABP 25 ± 1 mm Hg). This study also identified an MABP threshold of around 30 mm Hg, below which the CBF became pressure passive.[19] However, a definition of this lower threshold remains elusive. Victor et al. analyzed electroencephalography (EEG) patterns in 35 preterm infants

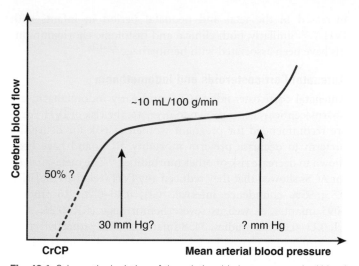

Fig. 43.1 Schematic depiction of the relationship between cerebral blood flow and mean arterial blood pressure. Note the autoregulatory plateau. The precise range of blood pressures in which this occurs for preterm neonates is unknown. (From Greisen G: Autoregulation of cerebral blood flow in newborn babies. Early Hum Dev 81:423-428, 2005.)

(median gestational age, 27 weeks) daily until day 4 of life.[20] Notably, four infants had abnormal EEGs, and the MABPs in these infants were significantly lower than those with normal EEGs (22 vs. 33 mmm Hg; $P < .001$). This suggests that the lower limit of MABP for autoregulation was in the range of 22 to 33 mm Hg in this cohort. Another study showed no difference in CBF between a group of preterm infants with an MABP of less than 30 mm Hg and another group with an MABP greater than 30 mm Hg.[21]

In summary, although cerebral autoregulation has been documented in the premature infant, it appears to function within a limited blood pressure range and is impaired or absent in the sick hypotensive preterm infant.[22-24] This vulnerable state places the developing brain at great risk for injury during times of hypotension and/or elevated blood pressures. This pressure passive state increases vulnerability to a variety of exposures that involve fluctuations of systemic blood pressures. Thus, CBF is one of the most important factors contributing to the major forms of preterm brain injury, as will be detailed subsequently.

BRAIN INJURY IN THE PRETERM INFANT

The most common forms of brain injury in the underdeveloped premature brain are periventricular-intraventricular hemorrhage (IVH; including periventricular hemorrhagic infarction [PVI]) and periventricular leukomalacia (PVL). These lesions are more likely to occur in the smallest, most immature infants with RDS requiring mechanical ventilation. The majority of permanent long-term neurologic sequelae in preterm infants are a result of these two forms of brain injury.[25,26]

Periventricular-Intraventricular Hemorrhage

The overall incidence of IVH and severe IVH has declined over the past few decades, although severe hemorrhage continues to be a significant morbidity in the increasing population of extremely preterm survivors.[27-29] The incidence and severity of IVH are inversely proportional to gestational age. For those

born below 29 weeks of gestation, 15% still have the most severe forms of hemorrhage, occurring in 37% of those born at 23 weeks and 24% in infants born at 24 weeks.[28]

The primary lesion in IVH is bleeding from the subependymal germinal matrix. This matrix is a transitional region of neuronal and glial precursor cells that migrate to other regions of the cerebrum. It is a highly cellular, richly vascularized structure and gelatinous in texture. It is located between the caudate nucleus and the thalamus at the level of, or slightly posterior to, the foramen of Monro. It begins to involute after 34 weeks, and by term gestation, it is essentially absent. Destruction of the germinal matrix may result in impairment of myelination, brain growth, and cortical development.[2]

Reviewing the vascular supply of the germinal matrix is crucial to understanding its propensity to bleed. The immature capillary network of the germinal matrix is supplied primarily by Heubner's artery, a branch of the anterior cerebral artery. Blood supply for the upper and middle regions of the matrix comes from the terminal branches of the lateral striate branches of the middle cerebral artery and the anterior choroidal artery[30] (see Fig. 43.2A). Venous drainage incorporates a system of medullary, choroidal, and thalamostriate veins that link to form the terminal vein. Where the terminal vein and the internal cerebral vein join, the venous flow makes a U-turn before continuing on to join the vein of Galen. This venous anatomy suggests that elevated venous pressure secondary to obstruction of the venous drainage may lead to venous distention and rupture (see Fig. 43.2B).[2] In addition, hypotension leading to decreased CBF probably also plays a role in the genesis of IVH in some infants. This likely occurs via a mechanism of ischemia-reperfusion with rupture of blood vessels upon reperfusion. Precise description of the vasculature of the germinal matrix has been elusive because the small capillaries, venules, and arterioles that populate the matrix are hard to distinguish from one another histologically because of their relatively simple endothelial wall structure.[30-32]

Physiologic Factors Contributing to Intraventricular Hemorrhage

The physiologic factors contributing to increased risk of IVH are complex and incorporate a combination of vascular, intravascular, and extravascular influences (see Table 43.1).[33,34] Intravascular factors, especially those that involve perturbations in CBF and volume, play a critical role in the development of hemorrhage. A pressure-passive circulation in the sick preterm brain leads to direct changes in CBF with changes in systemic blood pressure. Acute changes in blood pressure and cerebral perfusion are likely to lead to disruption of the vulnerable blood vessels in the germinal matrix.[23,35] Fluctuating CBF velocity in the very low birth weight (VLBW) infant also predisposes the infant to hemorrhage.[32,36] Physiologic increases in cerebral venous pressure exacerbate the already compromised venous drainage of the terminal vein. These physiologic disturbances may be from a variety of factors, such as the labor and delivery process and intrathoracic pressure changes induced by the ventilator or air leaks. Intrathoracic pressure is directly transmitted to cerebral vessels, and these fluctuations are applied to vessels probably already maximally dilated with little autoregulation.

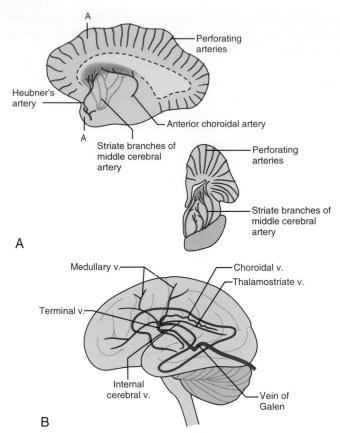

Fig. 43.2 **(A)** Arterial supply to the basal ganglia and periventricular areas in the preterm brain. (From Hambleton G, Wigglesworth JS: Origin of intraventricular haemorrhage in the preterm infant. Arch Dis Child 51:651-659, 1976.) **(B)** Schematic depiction of medullary veins draining into the terminal vein. Note the U-turn the terminal vein takes before draining into the internal cerebral vein, a potential site for increasing venous pressure. (From Volpe JJ, Volpe JJ: Volpe's Neurology of the Newborn. 6th ed. Philadelphia, PA, Elsevier, 2018.)

TABLE 43.1   Factors That Increase Risk of Brain Injury in the Preterm Infant

Intravascular factors	Hypotension, hypertension
	Blood pressure fluctuations
Extravascular factors	Poor vascular support
	Increased fibrinolytic activity
Cerebral factors	Vulnerable cerebral vascular bed
	Pressure-passive circulation
Respiratory factors	Respiratory distress syndrome
	Pneumothorax
	High mean airway pressure
	Hypocarbia, hypercarbia
	Hypoxia, hyperoxia
Perinatal factors	Chorioamnionitis
	Timing of cord clamping
Metabolic factors	Acidosis, alkalosis, hypernatremia

Inflammation and Intraventricular Hemorrhage

Another intravascular component that has been implicated in playing a role in IVH is inflammation, which has been correlated with increased risk of IVH.[37,38] Although precise mechanisms are unclear, increased interleukin (IL)-1β, IL-6, and IL-8; mononuclear cells; and other inflammatory markers have been

increased in the fetal and neonatal period in infants with IVH.[39-43] Similarly, both clinical and histologic chorioamnionitis have been associated with hemorrhage.[42,44-46]

Antenatal Corticosteroids and Indomethacin

Antenatal corticosteroids (ACSs) and early indomethacin are pharmaceutical agents shown to decrease the risk of IVH. ACSs are recommended for pregnant women at risk for delivering preterm to decrease preterm mortality, RDS, and have been shown to decrease risk of other morbidities.[47] The meta-analysis for ACSs showed that they reduced any IVH (relative risk [RR], 0.55; 95% confidence interval [CI], 0.40–0.76; 16 studies, 6093 infants), as well as severe hemorrhage (RR, 0.26; 95% CI, 0.11–0.60; six studies, 3438 infants).[48] The protective effect of steroids may in part be related to enhanced support for the fetal blood vessels within the germinal matrix.[33] The general vascular support of the germinal matrix capillaries is poor, with increased fibrinolytic activity and decreased glial stabilization. Finally, the germinal matrix capillaries themselves are quite tenuous, as they are in a constant state of involution and remodeling. Their vascular lining is deficient, and they reside in an end-arterial zone between the striate and the thalamic arterial distribution.[2]

Indomethacin is a prostaglandin synthetase inhibitor that has been used to promote closure of a patent ductus arteriosus (PDA). Its use as prophylaxis, before the PDA is hemodynamically significant, has been studied and was shown to decrease IVH. In a meta-analysis of those studies, there was a significant reduction of any IVH (RR, 0.88; 95% CI, 0.80–0.98; 14 trials, 2532 infants), as well as severe IVH (RR, 0.66; 95% CI, 0.53–0.82; 14 trials, 2588 infants).[49] Similar to ACSs, indomethacin is thought to promote maturation of microvessels in the germinal matrix.[50] It also helps attenuate the vascular hyperemia that occurs after hypoxia and hypercapnia.[51,52]

Delayed Cord Clamping

Delayed cord clamping has been shown to reduce the incidence of IVH in the preterm infant, likely because it allows for more stable transition to neonatal circulation. In a meta-analysis, there was a reduction in the risk of any IVH compared with immediate cord clamping (average RR, 0.83; 95% CI, 0.7–0.99; 15 studies, 2333 babies), without clear benefit in regard to severe IVH (average RR, 0.94; 95% CI, 0.63–1.39; 10 studies, 2058 babies).[53] Umbilical cord milking has been suggested as an alternative to delayed cord clamping, allowing rapid transfer of placental blood while providing earlier access for thermal and respiratory support for the preterm. However, a randomized study of cord milking as an alternative to delayed cord clamping in preterm infants was halted early because of a significant increase in severe IVH in the cord milking group (8% vs. 3%; 95% CI, 1%–9%; P = .02).[54]

Diagnosis of Intraventricular Hemorrhage

In most cases, the diagnosis of IVH is made with screening ultrasound. The most vulnerable period is the first few postnatal days, with greater than 50% occurring in the first 24 hours and 90% in the first 72 hours of life.[38] Risk factors associated with the development of IVH include low birth weight and

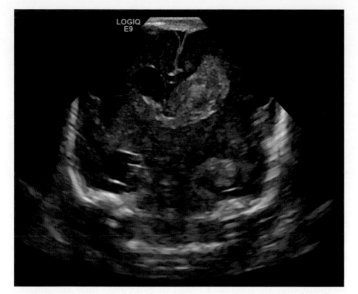

Fig. 43.3 Periventricular hemorrhagic infarction (also termed Grade 4 intraventricular hemorrhage). Coronal head ultrasound of a premature infant at 4 days of age—intraventricular hemorrhage/periventricular infarction. Note the increased echodense area in the left frontal white matter approximating the distribution of the medullary veins.

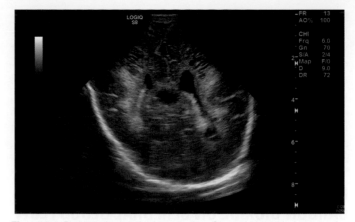

Fig. 43.4 Periventricular leukomalacia. Coronal head ultrasound—periventricular leukomalacia. Note the bilateral cystic areas within the periventricular white matter.

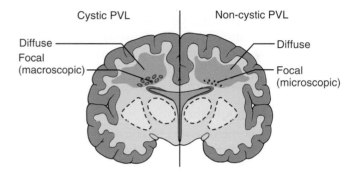

Fig. 43.5 Cystic and diffuse periventricular leukomalacia (*PVL*). (From Volpe JJ: The encephalopathy of prematurity – brain injury and impaired brain development of inextricably intertwined. Semin Pediatr Neurol 16(4):167-178, 2009.)

gestational age, maternal smoking, breech presentation, premature rupture of membranes, postnatal resuscitation and intubation, early-onset sepsis, RDS, pulmonary air leaks, metabolic acidosis, and rapid bicarbonate infusions.[55] Extremes of arterial $PaCO_2$ in the first 4 days of life are also associated with severe IVH (see later).[56]

Periventricular Hemorrhagic Infarction (Grade 4 Intraventricular Hemorrhage)

One of the complications of IVH is PVI, also termed Grade 4 IVH. PVI is a hemorrhagic venous infarction that is associated with severe and usually asymmetric bleeding. It occurs in about 15% of infants with IVH, particularly the smallest, most immature ones. On brain imaging, there is often a large, fan-shaped region of hemorrhagic necrosis in the periventricular white matter, invariably on the side with the larger amount of intraventricular blood (see Fig. 43.3). A variety of studies have shown that this lesion is not merely an extension of IVH. Instead, the likely mechanism is the obstruction of the medullary and terminal veins by the intraventricular and germinal matrix blood clot, leading to venous congestion in the periventricular white matter with subsequent hemorrhage and ischemia. PVI is associated with a high rate of mortality (40% to 60%), with survivors being at very high risk of cerebral palsy (CP) (66% in one study) and other neurologic abnormalities.[57,58]

Periventricular Leukomalacia and Diffuse White Matter Injury

Focal and diffuse white matter injury (WMI) may occur adjacent to the lateral ventricles with or without associated hemorrhage—a condition referred to as PVL (see Fig. 43.4).[25,59,60] The sonographic findings include cyst formation, ventriculomegaly, and diffuse WMI. Fig. 43.5 illustrates these forms of PVL, with diffuse WMI often manifesting with ventriculomegaly in the absence of cyst formation and occurring most commonly in premature infants who require prolonged ventilator support.[61]

Pathogenesis of White Matter Injury

The pathogenesis of WMI is complex and involves vascular factors, as well as the intrinsic vulnerability of oligodendrocytes to noxious substances. Vascular factors include the following: (1) the white matter resides in a border zone region,[62] which increases the likelihood of injury during periods of systemic hypotension; (2) the risk for injury to these regions is increased in the face of a pressure-passive circulation, as discussed earlier; and (3) there is a limited vasodilatory response to $PaCO_2$ of those vessels supplying the white matter.

The intrinsic vulnerability of the early differentiating oligodendrocyte has been established in studies that show that these cells are sensitive to injury secondary to the release of numerous factors, including free radicals, excitotoxins (glutamate), and cytokines, as well as a lack of growth factors.[25] The importance of intrinsic vulnerability is suggested from a report of 14 of 632 infants (2.3%) weighing less than 1750 g at birth who developed bilateral cystic PVL.[63] Overt hypotension occurred in only four of the babies with PVL, mostly in the immediate postnatal period. In the other 10 cases, PVL was seen in infants with mild to moderate lung disease without hypotension and was detected only on routine ultrasound screening. Two conditions were found to be significantly associated with the development of PVL in this cohort—chorioamnionitis and prolonged rupture of membranes. Other conditions that have been associated with the development of PVL include hypocarbia, meningitis, and recurrent severe apnea and bradycardia. Surviving preterm infants with PVL are at risk for CP (primarily spastic diplegia) and other motor deficits. Cognitive problems are also common, along with more subtle behavioral and attention disturbances.[2]

INFLUENCE OF OXYGEN CONCENTRATION AND CARBON DIOXIDE ON CEREBRAL BLOOD FLOW

As discussed earlier, abnormal CBF is one of the most important pathophysiologic factors in preterm brain injury. The cerebral circulation of the healthy newborn infant, and even in the very preterm infant, responds to physiologic stimuli in much the same way as in the adult. Cerebral blood vessels are sensitive to changes in $PaCO_2$, arterial oxygen concentration (CaO_2), and pH.[1] In pathologic situations, a pressure-passive state occurs and cerebral blood vessels may not react to chemical or metabolic stimuli. These infants are at increased risk for developing hemorrhagic and/or ischemic cerebral injury.

Oxygen and Hemoglobin

CBF increases when arterial oxygen tension decreases markedly in the human infant and in neonatal animal models.[1,3,25] CBF is regulated by CaO_2, which in turn is determined by hemoglobin concentration, oxygen affinity to hemoglobin, and PaO_2.[1,15] In preterm infants studied in the first 3 days of life, it has been shown that CBF increases by approximately 12% for every 1-mM decrease in hemoglobin concentration.[17] There is also a direct relationship of CBF with the relative proportion of fetal hemoglobin, probably because of the stronger affinity of fetal hemoglobin for oxygen.

Cerebrovascular dilation occurs within 30 to 60 seconds in response to hypoxia. At lower blood pressures, the vasodilator response to hypoxia may be impaired. Conversely, hyperoxia induces a fall in CBF in preterm infants through cerebral vasoconstriction.[1] Median reduction was found to be 0.06 cm/s for every 1-kPa increase in oxygen tension. When 80% oxygen was given during resuscitation at birth, preterm infants were subsequently shown to have a 25% reduction in CBF velocity versus those infants given room air.[64]

Carbon Dioxide

The fetal and neonatal brain remains sensitive to changes in $PaCO_2$; hypocarbia decreases CBF through vasoconstriction of cerebral arteries and hypercarbia has a relaxant effect.[1,3,65,66] The primary mediator linking arterial CO_2 tension and cerebral vasoreactivity may be pH. In one study performed on isolated dog cerebral arteries, hypercarbia-induced cerebral arterial relaxation was shown to be mediated mainly with a fall of extracellular pH.[67] Because CO_2 crosses the blood-brain barrier readily, abrupt changes in CO_2 tension may also cause a rapid change in vascular reactivity within 1 to 2 minutes. This acute effect is then actively regulated by perivascular pH, causing the vessel diameter to normalize gradually during the next 24 hours.[1]

In the healthy adult, CBF changes by a mean of approximately 30% for every 1-kPa change in $PaCO_2$. Similarly, in spontaneously breathing preterm infants studied at 2 to 3 hours after birth, CBF–carbon dioxide reactivity was shown to be approximately 30% per 1-kPa change in $PaCO_2$. In mechanically ventilated preterm infants, this reactivity was much less, that is, about 11% per 1-kPa change in $PaCO_2$ when studied shortly after birth, although it increased to near-adult levels by the second day of life. In infants in whom severe intracranial hemorrhage subsequently developed, there was a loss of CBF reactivity to changes in $PaCO_2$, implying an impairment of CBF regulation before hemorrhage.[17]

Linking Changes in Carbon Dioxide and Oxygen Concentration to Hemorrhagic–Ischemic Injury
Hypocarbia and White Matter Injury

Hypocarbia is a common occurrence in the ventilated preterm infant. It may be seen as a result of improved lung compliance and/or function or with aggressive ventilator support (either unintentional or intentional). Several studies have reported the association of hypocarbia with PVL, neurodevelopmental problems, and CP.[66,68,69] In one study, time-averaged $PaCO_2$ on the third day of life was lower in preterm infants who developed PVL than in those who did not develop PVL.[70] Others have supported a similar dose-dependent effect of hypocarbia, with longer and more frequent episodes of hypocarbia associated with more severe brain injury.[69,71] In full-term infants, hypocarbia following perinatal hypoxia-ischemia is associated with adverse outcomes, as evidenced by a retrospective study of nearly 250 newborns.[72] This was also noted in the National Institute of Child Health and Human Development Neonatal Research Network's trial of whole-body hypothermia.[73] When early blood gases were examined (from birth through 12 hours of hypothermia), infants with death or disability had significantly lower minimum PCO_2 concentrations (median, 22 vs. 26 mm Hg; $P = .15$), and this was a predictor of outcome.[74] This relationship also held true in those infants exposed to a higher cumulative duration of hypocarbia, as they also had worse outcomes. Despite these correlations, it remains unclear whether hypocarbia leads to brain injury or is merely an early marker of increased risk.

Hypercarbia and Intraventricular Hemorrhage

Permissive hypercarbia has been advocated as a ventilatory strategy to minimize barotrauma and volutrauma to the lungs of preterm infants and thus prevent evolution to chronic lung disease.[75] Although there may be beneficial effects in terms of lung injury, the risks of elevated $PaCO_2$ to the brain must not be ignored. As reviewed earlier, hypercarbia is associated with both an increase in CBF and an impairment of cerebral autoregulation in ventilated VLBW infants.[75] In a study undertaken in the first week of life in VLBW infants of gestational age 26.9 $\pm$ 2.3 weeks, increasing $PaCO_2$ resulted in increasing impairment of cerebral autoregulation.[76] Hypercarbia, defined by the maximum $PaCO_2$ recorded during the first 3 days of life, was also associated with severe IVH in a retrospective cohort study of 574 VLBW infants.[77] As maximum $PaCO_2$ increased from 40 to 100 mm Hg, the probability of severe IVH increased from 8% to 21%. A retrospective review of 849 infants weighing less than 1250 g suggested that extremes in $PaCO_2$, both hypocarbia and hypercarbia, as well as fluctuations in $PaCO_2$ during the first 4 days of life, increased the risk of severe IVH.[56] In this analysis, infants who developed severe IVH had higher maximum $PaCO_2$ (median, 72 vs. 59 mm Hg; $P < .001$), lower minimal $PaCO_2$ (median, 32 vs. 39 mm Hg; $P < .001$), and a greater range between maximum and minimum $PaCO_2$ values (median, 39 vs. 21 mm Hg; $P < .001$). This was reinforced in a reanalysis of data from the SUPPORT trial.[78,79] In over 1300 infants from 24 to 27 6/7 weeks, severe IVH was increased in those with $PaCO_2$ levels in the highest quartile. These infants were also at increased risk of neurodevelopmental impairment. Similarly, infants with a large range between maximum and minimum $PaCO_2$ (i.e., fluctuators) had increased incidences of neurodevelopmental impairment as well as bronchopulmonary dysplasia (BPD). Comparable results linking increased $PaCO_2$ fluctuations with IVH were shown in a retrospective analysis by Altaany et al.[80] Taken together, these studies indicate that extremes in $PaCO_2$ should be avoided during the period in which infants are at high risk of IVH.

Oxygen and Brain Injury

Fraction of inspired oxygen (FiO_2) is a parameter that must be chosen by the provider when respiratory support is initiated—this may range from room air to 100% O_2. Clinicians often use oxygen saturation (SpO_2) and PaO_2 to subsequently guide their administration, varying their targets based on factors such as gestational age, risk of retinopathy of prematurity, and heart and lung disease. Although the optimal saturation range of preterm infants is unclear, it is known that the extremes of both hypoxia and hyperoxia can have adverse effects on the developing brain.[81] Neonatal Oxygen Prospective Meta-analysis (NeOProM) Collaboration was formed to include five studies that randomized infants to SpO_2 targets of either 85% to 89% or 91% to 95% to address this question.[79] Although there were no differences in major disability at 18 to 24 months corrected age, the lower oxygen saturation group had an increased incidence of death (RR 1.16, 95% CI 1.03 to 1.31; 5 trials, 4873 infants) and the higher oxygen-saturation group had an increased incidence of severe retinopathy (RR 0.72, 95% CI 0.61 to 0.85, 5 trials, 4089 infants).

The effect of hyperoxia on the preterm infant has received considerable attention. As reviewed earlier, CaO_2 is a primary regulator of CBF. The preterm infant often has labile oxygen saturations and, therefore, CBF, which increases the risk of IVH. At a biochemical level, hyperoxia has also been shown to have deleterious effects on the preterm brain through mechanisms of inflammation, apoptosis, and oxidative stress.[82] Excess oxygen can lead to the generation of reactive oxygen species. These free radicals can be harmful to preterm infants because of their already low antioxidant defense compared to term infants. Of particular importance, premyelinating, or immature, oligodendrocytes are vulnerable to oxidative injury, which may be a potent contributor to PVL in a preterm infant receiving excessive oxygen therapy.[82,83]

In addition to SpO_2 and PaO_2, the measurement of regional tissue hemoglobin oxygen saturation ($rStO_2$) has been gaining popularity. Using NIRS, $rStO_2$ can be measured noninvasively in various circulatory regions (e.g., cerebral, splanchnic, etc.). A trial of 166 preterm infants of less than 28 weeks' gestation randomized subjects to visible or blinded cerebral NIRS monitoring for the first 3 days of life.[84] The visible NIRS subjects were managed with the goal of maintaining $rStO_2$ between 55% and 85% by targeting respiratory and circulatory parameters. Although the treatment group did maintain $rStO_2$ in the target range better than the control group, no significant differences in clinical outcomes were found.

In summary, both low and high blood oxygen concentrations have harmful effects on the brain. Pulse oximetry and PaO_2 are the mainstays of adjusting oxygen therapy, but new technologies, such as NIRS, may have a prominent role in the future.

MODE OF VENTILATION AND BRAIN INJURY

Mechanical factors related to the delivery of inhaled gas have also been implicated in causing brain injury. Driving gas via positive pressure into the lungs is fundamentally different from inhalation via negative pressure. Such pressure changes in the thorax can disrupt hemodynamics, increase venous pressure, and therefore alter CBF. This section focuses on the most common methods of respiratory support and how they relate to brain injury.

Continuous Positive Airway Pressure

Continuous positive airway pressure (CPAP) is a commonly used noninvasive mode of respiratory support that can improve ventilation and oxygenation by maintaining functional residual capacity. In a model of chronic lung disease in which preterm baboons were mechanically ventilated, Loeliger et al. weaned one group to CPAP at 24 hours of life and another at 5 days of life.[85] Both groups showed diffuse brain injury, but the early CPAP group had less severe injury. This link between longer duration of mechanical ventilation and worse neurologic outcome has also been shown in human studies.[86,87] Mechanical ventilation compared to CPAP has been associated with lower developmental scores, more disruptions in CBF, increased IVH, and a higher incidence of death.[86,87] However, infants receiving mechanical ventilation are likely to be sicker, and as a consequence, it is difficult to implicate ventilator support versus the underlying disease.

Conventional Mechanical Ventilation

Mechanical ventilation can affect CBF by impeding venous return or through changes in the acid-base balance (see earlier). Elevated mean airway pressure can increase central venous pressure, thereby decreasing superior vena cava return and increasing the risk for IVH. This will in turn decrease cardiac output, increasing the risk of cerebral hypoperfusion.[88,89] This puts the vulnerable areas of the premature brain, such as the periventricular white matter, at risk for injury.

Exposure to fluctuations of CBF with prolonged mechanical ventilation presumably results in repeated insults throughout the course of intensive care. Walsh et al. demonstrated that extremely low birth weight infants who are ventilated longer, probably representing the sickest of the cohort, have increased incidence of CP.[90] All surviving infants who were ventilated for 120 or more days had neurologic impairment.

High-Frequency Oscillatory Ventilation

Physiologically, continuous sustained lung inflation as seen with high-frequency oscillatory ventilation (HFOV) can lead to a higher mean airway pressure. The use of HFOV can avoid the large swings in pulmonary pressures in conventional mechanical ventilation. Its use is associated with an increased risk of venous distention, particularly to the medullary veins in the periventricular white matter (see earlier). However, when the lungs are poorly inflated, complications may result secondary to poor ventilation and low oxygenation. Thus, there is likely to be an optimal mean airway pressure to be achieved for each infant receiving high-frequency ventilation.

In a meta-analysis of 19 studies involving a total of 4096 preterm infants with RDS, the elective use of HFOV compared with conventional ventilation did not affect mortality, severe IVH, or PVL.[91] Although some studies have shown an increased risk of short-term neurologic morbidity with the use of HFOV, the overall meta-analysis showed no significant differences between HFOV and conventional ventilation.[91,92]

MEDICATIONS USED TO TREAT RESPIRATORY CONDITIONS

Surfactant

Before the widespread use of ACSs and surfactants, very preterm infants, especially those who developed a pneumothorax, had increased risk of IVH.[93-95] Because surfactants reduced the severity of RDS and the rate of pneumothorax, it was postulated that it would also lead to a substantial decrease in the rates of IVH. Although severe intracranial hemorrhage has declined in recent years for extremely preterm infants,[27,28] the specific contribution of surfactants has not been clearly demonstrated in multiple surfactant trials. A 2012 Cochrane review evaluated IVH as a secondary outcome when comparing prophylactic surfactant to CPAP with selective use of surfactants.[96] There was a trend toward decreased risk of IVH in those infants who received prophylactic surfactant (RR, 0.91; 95% CI, 0.82–1.0). Despite the many trials of surfactants and regardless of the type of intervention (prophylactic versus rescue), or the type of surfactant used (synthetic versus natural), no consistent effect on IVH has been observed.[97] This

lack of effect has been attributed to the impact of surfactant administration on fluctuations in CBF in sick preterm infants who have pressure-passive circulations and the rapid changes in $PaCO_2$ and PaO_2 that may subsequently lead to brain injury.[98] Multiple studies on the effects of intratracheal surfactant administration on CBF have been equivocal, with both human and animal data demonstrating conflicting results. More recently, less invasive surfactant administration (LISA) has shown some promise of being associated with decreased risk of intracranial hemorrhage.[99-101]

Methylxanthines

Methylxanthines have been used in neonatology as a respiratory stimulant since the 1970s, with caffeine being one of the most frequently prescribed medications in neonatal intensive care.[102,103] Caffeine has been found to decrease the frequency of apnea of prematurity as well as decrease the need for invasive ventilatory support. The mechanism of action is not fully elucidated, but it is likely related to an increase in chemoreceptor responsiveness, enhanced diaphragmatic contractility and function, and generalized central nervous system excitation.[104] The most likely pathway is a nonspecific inhibitor of adenosine receptors at multiple sites in the brain. There were initial concerns regarding the central nervous system effects of caffeine because adenosine is protective of the brain during experimental hypoxia and ischemia.[105]

The Caffeine for Apnea of Prematurity Trial Group reported on the short- and long-term effects of caffeine.[106-110] This randomized, placebo-controlled trial of over 2000 very preterm infants with birth weights of 500 to 1250 g showed that caffeine reduced the rate of death or survival with a neurodevelopmental disability at 18 to 21 months (40% vs. 46%; odds ratio [OR], 0.77; 95% CI, 0.64–0.93; $P = .008$). Caffeine also reduced the incidence of CP (4.4% vs. 7.3%; OR, 0.58; 95% CI, 0.39–0.87; $P = .0009$) and cognitive delay (33.8% vs. 38.3%; OR, 0.81; 95% CI, 0.66–0.99; $P = .04$) and even decreased the incidence of severe retinopathy of prematurity in the treatment group (5.1% vs. 7.9%; OR, 0.61; 95% CI, 0.42–0.89; $P = .01$).[107] The 5-year follow-up results of nearly 85% of these infants were not as notable.[108] At that time, 21% of caffeine-treated infants suffered death or disability versus 25% in the placebo group (OR, 0.82; 95% CI, 0.65–1.0; $P = .09$). In a secondary analysis of these infants, gross motor function was improved in the caffeine-treated infants (OR, 0.64; 95% CI, 0.47–0.88; $P = .006$) (see Table 43.2). Also, a subset of caffeine-treated infants

TABLE 43.2	Long-Term Effects of Caffeine Therapy			
	Outcome	Caffeine (n = 833)	Placebo (n = 807)	P value
18 months	Death or disability	307 (38.1%)	352 (45.1%)	0.006
	Cerebral palsy	33 (4.3%)	57 (7.7%)	0.006
	Severe cognitive delay[a]	88 (11.9%)	116 (16.2%)	0.02
5 years	Death or disability	176 (21.1%)	200 (24.8%)	0.09
	Motor impairment[b]	13 (1.6%)	21 (2.7%)	0.2
	Severe cognitive impairment[c]	38 (4.9%)	38 (5.1%)	0.89

[a]Mental developmental index <70.
[b]Gross motor function classification scale level >2.
[c]Full scale IQ <70.
(Data From: Schmidt B, et al. Survival without disability to age 5 years after neonatal caffeine therapy for apnea of prematurity. JAMA. 2012; 307(3):275-282.)

showed lower rates of developmental coordination disorder (11.3% vs. 15.2%; OR, 0.71; 95% CI, 0.52–0.97; $P = .03$), which has been associated with CP.[111] Overall, the striking differences in neurologic outcomes at 18 months did not persist at 5 years. By age 11 years, the caffeine-treated group was associated with reduced risk of motor impairment (19.7% vs. 27.5%; OR, 0.66; 95% CI, 0.48–0.90; $P = .009$),[109] without affecting general intelligence, attention, and behavior.[110]

Early caffeine (i.e., within the first 2–3 days of life) was associated with a combined reduction in death and BPD, but some studies reported a higher incidence of mortality in the early treatment group.[112-115] The clinical indication for caffeine varies among providers and centers but is often guided by gestational age and apneic events. The traditional practice is to prescribe caffeine for infants approaching extubation and/or those infants at high risk of apnea of prematurity. Some providers have expanded their use of caffeine beyond this as a potential neuroprotective agent—for example, prescribing early caffeine (at initiation of ventilator support or at <3 days of age) to a preterm infant who remains intubated and is not having apnea.[113,114,116] As described earlier, evidence supporting the benefits of early caffeine may be conflicting, so its risks and benefits must be considered. Overall, caffeine has an excellent safety profile, and thus, the risks are likely to be low in most cases.[105,117]

Inhaled Nitric Oxide

Inhaled nitric oxide (iNO) is an effective treatment in term infants with hypoxemic respiratory failure. Its use has expanded to preterm neonates for impaired oxygenation and has also been used prophylactically for those at increased risk for BPD. There has been some evidence regarding potential neurologic effects of nitric oxide, as it has been shown to be an important influence in both CBF and inflammation.[118]

Several studies on the use of iNO as a rescue treatment for hypoxic respiratory failure in preterm infants or as prophylaxis have shown conflicting results on IVH, severe IVH, or PVL.[119] A single-center study randomized 207 intubated preterm infants to receive iNO or placebo in the first 72 hours of life. Prophylaxis with iNO significantly reduced the risk of death or chronic lung disease (49% vs. 64%; RR, 0.76; 95% CI, 0.60–0.97; $P = .03$). In this study, the risk of severe IVH or PVL was significantly lower with iNO than with placebo (12% vs. 24%; RR, 0.53; 95% CI, 0.28–0.98; $P = .04$).[120] Other studies have shown no significant difference in severe IVH or PVL.[121] Some have even demonstrated a worsening of neurologic injury, including a multicenter study of 420 preterm infants with respiratory failure randomized to iNO or placebo treatment.[122] This study reported a post hoc analysis that indicated that severe IVH and mortality were higher in the iNO-treated infants who were 1000 g or less. A meta-analysis showed that among studies using iNO for hypoxic respiratory failure, there was a nonsignificant increase in the incidence of severe IVH or PVL (typical RR, 1.07; 95% CI, 0.88–1.33; eight studies, 901 infants). Meanwhile, of studies using iNO as prophylaxis in intubated preterm infants, there was a nonsignificant reduction in this outcome (typical RR, 0.9; 95% CI, 0.73–1.12; three studies, 1747 infants).[119]

Similarly, there have been conflicting results on the effects of iNO on long-term neurodevelopmental outcomes. In a meta-analysis, there was no significant difference in neurodevelopmental outcomes for those studies using iNO as rescue treatment.[119] For studies using iNO as prophylaxis, some studies showed a reduction in neurodevelopmental impairment. In the follow-up to the single-center prophylactic iNO study earlier,[120] a total of 138 children (82% of survivors) were assessed at 2 years of age.[123] Use of iNO was associated with a lower risk of abnormal neurodevelopmental outcome (disability or delay) compared with placebo (24% vs. 46%; RR, 0.53; 95% CI, 0.33–0.87; $P = .01$).[123] Meanwhile, the multicenter European Union Nitric Oxide Trial, which was a multicenter study randomizing preterm infants less than 29 weeks' gestation with moderate respiratory failure to iNO or placebo, showed no significant difference in BPD or neurodevelopmental outcomes.[121,124] There have been no effects on the incidence of CP with early iNO use.[119]

Postnatal Steroids

The use of postnatal systemic glucocorticoids, particularly high-dose dexamethasone, to prevent or treat chronic lung disease in the preterm infant has been shown to be associated with increased risk of CP and neurodevelopmental impairment.[125] Other strategies, such as lower dose dexamethasone for BPD, hydrocortisone for BPD, or short-course steroids for airway edema, may have fewer adverse effects, but current data are insufficient to provide specific recommendations.[125] The American Academy of Pediatrics' 2010 policy statement cited insufficient evidence to make recommendations regarding other steroid protocols.[126] Our practice is to reserve the use of systemic glucocorticoids to facilitate extubation of infants who cannot be weaned off mechanical ventilation beyond 3 to 4 weeks of life—that is, those at highest risk of developing BPD. This individualized decision should be made in conjunction with the family and involve a thorough analysis of the potential risks and benefits.

SUMMARY

The developing brain of the fetus and newborn is extremely vulnerable to injury in the form of IVH and/or PVL/WMI. Whereas the rate of severe brain injuries in preterm infants has decreased over time, they contribute to major morbidities (CP, cognitive impairment) in these survivors. There is an intimate relationship between neonatal respiratory disease and risk of brain injury in the premature infant.[36,70,127,128] Two major factors modulate this relationship (i.e., ACS, which has been shown to decrease IVH in a dose-dependent manner, and clinical/histologic chorioamnionitis and especially funisitis, which is associated with PVL/WMI). This respiratory relationship is a result of both the disease process, its complications, as well as the interventions that are used to treat these respiratory conditions. Factors that may increase the risk for brain injury include physiologic variables such as acid-base disturbances, imbalance in carbon dioxide or oxygen levels, positive-pressure mechanical ventilation, and commonly used respiratory medication. In the management of a sick newborn with respiratory distress, the risk and benefit of any intervention that is pursued for its benefit to the infant's respiratory state must be weighed against its potential to cause hemorrhagic-ischemic injury to the

TABLE 43.3 Potential Strategies That Decrease the Risk of Brain Injury in the Preterm Infant

Antenatal interventions	Prevention of premature delivery
	Antenatal corticosteroids
	Maternal transfer to perinatal center
Intrapartum interventions	Mode of delivery
	Delayed cord clamping
Postnatal interventions	Avoidance of hemodynamic fluctuations, e.g., sedation
	Synchronized mechanical ventilation
	Administration of surfactant (?)
	Minimize complications of RDS, e.g., pneumothorax
	Minimize mean airway pressure
	Minimize the hemodynamic effects of PDA
	Avoidance of extremes of $PaCO_2$
	Avoidance of metabolic disturbances, e.g., metabolic acidosis
	Minimize postnatal steroid use
	Use of early indomethacin
	Use of caffeine in apnea of prematurity

PDA, Patent ductus arteriosus; *RDS,* respiratory distress syndrome.

central nervous system (see Table 43.3). These considerations should be made to minimize such injury and thus improve long-term neurodevelopmental outcome.

KEY REFERENCES

2. Volpe JJ, Volpe JJ: Volpe's Neurology of the Newborn. 6th ed. Philadelphia, PA, Elsevier, 2018.

15. Pryds A, Tonnesen J, Pryds O, et al: Cerebral pressure autoregulation and vasoreactivity in the newborn rat. Pediatr Res 57(2):294-298, 2005.

23. Soul JS, Hammer PE, Tsuji M, et al: Fluctuating pressure-passivity is common in the cerebral circulation of sick premature infants. Pediatr Res 61(4):467-473, 2007.

35. Lou HC, Lassen NA, Friis-Hansen B: Impaired autoregulation of cerebral blood flow in the distressed newborn infant. J Pediatr 94(1):118-121, 1979.

36. Perlman JM, McMenamin JB, Volpe JJ: Fluctuating cerebral blood-flow velocity in respiratory-distress syndrome. Relation to the development of intraventricular hemorrhage. N Engl J Med 309(4):204-209, 1983.

39. Andrews WW, Goldenberg RL, Faye-Petersen O, et al: The Alabama Preterm Birth study: polymorphonuclear and mononuclear cell placental infiltrations, other markers of inflammation, and outcomes in 23- to 32-week preterm newborn infants. Am J Obstet Gynecol 195(3):803-808, 2006.

48. Roberts D, Brown J, Medley N, et al: Antenatal corticosteroids for accelerating fetal lung maturation for women at risk of preterm birth. Cochrane Database Syst Rev 3:CD004454, 2017.

98. Kaiser JR, Gauss CH, Williams DK: Surfactant administration acutely affects cerebral and systemic hemodynamics and gas exchange in very-low-birth-weight infants. J Pediatr 144(6): 809-814, 2004.

108. Schmidt B, Anderson PJ, Doyle LW, et al: Survival without disability to age 5 years after neonatal caffeine therapy for apnea of prematurity. JAMA 307(3):275-282, 2012.

119. Barrington KJ, Finer N, Pennaforte T: Inhaled nitric oxide for respiratory failure in preterm infants. Cochrane Database Syst Rev 1:CD000509, 2017.

126. Watterberg KL, American Academy of Pediatrics, Committee on Fetus and Newborn: Policy statement—postnatal corticosteroids to prevent or treat bronchopulmonary dysplasia. Pediatrics 126(4):800-808, 2010.

44

Pulmonary and Neurodevelopmental Outcomes Following Ventilation

Allison H. Payne, Monika Bhola, Gulgun Yalcinkaya, and Michele C. Walsh

KEY POINTS

- Bronchopulmonary dysplasia (BPD) remains an important consequence of very preterm birth, resulting in prolonged hospitalization and increased health care resource utilization and significant ongoing health challenges for survivors. The rate of BPD has changed little over the past two decades, with higher rate in boys compared to girls.
- In the first year of life, preterm survivors have higher rates of wheezing, are more likely to be rehospitalized for respiratory symptoms, and are more likely to be treated with bronchodilators. At early school age, these children have decreased peak expiratory flow and are more likely to have a diagnosis of wheezing.
- Pulmonary sequelae of extreme prematurity are also associated with increased rates of neurodevelopmental impairment.
- Pulmonary symptoms appear to stabilize in later childhood and early adulthood, but very long-term pulmonary outcome remains of concern as lung function begins its natural decline in later life.

INTRODUCTION

The outcomes of neonates after assisted ventilation are highly variable. Even among infants who require minimal respiratory support, predicting long-term lung and developmental outcomes is complex. Prematurity remains the strongest predictor of chronic lung disease and developmental delays. In this chapter, we will discuss the key drivers for long-term pulmonary morbidity among premature infants and the associated neurodevelopmental outcomes.

INCIDENCE AND DEFINITIONS OF BRONCHOPULMONARY DYSPLASIA

Prematurity, as defined by birth before 37 weeks' gestation, is an important risk factor for the development of lung disease. Despite significant advances in the respiratory care of neonates, bronchopulmonary dysplasia (BPD) remains the most common serious pulmonary morbidity in premature infants. Attempts at eliminating BPD have been largely unsuccessful. The incidence of BPD is widely variable among sites, even after adjusting for potential risk factors. Among Vermont Oxford Network (VON) sites, the rates of BPD range from 19% to over 40% among infants born at less than 32 weeks' gestation. As the neonatology community has attempted resuscitation of even more immature neonates at 22 to 23 weeks' gestation, the rates

of BPD have risen. Data from a 2018 VON report suggest that the incidence of BPD appears to have decreased very slowly over a 10-year period, with persistently higher rate in boys.[1] The absolute number of premature infants with BPD may be increasing because of improved survival of extremely preterm and extremely low birth weight (ELBW) infants, leading to an increase in the numbers of preterm infants who survive to be classified as having BPD.

The contemporary definitions, predictors, and outcomes of BPD have changed. BPD, as recognized and described by William Northway, a pediatric radiologist, was based largely on radiographic evidence of lung disease in infants who survived respiratory distress syndrome (RDS). Chest radiography demonstrated areas of diffuse heterogeneity and coarse opacities in the most severe of cases. Northway recognized that the key component was a history of mechanical ventilation, a technology not available only several years before Northway's observations. The infants were moderately to late premature infants, and the management of these infants included exposure to prolonged mechanical ventilation, high airway pressures, and oxygen. Histologically, characteristic areas of hyperinflation alternating with areas of focal collapse were found. Hyperplasia of the bronchial epithelium was present and extensive fibrosis was also noted.[2]

The current landscape in which BPD occurs is distinct from that of Northway. "Classic" or "old" BPD has now been replaced by a "new" form of the disease. "New" BPD is found primarily among extremely low gestational age neonates, defined as <28 weeks' gestational age, and ELBW (i.e., <1000 g birth weight) infants with a history of RDS. These infants are exposed to antenatal steroids and frequently treated with exogenous surfactant therapy. Even the most premature infants may receive only limited exposure to conventional mechanical ventilation but may be exposed to other noninvasive respiratory support such as nasal intermittent positive pressure ventilation (NIPPV), continuous positive airway pressure (CPAP), or high-flow nasal cannula. Between 2006 and 2016, infants born before 29 weeks were placed on CPAP as a primary support; this increased from 34% to 85%.[1,3] The trend in respiratory management has resulted in fewer days on positive pressure ventilation, less time on endotracheal intubation, and less exposure to supplemental oxygen. Chest radiography of new BPD is characterized by diffuse hazy opacities and minimal hyperinflation. In addition, the histology of new BPD shows a reduction in alveoli and capillaries, but minimal fibrosis.[4,5]

The definition of BPD has evolved as the disease itself has changed. The hallmark feature of BPD is the receipt of oxygen therapy or positive pressure for a period of time or on a specific day of life. There are three commonly used definitions: (1) receipt of oxygen at 28 days, (2) need for supplemental oxygen at 36 weeks' postmenstrual age (PMA), and (3) the physiologic definition. The first two definitions, although simple, are limited by the various developmental considerations of infants born at different gestational ages (i.e., 23 weeks vs 28 weeks), site variation in defining need for supplemental oxygen (i.e., oxygen targets), or the use of therapies targeted at reducing oxygen requirements (i.e., diuretics and steroids). A further complication is introduced by the evolution of respiratory care practices to include high-flow nasal cannulation—a treatment not accounted for in earlier definitions.

In 2000, a workshop to clarify the definition of BPD was held by the National Institute of Child Health and Human Development (NICHD). At that time, the NICHD recognized the importance of distinguishing BPD from the large heterogeneous group of chronic lung disease.[5] This workshop proposed a severity-based definition classifying BPD into mild, moderate, or severe based on either postnatal age or PMA (Table 44.1). Mild BPD was defined as a need for supplemental oxygen (O_2) for 28 days or more but not at 36 weeks' PMA or discharge; moderate BPD as O_2 for 28 days or more plus treatment with less than 30% O_2 at 36 weeks' PMA; and severe BPD as O_2 for 28 days or more plus 30% O_2 or more and/or positive pressure at 36 weeks' PMA. The severity-based definition of BPD was validated by Ehrenkranz et al.[6] by comparing it to the other commonly used definitions such as supplemental oxygen at 28 days and at 36 weeks' PMA. Overall, the NICHD consensus' severity-based scale identified infants most at risk for poor pulmonary outcomes as well as neurodevelopment impairment better than the common definitions[7] (Table 44.2).

The physiologic definition of BPD, as developed by Walsh, defines BPD at 36 weeks' adjusted age, using an oxygen reduction test. Unit-specific rates of BPD among premature infants weighing 501 to 1249 g were compared using the traditional oxygen at 36 weeks' PMA definition (15%–66%) and compared to rates of BPD using the physiologic definition (9%–57%). The physiologic definition reduces the between-center variability in the diagnosis of BPD and reduces the diagnosis as much as 10% at individual centers. The physiologic definition has also been validated and shown to be independently predictive of cognitive impairment in infants with BPD.[8] The physiologic definition is used in many clinical trials throughout the United States. Since the publication of the NICHD Neonatal Research Network *Early CPAP vs Surfactant in Extremely Preterm Infants Trial* in 2010, there is evidence that saturation targets have become more uniform among US centers.[9] This uniformity may decrease the utility of a physiologic room air challenge. In work in the National Heart, Lung, and Blood Institute (NHLBI) Prematurity and Respiratory Outcomes Program (PROP) Study, 43% of infants could not be classified on degree of BPD because of missing oxygen challenges.[10]

As respiratory care has evolved, so, too, must the definition of BPD. Jensen and colleagues compared 18 definitions of BPD among a contemporary cohort of 2677 infants born at less than 32 weeks' gestation. The definition that best predicted childhood

---

TABLE 44.1   National Institutes of Health Consensus Definition of Bronchopulmonary Dysplasia

	Respiratory Support at 28 Days of Age	Respiratory Support at 36 Weeks' PMA
No BPD	Room air	Room air
Mild BPD	Respiratory support	Room air
Moderate BPD	Respiratory support	Respiratory support (FiO_2 <30%)
Severe BPD	Respiratory support	Respiratory support (≥30%)

BPD, Bronchopulmonary dysplasia; *PMA*, postmenstrual age.
(Modified from Jobe AH, Bancalari E: Bronchopulmonary dysplasia. Am J Respir Crit Care Med 163:1723–1729, 2001.)

TABLE 44.2   Respiratory Outcomes of Infants at 18 to 22 Months' Corrected Age as Classified by the National Institutes of Health Consensus Definition of Bronchopulmonary Dysplasia[a]

BPD Definition	NICU Infants, *n* (%) (*n* = 4866)	Follow-up Infants, *n* (%) (*n* = 3848)	Pulmonary Medications (% of Follow-up[b])	Rehospitalized Pulmonary Cause (% of Follow-up[b])	RSV Prophylaxis (% of Follow-up[b])
Consensus					
None	1124 (23.1)	876 (22.8)	27.2	23.9	12.5
Mild	1473 (30.3)	1186 (30.8)	29.7	26.7	16.6
Moderate	1471 (30.2)	1143 (29.7)	40.8	33.5	19.2
Severe	798 (16.4)	643 (16.7)	46.6[c]	39.4[c]	28.4[c]

BPD, Bronchopulmonary dysplasia; *CXR*, chest x-ray; *NICU*, neonatal intensive care unit; *RSV*, respiratory syncytial virus.
[a]Missing data: 28 days–CXR, 17 infants (13 for follow-up cohort); 36 weeks–CXR, 12 infants (8 for follow-up cohort); pulmonary medications, 17; rehospitalizations for pulmonary causes, 35; RSV prophylaxis, 17.
[b]Cohort of infants who were seen at 18 to 22 months' corrected age.
[c]$P < .0001$, [d]$P < .001$ versus no BPD for the 28 days, 28 days–CXR, 36 weeks, and 36 weeks–CXR definitions, Mantel-Haenszel Π^2 for linear association across the categories of the consensus definition (none to severe), Mantel-Haenszel Π^2.
(Modified from Ehrenkranz RA, Walsh MC, Vohr BR, et al: Validation of the National Institutes of Health Consensus definition of bronchopulmonary dysplasia. Pediatrics 116:1353–1360, 2005.)

morbidity measured at 2 years of age was the mode of respiratory support at 36 weeks' PMA, regardless of level of oxygen supplementation.[11]

A major limitation of the physiologic definition of BPD is the reluctance of physicians or parents to undergo the challenge, despite the demonstrated safety of the exam.

Some clinicians have questioned whether all the definitions are needed. There is merit to the severity classification introduced with the National Institutes of Health (NIH) consensus definition, rather than a binary outcome of yes or no. There is also merit to the more objective criteria introduced by the physiologic definition with the room air challenge (Table 44.3).

PULMONARY OUTCOMES

Composite outcomes are frequently used in contemporary neonatal clinical trials. The value of such combined outcomes as death and BPD (or its counterpart, survival without BPD) becomes clear when considering an intervention that may increase the percentage of survivors without BPD by increasing mortality among the sickest or most vulnerable infants. Such composite outcomes also adjust for differences among centers in their willingness to withdraw support from infants with a poor neurodevelopmental prognosis.

Although BPD, as diagnosed near term gestation, cannot be considered a long-term outcome, the incidence of BPD remains a very relevant endpoint for clinical trials of respiratory management in preterm infants. BPD is an important cause of morbidity and mortality, has been associated with prolonged and recurrent hospitalizations, and is linked to higher rates of other serious complications of prematurity.[12] Its incidence is high, with 7000 to 10,000 new cases each year in the United States alone, and has not been reduced substantially by numerous interventions, including surfactant replacement therapy. The prevalence of BPD has actually increased since 2005 as more ELBW infants survive to discharge.[3]

Pulmonary Function Testing and Imaging

It would be desirable to directly assess an infant's functional respiratory status with bedside pulmonary function tests during the acute hospitalization. Such tests are currently feasible in intubated neonates and in older, nonintubated infants as young as 4 months of age and have revolutionized the care of neonates with cystic fibrosis.[13] Unfortunately, the currently available tests for nonintubated older infants require sedation and are appropriate only for those over 4 months of age. It would be highly desirable to develop such techniques to study nonintubated convalescent premature infants.

A rapid thoracic compression technique to evaluate pulmonary function in nonintubated infants has shown promise.[14] A working group convened by the American Thoracic Society concluded that "insufficient evidence exists to recommend incorporation of [pulmonary function testing] into routine diagnostic evaluation and monitoring of infants and young children with bronchopulmonary dysplasia."[15]

The primary pulmonary function abnormality in survivors of preterm lung disease is reduced forced flows and forced expiratory volume (FEV) in the presence of normal forced vital capacity, which did not normalize later in infancy in infants either with or without BPD.[16,17] Many investigators have documented limitations in airflow that may, in part, be reversible with bronchodilators.[17-20] In the original descriptions by Northway, persistent abnormalities were detected into adulthood.[2] However, more contemporary cohorts have demonstrated remarkable stability in FEV in preterm survivors with BPD between 10 and 18 years and 18 and 25 years of age, even in those with the most severe BPD.[21] This suggests an ability to augment alveolarization with continued development.

Narayanan and colleagues used magnetic resonance imaging (MRI) to demonstrate that former infants with BPD who were evaluated at 10 to 14 years of age had alveolar dimensions similar to those of term controls and of preterm infants without BPD.[22] One alternative to pulmonary function testing is the use of newer imaging modalities, including thoracic computed tomography (CT) scans and MRI. Several investigators have used high-resolution computerized tomography to evaluate the airways and parenchyma. Sarria and colleagues evaluated 38 survivors of preterm birth (25–29 weeks) and compared them to full-term infants who had sedated CT scans for nonpulmonary reasons.[23] They found structural differences in both airways and parenchyma. Increased heterogeneity within the parenchyma was seen in all survivors of BPD. Airway changes were the most marked, while reductions in lung volume were shown only among those with moderate or severe BPD. Further, they found that exposure to maternal smoking had a striking negative impact, with smaller airways in both BPD and control infants and toddlers. Additional information on the long-term impact of these airway and parenchymal changes is emerging.

TABLE 44.3 An Approach to Combining the National Institutes of Health Consensus Definition With the Physiologic Definition

Respiratory Support at 28 Days of Age	Respiratory Support at 36 Weeks' PMA	BPD Definition	
Room air	Room air	No BPD	
Any respiratory support	Room air	Mild BPD	
Any respiratory support	Respiratory support with FiO$_2$ <0.30	Room air challenge needed	Challenge passed, mild BPD Challenge failed, moderate BPD
Any respiratory support	Respiratory support with FiO$_2$ ≥0.30	Severe BPD	

BPD, Bronchopulmonary dysplasia; PMA, postmenstrual age.

Wong and colleagues studied 21 adult nonsmoking survivors of BPD with CT scan. All of those studied had parenchymal abnormalities, with some showing severe emphysematous changes (Figs. 44.1 and 44.2). These changes were correlated with reductions in pulmonary function tests.[24] Taken together, these findings raise concern about the future pulmonary function of survivors. The use of CT scans has limited utility because of concerns of exposure to high doses of ionizing radiation equivalent to up to 50 chest X-rays.

To avoid ionizing radiation, investigators have turned to MRIs to assess both airway and parenchyma. Higano and coworkers demonstrated the feasibility of performing MRIs in the neonatal intensive care unit (NICU). They assessed 42 neonates at term equivalent age and showed that increasing severity of abnormality on MRI correlated with the severity of BPD as defined by the NICHD classification score.[25]

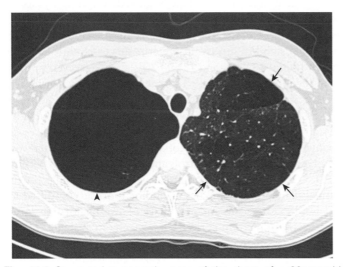

Fig. 44.1 Computed tomography scan of the chest of a 20-year-old nonsmoking male born at 28 weeks' gestation, showing severe emphysema and large bulla (*arrows*). (From Wong M, Lees AN, Louw J, et al: Emphysema in young adult survivors of moderate-to-severe bronchopulmonary dysplasia. Eur Respir J 32:321–328, 2008.)

Longer-Term Respiratory Morbidity

The disruption in the pulmonary function and respiratory outcomes of premature infants persists long after discharge from the NICU. Overall, preterm infants are at increased risk of wheezing-related illnesses as children and young adults, thought in part to be caused by an imbalance in the relationship between airway reactivity (smooth muscle structure and function) and airway compliance (connective tissues and parenchyma).[26] In the first year of life, preterm infants, compared to term infants, have higher rates of wheezing (44% vs 21%), are more likely to be rehospitalized for respiratory symptoms (25% vs 1.5%), and are more likely to receive an inhalation medication (13%).[27,28] At early school age, these differences result in decreased peak expiratory flow and high rates of wheezing diagnosis (36%) among former premature infants even without the diagnosis of BPD at hospital discharge. The prevalence of medication use for respiratory illnesses, wheezing events, and rehospitalizations was noted to decrease, however, from 30 months to 6 years.[29] Among ELBW children with a diagnosis of BPD at discharge, evaluation at 8 and 14 years showed that asthma medication use was unchanged (23%), although overall rates of asthma medication use increased among matched controls. This suggests a stability in wheezing prevalence among ELBW children as they age.[30] The long-term pulmonary morbidities of infants with BPD continue to evolve postdischarge. Hibbs et al. followed a cohort of 300 low-risk preterm infants and found an unexpected interaction between maternal race and vitamin D exposure. Vitamin D was protective for later respiratory morbidity in white infants but resulted in increased adverse outcomes in Black infants.[31]

HEALTH CARE UTILIZATION

Premature infants with BPD have a longer initial hospitalization than their peers without BPD,[32] and BPD remains a substantial lifelong burden. The costs of the disorder are both social and economic and are measured as impaired childhood health and quality of life, family stress and economic hardship,

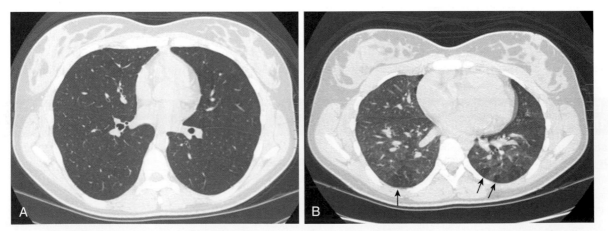

Fig. 44.2 Computed tomography scans (**A**, inspiratory; **B**, expiratory) of the chest of a 19-year-old nonsmoking female born at 25 weeks' gestation, showing minimal emphysema and moderate multilobar air trapping (*arrows*). (From Wong M, Lees AN, Louw J, et al: Emphysema in young adult survivors of moderate-to-severe bronchopulmonary dysplasia. Eur Respir J 32:321–328, 2008.)

and increased health care costs.[33-35] Lodha and colleagues documented that in a cohort of preterm infants of less than 1250 g birth weight, the use of respiratory medications and supplemental oxygen was significantly higher in infants who had BPD compared to those with no BPD.[36] Infants also had more physician visits and higher use of respiratory medications and supplemental oxygen continued through the third year of life. Alvarez-Fuente and coworkers showed the substantial economic impact of BPD in the first 2 years of life, even in a country with publicly funded health care.[37]

These findings must be taken in the context that even low-risk preterm infants without BPD have worse respiratory outcomes compared to a full-term cohort.[38]

Lapcharoensap and coauthors studied the costs of BPD survivors within the California Perinatal Quality Care Collaborative in infants born at less than 30 weeks' gestation between 2008 and 2011 in which 34% developed BPD. They found that the median cost of hospitalization in the first year per infant with BPD was $377,871, compared with $75,836 per infant without BPD.[39] These costs were driven by both longer hospitalizations and a higher likelihood of rehospitalization. Mowitz and colleagues analyzed health care claims of infants born at under 28 weeks' gestation between 2009 and 2015. They similarly found higher costs of care for infants with BPD compared to those without BPD. However, they also found that gestational age had a greater effect than the presence of BPD.[40]

NEURODEVELOPMENTAL OUTCOMES OF PRETERM INFANTS WITH BRONCHOPULMONARY DYSPLASIA

Infants with BPD have more neurodevelopmental sequelae in the forms of cognitive, language, motor, hearing, and vision deficits and cerebral palsy than matched gestational-age controls without BPD, even after controlling for confounding variables. Lodha and colleagues found that at 3 years of age, children with BPD, with or without need for chronic supplemental oxygen, had higher odds of neurodevelopmental disability compared to those without BPD (odds ratio, 1.9; 95% confidence interval [CI], 1.1–3.5).[41] These changes persist to 8 years of age, with 54% requiring special education classes compared with 37% of very low birth weight survivors without BPD.[42] De Mauro and coworkers showed that discharge home on oxygen was associated with a modest improvement in growth (which may not be clinically significant), with no improvement in neurodevelopmental impairment at 2 years of age. These infants did, however, have worsened pulmonary outcomes with increased rates of rehospitalization.[43] Early and middle school age studies suggest that BPD is associated with higher rates of subtle neurologic deficits and behavioral difficulties, as well as deficits in perceptual motor integration, motor coordination, and processing speeds.[44-46] In one of the first assessments of executive functioning in adult survivors of BPD, Gough and coworkers showed deficits in problem solving, awareness of behavior, and organization.[47] It is not clear whether BPD per se is responsible for these deficits or rather the prolonged illness and hospitalization, negative impact of medications such as corticosteroids and sedatives, and poor nutrition are the primary culprits.

Because inflammation has been shown to be a prominent component in BPD, there was great enthusiasm in the 1990s for the use of corticosteroids, especially dexamethasone, on the basis of several small case series. By 2001, numerous authors raised concern over neurotoxicity. Barrington completed a meta-analysis of available studies and concluded that the relative risk for developing cerebral palsy was 1.92 in those exposed to dexamethasone compared to controls.[48] By 2002, both the American Academy of Pediatrics and the Canadian Paediatric Society advised against the routine use of systemic dexamethasone.[49] Postnatal dexamethasone exposure has been associated with smaller total brain tissue volumes, which persist into adolescence.[50] There is concern, however, that the pendulum has swung too far with restricted use disadvantaging the highest-risk group. The use of an updated NICHD calculator to predict those at the highest risk of severe BPD may be helpful in guiding the choice of postnatal steroid use.[51]

A 2017 Cochrane review of late (>7 days) postnatal corticosteroids for chronic lung disease in preterm infants compiling data from 21 randomized trials showed that the composite outcomes of death or cerebral palsy and of death or major neurosensory disability were not significantly different between steroid and control groups.[52] These results may suggest a role for postnatal corticosteroids in preterm neonates over 1 week of age. The authors suggest that steroids be limited to those remaining on mechanical ventilation beyond 1 week of age.

Neonatologists continue to struggle to balance the risks of continued mechanical ventilation against the potential harm of corticosteroid exposure. Concerns have been raised that a high-risk subpopulation may benefit from lower dose and/or shorter courses of systemic steroids and that current practices have swung too far. Early or prophylactic use of low-dose courses of hydrocortisone in infants under 28 weeks has been shown to reduce risk of BPD[53] in the Premiloc study, with early data suggesting no adverse impact on neurodevelopmental outcomes at 2 years. In contrast to the beneficial findings of the Premiloc Trial, a similar trial of 3372 ventilator-dependent preterm infants treated with hydrocortisone between 7 and 14 days of age showed no change in the composite outcome of death or BPD at 36 weeks (adjusted risk difference, −36%; 95% CI, −12.7% to 5.4%).[54]

Inhaled corticosteroids are used in some units as they are thought to be safer than systemic steroids; however, systematic reviews of inhalation corticosteroids have found inadequate data to support these practices.[55] A more recent randomized trial by Bassler et al. showed a modest reduction in the composite outcome of death or BPD at 36 weeks (40% vs 46%; risk ratio [RR], 0.86; 95% CI, 0.75–1.00; $P = .05$) in infants assigned to the inhaled budesonide arm.[56] The apparent benefit was driven by a reduction in BPD in survivors (28% vs 38%; RR, 0.74; 95% CI, 0.60–0.90), with a trend toward higher mortality in inhaled the budesonide group (16.9% vs 13.6%; RR, 1.24; 95% CI, 0.91–1.69). A 2-year follow-up of this study showed that mortality was now significantly higher in the inhaled budesonide arm (19.9% vs 14.5%; RR, 1.37; 95% CI,

1.01–1.86),[57] which has dampened enthusiasm for this approach.

In attempts to more reliably deliver corticosteroids directly to alveoli of infants at risk of early lung injury, coadministration of budesonide with surfactant has been considered. Ye et al. have reported a significant decrease in the incidence of BPD or death in ventilated infants with severe RDS who received endotracheal budesonide.[58] Additional multicenter, randomized evaluation and follow-up studies of this practice are underway as of this writing.

OUTCOMES AFTER NEONATAL HYPOXIC RESPIRATORY FAILURE

Inhaled Nitric Oxide

The best studied pulmonary vasodilator used in hypoxic respiratory failure in term and late preterm infants is inhaled nitric oxide (iNO) (see Chapter 34). Fourteen randomized trials have been published with remarkably consistent findings.[59,60] The largest of these is the NINOS Trial conducted by the NICHD Neonatal Research Network in which 235 infants were randomized to iNO versus standard ventilator management.[61] The primary outcome was death or extracorporeal membrane oxygenation (ECMO). There was no difference in the occurrence of death, but there was a 40% reduction in the use of ECMO in those infants treated with iNO. Follow-up at 2 years of age showed similar neurodevelopmental outcomes in the two groups.[62] In a meta-analysis of the results from all 17 randomized trials, 50% of all infants treated responded to iNO, with an average increase in PaO$_2$ of 53 mm Hg.[63]

Lipkin and coworkers followed 133 full-term infants treated with iNO for respiratory failure to 1 year of age. There were no significant differences between the placebo and the iNO groups in any pulmonary or neurodevelopmental outcome. Rehospitalization occurred in 22% of the cohort. Forty-six percent of the cohort showed either neurodevelopmental or audiologic impairment. Major neurologic abnormalities occurred in 13%, cognitive delays in 30%, and hearing loss in 19% of infants.[64]

iNO has also been used in preterm infants. When used early in the course with severely ill preterm infants, there was a significantly increased rate of severe intraventricular hemorrhage (IVH) in the subgroup of infants weighing less than 1000 g (43% vs 33%; RR, 1.40; 95% CI, 1.03–1.88), as well as death (62% vs 48%; RR, 1.28; 95% CI, 1.06–1.54).[65] At the 18–22-month follow-up, moderate-severe cerebral palsy (CP) was slightly higher with iNO (RR, 2.41; 95% CI, 1.01–5.75), as was death or CP in infants weighing under 1000 g (RR, 1.22; 95% CI, 1.05–1.43).[66] Attempts to use iNO to prevent the development of BPD have been disappointing. In 2011, the NIH held a consensus conference that did not endorse the routine use of iNO.[67] However, they acknowledged that there might be individual situations, such as pulmonary hypoplasia, for which nitric oxide may be beneficial. A subanalysis of 12 infants with pulmonary hypoplasia related to prolonged rupture of membranes, nested within the Preemie Inhaled Nitric Oxide Trial (PINO), was led by Chock and colleagues.[68] Six infants were treated with iNO, and six with placebo. In this small series,

infants treated with iNO had a mean improvement of PaO$_2$ of 39 mm Hg, while control infants had a decrease of 11 mm Hg. Mortality was 33% in the iNO group versus 67% in controls, and BPD prevalence was 40% (2/5) versus 100% (2/2). Of note, in this selected subset, severe IVH or periventricular leukomalacia (PVL) was 20% in iNO-treated infants and 50% in control infants.

Baczynski and coauthors reported a retrospective cohort study over a 6-year period in which preterm infants with echocardiographic evidence of early pulmonary hypertension were selected. Forty-six percent of infants responded to iNO, with a 20% improvement in oxygenation. Responders showed improved survival free of disability (51% vs 15%; $P < .01$). Higher gestational age and a diagnosis of pulmonary hypertension in the setting of preterm prolonged rupture of membranes (PPROM) were independently associated with survival free of disability.[69] These findings are unlikely to be verified within a randomized trial and constitute the best evidence that iNO may be useful in preterm infants with pulmonary hypertension in the setting of PPROM.

Nitric oxide has been used in preterm infants in three separate contexts. Fifteen trials were analyzed by Barrington and Finer in the Cochrane Reviews.[70] They grouped the studies by the age of the infants at enrollment: early rescue treatment in the first 3 days of life, routine use over a prolonged interval with the intent to reduce BPD, and later treatment based on risk of BPD. Eight trials providing early rescue treatment for infants on the basis of oxygenation criteria demonstrated no significant effect of iNO on mortality or BPD (typical RR, 0.94; 95% CI, 0.87–1.01; 958 infants). Four studies examining routine use of iNO in infants with pulmonary disease reported no significant reduction in rates of death or BPD (typical RR, 0.94; 95% CI, 0.87–1.02; 1924 infants), although this small effect approached significance. Later treatment with iNO based on risk of BPD (three trials) revealed no significant benefit for this outcome in analyses of summary data (typical RR, 0.92; 95% CI, 0.85–1.01; 1075 infants). The authors concluded that "iNO does not appear to be effective as rescue therapy for the very ill preterm infant. Early routine use of iNO in preterm infants with respiratory disease does not prevent serious brain injury or improve survival without BPD. Later use of iNO to prevent BPD could be effective, but current 95% confidence intervals include no effect; the effect size is likely small (RR 0.92) and requires further study."[70]

Extracorporeal Membrane Oxygenation

According to the Extracorporeal Life Support Organization, as of early 2021, over 33,000 newborns have been treated with ECMO for respiratory failure, with an overall survival of 73% (see Chapter 28). Infants with meconium aspiration have the highest survival, at over 90%, contrasting with infants with congenital diaphragmatic hernia, whose survival is 51%.[71] Survivors of respiratory failure severe enough to be treated with ECMO are among the most severely ill infants treated by neonatologists. Early reports before the era of nitric oxide comparing those infants treated with ECMO to those who were "near misses" (i.e., not meeting criteria for ECMO cannulation) showed equivalent neurodevelopmental outcomes but worsened pulmonary outcomes in the conventionally treated group.[72,73] The largest randomized trial of ECMO enrolled 100 newborns in the UK Collaborative ECMO Trial. At 7 years of age, 90 of 100 survivors were assessed by a team masked to their intervention. Higher rates of respiratory morbidity were found in the conventionally treated group, with 32% having persistent wheezing compared with 11% of the ECMO-treated group.[74]

Within the first few years of life, cognitive scores and motor function for neonatal ECMO survivors overall are similar to those of healthy peers, although a subgroup analysis of ECMO—congenital diaphragmatic hernia survivors—suggests these specific infants have motor development indices significantly below age group norms.[75-78] At preschool ages, the UK ECMO Trial showed that 60% of ECMO-exposed children had neuromotor problems at age 4 years.[79] Furthermore, Glass et al.[80] and Dutch studies[81,82] showed gross motor, although not fine motor, skills to be poorer in ECMO-exposed 5-year-olds compared to healthy controls.

Moreover, at preschool ages, the UK ECMO Trial found cognitive scores within normal range in nearly two-thirds of the overall ECMO-exposed group.[75] While Glass et al.[80] also found ECMO-exposed survivors to have cognitive scores in the normal range, the mean scores were significantly lower than those of healthy peers (full-scale IQ 96 compared with 115).

However, cognitive scores alone do not give a complete picture, and ECMO survivors may be at risk of academic problems and school failure owing to noncognitive issues. With neuropsychological testing, Glass et al.[80] reported that about 30% of ECMO survivors with normal cognitive scores had problems in at least one domain. In particular, visuospatial ability,[74,81-83] working speed, and working memory[83-85] seem to be problematic. In a Dutch study, 8-year-old ECMO survivors were twice as likely to require either special education or adaptive mainstream education services compared to their peers. Potentially contributing to academic difficulties is an increase in risk of behavioral problems, particularly hyperactivity and attention deficits, in up to 35% of survivors by 5 years of age[74,79,83,86] (Table 44.4).

Additional information is emerging about adult survivors of neonatal ECMO. Madderom and coinvestigators assessed a cohort of 17–18-year-old survivors treated between 1991 and 1997 in the Netherlands.[87] Survivors performed more poorly on memory tasks compared to the norm population. Parents reported more organizational problems. Former patients reported more depressed behaviors and social problems. However, the former patients reported higher feelings of self-esteem and an average health status.

TABLE 44.4 Overview of Long-Term Outcomes Reported Following Neonatal ECMO Treatment

	Infancy (<2 years)	Preschool Age (2–5 years)	School Age (6–12 years)	Adolescence (>12 years)
Medical Outcome				
Lung function	Airflow obstruction,[7,8] normal lung volume,[7,8] and hyperinflation in CDH[9]	–	Airflow obstruction,[10,11,13] air trapping,[10,13] problems mainly in CDH patients[13]	Airflow obstruction and air trapping[10]
Exercise capacity	–	Decreased[14]	Decreased[11,14] to normal	Normal[10]
Growth	Normal[5,7] to slightly decreased weight[8] especially in CDH[9]	Normal[14]	Normal,[12,14] decreased height and weight in CDH[12]	–
SNHL	Prevalence ranging from 3% to 26%, in various studies over time[17-22,33]			
Chronic kidney disease	Abnormal urine protein/creatinine ratio or estimated glomerular filtration rate in 11%[31]			
[Neuro] Developmental Outcome				
Motor function	Normal in 84%[32]	Normal in 64%–73%[15,36]	Normal in 43%[39] and normal in 71% of CDH patients[36]	–
Cognition	Normal in 92%[32]	Normal average scores[15,33,38,45]	Normal in 68%[39] and normal average scores[43]	–
Neuropsychological tests	–	Decreased scores at verbal, reasoning, and spatial abilities,[22] and neuropsychological deficit at ≤1 domain in 11%[38]	Spatial ability scores below 10th percentile in 26%,[39] visuomotor integration below average in 20%,[43] memory problems in 26%–48%,[39] decreased working speed in 70%,[43] and decreased accuracy in 39%[43]	Memory problems in 46%–57%[36]
School performance	–	–	Special education 9%–20%[39,43]; extra support 20%–39%[39,43]	–
Behavior	–	Normal in 48.5%–65%,[45,47] more problems compared with controls in social, attention, and hyperactivity domains[38]	Clinical total problems 18%, social problems 5%, and attention problems 6%[43]	Self-reported externalizing problems 6%[36]

CDH, Congenital diaphragmatic hernia; *ECMO*, extracorporeal membrane oxygenation; *SNHL*, sensorineural hearing loss.
(From Ijsselstijn H, van Heijst AFJ: Long term outcome of children treated with neonatal extracorporeal membrane oxygenation: increasing problems with increasing age. Semin Perinatol 38:114–121, 2014.)

Engle led a group of US investigators in assessing 146 ECMO survivors (8.9% of available subjects) at a mean of 23.7 years of age.[88] Responses of ECMO survivors were compared to an age-matched data from a national sample in the Behavioral Risk Factor Surveillance System. The study is limited by the low response rate and evidence of selection bias skewing to more affluent and educated survivors. ECMO survivors were overall more satisfied with life (93% vs 84%) while also being more limited by physical, mental, or developmental problems (20% vs 11%). Learning problems occurred in 30% of the ECMO cohort.

CONCLUSION

Mechanical ventilation and the development of iNO and ECMO have been major therapeutic advances in neonatal care, particularly for term infants. Despite impressive improvements in survival, too many of these tiny patients carry both respiratory and neurologic morbidity that persists into school age and adolescence. Ongoing surveillance of these high-risk children is warranted to permit early detection of abnormalities and early intervention to reduce future impairments.

A complete reference list is available at https://expertconsult. inkling.com/.

KEY REFERENCES

6. Ehrenkranz RA, Walsh MC, Vohr BR, et al: Validation of the National Institutes of Health consensus definition of bronchopulmonary dysplasia. Pediatrics 116:1353–1360, 2005.

16. Friedrich L, Pitrez M, Stein RT, et al: Growth rate of lung function in healthy preterm infants. Am J Respir Crit Care Med 176:1269–1273, 2007.

17. Filbrun AG, Popova AP, Linn MJ: Longitudinal measures of lung function in infants with bronchopulmonary dysplasia. Pediatr Pulmonol 46:275–369, 2011.

18. Filippone M, Sartor M, Zacchello F, et al: Flow limitation in infants with bronchopulmonary dysplasia and respiratory function at school age. Lancet 361:753–754, 2003.

19. Fakhoury KF, Sellers C, Smith EO, et al: Serial measurements of lung function in a cohort of young children with bronchopulmonary dysplasia. Pediatrics 125:e1441–e1447, 2010.

21. Vollsæter M, Røksund OD, Eide GE, et al: Lung function after preterm birth: development from mid-childhood to adulthood. Thorax 68:767–776, 2013.

22. Narayanan M, Beardsmore CS, Owers-Bradley J, et al: Catch-up alveolarization in ex-preterm children: evidence from 3He magnetic resonance. Am J Respir Crit Care Med 187:1104–1109, 2013.

24. Wong M, Lees AN, Louw J, et al: Emphysema in young adult survivors of moderate-to-severe bronchopulmonary dysplasia. Eur Respir J 32:321–328, 2008.

25. Higano NS, Spielberg DR, Fleck RJ, et al: Neonatal pulmonary magnetic resonance imaging of bronchopulmonary dysplasia predicts short-term clinical outcomes. Am J Respir Crit Care Med 198:1302–1311, 2018.

29. Hennessy EM, Bracewell MA, Wood N, et al: Respiratory health in pre-school and school age children following extremely preterm birth. Arch Dis Child 93:1037–1043, 2008.

37. Álvarez-Fuente M, Arruza L, Muro M, et al: The economic impact of prematurity and bronchopulmonary dysplasia. Eur J Pediatr 176:1587–1593, 2017.

Gaps in Knowledge and Future Directions for Research

Tonse N.K. Raju, Payam Vali, and K. Suresh Gautham

> *Medicine, like all knowledge has a past as well as a present and future, and...*
> *in that past is the indispensable soil out of which improvement must grow.*
>
> *Alfred Stillé (1813–1900)[1]*

KEY POINTS

- With the possible exception of pediatric oncology, no other branch of medicine has seen such phenomenal advances as neonatal care over the past half-century, with significantly improved survival. These improvements are the result of improved high-risk obstetric and neonatal care and dramatic advances in assisted ventilation technology.

- A vast body of knowledge exists on the topic of neonatal ventilation—several thousand publications exist on this topic, with many more being added each month. In this chapter, we use selected aspects of this body of knowledge to describe the current state of knowledge and to highlight knowledge gaps that further research should address.

- After offering a brief historical note, we focus on issues related to study design, definitions, endpoints of research interventions, the techniques of assisted ventilation, surfactant therapy, and bronchopulmonary dysplasia and other conditions requiring assisted ventilation.

- We stress the importance of collaborative clinical trials and the value of engaging biomedical and bioengineering communities in developing noninvasive devices and instruments to facilitate neonatal care. Such efforts should lead to improved patient care and reduce chronic morbidities that still exist.

- We provide a list of ongoing clinical studies from around the world, downloaded from the ClinicalTrials.gov database.

INTRODUCTION

The first chapter of this volume offered a brief review of the historical aspects of neonatal respiratory physiology and assisted ventilation for newborn infants. Forty-four chapters later, the readers would have appreciated the great magnitude of advances accomplished over the past half century that contributed to more than 95% survival rates for all preterm infants through the first year of their lives. Many factors contributed to such improvements, summarized in Box 45.1 and excellently reviewed elsewhere.[2]

The goal of providing respiratory support today and new research in the future should not only improve survival but also reduce short- and long-term morbidity. Despite remarkable improvements in survival rates, the burden of morbidity still remains high, especially related to pulmonary, renal, special sensory, and neurological outcomes. This is partly because, as neonatal intensive care and respiratory support techniques improved, clinicians pushed the boundaries of "viability" to earlier gestation and began offering therapies for infants previously deemed incompatible with long-term survival, such as trisomy 18 and 13, and other complex congenital malformations.

In this chapter, we offer some lessons learned from the history of neonatology to guide the evolution and development of respiratory care for the future, addressing current gaps in knowledge and future directions for research. The chapter will be divided into five broad areas:

1. Development and application of new methods of generating knowledge;
2. Respiratory care, including delivery room management and assisted ventilation;
3. Management of specific respiratory and nonrespiratory conditions requiring assisted ventilation;
4. Development of devices;
5. Current ongoing research.

DEVELOPMENT AND APPLICATION OF NEW METHODS OF GENERATING KNOWLEDGE

A review of the vast history of generation of knowledge is beyond the scope of this chapter. Suffice to say that for centuries, empirical observations intermingled with an occasional experimental study were the primary means for the development of scientific knowledge, which was passed on to generations of students. Following the Renaissance, scientists relied upon experimental evidence to a greater extent that blossomed from the sixteenth through the nineteenth century with the towering examples of research studies by Robert Koch, Claude Bernard,[3] and Louis Pasteur, to name a few.

Likewise, the progress in the evolution of clinical trial designs and statistical methods has been long and tortuous.[4] Although a few notable trials were launched in the early twentieth century (e.g., the treatment of pulmonary tuberculosis designed by Sir

BOX 45.1 **Major Advances in Neonatal-Perinatal Medicine**

- Advances in the assessment of fetal well-being and increasing use of cesarean delivery
- Antibiotic prophylaxis to reduce group B streptococcus sepsis in the newborn
- Fetal surgery research, especially for meningomyelocele
- Widespread use of antenatal corticosteroids to enhance pulmonary maturity
- Magnesium sulphate for mothers at risk of preterm delivery to improve neurological outcomes
- The development of surfactant and refinements of its use
- Numerous technological advances in developing
  - Noninvasive ventilation and avoiding intubation and mechanical ventilation
  - High-frequency ventilators
  - Advanced methods of CPAP and nasal cannula oxygen therapies
- Reduction of severe Rhesus disease
- Improvements in neonatal cardiac surgery
- Regionalized perinatal care
- Long-term follow-up programs
- Point-of-care ultrasound and magnetic resonance imaging
- Parenteral nutrition
- Increasing understanding of feeding human milk (mothers' own or donated)
- Caffeine, probiotics, and inhaled nitric oxide
- Therapeutic hypothermia for hypoxic-ischemic encephalopathy
- Increasing number of multisite controlled clinical trials
- The growth of large databases (examples: Vermont-Oxford Network, NICHD Neonatal Research Network; Canadian Neonatal Network, and similar multi-site networks in the UK, Europe, Australia and New Zealand, Japan, and elsewhere)
- The evolution of systematic reviews (Cochrane Collaboration)

CPAP, Continuous positive airway pressure; *NICHD*, National Institute of Child Health and Human Development.
(Manley, B.J., et al., Fifty years in neonatology. J Paediatr Child Health, 2015. 51(1): p. 118-21.)

Braford Hill), clinical trials in neonatal assisted ventilation had to wait until the mid- to late-1950s and beyond. They were followed by a range of isolated efforts at resuscitation in the delivery room during the early decades of the twentieth century, some of which were spectacular failures.[5-10] Early cohort studies gradually changed to multicenter collaborative research efforts, brilliantly exemplified in the trials related to pulmonary surfactant of the 1980s and 1990s, a few trials of meconium aspiration, the trials involving high-frequency ventilation, and in the later decades of the twentieth and the early decades of the twenty-first centuries involving inhaled nitric oxide (iNO).

It is worth noting that among the early efforts to provide assisted ventilation were the encouraging reports by Donald and colleagues using "augmented respiration."[11,12] These studies were followed by concerted efforts by Stahlman,[13] Delivoria-Papadopoulos and Sweyer,[14-16] and Thomas and colleagues,[17] among others, to embark on prolonged assisted ventilation of newborn infants. Their attempts, however, resulted in a modest "success." Although some infants survived to be discharged, many died within a few hours to days after receiving assisted ventilatory support. Yet, those attempts were pioneering. The investigators had chosen patients considered as "terminal" or "near-terminal," in an era when such efforts were unthinkable. Besides, they earnestly urged others to begin assisted ventilation early in the course of respiratory distress.

As discussed in detail elsewhere in this book, the most common complication of neonatal assisted ventilation is bronchopulmonary dysplasia (BPD), a chronic lung disease first described by Northway et al. in 1967.[18] On the 25th anniversary of his landmark paper, Northway said, "...BPD is both a significant clinical problem associated with neonatal intensive care and a sign of the *success* of that care" (emphasis added).[19] Now, after nearly 70 years of neonatal assisted ventilation, we need to ask again: how do we define "success" and set meaningful endpoints of our approaches while treating neonatal respiratory conditions? Some of the pros and cons of these concepts are listed in Table 45.1.

Basic and Clinical Study Designs

Well-conducted, multicenter, prospective controlled trials remain the gold standard to provide conclusive evidence of the benefits or lack thereof of therapeutic interventions for patient care. However, the findings from clinical trials are only as good as the rigor of the study designs. A significant limitation of most neonatal studies has been a relatively small number of study participants recruited for clinical trials. Moreover, in most neonatal clinical trials, over half of the eligible participants cannot be recruited because of lack of parental consent. The demographics and risk profiles of the unrecruited participants could be much different from those recruited, and if so, the generalizability of the study findings from such trials will be limited. Although effective metaanalytical methods have evolved over the past two decades, conducting systematic review and metaanalyses would be challenging if one encounters several poorly conducted studies.[20-34] Besides, the heterogeneity of study designs would further limit systematic reviews to develop practice summaries. Some of the specific issues concerning study designs are summarized in Table 45.2.

RESPIRATORY CARE

Delivery Room Management

Inappropriate ventilatory techniques during neonatal resuscitation can initiate lung injury within a few minutes of birth through a cascade of events laying the foundations for permanent lung damage.[35-37] Despite this knowledge, many of the initial steps we undertake while resuscitating newborn infants require more robust evidence base.[38-42] The major gaps in knowledge concerning neonatal resuscitation include (1) methods to help clear lung fluid and help the lungs to expand uniformly; (2) methods to offer breathing support, such as positive end expiratory pressure (PEEP), continuous positive airway pressure (CPAP), or other noninvasive methods of assisted ventilation; (3) selecting the appropriate inspired oxygen concentrations; (4) umbilical cord clamping and milking issues; and (5) best methods for administering exogenous surfactant preparations.

Providing prolonged ("sustained") inflation into the liquid-filled lungs is an attractive approach to address the knowledge gap noted earlier.[43-49] However, the initial success of this approach could not be replicated in a large multicenter trial, Sustained Aeration of Infant Lung (SAIL). This trial was stopped

TABLE 45.1 Research Study Endpoints: Pros and Cons

Endpoints Used	Advantages	Limitations
Survival through hospital discharge (or equivalent to term PMA)	• No ambiguity in the definition and measurement	• Only a short-term outcome
Chronic lung disease with or without pulmonary hypertension at initial hospital discharge	• May be more relevant outcome related to intervention	• Difficult to define • Early death leads to undercount of the outcome
Pulmonary outcomes: 1. ER visits for pulmonary complications 2. Hospitalization for infections (RSV, pneumonia) or wheezing and/or respiratory failure 3. Asthma or hyperactive airway disease during infancy/childhood 4. Medication use during infancy/childhood	• Number of visits could be easy to count, or parents to keep track of • Hospitalization information can be obtained accurately from medical records • More meaningful impact on child's lifestyle • Can be counted easily, especially for inpatients, if they are filled-in by the hospital pharmacies	• Limitation as a result of loss of follow-up; accuracy of parental recollection • Other causes for hospitalization complicating measurement • Difficult to assess OTC medications • Prescription is not the same as usage
Pulmonary function test results 1. Work of breathing 2. Airway resistance 3. FEV$_1$ and other measures of pulmonary functions	• More meaningful outcomes. Pulmonary function determines the overall impact on lifestyle	• Difficult in smaller children • Need for sedation • Consenting and follow-up issues
Adolescence/adult outcomes 1. Exercise tolerance and endurance 2. Pneumonia and cardiopulmonary functions	• More meaningful measures of interventions • These outcomes may "matter" for the patients	• Difficult to conduct • Time gap between intervention and outcome studies • Time gap: loss to follow-up
Public health and family impact 1. Healthcare costs/cost savings 2. Impact on the family 3. Longevity	• Important at the public health and societal level • Policy changes possible • Longevity—measurable outcome	• Cost varies across countries and among health care policies • Difficult to quantify without accurate longitudinal registries

ER, Emergency room; *FEV$_1$*, forceful exhaled volume in 1 second; *OTC*, over the counter; *PMA*, postmenstrual age; *RSV*, respiratory syncytial virus.

TABLE 45.2 Study Design Issues

Issues	Advantages	Limitations
Multisite clinical studies	• Diverse cohort features • Quicker enrollment and study completion • Sharing of research burden • Variation in care practice, enhancing generalizability • If services are centralized, could be cost saving	• Difficulties in developing consensus on study design • Diverse range of patient care practices • Diverse pace of recruitment • Immeasurable site-specific effects • Could be expensive for funding agencies that have budgetary limits
Respiratory care practice during intervention	• Preset management criteria for the study duration might mitigate or prevent introducing new approaches	• New and evolving methods if followed by some care givers can introduce unexpected bias • Recruiting into original studies may be delayed
Study cohort characteristics	• Strict entry criteria help interpreting study results more precisely	• Might limit generalizability
Comparing complex interventions	• Simultaneous comparison of complex interventions can provide quicker answers	• Uniformity of management of complex interventions cannot be assured within, or across cohorts
National Registries	• Well-planned registries with large cohorts (example: The ECMO Registry) allow for detailed data mining • Relatively inexpensive • Help answer broad public health-level questions	• Owing to the heterogeneity of patient care information developing summary measures of treatment effect difficult • Effect of changing patient care over time (may not be uniform at all sites) complicates summarizing results
Inclusion of families in developing study design and in DSMB	• Endpoint selection choice by families may be very important • Unique perspective of DSMB members based on personal experience • Ethical fairness of research design process	• Selecting and training appropriate members from the "affected" families • Risk of bias based on personal success or failures • Issues of reimbursement for time and effort • Contractual and confidentiality issues

DSMB, Data safety monitoring board; *ECMO*, extracorporeal membrane oxygenation support.

after the enrollment of 460 infants out of the planned 600 by the Eunice Kennedy Shriver National Institute of Health and Human Development (NICHD) because of safety concerns raised by the Data and Safety Monitoring Board. An interim analysis of available data from 426 infants showed that although the primary study outcomes (death or BPD) were similar between the groups, the number of deaths occurring at less than 48 hours of age were higher in the SAIL intervention group compared to the standard care group: 16 infants (7.4%) versus 3 infants (1.4%), respectively.[50] Following these results, studies are underway to test if a more fine-tuned or "titrated" PEEP support as part of resuscitation could be more effective than sustained inflation of the infant lungs.[51-53]

Mechanical Ventilation

One of the earliest innovations to provide neonatal assisted ventilation was the development of time-cycled, pressure-limited ventilators. However, these were notoriously ineffective because they led to fluctuations in the delivered tidal volumes as the pulmonary compliance changed during the course of the infant's lung disease. By the mid-1970s, newer ventilator models were designed that could deliver volume-controlled breaths. Even these devices had many technological limitations, such as the inability to accurately measure small tidal volumes, a highly compliant circuit that increased compressible volume loss, an ineffective triggering system, a slow response time, and incompatibility with continuous flow during spontaneous breathing. Thus, clinicians stopped using this device.[54] By the end of the twentieth century, however, sophisticated technologies emerged that could incorporate microprocessing software allowing the introduction of newer ventilator models for use in extremely premature infants. For instance, the newest generation of ventilators provide feedback of respiratory mechanics and have proven to be more reliable than the ventilators of the prior decades.

What parameters need to be improved to achieve better ventilators? The answer would depend upon our definition of successful ventilation. Newly introduced equipment should be developed based on our understanding of the pathophysiological processes causing lung disease in the newborn leading to chronic lung injury. Northway and colleagues, who coined the phrase BPD, also astutely observed that the pathological changes were because of high positive pressure used during assisted ventilation.[18] Subsequent research studies shed light on the mechanisms of ventilator-induced lung injury (VILI; also referred to as ventilator-associated lung injury [VALI]). These topics are discussed elsewhere in this volume. But, briefly, four interrelated processes can explain the development of VALI. These are (1) damage caused by "volutrauma," or excessive tidal volume; (2) injury from "barotrauma," or excessive inflating pressure both of which cause distention of the alveoli and damage small airways; (3) "atelectrauma," or maldistribution of the tidal volume because of varying degrees of lung compliance causing repeated alveolar collapse and expansion (RACE) leading to shear stress–related injury to the alveolar units and small airways; and (4) "biotrauma," or damage from the inflammatory mediators released from pulmonary cells causing additional damage to the already injured lungs.

In an era where ventilator technology can sense the patients' respiratory efforts and continuously adjust flow to match desired tidal volumes, we may be in a position to study the interactions between mechanical ventilators and the patients, based on changing physiology. Although new ventilators are constantly appearing in the market, there is a need to evaluate their performance by conducting well-designed comparative clinical trials. This task is challenging because studies testing the performance of new ventilators need to consider not only the technological sophistication of the ventilator, but also the choice of patient population selected, as well as the skills of healthcare professionals using the newer models. These pragmatic issues should be included while designing studies to test the benefits of newer ventilator models.

Noninvasive Respiratory Support

In the early decades of the twenty-first century, the approach and philosophy in providing assisted ventilation dramatically shifted from one of "aggressive" to a "gentler" approach. The latter led to the idea of "noninvasive respiratory support" to mitigate VALI.

But these advances did not occur de novo. In 1968, Harrison and colleagues observed that the "grunting" maneuver was from the newborn's efforts to help maintain lung volume.[55] This seminal observation paved the way for Gregory et al. to develop CPAP offered through a "chamber device" in spontaneously breathing infants without an endotracheal tube.[56] Although later considered a landmark publication, this method of providing CPAP did not catch on immediately, perhaps because of somewhat cumbersome steps in adopting this method. Other CPAP methods appeared soon, including the face mask CPAP (securely attached to the infant's head by a Velcro band across the occiput), which was practiced at Toronto's Hospital for Sick Children mainly because the method did not require endotracheal intubation.[57] However, face mask CPAP caused changes in head shape (molding), and there were reports of higher rates of cerebellar hemorrhage with its use.[58] With increasing neonatal resuscitation training programs, more trainees and clinicians became adept at performing endotracheal intubation, noninvasive support using CPAP became less attractive, and invasive respiratory support became standard treatment for infants with significant respiratory distress.

By the late 1980s, the development of artificial surfactants and the availability of high-frequency ventilation added further enthusiasm to provide assisted ventilation rather than "gentler" forms of respiratory support, including CPAP. Quick endotracheal intubation followed by surfactant administration and ventilatory support became the unstated "standard of care," well into the early years of the twenty-first century.

In 2008, a large, groundbreaking, multicenter RCT led by Morley and colleagues from Australia demonstrated that infants randomized to nasal CPAP (nCPAP) had lower ventilation days and oxygen requirement at 28 days of age.[59] This was followed by the NICHD Neonatal Research Network study (called SUPPORT) and the Vermont Oxford Network Delivery Room Management Trial. The results of these studies provided strong evidence in support of initiating noninvasive ventilation in the delivery room.[60,61]

Although nCPAP has been shown to be an effective strategy to maintain adequate respiratory support starting in the delivery room, many premature infants require a higher level of support owing to worsening of respiratory distress syndrome (RDS) or developing apnea. Once intubated, clinicians make valiant efforts to wean and successfully extubate patients to avoid prolonged mechanical ventilation. Evidence is accumulating that bubble CPAP may provide better support compared to ventilator-CPAP[62,63] and can be successfully used in resource-limited environments. In vitro experiments on an infant lung model suggest that oscillations from bubbling may contribute to the gas exchange by delivering low-amplitude, high-frequency oscillations to the lungs.[64] A metaanalysis published in 2020 compared bubble CPAP to other forms of CPAP from 19 studies and showed that there were no improvements in mortality or BPD when using bubble CPAP.[65] They also noted methodological heterogeneity among studies, making generalizability of the results difficult. Many studies included in this systematic review had high or unclear risks of bias. Therefore, we believe that well-designed studies examining the benefits of bubble CPAP, if any, on lung development in premature infants is urgently needed.

Other common modes of noninvasive respiratory support include nasal intermittent positive pressure ventilation (NIPPV) and heated humidified high-flow nasal cannula. Despite extensive research on these topics, the optimal mode of noninvasive respiratory support remains unknown. Thus, as we write this review, we see no published results demonstrating the superiority of NIPPV in providing effective ventilation compared to various modes of CPAP therapy. The apparent benefit from NIPPV could be attributed to a higher mean airway pressure in this mode of ventilation compared to traditional CPAP methods. Newer modalities, such as noninvasive high-frequency ventilation (NIHFV)[66] and noninvasive neurally adjusted ventilation assist (NIV-NAVA),[67] are being increasingly used and their comparative advantage is a fruitful area for future research. Knowledge gaps concerning mechanical ventilation are listed in Box 45.2.

Exogenous Surfactant Administration

The history of the discovery of the role of surfactant in pulmonary biology began in 1929 when experiments on porcine lungs by von Neergaard led to the discovery that "surface tension is responsible for the greater part of total lung recoil compared to tissue elasticity."[68,69] Two decades later, Gruenwald concluded (by experiments on stillborn lungs) that resistance to neonatal lung aeration is as a result of surface tension and that surface-active substances decrease pressure to help aeration.[70] It would take another decade before Avery and Mead would show that RDS (formerly known as hyaline membrane disease) is caused by abnormal surface tension.[71] These discoveries, and the tragic death of prematurely born Patrick Bouvier Kennedy in 1963 (discussed in detail in Chapter 1 of this volume), helped increase the awareness of RDS, accelerating funding for research on neonatal lung diseases and development of therapies using exogenous surfactants.

Initial studies using synthetic surfactant (protein-free) administered by nebulization did not show significant beneficial

---

> **BOX 45.2 Mechanical Ventilation: Some Questions That Need to Be Addressed**
>
> - Choosing the method of respiratory support intervention based on:
>   - Infant age/size
>   - Underlining pathology
>   - Available expertise
>   - Pulmonary functions
> - Management of infants on assisted ventilation
>   - Monitoring changing pulmonary status to adjust ventilation parameters
>   - Predicting potential iatrogenic complications
> - Minimizing the complications associated with mechanical ventilatory support
>   - Mechanical issues (manufacturing issues)
>   - Quality control issues within the unit
>   - Training, and avoiding iatrogenic complications
> - Continued education
>   - With a constant change in high-tech ventilatory devices, caregivers need to be refreshed on a regular basis about the proper use of the new instruments and devices.
> - Emergency preparedness
>   - Example of COVID-19 pandemic

---

effects. However, early animal models studied using animal-derived surfactants (also called natural surfactants) were remarkably efficient. In preterm fetal rabbit lungs, the pressure–volume hysteresis was widened with the use of animal-derived surfactants.[72] Besides, premature lambs ($n = 10$) that received natural surfactant had 100% survival for 2 hours compared to control lambs ($n = 10$) that died within 60 minutes.[73] In 1980, Fujiwara and colleagues published the first clinical report where they directly instilled exogenous bovine surfactant into the lungs via the endotracheal tube in 10 premature infants with RDS. All treated infants had dramatic improvements.[74] More research followed, eventually leading to the commercial availability of animal-derived surfactant preparations by the late 1980s. Surfactant therapy has had a major impact on reducing neonatal mortality and morbidity. Exogenous surfactants have also been used for conditions where intrinsic surfactant may be inactivated, such as in meconium aspiration syndrome, pneumonia, and pulmonary hemorrhage.

In the past 30 years, exogenous surfactant therapy exemplifies the best evidence-based intervention to treat preterm infants suffering from RDS. Traditionally, exogenous surfactants were administered through an endotracheal tube followed by positive pressure inflations. This approach is gradually changing. To minimize need for prolonged ventilatory assistance and reduce the risks of VALI, many centers adopted the INtubation-SURfactant-Extubation (INSURE) method for administering exogenous surfactant preparations. Such an approach was promoted by Verder and colleagues from Denmark.[75,76] Because there is a potential for lung injury even with a few positive pressure inflations following endotracheal intubation, less invasive techniques, such as less invasive surfactant administration (LISA) or minimally invasive surfactant therapy (MIST), have evolved in recent years.

A thin catheter (i.e., gastric tube, umbilical catheter) is passed through the vocal cords using Magill forceps in LISA (also known as the Cologne method),[76,77] whereas in MIST, a stiff vascular catheter is used to intubate the trachea (also known as the Hobart method).[78] LISA/MIST techniques allow for spontaneous breathing during instillation of surfactant and do not require positive pressure ventilation. Complications and fluctuation in hemodynamic parameters associated with direct laryngoscopy, however, are not minimized using these approaches. Trials comparing INSURE to LISA/MIST have shown a reduction in BPD, but an important shortcoming of these trials is their relatively small size, especially of infants at gestational age under 28 weeks.[79,80]

Surfactant administration studies using supraglottic airway devices (laryngeal airway mask [LAM]) have shown promising results; however, the sizes of LAMs are the limitations for their use in infants under 1500 g. The development of efficient nebulization methods has led clinicians to revisit surfactant delivery through aerosolization. However, to overcome the limitations of the aerosolized surfactant preparation to be deposited predominantly in the trachea, improvements in nebulization technology and the development of new-generation surfactants need to occur.[81]

MANAGEMENT OF SPECIFIC RESPIRATORY AND NONRESPIRATORY CONDITIONS REQUIRING ASSISTED VENTILATION

Bronchopulmonary Dysplasia

Several components of BPD have been covered in other chapters in this manual. A few salient issues are discussed here, underscoring knowledge gaps related to the pathogenesis, prevention, and treatment strategies.

The concept of "new BPD"[82] has helped to define the condition as a result of a complex interplay between abnormal and interrupted growth and maturation of the immature airways, pulmonary alveoli, and pulmonary vasculature, superimposed by the consequences of the body's attempts at repairing the lung architecture. Furthermore, "new BPD" appears to be a milder form of lung morbidity during the neonatal period, yet despite being mild, a potential for prolonged morbidity into infancy and childhood persists.[83-86]

The challenges of developing a comprehensive definition have been reviewed extensively.[83,84,87-90] Box 45.3 summarizes the elements of such recent attempts proposed by experts participating in a 2017 workshop organized by NICHD.[91] Elsewhere in this volume and in earlier sections of this chapter, various knowledge gaps in neonatal resuscitation and mechanical ventilation have been addressed. Among these, comparative trials testing the best noninvasive methods of assisted ventilation for various neonatal conditions need the urgent attention of the research community. As noted in many excellent systematic reviews,[85,92-97] numerous knowledge gaps have been identified in the areas of the pathogenesis, diagnosis, and management aspects of BPD-associated pulmonary hypertension (PH).

The research efforts to identify biomarkers as potential predictors of BPD, BPD and/or death, and severe BPD have been generally disappointing until now because of their low predictive accuracy.[98-101] However, there is a potential for newer methods, such as

---

BOX 45.3 **National Institute of Health and Human Development Workshop–Proposed Definition of Bronchopulmonary Dysplasia**

Baseline items:
1. Gestational age at birth <32 weeks
2. 36 weeks of postmenstrual age at BPD designation
3. Persistent evidence of parenchymal lung disease, preferably confirmed radiologically
4. One of the following required for three consecutive days to maintain the pulse oximetry saturation ≥90%

Grading:
- Grade I
  - All baseline items noted earlier, plus one of the following
    - Oxygen hood percentage inspired O_2 concentration 30%
    - Nasal cannula with flow of <1 L/min and inspired O_2 concentration 21%–70%
    - Nasal cannula with flow of ≤3 L/min and inspired O_2 concentration ≥30%
    - nCPAP, NIPPV, or nasal cannula with flow ≥3 L/min, and inspired O_2 concentration 21%
- Grade II
  - All baseline items noted earlier, plus one of the following
    - Invasive IPPV, with an inspired O_2 concentration of 21%
    - Nasal cannula flow at 1–3 L/min, and inspired O_2 concentration ≥30%
    - nCPAP, NIPPV, or nasal cannula ≥3 L/min flow, and inspired O_2 concentration 22%–29%
- Grade III
  - All baseline items noted earlier, plus one of the following
    - Invasive IPPV with inspired O_2 concentration >21%
    - nCPAP, NIPPV, or nasal cannula ≥3 L/min flow, and inspired O_2 concentration ≥30%
- Grade III (A)
  - Death between postnatal age of 14 and 36 weeks of postmenstrual age, with evidence of pulmonary parenchymal disease and respiratory failure that cannot be attributed to other neonatal morbidities, such as necrotizing enterocolitis, intraventricular hemorrhage, redirection care, severe sepsis, etc.

BiPAP, Bilevel positive airway pressure; *BPD,* bronchopulmonary dysplasia; *IPPV,* intermittent positive pressure ventilation; *nCPAP,* nasal continuous positive airway pressure; *NIPPV,* nasal intermittent positive airway pressure ventilation.
(Higgins, R.D., et al., Bronchopulmonary Dysplasia: Executive Summary of a Workshop. J Pediatr, 2018. 197: p. 300-308)

---

multi-omic technologies, which may help define the cellular and humoral interactions that regulate normal as well as abnormal lung development and response to injury that are the hallmarks of BPD. For research in this field, several investigators are using gene expression in BPD lung tissue and in mouse models. Although many pathways have identified the involvement of lung development and repair pathways, such as CD44 and phosphorus oxygen lyase activities, additional molecules and pathways may be involved in the genetic predisposition to BPD.[85,102-105]

Numerous therapeutic agents have been used to prevent, treat, and/or reduce the severity of BPD, which have been reviewed extensively by many authors.[106-113] Some of the approaches include use of diuretics (furosemide, chlorothiazide, spironolactone), bronchodilators (albuterol, ipratropium, leval-buterol), inhaled corticosteroids (beclomethasone, budesonide, fluticasone), agents to treat PH (bosentan, sildenafil, treprostinil), and promotility or antireflux medications (erythromycin, lansoprazole, metoclopramide, omeprazole, ranitidine)—the strength and limitations have been excellently summarized by Abman et al.[92] Besides the steroidal agents noted earlier, other nonsteroidal antiinflammatory agents have been explored for reducing pulmonary inflammation and mitigate the severity of BPD.[114,115] The available literature clearly shows that most of these agents have no evidence base for their therapeutic efficacy, with a potential for significant untoward outcomes. Expert reviewers have cautioned that one needs to establish the risk versus benefit ratios and avoid drugs that have little efficacy and a high rate of toxicity.[87,92,109,116]

Although the effects of many interventions need to be tested prospectively, some investigators have compared the outcomes of available therapies reported from divergent trials and concluded that the primary use of noninvasive respiratory support, the application of surfactant without endotracheal ventilation, and the use of volume-targeted ventilation, early use caffeine citrate, and intramuscular vitamin A during the first 4 weeks of life may reduce BPD.[117]

Based on animal studies and early clinical trials, many studies have reported encouraging results of cell therapy, although many others have expressed caution while adapting this new, evolving, yet fascinating field of stem cell therapy.[118-126] The results of early clinical trials remain eagerly awaited. Because of the ease of extraction, some investigators contend that the use of mesenchymal stem cells is a promising therapy, particularly because of their low immunogenicity, antiinflammatory properties, and regenerative ability. The possible mechanism of action could be attributed to the paracrine effects of the stem cell–derived humoral factors, such as interleukin (IL)-6, IL-8, vascular endothelial growth factor, collagen, and elastin, rather than the multilineage and regenerative capacities of mesenchymal stem cells. Thus, it is possible that cell-free preparations derived from mesenchymal stem cells also may offer potential benefits. Although the phase 1 dose-escalation study was carried out in a limited number of newborn infants using umbilical cord blood–derived mesenchymal stem cell for BPD and showed to be effective and safe, we need more results from more ongoing clinical trials listed in Box 45.4.

Infants with BPD discharged from home may continue to experience pulmonary function abnormalities that may extend into childhood and adolescence, and in some cases even into adult age groups.[127] The epidemiology, medical needs, and various clinical phenotypes of pulmonary morbidity among BPD infants during posthospital discharge is an extremely important area that needs to be addressed.[128]

Other Conditions Requiring Ventilatory Support

The etiology of respiratory failure in newborns is vast, and depending upon the underlying pathogenesis of lung disease, specific ventilation strategies may be necessary to optimize respiratory support. Inherent differences in the lung and chest wall mechanics of premature and term newborns should also

---

> ### BOX 45.4 Bronchopulmonary Dysplasia: Selected Knowledge Gaps and Research Needs
>
> **Basic Science**
> - Animal models to better assess pathogenesis and pathophysiology and responses to treatment interventions
> - Developing new and testing the existing therapeutic agents being used for prevention and treatment
> - Identification of modifiable prenatal and postnatal risk factors
> - Developing biomarkers
>
> **Definition**
> - Severity of BPD as an accurate predictor of long-term respiratory outcomes
> - Defining specific criteria for parenchymal lung disease, including developing precise radiographic criteria
> - Better classification of BPD in small-for-gestational age infants and/or infants with intrauterine growth restrictions
> - Separating chronic lung disease seen in late preterm and term infants requiring long-term assisted ventilation and/or other respiratory care supports
> - Refining definition for grade I BPD (Box 45.3) by incorporating new and evolving respiratory support categories
> - Accounting for the competing outcome of early death of infants who have a high likelihood of developing BPD
> - Definition and classification of BPD severity based on measures of pulmonary functions, which can be correlated with ongoing lung pathology
>
> **Management**
> - Delivery room management: use of CPAP; cyclical sustained inflation; using appropriate inspired concentration of inspired oxygen
> - Early neonatal care for strategies to prevent chronic lung disease: use of equipment for servo-controlled inspired oxygen concentration and other ventilatory techniques, such as volume-targeted ventilation
> - Role of pharmacological agents for preventing BPD: steroid; iNO, caffeine; antioxidants (e.g., superoxide dismutase)
> - Strategies to prevent/minimize development of pulmonary hypertension
> - Rigorous research on inhalation therapies—most of the current inhalation therapies remain of questionable value.
> - Resolving the role of PDA on BPD
> - Managing established BPD beyond 36 weeks of PMA, including the management of severe BPD
> - Assessing and treating BPD-associated pulmonary hypertension
> - Improving nutritional support

Some content modified from the following references: 83,87,90–92,97, 105,115,116,146.
BPD, Bronchopulmonary dysplasia; *CPAP*, continuous positive airway pressure; *iNO*, inhaled nitric oxide; *PDA*, patent ductus arteriosus; *PMA*, postmenstrual age.

---

be considered when providing artificial ventilation. Some of these conditions are discussed here.

Congenital Diaphragmatic Hernia

Developmental defects in the diaphragm result in herniation of abdominal contents into the thoracic cavity and can lead to severe pulmonary hypoplasia, pulmonary vascular remodeling, as well as cardiac deformation and dysfunction. Severe hypoxic respiratory failure and persistent PH of the newborn (PPHN) often complicate the medical course of these patients. Recognizing the interdependence of the pulmonary and cardiovascular systems in the context of abnormal physiology is of paramount importance when providing medical management to congenital diaphragmatic hernia (CDH) patients.

The hypoplastic lungs in CDH are particularly sensitive to VALI. Gentle ventilation strategies using low tidal volumes (4 mL/kg), low mean airway pressures, and low PEEP (3–5 cm H_2O), thereby accepting permissive hypercapnia (CO_2 between 45 and 60 mm Hg), have shown to improve outcomes.[129] The only RCT comparing conventional to high-frequency ventilation (the VICI trial*) showed no difference in the primary outcome of death or BPD.[130] Patients who were randomized to the high-frequency oscillation ventilation (HFOV) group required more vasoactive drug and iNO therapy, a longer duration of mechanical ventilation, and more conversion to extracorporeal membrane oxygenation support (ECMO). However, given the susceptibility of the hypoplastic lungs to overdistention, the initial aggressive lung volume recruitment strategy used with HFOV may have been inappropriate. The mean airway pressures were set at 13 to 17 cm H_2O in the HFOV arm, in contrast to the gentle approach with conventional ventilation that employed mean airway pressures of 7 to 10 cm H_2O (PEEP 2–5 and peak inspiratory pressure [PIP] 20–25 cm H_2O). Based on experience from a single center in Salt Lake City, UT, USA, revisions to the CDH management guidelines have been published. The Utah experience demonstrated a significant decrease in the need for ECMO use and improved survival for CDH patients.[131] Their guidelines included initiating HFOV of respiratory support and decreasing the initial mean airway pressure from 13 to 15 cm H_2O down to 10 to 12 cm H_2O.

Despite our best efforts to adopt lung-protective strategies, the overall number of infants requiring ECMO has not changed over the past decade and CDH remains the most common indication for ECMO.[132] Emerging evidence suggests that cardiac dysfunction may be at the root of impending irreversible cardiopulmonary failure, more than the severity of PPHN.[133] Reduced left ventricular (LV) function leads to an increase in left atrial pressure with resultant pulmonary venous congestion and a rise in pulmonary venous pressure. Decreasing pulmonary arterial pressure in the setting of poor LV function can lead to pulmonary edema and exacerbate respiratory status. In CDH, supporting cardiac function is as imperative as managing PPHN. The role of milrinone (a pulmonary vasodilator with cardiac inotropic and lusitropic effects) is currently being evaluated in a randomized trial in participating centers of the NICHD Neonatal Research Network.[134] A concomitant European multicenter randomized controlled trial is investigating intravenous sildenafil and iNO incorporating cardiac function assessment (CoDiNOS trial—Eudra) (personal communication).

Experimental data suggest that delayed cord clamping reduces pulmonary vascular resistance (PVR) and significantly increases pulmonary blood flow in the lamb model of CDH.[135] A strategy combining ventilation with lower FiO_2 with an intact cord might be an effective approach during the delivery room resuscitation of CDH. The effects of delayed cord clamping are being investigated in a pilot trial for infants born with CDH.

Pulmonary Hypertension of the Newborn

PH in the neonatal period can be broadly categorized into two groups: (1) PPHN, defined as the failure of the elevated PVR to fall following birth, and (2) BPD-PH, development of PH as a consequence of severe pulmonary vascular disease in premature infants with BPD.[136] Several underlying pulmonary disorders can delay or prevent relaxation of the pulmonary vascular bed (CDH, meconium aspiration syndrome, pneumonia, RDS, retained fetal lung fluid, and very rarely from alveolar capillary dysplasia or mutations in surfactant protein B), and in approximately 10% of cases, no identifiable cause can be found (idiopathic). The goals of therapy in PPHN rely on adequate lung recruitment, relaxation of the pulmonary vascular bed, and optimizing oxygenation by avoiding hyperoxia (to minimize free radical injury and oxidative stress) and hypoxemia (known to increase PVR).

Achieving and maintaining optimal lung volume are of utmost importance in the management of hypoxic respiratory failure and PPHN. Underinflation or overinflation can increase PVR because of the mechanical effects on the extra-alveolar and intra-alveolar pulmonary blood vessels. Atelectasis can lead to V/Q mismatch, and worsening hypoxemia and overinflation can impede venous return to the heart and result in decreased cardiac output. Oxygen is a potent vasodilator and remains the mainstay therapeutic intervention in the management of PPHN. Knowledge gaps on the optimal oxygenation target lead to wide variations in practices and to excessive oxygen usage. Accepting a lower oxyhemoglobin saturation (SO_2) of around 90% to 92%, as appropriate, provides a buffer to preventing hypoxic pulmonary vasoconstriction and avoiding increases in SO_2 beyond 97%. This strategy could help minimize adverse effects from oxidative stress and optimizes pulmonary vasodilation.[137] The increased pulmonary pressure places a strain on the heart and echocardiography becomes an indispensable modality that can help estimate pulmonary arterial pressure and assess cardiac function. Patients with severe PPHN commonly require vasoactive agents to support systemic perfusion, but clinical evidence is lacking on which inotrope may be most beneficial in PPHN.

Birth asphyxia and hypoxic-ischemic encephalopathy are commonly associated with PPHN. Therapeutic hypothermia significantly decreases mortality and neurocognitive impairments but there is a risk that it can exacerbate PPHN.[138,139] Cumulative time spent with $PaCO_2$ values under 35 mm Hg has been shown to be associated with worse neurologic impairment in newborns with hypoxic ischemic encephalopathy (HIE).[140] $PaCO_2$ is a potent cerebral vasodilator, and hypocapnia can significantly reduce cerebral blood flow. However, it is unclear if the hypocapnia, which may be a normal physiologic compensatory mechanism in infants recovering from a hypoxic–ischemic insult, is the cause of the poor outcome or simply a marker of the severity of the metabolic acidosis that reflects the degree of asphyxia.[141] The optimal PCO_2 concentration to

---

* The acronym VICI is deducted from the words: HFO versus conventional ventilation in infants with congenital diaphragmatic hernia: an international randomised clinical trial.

ensure good clinical outcomes in neonates receiving respiratory support is unknown. How these optimal concentrations are modified by pH is also unknown. These are important topics to be addressed in future basic and clinical research.

ANCILLARY SUPPORT

Nutritional Support

One of the vexing problems in the care of infants requiring ventilatory care is the difficulty in providing optimal nutritional support. Born preterm, these infants are at risk of a low reserve of their mineral stores (Fe, calcium and phosphorus, zinc, and other essential nutrients). On top of this limitation, BPD infants continue to suffer from growth failure because of inadequate intake, and increased resting metabolic rates and energy expenditure. These deficits precede the development of BPD and persist postdischarge.[92,142-147]

Among the major gaps include diagnosing and treating specific nutritional deficiencies, including those of micronutrients and minerals, determining what should be deemed "optimal" growth, and providing macronutrients to meet the needs. For instance, besides calcium and phosphorous, zinc is an important metabolically active trace element in the human body, and it has a critical role in growth, through its actions on growth hormone, insulin-like growth factor 1 (IGF-1), insulin-like growth factor binding protein 3 (IGFBP-3), and bone metabolism. Prematurity is a risk factor for zinc deficiency because 60% of zinc accretion occurs in the third trimester. Impaired intake and absorption or excess excretion can further increase this risk. Finally, periods of rapid growth, as seen in preterm infants, increase the need for zinc. Zinc deficiency is defined by a serum zinc concentration of less than 55 mcg/dL. However, it is also known that the overall requirement of zinc is related to the needs of the growing infants, regardless of overall zinc status. Thus, preterm infants may have a subclinical deficiency despite serum zinc concentration. Thus, biomarkers are needed to diagnose zinc deficiency, which needs to be treated in infants with poor growth despite receiving adequate protein and calories.

Although it is established that human milk is the best source of nutrition, milk from mothers giving birth to preterm infants may not be sufficient to meet the needs of preterm infants on mechanical ventilation. Our understanding of appropriate human milk supplements during the hospital stay, after discharge, and during follow-up needs to be studied.

DEVELOPMENT OF DEVICES

Devices and instruments are the backbones of neonatal intensive care, especially for cardiopulmonary support of sick infants and children. Those that are developed for use in sick infants should be based on sound bioengineering principles and tested for safety, efficacy, and accuracy of functioning in the specific vulnerable target populations rather than miniaturized versions of those developed for use in adults, because of the inherent physiological or pathophysiological differences between these populations.

Despite major advances in biotechnology, research and development (R&D) efforts directed at introducing new and innovative pediatric devices and instruments (or improving existing ones) for use in newborn infants and small children have been limited. This shortage is in part caused by the lack of bioengineering expertise among the clinical caregiving experts (not knowing the infrequent collaboration between the clinical and bioengineering scientific communities for R&D in basic and translational efforts) to develop or improve pediatric devices and instruments. Successful R&D in this area requires close and innovative collaboration and partnership between scientists from different specialties, especially from small business concerns and clinical fields, as has been underscored by scientists participating in two NICHD-sponsored workshops.[148,149]

In addition, research endeavors need to focus on adapting recent biotechnology advances for developing products that can be used in the care of vulnerable populations. For example, leveraging advances in miniaturized computers and microcomputer chips; communication and ultrafast, high-resolution imaging methods, nanotechnology, and microfluidic methods; characterizing volatile products from epidermal layers; and information technology (M-Health) could be incorporated into developing devices that are safe and effective in the care of vulnerable populations.

Concerning continued collaboration between the experts in academic clinical medicine and academic and emerging bioengineering research, nothing is more urgent than those needed for neonatal and pediatric respiratory care—especially the cardiac and pulmonary devices and instruments. These include minimally invasive or noninvasive devices and instruments to measure pulmonary functions (e.g., pulmonary arterial pressures, gas exchange, airway pressure, lung volume, ventilation/perfusion ratios, PCO_2 and PO_2); improved systems for respiratory support and reducing air-leak interfaces for nCPAP that do not affect musculoskeletal development; synchronized ventilation; improved methods of patient-triggered ventilation and pulmonary perfusion; automated inspired oxygen control; airway secretion clearance devices (including but not limited to applications for children with cystic fibrosis); improved aerosol delivery systems targeting small airways for use in newborn infants and small children on and off ventilatory support; improved oxygen cannula tubing for infants during transportation; and diaphragm pacers for use in rapidly growing infants and children. Further improvements in safe radiographic (magnetic resonance imaging [MRI]) methods are needed for assessing pulmonary and cardiac structure and functions.

Similarly, cardiovascular functional changes are intimately connected to changes in respiratory care. Thus, there is a need for devices to help monitor and assess cardiovascular functions and treat cardiovascular conditions. These include noninvasive or minimally invasive devices, instruments, or methods for measuring and monitoring systemic blood pressure, such as advanced mathematical computations for analyzing cardiac pulse wave forms, devices to measure and monitor cardiac output and global tissue oxygen delivery, methods to assess blood volume and global and organ-specific tissue perfusion and oxygenation, and methods to assess cardiac electrophysiology. Also, there is a need for devices for use in cardiac surgery, interventional catheterization, and electrophysiology technologies for neonates and small children—improvements in these fields will impact postcardiac surgery ventilatory care.

CURRENT RESEARCH

Ongoing Clinical Trials Around the World

We have extracted a list of ongoing clinical trials around the world from the ClinicalTrials.gov database developed, by the US government.[150] Table 45.3 lists 49 trials related to BPD and Table 45.4 lists 58 trials related to neonatal assisted ventilation. These were extracted in February 2021, and because of the constant nature of updating of the information, the number of active trials in the ClinicalTrials.gov registry contains all privately and publicly funded clinical studies from around the world, entered and registered by the investigators. The registration requirement is mandatory for researchers receiving US federal government funds for the said research. For all others, it is an optional requirement. The list is constantly updated. The lists provided in Tables 45.3 and 45.4 are up to date as of February 10, 2021—the date we searched the database. The registry guidelines require that the investigators update the information when substantial changes occur in the study status and post the trial findings within 30 days of the study completion. The readers are encouraged to visit the website for updates on specific trials. If they wish, they can contact the investigators using the information provided on the website for trial updates.

CONCLUDING COMMENTS

Remarkable advances over the past seven decades in neonatal intensive care, in general, and ventilator support, in particular, are the reasons for the unimaginable improvements in neonatal mortality and morbidity in most countries of the world. Yet, much needs to be achieved. Besides the knowledge gaps noted previously, we need to understand the impact of care on the overall health of the population in general. Because more than 95% of preterm infants survive, and nearly 10% of all births are preterm, a large number of adults born at preterm gestations could be at higher risk for morbidities, even if the frequency of adverse outcomes are minimally higher among them compared to their term counterparts. Many countries have developed nationwide health registries, which are immensely valuable resources to track and understand the impact of neonatal care on long-term health of the population within communities.[151,152] If such registries could be developed in all countries, one can continually assess the global public health impact of neonatal interventions.

TABLE 45.3	Ongoing Clinical Trials Registered in ClinicalTrials.gov

Bronchopulmonary Dysplasia

Number	NCT Number	Title	Interventions	Enrollment #	Country
1	NCT04062136	Umbilical Cord Mesenchymal Stem Cells Transplantation in the Treatment of Bronchopulmonary Dysplasia	Combination product: stem cell transplantation	10	Vietnam
2	NCT03873506	Follow-up Study of Mesenchymal Stem Cells for Bronchopulmonary Dysplasia	Drug: transplantation of hUC-MSCs	30	China
3	NCT03558334	Human Mesenchymal Stem Cells for Bronchopulmonary Dysplasia	Drug: Transplantation of mesenchymal stem cell; Drug: No transplantation of mesenchymal stem cell	12	China
4	NCT03645525	Intratracheal Umbilical Cord–Derived Mesenchymal Stem Cell for the Treatment of Bronchopulmonary Dysplasia (BPD)	Drug: human umbilical cord–derived mesenchymal stem cell; Drug: placebo	180	China
5	NCT03378063	Stem Cells for Bronchopulmonary Dysplasia	Drug: transplantation of mesenchymal stem cell; Drug: no transplantation of mesenchymal stem cell	100	China
6	NCT03540680	p16Ink4a in Bronchopulmonary Dysplasia in Children	No intervention—collection of blood only	120	France
7	NCT03631420	Mesenchymal Stem Cells for the Treatment of Bronchopulmonary Dysplasia in Infants	Biological: human umbilical cord–derived mesenchymal stem cells	9	Taiwan
8	NCT03538977	Hydrotherapy in Premature Infants with Bronchopulmonary Dysplasia	Procedure: hydrotherapy; Procedure: conventional physiotherapy	24	Brazil
9	NCT04209088	Interest of Pulmonary Ultrasound to Predict Evolution Towards Bronchopulmonary Dysplasia in Premature Infants at Gestational Age Less Than or Equal to 34 Weeks of Gestation	Other: pulmonary ultrasounds	218	France

TABLE 45.3 Ongoing Clinical Trials Registered in ClinicalTrials.gov—cont'd

Bronchopulmonary Dysplasia

Number	NCT Number	Title	Interventions	Enrollment #	Country
10	NCT02443961	Mesenchymal Stem Cell Therapy for Bronchopulmonary Dysplasia in Preterm Babies	Biological: MSC therapy	10	Spain
11	NCT03774537	Human Mesenchymal Stem Cells For Infants at High Risk for Bronchopulmonary Dysplasia	Drug: transplantation of hUC-MSCs Drug: no transplantation of hUC-MSCs	20	China
12	NCT02921308	Pulmonary MRI of Ex-preterm Children with and Without BPD to Understand Risk of Emphysematous Changes		40	Canada
13	NCT03857841	A Safety Study of IV Stem Cell–Derived Extracellular Vesicles (UNEX-42) in Preterm Neonates at High Risk for BPD	Biological: UNEX-42 Biological: phosphate-buffered saline	18	United States
14	NCT03142568	Safety of Sildenafil in Premature Infants	Drug: sildenafil Other: placebo	120	United States
15	NCT02723513	Bronchopulmonary Dysplasia: From Neonatal Chronic Lung Disease to Early Onset Adult COPD	Other: hyperpolarized xenon-129	50	Canada
16	NCT03576885	Inhaled Nitric Oxide for Pulmonary Hypertension and Bronchopulmonary Dysplasia	Drug: inhaled nitric oxide Drug: placebo	138	United States
17	NCT03392467	PNEUMOSTEM for the Prevention and Treatment of Severe BPD in Premature Infants	Biological: PNEUMOSTEM Other: placebo	60	South Korea
18	NCT03532555	Enteral Zinc to Improve Growth in Infants at Risk for Bronchopulmonary Dysplasia	Dietary supplement: zinc acetate Other: no supplemental zinc	126	United States
19	NCT03475264	MRI of Lung Structure and Function in Preterm Children	Diagnostic Test: Lung MRI	21	Canada
20	NCT04003857	Follow up Study of Safety and Efficacy in Subjects Who Completed PNEUMOSTEM® Phase II (MP-CR-012) Clinical Trial	Biological: PNEUMOSTEM® Biological: normal saline	60	South Korea
21	NCT03542812	L-citrulline and Pulmonary Hypertension Associated with Bronchopulmonary Dysplasia	Drug: L-citrulline	36	United States
22	NCT03521063	Efficacy of Adding Budesonide to Poractant Alfa to Prevent Bronchopulmonary Dysplasia	Drug: budesonide Drug: poractant alfa Drug: saline	108	Mexico
23	NCT01897987	Follow-up Safety and Efficacy Evaluation on Subjects Who Completed PNEUMOSTEM® Phase-II Clinical Trial	Biological: PNEUMOSTEM® Biological: normal saline	70	South Korea
24	NCT03657693	MRI in BPD Subjects	Diagnostic test: NICU MRI Diagnostic test: polysomnography	160	United States
25	NCT01780155	Genes Associated with Bronchopulmonary Dysplasia and Retinopathy of Prematurity		3600	Argentina
26	NCT03613987	Randomized Control Trial: Synchronized Noninvasive Positive Pressure Ventilation Versus Non Synchronized Non Invasive Positive Pressure Ventilation in Extremely Low Birth Weight Infants	Device: NAVA technology to synchronize NIPPV	60	United States
27	NCT03946891	Nebulized Furosemide in Premature Infants with Bronchopulmonary Dysplasia—A Cross Over Pilot Study of Its Efficacy and Safety	Drug: inhaled furosemide Drug: intravenous furosemide	30	United States
28	NCT03961139	Continuous Versus Intermittent Bolus Feeding in Very Preterm Infants—Effect on Respiratory Morbidity	Other: method of feeding; continuous feeding OR bolus feeding	150	Singapore
29	NCT02729844	Neolifes Heart—Pulmonary Hypertension in Preterm Children		165	The Netherlands
30	NCT03808402	The Effect of Surfactant Dose on Outcomes in Preterm Infants with RDS		2600	United Kingdom
31	NCT03701074	Randomized Controlled Trial to Evaluate the Safety and Efficacy of Acetaminophen in Preterm Infants Used in Combination with Ibuprofen for Closure of the Ductus Arteriosus	Drug: ibuprofen and acetaminophen Drug: ibuprofen and placebo	80	United States

Continued

TABLE 45.3   Ongoing Clinical Trials Registered in ClinicalTrials.gov—cont'd

Bronchopulmonary Dysplasia

Number	NCT Number	Title	Interventions	Enrollment #	Country
32	NCT03086473	Early Caffeine in Preterm Neonates	Drug: caffeine citrate Drug: placebo (normal saline)	88	United States
33	NCT03938532	Feasibility and Impact of Volume Targeted Ventilation in the Delivery Room	Device: volume targeted ventilation (VTV) using the Philips Respironics NM3 monitor Device: tidal volume measurement using the Philips Respironics NM3 monitor	40	United States
34	NCT03782610	Early Prediction of Spontaneous Patent Ductus Arteriosus (PDA) Closure and PDA-Associated Outcomes		675	United States
35	NCT03717584	A Cohort Study of the Intestinal Microbiota of Premature Infants		300	United States
36	NCT03372525	Invasive Ventilation Strategies for Neonates with Acute Respiratory Distress Syndrome (ARDS)	Device: HFOV Device: CMV	400	China
37	NCT03649932	Enteral L Citrulline Supplementation in Preterm Infants—Safety, Efficacy and Dosing	Dietary supplement: enteral L-citrulline	42	United States
38	NCT03253263	A Clinical Efficacy and Safety Study of SHP607 in Preventing Chronic Lung Disease in Extremely Premature Infants	Drug: SHP607	600	United States
39	NCT03231735	Mid and Standard Frequency Ventilation in Infants With Respiratory Distress Syndrome	Device: midfrequency ventilation Device: Standard frequency ventilation	130	United States
40	NCT03797183	Genesis Electrical Impedance Tomography (EIT): A Preliminary Study		48	United States
41	NCT04068558	sNIPPV Versus NIV-NAVA in Extremely Premature Infants	Device: NIV-NAVA/sNIPPV Device: sNIPPV/NIV-NAVA	14	France
42	NCT03388437	Noninvasive Neurally Adjusted Ventilatory Assist Versus Nasal Intermittent Positive Pressure Ventilation for Preterm Infants After Extubation	Device: NI-NAVA Device: NIPPV	36	Saudi Arabia
43	NCT03775785	Targeted vs Standard Fortification of Breast Milk	Dietary supplement: tailored enteral nutrition	200	Poland
44	NCT03346343	Pulmonary Function Using Noninvasive Forced Oscillometry	Device: noninvasive forced airway oscillometry	1098	United States
45	NCT03876704	Effects of Fat-Soluble Vitamins Supplementation on Common Complications and Neural Development in Very Low Birth Weight Infants	Drug: high dose of fat-soluble vitamin Drug: conventional dose of fat-soluble vitamin	120	China
46	NCT03785899	Automatic Oxygen Control (SPOC) in Preterm Infants	Device: SPOCnew Device: 8s SpO2 averaging Device: SPOCold Device: 2s SpO2 averaging	24	Germany

The data are up to date as of May 1, 2020. The investigators who registered these trials are required to update them whenever significant changes occur in the study design and post the results and a simplified synopsis for the use by the general public of the results of the trial within 30 days of the assessment of the primary outcome data from the trial.

BPD, Bronchopulmonary dysplasia; CMV, conventional mechanical ventilation; COPD, chronic obstructive pulmonary disease; HOFV, high-frequency oscillation ventilation; hUC-MSC, human umbilical cord mesenchymal stem cell; MSC, mesenchymal stem cell; MRI, magnetic resonance imaging; NAV, neurally adjusted ventilation; NI-NAVA, noninvasive neurally adjusted ventilation assist; NIPPV, nasal intermittent positive pressure ventilation; NICU, neonatal intensive care unit; NIV-NAVA, noninvasive neurally adjusted ventilation assist; RDS, respiratory distress syndrome; sNIPPV, synchronized nasal intermittent positive pressure ventilation

The list provides ongoing clinical trials obtained from ClinicalTrials.gov[148]

TABLE 45.4 Ongoing Clinical Trials Registered in ClinicalTrials.gov Neonatal Assisted Ventilation

Number	NCT Number	Title	Conditions	Interventions	Country
1	NCT03591796	Invasive Ventilation for Neonates with Acute Respiratory Distress Syndrome (ARDS)	ARDS|conventional mechanical ventilation|HFOV	Device: HFOV Device: CMV	China
2	NCT03736707	Selective High Frequency Oscillatory Ventilation (HFOV) for Neonates	RDS|ARDS|HFOV	Device: selective HFOV Device: CMV	China
3	NCT03372525	Invasive Ventilation Strategies for Neonates With Acute Respiratory Distress Syndrome (ARDS)	ARDS|BPD|HFOV	Device: HFOV Device: CMV	China
4	NCT03422549	Diaphragmatic Electrical Activity in Preterm Infants on NonInvasive Ventilation	RDS, newborn|chronic lung disease of newborn (diagnosis)	Device: Drager VN500 Ventilator	Canada
5	NCT03938532	Feasibility and Impact of Volume Targeted Ventilation in the Delivery Room	Prematurity|BPD|RDS, newborn	Device: volume targeted ventilation (VTV) using the Philips Respironics NM3 monitor Device: tidal volume measurement using the Philips Respironics NM3 monitor	United States
6	NCT02849054	CDH—Optimisation of Neonatal Ventilation	Congenital diaphragmatic hernia	Device: Measurement of PTPdi Device: TTV at 4 mL/kg Device: TTV at 5 mL/kg Device: TTV at 6 mL/kg	United Kingdom
7	NCT04000568	Breathing Variability and NAVA in Neonates	Neonatal RDS|prematurity	Other: respiratory support: NAVA-NIV and PC-NIV	Italy
8	NCT03132428	Registry Evaluating Premature and Term-Near-Term Neonates with Pulmonary Hypertension Receiving Inhaled Nitric Oxide	Pulmonary hypertension of newborn	Drug: nitric oxide gas, for inhalation: observational study	United States
9	NCT02267018	Diaphragm Electrical Activity of Preterm Infants on nCPAP Versus NIHFV	RDS, newborn	Device: Drager VN500 ventilator	United States
10	NCT03181958	A Trial Comparing Noninvasive Ventilation Strategies in Preterm Infants Following Extubation	Intubated infants were intended to extubation using noninvasive ventilation strategies	Device: NHFOV Device: nCPAP Device: NIPPV	China
11	NCT04287907	Use of CO_2 Detectors to Help Provide Effective Breaths During Resuscitation of Preterm Newborns	Preterm birth	Device: monitor group	
12	NCT03226977	Nasal Intermittent Positive Pressure Ventilation (NIPPV) vs Continuous Positive Airway Pressure for Respiratory Distress Syndrome	NIPPV|nCPAP	Device: NIPPV Device: nCPAP	China
12	NCT03388437	Noninvasive Neurally Adjusted Ventilatory Assist Versus Nasal Intermittent Positive Pressure Ventilation for Preterm Infants After Extubation	Prematurity|respiratory failure|ventilator lung; newborn	Device: NI-NAVA Device: NIPPV	Saudi Arabia
14	NCT02858583	SI + CC Versus 3:1 C:V Ratio During Neonatal CPR	Heart arrest|birth asphyxia|bradycardia	Procedure: CC + SI Procedure: 3:1 C:V	
15	NCT04068558	sNIPPV Versus NIV-NAVA in Extremely Premature Infants	Premature birth|ventilator lung; newborn	Device: NIV-NAVA/sNIPPVDevice: sNIPPV/NIV-NAVA	France
16	NCT04326270	Crossover Comparison of Tidal Volume Delivery During Nasal Intermittent Positive Pressure Ventilation in Preterm Infants: Infant Cannula vs. Nasal Continuous Positive Airway Pressure Prongs	RDS in premature infant	Device: nasal interface	United States

Continued

TABLE 45.4 Ongoing Clinical Trials Registered in ClinicalTrials.gov Neonatal Assisted Ventilation—cont'd

Number	NCT Number	Title	Conditions	Interventions	Country
17	NCT03206489	Nasal High Frequency Oscillation for Respiratory Distress Syndrome in Twins Infants	Nasal HFOV	Device: NHFOV Device: nCPAP	China
18	NCT04244890	Feasibility of Uninterrupted Infant Respiratory Support Treatment	RDS, newborn|infant, newborn|respiratory insufficiency syndrome of newborn	Device: Uninterrupted CPAP for the first hours of life	Sweden
19	NCT04070560	Effects of Delayed Cord Clamping During Resuscitation of Newborn Near Term and Term Infants	Asphyxia neonatorum|resuscitation	Procedure: intact cord (≥ 180 seconds) resuscitation Procedure: early (≤ 60 seconds) cord clamping	Sweden
20	NCT04282369	Evaluation of the Efficacy of Four Different Noninvasive Ventilation Modes Performed in the Delivery Room	Respiratory disease|respiratory insufficiency	Device: HHHFNC Device: nCPAP Device: NIPPV Device: NHFO	Turkey
21	NCT03984175	Clinical Decision Support for Mechanical Ventilation of Patients with ARDS	ARDS	Procedure: implementation of processes	United States
22	NCT04221737	Early Use of Airway Pressure Release Ventilation (APRV) in ARDS	ARDS	Device: APRV. General Electric Healthcare Engstrom ventilator system Device: conventional. General Electric Healthcare Engstrom ventilator system	Mexico
23	NCT03764319	Low Frequency, Ultra-low Tidal Volume Ventilation in Patients with ARDS and VV-ECMO	ARDS |acute lung injury|extracorporeal membrane oxygenation|RDS|respiratory tract diseases|lung diseases|lung injury, acute	Other: ultraprotective ventilator settings Other: standard ventilator settings	Austria
24	NCT03558737	Nasal High-Frequency Jet Ventilation (nHFJV) Following Extubation in Preterm Infants	Infant, premature|respiratory failure|respiratory insufficiency|RDS in premature infant	Other: nHFJV Other: NIPPV	United States
25	NCT01770925	n-CPAP Versus n-BiPAP and NIPPV for Postextubation in RDS in Preterms	RDS	Device: nCPAP Device: n-BiPAP Device: NIPPV	Egypt
26	NCT03670732	CPAP vs. Unsynchronized NIPPV at Equal Mean Airway Pressure	Prematurity|RDS|apnea of prematurity	Other: continuous positive airway pressure Other: nasal intermittent positive pressure ventilation	United States
27	NCT03231735	Mid and Standard Frequency Ventilation in Infants with Respiratory Distress Syndrome	Ventilator-induced lung injury|RDS|BPD|Preterm Infant	Device: midfrequency ventilation Device: standard frequency ventilation	United States
28	NCT03424798	Measuring Heart and Lung Function in Critical Care	RDS, adult|critical illness|mechanical ventilation complication|hemodynamic instability|gas exchange impairment	Device: Inspiwave	United Kingdom
29	NCT02842190	NIPPV Versus Bi-level Nasal Continuous Positive Airway Pressure Following Extubation	Intubation complication|preterm birth	Device: NIPPV	Turkey

TABLE 45.4 Ongoing Clinical Trials Registered in ClinicalTrials.gov Neonatal Assisted Ventilation—cont'd

Number	NCT Number	Title	Conditions	Interventions	Country
30	NCT03709199	Long Term Follow up of Children Enrolled in the REDvent Study	RDS, adult|ventilator-induced lung injury|neurocognitive dysfunction|equality of life|respiration disorders	Diagnostic test: ventilation inhomogeneity Diagnostic test: diaphragm ultrasound Diagnostic test: respiratory inductance plethysmography Diagnostic test: spirometry Diagnostic test: functional residual capacity Diagnostic test: MIP/MEP Diagnostic test: 6-minute walk test Diagnostic test: Neurocognitive testing Diagnostic test: emotional health assessment Diagnostic Test: health-related quality of life Diagnostic Test: functional status Diagnostic Test: Respiratory Status Questionnaire	United States
31	NCT03613987	Randomized Control Trial: Synchronized Noninvasive Positive Pressure Ventilation Versus Non Synchronized Non Invasive Positive Pressure Ventilation in Extremely Low Birth Weight Infants	BPD	Device: NAVA technology to synchronize NIPPV	United States
32	NCT03086473	Early Caffeine in Preterm Neonates	BPD|apnea of prematurity|hemodynamic instability|intubation	Drug: caffeine citrate Drug: placebo (normal saline)	United States
33	NCT03650478	Assessment of NeuroBOX and NeuroPAP in Infants	Pediatric respiratory diseases|bronchiolitis |infant RDS	Device: NeuroPAP ventilation (2 hours) and NeuroBox monitoring (23 hours) Device: NeuroPAP ventilation (4 hours) and NeuroBox monitoring (25 hours)	Canada
34	NCT03808402	The Effect of Surfactant Dose on Outcomes in Preterm Infants with RDS	RDS|BPD		United Kingdom

The data are up to date as of May 1, 2020. The investigators who registered these trials are required to update them whenever significant changes occur in the study design and post the results and a simplified synopsis for the use by the general public of the results of the trial within 30 days of the assessment of the primary outcome data from the trial.

BiPAP, Bilevel positive airway pressure; *BPD,* bronchopulmonary dysplasia; *CC + SI,* chest compression + sustained inflation; *CPAP,* continuous positive airway pressure; *CMV,* conventional mechanical ventilation; *HFOV,* high-frequency oscillation ventilation; *HHHFNC,* heated humidified high flow nasal cannula; *MEP,* maximum expiratory pressure; *MIP,* maximum inspiratory pressure; *NAVA,* neutrally adjusted ventilation assist; *NAVA-NIV,* NAVA noninvasive ventilation; *NHFO,* nasal high frequency oscillation; *nCPAP,* nasal continuous positive airway pressure; *NHFOV,* noninvasive high-frequency oscillation ventilation; *NIHFV,* noninvasive high-frequency ventilation; *NIV-NAVA,* noninvasive neurally adjusted ventilation assist; *PC-NIV,* pressure control noninvasive ventilation; *PTPdi,* diaphragmatic pressure-time product; *RDS,* respiratory distress syndrome; *sNIPPV,* synchronized nasal intermittent positive pressure ventilation; *TTV,* targeted tidal volume; *VV-ECMO,* venovenous extracorporeal membrane oxygenation.

The list provides ongoing clinical trials obtained from ClinicalTrials.gov[148]

SELECTED READINGS

2. Manley BJ, Doyle LW, Davies MW, et al: Fifty years in neonatology. J Paediatr Child Health 51(1):118–121, 2015.

4. Lehigh Center for Clinical Research: The history of clinical trials. Cited 2021 February 10. Available from: www.lehighcenter.com/history/the-history-of-clinical-trials/.

6. O'Donnell CP, Gibson AT, Davis PG: Pinching, electrocution, ravens' beaks, and positive pressure ventilation: a brief history of neonatal resuscitation. Arch Dis Child Fetal Neonatal Ed 91(5):F369–F3673, 2006.

33. Relevo R, Balshem H: AHRQ Methods for Effective Health Care Finding Evidence for Comparing Medical Interventions, in Methods Guide for Effectiveness and Comparative Effectiveness

Reviews. Rockville, MD, Agency for Healthcare Research and Quality (US), 2008.

87. Abman SH, Bancalari E, Jobe A: The evolution of bronchopulmonary dysplasia after 50 years. Am J Respir Crit Care Med 195(4):421–424, 2017.

92. Abman SH, Collaco JM, Shepherd EG, et al: Interdisciplinary care of children with severe bronchopulmonary dysplasia. J Pediatr 181:12–28.e1, 2017.

99. Lal CV, Bhandari V, Ambalavanan N: Genomics, microbiomics, proteomics, and metabolomics in bronchopulmonary dysplasia. Semin Perinatol 42(7):425–431, 2018.

119. Ee MT, Thébaud B: The therapeutic potential of stem cells for bronchopulmonary dysplasia: "it's about time" or "not so fast"? Curr Pediatr Rev 14(4):227–238, 2018.

149. Raju TN: Developing safe and effective devices for neonatal intensive care. Pediatr Res 67(5):520, 2010.

151. Raju TNK, Buist AS, Blaisdell CJ, et al: Adults born preterm: a review of general health and system-specific outcomes. Acta Paediatr 106(9):1409–1437, 2017.

Appendices

Jay P. Goldsmith

APPENDIX 1

Lung Volumes in the Infant

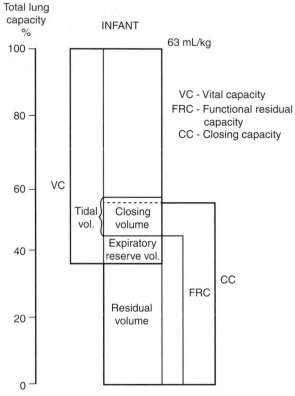

(Data from Smith CA, Nelson NM: The Physiology of the Newborn Infant. 4th ed. Springfield, IL, Charles C Thomas Publisher, 1976.)

APPENDIX 2

Changes in Respiratory System Dimensions With Growth[a]

	Newborn to 1 Month	Infant
Chest Diameter (cm)		
Transverse	10	14
Anteroposterior	7.5	9
Trachea, length (mm)	40/57	42/67
Diameter (mm)	4	5
CSA (mm^2)	26	34
Main Stem Bronchi		
Diameter (mm)	4	4
CSA, right/left (mm^2)	—	20/13
Bronchioles, diameter (mm)	0.3	0.4
CSA (mm^2)	0.07	0.12
Terminal Bronchioles		
Diameter (mm)	0.2	0.3
Internal diameter (mm)	0.1	0.12
CSA	0.03	0.07
Alveoli, diameter (mm)	0.05	0.06–0.07
Surface area (m^2)	2.8	6.5
Body length (cm)	50	–
Weight (kg)	3.4	–
Surface area (m^2)	0.21	0.3
Lung weight (g)	50	70
Dead space (mL)	7–8	–

[a]Values are from Engel (autopsy data) and Fearon and Whalen (living subjects; autopsy/living).
CSA, Cross-sectional area.
(Data from Scarpelli EM [ed]: Pulmonary Physiology of the Fetus, Newborn, and Child. Philadelphia, Lea & Febiger, 1975.)

APPENDIX 3

Effect of Age on Lung Size[a]

Age	No. of Cases Studied	Alveoli (10^6)	Respiratory Airways (10^6)	Air–Tissue Interface (m^2)	Body Surface Area (m^2)	Generations of Respiratory Airways
Birth	1	24	1.5	2.8	0.21	–
3 months	3	77	2.5	7.2	0.29	21
7 months	1	112	3.7	8.4	0.38	–
13 months	1	129	4.5	12.2	0.45	22
22 months	1	160	7.1	14.2	0.50	–
4 years	1	257	7.9	22.2	0.67	–
8 years	1	280	14.0	32.0	0.92	23
Adult		296	14.0	75.0	1.90	23
Approximate fold increase, birth to adult	–	10	10	21	9	–

[a]Values are from Dunnill MS.
(Data from Thibeault DW, Gregory GA [eds]: Neonatal Pulmonary Care. Menlo Park, CA, Addison-Wesley Publishing Co., 1979, pp. 217-236; and Scarpelli EM [ed]: Pulmonary Physiology of the Fetus, Newborn, and Child. Philadelphia, Lea & Febiger, 1975.)

APPENDIX 4

Normal Lung Function Data for Term Newborns During the Neonatal Period

Measurement	No. of Infants Studied	Mean	Standard Deviation	Range
Tidal volume (mL/kg)	266	4.8	1.0	2.9–7.9
Respiratory rate (bpm)	266	50.9	13.1	25–104
Minute volume (mL/kg/min)	266	232	61.4	
Dynamic compliance (mL/cm H_2O/kg)	266	1.72	0.5	0.9–3.7
Total pulmonary resistance (cm H_2O)/L/s)	266	42.5	1.6	3.1–171
Work of breathing (G·cm)	266	11.0	7.4	1.1–52.6
Expiratory time (s)	291	0.57	0.17	0.27–1.28
Inspiratory time (s)	291	0.51	0.10	0.28–0.87
Time to maximum expiratory flow/total expiratory time (s)	291	0.51	0.12	0.18–0.83
Static compliance (mL/cm H_2O/kg)	289	1.25	0.41	0.43–2.07
Respiratory system resistance (cm H_2O/L/s)	299	63.4	16.6	34.9–153.3
Time constant of respiratory system (s)	299	0.24	0.10	0.08–1.1
FRCpleth (mL/kg)	271	29.8	6.2	14.5–45.6

FRCpleth, Functional residual capacity by body plethysmography.
(Data from Greenough A, Milner AD [eds]: Neonatal Respiratory Diseases. 2nd ed. London, Arnold, 2003.)

APPENDIX 5

Allen's Test

Gently squeeze the hand to partially empty it of blood. Apply pressure to both the ulnar and the radial arteries. Then remove pressure from the hand and the ulnar artery. If the entire hand flushes and fills with blood, the ulnar artery can supply the hand with blood and the radial artery can be safely punctured or cannulated.

APPENDIX 6

Procedure for Obtaining Capillary Blood Gases

Equipment needed:
- 75-µL capillary tube (heparinized)
- Lancet device (3 mm)
- Alcohol sponge
- Metal stirrer and magnet
- Sealing wax

Procedure for obtaining capillary blood gases:
- Wash hands.
- Warm the infant's foot for 3 minutes with a commercially available warming pad; if not available, use water at body temperature or slightly warmer. Use a thermometer. Water temperature should not exceed 39° C (101°-104° F).
- Cleanse the heel with an alcohol sponge.
- Puncture with a lancet device.
- Wipe away the first drop of blood.
- Collect blood in a sample tube by holding the tube below the level of puncture and allowing blood to flow freely into the tube. Avoid squeezing the heel to fill the tube because this introduces serum and venous blood and renders the sample inaccurate. Avoid introducing air into the tube.
- Hold an alcohol sponge against the puncture site to stop the flow.
- Place a metal stirrer in the tube.
- Slide the magnet along the tube to move the stirrer and mix the blood.
- Seal the ends of the tube.
- Send to the laboratory for analysis.

APPENDIX 7

Normal Umbilical Cord Blood Gas Values

	Venous Blood Normal Range (Mean ± 2 SD)	Arterial Blood Normal Range (Mean ± 2 SD)
pH	7.25–7.45	7.18–7.38
P_{CO_2} (mm Hg)	26.8–49.2	32.2–65.8
(kPa)[a]	3.57–6.56	4.29–8.77
P_{O_2} (mm Hg)	17.2–40.8	5.6–30.8
(kPa)[a]	2.29–5.44	0.75–4.11
HCO_3^- (mmol/L)	15.8–24.2	17–27
BD[b] (mmol/L)	0–8	0–8

[a]1 kPa = 7.50 mm Hg; 1 mm Hg = 1.33 kPa.
[b]Estimated from data.
BD, Base deficit.
(Data from Yeomans ER, Hauth JC, Gilstrap LC, et al: Umbilical cord pH, P_{CO_2}, and bicarbonate following uncomplicated term vaginal deliveries. Am J Obstet Gynecol 151:798-800, 1985.)

APPENDIX 7A

Arterial Blood Gas Values in Normal Full-Term Infants[a]

		Umbilical Vein (Cord)	Umbilical Artery (Cord)	5–10 minutes	20 minutes	30 minutes	60 minutes	5 hours	24 hours	2 days	3 days	4 days	5 days	6 days	7 days
pH	$\bar{X}$	7.320	7.242	7.207	7.263	7.297	7.332	7.339	7.369	7.365	7.364	7.370	7.371	7.369	7.371
	SD	0.055	0.059	0.051	0.040	0.044	0.031	0.028	0.032	0.028	0.027	0.027	0.031	0.023	0.026
Pco_2 (mm Hg)	$\bar{X}$	37.8	49.1	46.1	40.1	37.7	36.1	35.2	33.4	33.1	33.1	34.3	34.8	34.8	35.9
	SD	5.6	5.8	7.0	6.0	5.7	4.2	3.6	3.1	3.3	3.4	3.8	3.5	3.6	3.1
Po_2 (mm Hg)	$\bar{X}$	27.4	15.9	49.6	50.7	54.1	63.3	73.7	72.7	73.8	75.6	73.3	72.1	69.8	73.1
	SD	5.7	3.8	9.9	11.3	11.5	11.3	12.0	9.5	7.7	11.5	9.3	10.5	9.5	9.7
Standard bicarbonate (mEq/L)	$\bar{X}$	20.0	18.7	16.7	17.5	18.2	19.2	19.4	20.2	19.8	19.7	20.4	20.6	20.6	21.8
	SD	1.4	1.8	1.6	1.3	1.5	1.2	1.2	1.3	1.4	1.4	1.7	1.7	1.9	1.3

$\bar{X}$ is the sample mean.

[a]Values are from Kcch and Wendel. Blood was obtained through the umbilical artery line. Po and Pco were measured with Clark and Severinghaus electrodes. (Data from Bancalari E: Pulmonary function testing and other diagnostic laboratory procedures. J Peds 110[3]:448–456, 1987; and Thibeault DW, Gregory GA (eds): Neonatal Pulmonary Care. Reading, MA, Addison-Wesley Publishing Co., 1979, p. 123, Table 7-4.)

APPENDIX 7B

Arterial Blood Gas Values in Normal Premature Infants[a]

		3–5 hours	6–12 hours	13–24 hours	25–48 hours	3–4 days	5–10 days	11–40 days
pH	$\bar{X}$	7.329	7.425	7.464	7.434	7.425	7.378	7.425
	SD	0.038	0.072	0.064	0.054	0.044	0.043	0.033
Pco_2 (mm Hg)	$\bar{X}$	47.3	28.2	27.2	31.3	31.7	36.4	32.9
	SD	8.5	6.9	8.4	6.7	6.7	4.2	4.0
Po_2 (mm Hg)	$\bar{X}$	59.5	69.7	67.0	72.5	77.8	80.3	77.8
	SD	7.7	11.8	15.2	20.9	16.4	12.0	9.6
Base excess (mEq/L)	$\bar{X}$	−3.7	−4.7	−3.0	−2.3	−2.9	−3.5	−2.1
	SD	1.5	3.1	3.3	3.0	2.3	2.3	2.2

$\bar{X}$ is the sample mean.

[a]Values from Orzalesi et al. Mean birthweight, 1.76 kg; gestational age, 34.5 weeks. Blood obtained from radial, temporal, or umbilical artery. Po$_2$ was measured with a Clark electrode, and Pco$_2$ was calculated with using the Siggaard-Andersen nomogram. (Data from Bancalari E. Pulmonary function testing and other diagnostic laboratory procedures. In: Thibeault DW, Gregory GA (eds): Neonatal Pulmonary Care. Reading, MA, Addison-Wesley Publishing Co., 1979, p. 123, Table 7-5.)

APPENDIX 8

Capillary Blood Gas Reference Values in Healthy Term Neonates

Variable	n	Mean ± SD	2.5 Percentile	97.5 Percentile
pH	119	7.395 ± 0.037	7.312	7.473
Pco₂ (mm Hg)	119	38.7 ± 5.1	28.5	48.7
Po₂ (mm Hg)	119	45.3 ± 7.5	32.8	61.2
Lactate (mmol/L)	114	2.6 ± 0.7	1.4	4.1
Hemoglobin (g/dL)	122	20.4 ± 11.6	14.5	23.9
Glucose (mg/dL)	122	69 ± 14	3.8	96
iCa (mmol/L)	118	1.21 ± 0.07	1.06	1.34

Samples were collected at 48 ± 12 hours of life.
iCa, Ionized calcium.
(Data from Cousineau J, Anctil S, Carceller A, et al. Neonate capillary blood gas reference values. Clin Biochem 38:906, 2005.)

APPENDIX 9

Blood Gas Values in Cord Blood and in Arterial Blood at Various Ages During the Neonatal Period

A. Oxygen Tension

		UV	UA	5–10 minutes	20 minutes	30 minutes	60 minutes	5 hours	24 hours	2 days	3 days	4 days	5 days	6 days	7 days
Po₂ (mm Hg)	X̄	15.9	27.4	49.6	50.7	54.1	63.3	73.7	72.7	73.8	75.6	73.3	72.1	69.8	73.1
	SD	3.8	5.7	9.9	11.3	11.5	11.3	12.0	9.5	7.7	11.5	9.3	10.9	9.5	9.7
	Range	7	15	33	31	31	38	55	54	62	56	60	56	55	57
		23	40	75	85	85	83	106	95	91	102	93	102	96	94

X̄ is the sample mean.
UA, Umbilical artery; *UV,* umbilical vein.
(Data from Koch G, Wendel H: Adjustment of arterial blood gases and acid-base balance in the normal newborn infant during the first week of life. Biol Neonat 12:136-161, 1968.)

B. Carbon Dioxide Tension

		UV	UA	5–10 minutes	20 minutes	30 minutes	60 minutes	5 hours	24 hours	2 days	3 days	4 days	5 days	6 days	7 days
Pco₂ (mm Hg)	X̄	49.1	37.8	46.1	40.1	37.7	36.1	35.2	33.4	33.1	33.1	34.3	34.8	34.8	35.9
	SD	5.8	5.6	7.0	6.0	5.7	4.2	3.6	3.1	3.3	3.4	3.8	3.5	3.6	3.1
	Range	35	26	35	31	28	28	29	27	26	26	27	28	28	30
		60	52	65	58	54	45	45	40	43	40	43	41	42	42

X̄ is the sample mean.
UA, Umbilical artery; *UV,* umbilical vein.
(Data from Koch G, Wendel H: Adjustment of arterial blood gases and acid-base balance in the normal newborn infant during the first week of life. Biol Neonat 12:136-161, 1968.)

C. pH

		UV	UA	5–10 minutes	20 minutes	30 minutes	60 minutes	5 hours	24 hours	2 days	3 days	4 days	5 days	6 days	7 days
pH	X̄	7.320	7.242	7.207	7.263	7.297	7.332	7.339	7.369	7.365	7.364	7.370	7.371	7.369	7.37
	SD	0.055	0.059	0.051	0.040	0.044	0.031	0.028	0.032	0.028	0.027	0.027	0.031	0.032	0.02
	Range	7.178	7.111	7.091	7.180	7.206	7.261	7.256	7.290	7.314	7.304	7.320	7.296	7.321	7.32
		7.414	7.375	7.302	7.330	7.380	7.394	7.389	7.448	7.438	7.419	7.440	7.430	7.423	7.43

X̄ is the sample mean.
UA, umbilical artery; *UV,* umbilical vein.
(Data from Koch G, Wendel H: Adjustment of arterial blood gases and acid-base balance in the normal newborn infant during the first week of life. Biol Neonat 12:136-161, 1968.)

D. Base Excess

		UV	UA	5-10 minutes	20 minutes	30 minutes	60 minutes	5 hours	24 hours	2 days	3 days	4 days	5 days	6 days	7 days
Base excess	X̄	−5.5	−7.2	−9.8	−8.8	−7.8	−6.5	−6.3	−5.2	−5.8	−5.9	−5.0	−4.7	−4.7	−3.2
	SD	1.2	1.7	2.3	1.9	1.7	1.3	1.3	1.1	1.2	1.2	1.1	1.1	1.1	0.6

X̄ is the sample mean.
UA, umbilical artery; *UV,* umbilical vein.
(Calculated from data in Koch G, Wendel H: Adjustment of arterial blood gases and acid base balance in the normal newborn infant during the first week of life. Biol Neonate 12:136-161, 1968. With permission from S. Karger, A.G. Basel.)

APPENDIX 10

Conversion Tables
A. Torr to Kilopascal

Torr	kPa
20	2.7
25	3.3
30	4.0
35	4.7
40	5.3
45	6.0
50	6.7
55	7.3
60	8.0
65	8.7
70	9.3
75	10.0
80	10.7
85	11.3
90	12.0
95	12.7
100	13.3
105	14.0
110	14.7
115	15.3
120	16.0
125	16.7
130	17.3
135	18.0

B. Kilopascal to Torr

kPa	Torr
2.5	19
3.0	22.5
3.5	26
4.0	30
4.5	34
5.0	37.5
5.5	41
6.0	45
6.5	49
7.0	52.5
7.5	56
8.0	60
8.5	64
9.0	67.5
9.5	71
10.0	75
10.5	79
11.0	82.5
12.0	90
12.5	94
13.0	97.5
13.5	101
14.0	105

APPENDIX 11

Siggaard-Andersen Alignment Nomogram

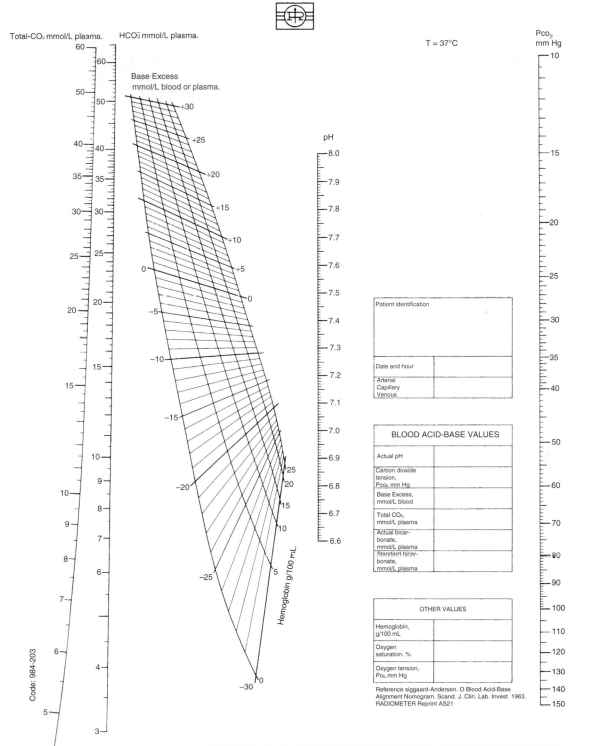

Blood acid–base alignment nomogram: scales for pH, pCO₂, base excess of whole blood of different hemoglobin concentrations, plasma bicarbonate, and plasma total CO₂.

APPENDIX 12

Systolic, Diastolic, and Mean Blood Pressure by Birth Weight and Gestational Age

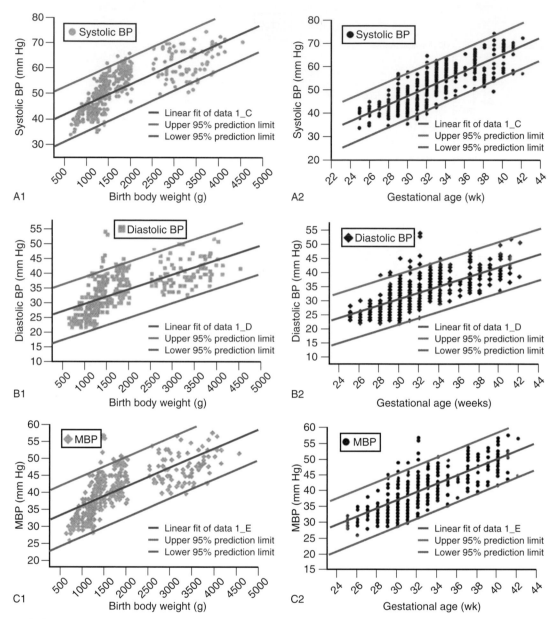

BP, Blood pressure; *MBP*, mean blood pressure. (Data from Pejovic B, Peco-Antic A, Marinkoviv-Eri J: Blood pressure in non-critically ill preterm and full-term neonates. Pediatr Nephrol 22:249-257, 2007.)

APPENDIX 13

Systolic and Diastolic Blood Pressure in the First 5 Days of Life

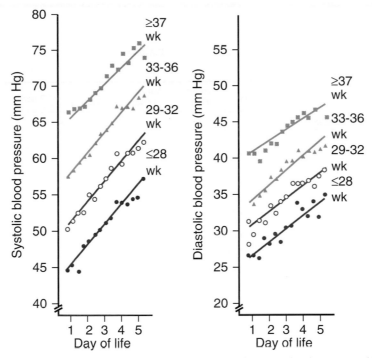

(From Zubrow AB, Hulman S, Kushner H, et al. Determinants of blood pressure in infants admitted to neonatal intensive care units: a prospective multicenter study. Philadelphia Neonatal Blood Pressure Study Group. J Perinatol 15:470, 1995.)

APPENDIX 14

Neonatal Resuscitation Record

Patient Name _____   Date _____

Est. Wt. _____ grams   Sex _____   Est. Gest. Age _____

Time of Birth _____ AM/PM

Time Resuscitation Procedures Initiated: _____

Time Resuscitation Procedures Completed: _____

Perinatal History:

	Min	Heart Rate	Muscle Tone	Reflex Irritability	Color	Resp. Effort	Total
A	1						
P	5						
G	10						
A	15						
R	20						
S	25						

Amniotic Fluid: ❑ Clear   ❑ Meconium Stained

PROCEDURES	START	END	BY WHOM	
UVC or UAC				UA/UV size: 3.5 5 8
Intubation				ETT Size: 2.5 3.0 3.5 4.0
Intubation w/Ventilation				
Intubation/Suctioning Only				
Cardiac Compressions				
Positive-Pressure Ventilation				
Free Flow Oxygen @ _____ L/min				
Suction				
O/G Tube In: ❑ Yes ❑ No				

DRUGS	TIME/AMT	TIME/AMT	ROUTE	FLUSH SOLUTIONS
Epinephrine 1:10000 0.1 - 0.3 mL/kg				_____ Normal saline + 1 unit heparin/cc
Volume Expander: 5% Albumin 10 mL/kg Normal saline Ringer's Lactate				_____ 1/2 Normal saline + 1 unit heparin/cc
Sodium Bicarbonate 0.5 mEq/mL 2 mEq/kg (4.2% solution)				_____ Other
Naloxone Hydrochloride 0.4 mg/mL or 0.1 mg/kg 1.0 mg/mL				
Blood Products				
Others				

BASE I.V. SOLUTION

_____ D_5W

_____ $D_{10}W$

LABS

_____ Glucose

Condition at Completion of Resuscitation: ❑ Good   ❑ Fair   ❑ Guarded   ❑ Expired

Transferred to: ❑ Newborn Nursery   ❑ NICU

Comments: _____
_____
_____

Resuscitation Personnel Signatures:

M.D. _____

NNP _____

R.N. _____

Recording R.N. _____

R.T. _____

APPENDIX 15

Effective FiO$_2$ Conversion Tables for Infants on Nasal Cannula

(T15-A-1 and T15-A-2)

1. The following tables are based on those used in the STOP-ROP trials.* The data were derived from Equations (3) and (4) in the paper by Benaron and Benitz (Maximizing the stability of oxygen delivered by nasal cannula. Arch Pediatr Adolesc Med 148:294-300, 1994).

2. These tables include assumptions made by Benaron and Benitz (that nasal flow is constant over the entire inspiratory cycle and that the upper airway does not act as a reservoir) plus the following assumptions made by the STOP-ROP investigators: inspiration time is 0.3 seconds, tidal volume is 5 mL/kg, and either inspiration is entirely nasal or cannula flow is sufficiently low such that on each inspiration the infant exhales all output from the cannula.

3. Example: What is the effective FiO$_2$ in a 2.0-kg infant on 100% cannula at a flow of 0.15 L/min?

   Answer: Use 2.0 and 0.15 L/min in Table 15.A1 to get a factor of 8. Then use Table 15.A.2 and the factor of 8% and 100% oxygen to yield an effective FiO$_2$ of 27%. Thus the effective oxygen concentration is less than 30% and the infant is eligible for the physiologic evaluation.

TABLE 15.A1 Factor as a Function of Flow and Weight[a,b]

Flow (L/min)	Flow (L/min)	WEIGHT (kg)								
		0.7	1.0	1.25	1.5	2	2.5	3	3.5	4
0.01		1	1	1	1	1	0	0	0	0
0.03	1/32	4	3	2	2	2	1	1	1	1
0.06	1/16	9	6	5	4	3	2	2	2	2
0.125	1/8	18	12	10	8	6	4	4	4	4
0.15		21	15	12	10	8	6	5	4	4
0.25	1/4	36	52	20	17	13	10	8	7	6
0.5	1/2	71	50	40	33	25	20	17	14	13
0.75	3/4	100	75	60	50	38	30	25	21	19
1.0	1.0	100	100	80	67	50	40	33	29	25
1.25		100	100	100	83	63	50	42	36	31
1.5		100	100	100	100	75	60	50	43	38
2.0		100	100	100	100	100	80	67	57	50

[a]Factor = 100 × min (1 U min/kg) (see Table 15.A2).
[b]Note: If your patient's exact values are not included in the table, round up or down to find the value closest to that of your patient. If the value is exactly halfway between the two values, round up.
(From the STOP-ROP Multicenter Study Group: Supplemental therapeutic oxygen for prethreshold retinopathy of prematurity (STOP-ROP): a randomized, controlled trial. I: Primary outcomes. Pediatrics 105:295-310, 2000.)

Table 15.A2 Effective FiO$_2$ ($\times$ 100) as a Function of Factor and Concentration[a]

Factor	CONCENTRATION (%)						
	21	22	25	30	40	50	100
0	21	21	21	21	21	21	21
1	21	21	21	21	21	21	22
2	21	21	21	21	21	22	23
3	21	21	21	21	22	22	23
4	21	21	21	21	22	22	24
5	21	21	21	21	22	22	25
6	21	21	21	22	22	23	26
7	21	21	21	22	22	23	27
8	21	21	21	22	23	23	27
9	21	21	21	22	23	24	28
10	21	21	21	22	23	24	29
11	21	21	21	22	23	24	**30**
12	21	21	21	22	23	24	**30**
13	21	21	22	22	23	25	31
14	21	21	22	22	24	25	32
15	21	21	22	22	23	25	33
17	21	21	22	23	24	26	34
18	21	21	22	23	24	26	35
19	21	21	22	23	25	27	36
20	21	21	22	23	25	27	37
21	21	21	22	23	25	27	38
22	21	21	22	23	25	27	36
23	21	21	22	23	25	28	39
25	21	21	22	23	25	28	41
27	21	21	22	23	25	29	42
28	21	21	22	24	26	29	43
29	21	21	22	24	27	29	44
30	21	21	22	24	27	30	45
31	21	21	22	24	27	31	47
33	21	21	22	24	27	31	47
36	21	21	22	24	28	31	49
38	21	21	23	24	28	32	51
40	21	21	23	25	29	33	53
42	21	21	23	25	29	33	53
43	21	21	23	25	29	33	55
44	21	21	23	25	29	34	56
50	21	21	23	25	30	35	60
55	21	21	23	26	31	37	64
57	21	22	23	26	32	38	66
60	21	22	23	26	32	38	68
63	21	22	24	27	33	39	71
67	21	22	24	27	34	40	74
71	21	22	24	27	34	42	77
75	21	22	24	28	35	43	80
80	21	22	24	28	36	44	84
83	21	22	24	28	37	45	87
86	21	22	24	29	37	46	89
100	21	22	25	30	40	50	100

[a]The shaded area signifies FiO$_2$ >3.0 (i.e., concentration >30%).

APPENDIX 16

Neonatal Indications and Doses for Administration of Selected Cardiorespiratory Drugs

Cardiorespiratory Pharmacopeia for the Newborn Period

Dosages and comments about these drugs are based on experience, consensus among neonatologists, and the limited evidence available from studies in neonates. Other styles of treatment are often acceptable and may be superior to those listed.

Administration Routes

ET—endotracheal
IM—intramuscularly
IT—intrathecally or intratracheally
IV—intravenously
PO—by mouth
PR—by rectum
SC—subcutaneously

Drug	Route and Dose	Contraindications and Cautions
Acetazolamide	IV, PO: 5 mg/kg/dose q6–8h; increase as needed to 25 mg/kg/dose (*temporarily effective*), max dose 55 mg/kg/day	Hyperchloremic metabolic acidosis, hypokalemia, drowsiness, paresthesias
Adenosine	Initial: 50 mcg/kg/dose IV as rapidly as possible (1–2 seconds) followed by saline flush of the line	Contraindicated in heart transplant patients; higher dosages needed in patients receiving methylxanthines; antidote for severe bradycardia is aminophylline 5–6 mg/kg over 5 minutes
	Increase dose by 50 mcg/kg/dose IV and repeat every 1–2 minutes if there is no response and no AV block	
Albumin, 5%	IV: 0.5–1 g/kg slowly	Hypervolemia, heart failure; monitor blood pressure
Albuterol	Aerosol: 0.5–1 mg/dose q2–6h	Tachycardia, arrhythmias, tremor, irritability
	PO: 0.1–0.3 mg/kg/dose q6–8h	
Aminophylline	See theophylline	See theophylline
Amiodarone	Loading dose: 5 mg/kg IV over 30–60 minutes, preferably by central venous catheter	Phlebitis, hypotension, bradycardia, liver enzyme elevations, increased and decreased thyroid function, photosensitivity, optic neuritis, pulmonary fibrosis in adults
	Maintenance: Infusion: 7–15 mcg/kg/min; PO: 5–10 mg/kg/dose q12h	
Amrinone	Initial: 0.75 mg/kg over 2–3 minutes	Fluid balance, electrolytes, renal function
	Maintenance: 3–5 mcg/kg/minutes	
Atropine	IV, IM, ET, SC: 0.01–0.03 mg/kg/dose, repeat q10–15 minutes prn; max total dose of 0.04 mg/kg	Bradycardia
Beractant (Survanta)	IT: *for prophylactic treatment*, give 4 mL/kg as soon as possible; may repeat at 6-hour intervals to a maximum of 4 doses in 48 hours	May give additional doses if infant still has respiratory distress and needs >30% FiO$_2$ to keep PAo$_2$ >50 mm Hg
	IT: *for rescue treatment*, give 4 mL/kg as soon as respiratory distress syndrome is diagnosed; may repeat at 6-hour intervals to a maximum of four doses in 48 hours	Administer each dose as four doses of 1 mL/kg each, giving each dose over 2–3 seconds and turning the newborn to a different position after each dose
		Watch for improved compliance or endotracheal plugging
Bumetanide	IV, PO: 0.005–0.05 mg/kg/dose q6–12h	Loop diuretic that also acts on proximal tubule; 40 times as potent as furosemide; less ototoxicity than furosemide; hypokalemia, hyponatremia, metabolic alkalosis
Caffeine citrate (Cafcit)	PO, IV: loading dose: 20–25 mg/kg; maintenance dose: 5–10 mg/kg/dose q24h	Restlessness, emesis, tachycardia; therapeutic plasma concentration 5–25 mcg/mL free base
Calcium chloride 10% (27 mg elemental Ca^{2+}/mL)	IV: 0.2 mL (9 mg Ca^{2+})/kg/dose for acute hypocalcemia; repeat q10min	Bradycardia if injected too quickly; necrosis from extravascular leakage

Continued

Drug	Route and Dose	Contraindications and Cautions
Calcium gluconate 10% (9.3 mg elemental Ca²⁺/mL)	IV: 1 mL (9 mg Ca²⁺)/kg/dose for acute hypocalcemia; repeat q10min PO: 3–9 mL/kg/day in two to four divided doses (28–84 mg Ca²⁺/kg/day) for chronic use	Bradycardia if injected too quickly; necrosis from extravascular leakage
Calfactant (Infasurf)	Initial: IT: 3 mL/kg divided into two aliquots repeated up to three times q12h	Do not shake or filter; ventilate for at least 30 seconds after dose until the infant is stable; administer at room temperature
Captopril	PO: 0.01–0.05 mg/kg/dose q6–24h; increase dose up to 0.5 mg/kg/dose to control blood pressure	High initial doses may cause hypotension and renal insufficiency
Chlorothiazide	PO: 5–15 mg/kg/dose q12–24h	Hypokalemia; hyponatremia decreases calcium excretion; hyperglycemia
Citric acid/sodium citrate	Dose according to degree of metabolic acidosis; each milliliter is equivalent to 1 mEq HCO_3 and contains 1 mEq sodium	Adds sodium and potassium and must be used carefully with renal dysfunction, hyperkalemia, or hypernatremia
Dexamethasone	IM, IV: for bronchopulmonary dysplasia, 0.25 mg/kg/dose q8–12h for 3–7 days; for severe chronic lung, 0.05–0.25 mg/kg/dose q12h IV or PO for 3–7 days	Delayed head growth and developmental delay associated with treatment for as few as 3 days; weigh risk and benefit
Diazepam	PO, IV, IM: as sedative, 0.02–0.3 mg/kg/dose q6–8h; for seizure, 0.1–0.2 mg/kg/dose slow IV push	Diluted injection may precipitate; IM absorption is poor; respiratory depression, hypotension
Digoxin	IV: Acute digitalization *Prematures* *Loading dose* <1.5 kg 10–20 mcg/kg 1.5–2.5 kg 20 mcg/kg *Term newborns* 30 mcg/kg *Infants (1–12 months)* 35 mcg/kg Maintenance dose: ⅛ loading dose q12h Begin 12 hours after last digitalization dose	Risk of arrhythmias is increased during digitalization; IV formulation is twice as concentrated as oral; conduction defects, emesis, ventricular arrhythmias
Dobutamine	IV: 2–20 mcg/kg/min by continuous infusion and titrate to desired effect	Tachycardia, hypotension
Dopamine	IV: 2–20 mcg/kg/min by continuous infusion and titrate to desired effect	Extravasation may lead to necrosis (phentolamine is an antidote); a high dose may constrict renal arteries, but the dose for this effect is uncertain in neonates
Enalapril (PO), enalaprilat (IV)	IV enalaprilat: for hypertension, 5–10 mcg/kg/dose q8–24h PO enalapril for CHF, 0.1 mg/kg/day each day to a max of 0.5 mg/kg/day	Reduce dose with renal failure; severe hypotension may occur, especially with volume depletion from diuretic treatment
Epinephrine	Resuscitation: IV 1:10,000: 0.01–0.03 mg/kg (0.1–0.3 mL/kg) q3–5 minutes; 0.1 mg/kg via ET if IV not available Hypotension: 0.01–0.1 mcg/kg/min by continuous infusion and titrate to desired effect	Tachycardia, arrhythmia
Fentanyl	IV, IM: 1–2 mcg/kg/dose, q4–6h prn, increase as needed	50–100 times the potency of morphine: muscle rigidity ("stiff man syndrome") may occur with rapid dose infusions; treat with muscle relaxants
Furosemide	IM, IV: 0.5–2 mg/kg/dose q12–24h PO: 1–2 mg/kg/dose q12–24h	Hypokalemia, hyponatremia, hypochloremia; half-life prolonged in premature newborns
Hydralazine	PO, IM, IV: 0.1–0.5 mg/kg q6h; increase as needed in 0.1-mg/kg increments up to 2 mg/kg/day Bioavailability reduced by cor pulmonale; may require higher dosages	Tachycardia, lupus-like reactions
Hydrochlorothiazide	PO: 2.0–4.0 mg/kg/day q12h	Hypercalcemia, hypokalemia, hyperglycemia
Hydrocortisone	Hypotension refractory to pressors, 1 mg/kg/dose IV; acute adrenal insufficiency, 0.25 mg/kg/dose q6h IV; physiologic replacement, 0.3 mg/kg/day IM	Treatment of more than 7–10 days requires gradual dosage reduction to avoid adrenal insufficiency; immunosuppression, hyperglycemia, growth delay, leukocytosis, gastric irritation
Ibuprofen lysine	Initial dose 10 mg/kg; second and third doses 5 mg/kg. Administer IV over 15 minutes at 24-hour intervals	GI perforation; renal impairment. Use cautiously in patients with active bleeding or renal or hepatic dysfunction Avoid in patients with ductal-dependent cardiac malformations

Drug	Route and Dose	Contraindications and Cautions
Indomethacin	PO, IV: 0.1–0.2 mg/kg/dose q12–24h for 2–7 days; 0.25 mg/kg/dose, >7 days	Transient renal dysfunction, decreased platelet aggregation; infuse over a minimum of 30–60 minutes to minimize reduction in CNS and mesenteric perfusion; avoid in patients with ductal-dependent cardiac malformations
Isoproterenol	IV: 0.05–0.5 mcg/kg/minutes by infusion	Arrhythmias, systemic vasodilation, tachycardia, hypotension, hypoglycemia
Lidocaine	IV: 1 mg/kg infused over 5–10 minutes; may be repeated q10min five times, prn; infusion dose 10–50 mcg/kg/min or 1 mg/kg/h	Monitoring of blood levels useful (therapeutic range 1–5 mcg/mL plasma); dilute for ET administration
Lorazepam	IV: 0.05–0.1 mg/kg infused over 2–5 minutes	Limited data in newborns, preparations may contain benzyl alcohol; dilute
Magnesium sulfate	IM, IV: 25–50 mg/kg q4–6h for three to four doses prn; use 50% solution IM, 1% solution IV	Hypotension, CNS depression; monitor serum concentration; calcium gluconate should be available as an antidote
Methyldopa	IV, PO: 2–3 mg/kg q6–8h; increase as needed at 2-day intervals; maximum dosage 12–15 mg/kg/dose	Sedation, fever, false-positive Coombs test, hemolysis; sudden withdrawal of methyldopa may cause rebound hypertension
Methylprednisolone	IV, IM: 0.1–0.4 mc/kg/dose, q6h	Hydrocortisone preferred for physiologic replacement
Metoclopramide	PO, IV: 0.1–0.2 mg/kg/dose q6–8h or before each feeding	Dystonic reactions, irritability, diarrhea, decreases glomerular filtration rate in adults Efficacy for GERD shown at >6 months
Midazolam	IV, IM, intranasal: 0.07–0.20 mg/kg/dose q2–4h prn for sedation; infusion dosing: <33 weeks, 30 mcg/kg/h; >33 weeks, 60 mcg/kg/h	Limited experience in newborns; respiratory depression, apnea Rapid infusion doses (<10 minutes) may cause tonic–clonic movements
Morphine sulfate	IV, IM, SC: 0.05–0.1 mg/kg/dose q2–6h prn; 0.1–0.2 mg/kg/dose PO q3–6h	Respiratory depression reversible with naloxone; local urticaria from histamine release
Naloxone	IV, IM, SC: 0.1 mg/kg/dose; may be repeated as necessary; delivery room minimum, 0.5 mg for term newborn	Onset of action may be delayed 15+ minutes after IM or SC administration; narcotic effects may outlast naloxone antagonism; dilute for ET administration
Neostigmine	IV: Test for myasthenia gravis, 0.02 mg/kg IM: Test for myasthenia gravis, 0.04 mg/kg PO: Treatment for myasthenia gravis, 0.33 mg/kg/day q3–6h	Cholinergic crisis atropine pretreatment is recommended
Nitroprusside	IV: Begin with dose of 0.25 mcg/kg/min and vary as needed up to 8 mcg/kg/min to control blood pressure	Profound hypotension possible; requires arterial line to monitor blood pressure; thiocyanate toxicity with long-term use or renal insufficiency
Omeprazole	PO: 0.5–1.5 mg/kg/dose each day	Hypergastrinemia; diarrhea; monitor gastric pH
Pancuronium	IV: 0.03–0.1 mg/kg/dose q1–4h prn; titrate to age and effect desired	Ensure adequate oxygenation and ventilation; tachycardia, bradycardia, hypotension, hypertension; potentiated by acidosis, hypothermia, neuromuscular disease, aminoglycoside antibiotics
Phentolamine	SC: Dilute to 0.5 mg/mL, inject 0.2 mL at five sites around α-adrenergic drug infiltration maximum, 2.5 mg total dose	Marked hypotension, tachycardia, arrhythmia Do not treat hypotension with epinephrine, because hypotension may worsen owing to α-adrenergic blockade
Fresh-frozen plasma	IV: 10 mL/kg; repeated prn	Volume overload, viral infection risk
Poractant alfa (Curosurf)	IT: 2.5 mL/kg/dose divided into 2 aliquots, followed by 1.25 mL/kg/dose q12h up to two additional doses if needed	Do not filter or shake; suction before administration; administer in two to four aliquots with positioning of infant to improve distribution within the lungs; ventilate for at least 30 seconds after dose until infant is stable
Prednisone	PO: 0.5–2 mg/kg/day q6h	Asystole, myocardial depression, anorexia, vomiting, nausea
Procainamide	IV: 1.5–2.5 mg/kg infused over 10–30 minutes; may be repeated in 30 minutes if needed; infusion: 20–60 mcg/kg/minutes PO: 40–60 mg/kg/day q4–6h	Blood level monitoring helpful (therapeutic range: procainamide, 3–10 mcg/mL; N-acetyl procainamide, 10–20 mcg/mL)
Propranolol	IV: 0.01 mg/kg initial dose and 0.01–0.15 mg/kg infused over 10 minutes; may be repeated in 10 minutes and then q6–8h to maximum of 0.15 mg/kg/dose PO: 0.05–2 mg/kg q6h	Relatively contraindicated in low-output congestive heart failure and patients with bronchospasm

Continued

Drug	Route and Dose	Contraindications and Cautions
Prostaglandin E1, alprostadil	IV: 0.03–0.1 mcg/kg/minutes; often, dose may be reduced by one-half after initial response; intra-arterial infusion offers no advantage	Apnea, seizures, fever, disseminated intravascular coagulation, diarrhea, cutaneous vasodilation, decreased platelet aggregation, cortical bone proliferation during prolonged infusion
Quinidine gluconate	PO, IM: 2–10 mg/kg/dose q2–6h until the desired effect or toxicity occurs	Check electrocardiogram before each dose; discontinue if the QRS interval increases 50% or more Maintain level of 2–6 mcg/mL; nausea, vomiting, diarrhea, fever, AV block
Sodium bicarbonate (0.5 mEq/mL)	IV route not recommended in neonates (dose is specific for the salt form) IV: 1–2 mEq/kg/dose infused slowly only if infant ventilated adequately	Intravascular hemolysis may be associated with rapid infusion
Sodium polystyrene sulfonate (Kayexalate)	PO, PR: 1 g/kg; approximately q6h	Usually administered as a solution with 20% sorbitol to prevent intestinal obstruction; 20% sorbitol solution may injure intestinal mucosa of very low birth weight newborns; may decrease serum calcium or magnesium
Spironolactone	PO: 1–3 mg/kg/day q8–12h	Contraindicated with hyperkalemia; onset of action delayed; drowsiness; nausea; vomiting; diarrhea; androgenic effects in females; gynecomastia in males
Theophylline	PO, IV: loading dose 5–6 mg/kg; maintenance dose 1–2.5 mg/kg/dose q6–12h; aminophylline (IV) dose = theophylline (IV) dose × 1.25	Blood level monitoring indicated (therapeutic range: *apnea, 7–12 mcg/mL; bronchospasm, 10–20 mcg/mL*); tachycardia at 15–20 mcg/mL; seizures at >40 g/mL; avoid rectal dosing because of variable absorption, clearance decreased by asphyxia and prematurity; tachycardia
Vecuronium	IV: 0.08–0.1 mg/kg/dose, repeat prn at 0.03–0.15 mg/kg/dose q1–2h; dose to effect	Neuromuscular blockade potentiated by calcium channel blockers such as verapamil and aminoglycoside antibiotics
Verapamil	IV: 0.1–0.2 mg/kg infused over 2 minutes; if response is inadequate, repeat in 30 minutes PO: 2–5 mg/kg/day in three divided doses	Monitor electrocardiogram during infusion; bradycardia, AV block, asystole; contraindicated in patients with second- or third-degree AV block during treatment with β-blockers

AV, Atrioventricular; *CHF,* congestive heart failure; *CNS,* central nervous system; *GERD,* gastroesophageal reflux disease; *GI,* gastrointestinal; *prn,* pro re nata (as needed).

(Data from Young TE, Mangum B: Neofax. 27th ed. Montvale, NJ, Thomas Reuters, 2014; and McClary J: Drug Dosing Table. In: Fanaroff AA, Fanaroff JM (eds). Klaus and Fanaroff's Care of the High Risk Neonate. 6th ed. Philadelphia, Elsevier, 2013.)

APPENDIX 17 APPS

Alveolar-Arterial Oxygen Gradient

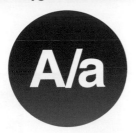

Name of the app: **Alveolar–Arterial Gradient (A/a)**

How to download the app:

iPhone: Go to the app store, search for "Alveolar-Arterial Gradient" and look for the icon, and tap to download.

Android: Go to the play store, search for "Alveolar–Arterial Gradient" and look for the icon, and tap to download.

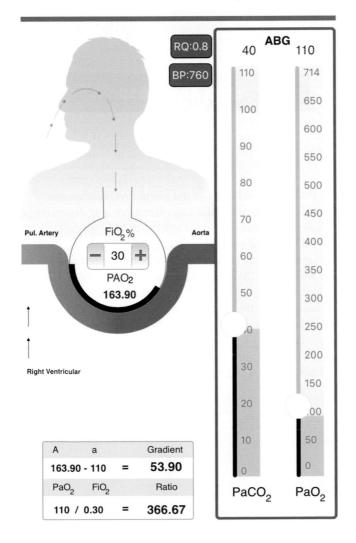

Enter:
FiO$_2$
PaCO$_2$

PaO$_2$

The app calculates A/a gradient and PaO$_2$/FiO$_2$ ratio.

RESPIRATORY QUOTIENT AND BAROMETRIC PRESSURE

Respiratory quotient (RQ): RQ can affect A/a gradient and PaO$_2$/FiO$_2$ ratio. The app calculates the correct value for a given RQ.

Barometric pressure (BP): The app can also calculate the correct A/a gradient and PaO$_2$/FiO$_2$ ratio. The app calculates the correct value for a given BP. This is especially useful if the baby has been airlifted.

INFORMATION ABOUT ALVEOLAR–ARTERIAL OXYGEN GRADIENT AND PAO$_2$/FIO$_2$ RATIO

The A/a oxygen gradient is a measure of oxygen transfer across the alveolar capillary membrane ("A" denotes alveolar and "a" denotes arterial oxygenation). It is the difference between the amounts of the oxygen in the alveoli and in the arteries.

PAO$_2$ is the alveolar oxygen tension.

PaO$_2$ is the arterial oxygen tension.

$$A/a\ oxygen\ gradient = PAO_2 - PaO_2.$$

PaO$_2$ is derived from the arterial blood gas (ABG) and PAO$_2$ is calculated as follows:

$$PAo_2 = [FiO_2 \times (P_{atm} - PH_2O)] - (PaCO_2 \div R),$$

where FiO$_2$ is the fraction of inspired oxygen (0.21 at room air), P$_{atm}$ is the atmospheric pressure (760 mm Hg at sea level), PH$_2$O is the partial pressure of water (47 mm Hg), PaCO$_2$ is derived from the ABG, and R is the respiratory quotient (the respiratory quotient is approximately 0.8 at normal physiological state).

The A/a gradient varies with age and can be estimated from the following equation, assuming the patient is breathing room air:

$$A/a\ gradient = 2.5 + 0.21 \times age\ in\ years.$$

The A/a gradient increases with higher FiO$_2$.

The PaO$_2$/FiO$_2$ ratio is a measure of oxygen transfer across the alveolar capillary membrane. The normal PaO$_2$/FiO$_2$ ratio is 300–500 mm Hg, with values less than 300 mm Hg indicating impaired gas exchange and values less than 200 mm Hg indicating severe hypoxemia.

Dr. Satish Deopujari, MD, DNB (Pediatrics)

Founder National Chairperson (Ex) Intensive Care Chapter, Indian Academy of Pediatrics

Professor of Pediatrics (Hon) LMH, Nagpur, India

deopujaris@gmail.com

deopujari@me.com

www.deopujari.com

COMPLETE ABG

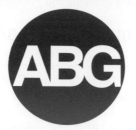

Name of the app: **Complete ABG**

How to download the app:

iPhone: Go to the app store, search for "Complete ABG" and look for the icon, and tap to download.

Android: Go to the play store, search for "Complete ABG" and look for the icon, and tap to download.

This dynamic arterial blood gas (ABG) app, assisted by clinical features, is designed to arrive at the complete ABG diagnosis. The app is simple to operate and is also helpful in learning the dynamic physiology of blood gas with all its details. The app is available free on Apple and Android smartphones. The internal consistency of the ABG is also checked by the app by confirming that the measured bicarbonate (shown by the app) corresponds to the depicted bicarbonate value in the ABG report.

At bedside the app also helps in calculations of alveolar/arterial oxygen gradient (A/aDO$_2$) difference and thus helps in evaluation of oxygenation status.

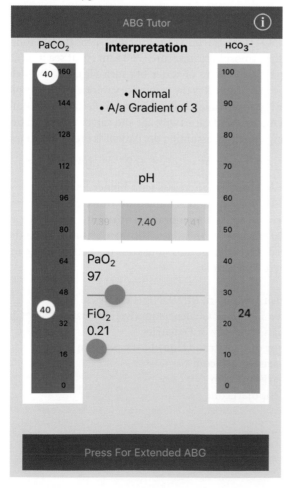

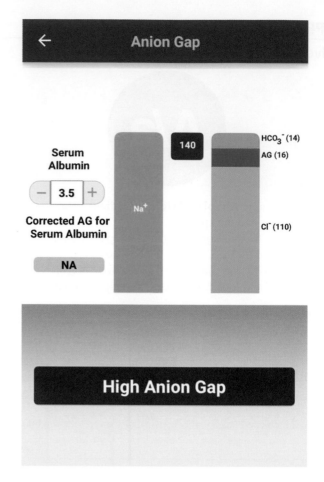

Enter PaCO$_2$ and pH and see the calculated bicarbonate.

Diagnosis is displayed under Interpretation, and depending on the diagnosis, the screen for extended ABG appears.

Enter PaO$_2$ and FiO$_2$ to get the A/a gradient.

Enter serum sodium, chloride, and albumin to obtain the value of anion gap (AG). Bicarbonate is pulled from the ABG calculations.

With high AG, further evaluation takes the user to Δ/Δ gap and osmolar gap and thus to the complete diagnosis of wide AG acidosis.

With normal AG, the evaluation leads to the diagnosis of renal tubular acidosis (RTA) and the subgroups.

For Metabolic Alkalosis

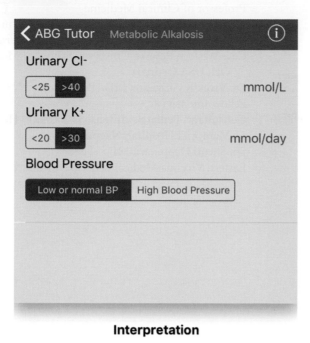

Interpretation

Gitelman Syndrome (low urinary calcium) or
Bartter Syndrome (high urinary calcium)

Press here for algorithm

Enter urinary chloride, potassium, and blood pressure as and when applicable for further workup of metabolic alkalosis.

App Information

Complete ABG: This app helps in the diagnosis of acid–base and oxygenation disorders and makes it easy to understand this complex subject.

It is designed as alphabet H and puts the Henderson–Hasselbalch (HH) equation at center stage.

From the ABG report, enter $PaCO_2$ and pH and see the calculated bicarbonate (do not try to move HCO_3; it is a calculated parameter and varies with $PaCO_2$ and pH). If the displayed bicarbonate does not correspond to that in the ABG report (±3), then the ABG report is not internally consistent.

On the first screen, it CLEARLY shows that bicarbonate is a calculated parameter.

Play with the app to understand this relationship between pH, $PaCO_2$, and bicarbonate and by doing this, you will actually understand the HH equation.

This app works in three steps:

1. Bedside ABG: This is useful for making decisions at the bedside (point of care). Simple and clear, it tells the user what matters at bedside. It calculates A/aDO_2, on the basis of the entered PaO_2 and FiO_2 values, considering an atmospheric pressure of 760 mm Hg and respiratory quotient of 0.8 (to learn more on A/aDO_2 use the A/a gradient).

2. Extended ABG: Extended interpretation is provided on the basis of AG, Δ/Δ, osmolar gap, urinary AG, and urinary potassium level.

3. Flowchart: This algorithm is available to learn the approach used by this app to arrive at the diagnosis.

This app works on the following equations:

1. HH equation: $\dfrac{\left[H^+\right]\left[HCO_3^-\right]}{PaCO_2} = 24.$

$$\left[H_+\right] = 10^{(9-pH)}$$

$$AG = (Na^+) - [(Cl^-) + (HCO_3^-)]$$

2. Corrected AG for serum albumin <3.5 = AG + [(3.5 − serum albumin) $\times$ 2.5]

$$\text{Delta Delta} = [(AG - 12) - (24 - HCO_3^-)].$$

3. Osmolar gap = measured osmolarity − calculated osmolarity

Calculated Osmolarity =

$$\left[(2\times Sr.\ Na)+\left(\frac{blood\ glucose}{18}\right)+\left(\frac{BUN}{2.8}\right)\right]$$

Urinary AG = Urinary Na^+ + Urinary K^+ − Urinary Cl^-.

Dr. Satish Deopujari, MD, DNB (Pediatrics)
Founder National Chairperson (Ex) Intensive Care Chapter, Indian Academy of Pediatrics
Professor of Pediatrics (Hon) LMH, Nagpur, India
deopujaris@gmail.com
deopujari@me.com
www.deopujari.com

Dr. Lawrence Martin, MD
Professor of Clinical Medicine
Author of the famous and most read book on ABG,
All You Really Need to Know to Interpret Arterial Blood Gases
Case Western Reserve University School of Medicine, Cleveland, OH, USA (retired)

Dr. Vivek K. Shivhare, MD (Pediatrics)
Fellow Intensivist
Consultant Pediatric Intensivist, CARE Hospital and Mure Memorial Hospital, Nagpur, India

Dr. Shruti Deopujari, MD
Eastern Virginia Medical School, Norfolk, VA, USA

ETCO₂ TUTOR

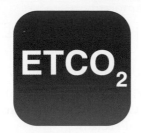

Name of the app: **ETCO₂ Tutor**
How to download the app:
iPhone: Go to the app store, search for "ETCO₂ Tutor" and look for the icon, and tap to download.
Android: Go to the play store, search for "ETCO₂ Tutor" and look for the icon, and tap to download.
ETCO₂ Tutor is a dynamic app and clearly explains the physiological background related to end-tidal CO_2 (ETCO₂) monitoring. Hyper- and hypoventilation affecting the ETCO₂ are clearly shown in the app by altering the respiratory rate. The app shows the various waveforms, in beautiful colors, and the related pathophysiology.

> Tap for breathing here and understand the concept of ETCO2

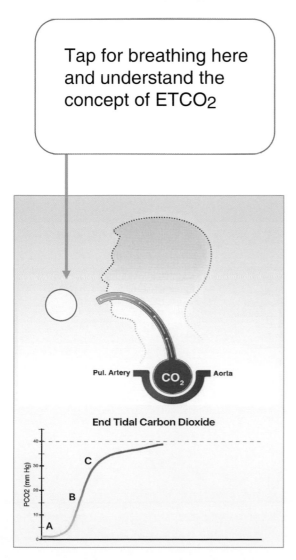

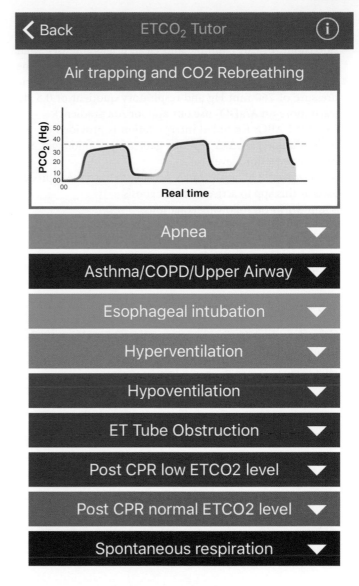

Clicking on the title shows the related graph.
Enter urinary chloride, potassium, and blood pressure as and when applicable for further workup of metabolic alkalosis.

◄─────── Press here for algorithm

App Information
Complete ABG: This app helps in the diagnosis of acid–base and oxygenation disorders and makes it easy to understand this complex subject.
It is designed as alphabet H and puts the Henderson–Hasselbalch (HH) equation at center stage.
From the arterial blood gas (ABG) report, enter PaCO₂ and pH and see the calculated bicarbonate (do not try to move HCO₃; it is a calculated parameter and varies with PaCO₂ and pH). If the displayed bicarbonate does not correspond to that in the ABG report (± 3), then the ABG report is not internally consistent.
On the first screen it CLEARLY shows that bicarbonate is a calculated parameter.
Play with the app to understand this relationship between pH, PaCO₂, and bicarbonate and by doing this you will actually understand the HH equation.

This app works in three steps
1. Bedside ABG: This is useful for making decisions at the bedside (point of care). Simple and clear, it tells the user what matters at bedside. It calculates A/aDO$_2$, on the basis of the entered PaO$_2$ and FiO$_2$ values, considering an atmospheric pressure of 760 mm Hg and respiratory quotient of 0.8 (to learn more on A/aDO$_2$ use our app for A/a gradient).
2. Extended ABG: Extended interpretation is provided on the basis of anion gap, Δ/Δ, osmolar gap, urinary anion gap, and urinary potassium level.
3. 🏛 Flowchart: This algorithm is available to learn the approach used by this app to arrive at the diagnosis.

This app works on following equations:

1. HH equation: $\dfrac{[H^+][HCO_3^-]}{PaCO_2} = 24$.

$[H_+] = 10^{(9-pH)}$

$AG = (Na^+) - [(Cl^-) + (HCO_3^-)]$

2. Corrected anion gap for serum albumin $<3.5 = AG + [(3.5 - serum\ albumin) \times 2.5]$

Delta Delta $= [(AG - 12) - (24 - HCO_3^-)]$.

3. Osmolar gap = measured osmolarity − calculated osmolarity

Calculated Osmolarity =
$$\left[(2 \times Sr.\ Na) + \left(\frac{blood\ glucose}{18} \right) + \left(\frac{BUN}{2.8} \right) \right]$$

Urinary AG = Urinary Na$^+$ + Urinary K$^+$ − Urinary Cl$^-$.

Dr. Satish Deopujari, MD, DNB (Pediatrics)
Founder National Chairperson (Ex) Intensive Care Chapter, Indian Academy of Pediatrics
Professor of Pediatrics (Hon) LMH, Nagpur, India
deopujaris@gmail.com
deopujari@me.com
www.deopujari.com
Dr. Lawrence Martin, MD
Professor of Clinical Medicine
Case Western Reserve University School of Medicine, Cleveland, OH, USA (retired)
Dr. Vivek K. Shivhare, MD (Pediatrics)
Fellow Intensivist
Consultant Pediatric Intensivist, CARE Hospital and Mure Memorial Hospital, Nagpur, India
Dr. Shruti Deopujari, MD
Eastern Virginia Medical School, Norfolk, VA, USA

Note: Page numbers followed by *f* indicate figures, *t* tables, *b* boxes.